ORTHOTICS and PROSTHETICS in REHABILITATION

ORTHOTICS and PROSTHETICS in REHABILITATION

Second Edition

Michelle M. Lusardi, PT, PhD
Associate Professor of Physical Therapy
Coordinator, Graduate Programs in Geriatrics
Department of Physical Therapy and Human Movement Science
College of Education and Health Professions
Sacred Heart University
Fairfield, Connecticut

Caroline C. Nielsen, PhD
Health Care, Education, and Research Consultant
Bonita Springs, Florida;
Former Associate Professor and Director
Graduate Program in Allied Health
University of Connecticut,
Storrs, Connecticut

Foreword by
Michael J. Emery, PT, EdD
Associate Professor and Chairman
Department of Physical Therapy and Human Movement Science
College of Education and Health Professions
Sacred Heart University
Fairfield, Connecticut

SAUNDERS

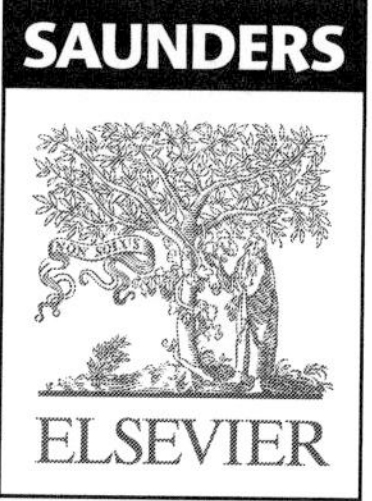

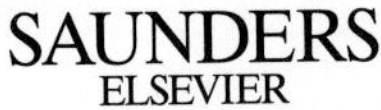

11830 Westline Industrial Drive
St. Louis, Missouri 63146

ORTHOTICS AND PROSTHETICS IN REHABILITATION

NOTICE

Neither the Publisher nor the Authors assume any responsibility for any loss or injury and/or damage to persons or property arising out of or related to any use of the material contained in this book. It is the responsibility of the treating practitioner, relying on independent expertise and knowledge of the patient, to determine the best treatment and method of application for the patient.

The Publisher

ISBN-13: 978-0-7506-7479-9
ISBN-10: 0-7506-7479-2

Acquisitions Editors: Marion Waldman, Kathy Falk
Developmental Editors: Marjory I. Fraser, Meghan Ziegler
Publishing Services Manager: Julie Eddy
Project Manager: Gail Michaels
Design Project Manager: Bill Drone

Printed in the United States of America

Last digit is the print number: 9 8 7 6 5 4 3 2

To Lawrence Mario Lusardi,
my husband and best friend
To love someone deeply gives you strength.
Being loved by someone deeply gives
you courage. —Lao Tzu

M.M.L

To Svend Woge Nielsen,
a true partner who nourishes
my spirit and achievements with his constant
understanding and belief in me

C.C.N.

Contributors

Noelle M. Austin, PT, MS, CHT
Owner
CJ Education and Consulting, LLC
Hand Therapist
The Orthopaedic Group
Woodbridge, Connecticut
Chapter 17: Orthotics in the Management of Hand Dysfunction

Edmond Ayyappa, MS, CPO
Director
National VA Prosthetics Gait Lab
Long Beach, California
Associate Clinical Professor
University of California, Irvine Medical School
Irvine, California
Department of Physical Medicine and Rehabilitation
Lecturer
California State University, Dominguez Hill
School of Allied Health, Department of Prosthetics and Orthotics
Long Beach, California
Chapter 3: Clinical Assessment of Pathological Gait
Chapter 25: Postsurgical Management of Partial Foot and Syme's Amputation

William J. Barringer, MS, CO
Associate Professor of Orthopeadic Surgery and Rehabilitation
Chief of Orthotics
University of Oklahoma Health Sciences Center
Oklahoma City, Oklahoma
Chapter 14: Orthotics in the Management of Musculoskeletal Impairment

Gary M. Berke, MS, CP, FAAOP
Private Practitioner
Redwood City, California
Adjunct Clinical Instructor
Department of Orthopaedic Surgery
Stanford University
Palo Alto, California
Chapter 26: Transtibial Prosthetic Options

Jennifer M. Bottomley, PT, MS, PhD
Core Faculty
Division on Aging, Harvard Medical School
Geriatric Rehabilitation Program Consultant
Geriatric Rehabilitation and Wellness
West Roxbury, Massachusetts
Chapter 8 Footwear: Foundation for Lower Extremity Orthoses

Donna M. Bowers, PT, MPH, PCS
Clinical Assistant Professor
Department of Physical Therapy and Human Movement Science
College of Education and Health Professions
Sacred Heart University
Fairfield, Connecticut
Chapter 5: Motor Learning and Motor Control in Orthotic and Prosthetic Rehabilitation
Chapter 12: Orthotics in the Management of Neuromuscular Impairments

James H. Campbell, PhD, CO
Director of Research and Development, Engineering and Technical Services
Becker Orthopedic
Troy, Michigan
Chapter 11: Knee-Ankle-Foot and Hip-Knee-Ankle-Foot Orthoses

Barbara Crane, PT, APT, PhD
Assistant Professor
Department of Physical Therapy
School of Education Nursing, and Health Professions
University of Hartford
West Hartford, Connecticut
Chapter 19: Adaptive Seating in the Management of Neuromuscular and Musculoskeletal Impairment

Thomas V. DiBello, BS, CO

President
Dynamic Orthotics and Prosthetics, Inc.
Houston, Texas
Chapter 11: Knee-Ankle-Foot and Hip-Knee-Ankle-Foot Orthoses

Joan E. Edelstein, PT, MA, FISPO

Special Lecturer
Program in Physical Therapy
College of Physicians and Surgeons
Columbia University
New York, New York
Chapter 31: Rehabilitation for Children with Limb Deficiencies

John Fergason, CPO

Director
Prosthetic-Orthotic Clinic
Brooke Army Medical Center
Fort Sam Houston, Texas
Chapter 24: Prosthetic Feet

Juan C. Garbalosa, PT, PhD

Associate Professor of Physical Therapy
College of Education, Nursing, and Health Professions
University of Hartford
West Hartford, Connecticut
Chapter 9: Functional Foot Orthoses

Thomas M. Gavin, CO

President and Director of Clinical Services
BioConcepts, Inc.
Burr Ridge, Illinois
Chapter 15: Orthotics in the Management of Spinal Dysfunction and Instability

Mark D. Geil, PhD

Academic Coordinator
Master of Science Program in Prosthetics and Orthotics
School of Applied Physiology
Georgia Institute of Technology
Atlanta, Georgia
Chapter 7: Principles Influencing Orthosis and Prosthesis Design: Biomechanics, Device-User Interface, and Related Concepts

Alexander J. Ghanayem, MD

Associate Professor and Chief
Division of Spine Surgery
Department of Orthopedic Surgery and Rehabilitation
Loyola University Medical Center
Maywood, Illinois
Chapter 15: Orthotics in the Management of Spinal Dysfunction and Instability

Thomas M. Harrigan, PT, CPO

Seacoast Rehabilitation Services
Orthotics and Prosthetics
Meadowbrook Offices
York, Maine
Chapter 16: Orthotics and Therapeutic Interventions in the Management of Scoliosis

Christopher F. Hovorka, MS, CPO

Clinical Coordinator
Master of Science Program in Prosthetics and Orthotics
School of Applied Physiology
Georgia Institute of Technology
Atlanta, Georgia
Chapter 7: Principles Influencing Orthosis and Prosthesis Design: Biomechanics, Device-User Interface, and Related Concepts

MaryLynn Jacobs, OTR/L, MS, CHT

Partner and Hand Therapist
Performance Rehabilitation of Western New England
Somers, Connecticut
Chapter 17: Orthotics in the Management of Hand Dysfunction

Carolyn B. Kelly, PT

Neuropathic Foot Program
Center for Wound Healing and Hyperbaric Medicine
Hartford Hospital
Hartford, Connecticut
Chapter 21: Conservative Management of the High-Risk Foot

John F. Knecht, PT, MA, ATC

Site Coordinator
Health South Physical Therapy and Sports Medicine Associates Willimantic
Willimantic, Connecticut
Chapter 13: Orthotic Options for Knee Instability and Pain

Géza F. Kogler, PhD, CO

Springfield Clinic Orthotic and Prosthetic Center
Springfield, Illinois
Chapter 2: Materials and Technology

Donald S. Kowalsky, PT, EdD

Assistant Professor and Chair
Physical Therapy Program
School of Health Sciences
Quinnipiac University
Hamden, Connecticut
Chapter 9: Functional Foot Orthoses

Robert S. Lin, CPO
Director of Pediatric Clinical Services and Academic Programs
Hanger Orthopedics Group at the Connecticut Children's Medical Center
Hartford, Connecticut
Chapter 10: Ankle-Foot Orthoses

Michelle M. Lusardi, PT, PhD
Associate Professor of Physical Therapy
Coordinator, Graduate Programs in Geriatrics
Department of Physical Therapy and Human Movement Science
College of Education and Health Professions
Sacred Heart University
Fairfield, Connecticut
Chapter 4: Energy, Exercise, and Aging in Orthotic and Prosthetic Rehabilitation
Chapter 5: Motor Learning and Motor Control in Orthotic and Prosthetic Rehabilitation
Chapter 6: An Evidence-Based Practice Approach to Orthotic and Prosthetic Rehabilitation
Chapter 7: Principles Influencing Orthosis and Prosthesis Design: Biomechanics, Device-User Interface, and Related Concepts
Chapter 12: Orthotics in the Management of Neuromuscular Impairments
Chapter 14: Orthotics in the Management of Musculoskeletal Impairment
Chapter 22: Determinants and Techniques of Amputation
Chapter 23: Postoperative and Preprosthetic Rehabilitation

John W. Michael, MEd, CPO, FISPO, FAAOP
Instructor, Allied Health Program
Century College
White Bear Lake, Minnesota
President, CPO Services, Inc.
Chanhassen, Minnesota
Chapter 30: Prosthetic Options for Persons with High-Level and Bilateral Amputation

Olfat Mohamed, PT, PhD
Associate Professor
Department of Physical Therapy
California State University
Long Beach, California
Chapter 3: Clinical Assessment of Pathological Gait

Caroline C. Nielsen, PhD
Health Care, Education, and Research Consultant
Bonita Springs, Florida
Former Associate Professor and Director
Graduate Program in Allied Health
University of Connecticut
Storrs, Connecticut
Chapter 1: Orthotics and Prosthetics in Rehabilitation: The Multidisciplinary Approach
Chapter 20: Etiology of Amputation

Roberta Nole, PT, MA, CPed
Stride Physical Therapy and Pedorthic Center
Middlebury, Connecticut
Chapter 9: Functional Foot Orthoses

Avinash G. Patwardhan, PhD
Professor, Chief, Section of Research
Department of Orthopedic Surgery and Rehabilitation
Loyola University Medical Center
Maywood, Illinois
Chapter 15: Orthotics in the Management of Spinal Dysfunction and Instability

Judith L. Pepe, MD
Department of Surgery, Hartford Hospital
Associate Professor
University of Connecticut School of Medicine
Hartford, Connecticut
Chapter 22: Determinants and Techniques of Amputation

Richard Psonak, MS, CPO
Director
Division of Prosthetics and Orthotics
Assistant Professor
Department of Orthopedic Surgery
School of Medicine
University of Mississippi Medical Center
Jackson, Mississippi
Chapter 28: Transfemoral Prostheses

Julie D. Ries, PT, MA, GCS
Assistant Professor of Physical Therapy
Marymount University
Arlington, Virginia
Chapter 27: Rehabilitation of Persons with Recent Transtibial Amputation

Anthony Rinella, MD
Instructor
Orthopedic Surgery and Rehabilitation
Department of Orthopedic Surgery and Rehabilitation
Maguire Center
Maywood, Illinois
Chapter 15: Orthotics in the Management of Spinal Dysfunction and Instability

Melvin L. Stills, CO
Chapter 14: Orthotics in the Management of Musculoskeletal Impairment

David M. Thompson, PT, PhD
University of Oklahoma Health Sciences Center
Oklahoma City, Oklahoma
Chapter 29: Rehabilitation for Persons with Transfemoral Amputation

Jesse M. VanSwearingen, PT, PhD
Associate Professor
Department of Physical Therapy
School of Health and Rehabilitation Sciences
University of Pittsburgh
Pittsburgh, Pennsylvania
Chapter 4: Energy, Exercise, and Aging in Orthotic and Prosthetic Rehabilitation

Victor G. Vaughan, PT, MS
Director of Rehabilitation
Sacred Heart University Sports Medicine and Rehabilitation Center
Fairfield, Connecticut
Chapter 27: Rehabilitation of Persons with Recent Transtibial Amputation

R. Scott Ward, PT, PhD
Associate Professor and Director
Division of Physical Therapy, University of Utah
Salt Lake City, Utah
Chapter 18: Splinting, Orthotics, and Prosthetics in the Management of Burns

Ellen Wetherbee, PT, MS, OCS
Clinical Assistant Professor
Department of Physical Therapy
University of Hartford
West Hartford, Connecticut
Chapter 13: Orthotic Options for Knee Instability and Pain

Margaret Wise, OTR, CHT, CVE, CCM
Upper Extremity Specialists
Dallas, Texas
Chapter 33: Rehabilitation for Persons with Upper Extremity Amputation

Rita A. Wong, PT, EdD
Professor and Chairperson of Physical Therapy
Marymount University
Arlington, Virginia
Chapter 6: An Evidence-Based Practice Approach to Orthotic and Prosthetic Rehabilitation

John R. Zenie, MBA, CPO
Clinical Director
Comprehensive Prosthetic Services
Guilford, Connecticut
Chapter 32: Prosthetic Options for Persons with Upper Extremity Amputation

Foreword

Today more than ever before, rehabilitation services are dependent upon access and utilization of the best available evidence to guide clinical decisions. The use of evidence in practice means that practitioners must know appropriate sources of evidence, have access to these within the context of clinical decision-making and value the importance of this evidence in making the best clinical decisions in collaboration with patients. *Orthotics and Prosthetics in Rehabilitation,* second edition, provides an excellent source of evidence for clinical decision-making, organized to correspond with typical patient problems and technical dilemmas in the prescription of orthotics and prosthetics. Part I of the revised text provides an overview of the bodies of knowledge that provide foundation for clinical decision-making in orthotics and prosthetics: effective interdisciplinary teaming, materials, and methods of orthotic/prosthetic fabrication, analysis of gait dysfunction, the cardiovascular/cardiopulmonary system's role as determinant of activity level, principles of motor learning and motor control, biomechanics and principles of orthotic/prosthetic design, and an exploration of footwear as the "base" for orthotic/prosthetic intervention. Part II expands on these principles by focusing on specific orthotic designs and the movement dysfunctions that they are meant to address. This includes special consideration of segmental structure and function and specific implications for common primary or secondary pathologies. Part III focuses on specific strategies and rationale for examination, evaluation, and rehabilitation/prosthetic intervention planning for individuals with amputation of various etiologies, at various points in the lifespan.

Education in the rehabilitation sciences has become increasingly case-based, as an enhancement of student learning. This case-based approach provides students with the opportunity to learn information needed in the clinical decision-making process, as well as to develop skill in applying the correct and most contemporary information to the appropriate cases. Students and clinical educators have reported that such case-based education improves students' understanding of new information and helps them to better apply this information in the clinical setting. The result is student clinicians who are more confident, skilled in clinical decision-making processes, and increasingly efficient in the clinical environment. This edition of *Orthotics and Prosthetics in Rehabilitation* has added a new student learning resource: the integrative case example. This new element of the text allows students to consider the newly learned knowledge in the context of a posed patient situation. A series of "questions to consider" in each case example raises issues and options that need to be considered, prompting the students to apply didactic information they have been reading. This provides several rich learning opportunities for faculty and their students.

Finally, education in the rehabilitation sciences has adopted the use of the disablement model as a framework for considering patient problems, setting priorities for intervention, and understanding the significance of risk factors and personal and environmental characteristics. In today's health care delivery system, identifying the major sources of disability as they affect a client's quality of life is the basis for determining a clinically effective patient intervention and demonstrates appropriate resource management. This text will assist the practitioner and student in determining the sources of disability, the options for intervention, and the methods to assess patient outcomes regarding prosthetics and orthotics use. Our rehabilitation professions possess a wide range of technologies, materials, and products that comprise the possible interventions to address the prosthetic or orthotic needs of the patient. Efficacy will be determined however, not by technology or materials but by the successful matching of the client's functional limitations with the most precisely prescribed clinical solutions. This text provides an approach to prosthetic and orthotic management that focuses on the patient's disability and the functional ramifications and thus helps the clinician to best consider quality-of-life issues within the available clinical solutions.

In *Prosthetics and Orthotics for Rehabilitation,* second edition, these three contemporary elements of rehabilitation science—evidence in practice, case-based education, and the disablement model—have provided a framework for organization and delivery of this body of knowledge. The text is a comprehensive and contemporary presentation of the pertinent science of orthotic and prosthetic management for the rehabilitation professional. It will serve as a useful organization of information for students new to this content, as well as a valuable resource for practicing clinicians as they each seek to bring the best evidence to patient care decision-making.

Michael J. Emery, PT, EdD

Preface

We have witnessed significant technological advances in the field of orthotics and prosthetics in the years since publication of the first edition of *Orthotics and Prosthetics in Rehabilitation* in 2000. A number of important changes in the health care delivery and reimbursement system both enhance and constrain the provision of effective interdisciplinary care to individuals whose function might be enhanced by an orthosis or prosthesis. We are challenged to provide care that is efficacious, as well as cost effective and efficient, since patients move through health care settings more quickly than ever. As with the first edition, our primary goal in preparing the second edition of this text is to provide an accessible, detailed, and current resource for students preparing to enter various rehabilitation disciplines, as well as a comprehensive and ready reference for clinicians actively involved in caring for patients of all ages.

The complexity of the rehabilitation process and the increasing range of technological developments pose an ongoing challenge for the health professional involved in rehabilitation. The expertise and input of many professional disciplines is necessary to best serve the needs of patients and their families. We hope that this work addresses this complexity by providing expertise from diverse perspectives. Our contributors are professionals from the fields of orthotics and prosthetics, physical and occupational therapy, and medicine and surgery. We present our work as an example of the value of collaborative and interdisciplinary patient care; readers will find an "interdisciplinary" thread woven through each chapter.

Each contributor has carefully researched recent developments in technology and patient management for the revised or new chapter presented in the second edition. We have asked the contributors to use an evidence-based practice approach to support the information they share with us and to help us develop our understanding of their content areas. We hope that this approach will provide a workable model, prompting each reader to critically appraise evidence from a variety of resources including the clinical research literature, integrate this material with their own expertise and that of others, and include the patient and family concerns, goals, and values when making clinical decisions.

We have added case examples in each of the orthotic and prosthetic chapters to illustrate the clinical decision-making process, especially when there are multiple options that might be considered. Each case example begins with a situational context, including current and past medical history, the social/family/developmental situation, and a realistic clinical problem to be solved. This narrative is followed by a series of questions that prompt the reader to use the information presented in the chapter to make recommendations for further examination or intervention. We deliberately do not provide "answers" to these questions but instead encourage readers to discuss and debate with colleagues and peers to sort out what options might be most appropriate. We seek to provide an opportunity to "practice" the process of evidence-based clinical decision making rather than prescribe an absolute recommendation or plan of care. To reflect the evolving roles and responsibilities of rehabilitation professionals, we have incorporated the perspective and language of the American Physical Therapy Association's *Guide to Physical Therapist Practice* and the World Health Organization's model of health and disablement, in the case examples and throughout the text.

As in the first edition, we have deliberately chosen to use "person first" language, to best reflect the humanity and value of the individuals we care for. Although phrases such as "person with amputation" or "person with stroke" may be a bit more cumbersome to read than the words "amputee" or "patient," we feel that the gentle reminder provided by the phrase is well worth the extra time and effort required.

We hope that these strategies will provide the student and the clinician with a foundation for comprehensive, individually oriented care.

Each chapter begins with a set of learning objectives, written to help readers understand the scope of the content and focus attention on key elements within the chapter and on the outcomes that the authors and editors intend.

The first part of the second edition is designed to provide a foundational understanding of the field of orthotics and prosthetics. This section includes updated discussions of the materials used and the prescription and fabrication process. Readers will recognize the importance of effective assessment of gait dysfunction as the foundation for orthotic and prosthetic prescription, intervention, and outcomes assessment. They will appreciate the significance that energy expenditure plays in the selection of an orthosis or prosthesis, especially for patients who have cardiopulmonary/cardiovascular impairment. We have added several new chapters to help readers apply current thinking about motor control and motor learning to orthotic and prosthetic rehabilitation and to provide an overview of the evidence-based approach to rehabilitative care and clinical decision making. The final chapter in this part helps readers understand the interplay of human kinesiology and the biomechanical characteristics of an orthosis or prosthesis.

The second part focuses on the use of orthoses in rehabilitation to enhance function and to prevent or correct deformity for persons with various musculoskeletal and neurological impairments. We begin with a consideration of footwear as the foundation for most lower extremity orthoses. Then, starting with the foot and moving upward through AFO, KAFO and HKAFO, and KO, we present a functional scheme for prescription of and training for the various lower extremity orthoses. We show the readers how to apply these strategies by discussing options for individuals with musculoskeletal and neuromuscular conditions most frequently encountered in the clinic. We present an overview of current splinting options for management of hand dysfunction and the role of orthoses and prostheses in the management of serious burn injuries. To complete Part II, a new chapter introduces the role of wheelchairs and adaptive seating to enhance mobility and function for persons with neuromuscular and musculoskeletal impairment.

Part III provides an overview of the rehabilitation process for individuals at risk of or with amputation. We begin with an overview of the various etiologies of amputation, the management of persons with vascular and neuropathic diseases that place them at risk of amputation and descriptions of the most commonly performed amputation surgeries. We present strategies for immediate postoperative care and early prosthetic fitting. We then provide descriptions of the prosthetic and rehabilitation alternatives for persons with amputations of the lower limb, with an emphasis on interdisciplinary teaming in both prosthetic and rehabilitative decision making. Chapters are organized so that the reader will develop an organizational schema for understanding design, alignment, and selection of appropriate components from among many available options. We present strategies for functional prosthetic training for patients with amputation, including gait assessment strategies to identify patient or prosthetic basis of gait dysfunction. We begin with distal amputations of the lower limb and move proximally through transtibial and transfemoral levels, considering the impact of joint loss on prosthetic control, stance phase stability, and energy expenditure during ambulation. We have added a new chapter about advanced training and athletics for persons with amputation. The book concludes with several chapters focusing on the needs of patients with high-level and bilateral lower extremity amputation, children with limb deficiency, and prosthetic options and rehabilitation for patients with upper extremity amputation.

Materials throughout all three parts have been updated to reflect new developments in technology and comprehensive contemporary practice. High-quality care in orthotic/prosthetic rehabilitation requires the resources of a variety of specialists working as collaborative health care teams. We hope that this text will enhance collaboration, mutual respect, and further understanding of the health care professionals involved in orthotic and prosthetic rehabilitation. This work is based on our belief that collaborative and interdisciplinary care enriches our clinical practice, our teaching, and especially our ability to care for our patients.

Michelle M. Lusardi
Caroline C. Nielsen

Acknowledgments

When we were asked to develop a second edition of *Orthotics and Prosthetics in Rehabilitation,* we knew we would once again need to rely on those colleagues who contributed so much to the first edition. We also needed their advice and expertise to meet the challenge of developing a text that addresses the needs of today's interdisciplinary rehabilitation team. We are grateful to those who were willing to work with us once again and to those who joined us in this venture for the first time. Without the willingness of professionals from many disciplines to participate and advance the field of orthotic and prosthetic rehabilitation, this book would not have been possible. This new, updated version is the result of their combined expertise and assistance, and we gratefully acknowledge their support:

- Colleagues from the Physical Therapy and Nursing programs at Sacred Heart University, who provided unwavering encouragement, valuable advice, and forgiveness for missed deadlines and short tempers during the lengthy manuscript preparation process. Special thanks to Michael Emery, Pam Levangie, Donna Bowers, Beverly Fein, Salome Brooks, Gary Austin, David Cameron, Linda Strong, and Julie Pavia.
- Colleagues from the Physical Therapy Program, the Graduate Program in Allied Health, and the Orthotics and Prosthetics certificate program at the University of Connecticut, who supported us through the preparation of the first edition of this text. Special thanks go to Pam Roberts, Rita Wong, Polly Fitz, and Priscilla Douglas for their belief in possibilities as we began this project.
- Robin C. Seabrook, Executive Director of the National Commission on Orthotic/Prosthetic Education, for her insight and continuing vision of the future of orthotic and prosthetic education and her ongoing support of this project; William Barringer for his efforts in developing and implementing this vision among the community of practitioners; and Ronald Altman for his initial creative thoughts on interdisciplinary education.
- Clinical colleagues who have helped us learn about orthotic and prosthetic care and who have willingly shared their expertise and energy with our students. Special thanks to Carolyn Kelly, John Zenie, David Knapp, Robert Lin, and Richard Psonak, among many others, for their commitment to clinical education and interdisciplinary patient care.
- The students from Sacred Heart University and the University of Connecticut who have explored the field of orthotics and prosthetics in our classrooms; their thirst for knowledge and desire for excellence in patient care have been the true catalyst for this project.
- Each of our contributors, for their willingness to meet the challenge of updating or creating their chapters, sharing their clinical experience and knowledge, and maintaining their enthusiasm for the project, as well as for their patience and perseverance during the long process.
- J.C. Bender, physical therapist and illustrator extraordinaire, who created most of the original illustrations for this work. His ability to turn our preliminary ideas and very rough sketches into an ideal illustration is miraculous.
- Our editors at Elsevier, Marjorie Fraser, Kathy Falk, Meghan Ziegler, Marion Waldman, and Gail Michaels, for their patience and expectancy, words of encouragement, technical assistance, and gentle reminders as this second edition moved from concept to reality, and Cynthia Mondgock for her assistance with the artwork and permissions. Thanks also to Mary Drabot, Leslie Kramer, and Barbara Murphy, who helped us to learn how to assemble a useful and accessible text and to believe we could and should attempt this project in the first place.
- And most important, to the members of our families who have steadfastly encouraged, graciously suffered, and joyfully celebrated with us during the writing and editing process:

  My mother, Elizabeth Ouellette Pullan, who by her loving example has taught me how much caring for others can be joyful work. My daughter, Tigre Karen, whose love of learning and celebration of difference enliven my spirit. And my husband, Lawrence, whose belief in me makes anything possible. —*M.M.L.*

  My husband, Svend, for his endless support and for contributing his expertise in pathology. And my children, Frederick, Elizabeth, and Caroline, who have not only endured but enthusiastically supported my endeavors. —*C.C.N.*

Contents

Part I
Building Baseline Knowledge

Part II
Orthotics in Rehabilitation

Part III
Prosthetics in Rehabilitation

I

Building Baseline Knowledge

1

Orthotics and Prosthetics in Rehabilitation: The Multidisciplinary Approach

CAROLINE C. NIELSEN

LEARNING OBJECTIVES

On completion of this chapter, the reader will be able to do the following:

1. Describe the role of the orthotist and the prosthetist in the rehabilitation of persons with movement dysfunction.
2. Compare and contrast the history of, development of, and interconnections among the professions of physical therapy, orthotics, and prosthetics.
3. Identify the key features of models of disability and their relevance for the rehabilitation team.
4. Justify why a team approach is important and effective in the rehabilitation of persons with movement dysfunction.
5. Determine the key characteristics of a successful interdisciplinary team.
6. Identify and suggest appropriate responses to the difficulties that might be encountered on an interdisciplinary rehabilitation team.

Today's health care environment emphasizes maximizing patient outcomes while containing costs. In addition, the ongoing development of evidenced-based practice and new definitions of disability affect the contemporary roles of the health care professional involved in rehabilitation. In this complex environment, current and evolving patterns of health care delivery focus on a team approach to the total care of the patient. Downsizing in health care, reorganization from traditional functional structures to patient-focused structures, and use of total quality management approaches that reward group participation over individual efforts have contributed to the increased emphasis on interdisciplinary team care.[1] Today, practicing allied health professionals are expected to collaborate in diverse health care settings to provide the most effective rehabilitation outcome for patients.

For a health care team to function effectively, each member must develop a positive attitude toward interdisciplinary collaboration. The collaborating health professional must understand the functional roles of each health care discipline within the team and must respect and value each discipline's input in the decision-making process of the health team.[2] Rehabilitation, particularly when related to orthotics and prosthetics, lends itself well to interdisciplinary teams because the total care of patients with complex disorders requires a wide range of knowledge and skills. The prosthetist, the orthotist, and the physical therapist are important participants in the rehabilitation team. Understanding the roles and professional responsibilities of each of these disciplines maximizes the ability of the rehabilitation team members to function effectively to provide comprehensive care for the patient.

Definitions of disability continue to evolve. Current definitions consider social, behavioral, and environmental factors that affect the person's ability to function in society. These definitions have considerably broadened the original pathology model in which disability was a function of a particular disease or group of diseases.[3] The current, more inclusive model requires expertise from many sectors in rehabilitative care. This chapter discusses the professions of orthotics and prosthetics, the history and development of the profession and the parallel development of physical therapy, and the development and relevance of models of disability and professional roles and attitudes in the team approach to rehabilitation.

ORTHOTISTS AND PROSTHETISTS

Every year approximately 150,000 people lose a limb to an accident or disease. Currently, more than 1.5 million people in the United States have had an amputation.[4] In addition, many other people require special devices to help

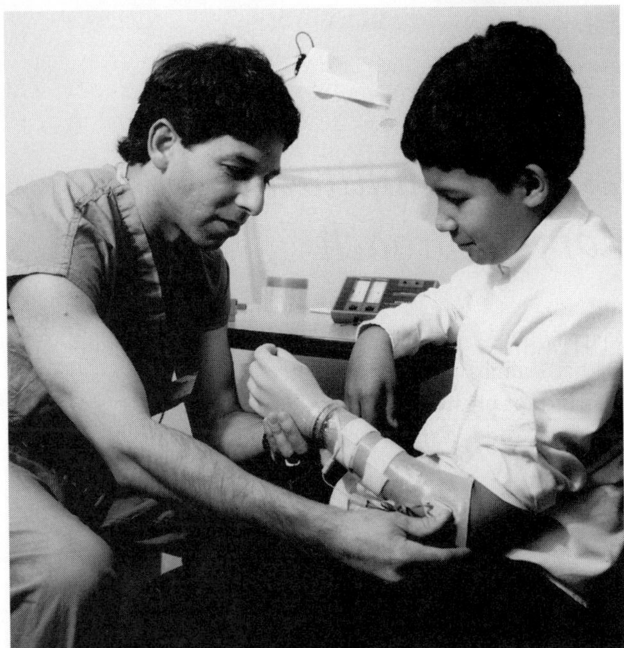

Figure 1-1
The prosthetist evaluates, designs, fabricates, and fits a prosthesis specific to a patient's functional needs. Here the prosthetist double-checks electrode placement sites for a myoelectrical upper extremity prosthesis in a child with amputation of the left forearm.

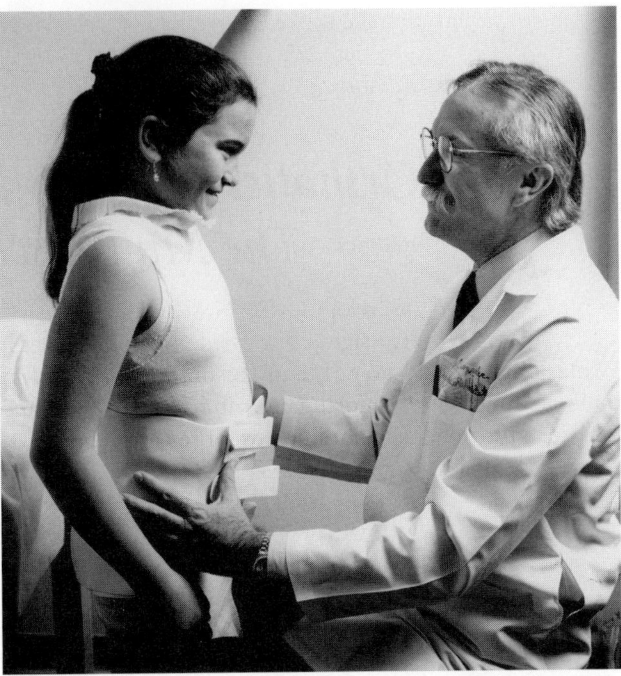

Figure 1-2
Once an orthosis has been fabricated, the orthotist evaluates its fit on the patient to determine if it meets prescriptive goals and can be worn comfortably during functional activities or if additional modifications are necessary. Here the orthotist is fitting a spinal orthosis and teaching his young patient about proper donning and wearing schedules.

them walk, regain active lives, or effectively participate in athletic activities.

Prosthetists and orthotists are allied health professionals who custom make and fit prostheses (artificial limbs) and orthoses (braces). Along with other health care professionals, including physical therapists and occupational therapists, they are integral members of the rehabilitation teams responsible for returning patients to productive and meaningful lives.

Definitions

Prosthetists provide care to patients with partial or total absence of limbs by designing, fabricating, and fitting prostheses, or artificial limbs. The prosthetist creates the design to fit the individual's particular functional and cosmetic needs; selects the appropriate materials and components; makes all necessary casts, measurements, and modifications (including static and dynamic alignment); evaluates the fit and function of the prosthesis on the patient; and teaches the patient how to care for it (Figure 1-1).

Orthotists provide care to patients with neuromuscular and musculoskeletal impairments that contribute to functional limitation and disability by designing, fabricating, and fitting orthoses, or custom-made braces. The orthotist is responsible for evaluating the patient's functional and cosmetic needs, designing the orthosis, and selecting appropriate components; fabricating, fitting, and aligning the orthosis; and educating the patient on appropriate use (Figure 1-2).

In 2006, more than 5469 certified prosthetists and orthotists were practicing in the United States (Table 1-1).[5] Approximately 14% of the current practitioners are women, although the number of women entering the field is increasing. An individual who enters the fields of prosthetics and orthotics today must complete advanced education (beyond an undergraduate degree) and residency programs before becoming

Table 1-1
Orthotists and Prosthetists Certified by the American Board for Certification Practicing in the United States in 1991 and 2006

	1991	*2006*
CP	864 (32.4%)	1364 (24.9%)
CO	1009 (37.8%)	2167 (39.6%)
CPO	795 (29.8%)	1938 (35.4%)
Total	2668 (100.0%)	5469 (100.0%)

Values are n (%).
CO, Certified orthotist; *CP,* certified prosthetist; *CPO,* certified prosthetist/orthotist.
From American Orthotic and Prosthetic Association, Alexandria, Va.: personal communication, July 2005.

eligible for certification. Registered assistants and technicians in orthotics or prosthetics assist the certified practitioner with patient care and fabrication of orthotic and prosthetic devices.

History

The emergence of orthotics and prosthetics as health professions has followed a course similar to that of the profession of physical therapy. Development of all three professions is closely related to three significant events in world history: World War I, World War II, and the onset and spread of polio in the 1950s. Unfortunately, it has taken war and disease to provide the major impetus for research and development in these key areas of rehabilitation.

Although the profession of physical therapy has its roots in the early history of medicine, World War I was a major impetus to its development. During the war, female "physical educators" volunteered in physicians' offices and army hospitals to instruct patients in corrective exercises. After the war ended, a group of these reconstruction aides, as they were called, joined together to form the American Women's Physical Therapy Association. In 1922, the association changed its name to the American Physical Therapy Association, opened membership to men, and aligned itself closely with the medical profession.[6]

Until World War II, the practice of prosthetics depended on the skills of individual craftsmen. The roots of prosthetics can be traced to early blacksmiths, armor makers, other skilled artisans, and even the individuals with amputations, who fashioned makeshift replacement limbs from materials at hand. During the Civil War, more than 30,000 amputations were performed on Union soldiers injured in battle; at least as many occurred among injured Confederate troops. At that time, most prostheses consisted of carved or milled wooden sockets and feet. Many were procured by mail order from companies in New York or other manufacturing centers at a cost of $75 to $100 each.[7] Before World War II, prosthetic practice required much hands-on work and craftsman's skill. D. A. McKeever, a prosthetist who practiced in the 1930s, described the process: "You went to [the amputee's] house, took measurements and then carved a block of wood, covered it with rawhide and glue, and sanded it." During his training, McKeever spent 3 years in a shop carving wood: "You pulled out the inside, shaped the outside, and sanded it with a sandbelt."[8]

The development of the profession of orthotics mirrors the field of prosthetics. Early "bracemakers" were also artisans such as blacksmiths, armor makers, and patients who used many of the same materials as the prosthetist: metal, leather, and wood. By the eighteenth and nineteenth centuries, splints and braces were also mass produced and sold through catalogues. These bracemakers were also frequently known as "bonesetters" until surgery replaced manipulation and bracing in the practice of orthopedics. "Bracemaker" then became a profession with a particular role distinct from that of the physician.[7]

World War II, and the period following, was a time of significant growth for the professions of physical therapy, prosthetics, and orthotics. During the war, many more physical therapists were needed to treat the wounded and rehabilitate those who were left with functional impairments and disabilities. The Army became the major resource for physical therapy training programs, and the number of physical therapists serving in the armed services increased more than sixfold.[9] The number of soldiers who required braces or artificial limbs during and after the war increased the demand for prosthetists and orthotists as well.

After World War II, a coordinated program for persons with amputations was developed. In 1945, a conference of surgeons, prosthetists, and scientists organized by the National Academy of Sciences revealed that little scientific effort had been devoted to the development of artificial limbs. A "crash" research program was initiated, funded by the Office of Scientific Research and Development and continued by the Veterans Administration. A direct result of this effort was the development of the patellar tendon-bearing prosthesis for individuals with transtibial (below-knee) amputation and the quadrilateral socket design for those with transfemoral (above-knee) amputation. This program also included educating prosthetists, physicians, and physical therapists in the skills of fitting and training of patients with these new prosthetic designs.[10] The needs of soldiers injured in the wars in Korea and Vietnam ensured continuing research, further refinements, and development of new materials. The development of myoelectrically controlled upper extremity prostheses and the advent of modular endoskeletal lower extremity prostheses occurred in the post–Vietnam War era. Amputation care and research gained an additional impetus from the Iraq conflict, with amputations among U.S. troops reaching twice the rate of past wars.[11]

The current term *orthotics* emerged in the late 1940s and was officially adopted by American orthotists and prosthetists when the American Orthotic and Prosthetic Association was formed to replace its professional predecessor, the Artificial Limb Manufacturers' Association. *Orthosis* is a more inclusive term than *brace* and reflects the development of devices and materials for dynamic control in addition to stabilization of the body. In 1948, the American Board for Certification in Orthotics and Prosthetics was formed to establish and promote high professional standards.

Although the polio epidemic of the 1950s played a role in the further development of the physical therapy profession, this epidemic had the greatest effect on the development of orthotics. By 1970, many new techniques and materials, some adapted from industrial techniques, were being used to assist patients in coping with the effects of polio and other neuromuscular disorders. The scope of practice in the field of orthotics is extensive, including working with children with muscular dystrophy, cerebral palsy, and spina bifida; patients of all ages recovering from severe burns or fractures; adolescents with scoliosis; athletes recovering from surgery or injury; and older adults with diabetes, cerebrovascular accident, severe arthritis, and other disabling conditions.

Like physical therapists, orthotists and prosthetists practice in a variety of settings. The most common setting is the private office, where the professional offers services to a patient on referral from the patient's physician. Many large institutions, such as hospitals, rehabilitation centers, and research institutes, have departments of orthotics and prosthetics with on-site staff to provide services to patients. The prosthetist or orthotist may also be a supplier or fabrication manager in a central production laboratory. In addition, some orthotists and prosthetists serve as full-time faculty in one of the eight programs that are available for orthotic and prosthetic entry-level training or in one of the programs available at the Master of Science level. Others also serve as clinical educators in a variety of facilities for the year-long residency program required before the certification examination.

Prosthetic and Orthotic Education

With rapid advances in technology and health care, the roles of the prosthetist and orthotist have expanded from a technologic focus to a more inclusive focus on being a member of the rehabilitation team. Patient evaluation, education, and treatment are now significant responsibilities of practitioners. Most technical tasks are completed by technicians who work in the office laboratory or at an increasing number of central fabrication facilities. The advent and availability of modifiable prefabrication systems have reduced the amount of time that the practitioner expends in crafting new prostheses and orthoses.[7]

Current educational requirements reflect these changes in orthotic and prosthetic practice. Entry into professional training programs requires completion of a bachelor's degree from an accredited college or university, with a strong emphasis on prerequisite courses in the sciences. Professional education in orthotics or prosthetics requires an additional academic year for each discipline. Along with the necessary technical courses, students study research methodology, kinesiology and biomechanics, musculoskeletal and neuromuscular pathology, communication and education, and current health care issues. Orthotics and prosthetics programs are most often based within academic health centers or in colleges or universities with hospital affiliations. After completion of the academic program, a year-long residency begins during which new clinicians gain expertise in the acute, rehabilitative, and long-term phases of pediatrics and adult care. On completion of the educational and experiential requirements, the student is eligible to sit for the certification examinations. Today, physical therapists, orthotists, and prosthetists must understand the language, roles, and concerns of all the potential members of the rehabilitation team, including orthopedic surgeons, neurologists, occupational therapists, social workers, nurses, and dietitians, as well as the patients and family members.

DISABILITY: DEFINITIONS AND MODELS

Historically, disability was considered a pathological process inherent in the afflicted individual. Over time, various conceptual frameworks have been developed to organize information about the process and effects of disability. The Nagi model was among the first to challenge the appropriateness of the traditional medical model. The four major elements of Nagi's theoretical formulation included *active pathology* (interference with normal processes at the level of the cell), *impairment* (anatomical, physiological, mental, or emotional abnormalities or loss at the level of body systems), *functional limitation* (limitation in performance at the level of the individual), and *disability*. *Disability* was defined as a "limitation in performance of socially defined roles and tasks within a sociocultural and physical environment."[3,12] This was among the first models of disability to consider the individual in a setting or personal environment.

In 1980, the World Health Organization (WHO) developed the International Classification of Impairments, Disabilities, and Handicaps to provide a standardized means to classify the consequences of disease and injury for the collection of data and the development of social policy. This document provided a framework for organizing information about the consequences of disease. However, it focused solely on the effects of pathological processes on the individuals' activity level. Disability was viewed as a result of an impairment and considered a "lack of ability to perform an activity in the normal manner."[12]

The Institute of Medicine enlarged Nagi's original concept in 1997 to include the individuals' social and physical environment (Figure 1-3). This revised model describes the environment as "including the natural environment, the built environment, culture, the economic system, the political system, and psychological factors." In this model, disability is not viewed as a pathosis residing in a person but instead is a function of the interaction of the person with the environment.[10]

The 2001 revision of the WHO classification document (International Classification of Functioning, Disability and Health) went even further, determining "functioning at the level of body/body part, whole person, and whole person in a social context."[12] This model helps in the description of changes in body function and structure, what people with particular health conditions can do in standard environments (their level of capacity), as well as what they actually do in their usual environments (their level of performance) (Figure 1-4). One of the major innovations of this model is the presence of an environmental factor classification that considers the role of environmental barriers and facilitators

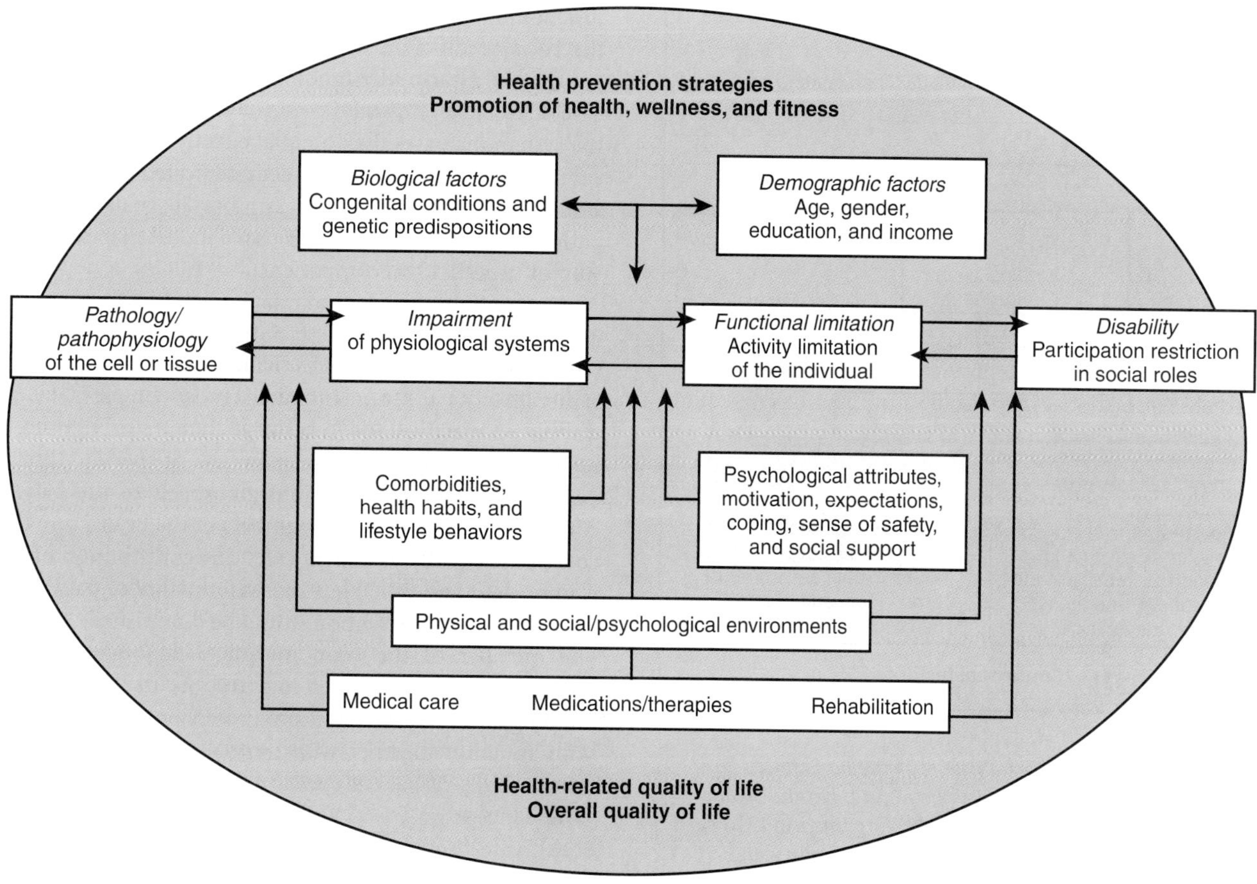

Figure 1-3

The revised Institute of Medicine/Nagi model of the disablement process considers the impact of pathological conditions and impairment as well as intraindividual and extraindividual factors that may influence functional limitation and disability affecting health-related and overall quality of life. (Modified from Guccione AA. Arthritis and the process of disablement. Phys Ther *1994;74[5]:410.)*

in the performance of tasks of daily living. Disability becomes an umbrella term for impairments, activity limitations, and participation restrictions. This model emphasizes health and functioning rather than disability, a radical shift from emphasizing a person's disability to focusing on the level of health. In the International Classification of Functioning, Disability and Health, disability and functioning are viewed as outcomes of interactions between health conditions (diseases, disorders, and injuries) and contextual factors.[13]

The contemporary models of disability guide the rehabilitation team to consider all these elements in rehabilitation and are at the core of physical therapy practice. Input from all members of the team is essential in addressing the pathosis or disease process, impairments, functional limitations, and disabilities. Interrelationships among all four of these elements are the focus of the rehabilitation team. The physical therapist, orthotist, and prosthetist work together to create the most effective outcome for the patient by identifying and addressing pathological processes, functional limitations, impairments, and disability. Implementation of this model of disability has been demonstrated to "improve considerably the quality of interdisciplinary work processes and contribute to a more systematic approach to rehabilitation tasks by the team members."[14]

CHARACTERISTICS OF INTERDISCIPLINARY HEALTH CARE TEAMS

Two issues are emerging in health care as health care professionals face the complexities of current patient care: the need for specialized health professionals and the need for collaboration. The enormous explosion of knowledge in health care, particularly in rehabilitation, has led to increasing specialization in many fields. The interdisciplinary health care team concept has evolved, in part, because no single individual or discipline can have all the necessary expertise and specialty knowledge required for high-quality care, especially the care of patients with complex disorders. Interdisciplinary health care teams provide this expertise, with members from

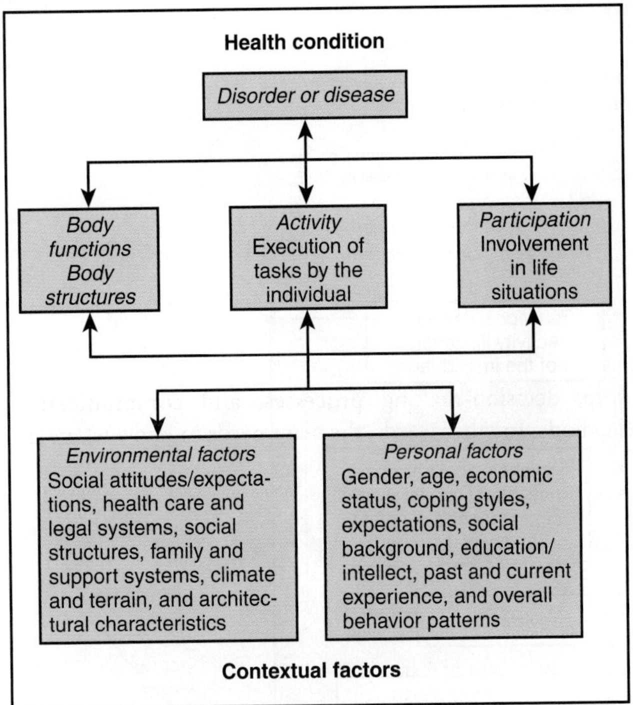

Figure 1-4

WHO uses a biopsychosocial model as the basis for its International Classification of Functioning, Disability and Health. (Modified from World Health Organization. Toward a Common Language for Functioning, Disability and Health. *Geneva: World Health Organization, 2002. pp. 9-10.)*

relevant professions working together, collaborating, and communicating closely to optimize patient care.[15]

Collaboration is defined as a joint communication and decision-making process with the goal of meeting the health care needs of a particular patient or patient population. Each participant on the team brings a particular expertise, and leadership is determined by the particular rehabilitation situation being addressed. The current emphasis on evidence-based practice enhances the role of the team. Evidence-based practice requires consideration and interpretation of research evidence, clinical expertise, and patient values.[16] Teams comprising a range of rehabilitation professionals can bring a wide perspective of expertise on particular rehabilitation issues. With this perspective, clinical decision making becomes a more inclusive process.

Effective team functioning begins during the education of each individual health professional. The rapid change that is occurring in health care practice reinforces the need for interdisciplinary education; in addition to discipline-specific skills and knowledge, students must be aware of the interrelationships among health professionals. Students must develop an understanding of and appreciation for the contributions of the other rehabilitation disciplines in the assessment and treatment of the patient and management of patient problems. One of the major barriers to effective team functioning is a lack of understanding or misconception of the roles of different disciplines in the care of the whole patient.[17] A clear understanding of the totality of the health care delivery system and the role of each professional within the system increases the potential effectiveness of the health care team. A group of informed, dedicated health professionals working together to set appropriate goals and initiate patient care to meet these goals uses a model that exceeds the sum of its individual components.[18]

Almost all health care today is provided in a team setting. This integrated approach facilitates appreciation of the patient as a person with individual strengths and needs rather than as a dehumanized diagnosis or problem. The diverse perspectives and knowledge that are brought to the rehabilitation process by the members of the interdisciplinary team provide insight into all aspects of the patient's concerns. Conceptually, all members of the health care team contribute equally to patient care. The contribution of each is important and valuable; otherwise, quality of patient care and efficacy of intervention would be diminished. Although one member of the team may take an organization or management role, decision making occurs by consensus building and critical discussion. Professionals with different skills function together with mutual support, sharing the responsibility of patient care.

Effective team-based health care assumes that groups of health care providers representing multiple disciplines can work together to develop and implement a comprehensive, integrated treatment plan for each patient. This requires professionals, who traditionally have worked independently and autonomously, to function effectively in interdependent relationships with members of other disciplines.[19] However, this may not be an easy task to accomplish because of the considerable potential for dysfunction.

The *Oxford English Dictionary* defines "team" as "beasts of burden yoked together." Pearson and Jones[19] define a team in more positive terms as "a small group of people who relate to each other to contribute to a common goal." A number of factors are important influences on health professionals' perception of team membership as either a hardship that transforms them into beasts of burden or an opportunity to contribute toward a common goal. Much of our understanding of team function is drawn from organization and management research literature, the theories of which provide insight and information on how interdisciplinary teams operate and the factors that facilitate or inhibit their effectiveness.

Values and Behaviors

Some of the factors that tend to limit the effectiveness of a work group are large group size, poor decision-making practices, lack of fit between group members' skills and task demands, and poor leadership.[21,22] Other factors that influence team dynamics are classified as *formal* (tangible or

Box 1-1 *Formal and Informal Factors That Influence Dynamics of the Multidisciplinary Work Group*

FORMAL (VISIBLE) INFLUENCES	INFORMAL (SUBMERGED) INFLUENCES
Policies of the group or institution	Informal relationships among team members
Objectives of the group	Communication styles of team members
Formal systems of communication	Power networks within the group
Job descriptions of group members	Individual values and beliefs
	Goals/norms of individuals in the group

Modified from Pearson P, Jones K. The primary health care non-team? Dynamics of multidisciplinary provider groups. *BMJ* 1994;309(6966):1387-1388.

visible) and *informal* (submerged). Formal factors include the policies and objectives of the group or its parent organization, the systems of communication available to the group, and the job descriptions of its members. Informal factors, which are often less obvious but equally influential on group process, include working relationships among team members; power networks within and external to the group; and the values, beliefs, and goals of individuals within the group (Box 1-1).[19] Team-building initiatives are often focused on the formal, or visible, areas, but informal communication, values, and norms play key roles in the functioning of the health care team.

A variety of characteristics and considerations also enhance the effectiveness of the interdisciplinary health care team. In addition to having strong professional backgrounds and appropriate skills, team members must appreciate the diversity within the group, taking into account age and status differences and the dynamics of individual professional subgroups.[23] The size of the team is also important: the most capable and effective teams tend to have no more than 12 members. Team members who know each other and are aware of and value each other's skills and interests are often better able to set and achieve goals. Clearly defined goals and objectives about the group's purpose and primary task, combined with a shared understanding of each member's roles and skills, increase the likelihood of effective communication.

Values and behaviors that facilitate the collaborative team care model include the following:

- Trust among members that develops over time as members become more familiar with each other
- Knowledge or expertise necessary for the development of trust
- Shared responsibility for joint decision making regarding patient outcomes
- Mutual respect for all members of the team
- Two-way communication that facilitates sharing of patient information and knowledge
- Cooperation and coordination to promote the use of skills of all team members
- Optimism that the team is indeed the most effective means of delivering quality care

In the early stages of development it is essential that the team spend some time developing goals, tasks, roles, leadership, decision-making processes, and communication methods. In other words, the team needs to know where it's going, what it wants to do, who is going to do it, and how it will get done.[24]

One of the most important characteristics of an effective health care team is the ability to accommodate personal and professional differences among members and to use these differences as a source of strength. The well-functioning team often becomes a means of support, growth, and increased effectiveness and professional satisfaction for the physical therapist and other health professionals who wish to maximize their strengths as individuals while participating in professional responsibilities.[25]

Rehabilitation Teams

The interdisciplinary health care team has become essential in the rehabilitation of patients whose function would be enhanced by an orthosis or prosthesis. The complexity of the rehabilitation process and the multidimensional needs of patients frequently require the expertise of many different professional disciplines. The rehabilitation team is often shaped by the typical needs and characteristics of the patient population that it is designed to serve. The professionals most often represented on the team include an orthopedic or vascular surgeon, neurologist, the patient's primary physician, a prosthetist and/or orthotist, nurses, a physical and/or occupational therapist, a dietitian, a social worker, a vocational counselor, and, most important, the patient (Figure 1-5). Each of the professionals has an important role to play in the rehabilitation of the patient. Patient education is often one of the primary concerns of the team; understanding the condition's process and prognosis and the available treatment options helps patients be active partners in the rehabilitation process rather than passive recipients of care. Patients and their families are best able to define their needs and concerns and communicate them to the other team members. Each member of the team has the responsibility to contribute to this education so that patients have the information needed for an effective partnership and positive outcome of rehabilitation efforts.

Research studies across a wide variety of medical conditions and health disciplines contain evidence that those

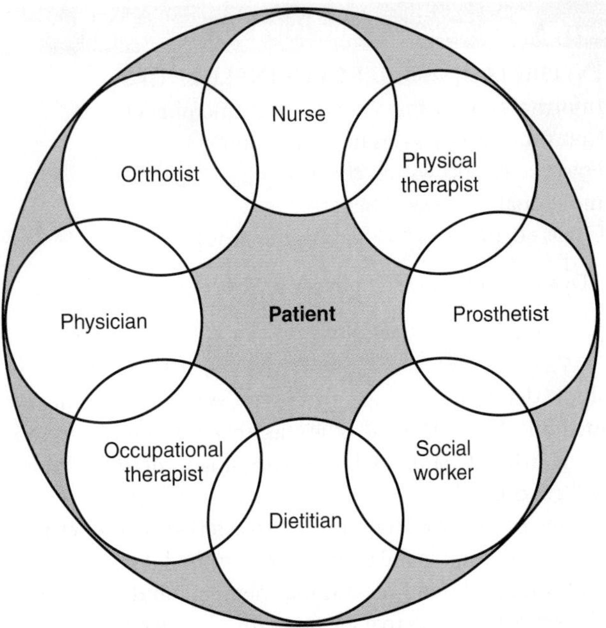

Figure 1-5
A key characteristic of the successful health care team is a clear understanding of the role, responsibilities, and unique skills and knowledge of each member of the rehabilitation team, combined with open and effective communication.

patients who feel prepared and informed are most likely to invest in and comply with recommended interventions and often have the most positive health outcome. Ideally, patient education about amputation and prosthetics begins in advance of, or at least immediately after, the amputation surgery.[26] A national survey of people with amputations (n = 109) revealed that information is often scarce at this crucial time.[27] Individuals with recent amputations are often caught in an information gap in the days between surgery and the initial process of prosthetic prescription and fitting. Only approximately 50% of patients with a new amputation received information about the timing and process of rehabilitation or about prosthetic options before or immediately after amputation.[27] Interestingly, the health professional most frequently cited as a provider of information at the time of amputation was the physical therapist (25%), followed by the physician (23%). The health professionals cited as most helpful after amputation were the prosthetist (65%) and the physical therapist (23%) (Table 1-2). Clearly, one of the most valued contributions of the physical therapist, in addition to the traditional role in facilitating a patient's mobility and independence, is as a provider of early information about the timing and process of the prosthetic fitting and training.

The respondents in this study desired to be active participants in treatment planning and rehabilitation decision making in partnership with the health care team. The keys to the patient's successful participation in the rehabilitation team are efforts to provide more information and opportunity for open communication; both are likely to enhance patient satisfaction and compliance and the achievement of a positive clinical outcome.

Table 1-2
Health Professionals Cited as Sources of Information to Persons with Amputations (n = 109)

Health Discipline	*Provided Information at Time of Amputation*	*Most Helpful After Amputation*
Physical therapist	24 (25%)	22 (23%)
Prosthetist	18 (19%)	63 (65%)
Surgeon/family physician	22 (23%)	28 (29%)
Others with amputation	21 (22%)	7 (7%)

Values are n (%).
Data from Nielsen CC: A survey of amputees: functional level and life satisfaction, information needs, and the prosthetist's role. *J Prosthet Orthot* 1991;3(3):125.

Coordinated care by a multidisciplinary team is just as essential for effective rehabilitation of children as it is for adults. For children with myelomeningocele or cerebral palsy, the broad knowledge base available through team interaction provides a stronger foundation for tailoring interventions to the ever-changing developmental needs of the child and family.[28,29] The optimal delivery of care to these children is best provided in the multidisciplinary setting in which the various specialists can provide a truly collaborative approach. Orthopedic surgeons, neurologists, orthotists, prosthetists, physical therapists, occupational therapists, nurses, dietitians, social workers, psychologists, and special education professionals may all be involved in setting goals and formulating and carrying out plans for intervention and outcomes assessment.

The concept of a multidisciplinary pediatric clinic team was formulated as World War II came to an end.[30] This structure has evolved further over the years and is particularly effective for the more complex orthotic and prosthetic challenges. A "mini-team" consisting of the patient's physician, a physical therapist, and a prosthetist or orthotist can usually be assembled, even in a small town with few facilities. Regardless of its size, an effective team views the child and family from a holistic perspective, with the input from each specialty being of equal value. Under these circumstances, the setting of treatment priorities, such as whether prosthetic fitting or training in single-handed tasks is most appropriate at a child's current age or developmental level, is made on the basis of the particular needs of the individual rather than on local custom.[31]

Clearly, the team is a diverse group of health care professionals, each with particular skills to address the needs of the patient. Each member of the team must understand the role and responsibilities of the other members. Clear and frequent communication is essential for this team to function effectively.

CASE EXAMPLE 1

Interdisciplinary Teams

P. G. is a 23-year-old man admitted to a level 3 trauma center 2 weeks ago after sustaining severe crush injuries to both lower extremities and a closed-head injury in an accident involving a motorcycle and an SUV. Initially unconscious with a Glasgow Coma Scale score of 8, P. G. was placed on life support in the Emergency Department. Radiographs revealed a severely comminuted fracture of the distal right femur and displaced fractures of the left tibia and fibula at midshaft. Examination revealed partial thickness "road burn" abrasions on left anterior thorax and thigh; these were thoroughly cleaned and covered with semipermeable dressings. A computed tomography scan of his cranium and brain revealed a subdural hematoma over the left sylvian fissure and moderate contusion of the anterior pole and undersides of the frontal lobes. Arteriography indicated rupture of the right femoral artery 4 inches above the knee. Given the extent of the crush injuries, the trauma team determined P. G. was not a candidate for reconstructive surgery to salvage his right limb.

P. G. was taken to surgery, where a standard length transfemoral amputation was performed on the right limb. Simultaneously, orthopedic surgeons performed an open-reduction internal fixation with an intramedullary rod in the tibia and used surgical plates and screws to repair the fibula. Neurosurgeons drained the subdural hematoma through a burr hole in his skull. P. G. was started on high-dose, broad-spectrum antibiotics in the operating room. He was transferred to the surgical intensive care unit for postoperative care.

P. G. has been weaned from his ventilator and is now functioning at a Rancho Los Amigos Scale level of 7. He is able to follow one- and two-step commands but becomes easily confused and angry in complex environments and when fatigued. His postoperative pain is currently being managed with Tylenol #3 with codeine as needed. His right lower extremity has been managed with soft dressings and elastic bandages; his residual limb is moderately bulbous, with resolving ecchymosis from the accident and surgery. Moderate serosanguineous drainage continues from the medial one third of the suture line. Although most of the skin abrasions show signs of regranulation, one area on his left thigh is red and hot, with yellowish drainage. When transferred (maximum assist of two) into a bedside recliner, P. G. tolerates 30 minutes in a 45-degree to 60-degree reclined position. He becomes lightheaded and has significant pain when sitting upright with his left lower extremity dependent. He has been referred to physical therapy for evaluation of rehabilitation potential and initiation of mobility activities.

Before his accident, P. G. was a graduate student in physics at a nearby university. He lived in a third-floor walk-up apartment with his fiancée and his golden retriever. Besides his motorcycle, his interests and hobbies included long-distance running and mountain climbing. His mother and father have traveled to be with him during the acute hospital stay.

Questions to Consider

- Given the extent of his injuries, what specialists and health professionals would best be part of the team involved in P. G.'s care? What are the priorities, specific roles, and responsibilities for each potential member of the team? How are these similar or different across the team?
- What environmental influences will affect team formation and functioning in a busy level 3 trauma center? What factors might facilitate team development? What factors might challenge the effectiveness of the team?
- What strategies might the members of the team use to enhance communication and decision making about P. G.'s condition and prognosis?
- As P. G. recovers from his injuries, how might the roles and responsibilities of the various team members change or evolve?

CASE EXAMPLE 2

Interdisciplinary Teams

E. L. is a 73-year-old woman with a 10-year history of adult onset (type 2) insulin-dependent diabetes mellitus. Two weeks before her most recent hospitalization, she and her husband (who is in the early stages of Alzheimer's disease) moved from their home of 50 years to an assisted-living complex in a neighboring town. Although the furniture is set up and functional, they have not had the chance to fully unpack and make the apartment their own.

Over the past 3 years, E. L. has been monitored by her team of physicians for progressive polyneuropathy of diabetes and for moderate peripheral vascular disease. She had a transmetatarsal amputation of her right forefoot 8 months ago because of nonhealing recurrent neuropathic ulcer. Despite wearing custom-molded shoes and accommodative orthoses, another ulcer of her first metatarsal head developed on the left foot 2 months ago. This new ulcer did not heal with conservative care and progressed to osteomyelitis 2 weeks ago. When vascular studies suggested inadequate circulation to heal the ulcer, E. L. underwent an elective transtibial amputation of her left lower extremity. Despite a short bout of postoperative delirium thought to be related to pain management with morphine, E. L. (5 days postoperatively) was adamant about returning to her new assisted-living apartment, using a wheelchair for mobility, and receiving home care until her residual limb is healed and ready for prosthetic fitting.

Currently she is able to ambulate 2 lengths of 15-foot-long parallel bars before needing to rest and has begun gait training with a "hop-to" gait pattern with a standard walker. She is able to transfer from sitting on a firm seating surface with armrests to standing with standby guarding and verbal cueing and needs minimal assistance from low and soft seats without armrests. She feels she and her husband will be able to manage at home because her bathroom has grab bars on the toilet, and a tub seat and handheld shower head are available from the "loaner closet" at her assisted-living facility.

At discharge, her new suture line had one small area of continued moderate drainage, requiring frequent dressing changes. She is unable to move her residual limb into a position for effective visual self-inspection of the healing surgical wound without significant discomfort. Her husband, although attentive, becomes confused with the routine of wound care. E. L.'s postoperative limb volume and edema are being managed with a total contact cast, which she is able to don and doff independently. She had one late evening fall, when she woke from a sound sleep having to go to the bathroom and was surprised when her left limb "wasn't really there" to stand on when she tried to get out of bed.

Since her amputation, E. L.'s insulin dosages have had to be adjusted frequently because of unpredictable changes in her blood sugar levels. She has lost 20 pounds (half of which can be attributed to her amputation) since admission.

Questions to Consider

- If you were involved in discharge planning for E. L and her husband, what types of services might you recommend be available to them on her return home? Are these services more likely to be coordinated from a central organization or "patchworked" together across a number of health care agencies and practices?
- What are the roles, priorities, and specific responsibilities of the various health care professionals who are likely to be involved in her care?
- What are the major challenges facing the likely informal team of care providers involved in the postoperative, preprosthetic care of E. L and her husband? How are these similar to or different from the trauma center team previously considered? What strategies are currently in place or must be developed to ensure that E. L.'s care at home is comprehensive and coordinated?
- In what ways will the decision making in E. L.'s case likely to be different than the decision making in the previous case (P. G.)? How will the roles and responsibilities of the team members evolve and change as she recovers from her surgery and is ready to begin prosthetic use?

CASE EXAMPLE 3
Interdisciplinary Teams

M. S. is a 12-year-old girl with myelomeningocele (spina bifida) in whom significant scoliosis has developed over the last year during a growth spurt. Concerned about the rate of increase in her S-shaped thoracolumbar curve, her parents sought the advice of an orthopedic surgeon who has been involved as a consultant in her care since birth. The surgeon recommends surgical stabilization of M. S.'s spine with Harrington rods and bony fusion to (1) prevent further progression of the curve and rib hump so that secondary impairment of the respiratory system will be minimized as she grows and (2) provide more efficient upright sitting posture for wheelchair propulsion in the years ahead.

M. S. currently attends special education classes in her neighborhood middle school and is monitored by a school-based physical therapist. Until 2 years ago, she ambulated for exercise by using a reciprocal gait orthosis during gym periods at school, but with recent spurts in growth the use of a manual wheelchair is more efficient for mobility (to keep up with her classmates). She is also followed up on a regular basis by a neurologist who monitors the operation of her ventriculoperitoneal shunt (commonly used in the management of hydrocephalus associated with myelomeningocele).

In addition to their concerns about the risk of the surgical procedure, M. S.'s parents are quite concerned about how the anticipated 4-month postoperative immobilization in a thoracolumbosacral orthosis will affect her capacity for self-care and independent wheelchair mobility. They are also concerned about how the surgery and postoperative period will potentially interrupt the effective bowel and bladder management routine for which M. S. has just begun to assume responsibility. As witnesses to their daughter's deconditioning and loss of stamina over the last 6 months, they are concerned that she might not be "physically ready" for the surgery and postoperative rehabilitation. They also are asking questions about whether this spinal surgery will ultimately improve the prognosis of a successful return to ambulation with her reciprocal gait orthosis.

Questions to Consider

- What are the priorities, roles, and responsibilities of the health professionals involved in the care of this child and her family? In what ways is the composition of M. S.'s team similar to or different from that of P. G.'s and E. L.'s teams? How many different care systems are likely to play a role in the decision-making process? How many different care systems are likely to be involved in postoperative rehabilitation?
- How are the goals and priorities of the family system, the educational system, and the health care system

going to interact? What constraints exist for effective communication and coordination of care across these systems?

- Given the complexity of her condition and the expected length of recovery, how many different rehabilitation service organizations are M. S. and her family likely to interact with during her rehabilitation and eventual return to school? How will the priorities, roles, and responsibilities of these rehabilitation service organizations evolve as M. S. recovers from her surgery?

SUMMARY

The development of interdisciplinary teams in health care practice today is prevalent and often required. The use of teams has evolved in part because no one person or discipline can have expertise in all the areas of specialty knowledge required for high-quality care. This situation is particularly true in orthotic and prosthetic rehabilitation, in which complex issues require the resources of a variety of specialists. For health professionals to work together in a collaborative and cooperative manner, particular attitudes and attributes are essential. These attitudes include the following:

1. Openness and receptivity to the ideas of others
2. An understanding of, value of, and respect for the roles and expertise of other professionals on the team
3. Interdependence and acceptance of a common commitment to comprehensive patient care
4. Willingness to share ideas openly and to take responsibility[23]

This chapter has explored the influence of these attitudes on the team approach to rehabilitation. The contributions of a physical therapist as an integral member of the rehabilitation team to the holistic care of the patient can be enhanced by an understanding of orthotics and prosthetics. Collaboration, mutual respect, and an understanding of the roles and responsibilities of colleagues engender productive teamwork and improved outcomes for the rehabilitation patient.

REFERENCES

1. Fitz PA, Smey JW, Douglas PD, et al. A case study in core curriculum: twenty years and counting. In *Core Curricula in Allied Health.* Washington, DC: Pew Health Professions Commission, 1995. pp. 139-164.
2. Stubblefield C, Houston C, Haire-Joshu D. Interactive use of models of health-related behavior to promote interdisciplinary collaboration. *J Allied Health* 1994;23(4):237-243.
3. National Institute on Disability and Rehabilitation Research. Dimensions of disability. In *Proposed Long-Range Plan for Fiscal Years 1999-2004.* Washington, DC: Federal Register, 1998.
4. Limb Loss Research and Statistics Program, vol. 1, no. 1, Summer, 2000. pp.1-5.
5. American Orthotic and Prosthetic Association, Alexandria, VA: personal communication, March 2006.
6. Myers RS. Historical perspective, assumptions, and ethical considerations for physical therapy practice. In Myers RS (ed), *Saunders Manual of Physical Therapy Practice.* Philadelphia: Saunders, 1995. pp. 3-7.
7. Shurr DG, Michael JW. *Prosthetics and Orthotics,* 2nd ed. Norwalk, CT: Appleton & Lange, 2002. pp. 1-5.
8. Retzlaff K. AOPA celebrates 75 years of service to O&P. *Orthotics and Prosthetics Almanac* 1992;Nov:45.
9. Hazenhyer IM. A history of the American Physiotherapy Association. Part IV: maturity, 1939-1946. *Phys Ther Rev* 1946;26:174-184.
10. Wilson BA. History of amputation surgery and prosthetics. In Bowker JH, Michael JW (eds), *Atlas of Limb Prosthetics: Surgical, Prosthetic and Rehabilitation Principles.* St. Louis: Mosby–Year Book, 1992. pp. 3-15.
11. Mishra R. Amputation rate for U.S. troops twice that of past wars, *Boston Globe*, December 9, 2004.
12. Guide to physical therapy practice: on what concepts is the guide based? *Phys Ther* 2001;81(1):27-33.
13. World Health Organization. *Towards a Common Language for Functioning, Disability and Health.* Geneva: World Health Organization, 2002.
14. Rentsch HP, Bucher P, Dommen Nyffeler I, et al. The implementation of the International Classification of Functioning, Disability and Health (ICF) in daily practice of neurorehabilitation: an interdisciplinary project at the Kantonsspital of Lucerne, Switzerland. *Disabil Rehabil* 2003;25(8):411-421.
15. Hall P, Weaver L. Interdisciplinary education and teamwork: a long and winding road. *Med Educ* 2001;35(9):867-875.
16. Lusardi M, Levangie P, Fein B. A problem-based learning approach to facilitate evidence-based practice in entry-level health professional education. *JPO* 2002;14(2):40-50.
17. Strasser DC, Falconer JA, Martino-Saltzmann D. The rehabilitation team: staff perceptions of the hospital environment, the interdisciplinary team environment, and interprofessional relations. *Arch Phys Med Rehabil* 1994;75(2):177-182.
18. Douglas PD. The core concept. In Farber NE, McTernan EJ, Hawkins RO (eds), *Allied Health Education.* Springfield, IL: Thomas, 1989. pp. 87-97.
19. Alexander JA, Lichtenstein R, Jinnet K, et al. The effects of treatment team diversity and size on assessment of team functioning. *Hospital and Health Services Administration* 1996;41(1):37.
20. Pearson P, Jones K. The primary health care non-team? Dynamics of multidisciplinary provider groups. *BMJ* 1994;309(6966):1387-1388.
21. Hackman JR. *Groups That Work (& Those That Don't): Creating Conditions for Effective Team Work.* San Francisco: Jossey-Bass, 1990.
22. Goodman PS, Devadas RA, Hughson TLG. Groups and productivity: analyzing the effectiveness of self-managing teams. In Campbell JP, Campbell JR (eds), *Productivity in Organizations.* San Francisco: Jossey-Bass, 1988. pp. 295-327.
23. Fried B, Rundall T. Group and teams in health services organizations. In Shortell SM, Kaluzny AD (eds), *Health Care*

Management, Organization, Design and Behavior, 3rd ed. Albany, NY: Delmar, 1994.

24. Area Health Education Center, DC. *Models of Team Practice-Interdisciplinary Health Care Team Practice, Session 3.* Washington, DC, 2003.
25. Lopopolo RB. The relationship of role-related variable to job satisfaction and commitment to the organization in a restructured hospital environment. *Phys Ther* 2002;82(10):984-999.
26. Nielsen CC. Factors affecting the use of prosthetic services. *J Prosthet Orthot* 1989;1(4):242-249.
27. Nielsen CC. A survey of amputees: functional level and life satisfaction, information needs, and the prosthetist's role. *J Prosthet Orthot* 1991;3(3):125-129.
28. Banta JV, Lin RS, Peterson M, et al. The team approach in the child with myelomeningocele. *J Prosthet Orthot* 1990;2(4):365-375.
29. Wiart L, Darrah J. Changing philosophical perspectives on the management of children with physical disabilities: their effect on the use of powered mobility. *Disabil Rehabil* 2002;24(9):492-498.
30. American Academy of Orthopedic Surgeons. *Atlas of Limb Prosthetics.* St. Louis: Mosby, 1981. p. 493.
31. Michael J. Pediatric prosthetics and orthotics. *Phys Occup Ther Pediatr* 1990;10(2):123-146.

2

Materials and Technology

GÉZA F. KOGLER

LEARNING OBJECTIVES

On completion of this chapter, the reader will be able to do the following:

1. Compare and contrast the materials most often used in current orthoses and prostheses.
2. Describe how the basic mechanical properties of commonly used materials determine how they will be used in orthotic and prosthetic devices.
3. Describe the process of, and measures used in, the formulation of a biomechanically appropriate orthotic or prosthetic prescription that will address a patient's functional deficits.
4. Describe how a prosthetist or orthotist determines the appropriate prosthetic or orthotic controls needed for the management of a patient's impairments or functional limitations.
5. Delineate the steps in the fabrication or production of a custom orthosis or prosthesis.
6. Discuss the use of CAD/CAM in the measurement for and fabrication of orthoses and prostheses.
7. Describe the factors influencing the development of central fabrication centers and the manufacture of prefabricated components, orthoses, and prostheses.

A fundamental concept and common goal within the professions of orthotics, prosthetics, and rehabilitation is the restoration of normal form and function after injury or disease. To accept this challenge, the fields of orthotics and prosthetics have evolved into uniquely specialized professions. In addition to training in the basic biological and medical sciences, orthotists and prosthetists have an understanding of biomechanics, kinesiology, and the material sciences complemented by highly developed technical skills. Knowledge of the physical properties of materials and the techniques to manipulate and use them is essential to the design and fabrication of orthoses and prostheses. However, the subject of material science and technology as it relates to orthotics and prosthetics is exhaustive and could not possibly be given justice within the scope of this text. The topic is presented here as a general overview so that the rehabilitation clinician can develop a basic understanding of current design and fabrication processes used by orthotists and prosthetists.

ORTHOTICS AND PROSTHETICS IN THE TWENTIETH CENTURY

Orthotics and prosthetics have a rich history of research and development. Many innovative devices have been designed to restore function and provide relief from various medical ailments. Although progress can be documented throughout human history, the most significant contributions to orthotics and prosthetics were made in the twentieth century, stimulated by the aftermath of the world wars. Injured veterans who returned home from battle with musculoskeletal and neuromuscular impairments or traumatic amputation dramatically increased the demand for orthotic and prosthetic services. Although World War I stimulated some clinical progress in the two disciplines, notable scientific advancements did not occur until World War II. To improve the quality and performance of assistive devices at the end of World War II, particularly for veterans with amputation, the U.S. government sponsored a series of research and development projects under the auspices of the National Academy of Sciences (NAS) that would forever change the manner in which orthotics and prosthetics would be practiced.[1]

An extensive research effort was initiated by the NAS in late 1945, when a consensus conference revealed that few modern scientific principles or developments had been introduced in prosthetics.[2] Research and educational committees were formed between 1945 and 1976 to advise and work with the research groups. Universities, the Veterans

Administration, private industry, and other military research units were subcontracted to conduct various prosthetic research projects. In summarizing the most notable achievements in prosthetics during this period, Wilson[3] cites the development of the total contact transfemoral socket; the quadrilateral socket design and hydraulic swing-phase knee-control units for the transfemoral prosthesis; the patellar tendon-bearing (PTB) transtibial prosthesis; the solid-ankle, cushioned-heel prosthetic foot; several new designs for the Syme's prosthesis; and the Canadian hip-disarticulation prosthesis. He also notes the implementation of immediate postsurgical and early fitting as having a significant impact on the rehabilitation process for persons with lower extremity amputation. The most notable improvements in upper extremity prosthetics were the lyre-shaped three-jaw chuck terminal device and more efficient harnessing systems. In addition, modular components and advances in bioengineering have permitted increased use and availability of the myoelectric prosthesis since it was first proposed in 1950.[4]

Of the wealth of scientific advances made during this intensive research period, the most important is the greater attention paid to the biomechanics of prosthetic alignment and socket design.[5] According to Wilson,[2] "The introduction of socket designs based on sound biomechanical analyses to take full advantage of the functions and properties of the stump in conjunction with the rationale for alignment undoubtedly represents the greatest achievement in prosthetics since World War II."

Although the focus of the NAS Artificial Limb Program was in prosthetics, it was anticipated that these efforts would also benefit orthotics. A formal research directive in orthotics did not begin until 1960. Biomechanical principles developed for the PTB prosthesis were immediately introduced in orthotics at the Veterans Administration Prosthetic Center, with the PTB orthosis to unload the foot-ankle complex axially.[6] The concept of fracture bracing or cast bracing began at approximately the same time and is now common practice for orthopedic management of fractures.[7,8] Clinical aspects of orthotic practice were also considered; a systematic approach to prescription formulation was established with the development of the technical analysis forms. Nomenclature to describe orthoses and their functions was standardized to identify the body segments they encompassed with the desired biomechanical control mechanisms.[9]

The introduction of new materials led to further advances in the field shortly after World War II. The use of thermosetting plastics in prosthetics permitted the development of the suction socket suspension system.[10] Transparent plastics offered a new approach to diagnostic and fitting evaluation techniques, such as the transparent prosthetic socket (test socket) and the transparent face mask for patients with thermal injuries. In orthotics, the addition of thermoplastics led to numerous innovative designs of ankle-foot orthoses (AFOs) in the 1960s and 1970s. The custom plastic AFO was an important technological advance in lower extremity orthotics. The physical characteristics of thermoformable plastics allowed biomechanical controls to match the prescription for improved function. The mechanical properties of an orthosis could be controlled by the layout of the trimlines of a device or structural reinforcements through specially placed corrugations that could be incorporated into its surface geometry. Advances have been steady in the area of material engineering and continue to have an impact on orthotics and prosthetics. Numerous prosthetic feet have been introduced as elite athletes demand increased performance capabilities from their prosthetic components. Innovative designs for some prosthetic feet have been possible in part because of the diversity of carbon composite technology complemented by sound engineering design.

The development of computer-aided design/computer-aided manufacture (CAD/CAM) systems for orthotics and prosthetics, which began in the 1970s, was another major technological advance, considering the long tradition of custom hand-crafted devices in the profession. In the late 1980s and early 1990s, as computers became more economical, facilities began to integrate CAD/CAM systems into their practices. CAD/CAM systems have now been designed for most orthotic and prosthetic applications, often with specialized digitizers, scanners, and milling equipment to accommodate the unique needs of a particular device. The current trend within the profession is that orthotists and prosthetists use the CAD portion to digitize and manipulate the data, then subcontract the production of a device from a central fabrication company for the CAM portion. The art and workmanship that have distinguished the orthotists and prosthetists from other health professionals for most of the twentieth century continue to evolve as CAD/CAM technologies improve the design, manufacture, and diagnostic aspects of the field.

Orthotics and prosthetics have played an important historical role in the development of medical and surgical orthopedics and rehabilitation. Fundamental concepts that evolved from orthotic and prosthetic advancements are now basic principles in rehabilitation. Orthotics and prosthetics have evolved as sister professions because the technical skills and knowledge base to prescribe, fabricate, and fit the respective mechanical devices are similar. Because of this, material and technological advancements have been shared between these two rehabilitation specialties.

MATERIALS

In the first part of the twentieth century, orthoses were constructed primarily of metal, leather, and fabric, and prostheses were manufactured from wood and leather. In the last 60 years, however, tremendous technological advancements have been made in the material sciences. The demand for strong and lightweight components in the aerospace and marine industries has produced a variety of new materials that possess mechanical properties suitable for use in the construction of orthoses and prostheses. New plastics have led to revolutionary advancements in the profession, permitting increased durability and strength and significant cosmetic improvements. Although a multitude of materials are now available, traditional ones are still in wide use; material selection depends in part on the individual needs of each patient. In a rehabilitation team setting, the orthotist and prosthetist are responsible for choosing the appropriate materials and components for fabrication because their experience and training are specialized in this area.

This chapter presents an overview of the general types of materials used in orthotics and prosthetics for rehabilitation professionals. Publications by the American Society for Testing and Materials contain specific technical information.[11] Industry standards established by the International Organization for Standardization for consumer and patient protection give the strength requirements for orthotic and prosthetic components.[12]

The types of materials used most commonly in current orthotic and prosthetic practice include leather, metal, wood, thermoplastic and thermosetting materials, foamed plastics, and viscoelastic polymers. In deciding which materials are most appropriate for a patient, the orthotist or prosthetist considers the five important characteristics of materials: strength, stiffness, durability, density, and corrosion resistance. [13]

A material's *strength* is determined by the maximum external load that the material can support or sustain. Strength is especially important in lower limb devices, in which loading forces associated with gait can be very high, or when heavy use of the orthotic or prosthetic device is anticipated.

Stiffness is the amount of bending or compression that occurs when a material is loaded (stress/strain or force/displacement ratios). The stiffer a material, the less flexible it is and the less likely that deformation will occur during wear. When significant external stability is desirable (e.g., in a fracture brace or a rigid prosthetic frame), a stiff material is often chosen. When conformation to body segments is necessary (for example, in a posterior leaf-spring AFO or a flexible transfemoral prosthetic socket), a more flexible material is used.

The *durability* (fatigue resistance) of a material is determined by its ability to withstand repeated cycles of loading or unloading during functional activities. Repeated loading compromises the material's strength and increases risk of failure or fracture of the material. Fatigue resistance is especially problematic in the interface of materials with different characteristics.

Density is the material's weight per unit of volume, a prime determinant of energy cost during functional activities while a patient wears a prosthetic or orthotic device. Although the goal is to provide as lightweight a device as possible, strength, durability, and fatigue resistance needs may necessitate a denser material.

Corrosion resistance is the degree to which the material is susceptible to chemical degradation. Many of the materials used for orthoses or prostheses retain heat, making perspiration a problem. For some patients who require lower extremity devices, incontinence may also be a concern. Materials that are impervious to moisture are easier to clean than porous materials.

The ease of fabrication is also an important consideration for materials. Certain materials can be easily molded or adjusted for a custom fit; others require special equipment or techniques to shape the material.

Leather

Leather is manufactured from the skin and hides of various animals. Tanning methods and the type of hide determine the final characteristics of the leather. As an interface material for an orthosis or a prosthesis, vegetable-tanned leather is used to protect the skin from irritation. Chrome-tanned leather is used for supportive purposes when strength and resiliency are needed. Additional chemical processes can be incorporated during manufacturing to produce leathers that are waterproof, porous, flexible, or stiff. Useful qualities of leather include its dimensional stability, porosity, and water vapor permeability.[14] These features have made leather a frequently used material within orthopedics, and it continues to be a material of choice in many current devices. Today, leather is used for supportive components such as suspension straps, belts, and limb cuffs. Leather is also used to cover metallic structures such as pelvic, thigh, and calf bands. For foot orthoses and shoe modifications, leather is often preferred over synthetic substitutes because of its superior "breathability" characteristics.

Another important attribute of leather is its moldability. Although numerous techniques are available to mold leather, the most common one in orthotics and prosthetics is to stretch it over a plaster cast after it has been mulled (dampened or soaked) in water. When the water evaporates from the molded leather, its dried shape is maintained, and the leather can be trimmed to the desired dimensions. To increase strength and durability, leather can be reinforced by lamination with plastics or other leathers. Similarly, if padding is desired over bony regions of the body, foamed plastics or felt can be sandwiched between layers of leather for comfort or to distribute applied forces over a larger surface area. Three basic skills are required for crafting orthotic or prosthetic components of leather: cutting, sewing, and molding. A technique specific to leather work is that of skiving, or thinning the edge on the flesh side of the hide. Finishing methods such as these contribute to the final appearance of the leather work and the device.

Metals

The types of metal used in the fabrication of orthoses and prostheses can be categorized into three groups: steel and its alloys, aluminum, and titanium or magnesium alloys. These metals may or may not share similar characteristics. If metals are incorporated into an orthosis or prosthesis, the choice of metal is determined by the needs and preferences of the particular patient.

Steel

The general term *steel* refers to any iron-based alloy material. Carbon alloys have carbon added to the composition of steel. The term *alloy steel* is used when other materials are included in the material manufacture. Alloy steels are further defined as low-alloy or high-alloy steels. Steels are strong, rigid, ductile, and durable, but their high density (weight) and susceptibility to corrosion are major disadvantages. Many different types of steel are available to meet various engineering needs. To assist in identifying the composition and type of material, the American Iron Steel Institute–Society of Automotive Engineers has established a four-digit numbering system. The first two digits in the number indicate the type of steel, and the last two digits identify the carbon content. For alloy steels, the first digit identifies the major alloy and the second digit indicates the percentage of the major alloying element.

The carbon content of steel is the major determinant of its ductility and yield strength characteristics. Yield strength is an offset measure in a stress-strain curve in which strain occurs without an increase in stress. Ductility is the property of a material to deform in the inelastic or plastic range. Low carbon content (0.05% to 0.10%) produces high ductility and a low yield strength.[15] As the carbon concentration increases, yield strength increases and ductility is reduced. Heat treatments can alter the properties of carbon steel by increasing yield strength and reducing ductility. The mechanical properties of low-alloy steels fall between those of carbon steels and high-alloy steels. High strength/weight ratios are possible with the high-alloy steels, an important characteristic for repetitive loading situations. These types of steels are used for some orthotic and prosthetic joint components. High-alloy steels are not very resistant to corrosion and are often more difficult to fabricate.

Stainless steel is a steel alloy that contains 12% or more of chromium, a material that increases resistance to corrosion and oxidation. Chromium produces a light oxide film on the surface that deters deterioration of the base metal. Because durability and protection from corrosion are highly desirable, stainless steels are used extensively within orthotics and prosthetics to enhance longevity of devices. Two types of stainless steel, martensitic steel and ferretic steel, have chromium as the predominant alloying element, but martensitic steel is the only one used in orthotics and prosthetics because it can be hardened by heat treatment. Stainless steels are used for orthotic and prosthetic joints, support uprights, and band material.

Aluminum

Aluminum alloys are well suited for orthotics and prosthetics because of their high strength/weight ratio and resistance to corrosion. As with steels, the properties of aluminum depend on alloying compositions, heat treatments, and cold working. *Wrought* and *cast* are terms used to describe the two major types of aluminum alloys. Alloys are further subdivided into those that are heat treatable and those that are not. The low ductility and low strength of cast aluminum are ideal for prefabricated prosthetic components and in some assemblies for moving parts. Wrought aluminum alloys are used in orthotics and prosthetics for structural purposes such as prosthetic pylons, orthotic uprights, and upper extremity devices. The high-compression bending stresses of lower extremity prosthetics are well suited to the use of wrought aluminum alloys.

Although aluminum alloys are very resistant to atmospheric and some chemical corrosion, the acids and alkalis in urine, perspiration, and other bodily fluids deteriorate the natural protective oxides on the material's surface, making the aluminum susceptible to corrosion. To deter corrosion in aluminum and to resist abrasive wear, various hard coatings, such as anodic or oxide finishes, can be applied. Mechanical finishes, such as polishing, buffing, and sandblasting, offer attractive cosmetic appearances for devices.

Titanium and Magnesium

Components made of titanium alloys have become more prevalent in prosthetics but are rarely used in orthotics. Although titanium alloys are stronger than those of aluminum and have comparable strength to some steels, their density is 60% that of steel.[16] Because prosthetic components made of titanium are lighter in weight that steel counterparts, they require less energy expenditure by the patient during use. Titanium alloys are also more resistant to corrosion than are aluminum and steel. It is important to note, however, that titanium alloys are often more difficult to machine and fabricate. Because of this, titanium is most often used in prefabricated prosthetic components, when strength and light weight are of concern. Titanium is also more expensive than aluminum and steel, which has been a limiting factor for its use.

Magnesium alloys are lighter than those of aluminum and titanium, are corrosion resistant, and have a lower modulus of elasticity than does aluminum. The modulus of elasticity (Young's modulus) is defined as the ratio of unit stress to unit strain in a stress-strain curve's elastic range; materials with low modulus values are associated with lower rates of fatigue under conditions of repeated stress. Although some of these features are promising, magnesium alloys have not yet been widely used in orthoses and prostheses.

Wood

Wood possesses many desirable characteristics for use in prosthetics. Its wide availability, strength, light weight, and ability to be shaped easily have continued to be of benefit in prosthetics socket and component construction, even with the introduction of thermoplastics. The wood used in prosthetics must be properly cured, free of knots, and relatively strong. Yellow poplar, willow, basswood (linden), and balsa are most commonly used. Hardwoods have been reserved for prosthetic applications in which structural strength is essential, most often in certain types of prosthetic feet or as reinforcement for knee units. The keel prosthetic foot is fabricated of maple and hickory. The solid-ankle, cushioned-heel prosthetic foot has a hardwood keel that is bolted to the prosthetic shank, creating a solid structural unit for standing and ambulation.

Plastics

One of the most important production-related characteristics of an orthotic or prosthetic material is its ability to be molded over a positive model. Because plastics can be readily formed, they are a very popular, widely used material for orthoses and prostheses. Plastics are grouped into two categories: thermoplastics and thermosetting materials.[17-19]

Thermoplastics

Thermoplastic materials are formable when they are heated but become rigid after they have cooled. Thermoplastics are classified as either low-temperature or high-temperature materials, depending on the temperature range at which they become malleable. Low-temperature thermoplastics become moldable at temperatures less than 149° C and often can be molded directly on the patient's limb, whereas high-temperature materials require heating to much higher temperatures and must be molded over a positive model of the patient's limb.[18] One advantage of thermoplastic materials is that they can be reheated and shaped multiple times, making possible minor adjustments of an orthosis or prosthesis during fittings. Thermoplastics are the material of choice for "shell" designs in which structural strength is required. Some of the more popular materials used are acrylic, copolymer, polyethylene, polypropylene, polystyrene, and a variety of vinyls.

Certain low-temperature thermoplastics, those moldable at temperatures less than 80° C, can be applied and shaped directly to the body. Some of the most commonly available materials include Kydex (Kleerdex, Aiken, S.C.), Orthoplast (Johnson & Johnson, Raynham, Mass.), and Polysar (Bayer, Pittsburgh, Pa.). These materials are most often reserved for orthotic devices that are designed to provide temporary support and protection. Their susceptibility to repetitive stress, high loads, and temperature changes usually limits their use to spinal and upper extremity orthoses. Because these devices are molded directly on the patient, no casting is necessary, and the time required from measurement to finished product is greatly reduced. Another important convenience of low-temperature thermoplastic materials is that no special equipment is required; hot water heated in an electric frying pan, a heat gun, and sharp scissors are all that are necessary to produce a functional splint or orthosis.

High-temperature plastics are frequently used in the production of orthotics and prosthetics. The most commonly used materials include polyethylene, polypropylene, polycarbonate, acrylic, acrylonitrile butadiene styrene, acrylics, polyvinyl acetate, polyvinyl chloride, and polyvinyl alcohol.

Polypropylene is a rigid plastic material that is relatively inexpensive, lightweight, and easy to thermoform. Polypropylenes, which can be further characterized as homopolymers or copolymers, are one of the most widely used plastics in orthotics. The material has a white, opaque color and is available in sheets of various thicknesses, from 1 mm to 1 cm. Polypropylene is impact resistant and can endure several million cycles of repetitive flexes. This attribute has been extremely useful in orthotics for hinge joints and spring assists in AFOs. The material is, however, susceptible to ultraviolet light and extreme cold and is sensitive to scratches and nicks. In prosthetics, the light weight of polypropylene makes it ideal for components such as sockets, pelvic bands, hip joints, or knee joints. Polypropylene is commonly used for prefabricated AFOs and preformed modular orthotic systems.

The long fatigue life of polyethylene during repeated loading situations makes this material suitable for a number of orthotic and prosthetic applications. Prosthetic sockets, orthotic hinge joint components, and compression shells for clamshell design orthoses are common uses of polyethylene plastics. Several densities of polyethylene are available from various manufacturers. Low-density polyethylene is used for upper extremity and spinal orthoses under the trade names Vitrathene (Stanley Smith & Co, Ltd, Isleworth, United Kingdom) and Streifen (FG Streifeneder KG, Munich, Germany). High-density polyethylene, Subortholen (Wilhelm Julius Teufel GmbH, Stuttgart, Germany), is used for spinal and lower extremity orthoses. The ultra-high-density polyethylenes such as Ortholen (Wilhelm Julius Teufel) are used principally for lower extremity orthoses.

Thermosetting Materials

Thermosets are plastics that are applied over a positive model in liquid form and then chemically "cured" to solidify and maintain a desired shape. To enhance their structural properties, thermosets are often impregnated into various fabrics by a process of lamination. Although this group of plastics has inherent structural stability, their rigidity precludes modification by heat molding; their shape can only be changed by grinding. Thermosetting plastics cannot be reheated without destroying their physical properties. Some of the most common thermoset resins used to produce rigid orthoses are acrylic, polyester, and epoxy. Because acrylic resins are strong, lightweight, and somewhat pliable, they offer a different set of characteristics than those of polyester resins. With lamination, acrylic resin can create a thin but strong structural wall for a prosthetic socket or component of an orthotic. If frequent adjustments are anticipated, however, thermoforming plastics are chosen instead. Fiberglass, nylon, aramid fiber (Kevlar, DuPont, Wilmington, Del.), and carbon graphite are the materials used in conjunction with the thermoset plastic to give it added strength. Collectively, they are often referred to as *composites* or *laminates*. Thermosets are used more frequently in prosthetics than in orthotics, for which the advantages of thermoforming plastics have significantly decreased the use of thermosets.

Foamed Plastics

Foamed plastics can be used as a protective interface between the orthotic or prosthetic and the skin, especially over areas that are vulnerable to pressure, such as bony prominences. Foamed plastics are grouped into two classes: open and closed cell. Cells are created in rubber or polymers in a high-pressure gassing process.[18] The microcell structure allows the foamed plastic material to be displaced in several planes, which is an ideal physical property for the reduction of shear forces. In an open-cell foam, the cells are interrelated (as in a kitchen sponge); in a closed-cell foam, the cells are separate from each other. Because closed-cell foams are impervious to liquids, they are less likely to absorb body fluids such as perspiration or urine; however, they do act as insulators and can be hot when worn for extended periods.

An orthopedic grade of polyethylene foam was introduced in the 1960s by a British subsidiary of the Union Carbide Company.[20] These closed-cell foams are available in a wide array of durometer hardnesses. (Durometer refers to a spring indenture post instrument that is used to measure the resistance to the compression/hardness of a material.) Polyethylene foams are commercially available under trade names such as Plastazote (Hackettstown, N.J.), Pe-Lite, Evazote (Bakelite Xylonite Ltd., Croydon, United Kingdom), and Aliplast (Alimed Inc., Dedham, Mass.). Various polyethylene foams are used in the manufacture of soft and rigid orthoses, depending on the density of the material. Plastazote is a low-temperature, heat-formable foam that has been used successfully in the treatment and prevention of neuropathic foot lesions.[21-24] Its light weight and forgiving quality to bony prominences make it a desirable interface for the insensate foot. See Hertzman[21] for a complete review of the use of Plastazote in lower limb orthotics and prosthetics.

Closed-cell foams are also made with synthetic rubbers or polychloroprenes. Neoprene is available in various densities, making the low-durometer versions suitable as liners for orthoses, whereas the firmer materials are used for posts or soling for shoes. Spenco (Spenco Medical Corp., Waco, Tex.) is a microcellular neoprene foam that reduces shear forces to the foot's plantar surface and the occurrence of foot blisters in athletes.[25] The nylon (polyamide)-covered neoprene acts as a shock absorber while also reducing friction on the foot's plantar surface.[20] Although few of these materials are heat moldable, most can be conformed without difficulty to the shallow contours of foot orthoses. Lynco (Apex Foot Health Industries, Teaneck, N.J.) is an open-cell neoprene foam that dissipates heat more efficiently than its closed-cell cousin; however, it does not attenuate shock as well as Spenco.[20]

Polyurethane open-cell foams are alternatives for top covers for foot orthoses. They provide good shock absorption and dissipate heat well. Some of the commercially available open-cell polyurethane foams include Poron (Rogers Corporation, Rogers, Conn.), PPT (Professional Protective Technology, Deer Park, N.Y.), and Vylite (Steins Foot Specialties, Newark, N.J.).

Several studies that compare materials used to fabricate orthoses have been conducted.[26-32] In 1982, Campbell et al[26] conducted compression tests on 31 materials to determine their suitability for insoles in shoes. Materials were classified according to stiffness into the categories "very stiff," "moderately deformable," and "highly deformable." The moderately deformable group of plastics, which included 19 of the tested foamed plastics, was deemed the most beneficial as an insole material. Campbell et al[26] concluded that these materials could relieve stress from bony prominences and transfer the loads to the adjacent soft tissues more effectively than could the very stiff or highly deformable materials. Studies evaluating shoe insole materials also report them to be effective at attenuating shock during walking in various ways.[32]

Viscoelastic Polymers

A viscoelastic solid is a material that possesses the characteristics of stress relaxation and creep. Stress relaxation occurs when a material that is subjected to a constant deformation requires a decreasing load with time to maintain a steady state.[33] Creep refers to the increase in deformation with time to a steady state as a constant load is applied.[33] Sorbothane (Sorbothane, Inc., Kent, Ohio), widely used as an insole material, is made of a noncellular polyurethane derivative that possesses good shock-attenuating characteristics.[33] Viscolas (Viscolas Corp., Soddy Daisy, Tenn.), another type of viscoelastic solid, has been found to attenuate skeletal shock at heel strike in the tibia to half the normal load.[15,34] Two other viscoelastic polymers used to fabricate orthotic prosthetic components are Viscolite (Polymer Dynamics, Inc., Allentown, Pa.) and PQ (Riecken's Orthotic Laboratories, Evansville, Ind.).

PRESCRIPTION GUIDELINES

The formulation of a prescription for an orthosis or prosthesis greatly influences the potential functional outcome for the patient. It is critical that rehabilitation objectives and design criteria be carefully considered. Physicians, therapists, orthotists, and prosthetists who are involved in developing a prescription for an orthotic or prosthetic device must have a sound understanding of orthotics and prosthetics to be successful in effectively treating patients with these devices.

Assessment of functional deficit includes a thorough evaluation of the patient's present physical status, including muscle strength testing, range of motion measures, and documentation of other physical impairments that would affect the fit or performance of the device. Equally important to the physical examination is the consideration of any individual needs of the patient and an understanding of how the treatment will affect daily activities. To increase the success of treatment, the patient and other rehabilitation team members must reach a consensus on the type of device and the associated training and education required for optimal functional outcome.

Orthotic Prescription

The Committee on Prosthetics and Orthotics of the American Academy of Orthopaedic Surgeons developed a technical analysis form to standardize the process of patient evaluation. This evaluation protocol documents the biomechanical deficits of the patient and provides the basic information needed for orthotic prescription formulation. This systematic approach has two major objectives: to define the anatomical segments that the orthosis will encompass and describe accurately the biomechanical controls needed for treatment. The underlying principle of this assessment is that orthoses should be designed to control only those movements considered abnormal while permitting free motion in anatomical segments that are not impaired.

Technical analysis forms were developed for three general regions of the body: the upper limb, lower limb, and spine. The forms are four pages long with the same basic approach for formulating an orthotic prescription. The first page has sections for recording general patient information and noting major physical impairments (Figure 2-1). The major impairment section characterizes any functional limitations, such as skeletal structure, sensation, or joint contracture. This information provides an overview of the patient's clinical presentation.

The second and third pages of the technical analysis form (Figure 2-2) contain diagrams of the respective anatomical (limb or trunk) segments for which an orthotic prescription is being considered. Each skeletal region is represented in three planes of motion: coronal, sagittal, and transverse. On either side of the figures, square boxes at the level of the joints are used to note volitional force, hypertonicity, proprioception, and range of motion. The fourth page consists of a summary of the functional disability, treatment objectives, orthotic recommendation, and a key for the biomechanical controls of function.

Voluntary movements of muscles are assessed by conventional muscle testing techniques. Muscle strength can be recorded with either the standard descriptive or numeric muscle grading systems, depending on regional preferences.

Two types of joint (limb) motion are recorded on the forms: rotary and translatory. According to McCollough,[35] all points of the distal segment move in the same direction, following the same path shape and distance during translatory motion. During rotary motion, one point of the distal segment (or its imaginary extension) remains fixed while other points move in an arc around it. Translatory motion is recorded with linear arrows in the direction of the distal segment's movement relative to its proximal counterpart. The linear arrows are placed below the circle (representing the joint axis) for translatory motion. If translatory force acts in the vertical axis, the linear arrow is placed to the side of the circle. Rotary motion and the related degree of range of motion are documented by an arrow within a protractor-type arrangement for each joint. The established normal range of motion for each joint is shaded on the form for comparative reference. If a fixed contracture or fusion of the joint is present, a double linear arrow is used.

Hypertonicity of muscle groups in each of the body segments is described by a functionally based letter scale.[35] A designation of *mild tonicity* is given when any hypertonus that is present is thought to be functionally insignificant. *Moderate tonicity* indicates that tone might have some functional value, such as assisting the patient in holding an item during minor tasks. A designation of *severe tonicity* indicates that normal function is not possible. The patient's proprioceptive ability is described in a similar way, as *absent, impaired,* or *normal* for each of the body segments of interest.

The final page of the technical analysis form (Figure 2-3) contains space for an overview of functional impairments, a checklist of the orthotic treatment objectives, and a chart that details the orthotic recommendation. The desired orthotic control for each body segment is indicated by a specific letter; as many as seven types of orthotic controls can be incorporated into the design of an orthosis. The terms and descriptions of these controls are indicated in the key. If the orthotic recommendation section is completed correctly, the chart will indicate the body segments that the device will encompass and the desired biomechanical control of function needed. Any comments on the specific design requirements or materials, or both, can be detailed in the remarks section of the form.

For the orthotist, the prescription is the blueprint from which the design of a device is based. It specifies the force system requirements needed to achieve the treatment objectives independent of material selection or production processes. Although an in-depth biomechanical assessment may not always be necessary, a system based on these principles is a logical and objective method for formulating an orthotic prescription.

Prosthetic Prescription

The formulation of a prosthetic prescription requires a different evaluative process. Prosthetic prescription depends on an in-depth understanding of components and materials as well as their indications and contraindications for use. Ideally, prosthetic prescription begins before amputation surgery, so that the residual limb is of appropriate length and

Technical Analysis Form **Lower Limb** **Revised March 1973**

Name ______________________ No. ________ Age ________ Sex ________

Date of onset ______________ Cause ______________________

Occupation ______________ Present lower-limb equipment ______________

Diagnosis ____

Ambulatory ☐ Nonambulatory ☐

Major impairments:

A. Skeletal
1. Bone and joints: Normal ☐ Abnormal ______________
2. Ligaments: Normal ☐ Abnormal ☐ Knee: AC ☐ PC ☐ MC ☐ LC ☐
   Ankle: MC ☐ LC ☐
3. Extremity shortening: None ☐ Left ☐ Right ☐
   Amount of discrepancy: ASIS-Heel ________ ASIS-MTP ________ MTP-Heel ________

B. Sensation: Normal ☐ Abnormal ☐
1. Anesthesia ☐ Hypesthesia ☐ Location: ______________
   Protective sensation: Retained ☐ Lost ☐
2. Pain ☐ Location: ______________

C. Skin: Normal ☐ Abnormal: ______________

D. Vascular: Normal ☐ Abnormal ☐ Right ☐ Left ☐

E. Balance: Normal ☐ Impaired ☐ Support: ______________

F. Gait deviations: ______________

G. Other impairments: ______________

Legend

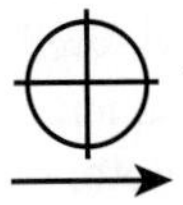

= Direction of translatory motion

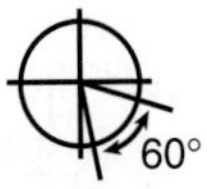

= Abnormal degree of rotary motion (60°)

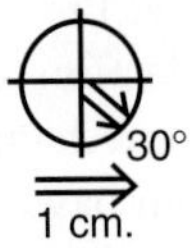

= Fixed position (30°, 1 cm.)

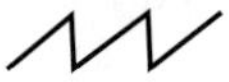

= Fracture

Volitional force (V)
N = Normal
G = Good
F = Fair
P = Poor
T = Trace
Z = Zero

Hypertonic muscle (H)
N = Normal
M = Mild
Mo = Moderate
S = Severe

Proprioception (P)
N = Normal
I = Impaired
A = Absent

D = Local distension or enlargement

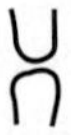

= Pseudarthrosis

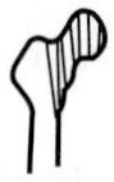

= Absence of segment

Figure 2-1

The technical analysis form provides a systematic method of data collection for the development of prescriptions for lower extremity orthoses. The first page of the form is used to record the patient's history and current impairments. AC, *Anterior cruciate ligament;* ASIS, *anterior superior iliac spine;* LC, *lateral collateral ligament;* MC, *medial collateral ligament;* MTP, *medial tibial plateau;* PC, *posterior cruciate ligament. (From Committee on Prosthetics Research and Development.* Report of the Seventh Workshop Panel on Lower Extremity Orthoses of the Subcommittee on Design and Development. *Washington, D.C.: National Research Council–National Academy of Sciences, 1970; and McCollough NC III. Biomechanical analysis systems for orthotic prescription. In American Academy of Orthopaedic Surgeons,* Atlas of Orthotics: Biomechanical Principles and Application, *2nd ed. St. Louis: Mosby, 1985. pp. 35-75.)*

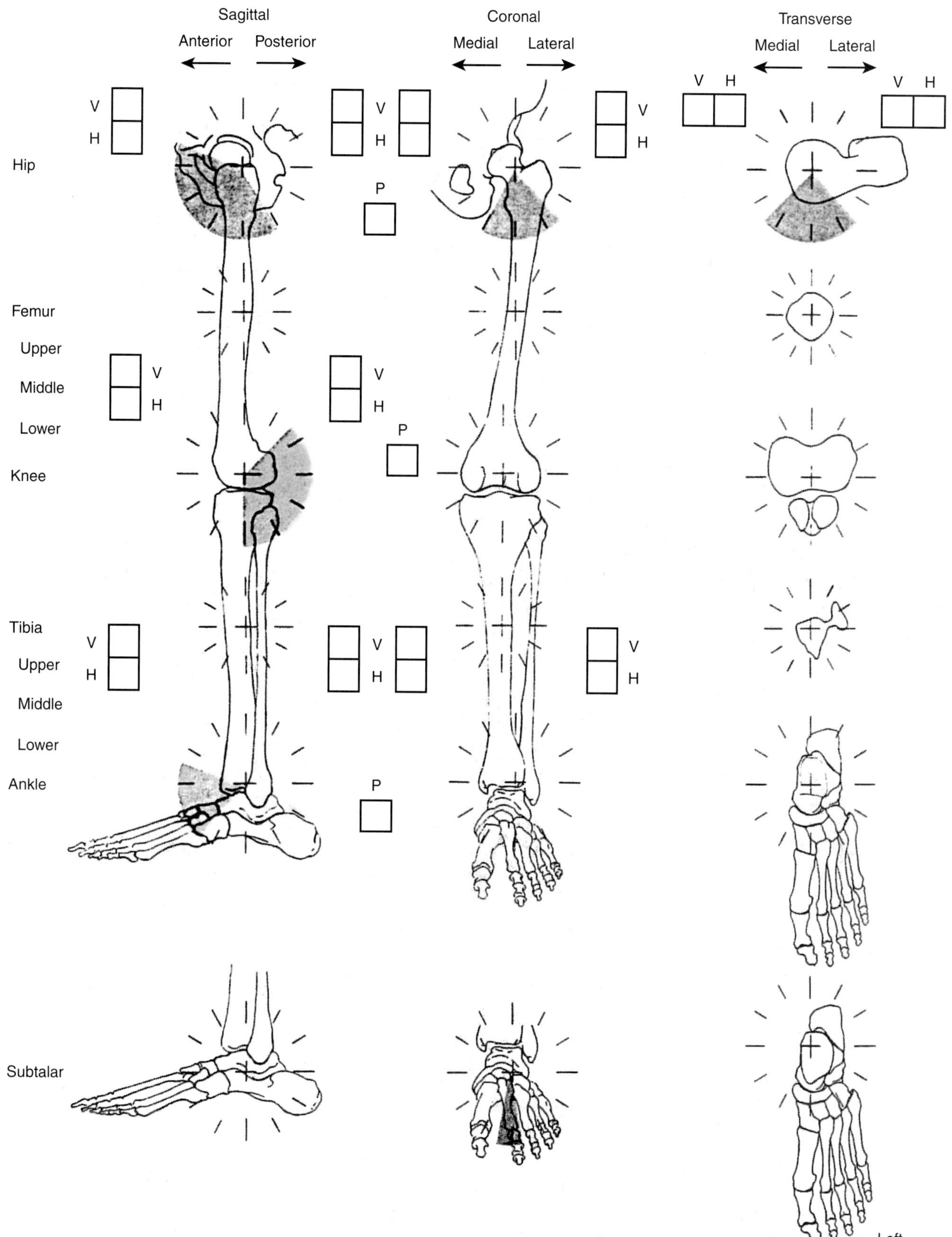

Figure 2-2

Subsequent pages of the technical analysis form are used to detail characteristics of each limb or body segment for which the orthosis or prosthesis will be made. Information recorded on these pages includes existing deformity, proprioceptive capacity (P), *restriction or hypermobility of joint rotary and translatory range of motion in all three planes of movement, volitional strength* (V), *and the level of hypertonicity* (H). *(From Committee on Prosthetics Research and Development.* Report of the Seventh Workshop Panel on Lower Extremity Orthoses of the Subcommittee on Design and Development. *Washington, D.C.: National Research Council–National Academy of Sciences, 1970; and McCollough NC III. Biomechanical analysis systems for orthotic prescription. In American Academy of Orthopaedic Surgeons,* Atlas of Orthotics: Biomechanical Principles and Application, *2nd ed. St. Louis: Mosby, 1985. pp. 35-75.)*

Summary of functional disability ______________________________

____

____

____

____

____

Treatment objectives:

Prevent/correct deformity	☐	Improve ambulation	☐
Reduce axial load	☐	Fracture treatment	☐
Protect joint	☐	Other ______________	

Orthotic Recommendation

Lower limb		Flex	Ext	Abd	Add	Rotation Int	Rotation Ext	Axial load
HKAO	Hip							
KAO	Thigh							
	Knee							
AFO	Leg							
	Ankle	(Dorsi)	(Plantar)					
FO Foot	Subtalar					(Inver)	(Ever)	
	Midtarsal							
	Met-phal							

Remarks:

Signature ______________ Date ______________

Key: Use the following symbols to indicate desired control of designated function:

F = Free	Free motion
A = Assist	Application of an external force for the purpose of increasing the range, velocity, or force of a motion
R = Resist	Application of an external force for the purpose of decreasing the velocity or force of a motion
S = Stop	Inclusion of a static unit to deter an undesired motion in one direction
v = Variable	A unit that can be adjusted without making a structural change
H = Hold	Elimination of all motion in prescribed plane (verify position)
L = Lock	Device includes an optional lock

Figure 2-3

The final page of the technical analysis form details the goals for the orthosis and the specific prescription for the desired device. Once the prescription is developed, the form serves as a guideline for fabricating and fitting the orthosis. FO, Foot orthosis; HKAO, *hip-knee-ankle orthosis; V, volitional force. (From Committee on Prosthetics Research and Development.* Report of the Seventh Workshop Panel on Lower Extremity Orthoses of the Subcommittee on Design and Development. *Washington, D.C.: National Research Council–National Academy of Sciences, 1970; and McCollough NC III. Biomechanical analysis systems for orthotic prescription. In American Academy of Orthopaedic Surgeons,* Atlas of Orthotics: Biomechanical Principles and Application, *2nd ed. St. Louis: Mosby, 1985. pp. 35-75.)*

healing is adequate for optimal prosthetic use. Factors such as vascular supply, anticipated activity level, intelligence, vocation, and age are also important to consider. Range of motion, flexible and fixed contracture, functional strength, skin condition, girth measurements, pain, and sensation of the residual limb and the intact limb are evaluated.

An important part of prosthetic prescription is component selection. The diversity of prosthetic foot-ankle units and knee mechanisms for lower extremity prosthetics, and the variety of terminal devices for the upper extremity, can present difficult decisions for those who are unfamiliar with their intended application. Therefore, prosthetists are often relied on for recommendations on components because they are usually most familiar with the specifications and limitations. Many prosthetic teams have developed data collection forms to standardize the prosthetic prescription process. Redhead[36] suggests that the prescription for a prosthesis consider each of the major "prescription options." Examples of the specifications delineated by Redhead for a transfemoral prosthesis are type of limb, socket material and design, suspension, knee joints, knee controls, ankle joints, feet, and cosmesis.

FABRICATION PROCESS

Once a prescription for a custom orthosis or prosthesis has been created, the fabrication process begins. The traditional fabrication process is composed of six steps. The process begins with making accurate measurements of the limb, followed by taking a negative impression (cast). Next, a three-dimensional positive model of the limb or body segment is created and then modified to incorporate the desired controls. The orthosis or prosthetic socket is then created around the positive model. The final step is the fitting of the device to the patient. In some instances, further modification or adjustment is necessary to achieve optimal fit and function of the device.

Measurement

Measurements are most often referenced from readily palpable bony landmarks. Important measurements include the length, successive circumferences, and mediolateral and anteroposterior dimensions of the body segment for which the orthotic or prosthetic device is being created. Although many measurements can be obtained with simple tools such as a tape measure, specialized measurement devices such as electronic scanning devices have been developed to enhance accuracy and reproducibility. Measurements are recorded on forms that are specific to the body segment being treated, such as the technical analysis form previously described. These measurements are used in two ways: as a reference when modifications to the positive cast are needed and as the way to determine the placement of the perimeter trimlines of the device.

Negative Mold

A negative impression is a mold taken of an actual body part that is used to create the three-dimensional positive cast or model necessary for fabrication of the orthosis or prosthesis. This negative impression is most often taken with a plaster of Paris bandage or fiber resin tape, although in some instances direct impressions are used as an alternative. Creation of a negative impression has four steps. First, a layer of tubular stockinet or a stocking is placed over the skin to create a protective interface and control the position of soft tissue structures within the cast (Figure 2-4). Tubular stockinette is available in sizes that range from small diameter for the pediatric limb to large diameter for the adult torso. When a direct impression technique is being performed, a topical separator such as petroleum jelly can be used as an interface to minimize the risk of capturing cuticle hair in the impression. Second, bony prominences or other important guiding landmarks are marked on the body segment with indelible ink. These marks transfer to the inside of the negative mold and from there to the surface of the positive model.

Once the limb or body segment has been prepared, a thin layer of plaster of Paris or fiber resin tape is applied (see Figure 2-4, *B*). This procedure differs from that of fracture casts in one important way: the goal is to achieve an "intimate" fit that captures the actual contours of the limb or body segment so that no protective padding is required. Rolls of elasticized plaster can be wrapped circumferentially in no more than two or three layers. Alternatively, strips of the material can be laid along the length of the limb or body segment. Most impression casting materials are readily available in roll form, although special versions have been produced for specific types of impression procedures, such as the fiber resin sock for an AFO. As the molding material is applied, the clinician smoothes the surface, following the normal shape of the limb. While the mold hardens, the clinician supports the limb or segment in the desired position, sometimes applying a light corrective force. As an example, the desired limb position of an orthosis incorporating the ankle joint might be in subtalar and talocrural neutral. If a PTB socket design is desired for a transtibial prosthesis, an extra force applied just distal to the patella marks its desired location on the resulting positive mold.

Once the cast is hardened sufficiently, it is carefully removed from the limb segment, preserving its shape and contours, and checked for alignment (see Figure 2-4, *C* and *D*).

It is essential that the clinician who takes the negative impression has a thorough understanding of the forces that will be applied to the anatomical segments involved to ensure optimal fit and function of the orthosis or prosthesis. Estimates of soft tissue compression and skeletal alignment changes need to be carefully considered during the negative impression procedure. A skilled and experienced professional uses clinical judgment to create a negative impression,

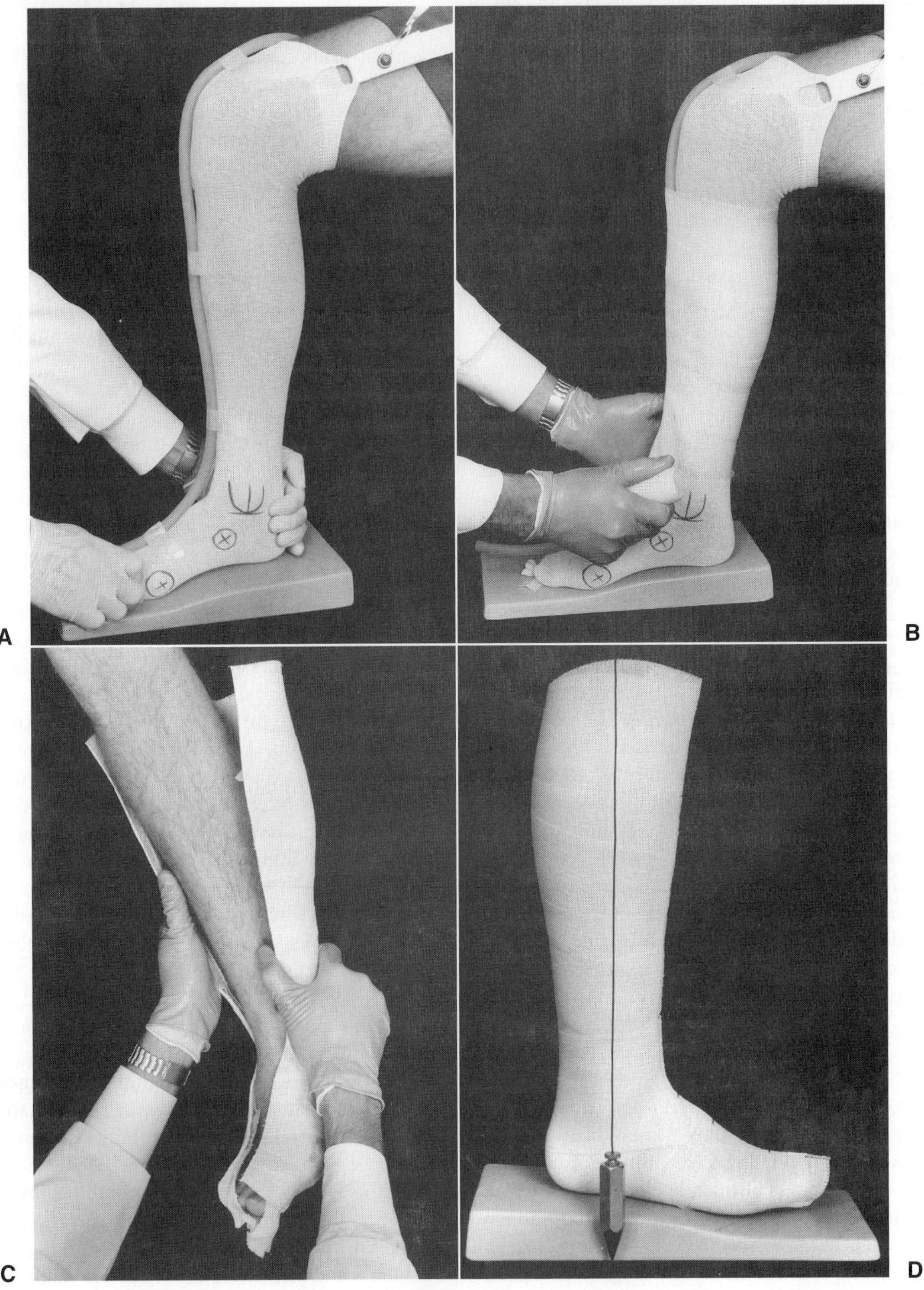

Figure 2-4

*The procedure for taking a conventional negative impression begins with placing a layer of cotton stockinette over the limb and marking bony prominences with an indelible water-soluble transfer pencil (**A**). Surgical tubing is positioned on the anterior aspect of the limb to serve as a guideline for cast removal and to protect the shin. The limb is positioned on a shoe "last" impression in preparation for circumferential application of a plaster of Paris bandage or fiber resin casting tape (**B**). The impression board allows the foot to assume the contours of a shoe during molding for an optimal foot/shoe/AFO interface. Once the cast is "set," a cast saw is used to open the front of the cast (**C**), and the negative impression is carefully removed from the limb. The anterior edges are closed, and the ankle-foot alignment of the negative impression is verified with a plumb line (**D**).*

not only to capture the shape of the anatomical segment but also to apply an efficient force system to improve or maximize function. Basic design decisions must be made before the impression procedures so that any special accommodations required for the desired functional outcome can be incorporated.

Special negative impression techniques have been developed for specific purposes. Polystyrene foam impression blocks are one of the common methods of acquiring an impression of the plantar surface of the foot.[37] For patients who are recovering from facial burns, fabrication of a facial orthotic designed to deliver even, steady pressure during the period of scar maturation requires a highly detailed mold of the face. Alginate impressions, also referred to as *moulage techniques*, similar to those used in dentistry, are often used.

Fabricating and Modifying the Positive Model

Conventional methods for creating a positive cast are well established. The negative impression is prepared by sealing the mold so that it can accept liquid plaster of Paris. A separator material (e.g., silicone, soap) is added to the inner walls of the mold before the plaster of Paris is poured so that it can be removed more easily once the positive model has set. Once the cast has solidified, the negative impression is stripped away and discarded. The anatomical landmarks and reference points marked on the limb or body segment with indelible pencil and transferred from the patient to the negative impression are again transferred to the positive model. A mandrel (post) is embedded into the setting plaster of the positive model. This mandrel is used to hold the model for cast rectification and the rest of the production processes.

Model rectifications remove artifacts produced during the molding or impression process and bring the cast to specification of the measured values taken from the patient. Once the positive model has been rectified, further modifications can be made on the basis of the design of the orthosis or prosthesis being fabricated. During the negative impression procedure, soft tissue may have been manipulated for specific applications of force or pressure to be incorporated into the final orthosis or prosthesis. Although the positive model represents a three-dimensional shape of a respective body segment, it cannot relay information about the density of the tissue that it will interface. In general, additional plaster is added where relief of pressure is desired (e.g., over bony prominences) (Figure 2-5) or is removed where additional forces are to be applied. When the orthosis or prosthesis is formed over the model, an area of relief for a more intimate fit is achieved. Although some guidelines have been established regarding the amount of material to be removed or added to the positive model, the clinical experience of the prosthetist or orthotist is essential in this stage of the process. The positive model can also be modified to reconfigure surface geometry to improve the strength of the finished product.

Once design changes have been incorporated into the model, its surface is prepared for component production. This involves removing any surface imperfections with abrasive tools and abrasive sanding screen to ensure that the surface in contact with skin will be smooth. The positive cast is then ready to be used as a form from which different materials can be shaped to produce an interface component.

Fabricating the Orthosis or Prosthetic Socket

The fabrication process used with the positive model depends on the material selected for the device. Thermoforming is a common production method used in orthotics and prosthetics. Thermoplastic sheet material is heated in an oven until it has reached its "plastic" state, then shaped over a positive model by changing the air pressure difference across its surface (vacuum forming) (Figure 2-6). Once the plastic has cooled and returned to its solid state, trimlines are delineated on the formed plastic before the edges are finished and smoothed.

CAD/CAM

In the 1960s, an alternative method of prosthetic fabrication that used computers was first introduced. Early CAD/CAM methods used stereophotography and digitization to create a numerical model, which guided a milling machine in the creation of a positive model of the residual limb.[2] A more complete concept of fabrication and manufacture of a prosthesis was developed at the University College London in the late 1970s and early 1980s.[38] After establishing a system for automated production of a prosthesis called Rapidform, the London research group conceived a completely automated fabrication process that used appropriate prosthetic alignment data.[39]

In the United States, the Veterans Administration began funding research projects in the 1980s to investigate the potential of CAD/CAM in orthotics and prosthetics. Advances were also made in private industry as the availability of personal computers became widespread. Beginning in the late 1980s, manufacturers have designed a multitude of CAD/CAM systems for various applications in orthotics and prosthetics. Advances in computer hardware, processors, and software have made CAD/CAM systems fast and efficient as well as an economical alternative for fabrication of devices for many orthotic and prosthetic practices.

Today, most CAD systems use a scanning device to record digital information of a body segment for CAM. The primary components of a CAD/CAM system consist of a digitizing device, computer, and milling machine. Surface contours of the anatomical segment are recorded with various digitization devices: optical-laser scanners, surface-contacting stylus, and pneumatically operated mechanical posts. Digital information acquired from a scan of a body segment is processed by the computer and translated into a triordinate data point

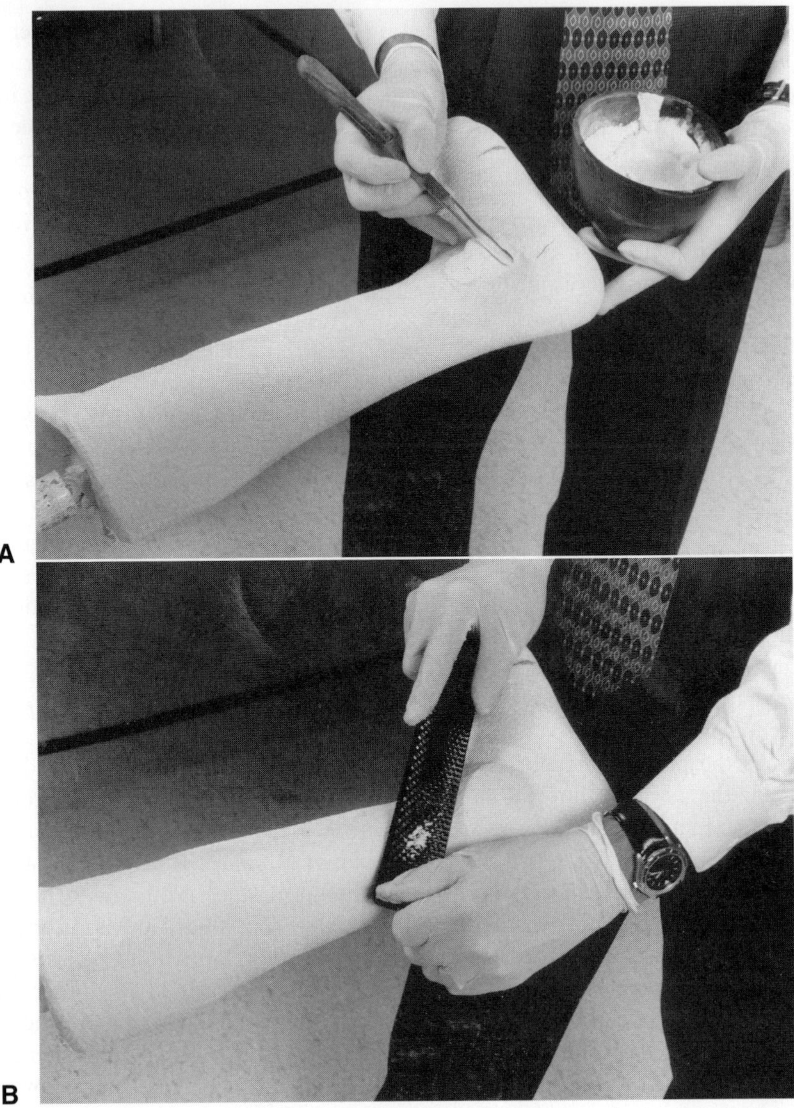

Figure 2-5

*In the rectification of a positive model, plaster of Paris added over pressure-sensitive areas, such as the lateral malleolus (**A**), results in a "relief" in the finished orthosis. Modification of the positive model by removal of material with a plaster rasp over pressure-tolerant areas (**B**) increases intimacy of fit for better loading or stabilizing of the limb.*

file. This file is used by the computer to create a graphic image in the form of a surface contour plot.[40] The data are then relayed to a milling unit to carve an orthosis or prosthesis for a positive model.

Data Acquisition

Each of the many digitizers used for data acquisition is designed for a specific task or to handle certain anatomical regions. Noncontact laser digitizers capable of circumferential scanning are well suited for measurement of cylindrical shapes such as those found in limb prosthetics or spinal orthotics. An optical-laser camera mechanism images the surface topography of the body segment and records the measured data points in a computer. Special holding fixtures and bars to aid in patient comfort and safety are part of each system. An apparatus designed to scan the torso for a spinal orthosis usually requires a different setup than that of a limb prosthesis. Some scanners are capable of digitizing directly from the patient's body segment, whereas other systems take measurements from a negative impression or mold of the segment (Figure 2-7). Compact, handheld contact digitizers have been introduced by several CAD/CAM manufacturers. These units allow the clinician to digitize a body segment by direct contact with the skin. Handheld contact digitizers are described as a wand, pen, stylus, or pointer. Contact digitizers often have special attachments to scan certain shapes or measurement tools, such as calipers, for acquiring anteroposterior or mediolateral dimensions. Their versatility permits data acquisition of complex shapes. In some

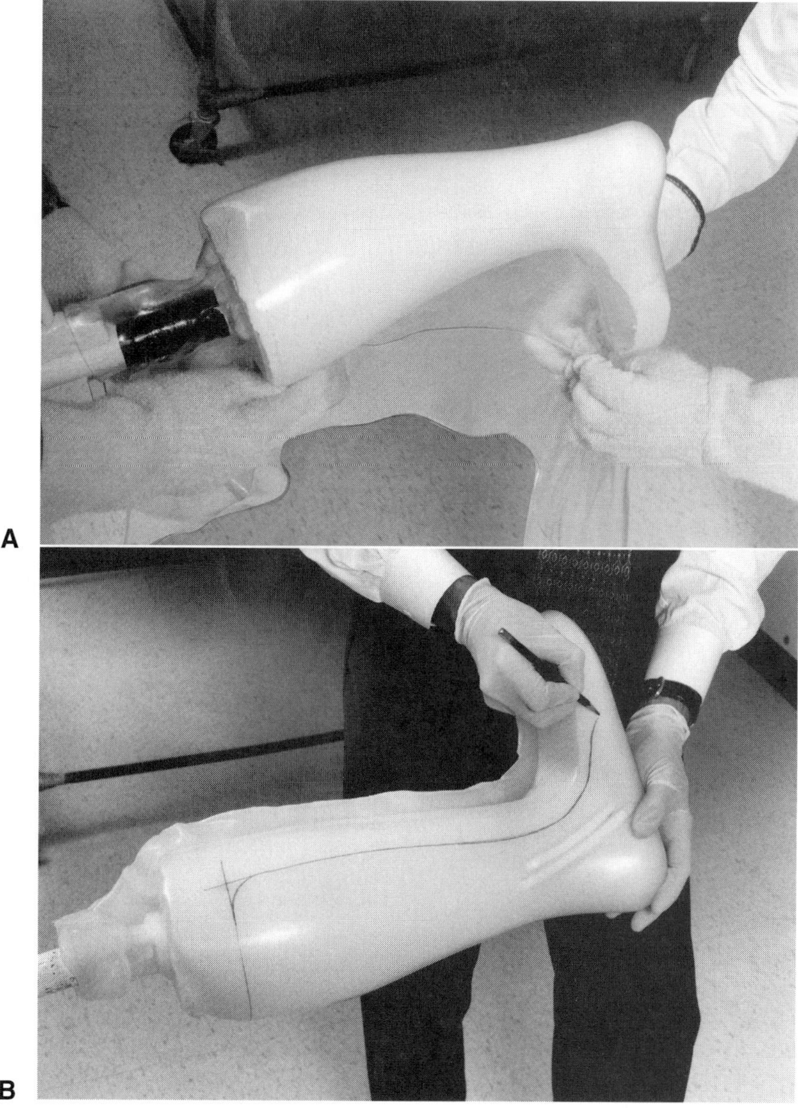

Figure 2-6

*Once a sheet of thermoplastic material has been heated, it is dropped over the rectified positive model (**A**) and the edges of the thermoplastic are sealed. Negative pressure created by a vacuum pump removes any trapped air and draws the polypropylene to the surface of the positive model. When the material has cooled, trimlines are drawn on the formed plastic (**B**) by using measurements taken during the initial evaluation and bony landmarks as guides. Note the corrugations incorporated to strengthen the orthosis at the ankle.*

systems, handheld digitizers can be used in conjunction with a laser scan.

The use of digitizers in the production of foot orthoses is also becoming more common. Several systems based on differences in technique and philosophy in foot orthosis design have been developed for data acquisition of the foot. For full weight-bearing or partial weight-bearing techniques, pneumatically operated mechanical posts are used to digitize the foot's plantar surface (Amfit Corp, Vancouver, Wash.). Orthotic contoured shapes such as metatarsal domes can be evaluated during the digitization procedure to determine optimal position and comfort before fabrication. An optical-laser scanner situated under an acrylic platform has also been used for scanning the foot when a weight-bearing technique is desired (Bergmann Orthotics Lab, Northfield, Ill.). Because this system is also capable of scanning the foot with non–weight-bearing methods without the platform, it is quite versatile in clinical practice.

In many instances, orthotists and prosthetists are restricted to surface geometry and palpation of underlying anatomical structures to interpret the position of skeletal and soft tissue structures of the body segment. Magnetic resonance imaging and computed tomography have been used to create a three-dimensional computer model and assist in making design decisions for a mechanical device (Figure 2-8). Data from these scans are converted to a working format for specific

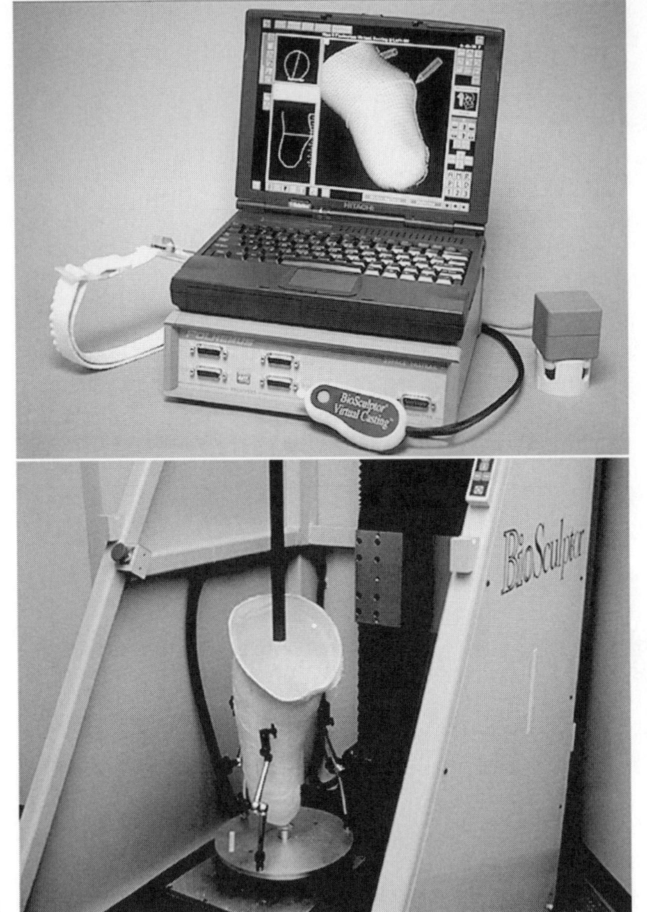

Figure 2-7

*Examples of CAD/CAM data acquisition systems. A digital model of the residual limb (**A**) can be captured by a laptop computer, appropriate signal processor components, and a handheld digitizer. Laser digitization (**B**) can be used to capture accurately the contours of a conventional negative impression of a residual limb. (Courtesy BioSculptor Corporation, Hialeah, Fla.)*

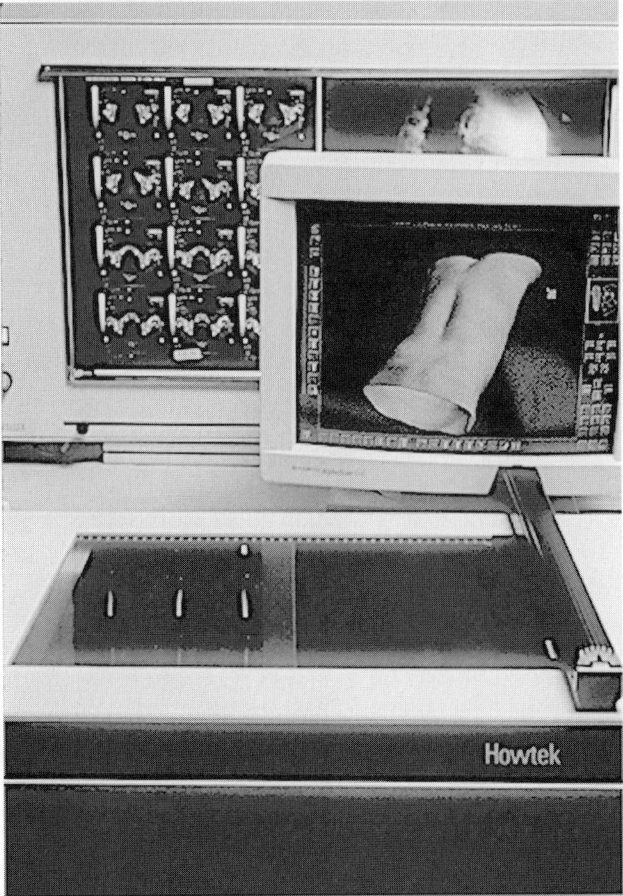

Figure 2-8

Computed tomographic or magnetic resonance images can be used to create a digitized computer model of a body segment for various orthotic or prosthetic CAD/CAM applications. The components of this type of system include an image scanner (foreground), *a computer monitor for display of digitized images (e.g., the torso;* center right*), and the computed tomographic or magnetic resonance images being used* (background). *(Courtesy BioSculptor Corporation, Hialeah, Fla.)*

graphic and modeling programs. Although this capability may not be practical for all applications, it may offer insight into areas of further research and development in the field.

Shape-Manipulation Software

The ability to modify the three-dimensional model of a patient's body segment permits the clinician to incorporate the desired biomechanical controls into an orthosis or prosthesis. The amount of force applied to a specific area depends in part on manipulation of the digital three-dimensional model. Software packages are now available to assist orthotists and prosthetists in designing the most appropriate modifications for a given patient. Generic modification templates or custom-designed templates can be used to make a wide range of revisions to the data. The clinician can incorporate reliefs for bony prominences of the limb or trunk or can change the geometry of the shape to enhance structural strength characteristics in the final orthosis or prosthesis. Trimlines can be delineated so that technicians who are involved in the assembly of components can complete a device without further instruction.

Milling and Production

Once the digital model is in place, the milling apparatus creates the actual orthotic or prosthetic device. Because each type of orthosis or prosthesis usually has specific milling parameters, a different setup may be required for each. For instance, the long, rounded shape of a transtibial or transfemoral socket is often manufactured with a lathe-type

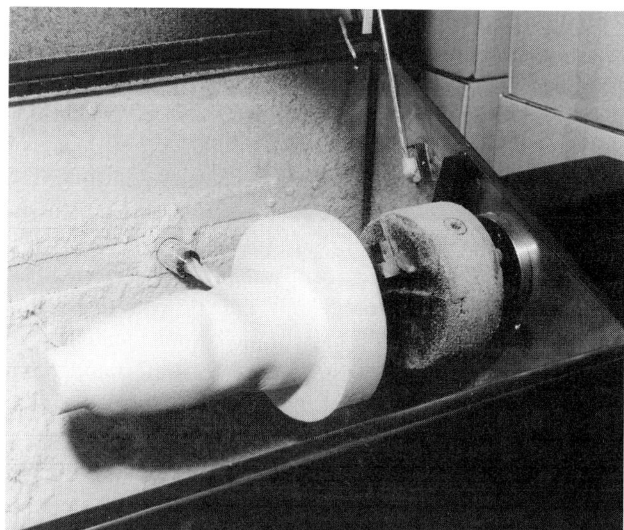

Figure 2-9
A positive model for a transtibial prosthetic socket being carved on a computer-controlled milling/lathe machine. (Courtesy Prosthetic Design, Inc., Clayton, Ohio.)

milling machine (Figure 2-9). In contrast, foot orthoses are manufactured by an end mill setup because their platelike structure and production processes create different finishing needs. The production laboratory needs to be large enough to have separate milling stations for each type of orthosis or prosthesis. This manufacturing limitation has led to the establishment of laboratory production companies that mill the positive models and manufacture the orthoses or prostheses from computer data transmitted by modem. Computer production networks can often reduce fabrication time and decrease production times, making the use of CAD/CAM economically feasible even for small orthotic/prosthetic facilities. Special production equipment is available that partially automates the thermoforming processes of some components. In the thermoforming machine for prosthetic sockets, a preformed polypropylene shell travels upward on a mechanical platform to an oven that heats the plastic to its formable temperature. The heated shell is then lowered over the positive model of the residual limb and vacuum formed for an intimate fit.

CAD/CAM in orthotics and prosthetics will play an important role in clinical and research settings. Although the development of CAD/CAM in orthotics and prosthetics has a history that spans more than two decades, only since the 1990s has it become an integral part of some clinical practices. Systems that have been designed for virtually all prosthetic and orthotic applications can be integrated with computed tomography, magnetic resonance imaging, and other medical imaging technologies. The technological advancements of CAD/CAM offer orthotists and prosthetists an additional clinical fabrication and research tool. Although this sophisticated equipment can contribute greatly to certain clinical and manufacturing tasks, successful fitting of a device depends on proper data input and prescription formulation.

CENTRAL FABRICATION AND MASS PRODUCTION

The techniques and processes associated with the fabrication of orthoses and prostheses described in this chapter can be relatively labor intensive and expensive. As managed care and insurance companies strive to reduce medical costs, the profession is under greater pressure to remain competitive by finding alternative production methods that are cost effective. One option is to maximize the clinical productivity of orthotists and prosthetists and limit their technical responsibilities. Central fabrication operations allow practitioners to develop clinical practices that do not require large technical facilities and space. Depending on the size of the practice, outsourcing the production portion of the business can be a more economical way to run an orthotic/prosthetic clinic. Some practitioners do not want to manage in-house technical operations that include additional technical staff, specialized equipment, and increased space requirements. Another advantage is that central fabrication may offer improvements in consistency and quality of devices.

Central Fabrication Facilities for Custom Devices

Central fabrication facilities typically specialize in the manufacture of custom orthoses and prostheses, often serving a large number of orthotic and prosthetic practices. These manufacturing services are available to produce almost every kind of orthosis and prosthesis, with many companies specializing in a specific area (e.g., spinal orthoses, knee orthoses, transtibial prosthetics). Some central fabrication operations offer the advantage of producing a device without the need for a negative impression, an additional cost savings in time and materials. A series of conventional measurements of patients combined with height and weight data is entered into a computer to generate a milled positive model for production. Orthotic systems in particular have been refined to produce excellent fitting devices that are comparable in function to custom-molded orthoses produced from a patient model. Although there will always be a need for custom-molded devices, technological advancements in human factors, ergonomics, and computer modeling will improve generic sizing and contoured interface systems, permitting a larger portion of the population to be fit with prefabricated devices and components. Modular components of varying material properties are already a part of general practice in prosthetics.

Mass Production

Mass-produced, prefabricated orthoses outnumber custom-molded orthoses fitted to patients for rehabilitative purposes.

Orthopedic companies continue to develop orthotic and prosthetic products whose fit and performance approach that of custom-molded devices through diverse sizing systems and modular components. In the future, prefabricated modular component systems may bridge the gap between prefabricated and custom-molded devices by improving performance outcomes with custom-fitted systems and expanding their use in clinical practice. Although these advances in fit and function are possible for some problems, certain deformities and pathological conditions will almost always require custom-molded or measured orthoses and prostheses made by traditional or CAD/CAM methods of production.

MAINTENANCE OF ORTHOSES AND PROSTHESES

Routine care and maintenance of orthoses and prostheses are important for proper function and long-term use of a device. An orthotic or prosthetic maintenance program usually includes servicing by the orthotist or prosthetist and the patient. The service schedule depends on the specific orthosis or prosthesis, the materials from which it is made, the durability of the components, and the knowledge and ability of the patient and caregivers. Patient instructions for the daily care of an orthosis or prosthesis should include cleaning and inspection. Proper patient education of basic fitting criteria and instructions on donning and doffing a device allow the patient to evaluate the fit of a device during routine use.

Orthoses and prostheses should be inspected weekly for any defects, stress risers (nicks, scratches), loose screws, or weakened rivets. Any device that has mechanical components and moving parts and is subjected to repetitive loading requires periodic servicing; it is less expensive to recognize and fix early signs of a problem than it is to replace a device that has failed because of a lack of proper maintenance. Informing patients of potential problems associated with the use of their orthoses or prostheses and how to resolve these problems can prevent serious problems from arising.

Most plastic components should be cleaned with a mild antibacterial soap and rinsed thoroughly with cold water. Extra moisture should be absorbed with a towel, and the orthosis or prosthesis air dried. Heat can distort some plastics; patients should be warned not to use electric hairdryers to dry their devices. Similarly, devices should not be left near direct heat sources, such as radiators, wood stoves, or any appliance that generates heat when running. They must also be protected from intense direct sunlight.

Leather liners and covers are cleaned weekly with a leather "saddle" soap. Leather softeners should not be used unless directed by the orthotist because they can compromise function of some straps and cuffs. Water-repellent treatments and protectants for leather often contain skin irritants and should not be used on leather components that have direct contact with the body.

Most orthoses and prostheses are designed to apply a corrective or stabilizing force to a body segment during wear. For some patients, especially those with fragile skin or scarring, this pressure may increase the risk of skin irritation or damage. The risk of skin problems differs from device to device and depends on the general health and skin condition of the individual who is wearing the orthosis or prosthesis. To minimize problems with skin intolerance of these extra forces, most new orthotic or prosthetic users begin with an intermittent wearing schedule. A treatment plan that incorporates a gradual buildup of orthotic or prosthetic use can avert complications such as excessive redness, chafing, and blisters. For a patient with a high risk or a history of skin problems, a variety of preventive measures (e.g., foam or silicone interface liners) can be incorporated into the orthotic or prosthetic system.

Most custom orthoses or prostheses are designed to achieve a very intimate fit with the body segments that they encompass. Changes in the physical condition of a patient can significantly alter the fit and function of a device. Compromised fit occurs most often when the patient has had significant growth, weight gain or loss, muscle atrophy, edema, structural degeneration, or trauma. Periodic evaluations are necessary to ensure that fit and function are maintained in the months and years after the initial fitting. Semiannual or annual checkups should be part of the treatment plans for definitive orthotic and prosthetic devices.

To maintain proper function of a lower extremity prosthesis, special attention is needed in several areas. The alignment of a prosthesis is usually based on a specific heel height; variation from the prescribed heel height (when footwear is changed) often leads to functional problems during gait. In the same way, moderate to excessive wear of the shoe at the heel also compromises performance. The condition of footwear must be carefully and frequently monitored. The prosthesis should be free of dirt, sand, and other debris to ensure that joint mechanisms and their movements are not inhibited. Socket attachment and suspension systems need daily attention because they are usually prone to accumulation of lint, dirt, and other debris. If the prosthesis or any of its components are subjected to water, the device should be thoroughly dried to prevent permanent damage. Rubber bumpers in prosthetic feet deteriorate over time and with use and must be replaced regularly. The prosthetist can advise patients on specific parts that require regular maintenance.

The socket portion of a prosthesis should be faithfully cared for to avoid potential skin problems, especially infection, on the residual limb. When a special liner is used with a prosthesis, specific instructions for cleaning are necessary because materials used vary greatly. For patients who are fitted with suction sockets or special socket attachment mechanisms, the joining components or threads should be cleaned with a soft brush or rag to remove debris.

SUMMARY

This chapter explores the materials and methods most commonly used in the prescription, measurement, and production of orthoses and prostheses. The type of design, materials, and components are selected to best facilitate the functional goals of the patient. The foundation for effectiveness of the orthosis or prosthesis is careful measurement of the body segment (by casting or by CAD/CAM) and careful modification of the resulting model for optimal fit. For an individual who is being fit for his or her initial orthosis or prosthesis, shared decision making of the rehabilitation team, including the patient and caregivers, is essential. An orthosis or prosthesis that is difficult to don or is uncomfortable to wear is more likely to be found standing in a closet or pushed under a bed than on the patient for daily use.

REFERENCES

1. Committee on Artificial Limbs. *Terminal Research Reports on Artificial Limbs (Covering the Period from April 1, 1945 through June 30, 1947).* Washington, DC: National Research Council, 1947.
2. Wilson AB. History of amputation surgery and prosthetics. In Bowker JH, Michael JW (eds), *Atlas of Limb Prosthetics: Surgical, Prosthetic, and Rehabilitation Principles,* 2nd ed. St. Louis: Mosby, 1992. pp. 3-15.
3. Wilson AB. Prosthetics and orthotics research in the U.S.A. In *International Conference on Prosthetics and Orthotics.* Cairo: S.O.P. Press, 1972. pp. 268-273.
4. Rang M, Thompson GH. History of amputations and prostheses. In Kostuik JP, Gillespie R (eds), *Amputation Surgery and Rehabilitation: The Toronto Experience.* New York: Churchill Livingstone, 1981. pp. 1-12.
5. Eberhart HD, Inman VT, Dec JB, et al. *Fundamental Studies of Human Locomotion and Other Information Relating to the Design of Artificial Limbs. A Report to the National Research Council.* Berkeley, CA: University of California, 1947.
6. Kay HW. Clinical applications of the Veterans Administration Prosthetic Center patellar tendon-bearing brace. *Artif Limbs* 1971;15(1):46-67.
7. Mooney V, Nickel VL, Harvey JP, et al. Cast-brace treatment for fractures of the distal part of the femur. *J Bone Joint Surg Am* 1970;52A(8):1563-1578.
8. Sarmiento A, Sinclair WF. *Tibial and Femoral Fractures—Bracing Management.* Miami: University of Miami, 1972.
9. Committee on Prosthetics Research and Development. *Report of the Seventh Workshop Panel on Lower Extremity Orthoses of the Subcommittee on Design and Development. Washington, DC: National Research Council–National Academy of Sciences,* 1970.
10. Eberhart HD, McKennon JC. Suction-socket suspension of the above-knee prosthesis. In Klopsteg PE, Wilson PD (eds), *Human Limbs and Their Substitutes.* New York: McGraw-Hill, 1954.
11. American Society of Testing and Materials (ASTM). *Standards.* Philadelphia: ASTM; 2001.
12. International Organization for Standardization (ISO). *Prosthetics-Orthotics.* Paramus, NJ: ILI Infodisk, 2000.
13. Shurr DG, Michael JW. Methods, materials, and mechanics. In *Prosthetics and Orthotics,* 2nd ed. Norwalk, CT: Appleton & Lange, 2002. pp. 2137.
14. O'Flaherty F. Leather. In *American Academy of Orthopaedic Surgeons, Orthopaedic Appliances Atlas.* Ann Arbor, MI: JW Edwards, 1952. pp. 17-28.
15. Redford JB II. *Orthotics Etcetera,* 3rd ed. Baltimore: Williams & Wilkins, 1986.
16. Murphy EF, Burnstein AH. Physical properties of materials including solid mechanics. In *American Academy of Orthopaedic Surgeons, Atlas of Orthotics: Biomechanical Principles and Application,* 2nd ed. St. Louis: Mosby, 1985. pp. 6-33.
17. Compton J, Edelstein JE. New plastics for forming directly on the patient. *Prosthet Orthot Int* 1978;2(1):43-47.
18. Lockard MA. Foot orthoses. *Phys Ther* 1988;68(12):1866-1873.
19. Peppard A, O'Donnell M. A review of orthotic plastics. *Athletic Training* 1983;18(1):77-80.
20. Levitz SJ, Whiteside LS, Fitzgerald TA. Biomechanical foot therapy. *Clin Podiatr Med Surg* 1988;5(3):721-736.
21. Hertzman CA. Use of Plastizote in foot disabilities. *Am J Phys Med* 1973;52(6):289-303.
22. Jopling UH. Observation on the use of Plastizote insoles in England. *Lepr Rev* 1969;40:175-176.
23. Mondl AM, Gardiner J, Bisset J. The use of Plastizote in footwear for leprosy patients. A preliminary report. *Lepr Rev* 1969;40(3):177-181.
24. Tuck UH. The use of Plastizote to accommodate foot deformities in Hansen's disease. *Lepr Rev* 1969;40(3):171-173.
25. Spence WR, Shields MN. Insole to reduce shearing forces on the soles of the feet. *Arch Phys Med Rehabil* 1968;49(8): 476-479.
26. Campbell G, Newell E, McLure M. Compression testing of foamed plastics and rubbers for use as orthotic shoe insoles. *Prosthet Orthot Int* 1982;6(1):48-52.
27. Campbell G, McLure M, Newell EN. Compressive behavior after simulated service conditions of some foamed materials intended as orthotic shoe insoles. *J Rehab Res* 1984;21(2):57-65.
28. Leber C, Evanski PM. A comparison of shoe insole material in pressure relief. *Prosthet Orthot Int* 1986;10(3):135.
29. Pratt DJ, Rees PH, Rodgers C. Assessment of some shock absorbing insoles. *Prosthet Orthot Int* 1986;10(1):43.
30. Rome K. Behavior of orthotic materials in chiropody. *J Am Podiatry Assoc* 1990;80(9):471-478.
31. Foto JG, Birke JA. Evaluation of multidensity orthotic materials used in footwear for patients with diabetes. *Foot Ankle Int* 1999;20(2):143.
32. Gillespie KA, Dickey JP. Determination of the effectiveness of materials in attenuating high frequency shock during gait using filter bank analysis. *Clin Biomech* 2003;18(1)50-59.
33. Cinats J, Reid DC, Haddow JB. A biomechanical evaluation of sorbothane. *Clin Orthop* 1987;Sep(222):281-288.
34. MacLellan GE, Bybyan B. Management of pain beneath the heel and Achilles tendonitis with visco-elastic heel insert. *Br J Sports Med* 1981;15(2):117.
35. McCollough NC III. Biomechanical analysis systems for orthotic prescription. In *American Academy of Orthopaedic Surgeons, Atlas of Orthotics: Biomechanical Principles and Application,* 2nd ed. St. Louis: Mosby, 1985. pp. 35-75.

36. Redhead RG. Prescription criteria, fitting, check-out procedures and walking training for the above-knee amputee. In Murdoch G, Donovan RG (eds), *Amputation Surgery and Lower Limb Prosthetics.* Oxford: Blackwell Scientific, 1988.
37. Schuster RO. Neutral plantar impression cast: methods and rationale. *J Am Podiatry Assoc* 1976;6(66):422-426.
38. Davies RM, Lawrence RB, Routledge PE, et al. The Rapidform process for automated thermoplastic production. *Prosthet Orthot Int* 1985;9(1):27-30.
39. Davies RM. Computer aided socket design: the UCL system. In Davies RM (ed), *Annual Report of the Bioengineering Centre.* Roehampton, England: The Bioengineering Centre; 1986. pp. 9-12.
40. Davis FM. In-office computerized fabrication of custom foot supports. The AMFIT system. *Clin Podiatr Med Surg* 1993;10(3):393-401.

3

Clinical Assessment of Pathological Gait

EDMOND AYYAPPA AND OLFAT MOHAMED

LEARNING OBJECTIVES

On completion of this chapter, the reader will be able to do the following:

1. Describe the major tasks of the gait cycle and their corresponding determinants.
2. Identify muscular activity, ground reaction force, and joint motion during each of the phases of the gait cycle.
3. Define each of the time and distance parameters used to describe and assess normal gait.
4. Describe common "pathological gait patterns," including contributing factors, primary and compensatory deviations, and the part of the gait cycle when the pathological pattern is most likely to occur or be observed.
5. Compare and contrast the type and quality of information gathered in various quantitative, qualitative, instrumented, and function-based gait assessment strategies.
6. Differentiate pathological and compensatory gait characteristics typically observed in patients with lower motor neuron disease, hemiplegia, spastic diplegic cerebral palsy, and spina bifida.
7. Discuss how prosthetic components and alignment influence the efficacy and quality of gait for individuals with amputation at transtibial and transfemoral levels.

WHY DO WE ANALYZE GAIT?

The first attempts to analyze gait, recorded in the *Rig Veda* more than 3500 years ago, most likely reflect attempts to enhance mobility through early orthotic or prosthetic intervention. This classic prose chronicles the story of Vispala, a fierce female warrior whose leg, lost in battle, was replaced by an iron prosthesis that enabled her return to the front to fight again.[1]

Gait assessment is used to describe the patterns of movement that control progression of the body in walking. Bipedal gait requires a combination of automatic and volitional postural components. This can result in either asymmetric reciprocal movements of the lower limbs (seen in walking or running) or symmetric, simultaneous two-legged hopping. Kangaroos are bipeds that are successful two-legged hoppers.[2] Homo sapiens have reached the zenith of movement efficiency in bipedal walking and running by using reciprocal patterns of motion.

The integration of numerous physiological systems is needed for successful locomotion. Normal walking requires stability to provide antigravity support of body weight in stance, mobility of body segments, and motor control to sequence multiple segments while transferring body weight from one limb to the other. Gait characteristics are influenced by the shape, position, and function of neuromuscular and musculoskeletal structures and by the ligamentous and capsular constraints of the joints. The primary goal in gait is energy efficiency in forward progression by using a stable kinetic chain of joints and limb segments working congruently to transport its passenger unit (the head, arms, and trunk).

Understanding the process of walking can help improve the performance efficiency of persons with musculoskeletal and neuromuscular impairments. Gait assessment in orthotic and prosthetic intervention provides an accurate description of walking patterns for a given patient. Assessment also identifies primary or pathological gait problems and helps differentiate them from compensatory strategies. Skilled gait assessment is necessary for selection of appropriate orthotic or prosthetic components, alignment parameters, and identification of other variants that might enhance an individual's ability to walk. Clinical gait assessment contributes to the development of a comprehensive treatment plan, with the ultimate goal of optimal energy efficiency and appropriate pathomechanical controls during walking, balancing cosmesis with overall function.

KINEMATIC DESCRIPTORS OF HUMAN WALKING

Step length, stride length, cadence, and velocity are important, interrelated, and quantitative kinematic measures of gait. Step length and stride length are not synonymous. *Step length* is the distance from the floor-contact point of one (ipsilateral, originating) foot in early stance to the floor-contact point of the opposite (contralateral) foot: the distance from right heel contact to left heel contact. *Stride length* is the distance from floor contact on one side to the next floor contact on that same side: the distance from right heel contact to the next right heel contact. Stride length contains a left and a right step length. A reduction in functional joint motion or the presence of pain or muscle weakness can result in reduction in stride or step length, or both. Pathological gait commonly produces asymmetries in step length between the two lower limbs.

Cadence is defined as the number of steps taken in a given unit of time, most often expressed in steps per minute. *Velocity* is defined as the distance traveled in a given unit of time (the rate of forward progression) and is usually expressed in centimeters per second or meters per minute. Velocity is the best single index of walking ability. Reductions in velocity correlate with joint impairments and with many acute pathological conditions. Velocity can also be qualitatively described as free, slow, or fast. Free walking speed is an individual's normal self-selected (comfortable) walking velocity. Fast walking speed describes the maximum velocity possible for a given individual. Slow walking speed describes a velocity below the normal self-selected walking speed. For healthy individuals, fast walk velocity may be as much as 44% faster than free walking speed.[3] In people with musculoskeletal and neuromuscular impairment that affects gait, often much less difference is found between free and fast gait velocity.

Double limb support is the period of time when both feet are in contact with the ground. It occurs twice during the gait cycle, at the beginning and the end of each stance phase. As velocity increases, double limb support time decreases. When running, the individual has rapid forward movement with little or no period of double limb support. Individuals with slow walking speeds spend more of the gait cycle in double support.

Step width, or width of the walking base, typically measures between 5 and 10 cm from the heel center of one foot to the heel center of the other foot. A wide walking base may increase stability but also reduces energy efficiency of gait. The *ground reaction force (GRF) vector* is the mean load-bearing line, which takes into account both gravity and momentum. It has magnitude as well as directional qualities. The spatial relation between this line and a given joint center influences the direction in which the joint tends to rotate. The rotational potential of the forces that act on a joint is called a *torque* or *moment*.

GAIT CYCLE

A variety of conceptual approaches have been used to understand the walking process. Saunders and colleagues[4] and Inman and colleagues[5] define the functional task of walking as translation of the center of gravity through space in a manner that requires the least energy expenditure. They identify six determinants, or variables, that affect energy expenditure in sustained walking: pelvic rotation, pelvic tilt, knee flexion in stance phase, foot interaction with the knee, ankle interaction with the knee, and lateral pelvic displacement. Individually and collectively, these determinants have an impact on energy expenditure and the mechanics of walking. Although they help us understand the process of walking, the determinants do not themselves offer a practical clinical solution to address the problems of assessment of pathological gait.

A comprehensive system that is useful in describing normal and abnormal gait has been developed by the Pathokinesiology and Physical Therapy Departments at Rancho Los Amigos Medical Center over the last several decades.[6-8] The Rancho Los Amigos system serves as the descriptive medium for this chapter (Figure 3-1). Because velocity affects many parameters of walking, the description of normal gait assumes a comfortable self-selected velocity. At free walking velocity, the individual naturally enlists the mannerisms and the speed that provide maximum energy efficiency for their physiological system.

The gait cycle is considered to be the period between any two identical events in the walking cycle. Initial contact is traditionally selected as the starting and completing event of

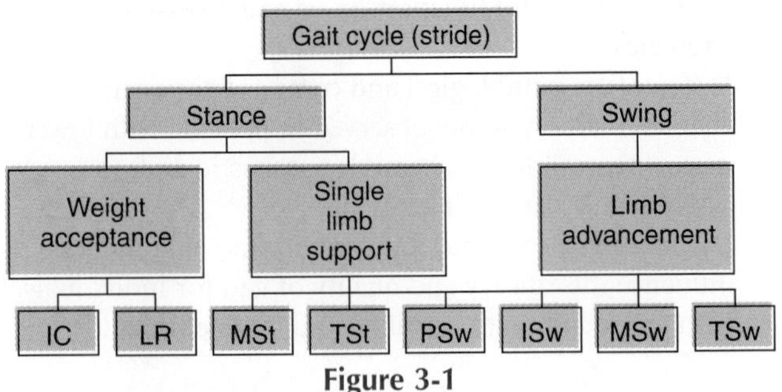

Figure 3-1

A complete gait cycle can be viewed in terms of the three functional tasks of weight acceptance, single limb support, and limb advancement. The gait cycle can also be described in phasic terms of IC, LR, MSt, TSt, PSw, ISw, MSw, and TSw. The PSw phase is a transitional phase between single limb support and limb advancement. IC, *Initial contact;* LR, *loading response;* MSt, *midstance;* TSt, *terminal stance;* PSw, *preswing;* ISw, *initial swing;* MSw, *midswing;* TSw, *terminal swing.*

a single cycle of gait. Each cycle is divided into two periods: stance phase and swing phase. *Stance* is the time when the foot is in contact with the ground; it constitutes approximately 60% of the gait cycle. *Swing* denotes the time when the foot is in the air; it constitutes the remaining 40% of the gait cycle. There are five subphases within the stance period: initial contact (IC), loading response (LR), midstance (MSt), terminal stance (TSt), and preswing (PSw). Swing phase is divided into three subphases: initial swing (ISw), midswing (MSw), and terminal swing (TSw). Because PSw prepares the limb for swing advancement, many consider PSw to be a preparatory component of swing phase.

Three functional tasks are achieved during these eight gait phases: weight acceptance in early stance, single limb support in mid- to late stance, and limb advancement during swing.

Functional Task 1: Weight Acceptance

IC and LR are the subphases of stance involved in the task of weight acceptance. Effective transfer of body weight onto the limb as soon as it makes contact with the ground requires initial limb stability and shock absorption and the preservation of forward momentum.

Initial Contact

IC is the instant that the foot of the leading lower limb touches the ground. Most motor function during IC is preparation for LR. At IC, the ankle is in neutral position, the knee is close to full extension, and the hip is flexed 30 degrees. The sagittal plane GRF vector lies posterior to the ankle joint, creating a plantar flexion moment (Figure 3-2). Eccentric contraction of the pretibial muscles (tibialis anterior and long toe extensors) holds the ankle and subtalar joint

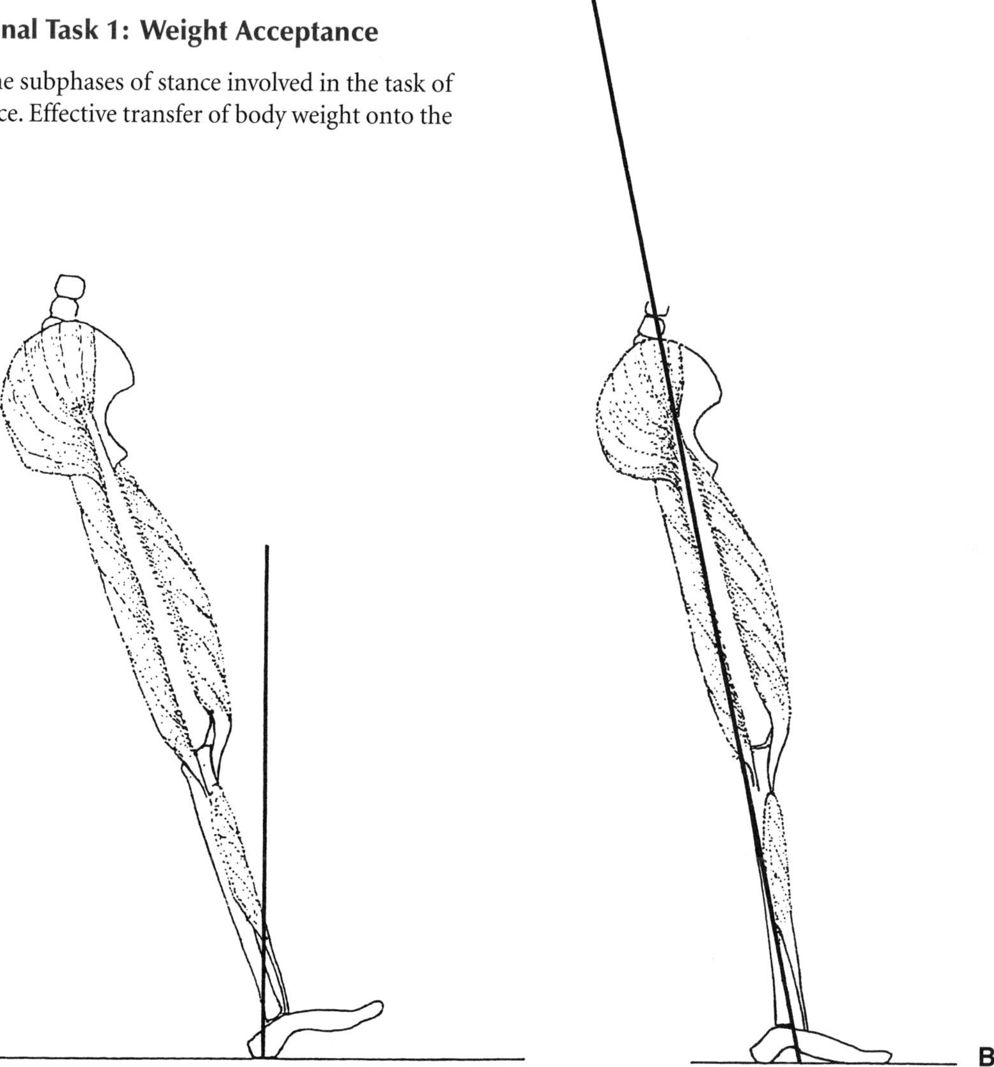

Figure 3-2
The two subphases of gait involved with the functional task of weight acceptance are IC and LR. ***A,*** *At IC, the GRF line is posterior to the ankle and anterior to the knee and hip with activation of pretibial, quadriceps, hamstring, and gluteal muscles. Note that the length of the GRF line represents its magnitude.* ***B,*** *The LR phase results in an increased magnitude of the vertical force, which ultimately exceeds body weight. Activity of the same muscle groups elicited at IC increases steadily with the vertical force.* IC, *Initial contact;* LR, *loading response;* GRF, *ground reaction force.*

in neutral position. At the knee, the GRF vector is anterior to the joint axis, which creates a passive extensor torque. Muscle contraction activity of the quadriceps and hamstring muscle groups continues from the previous TSw to preserve the neutral position of the knee joint. A flexion moment is present around the hip joint because the GRF vector falls anterior to the joint axis. Gluteus maximus and hamstring muscles are activated to restrain the resultant flexion torque.

Loading Response

LR occupies approximately 10% of the gait cycle and constitutes the period of initial double limb support (see Figure 3-2, *B*). Two functional tasks occur during LR: controlled descent of the foot toward the ground and shock absorption as weight is transferred onto the stance limb.

The momentum generated by the fall of body weight onto the stance limb is preserved by the *heel rocker* (first rocker) of the stance phase. Normal IC at the calcaneal tuberosity creates a fulcrum about which the foot and tibia move. The bony segment between this fulcrum and the center of the ankle rolls toward the ground as body weight is dropped onto the stance foot, preserving the momentum necessary for forward progression. Eccentric action of the pretibial muscles regulates the rate of ankle plantar flexion, and the quadriceps contract to limit knee flexion. The action of these two muscle groups provides controlled forward advancement of the lower extremity unit (foot, tibia, and femur). During the peak of LR, the magnitude of the vertical GRF exceeds body weight. To absorb the impact force of body weight and preserve forward momentum, the knee flexes 15 to 18 degrees and the ankle plantar flexes to 10 degrees. The hip maintains its position of 30 degrees of flexion. Contraction of the gluteus maximus, hamstrings, and adductor magnus prevents further flexion of the hip joint.

Functional Task 2: Single Limb Support

Two phases are associated with single limb support: MSt and TSt. During this period the contralateral foot is in swing phase, and body weight is entirely supported on the stance limb. Forward progression of body weight over the stationary foot while maintaining stability must be accomplished during these two subphases of stance.

Midstance

MSt begins when the contralateral foot leaves the ground and continues as body weight travels along the length of the stance foot until it is aligned over the forefoot, approximately 20% of the gait cycle (Figure 3-3). This pivotal action of the *ankle rocker* (second rocker) advances the tibia over the stationary foot. Forward movement of the tibia over the foot is controlled by the eccentric contraction of the soleus, assisted by the gastrocnemius.

During this phase, the ankle moves from its LR position of 10 degrees of plantar flexion to approximately 7 degrees of dorsiflexion. The knee extends from 15 degrees of flexion to a neutral position. The hip joint moves toward extension, from 30 to 10 degrees of flexion. With continued forward progression, the body weight vector moves anterior to the ankle, creating a dorsiflexion moment. Eccentric action of the plantar flexors is crucial in providing limb stability as the contralateral toe-off transfers body weight onto the stance foot. By the end of MSt, the body weight vector moves anterior to the knee (creating passive stability of the limb) and posterior to the hip (reducing the demand on the hip extensors). The gluteus maximus, active in early MSt, yields to this passive hip extension as the hip nears vertical alignment over the femur. Vertical GRF is reduced in magnitude at MSt because of the upward momentum of the contralateral swing limb. In the coronal plane, activity of hip abductors during MSt is essential to provide lateral hip stability and a level pelvis.

Terminal Stance

TSt, the second half of single limb support, begins with heel rise of the stance limb and ends when the contralateral foot makes contact with the ground. As the body vector approaches the metatarsophalangeal joint, the heel rises and the phalanx dorsiflexes (extends). The metatarsal heads serve as an axis of rotation for body weight advancement (see Figure 3-3, *B*). This is referred to as the *forefoot* or *toe rocker* (third rocker of gait). The forefoot rocker serves as an axis around which progression of the body vector advances beyond the area of foot support, creating the highest demand on calf muscles (gastrocnemius and soleus) of the entire gait cycle. During TSt, the ankle continues to dorsiflex until it reaches 10 degrees of dorsiflexion. The knee is fully extended, and the hip moves into slight hyperextension. Forward fall of the body moves the vector further anterior to the ankle, creating a large dorsiflexion moment. Stability of the tibia on the ankle is provided by the eccentric action of calf muscles.

The trailing posture of the limb and the presence of the vector anterior to the knee and posterior to the hip provide passive stability at hip and knee joints. The tensor fascia lata serves to restrain the posterior vector at the hip. At the end of TSt, the vertical GRF reaches a second peak greater than body weight, similar to that which occurred at the end of LR.

Functional Task 3: Limb Advancement

Four phases contribute to limb advancement: PSw, ISw, MSw, and TSw. During these phases the stance limb leaves the ground, advances forward, and prepares for the next IC.

Preswing

PSw, the second period of double limb support in gait, comprises the last 10% of the stance phase. It begins when the contralateral foot makes contact with the ground and ends with ipsilateral toe-off. During this period the stance

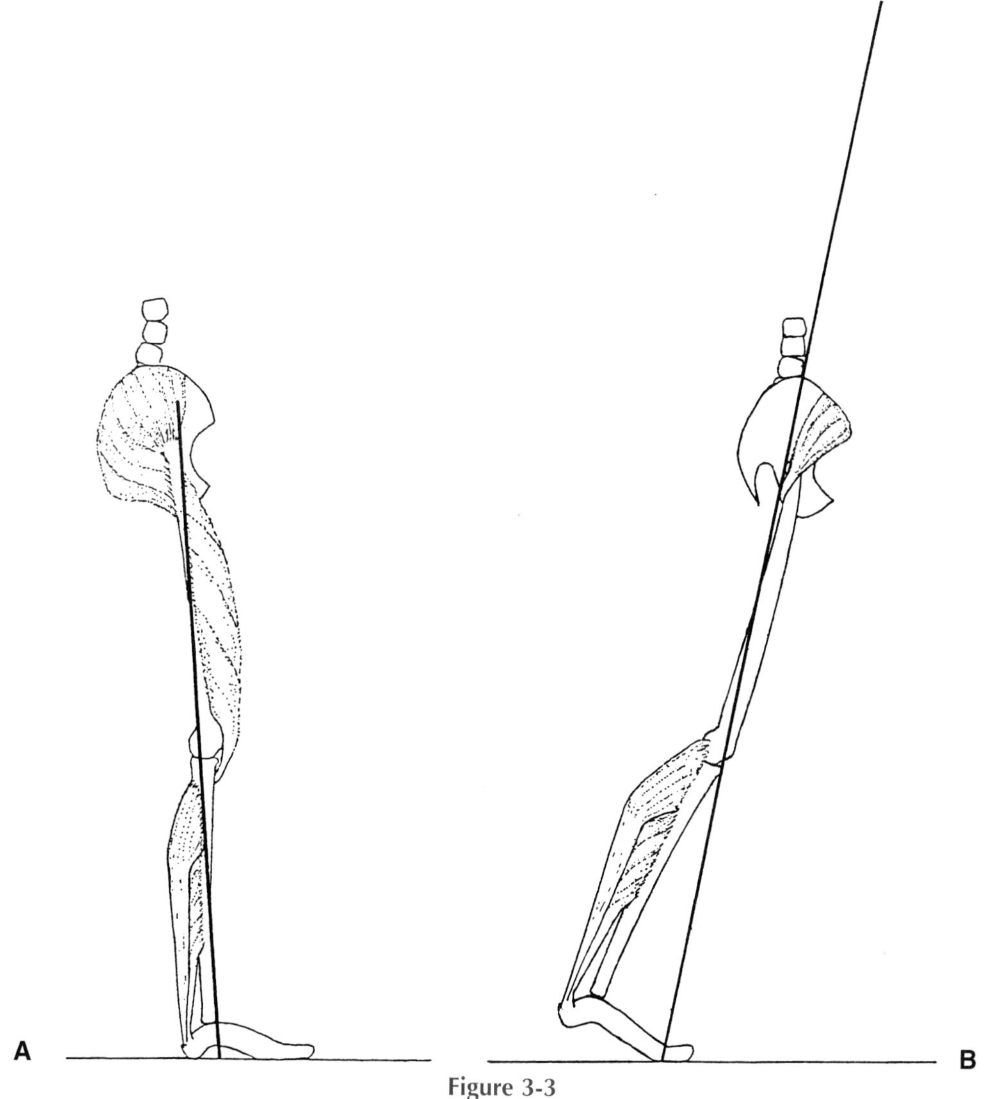

Figure 3-3
The subphases of gait involved in the functional task of single limb support are MSt and TSt. ***A,*** *In early MSt, the vertical force begins to decrease and the triceps surae, quadriceps, and gluteus medius and maximus are active.* ***B,*** *During TSt, there is a second peak in vertical force, exceeding body weight, with high activity of the triceps surae, which maintain the third rocker. The tensor fascia lata restrains the increasing posterior hip vector.* MSt, *Midstance;* Tst, *terminal stance.*

limb is unloaded and body weight is transferred onto the contralateral limb (Figure 3-4). The ankle moves rapidly from its TSt position of dorsiflexion into 20 degrees of plantar flexion. During this subphase, plantar flexor muscle activity decreases as the limb is unloaded. Toward the end of PSw, the vertical force is diminished such that plantar flexors are quiescent. There is no active muscle contraction for "push off" in normal reciprocal free walk bipedal gait.[6] The knee also flexes rapidly to achieve 35 to 40 degrees of flexion by the end of PSw. The GRF vector is at the metatarsophalangeal joints and posterior to the knee, and the resultant knee flexion is mainly passive. Knee flexion during this phase prepares the limb for toe clearance in the swing phase. PSw hip flexion is initiated by the rectus femoris and the adductor longus, which also decelerates the passive abduction created by contralateral body weight transfer. The sagittal vector extends through the hip as the hip returns to a neutral position.

Initial Swing

Approximately one third of the swing period is spent in ISw. It begins the moment the foot leaves the ground and continues until maximal knee flexion occurs, when the swinging extremity is directly under the body (see Figure 3-4, *B*). Concentric contraction of pretibial muscles begins to lift the foot toward dorsiflexion from its initial 20 degrees to 5 degrees of plantar flexion. This is necessary for toe and foot clearance as the swing phase begins. Knee flexion,

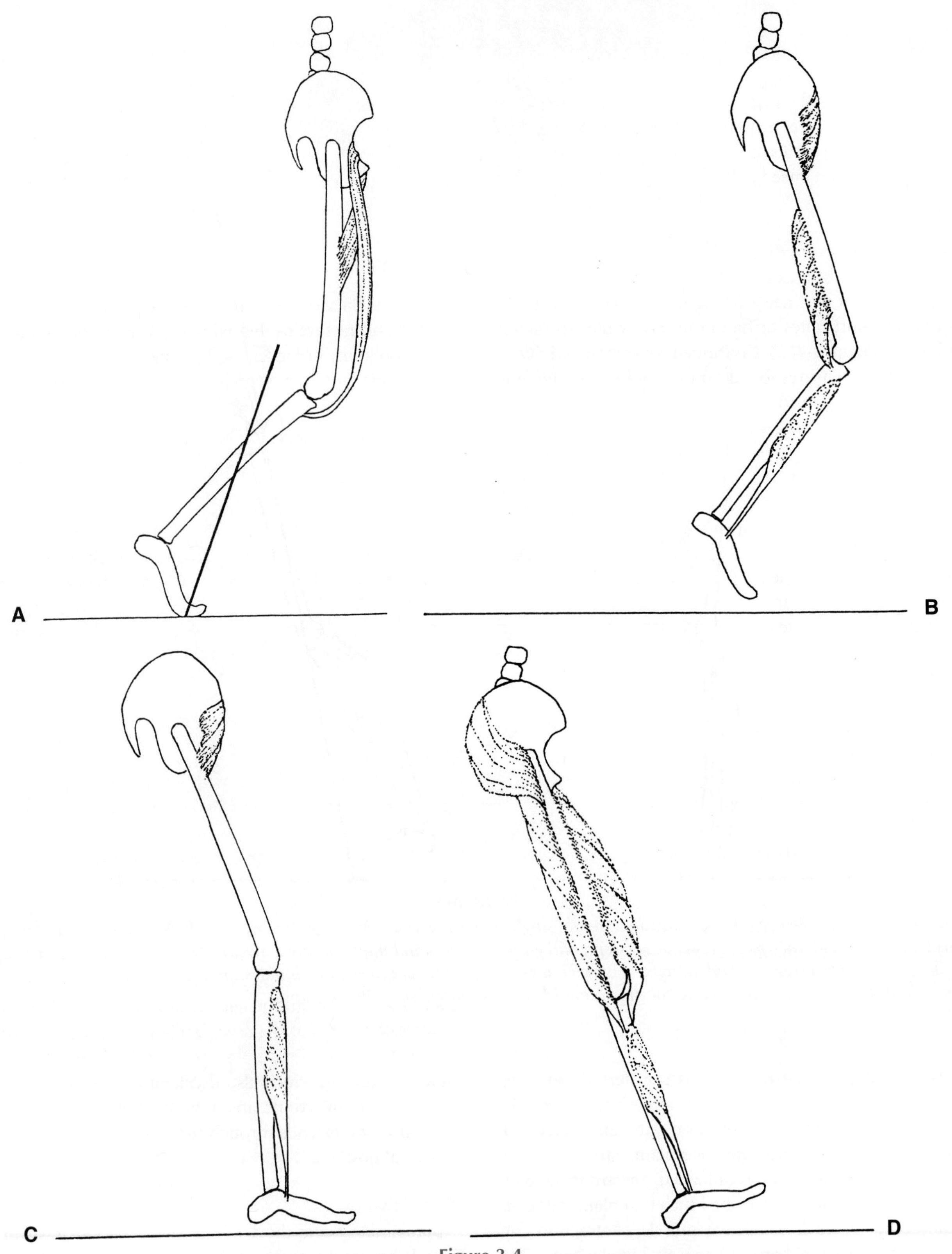

Figure 3-4

The subphases of gait involved in the functional task of swing limb advancement include PSw, ISw, MSw, and TSw. **A,** *During PSw, contralateral loading results in limited muscle activity in the limb transitioning from stance to swing. The rectus femoris and adductor longus initiate hip flexion. Knee flexion is passive, resulting from the planted forefoot and mobile proximal segments.* **B,** *During ISw, the pretibial muscles, short head of the biceps femoris, and iliacus are active in initiating limb advancement and providing swing clearance.* **C,** *A vertical tibia signals the end of the period of MSw. Here contraction of the iliacus preserves hip flexion while pretibial muscle activity maintains foot clearance.* **D,** *At TSw, the gluteus maximus, hamstrings, quadriceps, and pretibial muscles are active to prepare for limb placement and the ensuing LR.* PSw, *Preswing;* ISw, *initial swing;* MDs, *midswing;* TSw, *terminal swing.*

resulting from action of the short head of the biceps femoris, also assists in toe clearance. The knee continues to flex until it reaches a position of 60 degrees of flexion. Contraction of the iliacus brings the hip into 20 degrees of flexion. Contraction of the gracilis and sartorius muscles during this phase assists hip and knee flexion.

Midswing

During MSw, limb advancement and foot clearance continue. MSw begins at maximum knee flexion and ends when the tibia is vertical. Knee extension, coupled with ankle dorsiflexion, contributes to foot clearance while advancing the tibia (see Figure 3-4, *C*). Continued concentric activity of pretibial muscles ensures foot clearance and moves the foot toward the neutral position. Momentum creates an extension moment, advancing the lower leg toward extension from 60 degrees to 30 degrees of flexion, with the quadriceps quiescent. Mild contraction of hip flexors continues to preserve the hip flexion position.

Terminal Swing

In the final phase, TSw, the knee extends fully in preparation for heel contact (see Figure 3-4, *D*). Eccentric contraction of the hamstrings and gluteus maximus decelerates the thigh and restrains further hip flexion. Activity of the pretibial muscles maintains the ankle at neutral to prepare for heel contact. In the second half of TSw, the quadriceps become active to facilitate full knee extension. Hip flexion remains at 30 degrees.

DESCRIBING PATHOLOGICAL GAIT

Clinicians often use qualitative descriptive terms to characterize the gait deviations and compensations of pathological gait. Some of these terms help identify specific primary problems. Others describe compensatory strategies used by patients to solve gait difficulties created by various primary problems.

Gait Deviations Observed during Stance

Trendelenburg's gait occurs in the stance phase, when the trunk leans to the same side as the hip pathosis (ipsilateral lean). This is a compensatory strategy used when the gluteus medius muscle and its synergists (gluteus minimus and tensor fascia lata) cannot adequately stabilize the pelvis during stance.[9] Normally, the drop of the contralateral pelvis is limited to 5 degrees by the strong response of the hip abductor musculature. To support the pelvis, the hip abductor muscles must generate a force that is 1.5 times the body weight.[10] A weak or absent gluteus medius leads to postural substitution of trunk lean over the weight-bearing hip joint. This reduces the external varus moment created by a GRF line that falls medial to the joint center. Without this postural compensation, clearance becomes a problem for the swinging contralateral limb. Rarely, Trendelenburg's gait is caused by overactive hip adductors (adductors longus, magnus, brevis, and gracilis).

Vaulting is exaggerated heel elevation of the stance foot, sometimes in combination with increases in stance limb hip and knee extension, with the goal of raising the pelvis to clear the contralateral swing limb. It occurs when the functional length of the swing limb is relatively longer than that of the stance limb. It also occurs when swing limb advancement is impaired or delayed by inadequate motor control of hip or knee flexion, or both, or in the presence of a plantar flexion contracture of the swing leg. It may compensate for pelvic obliquity or leg length discrepancy.

Antalgic gait is a strategy used to avoid pain during walking. It is frequently seen at LR when the patient reduces single limb support time on the affected limb. If the pain occurs during a particular period in stance, that specific time period is diminished. Antalgic gait caused by pain that originates around the hip might translate into a lateral lean to permit the patient to get the center of gravity over the support point, the head of the femur. If the pain occurs during the extreme end range of a particular joint motion, that motion is diminished. For example, if full extension produces pain, the knee would be maintained in slight flexion throughout the gait cycle.

Gait Deviations Observed during Swing

The *circumducted gait* is a swing phase deviation in which hip abduction is combined with a wide arc of pelvic rotation, most often occurring as a compensatory pattern when there is a relatively longer swing limb compared with the stance limb. This action is most likely to happen when there is limitation in range of motion or impaired motor control in ankle dorsiflexion, knee flexion, or hip flexion. A plantar flexion contracture at the foot or a stiff knee or hip joint can also lead to the use of a circumduction pattern during swing in an effort to achieve toe and foot clearance. This combination of abduction and pelvic rotation can provide a compensatory method of the usual limb advancement process.

Circumduction can be observed as a lateral arc of the foot in the transverse plane that begins at the end of PSw and ends at IC on the same limb. The arc reaches the apex of its lateral movement at MSw. The typical pattern is a mixture of a wide base of support with the foot abnormally outset and may include an ipsilateral pelvic drop. It is possible for a contracture of the contralateral adductors to create this deviation by pulling the pelvis toward the contralateral femur and demanding a compensatory ipsilateral abducted position relative to the pelvis. A severe leg length discrepancy can result in an exaggerated pelvic tilt from the contralateral stance leg, which obligates the swing limb to an increased abduction position. Circumduction and abduction create a significant energy cost penalty, increasing lateral displacement of the center of gravity.

Gait Deviations Associated with Abnormal Tone

A variety of abnormal gait patterns are associated with abnormal muscle tone (spasticity, rigidity, hypotonicity) or muscle weakness. *Scissors gait* describes a pattern of poor control in limb advancement or tracking of the swing leg and is characterized by the crossing, or scissoring, of the lower limbs. It is most often observed in patients with spastic or paretic pathological conditions, such as hemiplegia, or spastic quadriplegic cerebral palsy. *Steppage gait* occurs when weakness or paralysis of the dorsiflexor musculature, such as peroneal palsy or a neuropathy, demands exaggerated hip and knee flexion of the proximal joints to accomplish swing clearance. It is most easily observed in late MSt.

In *crouch gait* exaggerated knee and hip flexion occurs throughout the gait cycle. Crouch gait is often seen in combination with a toe-walking stance in children and adults with spastic diplegic cerebral palsy. It has been attributed to a combination of overactivity of the hamstrings and weakness of calf muscles. Although use of an orthosis can successfully control abnormal motion in the sagittal plane (for example, in steppage gait), orthoses are less effective in controlling the abnormal transverse, rotational, or coronal limb placement problems observed in scissors or crouch gait.

In *ataxic gait* there is a failure of coordination or irregularity of muscular action of the limb segments. It may be caused by cerebellar dysfunction or loss of joint proprioception. Ataxia often becomes accentuated when the eyes are closed or vision is otherwise impaired.

METHODS OF QUANTITATIVE GAIT ANALYSIS

Quantitative analysis seeks to understand the process of walking with measurable parameters collected through instrumentation. Perhaps the potential to assess gait through quantified measurement emerged prehistorically with the sunrise-to-sunset movement of a lone traveler on foot or with the hailing chant of each advancing step of a marching army. Such basic techniques would have enabled measurement of walking velocity (distance traversed per unit of time) and cadence (steps per unit of time). Marks,[11] a New York City prosthetist, offered a more precise qualitative description of pathological gait in 1905, when he described the gait process in eight organized phases and discussed the implications of prosthetic component design on the function of walking. Marks praised "kinetoscopic" photography as a potential diagnostic tool for optimizing pathological gait.

Today we record gait parameters with instruments as common as a stopwatch or as complex as the simultaneous integration of three-dimensional kinematics, kinetics, and electromyographic (EMG) methods. The primary emphasis of clinical assessment has been on the use of accessible techniques and inexpensive technologies. A simple, inexpensive footprint mat has been used for decades to record barefoot plantar pressures. Individual or multiple mats have been used in the clinic to record step and stride length as well as walking base width. Early on, video technology with slow-motion capabilities made more precise qualitative description of the gait cycle possible, but the recent development of inexpensive video gait assessment software has made clinical quantitative applications as well. Most quantitative and qualitative video systems measure joint angles in two dimensions. Because walking is a three-dimensional function, however, these systems may have limited value for comprehensive assessments and as a research tool.

Technology in Gait Assessment

Perhaps the most user-friendly and economically accessible family of measurement tools with broad clinical application is the emerging pressure technologies. A thin plastic array can slip nearly unnoticed between the plantar surface of the foot and an orthosis or the insole of the shoe (Figure 3-5). This array, connected to a computer by a lead wire, can measure dynamic pressure patterns and record critical events throughout the walking cycle. A prosthetic version can provide pressure measurements at 60 individual sites within a socket and record those measurements during multiple events of the gait cycle. The clinical relevance lies in identifying critical gait events, temporal measurements, and skin-loading pressure patterns. Because of the ease in collection of temporal and plantar pressure readings and relatively modest cost, this approach may replace microswitch technologies in the future and be increasingly accessible to therapists, prosthetists, and orthotists for clinical use.

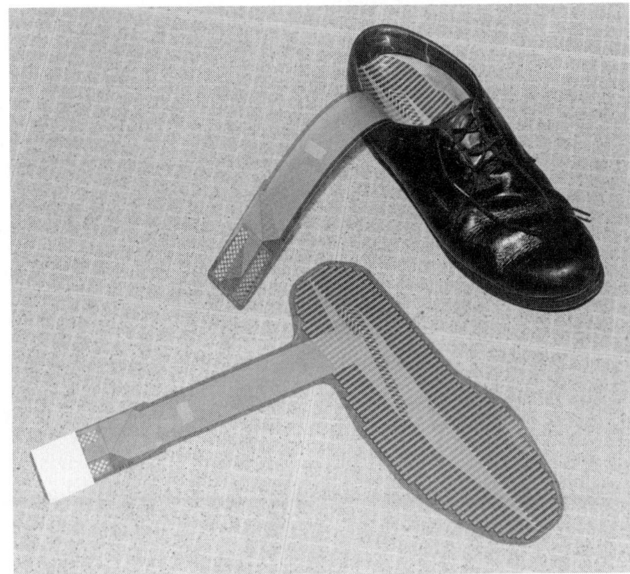

Figure 3-5
An in-shoe pressure-sensing array can help identify areas of high pressure concentration. This information assists in the design of an orthosis to modify pressure dynamics during the stance phase of gait.

The high-tech side of quantitative gait analysis has traversed a surprisingly long road. The birth of instrumented kinematic, EMG, and temporal performance analysis began in the 1870s with E. J. Marey, who first performed movement analysis of pathological gait with photography.[12] He also developed the first myograph for measuring muscle activity and the first foot-switch collection system for measuring gait events related to time and difference (temporal). The foot-switch system was an experimental shoe that measured the length and rapidity of the step and the pressure of the foot on the ground. Eadweard Muybridge,[13] working at Stanford University in the 1880s, used synchronized multiple camera photography with a scaled backdrop to capture on film and assess the motion of subjects walking. Other major advances in instrumented gait analysis were made by Scherb, who performed hand muscle palpation with a treadmill in 1920, and Adrian, who in 1925 advocated the use of EMG to study the dynamic action of muscles.[14]

Modern gait technology began in 1945, when Inman and colleagues initiated the systematic collection of gait data for individuals without impairment and with amputation in the outdoor gait laboratory at the University of California at Berkeley. Since then, researchers and clinicians have increasingly used the growing array of gait technologies to measure the parameters of human performance in normal and pathological gait. A full-service gait laboratory gathers information on six performance parameters in walking: temporal, metabolic, kinematic, kinetic, EMG, and pressure.[15]

Measuring Temporal and Distance Parameters

Temporal (time-distance) parameters enable the clinician to summarize the overall quality of a patient's gait. In the gait laboratory, temporal data can be collected with microswitch-embedded pads taped to the bottom of a patient's shoes or feet that record the amount of time that the patient spends on various points of the sole over a measured distance. A number of portable pressure-sensitive gait mats connected to laptop computers with gait analysis software for time and distance gait parameters are also commercially available to use in clinical settings (Figure 3-6).[16,17] Stride length, velocity,

A

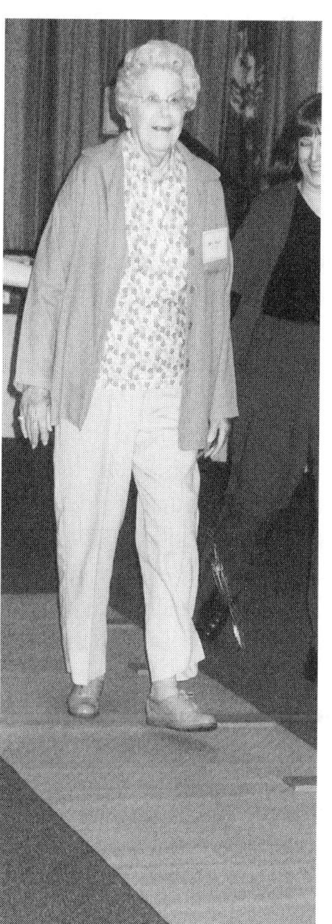

B

Parameters

Distance (cm)	281.9
Ambulation time (sec)	2.50
Velocity (cm/sec)	112.7
Mean normalized velocity	1.44

Functional ambulation profile: 99

Cadence (steps/min)	120.0
Step time differential (sec)	0.01
Step length differential (cm)	0.36
Cycle time differential (sec)	0.01

Walk # / footfall #	L/R	Mean (%CV)	All ages
Step time (sec)	L	0.494 (2)	
	R	0.504 (3)	0.53 0.59
Cycle time (sec)	L	0.994 (3)	
	R	1.007 (1)	1.06 1.18
Swing time (sec)	L	0.356 (2) /35.8	
/ %GC	R	0.382 (2) /37.9	36 44
Stance (sec)	L	0.638 (3) /64.2	
/ %GC	R	0.625 (0) /62.1	56 64
Single support (sec)	L	0.382 (2) /38.4	
/ %GC	R	0.356 (2) /35.4	38 42
Double support (sec)	L	0.269 (3) /27.1	
/ %GC	R	0.269 (3) /26.7	16 24
Step length (cm)	L	56.587 (5)	
	R	56.229 (3)	58 85
Stride length (cm)	L	113.665 (2)	
	R	112.429 (1)	116 170
Base of support (cm)	L	9.56 (36)	
	R	11.41 (17)	
Toe in / out (deg)	L	7 (33)	
	R	11 (13)	

Figure 3-6

A, *An example of a portable pressure-sensitive walkway used to assess temporal and distance parameters of gait.* ***B,*** *The walkway is connected to a laptop computer, and the operator is able to quickly generate values for velocity, stride and step lengths, cadence, time and percent of cycle spent in stance, single and double limb support, and swing. (Courtesy the Motion Analysis Laboratory, Department of Physical Therapy and Human Movement Science, Sacred Heart University, Fairfield, Conn.)*

cadence, percentage of the gait cycle spent in single and double limb support, and general stance progression patterns can be measured and assessed. Tendencies toward excessive inversion, eversion, or prolonged heel-only time can be noted and may suggest modifications to alignment or components of prostheses or orthoses to normalize such gait patterns. A temporal data collection system is particularly cost efficient, clinically meaningful, and affordable. Temporal data can be, and often are, part of another system such as EMG or motion analysis.

Assessing the Energy Cost of Walking

Metabolic data reflect the physiological "energy cost" of walking. The traditional measures of energy cost are oxygen consumption, total carbon dioxide generated, and heart rate. Other relevant factors include volume of air breathed and respiration rate. All these parameters are viewed in terms of velocity and distance walked over the collection period. Historically, metabolic data were collected while the patient walked on a treadmill, wearing umbilical devices. In recent years, because of the known influence of treadmill collection in altering normal gait velocity, energy cost data are more likely to be obtained on an open track of a measured distance with the patient ambulating in a free walk or natural cadence (Figure 3-7). The primary limitation of energy cost as an assessment tool is that, although it can inform the investigator about body metabolism relative to the patient's gait, it cannot explain why or how an advantage or disadvantage was obtained. Waters[18] demonstrated that an individual with Syme's level amputation uses less oxygen to traverse a given distance than someone with a transtibial amputation but could not explain why. For that explanation, other gait parameters must be examined. Energy cost measures cannot easily identify widely variant prosthetic foot designs worn by the same patient, whereas kinematic, kinetic, and EMG data typically can.[19]

Perhaps the best-kept secret in the energy cost arsenal is the *physiological cost index* (PCI). It is easily calculated as follows:

PCI = (Walking pulse – Resting pulse)/Gait speed

The PCI is one of the most sensitive indicators of energy cost of gait. Winchester et al,[20] who compared two different orthotic designs by measuring a wide variety of metabolic parameters, used the PCI to identify a statistically significant difference between the two devices when all other measures failed to produce such differences. Pulse and respiratory rate taken at rest and after timed intervals during normal comfortable gait can also help assess exertion levels.

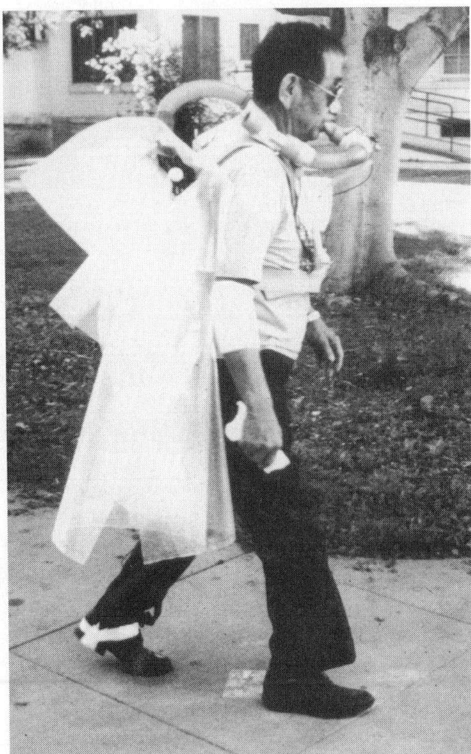

Figure 3-7

The Douglas bag method collects exhaled gases for later analysis as the patient walks in a circular walkway. Heart rate and other metabolic variables are monitored by radio telemetry.

Kinematic and Kinetic Systems

Most *kinematic* systems provide joint and body segment motion in graphic form. This information includes sagittal, coronal, and transverse motions that occur at the ankle, knee, hip, and pelvis. The patient is instrumented with reflective spheres that are placed on well-recognized anatomical landmarks (Figure 3-8). Typically, an infrared light source is positioned around each of several cameras. This light is directed to the reflective spheres, which in turn are reflected into the cameras. Each field of video data is digitized, the markers are manually identified by an operator, and the coordinates of the geometric center of each marker are calculated with computer software. Resultant data are displayed as animated stick figures that represent the actual motions produced by the patient. The operator can freeze any frame and enlarge the image at any joint to examine gait patterns in greater depth. The operator can extract raw numbers that represent joint placement and motion in space or produce a printout showing joint motion in all planes plotted against the percentage of the gait cycle (Figure 3-9). Angular velocities, accelerations, and joint and segment linear displacements can be calculated. Data from other systems (force platforms and EMG) collected during the same time sequence as the motion data are often integrated with the kinematics.

Kinetic information is obtained from one or more force platforms, which collect data on vertical force, fore-aft shear, and mediolateral shear (Figure 3-10). The contribution of kinetic data can be profound. Fore-aft shear is quite useful in establishing appropriate transtibial prosthetic alignment in the sagittal plane. For this purpose the analyst would anticipate a balanced magnitude and timing of the braking and propulsive patterns. Collection of data from two consecutive steps requires dual force plates. The typical force platform system can obtain power calculations or center of pressure graphs or can be combined with kinematic data to show joint moments. This system is useful in measuring the dynamic joint control of an individual throughout stance. Some kinetic software offers specialized programs for specific purposes such as stability analysis, which provides information about center of gravity shift relative to time.

Electromyography

EMG data may be the single most important technology in terms of understanding the direct physiological effect of gait variants. Patterns of muscle activity in patients with abnormal gait are compared with well-established norms. Knowledge of the timing and intensity of the muscle activity throughout the gait cycle may guide gait training, orthotic or prosthetic prescription, and dynamic orthotic or prosthetic alignment aimed at reduction of excessive, ill-timed, or prolonged muscle activity. EMG data are also helpful in guiding decisions about surgical intervention (dorsal rhizotomy, tendon lengthening, or osteotomy) in children with cerebral palsy.

Pressure-Sensing Technology

Pressure-sensing technologies offer the clinician tremendous insights into the treatment of patients at risk for amputation because of vascular disease and diabetic neuropathy and can assist vascular surgeons and orthopedic foot specialists in limb salvage through more appropriate custom-designed prophylactic orthoses. This area is one of the more recent and clinically promising technologies for the assessment team.

Over the last several decades, technologies have significantly improved understanding of pathological gait, offered strong evidence for the efficacy of various treatment approaches, and enhanced patient care. Advocates of a more universal application of the high-end technologies in the clinical setting, however, have yet to make a compelling case, particularly in the current climate of cost containment. Perhaps the strongest argument for gait technology in our present era lies in its use for outcome measurement in the justification of legitimate therapeutic treatment approaches as well as orthotic and prosthetic applications.

QUALITATIVE GAIT ASSESSMENT

Qualitative methods for identification and recording of gait deviation have played a role in patient care for decades. In 1925, Robinson[21] described 11 pathological gait patterns and attempted to correlate them with specific disease processes. In 1937, Boorstein[22] identified 14 disease processes that could be diagnosed with the help of gait assessment. He described seven major gait deficit groups, attributing the term *steppage gait* to the French physician Charcot and the identification of *waddling gait* in hip dysplasia to Hippocrates. In the late 1950s, Blair Hangar, the founder of Northwestern University's School of Prosthetics and Orthotics, and Hildegard Myers, a physical therapist at Rehabilitation Institute of Chicago, collaborated to develop the first comprehensive system of clinical gait analysis for persons with transfemoral amputation.[23] They identified 16 gait deviations and suggested numerous patient and prosthetic causes for each. Their work, developed into an educational film and handbook in 1960, has been a model for subsequent instructional videos and assessment systems in prosthetics.[24] Brunnstrom's[25] comprehensive gait analysis form for hemiplegic gait, published in 1970, is a checklist of 28 deviations seen at the ankle, knee, and hip that are common after stroke.

Early work in observational gait analysis received a significant impetus from Perry[26] as an outgrowth of basic research data published in 1967. In the late 1960s, Perry and a group of physical therapists from the Rancho Los Amigos

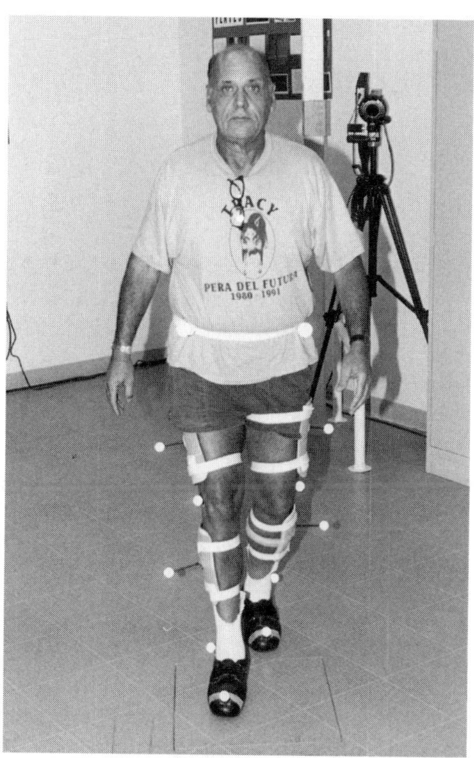

Figure 3-8
This individual is wearing reflective spheres. An infrared camera system can track limb segment motion as the patient walks across the field of view.

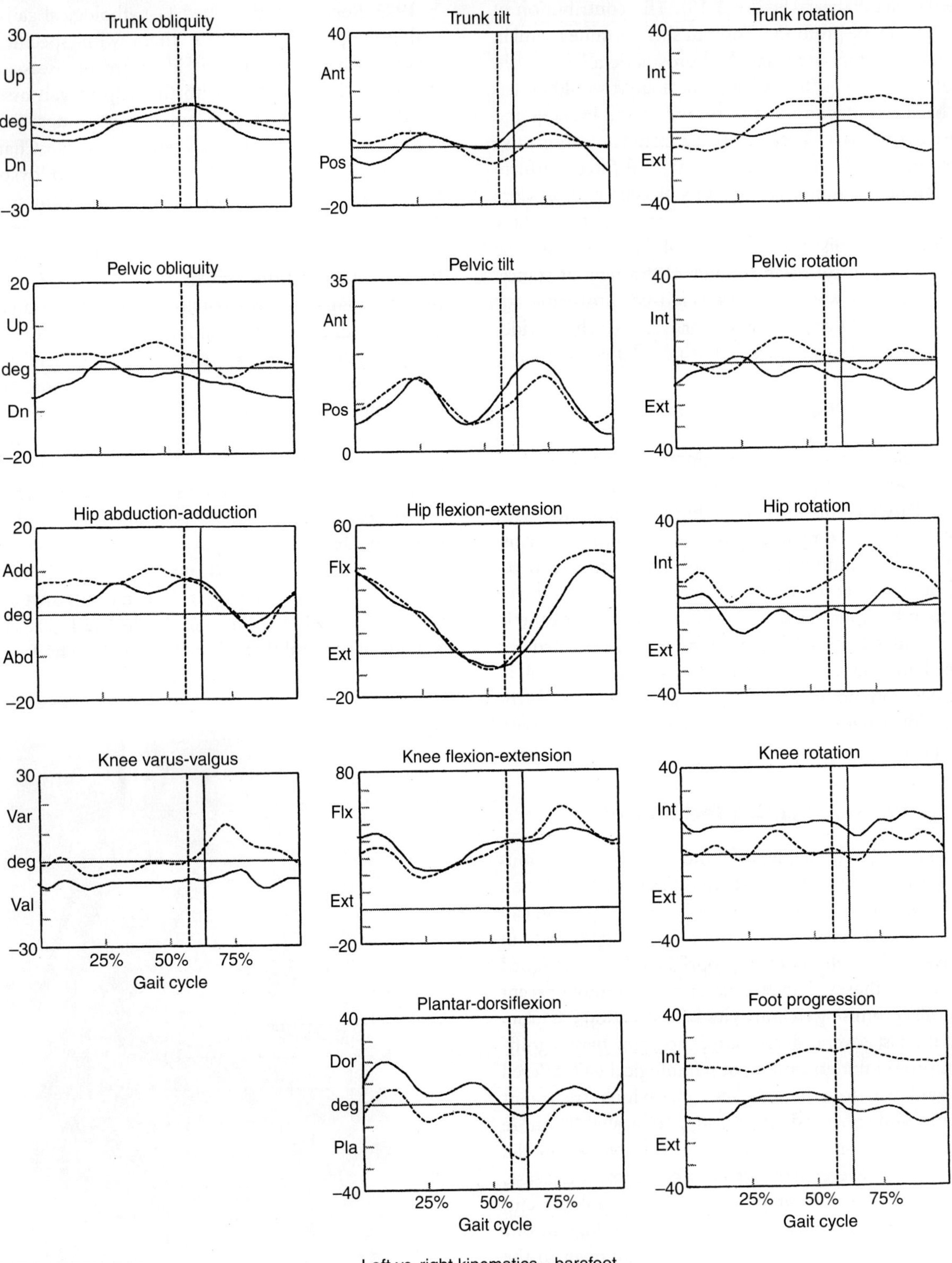

Figure 3-9

The output generated by a computer-based motion analysis system includes graphs of the mean range of motion at each body segment or joint (trunk, pelvis, hip, knee, and ankle) in coronal (left column), sagittal (middle column), and transverse (right column) planes as the individual being evaluated progresses through multiple gait cycles. This is the output of an 8-year-old child with spastic diplegic cerebral palsy. (Courtesy the Center for Motion Analysis, Connecticut Children's Medical Center, Hartford, Conn.)

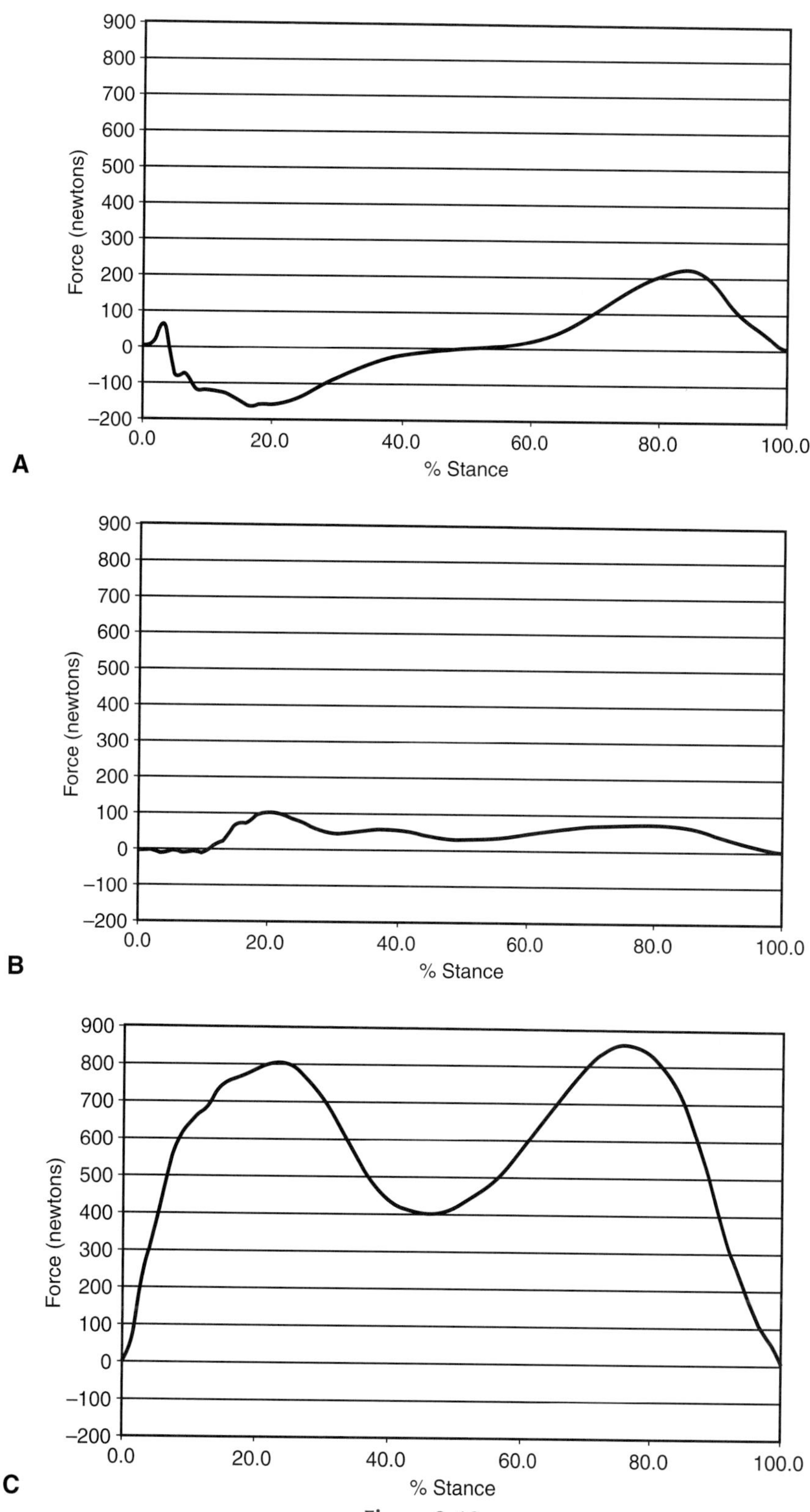

Figure 3-10

Example of output generated by a forceplate as the individual being tested progresses through stance phase. ***A,*** *The anterior-posterior component of the ground reaction force (GRF);* ***B,*** *the medial lateral component of the GRF; and* ***C,*** *the vertical component of the GRF. (Output courtesy the Motion Analysis Laboratory, Department of Physical Therapy and Human Movement Science, Sacred Heart University, Fairfield, Conn.)*

Medical Center Physical Therapy Department developed an organized format for systematically applied observational gait analysis. Their work initially focused on the development of an in-house training program for students and personnel who were new to the rehabilitation hospital. The first Normal and Pathological Gait Syllabus was published by the Professional Staff Association of Rancho Los Amigos Hospital in 1977.[7] Subsequent revisions have included additional basic gait data and gait interpretation.[27] This syllabus uses parameters of normal gait as a comparative standard for abnormal or pathological gait. It focuses on identifying gait deviations that affect the three functional tasks of walking: weight acceptance, single limb support, and swing limb advancement. A form listing the most commonly occurring gait deviations in each subphase of gait is used to record any observed gait deviations that interfere with these functional tasks (Figure 3-11). Problems in each of the six major body segments are noted with a check in one of the boxes, beginning with the toes, then the ankle, knee, hip, pelvis, and trunk. This format allows the clinician to consider systematically the following questions:

Are the toes up, inadequately extended, or clawed?

- Is there forefoot-only contact (toe walking), foot-flat contact, foot slap, excess plantar flexion, or dorsiflexion? Is heel off, foot drag, or contralateral vaulting present?
- Is knee flexion adequate, absent, limited, or excessive? Is extension inadequate? Does the knee wobble, hyperextend, or produce an extension thrust (recurvatum)? Is varum or valgum present, or is excessive contralateral flexion seen?
- Is hip flexion adequate, absent, limited, or excessive? Is adequate extension seen? Is retraction of the thigh during TSw from a previously attained degree of flexion seen? Can internal or external rotation, abduction, or adduction be observed?
- Does the pelvis hike? Does it tilt anteriorly or posteriorly? Is forward or backward rotation seen? Does it drop to the ipsilateral or contralateral side?
- Does the trunk lean or rotate backward or forward? Does it lean laterally to the right or left?

Qualitative gait assessment is an important component of preorthotic assessment because it assists the clinician in identifying the functional task and the subphase of gait that are problematic and can be addressed with orthotic intervention. Similarly, findings of observational gait analysis can identify the need for adjustment of prosthetic alignment.

FUNCTION-BASED ASSESSMENT

Holden and colleagues[28] suggest that gait performance goals for patients with neurological impairments are best measured against values from impaired rather than healthy subjects. Treatment goals are adjusted for the individual patient's diagnosis, etiologic factor, ambulation aid, and functional category. In separate studies, Brandstater and colleagues[29] and Holden and colleagues[28] found that patients with the greatest number of gait deviations did not have the lowest temporal gait values. A great deal of energy is often expended by physical therapists, prosthetists, and orthotists in an attempt to achieve gait patterns of "optimal quality." Holden and colleagues[28] suggest that hard-won qualitative gait improvements may bring with them secondary losses in time-distance parameters, such as slower velocity and reduced step length. The fundamental issue is whether temporal gait efficiency or cosmesis should be the preferred goal. Certainly, in cases in which patients are nominal walkers and in which therapy, surgery, and orthotics or prosthetics have been maximized, general gait efficiency is far more important than reduction in compensatory gait deficits.

In the past, symmetry and reciprocity have been significant treatment goals. Wall and Ashburn[30] maintain that "an ideal objective in the functional rehabilitation of hemiplegia is the reduction of the asymmetrical nature of movement patterns." Measuring pathological gait against normal gait values is a useful means of providing an overall clinical picture. In setting treatment goals, however, measuring a patient's performance against that patient's own best possible outcome is more reasonable. How can a given patient's best possible outcome be anticipated? This requires collection of accurate data to establish pretreatment and posttreatment profiles for a wide variety of involvement levels within each pathological condition. Olney and Richards[31] suggest that large groups of instrumented studies be undertaken to identify clusters of biomechanical features associated with functional performance during walking.

Time-distance parameters have enormous potential for setting outcome goals. Variations in time-distance values are often specific to pathological condition. Asymmetries in hemiplegia, for example, are obviously greater than in most other types of pathological conditions. Variables that are reported to affect temporal measurements in normal healthy subjects include age, sex, height, orthotic use, or type of assistive device. In separate studies of patients with pathological conditions, Brandstater and colleagues[29] and Holden and colleagues[28] found no significant difference in temporal performance based on sex or age.

Corcoran and colleagues[32] measured temporal parameters of subjects with hemiplegia under two gait conditions: with and without their ankle-foot orthosis (AFO). Patients with hemiplegia had significantly faster gait velocity when wearing their orthoses than when walking without them.[32] A similar study of healthy unimpaired subjects wearing AFOs found reduced step length. Apparently subjects without central nervous system pathosis altered their movement strategy to decrease movements at the knee in an effort to minimize shearing forces in the AFO.[33] Reduced step length can minimize force exerted by the brace along the posterior aspect of the calf band.[34]

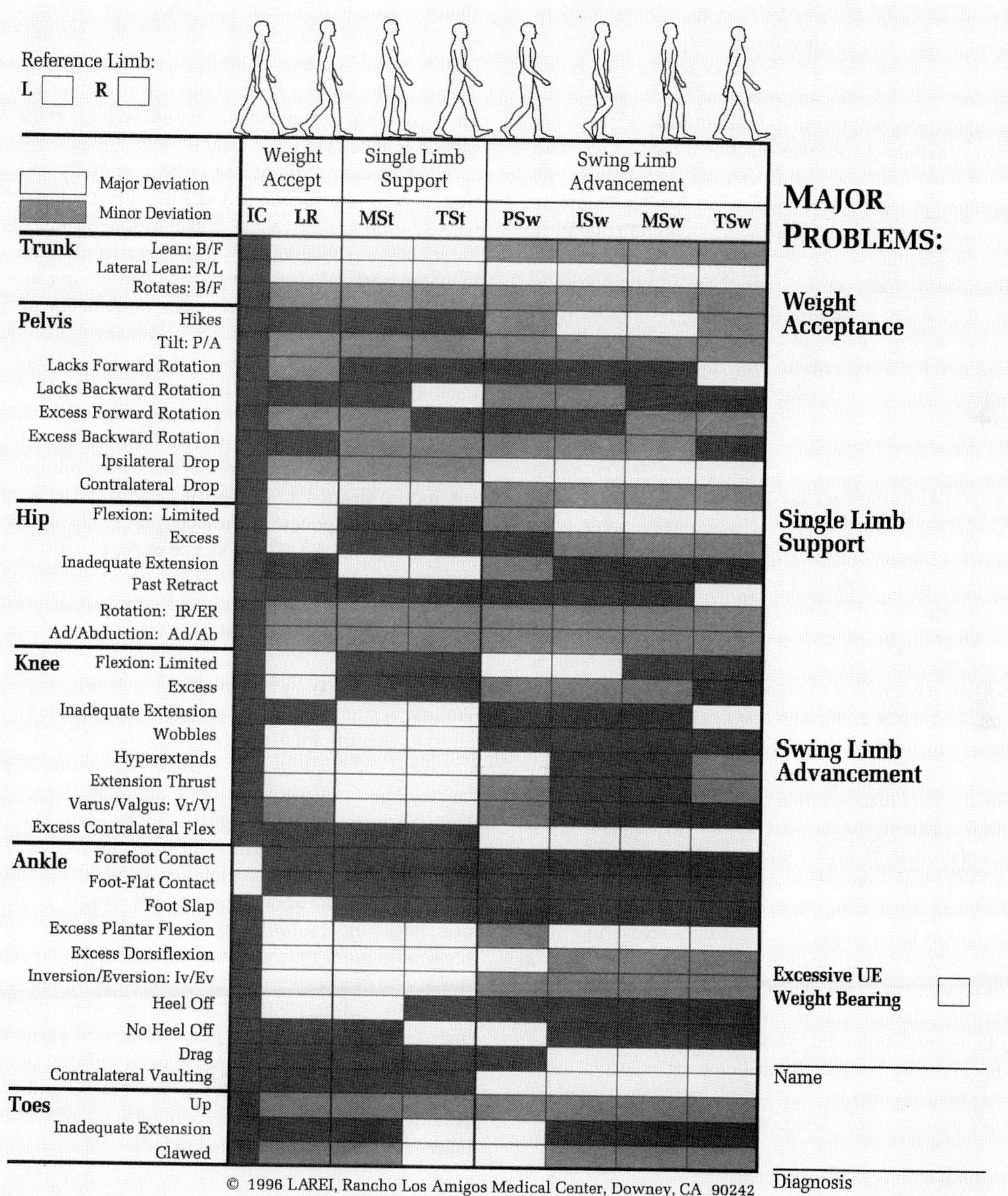

GAIT ANALYSIS: FULL BODY

RANCHO LOS AMIGOS MEDICAL CENTER
PHYSICAL THERAPY DEPARTMENT

Reference Limb:
L ☐ R ☐

☐ Major Deviation
▒ Minor Deviation

		Weight Accept		Single Limb Support		Swing Limb Advancement			
		IC	LR	MSt	TSt	PSw	ISw	MSw	TSw
Trunk	Lean: B/F								
	Lateral Lean: R/L								
	Rotates: B/F								
Pelvis	Hikes								
	Tilt: P/A								
	Lacks Forward Rotation								
	Lacks Backward Rotation								
	Excess Forward Rotation								
	Excess Backward Rotation								
	Ipsilateral Drop								
	Contralateral Drop								
Hip	Flexion: Limited								
	Excess								
	Inadequate Extension								
	Past Retract								
	Rotation: IR/ER								
	Ad/Abduction: Ad/Ab								
Knee	Flexion: Limited								
	Excess								
	Inadequate Extension								
	Wobbles								
	Hyperextends								
	Extension Thrust								
	Varus/Valgus: Vr/Vl								
	Excess Contralateral Flex								
Ankle	Forefoot Contact								
	Foot-Flat Contact								
	Foot Slap								
	Excess Plantar Flexion								
	Excess Dorsiflexion								
	Inversion/Eversion: Iv/Ev								
	Heel Off								
	No Heel Off								
	Drag								
	Contralateral Vaulting								
Toes	Up								
	Inadequate Extension								
	Clawed								

MAJOR PROBLEMS:

Weight Acceptance

Single Limb Support

Swing Limb Advancement

Excessive UE Weight Bearing ☐

Name

Diagnosis

Figure 3-11

The Rancho gait analysis system seeks to identify and record any observable activity that interferes with the three functional tasks of walking: weight acceptance, single limb support, and swing limb advancement. (From Los Amigos Research and Education Institute, Rancho Los Amigos Medical Center. Observational Gait Analysis Handbook. Downey, CA: Los Amigos Research and Education Institute, Rancho Los Amigos Medical Center, 1989. p. 55.)

Functional Measures

A variety of functional measures have been developed, each intended to provide information about change in status of ambulatory ability for individuals with neuromuscular, musculoskeletal, cardiorespiratory, or metabolic diseases. Most of these measures are designed to be completed in clinical settings without specialized equipment or instrumentation. Examples of such measures are the Functional Ambulation Classification System (FAC), the Functional Independence Measure (FIM) locomotion and mobility subscales , the Gait Abnormality Rating Scale (GARS), and the Timed Up and Go Test (TUG). These measures are intended to provide information about how gait impairments affect function in an individual's environment, rather than about specific gait problems or deviations. The extent to which functional measures have been psychometrically evaluated to assess reliability and validity of the measure within and across testers and patient groups with different diagnoses varies. Most require some degree of practice or training so that testers develop accuracy in using the tool. Few have been used to assess efficacy of orthotic or prosthetic intervention specifically.

Functional Ambulation Classification

Holden and colleagues[28] suggest that grouping subjects by motor ability or functional category is more important than grouping by other indicators of gait. They have developed the Massachusetts General Hospital (MGH) FAC.[35] Six functional categories are defined in their system. A score of 1 indicates nonfunctional ambulation. Patients who require the assistance of another for support and balance are scored with a 2. A score of 3 indicates that light touch assistance is required, and 4 means that the patient needs verbal cueing or occasional safety assistance. To be scored as a 5, the patient must be independent in ambulation on level surfaces, and a score of 6 means the patient is independent in ambulation on all surfaces, including stairs and inclines.

The FAC has been used most extensively in the assessment of functional locomotion and efficacy or outcomes of rehabilitation intervention for individuals recovering from stroke.[36-38] In a Rausch analysis of discriminant validity of measures used to assess outcome of stroke rehabilitation intervention, however, FIM motor scores and gait speed were better discriminators of outcome than FAC scores.[39] The FAC has also been used to help assess concurrent reliability of new mobility measures in stroke rehabilitation and portable instrumented pressure-sensitive monitors.[40,41]

Functional Independence Measure

Initially developed to assess burden of care for staff caring for patients in acute care settings,[42] the FIM is a multidimensional scale that assesses locomotion as one dimension of overall functional status. In the last decade, it has come into wide use as a tool to assess outcomes of rehabilitation interventions for patients with musculoskeletal conditions such as hip fracture and total joint replacement and for those with neuromuscular conditions such as spinal cord injury, myelopathy from spinal stenosis, and stroke.[43-49] The WeeFIM is a version of the FIM intended for use with children with cerebral palsy and other developmental disabilities, acquired brain injury, and other neuromuscular and musculoskeletal impairments.[50-53] The reliability and validity of the FIM have also been assessed in home care and assisted living settings for frail and disabled older adults.[54,55] There is both a performance-based and interview-based version of the FIM.[56,57]

The FIM has two domains of function: motor and cognitive.[56] The motor subscale has four dimensions: *self-care* (eating, grooming, bathing, dressing upper body, dressing lower body, and toileting), *sphincter control* (bladder and bowel management), *ability to transfer* (bed-chair-wheelchair, toilet, tub or shower), and *locomotion* (ambulation or wheelchair use, stair management). The cognitive subscale includes *communication* (comprehension and expression) and *social cognition* (social interaction, problem solving, and memory). Possible scores for each component of the subscales range from 1 (total assistance required) to 7 (completely independent without any assistive device). Each component has specifically defined criteria. The scoring criteria for the ambulation component of the locomotion subscale are summarized in Table 3-1. The evidence of the measure's validity is strongest when a composite FIM score or motor/cognitive subscale scores are used, although component scores are sometimes used in documentation and record keeping.[55]

Gait Abnormality Rating Scale

Wolfson and colleagues[58] developed the original GARS in an effort to quantify abnormal gait performance of frail institutionalized older adults and identify those most at risk of falling. The scale has since been modified (GARS-M) by VanSwearingen and colleagues[59] for use in community settings.

In the GARS-M, a videotape of a patient walking on a level surface is scored on 7 dimensions: variability, guardedness, staggering, foot contact, hip range of motion, shoulder range of motion, and synchrony of arm movement and heel strike. The measure uses a four-point criterion-based rating scale (0 to 3). Total GARS-M scores range from 0 to 21, with high scores indicating less efficient or safe performance. Evidence of interrater and intrarater reliability, as well as concurrent validity (compared with temporal and distance parameters of gait) and discriminate validity (between fallers and nonfallers) has been reported.[59,60]

Timed Up and Go

In the original "get up and go" test and the TUG test, patients are asked to rise from a seated position in a standard height chair, walk 3 meters on a level surface, turn, walk back to the chair, and return to a seated position, moving as quickly as

Table 3-1
Scoring Criteria for the Locomotion Component of the FIM

Score	*Score Criteria*
7	Able to walk at least 150 feet (50 m) *completely independently*, without any type of assistive device or wheelchair, safely and within in a reasonable (functional) period of time
6	Able to walk at least 150 feet (50 m) *independently, but requires an assistive device* (orthosis, prosthesis, wheelchair, special shoes, cane, crutches, walker), or takes more than reasonable time, or has safety concerns
5	Requires *standby supervision*, cuing, or coaxing to walk or propel wheelchair at least 150 feet (50 m)
4	Requires *minimum contact assistance* (patient contributes 75% effort) to walk or propel wheelchair at least 150 feet (50 m)
3	Requires *moderate assistance* (patient contributes 50% to 74% effort) to walk or propel wheelchair a minimum of 150 feet (50 m)
2	Requires *maximal assistance* of one person (patient contributes 25% to 49% effort) to walk or propel wheelchair 50 feet (17 m)
1	Requires *total assistance* (patient contributes less than 25% effort) or requires assistance of more than one helper, or is unable to walk or propel wheelchair at least 50 feet (17 m)

they are safely able. Although the original get up and go test used a somewhat subjective 0 to 5 rating to score each component of the task,[61] performance is now based on total time to complete the task.[62] In both versions, individuals being evaluated are instructed to move as quickly as they are safely able to move. Importantly, the TUG is a measure of overall functional mobility, assessing the ability to transfer, walk, and change direction.

Normative data for TUG in healthy community-living adults 65 years and older have been reported; less information is available for TUG performance in children and younger adults. Although TUG times increase with age, most community-living older women between 65 and 85 years are able to complete the TUG task in fewer than 12 seconds.[63-65] Although TUG times increase when healthy elders are testing without and then with an assistive device, the impact on TUG times of assistive device use by those who typically use these devices has not been investigated.[66,67] Higher TUG times are associated with functional impairment in individuals with arthritis, amputation, hip fracture, and Parkinson's disease.[68-74]

CHOOSING AN ASSESSMENT STRATEGY

Recognizing similarities and differences in purpose and design of the various gait assessment methods is important. Gait-based methods, such as the Rancho Los Amigos observational gait assessment, seek to identify and differentiate pathological versus compensatory mechanisms and therefore guide the specific surgical, therapeutic, orthotic, or prosthetic interventions for a particular patient. Functional indexes, such as the MGH FAC, the FIM, or the TUG, may be a means of evaluating treatment efficacy, disease-related decline, or improvement over time. The cost of gait assessment through comprehensive instrumented procedures often precludes its general use in the clinical arena. Observational analysis through gait-based assessment will remain a viable and important contribution to clinical care for many years to come.

CASE EXAMPLE 1

A Patient with Flaccid Paralysis of Pretibial Muscles

J. J. is a 37-year-old man with inherited sensorimotor neuropathy (Charcot-Marie-Tooth disease) who has been referred to the gait assessment clinic for evaluation of his orthotic intervention. Examination of muscle function and strength reveals relatively symmetric distal impairment. Manual muscle test scores include "trace" activity of dorsiflexion muscles bilaterally, "poor" plantar flexion on the left, and "fair+" plantar flexion on the right. Knee and hip strength is "normal."

Questions to Consider

- Given J. J.'s pattern of weakness, what types of primary difficulties or deviations might you predict during the functional task of weight acceptance (IC and LR)? Of single limb support (MSt and TSt)? Of swing limb advancement (PSw, ISw, MSw, and TSw)?
- Given J. J.'s pattern of weakness, what compensatory strategies (pathological gait deviations) might he use to accomplish these functional tasks of gait?
- What quantitative measures, indicators of energy cost, qualitative measures, or function-based assessments would you use to determine if a change in orthoses would be warranted? Why would you select those measures?

Examination and Evaluation

For foot-switch stride analysis, J. J. walks without his usual orthoses. In the trailing left limb, the posterior compartment fails to support the forefoot lever arm so that the tibia progresses forward with limited heel off in late stance (Figure 3-12). This creates excessive knee flexion and limits the step length of the contralateral limb. The net effect of this inadequate forefoot rocker is a reduction in velocity. Lack of support of the trailing forefoot allows depression of the center of gravity. At the same time, dorsiflexion weakness on the right creates early, abrupt plantar flexion (foot slap) with premature contact of the first metatarsal. The variance between plantar flexor strength of the left and right limbs is demonstrated by difference in single-limb support times. The stronger right calf participates in 39.8% (0.416 seconds) of the gait cycle, whereas the weaker left calf commits itself to only 31.4% (0.328 seconds). This subtle timing discrepancy in gait was not readily identifiable in observational analysis.

In right MSw, while the left foot is in a supporting posture, the classical steppage gait characteristics of a flail forefoot are observed: Compensatory swing clearance is accomplished through excessive hip and knee flexion (see Figure 3-12, *B*).

When J. J. wears his orthoses (a dorsiflexion assist thermoplastic AFO on the right and a dorsiflexion stop–plantar flexion resist thermoplastic AFO on the left), results of foot-switch temporal analysis are quite different. Velocity, cadence, and stride length increase slightly. The asymmetry between right and left single limb support times decreases because the AFO provides external support of the trailing left limb. The energy-inefficient steppage gait and unsightly foot slap are diminished as well.

Questions to Consider

- What specific problems do the examination and evaluation identify in each of the functional tasks of gait: weight acceptance (IC and LR), single limb support (MSt and TSt), and swing limb advancement (PSw, ISw, MSw, and TSw)?
- In what ways do J. J.'s orthoses address the functional problems observed when he walks without his orthoses in each of the functional tasks of the gait cycle: weight acceptance (IC and LR), single limb support (MSt and TSt), and swing limb advancement (PSw, ISw, MSw, and TSw)? In what ways do his orthoses potentially limit each of the functional tasks of gait? Do the benefits outweigh the limitations?

Clinical Characteristics of Gait in Hemiplegia

For most patients who are recovering from stroke (cerebrovascular accident [CVA]), improvement in the quality of gait is related to the natural history of the pathological process and the impact of gait retraining in rehabilitation. In the week immediately after CVA, only 24% to 38% of patients are able to ambulate independently.[75] After weeks of rehabilitation, more than 50% are able to walk without assistance, especially if using an appropriate AFO and assistive device.[76] At the 6-month mark, more than 80% of patients with CVA are functionally independent in ambulation.[77]

The many variations of limb control observed during the gait of patients who are recovering from a CVA can be explained by one or more of the following factors: primitive locomotor patterns, impaired postural responses, abnormal postural tone with various degrees of spasticity and rigidity, inappropriately timed muscle contractions, and diminished muscle strength. One of the primary determinants of gait dysfunction in post-CVA hemiplegia is whether the patient has some degree of selective control of specific muscles rather than activation of abnormal synergy patterns (mass flexion or extension). Patients with hemiplegia often have difficulty grading the magnitude of a particular muscle contraction with respect to other muscle contractions. Because of hyperactivity of muscle spindle/stretch reflex in the presence of spasticity, the ability to move toward dorsiflexion with forward progression of the tibia during stance may be counteracted by contraction of plantar flexors into a position of equinus. Spasticity, although difficult to measure, can be described for clinical purposes with the Ashworth Spasticity Scale.[78] The baseline level 0 indicates no measurable tone. A designation of level 1, mild tone, is given when a muscle "catches" with an abrupt passive movement into flexion or extension. A level 2 designation indicates marked abnormal tone but flexible range of motion, and level 3 is characterized by pronounced tone and difficult passive movement. Level 4 denotes a limb that is held rigidly in either flexion or extension.

The orthotic goal for patients with hypertonicity of the lower extremity after a CVA is to control ankle motion and preposition for tibial advancement. Two orthotic strategies are commonly used: (1) provision of an AFO with a locked ankle component set in slight dorsiflexion or (2) use of an articulated AFO that allows slight ankle motion around the neutral position. When ankle joint motion is limited or blocked by an orthosis, stability in stance improves; however, forward progression of the tibia is compromised, and step length is reduced. Modifications to the shoe, such as application of a rocker bottom sole or elevation of the heel, can compensate by mimicking the second rocker of gait.

Over the course of rehabilitation, the patient with hemiplegia often experiences changes in tone, joint flexibility, pain or discomfort, fear or confidence, motor strength or weakness, and quality of proprioception. Six stages of motor recovery in hemiplegia have been identified by Brunnstrom.[79] In the first stage, no voluntary movement of limbs is present. In the second, movement reappears but is limited by pronounced muscle weakness or spasticity, or both. The patient is usually not yet ready for functional ambulation. In the third stage, spasticity coexists with limb synergy motion.

Typically a mass extensor pattern is seen in the lower limb. As the patient continues to improve in the fourth stage, spasticity may be reduced as the patient begins to move out of stereotypical synergy patterns. In stage 5, selective control outside mass synergy patterns becomes more consistent and more functional. With recovery complete, in stage 6 the patient may achieve coordinated controlled movement. Because of the dynamic nature of the recovery process, the ability to adjust or alter orthotic alignment or characteristics is very desirable. It is not unusual that an orthosis prescribed early in rehabilitation becomes inappropriate or creates further gait dysfunction at a later stage. Once rehabilitation is complete and the patient has achieved stability in walking patterns, definitive biomechanical needs are identified and the adjustability of the orthosis is less important.

The extension synergy pattern places the lower extremity in excessive extension at the hip and knee and the foot in equinovarus. This reduces the amount of knee flexion and dorsiflexion during swing, necessitating a compensatory strategy, such as circumduction, to provide swing phase clearance.[80] The rigidity of the ankle leaves the patient with inadequate dorsiflexion mobility as well as vastly reduced plantar flexion excursion during PSw and early swing. Stance time is considerably reduced on the hemiplegic/paretic side, and the quadriceps, gastrocnemius, gluteus maximus, and semitendinous muscles are inappropriately active throughout stance.[81] The activity of most lower limb muscle groups on the hemiplegic/paretic side is increased compared with normal patterns of muscle activation. Excessive hip flexion at MSt on the hemiplegic/paretic side shifts the GRF line anteriorly, producing a knee extension moment that interferes with forward progression. The hemiplegic/paretic side also displays less hip adduction in single limb support, which compromises lateral shift toward the affected side.[82]

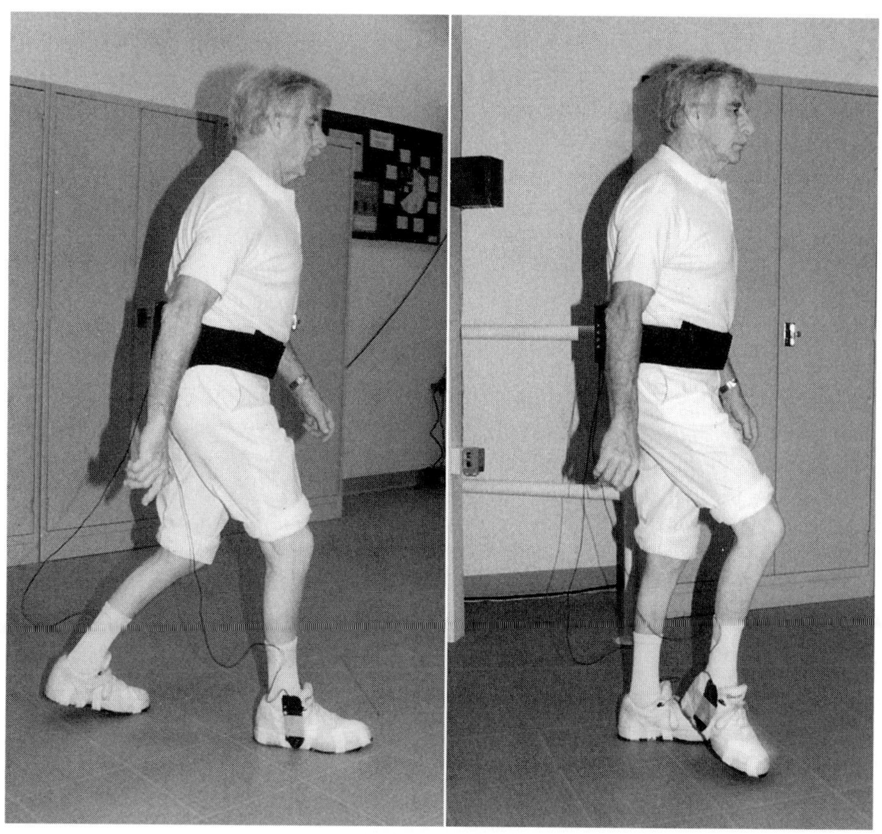

Figure 3-12

*This individual with Charcot-Marie-Tooth disease demonstrates shortened right stride length because of inadequate support at the foot and ankle in late stance of the left limb (**A**) and the use a compensatory steppage gait to ensure swing clearance in the presence of dorsiflexion weakness (**B**).*

Brandstater and colleagues[29] describe reduced velocity, cadence, stride length, and single limb support time on the affected side, with consequent increased single limb support and reduced step length on the sound side. Hirschberg and Nathanson[81] demonstrated that an appropriate AFO improves the quality of gait by increasing step length and stance time as well as reducing swing time of the affected side. Velocity of gait improves when the AFO is placed in slight dorsiflexion. When spasticity is not problematic, an AFO that permits some plantar flexion normalizes IC to LR timing and prevents an unstable knee flexion moment in early stance. Because knee extensor strength often equals or exceeds hip extensor strength after CVA, most patients with hemiplegia can be effectively managed with an AFO rather than a knee-ankle-foot orthosis.[82] Muscle strengthening is less important in achieving improved walking characteristics in hemiplegia than is the retraining of normal movement patterns in gait.[83]

CASE EXAMPLE 2

A Patient with Hemiplegia

M. G. is a 67-year-old man referred to the gait laboratory for evaluation 13 months after a CVA damaged the sensorimotor cortex of the left hemisphere. Currently he is a community ambulator (MGH functional ambulation classification level 6) who walks with the aid of an AFO and quad cane (FIM locomotion score 6). In the clinical examination, his spasticity becomes apparent when his ankle moves toward a neutral position (Ashworth spasticity scale level 3). The orthosis he received early in rehabilitation, and continues to use, is a traditional double upright, which locks his ankle in slight plantar flexion. Although this ankle angle delays tibial advancement and forward progression in stance, the patient has come to rely on its contribution to stability at proximal joints.

Questions to Consider

- Given M. G.'s pattern of spasticity and weakness, what types of primary difficulties or deviations might you predict, when he is not wearing his orthosis, during the functional task of weight acceptance (IC and LR)? Of single limb support (MSt and TSt)? Of swing limb advancement (PSw, ISw, MSw, and TSw)?
- Given M. G.'s pattern of spasticity and weakness, what compensatory strategies (pathological gait deviations) might he use to accomplish these functional tasks of gait?
- What additional quantitative measures, indicators of energy cost, qualitative measures, or function-based assessments would you use to determine if a change in orthosis would be warranted? Why would you select those measures?

Examination and Evaluation

M. G.'s gait with the AFO is evaluated by foot-switch testing. Extensor synergy patterns contribute to function by providing a degree of stability in stance but also reduce efficiency of gait by limiting normal stance progression beginning with the first rocker period (Figure 3-13). Duration heel-only time of the first rocker (IC to the foot-flat position at the end of LR) is approximately one sixth of a second on the hemiplegic side, significantly less than normal heel-only time. Heel-only time on the intact side is roughly three times greater than that on the hemiplegic side. Forward progression during MSt is halted at the second rocker when spasticity prevents the necessary dorsiflexion of the ankle (see Figure 3-13). As M. G. moves into TSt, when metatarsophalangeal break (concurrent with heel off) should allow progression onto the forefoot, the third rocker is also relatively blocked. This lack of mobility of the metatarsophalangeal joints and inadequate third rocker result in a loss of knee flexion, necessary for an effective PSw, for which the patient is unable to compensate. Of the 60 degrees of knee flexion necessary for the swing phase clearance, 35 degrees should be achieved passively during PSw. For patients with hemiplegia, the loss of this positional flexion is an additional challenge to clearance, beyond that produced by the equinus position of the ankle. Any attempts to compensate by "hip hiking" are likely to be inefficient and unsuccessful. These rocker limitations reduce step length of the sound side, leading to premature double limb support. The corresponding MSw knee flexion on the hemiplegic side is also reduced. M. G. demonstrates a much reduced stance time on the affected side (62% gait cycle) versus the sound side (71% gait cycle) and a reduced single limb support time on the affected side (28% gait cycle) versus the sound side (38% gait cycle).

Questions to Consider

- What specific problems has the examination and evaluation identified in each of the functional tasks of gait: weight acceptance (IC and LR), single limb support (MSt and TSt), and swing limb advancement (PSw, ISw, MSw, and TSw)? How do these problems relate to his abnormal tone and motor control?
- In what ways does M. G.'s orthosis address or constrain each of the functional tasks of the gait cycle: weight acceptance (IC and LR), single limb support (MSt and TSt), and swing limb advancement (PSw, ISw, MSw, and TSw)?

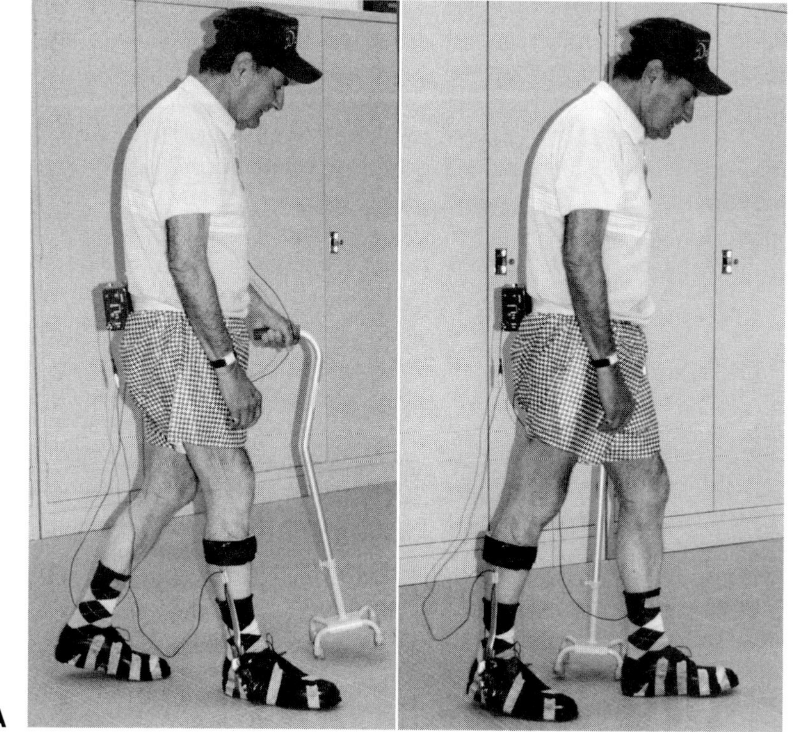

Figure 3-13

*In this patient with hemiplegia after CVA, the first rocker from IC to foot flat (**A**) is abrupt as a result of extensor patterns and limb rigidity. Extensor pattern at the ankle (**B**) translates into a failure to yield into dorsiflexion toward the end of the second rocker. Third rocker heel elevation will also be reduced, and lack of mobility reduces the step length of the contralateral limb.*

Clinical Characteristics of Gait in Spastic Diplegic Cerebral Palsy

Children with spastic diplegic cerebral palsy often have significant spasticity and marked weakness of the antigravity muscles in both lower extremities. This combination is a precursor of joint contracture. The clinical term often used to describe the typical gait of a patient with diplegia is *crouch gait*. In crouched gait marked internal rotation of the femur and tibia occurs throughout the gait cycle, the knees remain in flexion throughout stance, and the ankles remain in plantar flexion during stance (toe walking) and swing. Gage[84] clearly documented the high energy cost of flexed knee gait. The pathological combination of an equinus ankle, positive Trendelenburg's hip, and stiff knee gait often produces various combinations of compensatory hiking of the pelvis, external rotation of the foot, and circumduction of the swing limb. This pattern has been attributed to tightness and overactivity of the distal hamstrings, alone or in combination with the hip flexors.[85]

Some patients with diplegia ambulate with a *jump gait* pattern, using somewhat less hip and knee flexion than do patients with crouch gait but with prolonged ankle dorsiflexion rather than plantar flexion. Jump gait is often a postoperative manifestation of bilateral Achilles tendon lengthening without concurrent release of hip and knee contractures. Common compensatory strategies in jump gait include vaulting and circumduction. In crouch and jump gait, the GRF line falls progressively behind the knee joint center during single limb support of the stance phase. This creates an excessive demand on the quadriceps for stance phase stability. One surgical strategy used to correct jump gait combines hip flexion releases, hip flexion release lengthening of the distal hamstrings, and correction of external rotation. Postoperatively, the patient is fitted for floor reaction AFOs.[86] Ideally, the Achilles tendon is lengthened to neutral dorsiflexion position and the patient protected in AFOs for 1 year postoperatively.

The *scissoring* pattern, which is also a common gait deviation in children with diplegia, is aggravated by spastic hip flexors and adductors because the widened base of support reduces the efficiency of their line of pull. Orthotic solutions provide limited assistance in limb tracking and rotational control. Those that attempt to control rotation must cross the hip joint, adding significant weight and bulk and increasing difficulty in donning and doffing.

CASE EXAMPLE 3

A Patient with Spastic Diplegic Cerebral Palsy

K. E. is a 10-year-old boy with spastic diplegic cerebral palsy who has been referred to the gait laboratory for evaluation to assist his orthopedist in deciding whether corrective surgery is indicated. The boy currently ambulates independently, without assistive devices, wearing bilateral solid ankle AFOs (WeeFIM locomotion score of 6).

Questions to Consider

- Given K. E.'s pattern of spasticity and weakness, what types of primary difficulties or deviations might you predict when he is not wearing his orthoses during the functional task of weight acceptance (IC and LR)? Of single limb support (MSt and TSt)? Of swing limb advancement (PSw, ISw, MSw, and TSw)?
- Given K. E.'s pattern of spasticity and weakness, what compensatory strategies (pathological gait deviations) might he use to accomplish these functional tasks of gait?
- What additional quantitative measures, indicators of energy cost, qualitative measures, or function-based assessments might help determine if surgical orthopedic intervention is warranted? Why would you select those measures?

Examination and Evaluation

K. E. is fitted with reflective markers for three-dimensional motion analysis of this gait. A typical crouch gait pattern is observed during observational gait analysis while his gait is being recorded for more detailed kinematic and kinetic analysis by computer software. Footswitch analysis confirms diminished heel contact with no heel-only time on the left and no heel contact at all on the right.

Clinical examination of K. E.'s lower extremity function reveals a combination of overactive hamstrings and weak gastrocnemius and soleus (Figure 3-14). The flexion of hips and knees increases the need for proximal stabilization, resulting in compensatory hyperextension of the trunk and posterior arm placement (see Figure 3-14, *B*). Because the ankles are held in equinus, the final rocker propels tibial advancement despite limitation in ankle mobility. K. E. spends most of the stance phase in TSt and PSw; consequently, double limb support time is vastly increased.

K. E. has not had previous surgical release of his gastrocnemius muscles. Even with surgery, impairment of motor control may continue to be problematic, so that dorsiflexion may not work in concert with the knee flexion to provide a heel-toe gait pattern. Gastrocnemius release without concurrent release of the hip and knee contractures usually leads to short step lengths with a compensatory increase in cadence. Spastic hip flexors, also serving as adductors, create a mild scissors effect during each swing limb advancement. Ambulation with bilateral AFOs, which the patient prefers, increases step length and reduces knee flexion compared with ambulation with no orthosis.

Questions to Consider

- What specific problems does the examination and evaluation identify in each of the functional tasks of gait: weight acceptance (IC and LR), single limb support (MSt and TSt), and swing limb advancement (PSw, ISw, MSw, and TSw)? How do these problems related to K. E.'s abnormal tone and motor control?
- In what ways do K. E.'s orthoses address or constrain each of the functional tasks of the gait cycle: weight acceptance (IC and LR), single limb support (MSt and TSt), and swing limb advancement (PSw, ISw, MSw, and TSw)? What is the interaction of his abnormal tone and impaired motor control with his orthoses on the efficacy and energy cost of his walking?

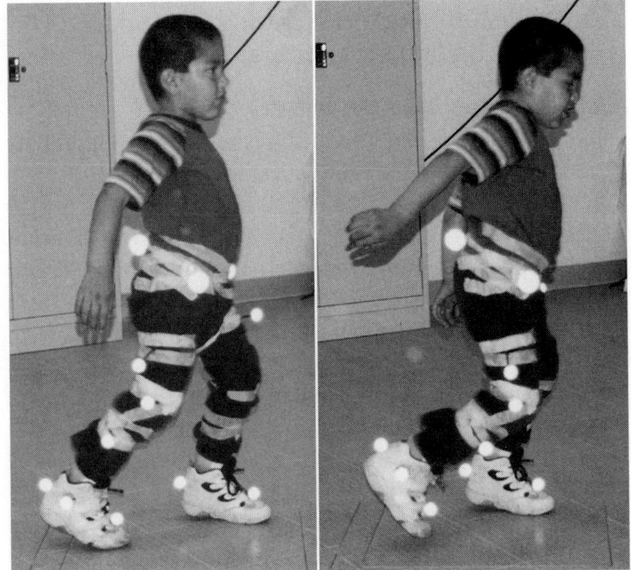

Figure 3-14

*In children with spastic diplegia, classic crouch gait (**A**) is characterized by increased hip and knee flexion in combination with toe walking. Postural substitutions in crouch gait (**B**) may include increased lumbar lordosis, trunk extension, and posterior arm placement.*

Clinical Characteristics of Gait in Children with Spina Bifida

Spina bifida (myelomeningocele) occurs when vertebral arches fail to unite very early in gestation. Clinically, this leads to partial or complete paralysis at or below the level involved. The most common impairment is a flaccid paralysis, with loss of proprioception and exteroception (pain, temperature sensation, light touch, and pressure sensation). Many children with spina bifida have significant ambulatory deficiencies; more than 50% require an orthosis of some kind to ambulate.[87] Assessment for orthotic support begins as soon as the child attempts to gain an erect posture.

Severity of gait dysfunction depends on the level of involvement of the spinal cord. When the L-5 and S-1 nerve roots are affected, the gluteus maximus, hip abductors, and triceps surae are lost; the hamstrings are present but weak; and sensory loss is limited to the plantar surface of the feet. The plantar flexor deficit requires setting limits to dorsiflexion range of motion through orthotic joint control. This limitation of dorsiflexion allows the patient to establish hip stability through hip extension accomplished with exaggerated trunk lordosis. Without it, the patient would fall forward unopposed. Lateral stability is achieved through crutches and a wide walking base.

When the L-3 and L-4 root nerves are affected, hamstring function, hip extension, knee flexion, plantar flexion, and dorsiflexion are completely lost. The resulting foot drop cannot be adequately compensated for in swing by knee flexion. Hip flexion, adduction, and knee extension are intact but may be weak. At the L-3 level weak knee flexion from the gracilis may also be present. These children benefit early from standing frames; later, they often are able to ambulate with orthotic assistance (see Chapter 11 for more information about standing frames and other hip-knee-ankle-foot orthoses for children with myelomeningocele). Adequate stabilization of the foot and ankle is achieved through orthotic application of a locked ankle in neutral or slight dorsiflexion. Trunk lordosis is a compensatory strategy used to stabilize the hip during stance. The muscular imbalance at the hip increases the likelihood of flexion contracture, which in turn amplifies the need for even more compensatory lordosis. Extreme hip flexion contracture may ultimately preclude ambulation. If contractures at the hip, knee, and ankle are minimal and the child gains trunk control, he or she will be able to stand erect but will rely on trunk alignment for static balance and forearm crutches for further stability.

A child with lesions that involve L-1 and L-2 levels has little lower limb function other than weak hip flexors. Such children often begin upright function with a parapodium or swivel walker and can later progress to reciprocal gait orthoses (see Chapter 11). The swing-through gait with bilateral hip-knee-ankle-foot orthosis has been shown to be less efficient than a reciprocal gait orthosis for thoracic level spina bifida.[88]

CASE EXAMPLE 4

A Child with Spina Bifida

N. P. is an active 9-year-old boy with myelomeningocele at L-5 who returns to the gait laboratory as part of an ongoing research study to document changes in gait characteristics over time. He currently ambulates wearing bilateral AFOs set in a neutral ankle position, using Loftstrand crutches in a four-point reciprocal gait pattern.

Questions to Consider

- Given N. P.'s pattern of weakness and sensory loss, what types of primary difficulties or deviations might you predict when he is not wearing his orthoses, during the functional task of weight acceptance (IC and LR)? Of single limb support (MSt and TSt)? Of swing limb advancement (PSw, ISw, MSw, and TSw)?
- Given N. P.'s pattern of weakness and sensory loss, what compensatory strategies (pathological gait deviations) might he use to accomplish these functional tasks of gait?
- What additional quantitative measures, indicators of energy cost, qualitative measures, or function-based assessments might help determine if surgical orthopedic intervention is warranted? Why would you select those measures?

Examination and Evaluation

Comparative foot-switch testing reveals that, without crutches, stride length and velocity are reduced. External rotation of both limbs is present throughout the gait cycle (Figure 3-15). With or without crutches, N. P. has no measurable fifth metatarsal or toe contact on either limb in his typical stance phase weight-bearing patterns. Passive external rotation is present at the hip as well as abducted limb placement as he advances over the forefoot. His abducted limb placement and wide-based gait provide increased stability at a cost of excessive loading on the posteromedial aspect of the feet (see Figure 3-15, *B*). Like many children with spina bifida, he spends excessive time in heel contact, largely to the exclusion of lateral forefoot weight bearing. This loading and shear pattern often leads to callusing and eventual neuropathic breakdown in adult life. His fastest gait velocity (55 m/min) is approximately 60% of normal free-gait velocity. During swing phase, external rotation of the limb is marked. The flail foot is held in slight dorsiflexion during TSw through the support of the AFO.

Questions to Consider

- What specific problems does the examination and evaluation identify in each of the functional tasks of gait: weight acceptance (IC and LR), single limb support (MSt and TSt), and swing limb advancement (PSw, ISw, MSw, and TSw)? How do these problems related to N. P.'s flaccid paralysis and sensory impairment?
- In what ways do N. P.'s orthoses address or constrain each of the functional tasks of the gait cycle: weight acceptance (IC and LR), single limb support (MSt and TSt), and swing limb advancement (PSw, ISw, MSw, and TSw)? What is the interaction of his flaccidity and sensory with his orthoses on the efficacy and energy cost of his walking?

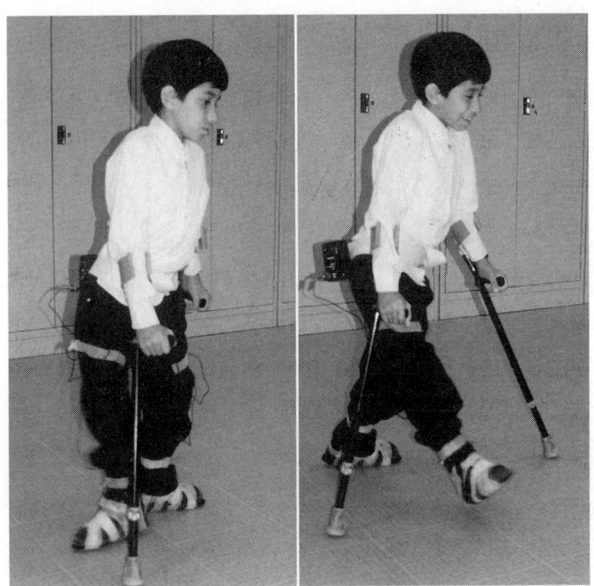

Figure 3-15
*In this child with myelomeningocele, weakness at the hip results in external rotation of the limbs in both stance and swing phase (**A**), which contributes to altered forward progression from the heel to the medial forefoot, with minimal weight bearing on the lateral foot (**B**).*

GAIT PATTERNS IN INDIVIDUALS WITH AMPUTATION

Qualitative observational gait analysis is a broadly accepted approach to achieving a clinically optimal gait in individuals with amputation. Instrumented gait analysis provides a more repeatable accurate assessment of prosthetic function. In its broadest scope, the data derived increasingly serve as foundation guidelines for both prosthetic design and clinical application. The daily practice of assessment and management of prosthetic gait, however, depends on the subjective skills of the prosthetist and the targeted treatment protocol of the therapist.

The University of California at Berkeley prosthetic project, which began in the mid 1950s, represented the most concentrated period of prosthetic advancement. The comprehensive basic gait studies and their application to the biomechanics of amputee gait for transtibial and transfemoral amputations established fundamental design criteria.[89] Contributions of subsequent investigators continue to be largely based on the Berkeley criteria.

Extensive calculations and interpretations were required to relate normal and prosthetic gait data to the problems of prosthetic design. Data reduction was a slow process before relatively recent technological advancements because all motion measurements had to be performed by hand. There were no automated film analyzers to identify the motion patterns and no computers to perform rapid data processing. Therefore, the number of subjects studied was limited. The project also had the additional depth of considering all three planes of motion, in contrast to prior studies that analyzed only the sagittal plane of gait progression.[5,90] Subsequent investigators, with the aid of more advanced instrumentation, have replicated and expanded the Eberhart-Inman work but have not found it in error.

Transtibial Prosthetic Gait

In 1957 the Berkeley project was specifically commissioned to reconsider transtibial prosthetic gait and biomechanics; with that goal, an advisory conference was held.[91] The basic transtibial prosthesis at that time was attached to the limb with a thigh lacer that included articulated knee joints and a foot with an articulated ankle. Detailed review of the normal and transtibial amputee-gait data resulted in a totally new approach that led to two developments: the patellar tendon-bearing (PTB) prosthesis and the solid-ankle, cushion heel foot.[92-94] The improved transtibial socket was a PTB design that closely followed the contours of the proximal tibia.[95] The PTB prosthesis replaced the thigh lacer with supracondylar fixation, again with the advantage of anatomical contour and total contact.

Prosthetic Feet during Stance

Compressible heel prosthetic feet have a solid plastic keel embedded in the proximal portion of a stiff foam foot that allows a slight degree of forefoot flexibility while the cushion heel lessens the impact of initial floor contact and through vertical compression simulates articulated ankle plantar flexion. Material compressibility replaced the mechanical joint of the single-axis foot. Foot contour, alignment, and elasticity facilitated progression onto the forefoot. This design followed careful analysis of the essential degrees of mobility. The compressible heel foot has become the standard terminal device for most individuals with amputation, though hybrids incorporating both low- and high-performance feet with multidirectional articulated ankles hold a significant place in clinical use as well (see Chapter 24 for detailed information about prosthetic feet.)

Transtibial Alignment

The positional relation between the socket and prosthetic foot is critical to achieve optimal progression in stance, yet also highly subjective (see Chapter 26 for additional information on transtibial prosthetic alignment and gait assessment). The goal is to encourage tibial progression in stance and place the knee in a stable (minimally flexed) weight-bearing posture without causing hyperextension in late stance and to have the lower limb follow a normal path of motion in swing.

Static, or "bench," alignment uses the subcutaneous crest of tibia (tibial blade) to establish alignment of the residual limb within the prosthesis. In the sagittal plane this landmark, at its origin at the tibial tubercle, is typically angled approximately 5 degrees forward of the perpendicular to the tibial plateau that serves as the supporting surface for the knee joint. Hence, if the socket is aligned by the tibial blade, the socket is set so that the tibia is tilted slightly forward to avoid a backward thrust during stance. This angular posture of the prosthetic socket, in conjunction with a deliberate anterior displacement (translation) of the socket relative to the foot, generally succeeds in encouraging tibial progression.

Even with this alignment, the individual with dysvascular transtibial amputation who typically exhibits some degree of weakness will shift the weight line anterior to the knee by simply leaning forward during LR in a postural movement akin to a quad avoidance gait. This results in reduced knee flexion throughout stance phase and delayed flexion in swing (Figure 3-16). A hesitation of stance progression (the MSt dead spot) is a common phenomenon. A delay in the rollover pattern, common to the dysvascular transtibial amputee, is reflected in the shear pattern (see Figure 3-16, *B*)

Final positioning of the socket-foot relation is determined by observational analysis of the subject's gait and feedback from the individual with amputation. This process, referred to as dynamic alignment, examines smoothness of the rollover pattern and medial-lateral verticality of the foot, avoiding both extremes of inversion or eversion during progression. The absence of abnormal motions in swing such as a whip, compensatory motions to avoid scuffing the foot in swing (such as degree of pelvic elevation or vaulting), and an erect trunk posture are additional observational criteria used for assessment. Comfort and ease of walking are criteria of the individual with amputation. A one-subject study of repeated realignment by an experienced prosthetist over a 2-year period documented inconsistencies in the alignment accepted as being good, a decision confirmed each time by three other prosthetists.[96,97] A range of alignment variation satisfactory to both the prosthetist and amputee was defined.

In optimizing the alignment in the coronal plane, there is an attempt to mimic the slight varus moment seen at the knee during MSt of normal human locomotion. This moment is usually achieved by a slight medial inset of the prosthetic foot relative to the socket, taking advantage of the good weight-bearing areas in the proximal-medial and lateral-distal regions of the residual limb. Pressure in these areas is well tolerated. Inadequate inset of the foot, or worse, outset of the foot, will generally result in excessive pressure on the very superficial cut end of the tibia (medial-distal) and the perineal nerve and bony prominence of the head of the fibula (lateral-proximal). Although observational analysis is appropriate for general clinical care, the alignment of individuals with amputation with complex fitting problems is best resolved through objective confirmation with forceplate and motion data.

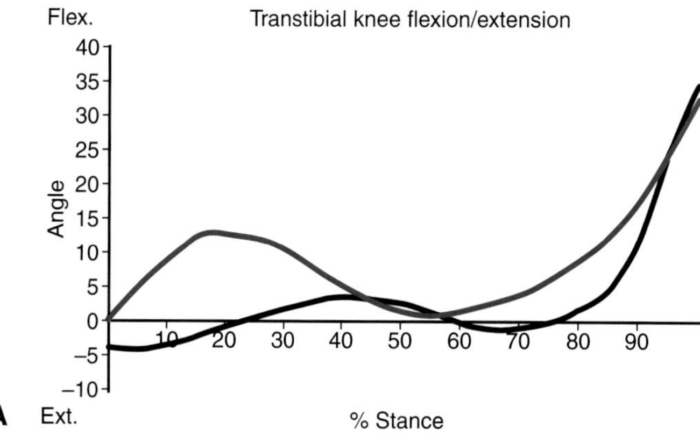

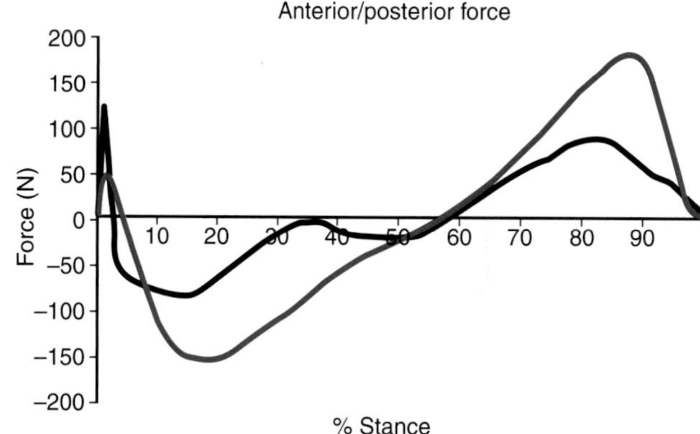

Figure 3-16

A, Individuals with dysvascular transtibial amputation typically shift the weight line anterior to the knee early in stance, which results in reduced knee flexion throughout stance phase and delayed flexion in swing. B, Typical midstance hesitation in the progression of rollover is reflected in the shear pattern. Black line indicates affected; maroon line indicates sound. (Courtesy VA Long Beach Gait Laboratory.)

Studies of Transtibial Prosthetic Gait

Most instrumented studies of individuals with transtibial amputation have focused on foot design, with the general exclusion of alignment. Prosthetic foot designers attempt to passively reproduce, by material quality, the normal dynamic functional balance between mobility and stability provided by the anatomical foot. The greatest difference is between the relatively rigid compressible heel–type feet and the mobile hinge of the single-axis foot.[98] Motion analysis has shown that the articulated ankle improves weight acceptance stability by providing significant plantar flexion, allowing an earlier foot flat posture[99]; however, the arc of knee flexion and the timing and intensity of the quadriceps do not differ from that of the compressible heel–type foot.[100] Stance phase limb progression is enhance by an articulating ankle in two ways. In footswitch analysis, the mobile ankle had a longer period of single limb stance time, whereas total stance time was shorter compared with solid-ankle designs.[101] In addition, there was more prolonged hamstring action with the compressible heel foot; this implies that a forward lean was used to improve progression over the less yielding foot. These functional advantages of a mobile prosthetic foot would be significant in a marginal walker, but the heaviness of a single-axis foot creates an energy-cost penalty that also must be considered.

Beginning in the 1980s, the use of elastic materials and designs has been increasingly applied to prosthetic feet. The initial objective was to facilitate running because the presence of normal knee control gives the transtibial individuals with amputation considerable functional potential.[101] All the foot designs emphasize controlled dorsiflexion mobility for greater push-off. It has been assumed that these dynamic, elastic prosthetic feet would be advantageous for the average walker by reducing the greater-than-normal energy cost currently experienced by individuals with amputation.[102] The most mobile designs, in terms of dorsiflexion range, are those with a long-bladed shaft such as the Flexfoot and Springlite. These bladed shaft designs have not lessened the muscular demands of weight acceptance. Their simulated "ankle plantar flexion" during limb loading is no better than the solid-ankle, cushion-heel foot. Both result in a plantar flexion that is markedly less than the normal controlled, yet rapid, ankle plantar flexion of 12 degrees used to reduce the propulsive effect of the heel rocker by allowing early forefoot contact. Both prosthetic feet cause a significant delay in attaining the stability of foot flat.[103]

The intact limb uses a modest arc (15 to 20 degrees) of knee flexion to absorb the shock of floor contact.[6] Prosthetic feet rely on a cushion heel. The time needed for adequate cushion compression delays the drop of the forefoot to the floor. This perpetuates an unsteady, heel-only source of support that requires increased active muscular control of the knee and hip to ensure weight-bearing stability. This subtle source of instability is obscured by two findings. Displacement of the customary heel marker gives a false reading of plantar flexion.[104] Heel cushion compression delays the rate of initial tibial advancement, resulting in reduced weight acceptance knee flexion for the transtibial amputee compared with normal. This difference is reflected in calculations of subnormal moments and powers.[105,106] These findings have been interpreted as a sign of reduced muscle demand, and a corresponding conservation of energy has been attributed to the dynamic elastic-response feet. Direct EMG recordings, however, show significantly higher than normal muscle demand for five different feet tested.[107]

Transfemoral Prosthetic Gait

Initial research of transfemoral amputation by the Berkeley researchers emphasized the function of unilateral amputation because the problems of this group appeared more critical at that time.[90]

Motion analysis showed a fully extended knee starting in TSw and continuing through stance. The inadequate ankle plantar flexion that followed heel strike and threatened knee stability was attributed to dependence on an ankle bumper in place of the lost pretibial muscle control. Active ipsilateral thigh control and postural adaptation by the sound limb and trunk were identified as the variable mechanisms used by the individual with transfemoral amputation to ensure knee extension stability. Rotation of the fully extended limb rolling over the ankle before heel rise causes a maximum rise of the hip (and thus center of gravity), which was interpreted as vaulting. Compensatory actions by the sound limb were identified.

In swing, the inability of the prosthetic foot to generate a propelling force to initiate limb advancement was interpreted as a need to restrict the weight of the prosthesis so that the work of hip flexors would not be excessive. The individual with transfemoral amputation also demonstrated rapid hip extension in TSw to use tibial inertia as a means of completing knee extension in preparation for stance. These findings of excessive knee extension in stance and excessive hip action in swing formed the basis for others to design more sophisticated knee joints to replace the then-dominant single-axis constant friction joint.

The biomechanical response to the problem of residual limb discomfort was twofold. Torque absorbers were designed, but the solution was the combination of improved socket design in addition to more normal joint mechanics. The loss of knee control creates compensatory kinematic and kinetic changes that result in asymmetries reflected in a variety of gait parameters. As the individual wearing a transfemoral prosthesis with a compressible heel-type foot levers over the heel rocker during LR, the knee may be at an increased risk of destabilization. When challenged by the potential for knee instability, the prosthetic wearer will attempt to preposition the hip before LR with a change in body mechanics to shift the GRF to a more anterior position. These typical compensatory patterns can be measured directly through EMG, kinematics, or kinetics or inferred by measuring heel-only load-bearing time through a temporal analysis.

Temporal Values

There are several temporal values for which individuals with transfemoral amputation differ compared with those without amputation. A retrospective footswitch gait study conducted at the National VA Prosthetics Gait Lab, Long Beach, California, measured the self-selected velocity in 10 individuals with traumatic transfemoral amputation and compared it with the self-selected velocity of individuals without amputation. The individuals with amputation demonstrated a mean stride length of 1.16 meters compared with an average of 1.59 meters for individuals without amputation.[108] The overall timing of the transfemoral prosthetic gait cycle was slower for the individuals with amputation, requiring a mean of 1.25 seconds from IC to subsequent IC compared with 1.08 seconds for individuals without amputation. The mean velocity of the individuals with amputation was 55.8 m/min versus 88.3 m/min for individuals without amputation. James et al[109] found that a longer, slower gait cycle on the prosthetic side combined with a reduced step length on the sound side resulted in a velocity that was only 38% of nonamputee velocity. Stride length was significantly less for those with transfemoral amputation, who averaged 1.16 meters per stride compared with 1.59 meters per stride for those without amputation. As profound as these differences are, they are probably still subtle enough to remain unremarkable in a typical clinical environment. Murray[110] measured transfemoral gait with a younger group of individuals with amputation and found similar but slightly more subtle differences between individuals with amputation and those without amputation.

Initial Contact and Loading Response

The initiation of heel contact at the beginning of stance phase in transfemoral gait has been reported to be characteristically delayed on the prosthetic side, which typically demonstrates a slower swing phase.[110] Contemporary hydraulic knee units, particularly those that provide a programmable chip that can establish optimal swing phase timing characteristics, have the potential to overcome this limitation. However, probably because of cost, they do not represent typical prosthetic use (see Chapter 28 for more information on prosthetic knee units and alignment issues). Early gait studies of single-axis prosthetic feet showed that as the prosthetic limb made contact with the ground and began to load, an exaggerated knee extension was seen in the prosthetic limb that continued throughout early stance.[110] Obviously this phenomena depends somewhat on knee design. There is little evidence that polycentric knees, such as four- and six-bar linkage knee units, and others that have been designed to be stable with a few degrees of built-in flexion compliance during stance, provide normal kinematics of the knee in stance. Most individuals with transfemoral amputation who use the polycentric designs walk with a nearly extended knee.

The total vertical forces occurring on the prosthetic side are less during the initial double limb support period than on the contralateral side during the terminal double limb support period. It has been theorized that this loading restraint requires costly compensations of the sound limb.[111] Knee instability, which produces these costly compensations, generally results from inappropriate positioning of the knee joint relative to the socket and prosthetic foot. The individual with transfemoral amputation relies on hip extensor strength and the reduced lever arm of the transected femur to stabilize the prosthetic knee by restraining the limb during LR. Profound hip extensor weakness can be catastrophic and preclude functional ambulation. Anterior translation of the prosthetic socket relative to the knee and foot has the effect of shifting the GRF anterior to the knee joint axis, thereby increasing stability. Socket flexion affects knee stability as well. Because efficient use of the gluteus maximus as a hip extensor requires the muscle group to be on stretch, the prosthetist deliberately places the socket in a position of flexion. Five degrees of socket flexion are generally considered clinically optimal in a patient with no contracture at the hip. In cases of hip contracture, the amount of flexion is limited by the length of the femoral remnant.[89]

Stability of the knee joint is unquestionably the most important factor in considering a knee unit. Uncontrolled knee flexion renders an otherwise perfect prosthesis useless. Thiele and colleagues[112] investigated possible neurophysiological reasons for weakness in individuals with transfemoral amputation by recording EMG activity of the quadriceps during gait. His team did not find abnormal recordings and concluded that muscle weakness is caused by biomechanical, rather than neurophysiological, factors. This supports the long-held clinical view that apart from the patient's general muscle tone, residual limb length is a crucial factor because of its effect as a lever arm against the socket wall and as a result of intact or ablated insertions of the hamstring tendons and their obvious detrimental effect on extensor strength. A slight degree of socket flexion is also a factor affecting stability because socket flexion slightly elongates hip extensors, rendering them more effective. The relative positions of the prosthetic foot, knee, and socket to this line significantly affect stability of the knee when the patient walks. When the ground reaction line passes posterior to the knee center, the knee will collapse unless resisted by another force, usually the hip extensors forcing the femur against the socket wall.

Another potential destabilizing factor is limitation of free plantar flexion at heel contact, which may tend to produce a knee flexion moment in early stance. This is why an articulated prosthetic foot (as opposed to a prosthetic foot, which attains a plantar grade position by means of heel compression) provides increased stability for those with transfemoral amputation. A general clinical guideline on a patient who demonstrates nominal knee stability is that the prosthetic foot should reach foot-flat position (mimicking plantar flexion during LR) as quickly as possible, short of demonstrating an uncosmetic foot slap. As soon as the foot plantarflexes fully during stance phase, the ground reaction line moves anteriorly from the point of foot-floor contact at the heel to approximately midfoot, enhancing stability at the knee. Because of this, a single or multiaxis foot with a soft plantar flexion bumper is preferred for those with a short transfemoral residual limb, who have limited muscular control for knee stability. At times, the single-axis function can be combined with that of dynamic response, such as with the College Park foot.

Midstance

As the individual using a transfemoral prosthesis moves into MSt, sound side hip elevation and trunk lean toward the affected side provide balance, limit the force on the lateral aspect of the residual limb, and reduce the demands of the residual limb abductors. The transition from braking to propulsive shear on the ipsilateral limb is characteristically delayed and unsteady (Figure 3-17).

When both limbs are intact, the momentum of the contralateral swing limb results in a reduced vertical force at MSt of the stance limb. This is not so, however, for those with dysvascular transfemoral amputation, in which the reduced upward velocity and momentum of the contralateral swing limb does not have the vigor necessary to decrease vertical force of the prosthetic limb during MSt (see Figure 3-17, *B*). Even in those with traumatic amputation, maximum knee flexion of the sound side during swing phase reaches only 51 degrees, approximately 10 degrees less than normal gait.[113]

Stance phase knee flexion of the affected side is significantly reduced throughout stance (see Figure 3-17, *C*). During PSw, delayed and reduced knee flexion, and consequent reduced heel rise on the ipsilateral limb, are characteristic of the transfemoral amputee. Except in the case of those fitted with microprocessor stance control knees, it can be anticipated that many individuals with transfemoral amputation will progress through MSt with a nearly extended knee. Microprocessor-controlled hydraulic knees, particularly the Otto Bock version, have shown a trend toward improvements in stance knee flexion as well as increased velocity in stair descent.[114,115] This is an important development because it may provide increased energy efficiency in gait and avoid compensatory mechanisms such as prepositioning of the femur before LR and MSt.

Terminal Stance

TSt on the prosthetic limb is noted for its premature cessation. The prosthetic side generally shows a decrease in single-limb support time, whereas the sound side shows a concurrent increase in single-limb support time.[113] There is a persistence of knee extension on the prosthetic limb during contralateral sound side deceleration.[116] Delayed and reduced knee flexion, and consequent reduced heel rise on

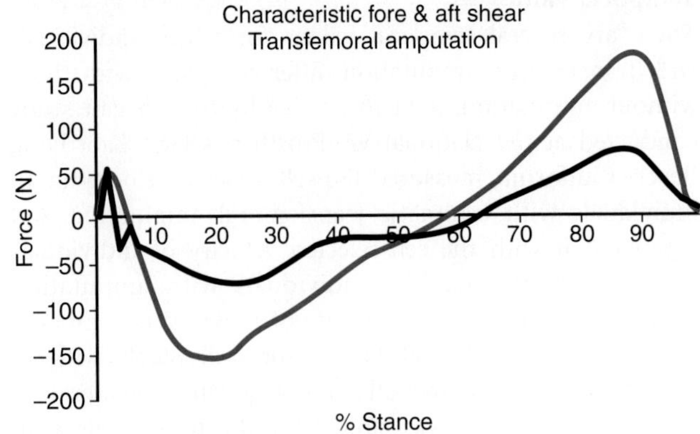

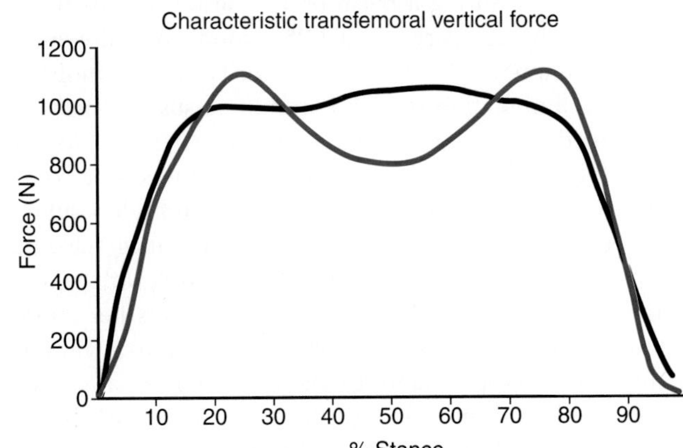

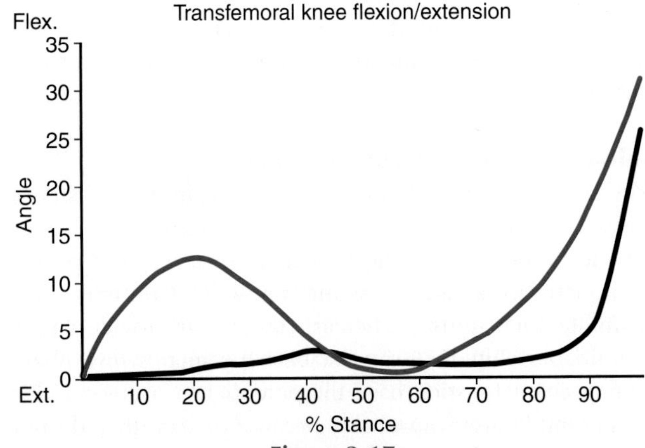

Figure 3-17

A, *The transition from braking to propulsive shear on the ipsilateral limb during transfemoral prosthetic gait is characteristically delayed and unsteady.* ***B,*** *Although there is a reduction in vertical force at midstance of the sound limb as the prosthetic limb advances in swing, the prosthetic transfemoral limb demonstrates reduced upward velocity because the momentum of the contralateral swing limb lacks the vigor to lessen the vertical force of the affected stance limb during midstance.* ***C,*** *Knee flexion of the transfemoral prosthetic limb is reduced throughout stance. During preswing, delayed and reduced knee flexion and consequent reduced heel rise on the ipsilateral limb is characteristic. Black line indicates affected; maroon line indicates sound. (Courtesy VA Long Beach Gait Laboratory.)*

the ipsilateral limb, are characteristic of transfemoral prosthetic gait (see Figure 3-17, *C*). A failure to limit dorsiflexion in a single-axis foot at this juncture will have a destabilizing effect on the prosthetic knee joint during TSt. Without an appropriately placed dorsiflexion stop, nothing will dampen the forward progression of the tibia and the tibial section may continue its anterior progression to the point of knee collapse.

Preswing

During PSw in transfemoral gait, the vertical force of the sound side is abnormally high and greater than that of the prosthetic side.[111] An abrupt reversal from hip extension to hip flexion occurs because some hip extension is required for knee stability until the moment when the prosthetic knee has to flex to initiate swing. In normal gait, half the knee flexion required for swing phase is obtained passively during PSw.

During prosthetic PSw, inadequate forefoot support can lead to costly compensations in the double limb support period.[111] PSw is characterized by a rapid transfer of body weight to the contralateral limb. In normal gait this transfer begins at 50% of the gait cycle and continues until the end of stance phase (approximately 62% of the gait cycle).

Individuals with transfemoral amputation often have a shortened sound side step length. This may be aggravated by insufficient socket flexion because the individual with transfemoral amputation uses any and all available lumbar lordosis to advance the sound limb. Failure to place the socket in flexion limits the availability of lumbar lordosis and prohibits a sound side step length that is at least somewhat close to normal. Even in an optimal prosthetic gait, typical sound side step length is reduced compared with the prosthetic side or the normal side.

Swing Phase

Gait characteristics during swing phase when wearing a transfemoral prosthesis can be profoundly influenced by prosthetic alignment and design variations. The most challenging factor in achieving a functional swing phase is the lack of active dorsiflexion in most prosthetic designs. The Stewart-Vicars knee developed in 1947 and the more recent Hydracadence knee couple knee flexion with ankle dorsiflexion. However, this design concept has been largely ignored in recent years. With the prosthetic incorporation of active dorsiflexion in early swing, many costly postural substitutions, including vaulting and abducted or circumducted gait, could be minimized.

The swing velocity of the prosthetic limb is often slower than that of the sound limb.[109] Obviously the presence or lack of fluid control mechanisms, variations in alignment stability, extension assist, and joint friction alignment mechanisms can all influence swing phase timing. During MSw, the individual with transfemoral amputation demonstrates exaggerated hip elevation of the prosthetic side to enable swing clearance. In TSw, prosthetic swing time is much greater than sound limb swing time or normal swing time.[116] Excessive prosthetic swing flexion is one of the commonly reported transfemoral prosthetic gait deviations.[116] Zuniga,[113] however, reports that prosthetic knee flexion reaches a mean of only 45 degrees. This contradiction in results can easily be attributed to the wide variety of prosthetic dampening and extension assist designs as well as other variations in prosthetic adjustment.

James and colleagues[109] and Murray[116] performed gait laboratory investigations of transfemoral stride parameters and their relation to knee flexion-extension angles at various cadences. They confirmed stance and swing phase asymmetry between the prosthetic and sound side, regardless of the speed of walking. Zuniga[113] used electrogoniometers attached to the knee and foot to document asymmetry during stance and swing phases, comparing prosthetic and sound limbs. A lack of symmetrical cadence response on the prosthetic side is seen as partially responsible. Most prosthetic designs permit only one walking speed. No matter how fast the patient walks, the prosthetic wearer must wait for the leg to return from the normal 65 degrees of swing phase flexion to full extension before safely loading the prosthesis for weight bearing in stance.

Common Gait Deviations in Transfemoral Prosthetic Gait

Our understanding of transfemoral prosthetic gait deviations and the dynamic alignment process has evolved over many decades. The important early work of Inman,[5] described previously, served as a basis for subsequent development. In 1951, New York University published a method for observing amputee gait and described eight commonly seen gait deviations.[117] Several years later, Hangar and associates[23] at Northwestern University, under a grant from the Veterans Administration, developed an educational film that incorporated the eight deviations defined by NYU and expanded upon these. A brief description of each of these transfemoral gait deviations is found in Table 3-2. Addition information on recognizing and addressing gait deviations in transfemoral gait can be found in Chapter 28.

SUMMARY

The examples of gait deficiencies typical of neuromuscular conditions and in prosthetic gait that we have considered demonstrate the complexity and variety that challenge orthotists, prosthetists, and physical therapists working with individuals with gait problems. Each patient presents unique combinations of pathological and compensatory deficits, which require a combination of the essential tools of simple quantitative measure (cadence and velocity, step length, stride length and width, and double support time), systematic qualitative gait analysis (Rancho Los Amigos

Table 3-2
Common Deviations in Transfemoral Prosthetic Gait

Deviation	*Description*
Foot slap	Rapid, uncosmetic plantar flexion movement at heel contact. Most commonly caused by insufficient plantar flexion resistance.
Knee instability	Uncontrollable knee flexion at LR. May be caused by anteriorly placed knee unit, excessive durometer of cushion heel or plantar flexion bumper, or weakness of hip extensors.
Delayed progression	Hesitation or delay in rollover of prosthetic forefoot between MSt and TSt. May be the result of a long toe lever, a plantarflexed prosthetic foot, or shoes with low heel.
Unequal step length	Sound side step length is visibly shorter than the prosthetic step length. May be caused by inadequate preflexion of socket, hip flexion contracture. Associated with excessive lumbar lordosis and low back pain.
External rotation	Foot externally rotates at heel contact. May be caused by excessively firm heel cushion or a tight prosthetic socket (especially on a residual limb with extra soft tissue).
Lateral trunk bend	Significant leaning of the body over the hip during prosthetic MSt. Often caused by excessively outset prosthetic foot, distal lateral femoral discomfort, short prosthesis, excessively abducted socket, or gluteus medius weakness.
Abducted gait	Wide walking base throughout the gait cycle, often caused by pressure or discomfort on medial pubic ramus, small socket, or excessively long prosthesis.
Pelvic elevation	"Hip hiking" on prosthetic side from ISw to MSw, associated with increased energy cost of gait. Often caused by long prosthesis or inadequate knee flexion as swing begins.
Knee hyperextension	Seen at MSt to compensate for perceived knee instability. Often caused by short forefoot lever or dorsiflexed prosthetic foot.
Lateral whip	The heel of the prosthetic foot moves in a lateral arc as swing begins, often caused by excessive internal rotation of the knee bolt.
Medial whip	The heel of the prosthetic foot moves in a medial arch as swing begins, often from excessive external rotation of the knee bolt or improper donning of prosthesis.
Excessive heel rise	Prosthetic foot rises abnormally upward during ISw, typically a result of inadequate resistance to knee flexion.
Inadequate heel rise	Heel off is diminished in ISw, usually because of excessive knee flexion resistance.
Circumduction	A wide lateral arch of the prosthetic limb during swing phase. Often the result of inadequate knee flexion, excessive medial brim pressure, or long prosthesis.
Pistoning	A sense that residual limb slips slightly out of the socket in swing and descends into the socket in stance. Often the result of inadequate fit or suspension.
Vaulting	Rising up on the sound forefoot during MSt in an effort to enhance prosthetic swing limb clearance. May result from a long prosthesis, excessive knee friction, or fear of letting the knee flex.
TSw impact	An audible click at the end of TSw as knee unit fully extends with insufficient resistance or by forceful knee extension by the prosthetic wearer.
Reduced velocity	An adaptation typically observed during initial training or with new components, often related to pain, fear, or insecurity.

observational gait assessment protocol), measures of energy cost (PCI), level of assistance (the FAC or FIM), and functional measures (the TUG or GAR-M). These tools help the clinician to differentiate primary pathological conditions from secondary compensations, guide orthotic prescription and therapeutic intervention, and assess efficacy of treatment. Instrumented gait assessment is an important part of preoperative assessment and research in orthotic and prosthetic design. In addition, the data collected in gait laboratories are building a database that can provide information necessary to build accurate outcome estimations for many groups of patients. The current challenge is for the clinic team to gain the broadest possible knowledge base in analytical gait assessment and to serve the patient as a team, considering each patient as an individual.

ACKNOWLEDGMENTS

The authors are grateful to Sue Rouleau, PT, and the Physical Therapy Department of Rancho Los Amigos Medical Center for assistance in identifying patient models and to Jacquelin Perry, MD, and Los Amigos Research and Education Institute for permission to duplicate the Rancho full-body gait analysis form.

REFERENCES

1. Shastri JL (ed). *Hymns of the Rig Veda.* Griffith RTH (trans). Varanasi, India: Motilal Banarsidas, 1976. pp. 72-80.
2. McMahon TA. *Muscles, Reflexes, and Locomotion.* Princeton, NJ: Princeton University Press, 1984. pp. 168-171.
3. Finley FR, Cody K, Finizie R. Locomotive patterns in elderly women. *Arch Phys Med Rehabil* 1969;50(3):140-146.
4. Saunders JB, Inman VT, Eberhart HD. The major determinants in normal and pathological gait. *J Bone Joint Surg* 1953;35A:543-558.
5. Inman V, Ralston HJ, Todd F. *Human Walking.* Baltimore: Williams & Wilkins, 1981.
6. Perry J. *Gait Analysis: Normal and Pathological Function.* Thorofare, NJ: Slack, 1992.
7 Los Amigos Research and Education Institute. *Observational Gait Analysis Handbook.* Downey, CA: Professional Staff Association of Rancho Los Amigos Medical Center, 1989. pp. 1-55.
8. Perry J. Integrated function of the lower extremity including gait analysis. In Cruess RL, Rennie WA (eds), *Adult Orthopedics.* New York: Churchill Livingstone, 1984. pp. 1161-1207.
9. Winter DA. Energy generation and absorption at the ankle and knee during fast, natural, and slow cadences. *Clin Orthop* 1983;May(174);147-154.
10. Merchant AC. Hip abductor muscle force. An experimental study of the influence of hip position with particular reference to rotation. *J Bone Joint Surg* 1965;47A:462-476.
11. Marks AA. *Manual of Artificial Limbs.* New York: AA Marks, 1905. pp. 17-20.
12. Braun M. *Picturing Time, Work of Etienne-Jules Marey, 1830-1904.* Chicago: University of Chicago Press, 1995. pp. 24-84.
13. Muybridge E. *Muybridge's Complete Human and Animal Locomotion.* New York: Dover, 1887. pp. 20-78.
14. Sutherland DH. Historical perspective of gait analysis (lecture handouts). *Interpretation of Gait Analysis Data,* San Diego: Children's Hospital and Health Center, Oct 17, 1994. pp. 1-2.
15. Ayyappa E. Gait lab technology: measuring the steps of progress. *Orthot Prosthet Almanac* 1996;45(2);28-56.
16. Cutlip RG, Mancinelli C, Huber F, et al. Evaluation of an instrumented walkway for measurement of the kinematic parameters of gait. *Gait Posture* 2000(2);12:134-138.
17. Bilney B, Morris M, Webster K. Concurrent related validity of the GAITRite walkway system for quantification of the spatial and temporal parameters of gait. *Gait Posture* 2003;17(1):68-74.
18. Waters RL. Energy expenditure. In Perry J (ed), *Gait Analysis.* Thorofare, NJ: Slack, 1992. pp. 443-489.
19. Torburn L, Perry J, Ayyappa E, et al. Below-knee amputee gait with dynamic elastic response prosthetic feet: a pilot study. *J Rehab Res Dev* 1990;27(4):369-384.
20. Winchester PK, Carollo JJ, Parekh RN, et al. A comparison of paraplegic gait performance using two types of reciprocating gait orthoses. *Prosthet Orthot Int* 1993;17(2):101-106.
21. Robinson GW. A study of gaits. *J Kansas Med Soc* 1925;25(12),402-406.
22. Boorstein SW. Abnormal gaits as a guide in diagnosis. *Hebrew Physician* 1937;1:221-227.
23. Northwestern University Prosthetic Orthotic Center. Gait analysis instructional film. Chicago: Northwestern University, 1960. (Handbook published by Ideal Picture Co, Chicago.)
24. Hangar HB. Personal communication, July 1994.
25. Brunnstrom S. *Movement Therapy in Hemiplegia: Neurophysiological Approach.* New York: Harper & Row, 1970.
26. Perry J. The mechanics of walking: a clinical interpretation. *Phys Ther* 1967;47(9):777-801.
27. Los Amigos Research and Education Institute. *Observational Gait Analysis.* Downey CA: Los Amigos Research and Education, 2001.
28. Holden MK, Maureen K, Gill KM, et al. Gait assessment for neurologically impaired patients; standards for outcome assessment. *Phys Ther* 1986;66(10):1530-1539.
29. Brandstater M, deBruin H, Gowland C. Hemiplegic gait: analysis of temporal values. *Arch Phys Med Rehabil* 1983;64(12):583-587.
30. Wall JC, Ashburn A. Assessment of gait disabilities in hemiplegics: hemiplegic gait. *Scand J Rehabil Med* 1979;11(3):95-103.
31. Olney SJ, Richards C. Hemiparetic gait following stroke. Part 1: characteristics. *Gait Posture* 1996;4(1):136-148.
32. Corcoran PJ, Jebsen RH, Brengelmann GL. Effects of plastic and metal leg braces on the speed and energy cost of hemiparetic ambulation. *Arch Phys Med Rehabil* 1970;51(2):69-77.
33. Lehmann JF, Condon SM, Price R, et al. Gait abnormalities in hemiplegia: their correction by ankle-foot orthoses. *Arch Phys Med Rehabil* 1987;68(11):763-771.

34. Lee K, Johnston R. Effect of below-knee bracing on knee movement: biomechanical analysis. *Arch Phys Med Rehabil* 1974;55(4):179-182.
35. Holden MK, Gill KM, Magliozzi MR. Clinical gait assessment in the neurologically impaired: reliability and meaningfulness. *Phys Ther* 1984;64(1):35-40.
36. Nilsson L. Walking training of patients with hemiparesis at an early stage after stroke: a comparison of walking training on a treadmill with body weight support and walking training on the ground. *Clin Rehabil* 2001;15(5):515-527.
37. Sanchez-Blanco I. Predictive model of functional independence in stroke patients admitted to a rehabilitation program. *Clin Rehabil* 1999;13(6):464-475.
38. Stevenson TJ. Using impairment inventory scores to determine ambulation status in individuals with stroke. *Physiother Can* 1999;51(3):168-174.
39. Brock KA. Evaluating the effectiveness of stroke rehabilitation: choosing a discriminative measure. *Arch Phys Med Rehabil* 2002;83(1):92-99.
40. Simondson J, Goldie P, Greenwood KM. The mobility scale for acute stroke patients: concurrent validity. *Clin Rehabil* 2003;17(5):558-563.
41. Roth EJ. The time logger communicator gait monitor: recording temporal gait parameters using a portable computerized device. *Int Disabil Stud* 1990;12(1):10-16.
42. Functional Independence Measure. In *Uniform Data System for Medical Rehabilitation,* Buffalo, NY: Research Foundation of SUNY, 1990.
43. Mendelsohn ME. Specificity of functional mobility measures in older adults after hip fracture: a pilot study. *Am J Phys Med Rehabil* 2003;82(10):766-774.
44. Hannan EL. Mortality and locomotion 6 months after hospitalization for hip fracture: risk factors and risk-adjusted hospital outcomes. *JAMA* 2001;285(21):2736-2742, 2793-2794.
45. Stratford PW. Validation of the LEFS on patients with total joint arthoplasty. *Physiother Can* 2000;52(2):97-105.
46. Bahlberg A. Functional independence in persons with spinal cord injury in Helsinki. *J Rehabil Med* 2003;35(5):217-220.
47. Grey N. The Functional Independence Measure: a comparative study of clinician and self-ratings. *Paraplegia* 1993;31(7):457-461.
48. McKinley WO. Rehabilitation outcomes of individuals with nontraumatic myelopathy resulting from spinal stenosis. *J Spinal Cord Med* 1998;21(2):131-136.
49. Hamilton BB. Disability outcomes following inpatient rehabilitation for stroke. *Phys Ther* 1994;74(5):494-503.
50. Ziviani J. Concurrent validity of the Functional Independence Measure for children (WeeFIM) and the Pediatric Evaluation of Disability Inventory in children with developmental disabilities and acquired brain injury. *J Phys Occup Ther Pediatr* 2001;21(2/3):91-101.
51. Azuali M. Measuring functional status and family support in older school aged children with cerebral palsy: comparison of three instruments. *Arch Phys Med Rehabil* 2000;81(3): 307-311.
52. Ottenbacher KJ. Interrater agreement and stability of the Functional Independence Measure for Children (WeeFIM): use in children with developmental disabilities. *Arch Phys Med Rehabil* 1997;78(12):1309-1315.
53. Ottenbacher KJ. The stability and equivalence reliability of the functional independence measure for children. *Dev Med Child Neurol* 1996;38(10):907-916.
54. Bohannon RW, Scoring transfer and locomotion independence of home care patients: Barthel Index versus Functional Independence Measure. *Int J Rehabil Res* 1999;22(1):65-66.
55. Pollack N. Reliability and validity of the FIM for persons aged 80 and above from a multilevel continuing care retirement community. *Arch Phys Med Rehabil* 1996;77(10):1056-1061.
56. Granger CV. Performance profiles of the functional independence measure. *Am J Phys Med Rehabil* 1993;72(2):84-89.
57. Daving Y. Reliability of an interview approach to the Functional Independence Measure. *Clin Rehabil* 2001;15(3):301-310.
58. Wolfson L, Whipple R, Amerman R, et al. Gait assessment in the elderly: a gait abnormality rating scale and its relation to falls. *J Gerontol* 1990;45(1):M12-M19.
59. VanSwearingen JM, Paschal KA, Bonino P, et al. The modified gait abnormalities rating scale and recognizing recurrent fall risk of community-dwelling frail older veterans. *Phys Ther* 1996;76(9):994-1002.
60. VanSwearingen JM, Paschal KA, Bonino P, et al. Assessing recurrent fall risk of community dwelling frail veterans using specific tests of mobility and the Physical Performance Test of Function. *J Gerontol* 1998;53:M457-M464.
61. Mathias S, Nayak US, Isaacs B. Balance in elderly patients: the "get up and go" test. *Arch Phys Med Rehabil* 1986;67(6): 387-389.
62. Posdiadlo D, Richardson S. The "timed up and go"; a test of functional mobility for frail elderly persons. *J Am Geriatr Soc* 1991;39(2):142-148.
63. Steffen TM, Hacker TA, Mollinger L. Age- and gender-related test performance in community dwelling elderly people: six minute walk test, Berg Balance Scale, Timed up and Go, and gait speed. *Phys Ther* 2002;82(2):128-137.
64. Lusardi MM, Pellecchia GL, Schulman G. Functional performance in community living older adults. *J Geriatr Phys Ther* 2003;26(3):14-22.
65. Biscoff HA. Identifying a cut-of point of normal mobility; a comparison of the timed up and go testing in community dwelling and institutionalized elderly women. *Age Ageing* 2003;32(3):315-320.
66. Thomas SG. Physical activity and its relationship to physical performance in patients with end stage knee osteoarthritis. *J Orthop Sports Phys Ther* 2003;33(12):745-754.
67. Thompson M. Performance of community dwelling elderly on the timed up and go test. *Phys Occup Ther Geriatr* 1995;13(3):17-30.
68. Medley A. The effect of assistive devices on the performance of community dwelling elderly on the time up and go test. *Issues Aging* 1997;20(1):3-7.
69. Matjacic Z. Dynamic balance training during standing in people with transtibial amputation; a pilot study. *Prosthet Orthot Int* 2003;27(3):214-220.
70. Schoppen T. Physical, mental, and social predictors of functional outcome in unilateral lower limb amputees. *Arch Phys Med Rehabil* 2003;84(6):803-811.

71. Ingemarsson AH. Walking ability and activity level after hip fracture in the elderly—a follow-up. *J Rehabil Med* 2003;35(2):76-83.
72. Crotty M. Patient and caregiver outcomes 12 months after home-based therapy for hip fracture: a randomized controlled trial. *Arch Phys Med Rehabil* 2003;84(8):1237-1239.
73. Campbell CM. The effect of cognitive demand on timed up and go performance in older adults with and without Parkinson disease. *Neurol Rep* 2003;27(1):2-7.
74. Morris S, Morris ME. Reliability of measurements obtained with the timed up and go test in people with Parkinson disease. *Phys Ther* 2001;81(2):810-818.
75. Von Schroeder HP, Coutts RD, Lyden PD, et al. Gait parameters following stroke: a practical assessment. *J Rehabil Res Dev* 1995;32(1):25-31.
76. Burdett RG, Borello-France D, Blatchly C, et al. Gait comparison of subjects with hemiplegia walking unbraced, with ankle foot orthosis, and with air-stirrup brace. *Phys Ther* 1988;68(8):1197-1203.
77. Wade DT, Wood VA, Helleer A, et al. Walking after stroke: measurement and recovery over the first 3 months. *Scand J Rehabil Med* 1987;19(1):25-30.
78. Ashworth B. Preliminary trial of carisoprodol in multiple sclerosis. *Practitioner* 1964;192(4):540-542.
79. Brunnstrom S. *Movement Therapy in Hemiplegia: Neurophysiological Approach.* New York: Harper & Row, 1970. pp. 34-55.
80. Lehmann JF, Warren CG, Hertling D, et al. Craig-Scott orthosis: a biomechanical and functional evaluation. *Arch Phys Med Rehabil* 1976;57(9):438-442.
81. Hirschberg GG, Nathanson K. Electromyographic recording of muscular activity in normal and spastic gaits. *Arch Phys Med Rehabil* 1952;33:217.
82. Perry J. Lower extremity bracing in hemiplegia. *Clin Orthop* 1969;63(4):32-38.
83. Bobath K. The facilitation of normal postural reactions and movements in the treatment of cerebral palsy. *Physiotherapy* 1964;50:246.
84. Gage JR. *Gait Analysis in Cerebral Palsy.* New York: Cambridge University Press, 1991.
85. Ounpuu S, Muik E, Davis RB, et al. Rectus femoris surgery in children with cerebral palsy. Part 1: the effect of rectus femoris transfer location on knee motion. *J Pediatr Orthop* 1993;13(3):325-330.
86. Sutherland DH. Common gait abnormalities of the knee in cerebral palsy. *Clin Orthop* 1993;March(288):139-147.
87. Knutsson E, Richards C. Different types of disturbed motor control in gait of hemiparetic patients. *Brain* 1979;102(2):405-430.
88. Mazur JM, Sienko-Thomas S, Wright N, et al. Swing-through versus reciprocating gait patterns in patients with thoracic-level spina bifida. *Z Kinderchirurgie* 1990;1(12):23-25.
89. Radcliffe CW. Functional considerations in the fitting of Trans-Femoral prostheses. In *Selected Articles from Artificial Limbs,* Huntington, NY: Krieger Publishing, 1970. pp. 5-30.
90. Eberhart H, Elfman H, Inman V. The locomotor mechanism of the amputee. In Klopsteg P, Wilson P (eds). *Human Limbs and Their Substitutes,* New York: Hafner, 1968. pp. 472-480.
91. Wilson AB. Recent advances in artificial limbs. *Artif Limbs* 1969;13:1-12.
92. Radcliffe CW, Foort J. *The Patellar Tendon Bearing Below Knee Prosthesis,* Berkeley, CA: University of California Biomechanics Laboratory, 1961.
93. Wilson AB. The prosthetic and orthotic programs. *Artif Limbs* 1970;14:1-8.
94. Ayyappa E: *Prosthetics Desk Reference: Physiatry Prosthetic Program Manual,* Irvine, CA: University California, 2004.
95. Foort J. The patellar tendon bearing prosthetis for below-knee amputees: a critical review of technique and criteria. In *Committee on Prosthetic Research and Development, Selected articles from Artificial Limbs (1/54-2/66),* Huntington, NY: Krieger, 1970. pp. 353-362.
96. Hannah RE, Morrison JB. Prostheses alignment: effect on gait of persons with below-knee amputation. *Arch Phys Med Rehabil* 1984;65:159-162.
97. Zahedi MS, Spence WD, Solomonidis SE, et al. Alignment of lower-limb prostheses. *J Rehabil Res Dev* 1986;23:2-19.
98. Goh JCH, Solomonidis SE, Spence WD, et al. Biomechanical evaluation of SACH and uniaxial feet. *Prosthet Orthot Int* 1984;8:147-154.
99. Doane NE, Holt LE. A comparison of the SACH and single axis foot in the gait of unilateral below-knee amputees. *Prosthet Orthot Int* 1983;7:33-36.
100. Culham EG, Peat M, Nowell E. Below-knee amputation: A comparison of the effects of the SACH foot and the single axis foot on electromyographic patterns during locomotion. *Prosthet Orthot Int* 1986;10:15-22.
101. Burgess EM, Hittenberger DA, Forsgren SM, et al. The Seattle prosthetic foot—a design for active sports: preliminary studies. *Orthot Prosthet* 1983;37(1):25-31.
102. Waters RL, Antonelli D, Hislop H. Energy cost of walking of amputees: the influence of level of amputation. *J Bone Joint Surg* 1976;58A:42-46.
103. Wagner EM, Sienko S, Supan T, et al. Motion analysis of SACH vs. Flexfoot in moderately active below-knee amputees. *Clin Prosthet Orthot* 1987;11:55-62.
104. Torburn L, Perry J, Ayyappa E. Below knee amputee gait with dynamic elastic response prosthetic feet: a pilot study. *J Rehabil Res Dev* 1990;27(4):369-384.
105. Barth D, Schumacher L, Sienko TS. Gait analysis and energy cost of below-knee amputees wearing six different prosthetic feet. *J Prosthet Orthot* 1992;4(2):63-75.
106. Gitter A, Czerniecki JM, DeGroot DM. Biomechanical analysis of the influence of prosthetic feet on below-knee amputee walking. *Am J Phys Med Rehabil* 1990;70:142-148.
107. Powers CM, Torburn L, Perry J, et al. Influence of prosthetic foot design on sound limb loading in adults with unilateral below-knee amputations. *Arch Phys Med Rehabil* 1994;75:825-829.
108. Farivar S, Ayyappa E. Time-distance parameters of trans-femoral amputees. Proceedings of the 23rd Annual Meeting and Scientific Symposium, American Academy of Orthotists and Prosthetists, Orlando, March 5-9, 1996.
109. James U, Oberg K. Prosthetic gait patterns in unilateral above-knee amputees. *Scand J Rehab Med* 1973;5:35-50.
110. Murray MP, Mollinger LA, Sepic SB, et al. Gait patterns in trans-femoral amputee patients: hydraulic swing control vs. constant-friction knee components. *Arch Phys Med Rehabil* 1983;64(8):339–45.

111. Suzuki K. Force plate study on artificial limb gait. *J Jap Orthop Assoc* 1972;46:503-516.
112. Thiele B, James U, Stalberg E. Neurophysiological studies on muscle function in the stump of transfemoral amputees. *Scand J Rehab Med* 1983;15:67-70.
113. Zuniga EN, Leavitt LA, Calvert JC, et al. Gait patterns in Trans-Femoral amputees. *Arch Phys Med Rehabil* 1972;53:373-382.
114. Ayyappa E. *Gait and Limb Technology: Microprocessor Knees, Capabilities,* vol II, no 2, Chicago: Northwestern University, 2002.
115. Kaufman K. Instrumented Comparison Between Mauch SNS Hydraulic Knee and the Otto Bock C-Leg. Proceedings of 4th Annual National VA Conference on Prosthetic & Orthotic Rehabilitation, Long Beach, CA, January 15-16, 2004.
116. Murray MP, Sepic SB, Gardner GM, et al. Gait patterns of Trans-Femoral amputees using constant-friction knee components. *Bull Prosthet Res* 1980;13(2):35-45.
117. *Evaluation of Gait of Unilateral AK Individuals with amputation.* New York: NYU College of Engineering, 1951. pp. 10-13.

4

Aging and Activity Tolerance: Implications for Orthotic and Prosthetic Rehabilitation

MICHELLE M. LUSARDI AND JESSIE M. VANSWEARINGEN

LEARNING OBJECTIVES

On completion of this chapter, the reader will be able to do the following:

1. Describe the role of the cardiopulmonary and cardiovascular systems as "effectors" for goal-driven functional motor activity.
2. Define the key components of cardiopulmonary and cardiovascular systems as they relate to energy expenditure during functional activity.
3. Describe the functional consequences of age-related change in cardiopulmonary and cardiovascular structures, especially with respect to exercise and activity tolerance.
4. Apply principles of cardiopulmonary/cardiovascular conditioning to rehabilitation interventions for older or deconditioned individuals, or both, who will be using a prosthesis or an orthosis.
5. Weigh the benefits and limitations, with respect to energy cost and facilitation of daily function, in selecting an appropriate orthosis or prosthesis for an older or deconditioned individual.

Many individuals who rely on orthotic or prosthetic devices in order to walk or to accomplish functional tasks have impairments of the musculoskeletal or neuromuscular systems that limit the efficiency of their movement and increase the energy cost of their daily and leisure activities. The separate and interactive effects of aging, inactivity, and cardiac or pulmonary disease can also compromise the capacity for muscular "work," tolerance of activity, and ability to function.

Consider this example: a 79-year-old woman with insulin-controlled type 2 diabetes has been referred for physical therapy evaluation after transfemoral amputation following a failed femoral-popliteal bypass. She has been on bed rest for several weeks because of her multiple surgeries. The physical effort required by rehabilitation and prosthetic training may initially feel overwhelming to this woman. In her deconditioned state, preprosthetic ambulation with a walker is likely to increase her heart rate (HR) close to the upper limits of a safe target HR for aerobic training. What, then, is her prognosis for functional use of a prosthesis? What are the most important issues to address in her plan of care? What intensity of intervention is most appropriate given her deconditioned state? In what setting and for how long will care be provided? These are questions without simple answers.

The physical therapist, orthotist, and prosthetist must recognize factors that can be successfully modified to enhance performance and activity tolerance when making decisions about prescription and intervention strategies. Aerobic fitness should be a key component of the rehabilitation program for those who will be using a prosthesis or orthosis for the first time. Finally, it is important that rehabilitation professionals recognize and respond to the warning signs of significant cardiopulmonary or cardiovascular dysfunction during treatment and training sessions.

Although the anatomical and physiological changes in the aging cardiopulmonary system are important to our discussion, our focus is on the contribution of cellular and tissue-level changes to performance of the cardiopulmonary and cardiovascular systems and, subsequently, on the individual's ability to function. This view provides a conceptual framework for answering four essential questions:

- Is this individual capable of physical work?
- If so, what is the energy cost of doing this work?
- Is it possible for this individual to become more efficient or more able to do physical work?
- What impact does the use of an orthosis or prosthesis have on energy use and cost during functional activities for this person?

OXYGEN TRANSPORT SYSTEM

The foundation for the functional view of the cardiopulmonary system is the equation for the oxygen transport system (Figure 4-1). Aerobic capacity (VO_2max) is the body's ability to deliver and use oxygen (maximum rate of oxygen consumption) to support the energy needs of demanding physical activity. VO_2max is influenced by three factors: the efficiency of ventilation and oxygenation in the lungs, how much oxygen-rich blood can be delivered from the heart (cardiac output, or CO) to active peripheral tissues, and how well oxygen is extracted from the blood to support muscle contraction and other peripheral tissues during activity (arterial-venous oxygen difference, or AVO_2diff).[1-3] Aerobic capacity can be represented by the following formula:

$$VO_2max = CO \times AVO_2diff$$

The energy cost of doing work is based on the amount of oxygen consumed for the activity, regardless of whether the activity is supported by aerobic (with oxygen) or anaerobic (without oxygen) metabolic mechanisms for producing energy. VO_2max provides an indication of the maximum amount of work that can be supported.[1-3]

CO is the product of two elements. The first is the HR, the number of times that the heart contracts, or beats, per minute. The second is stroke volume (SV), the amount of blood pumped from the left ventricle with each beat (measured in milliliters or liters). Cardiac output is expressed by the following formula:

$$CO = HR \times SV$$

As a product of HR and SV, CO is influenced by four factors: (1) the amount of blood returned from the periphery through the vena cava, (2) the ability of the heart to match its rate of contraction to physiological demand, (3) the efficiency or forcefulness of the heart's contraction, and (4) the ability of the aorta to deliver blood to peripheral vessels. The delivery of oxygen to the body tissues to be used to produce energy for work is, ultimately, a function of the central components of the cardiopulmonary system.[1-3]

The second determinant of aerobic capacity, the AVO_2diff, reflects the extraction of oxygen from the capillary by the surrounding tissues. The AVO_2diff is determined by subtracting the oxygen concentration on the venous (postextraction) side of the capillary bed (C_vO_2) from that of the arteriole (preextraction) side of the capillary bed (C_aO_2), according to the formula:

$$AVO_2diff = C_aO_2 - C_vO_2$$

The smaller vessels and capillaries of the cardiovascular system are involved in the process of extraction of oxygen from the blood by the active tissues. Extraction of oxygen

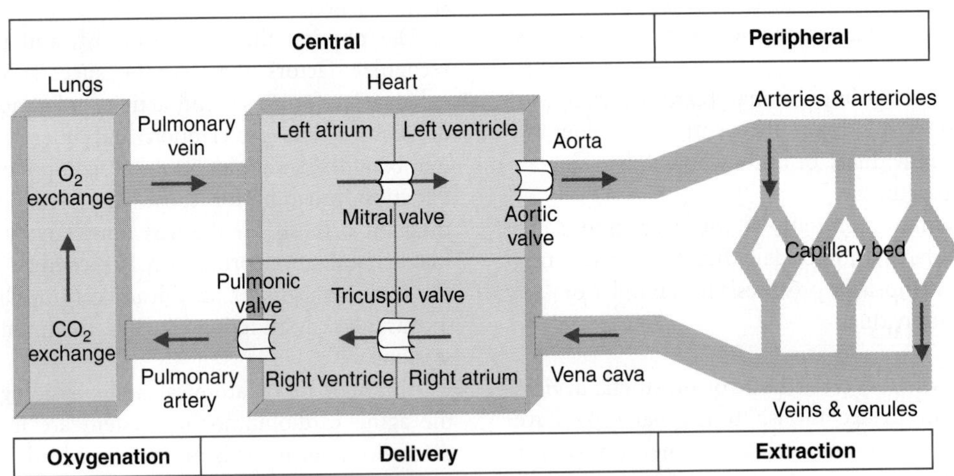

Figure 4-1

Work capacity: $VO_2max = CO \times AVO_2diff$
$(HR \times SV) \times (C_aO_2 - C_vO_2)$

Functional anatomy and physiology of the cardiorespiratory system. After blood is oxygenated in the lungs, the left side of the heart contracts to deliver blood, through the aorta and its branches, to active tissues in the periphery. Oxygen must be effectively extracted from blood by peripheral tissues to support their activity. Deoxygenated blood, high in carbon dioxide, returns through the vena cava to the right side of the heart, which pumps it to the lungs for reoxygenation. Aerobic capacity (VO_2max) is the product of how well oxygen is delivered to cardiac output (CO) and extracted by arterial-venous oxygen difference (AVO_2diff) active tissues. (*HR, Heart rate; SV, stroke volume.*)

from the blood to be used to produce energy for the work of the active tissues is a function of the peripheral components of the cardiopulmonary system.[1-3]

During exercise or a physically demanding activity, CO must increase to meet the need for additional oxygen in the more active peripheral tissues. This increased CO is the result of a more rapid HR and a greater SV: As the return of blood to the heart increases, the heart contracts more forcefully and a larger volume of blood is pumped into the aorta by the left ventricle. Chemical and hormonal changes that accompany exercise enhance peripheral shunting of blood to the active muscles, and oxygen depletion in muscle assists transfer of oxygen from the capillary blood to the tissue at work.[3,4]

The efficiency of central components, primarily of CO, accounts for as much as 75% of VO_2max. Peripheral oxygen extraction (AVO_2diff) contributes the remaining 25% to the process of making oxygen available to support tissue work.[5] In healthy adults, under most conditions, more oxygen is delivered to active tissues (muscle mass) than is necessary.[3,5] For those who are significantly deconditioned or who have cardiopulmonary or cardiovascular disease, the ability to deliver oxygen efficiently to the periphery as physical activity increases may be compromised. With normal aging, there are age-related physiological changes in the heart itself that limit maximum attainable HR. Because of these changes, it is important to assess whether and to what degree SV can be increased effectively if rehabilitation interventions are to be successful.[6]

THE AGING HEART

The ability to plan an appropriate intervention to address cardiovascular endurance and conditioning in older adults who may need to use a prosthesis or orthosis is founded on an understanding of "typical" age-related changes in cardiovascular structure and physiology, as well as on the functional consequences of these changes.

Cardiovascular Structure

Age-related structural changes in the cardiovascular system occur in five areas: myocardium, cardiac valves, coronary arteries, conduction system, and coronary vasculature (i.e., arteries)[6-9] (Table 4-1). Despite these cellular and tissue level changes, a healthy older heart can typically meet energy demands of usual daily activity. Cardiovascular disease, quite prevalent in later life, and a habitually sedentary lifestyle can, however, significantly compromise activity tolerance.[10]

Table 4-1
Age-Related Changes in the Cardiovascular System

Structure	*Change*	*Functional Consequences*
Heart	Deposition of lipids, lipofuscin, and amyloid within cardiac smooth muscle Increased connective tissue and fibrocity Hypertrophy of left ventricle Increased diameter of atria Stiffening and calcification of valves Fewer pacemaker cells in sinoatrial and atrioventricular nodes Fewer conduction fibers in bundle of His and branches Less sensitivity to extrinsic (autonomic) innervation Slower rate of tension development during contraction Prolonged	Less excitability Diminished cardiac output Diminished venous return Susceptibility to dysrhythmia Reduction in maximal attainable heart rate Less efficient dilation of cardiac arteries during activity Less efficient left ventricular filling in early diastole, leading to reduced stroke volume Increased afterload, leading to weakening of heart muscle
Blood vessels	Altered ratio of smooth muscle to connective tissue and elastin in vessel walls Decreased baroreceptor responsiveness Susceptibility to plaque formation within vessel Rigidity and calcification of large arteries, especially aorta Dilation and increased tortuosity of veins	Less efficient delivery of oxygenated blood to muscle and organs Diminished cardiac output Less efficient venous return Susceptibility to venous thrombosis Susceptibility to orthostatic hypotension

Modified from Thompson LV. Physiological changes associated with aging. In Guccione AA (ed), *Geriatric Physical Therapy*, 2nd ed. St. Louis: Mosby, 2000. p. 33.

Myocardium

With advanced age, cells of the myocardium show microscopical signs of degeneration including the accumulation of lipid deposits and lipofuscin[8]; however, these deposits have not been associated with abnormalities of heart function.[11] Unlike aging skeletal muscle cells, there is minimal atrophy of cardiac smooth muscle cells. More typically, there is hypertrophy of the left ventricular myocardium, increasing the diameter of the left atrium.[12-14] These changes have been attributed to cardiac tissue responses to an increased systolic blood pressure (SBP) and to reduced compliance of the left ventricle and are associated with an increase in weight and size of the heart.[13-17]

Valves

The four valves of the aged heart often become fibrous and thickened at their margins, as well as somewhat calcified.[18] Calcification of the aorta at the base of the cusps of the aortic valve (aortic stenosis) is clinically associated with the slowed exit of blood from the left ventricle into the aorta.[2,8,19] Such aortic stenosis contributes to a functional reduction in CO. A baroreflex-mediated increase in SBP attempts to compensate for this reduced CO.[20-22] Over time, the larger residual of blood in the left ventricle after each beat (increased end systolic volume, ESV) begins to weaken the left ventricular muscle.[23] The ventricular muscle must work harder to pump the blood out of the ventricle into a more resistant peripheral vascular system.[24,25]

Calcification of the annulus of the mitral valve can restrict blood flow from the left atrium into the left ventricle during diastole.[24] As a result, end diastolic volume (EDV) of blood in the left ventricle is decreased because the left atrium does not completely empty. Over time, this residual blood in the left atrium elongates the muscle of the atrial walls and increases the diameter of the atrium of the aged heart.[24-26]

Coronary Arteries

Age-related changes of the coronary arteries are similar to those in any aged arterial vessel: an increase in thickness of vessel walls and tortuosity of its path.[7,9,11,25] These changes tend to occur earlier in the left coronary artery than in the right.[24,27] When coupled with atherosclerosis, these changes may compromise the muscular contraction and pumping efficiency and effectiveness of the left ventricle during exercise or activity of high physiological demand.[2,3,28]

Conduction System

Age-related changes in the conduction system of the heart can have substantial impact on cardiac function.[7,11] The typical 75-year-old has less than 10% of the original number of pacemaker cells of the sinoatrial node.[29,30] Fibrous tissue builds within the internodal tracts as well as the atrioventricular node, including the bundle of His and its main bundle branches.[29,30] As a consequence, the exquisite ability of the heart to coordinate the actions of all four of its chambers may be compromised.[24,25,29] Arrhythmias are pathological conditions that become more common in later life; they are managed pharmacologically or with implantation of a pacemaker/defibrillator.[31] Rehabilitation professionals must be aware of the impact of medications or pacemaker settings on an individual's ability to physiologically respond to exercise and to adapt to the intervention, whether it be a conditioning program or early mobility after a medical/surgical event, accordingly.[32]

Arterial Vascular Tree

Age-related changes in the arterial vascular tree, demonstrated most notably by the thoracic aorta and eventually the more distal vessels, can disrupt the smooth flow of blood from the heart toward the periphery.[6,31,33] Altered alignment of endothelial cells of the intima creates turbulence, which increases the likelihood of deposition of collagen and lipid.[34] Fragmentation of elastic fibers in the intima and media of larger arterioles and arteries further compromises the functionally important "rebound" characteristic of arterial vessels.[6,9,35] Rebound normally assists directional blood flow through the system, preventing the backward reflection of fluid pressure waves of blood.[8,25] This loss of elasticity increases vulnerability of the aorta, which, distended and stiffened, cannot effectively resist the tensile force of left ventricular ejection.[6,11,25] Not surprisingly, the incidence of abdominal aortic aneurysms rises sharply among older adults.[36]

Cardiovascular Physiology

Although the physiological changes in the cardiovascular system are few, their impact on performance of the older adult can be substantial. The nondiseased aging heart continues to be an effective pump, maintaining its ability to develop enough myocardial contraction to support daily activity. The response of cardiac muscle to calcium (Ca^{++}) is preserved, and its force-generating capacity maintained.[11,25] Two aspects of myocardial contractility do, however, change with aging: the rate of tension development in the myocardium slows, and the duration of contraction and relaxation is prolonged.[24,25]

Beta-Adrenergic Sensitivity

One of the most marked age-related changes in cardiovascular function is the reduced sensitivity of the heart to sympathetic stimulation, specifically to the stimulation of beta-adrenergic receptors.[8,25,37] Age-related reduction in beta-adrenergic sensitivity includes a decreased response to norepinephrine and epinephrine released from sympathetic nerve endings in the heart, as well as a decreased sensitivity to any of these catecholamines circulating in the blood.[37,38] Normally, norepinephrine and epinephrine are potent stimulators of ventricular contraction.

An important functional consequence of the change in receptor sensitivity is less efficient cardioacceleratory response, which leads to a lower HR at submaximal and maximal levels of exercise or activity.[8,39] The time for HR rise to the peak rate is prolonged, so more time is necessary to reach the appropriate HR level for physically demanding activities. A further consequence of this reduced beta-adrenergic sensitivity is less than optimal vasodilation of the coronary arteries with increasing activity.[37,40] In peripheral arterial vessels, beta-adrenergic receptors do not appear to play a primary role in mediating vasodilation in the working muscles.[41]

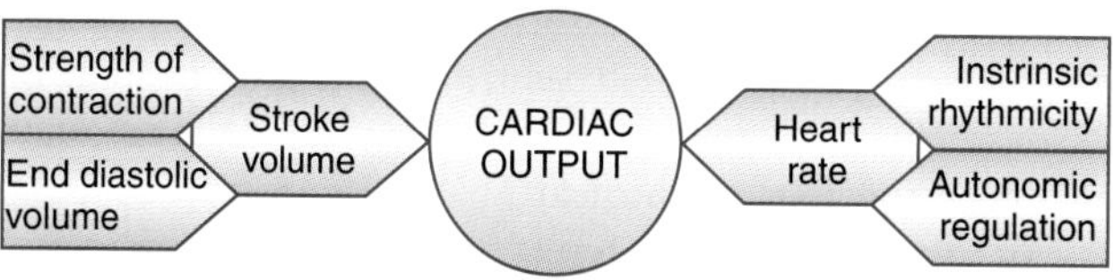

Figure 4-2

Factors affecting cardiac output are influenced by the aging process: If strength of contraction decreases and end diastolic volume increases, stroke volume is reduced. Coupled with alterations in heart rate response to increasing workload, activities that were submaximal in intensity at a younger age may become more physiologically demanding in later life.

Baroreceptor Reflex

Age-related change in the cardiovascular baroreceptor reflex also contributes to prolongation of cardiovascular response time in the face of an increase in activity (physiological demand).[40] The baroreceptors in the proximal aorta appear to become less sensitive to changes in blood volume (pressure) within the vessel. Normally, any drop in proximal aortic pressure triggers the hypothalamus to begin a sequence of events that leads to increased sympathetic stimulation of the heart. Decreased baroreceptor responsiveness may increase an older individual's susceptibility to orthostatic (postural) and postprandial (after eating) hypotension or compromise their tolerance of the physiological stress of a Valsalva maneuver associated with breath holding during strenuous activity.[42,43] Clinically, this is evidenced by lightheadedness when rising from lying or sitting, especially after a meal, or if one tends to hold one's breath during effortful activity.

The consequences of age-related physiological changes on the cardiovascular system can often be managed effectively by routinely using simple lower extremity warm-up exercises before position changes. Several repetitions of ankle and knee exercises before standing up, especially after a prolonged time sitting (including for meals) or lying down (after a night's rest), help to maximize blood return to the heart (preload), assisting cardiovascular function for the impending demand. In addition, taking a bit more time in initiating and progressing difficulty of activities may help the slowed cardiovascular response time to reach an effective level of performance. Scheduling physical therapy or physical activity remote from mealtimes might also be beneficial for patients who are particularly vulnerable to postprandial hypotension.

Functional Consequences of Cardiovascular Aging

What are the functional consequences of cardiovascular aging for older adults participating in exercise or rehabilitation activities? This question can best be answered by focusing on what happens to the CO (Figure 4-2). The age-related structural and physiological changes in the cardiovascular system give rise to two loading conditions that influence CO: cardiac filling (preload) and vascular impedance (afterload).[3,7,20]

Preload

Cardiac filling/preload determines the volume of blood in the left ventricle at the end of diastole. The most effective ventricular filling occurs when pressure is low within the heart and relaxation of the muscular walls of the ventricle is maximal.[1,5] Mitral valve calcification, decreased compliance of the left ventricle, and the prolonged relaxation of myocardial contraction can contribute to a less effective filling of the left ventricle in early diastole.[44] Doppler studies of the flow of blood into the left ventricle in aging adults demonstrate decreased rates of early filling, an increased rate of late atrial filling, and an overall decrease in the peak filling rate.[5,23,44] When compared with healthy 45- to 50-year-old adults, the early diastolic filling of a healthy 65- to 80-year-old is 50% less.[5,23,45] This reduced volume of blood in the ventricle at the end of diastole does not effectively stretch the ventricular muscle of the heart, compromising the Frank-Starling mechanism and the myocontractility of the left ventricle.[46] The functional outcome of decreased early diastolic filling and the reduced EDV is a comparative decrease in SV, one of the determinants of CO and, subsequently, work capacity (VO_2max).[5,22,25]

Afterload

High vascular impedance and increased afterload disrupts flow of blood as it leaves the heart toward the peripheral vasculature. Increased afterload is, in part, a function of age-related stiffness of the proximal aorta, an increase in systemic vascular resistance (elevation of SBP, hypertension), or a combination of both factors.[6,8,25,47] Ventricular contraction that forces blood flow into a resistant peripheral vascular system produces pressure waves in the blood. These pressure waves reflect back toward the heart, unrestricted by the stiffened walls of the proximal aorta. The reflected pressure waves, aortic stiffness, and increased systemic vascular resistance collectively contribute to an increased afterload in the aging heart.[9,24,47] Increased afterload is thought to be a major factor in the age-associated decrease in maximum SV, hypertrophy of the left ventricle, and prolongation of myocardial relaxation (e.g., slowed relaxation in the presence of a persisting load on the heart).[6,9]

An unfortunate long-term consequence of increased afterload is weakening of the heart muscle itself, particularly of the left ventricle. Restricted blood flow out of the heart results in a large residual volume (RV) of blood in the heart at the end of systole when ventricular contraction is complete. Large ESVs gradually increase the resting length of ventricular cardiac muscle, effectively weakening the force of contraction.[2,6,9,23,48]

Left Ventricular Ejection Fraction

Left ventricular ejection fraction (LVEF) is the proportion of blood pumped out of the heart with each contraction of the left ventricle, which is expressed by the following equation:

$$\text{LVEF} = (\text{EDV} - \text{ESV}) \div \text{EDV}$$

At rest the LVEF does not appear to be reduced in older adults. Under conditions of maximum exercise, however, the

Healthy young adult	Healthy older adult	Sedentary older adult	Older adult with disease
Reserve capacity	Age-related loss	Age-related loss	Age-related loss
	Reserve capacity	Impact of inactivity	Impact of inactivity
		Reserve capacity	Impact of disease
			Reserve capacity
ADLs	ADLs	ADLs	ADLs
At rest	At rest	At rest	At rest

Figure 4-3

Comparison of the effects of aging, inactivity, and cardiopulmonary disease on functional reserve capacity, expressed as cardiac output (CO; liters per minute). At rest, the heart delivers between 4 and 6 L of blood per minute to peripheral tissues. This may double during many activities of daily living. In a healthy young person, the CO may increase to as much as 24 L/min to meet metabolic demands of sustained exercise. This reserve capacity decreases to approximately 18 L/min in healthy, fit elders after the age of 60. A sedentary lifestyle decreases functional reserve capacity further. Superimposed cardiopulmonary disease further limits the ability to do physical work, in some cases approaching or exceeding cardiopulmonary reserve capacity. (Modified from Irwin SC, Zadai CC. Cardiopulmonary rehabilitation of the geriatric patient. In Lewis CB [ed], Aging: the Health Care Challenge. *Philadelphia: F.A. Davis, 1990. p. 190.)*

rise in LVEF is much less than in younger adults.[22,49,50] This reduced rise in the LVEF with maximal exercise clearly illustrates the impact that preload and afterload functional cardiovascular age-related changes have on performance. A substantial reduction in EDV, an expansion of ESV, or a more modest change in both components may account for the decreased LVEF of the exercising older adult:

$$\downarrow \text{EDV} = \downarrow \text{LVEF}$$

$$\uparrow \text{ESV} = \downarrow \text{LVEF}$$

When going from resting to maximal exercise conditions, the amount of blood pumped with each beat for young healthy adults increases 20% to 30% from a resting LVEF of 55% to an exercise LVEF of 80%. For a healthy older adult, in contrast, LVEF typically increases less than 5% from rest to maximal exercise.[49,51] The LVEF may actually decrease in adults who are 60 years of age and older.[49,52] As LVEF and CO decrease with aging, so does the ability to work over prolonged periods (functional cardiopulmonary reserve capacity) because the volume of blood delivered to active tissue decreases (Figure 4-3). Functional reserve capacity is further compromised by the long-term effects of inactivity and by cardiopulmonary pathology.[22,28,53,54] The contribution of habitual exercise to achieving effective maximum exercise LVEF is not well understood but may be important: Rodeheffer and colleagues[22] report that the decline in maximum exercise LVEF may not be as substantial for highly fit older adults.

PULMONARY FUNCTION IN LATER LIFE

Several important age-related structural changes of the lungs and of the musculoskeletal system have a significant impact on pulmonary function.[55,56] These include change in the tissues and structures making up the lungs and airways, alteration in lung volume, reduced efficiency of gas exchange, and a mechanically less efficient ventilatory pump related to changes in alignment and posture[57] (Table 4-2). Although a healthy adult at midlife uses only 10% of the respiratory system capacity at rest, aging of the pulmonary system, especially when accompanied by chronic illness or acute disease, negatively affects the ability of the lungs to respond to increasing demands of physical activity[58] (Figure 4-4). Age-related changes in the pulmonary and musculoskeletal systems also contribute to an increase in the physiological work of breathing.

Changes within the Lung and Airway

The production of elastin, which is the major protein component of the structure of the lungs, decreases markedly in late life. The elastic fibers of the lung become fragmented, and, functionally, the passive elastic recoil or rebound important for expiration becomes much less efficient.[59] The

Table 4-2

Summary of Age-Related Changes in the Cardiopulmonary System and Functional Consequences

Anatomical Changes	*Physiological Changes*	*Consequences*	*Change in Lung Function Tests*
Rearrangement and fragmentation of elastin fibers Stiffened cartilage in articulation of ribs and vertebrae Increasing stiffness and compression of annulus fibrosis in intervertebral disks Reduction of strength and endurance of respiratory musculature	Less elastic recoil for expiration Greater compliance of lung tissue More rigid thoracic cage Decreased volume of maximum voluntary ventilation and maximum sustained ventilatory capacity Greater mismatch between ventilation and perfusion within lung	Greater airspace within alveoli, less surface area for O_2/CO_2 exchange Shorter, less compliant thoracic cage Increased work of breathing Less force during inspiration Less efficient cough Diminished exercise tolerance Reduced resting PaO_2	Increased functional residual capacity and residual volume Decreased vital capacity, forced vital capacity, and forced expiratory volume in 1 second (FEV_1) Decreased maximum inspiratory pressure, maximum expiratory pressure, and maximum voluntary ventilation

Modified from Bourgeois MC, Zadai CC. Impaired ventilation and respiration in the older adult. In Guccione AA (ed), *Geriatric Physical Therapy.* St. Louis: Mosby, 2000. p. 231.

elastic fibers that maintain the structure of the walls of the alveoli also decrease in number. This loss of elastin means loss of alveoli and consequently less surface area for the exchange of oxygen, as well as an increase in residual volume associated with more "dead space" within the lung where air exchange cannot occur.[57,58] There may be as much as a 15% decrease in the total number of alveoli per unit of lung volume by the age of 70 years.[60]

With aging, there is also an increase in diameter of major bronchi and large bronchioles, as well as a decreased diameter of smaller bronchioles, often leading to a slight increase in resistance to air flow during respiration.[60] This contributes to greater physical work to breathe as age advances.

Starting at midlife and continuing into later life, there tends to be a growing mismatch between lung area ventilated with each breath and lung area perfused by pulmonary arterioles and capillaries,[61] attributed to alteration in alveolar surface, vascular structures, and posture. Such a mismatch compromises the efficiency of diffusion of oxygen across the alveoli into the capillary bed (i.e., decreasing arterial oxygen tension) within the lung becomes less efficient from midlife into later life.[57,61]

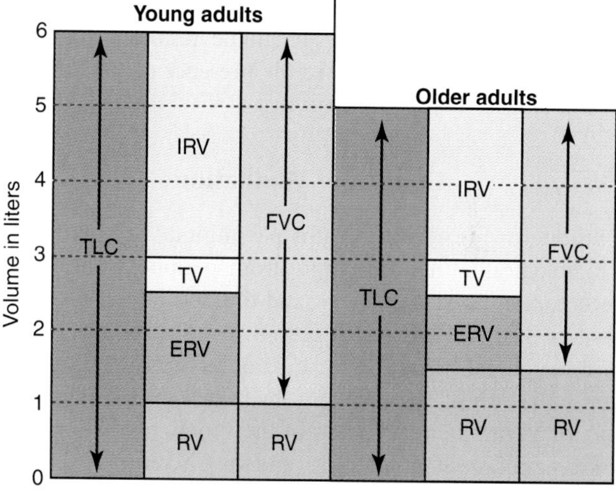

Figure 4-4

Changes in the distribution of air within the lungs (volume) have an impact on an older adult's efficiency of physical work. Loss of alveoli and increasing stiffness of the rib cage result in a 30% to 50% increase in residual volume (RV) and a 40% to 50% decrease in forced vital capacity (FVC). FVC includes three components: Inspiratory reserve volume (IRV) and expiratory reserve volume (ERV) tend to decrease with aging, whereas resting tidal volume (TV), the amount of air in a normal resting breath, tends to be stable over time. Total lung capacity (TLC) and inspiratory capacity (IRV + TV) also tend to decrease. Over time, the physiological consequences of these changes make the older adult more vulnerable to dyspnea (shortness of breath) during exercise and physically demanding activity.

Changes in the Musculoskeletal System

The decreasing elastic recoil and alveolar surface area for oxygen exchange may be further compounded by increased stiffness (loss of flexibility), "barreling" of the thoracic rib cage that houses the lungs, and decrease in height as intervertebral disks narrow and stiffen.[62] Much of the stiffness is attributed to changes in the articulation between rib and vertebrae, as well as decreased elasticity of intercostal muscle and soft tissue.[63] Although the stiffened rib cage may be as much a consequence of a sedentary lifestyle as of advancing age, lack of flexibility compromises inspiration and also decreases elastic recoil of expiration.[64,65] In addition, the forward head and slight kyphosis that tend to develop with aging alter rib and diaphragm position, decreasing mechanical efficiency of inspiration.[58,62,65] The net effect of a stiffer thoracic cage is an increase in the work of taking a breath; muscles of respiration must work harder during inspiration to counteract the stiffness.[58]

The striated muscles of respiration are composed of a combination of type I (slow twitch, fatigue resistant, for endurance) and type II (fast twitch, for power) fibers and are susceptible to the same age-related changes in strength and endurance that have been observed in muscles of the extremities.[66] Normally, type I muscle fibers are active during quiet breathing; recruitment of type II fibers is triggered by increasing physiological demand as activity increases. Age-related decrement in the strength and efficiency of the diaphragm, intercostals, abdominal muscles, and other accessory muscle of respiration affects the effectiveness and work of breathing.[58,67] Altered posture and higher residual volume within the lung also contribute to an increased work of breathing; when the diaphragm rests in less than optimal configuration for contraction, accessory muscles become active sooner, as physiological demand increases. Oxygen consumption in respiratory muscles, as in all striated muscle, decreases linearly with age, making older muscle more vulnerable to the effects of fatigue in situations of high physical demand, especially in the presence of lung disease or injury.[57]

Control of Ventilation

The rate of breathing (breaths per minute) is matched to physiological demand by input from peripheral mechanoreceptors in chest wall, lungs, and thoracic joints, as well as centers in the brainstem of central nervous systems (CNS) and peripheral aortic and carotid bodies that are sensitive to concentration of CO_2, O_2, and hydrogen ions (pH) in the blood.[68] With aging, stiffness of the thorax tends to reduce efficiency of mechanoreceptors, and the CNS and PNS centers that monitor CO_2, O_2, and pH to detect hypoxia during activity slowly begin to decline.

Gradual loss of descending motor neurons within the CNS also occurs, with less efficient activation of neurons innervating muscles of respiration via phrenic nerve to diaphragm for inspiration and of spinal nerves to intercostals for expiration.[61] These three factors combine to compromise the individual's ability to quickly and accurately respond to increasing physiological demand and increase the likelihood of dyspnea during activity.

Functional Consequences of Pulmonary Aging

With less recoil for expiration and reduced flexibility for inspiration, the ability to work is compromised in two ways (see Figure 4-4). First, vital capacity (VC), the maximum amount of air that can be voluntarily moved in and out of the lungs with a breath, is decreased by 25% to 40%. Second, RV, the air remaining in the lungs after a forced expiration, is increased by 25% to 40%.[57] This combination of reduced movement of air with each breath and increased air remaining in the lung between breaths leads to higher lung-air carbon dioxide content and, eventually, lower oxygen saturation of the blood after air exchange.[69] The increase in RV also affects the muscles of inspiration: the dome of the diaphragm flattens, and the accessory respiratory muscles are elongated. As a result of these length changes, the respiratory muscles work in a mechanically disadvantageous range of the length-tension curve, and the energy cost of the muscular work of breathing rises.[58]

Functionally, the amount of air inhaled per minute (minute ventilation) is a product of the frequency of breathing times the tidal volume (volume of air moving into and out of the lungs with each usual breath). In healthy individuals, the increased ventilatory needs of low-intensity activities are usually met by an increased depth of breathing (i.e., increased tidal volume).[70] Frequency of breathing increases when increased depth alone cannot meet the demands of activity, typically when tidal volume reaches 50% to 60% of the VC.[70] For the older adult with reduced VC who is involved in physical activity, tidal volume can quickly exceed this level so that frequency of breathing increases much earlier than would be demonstrated by a young adult at the same intensity of exercise.[71] Because the energy cost of breathing rises sharply with the greater respiratory muscle work associated with an increased respiratory rate, an important consequence of increased frequency of breathing is fatigue.[72] This early reliance on an increased frequency of breathing, combined with a large RV and its higher carbon dioxide concentration in lung air, results in a physiological cycle that further drives the need to breathe more often. Overworked respiratory muscles are forced to rely on anaerobic metabolism to supply their energy need, resulting in a buildup of lactic acid. Because lactic acid lowers the pH of the tissues (acidosis), it is also a potent physiological stimulus for increased frequency of breathing.[72-74] The older person can be easily forced into a condition of rapid, shallow breathing (shortness of breath) to meet the ventilatory requirements of seemingly moderate-intensity exercise.

IMPLICATIONS FOR INTERVENTION

Rehabilitation professionals must consider two questions about the implications of age-related changes in the cardiovascular and cardiopulmonary systems on an older person's ability to do physical work. First, what precautions should be observed to avoid cardiopulmonary and cardiovascular complications? Second, what can be done to optimize cardiopulmonary and cardiovascular function for maximal physical performance?

Precautions

Because of the combined effects of the age-related changes in the cardiovascular and cardiopulmonary systems, the high incidence of cardiac and pulmonary pathologies in later life, and the deconditioning impact of bed rest and inactivity, older patients who require orthotic or prosthetic intervention may be vulnerable if exercise or activity is too physiologically demanding. Although most older adults can tolerate and respond positively to exercise, exercise is not appropriate in a number of circumstances (Table 4-3).

Estimating Workload: Heart Rate and Rate Pressure Product

One of the readily measurable consequences of the reduced response of the heart to sympathetic stimulation in later life is a reduction in the maximal attainable HR.[24,68,75] This reduction in maximal HR also signals that an older person's HR reserve, the difference between the rate for any given level of activity and the maximal attainable HR, is limited as well. For older patients involved in rehabilitation programs, the distance between resting and maximal HR is narrowed. One method of estimating maximal (max) attainable HR is the following[5]:

$$\text{Max HR} = 220 - \text{age}$$

For healthy individuals, the recommended target HR for aerobic conditioning exercise is between 60% and 80% of maximal attainable HR. For many older adults, especially those who are habitually inactive, resting HR may be close to the recommended range for exercise exertion.[76] Consider an 80-year-old individual with a resting HR of 72 beats per

Table 4-3
Signs and Symptoms of Exercise Intolerance

Category	*Cautionary Signs/Symptoms*	*Contraindications to Exercise*
Heart rate	<40 bpm at rest >130 bpm at rest Little HR increase with activity Excessive HR increase with activity Frequent arrhythmia	Prolonged at maximum activity Prolonged arrhythmia or tachycardia
ECG	Any recent ECG abnormalities	Exercise-induced ECG abnormalities Third-degree heart block
Blood pressure	Resting SBP >180 mm Hg Resting DBP >100 mm Hg Lack of SBP response to activity Excessive BP response to activity	Resting SBP >200 mm Hg Resting DBP >110 mm Hg Drop in SBP >20 mm Hg in exercise Drop in DBP during exercise
Angina	Low threshold for angina	Prolonged/intense angina in activity New jaw, shoulder, or left arm pain
Respiratory rate	Dyspnea >35 breaths/min	Dyspnea >45 breaths/min
Blood gas values	O_2 saturation <90%	O_2 saturation <86%
Other symptoms	Mild to moderate claudication Onset of pallor Facial expression of distress Lightheadedness or mild dizziness Postactivity fatigue >1 hr Slow recovery from activity	Severe, persistent claudication Cyanosis, severe pallor, or cold sweat Facial expression of severe distress Moderate to severe dizziness, syncope Nausea, vomiting Onset of ataxia, incoordination Increasing mental confusion
Acute illness	Fever >100°F Recent mental confusion Abnormal electrolytes (potassium)	<2 days after myocardial infarction <2 days after pulmonary embolism Acute thrombophlebitis Acute hypoglycemia Digoxin toxicity

bpm, beats per minute; *DBP,* diastolic blood pressure; *ECG,* electrocardiogram; *HR,* heart rate; *SBP,* systolic blood pressure. Modified from Hillegass EA, Sadowsky HS. *Essentials of Cardiopulmonary Physical Therapy.* Philadelphia: Saunders, 1994. p. 166; and Watchie J. *Cardiopulmonary Physical Therapy: A Clinical Manual.* Philadelphia: Saunders, 1995. p. 16.

minute. His maximal attainable HR is approximately 140 beats per minute (220 – 80 years). A target HR for an aerobic training level of exertion of 60% of maximal HR would be 84 beats per minute. His resting HR is within 12 beats of the HR for aerobic training. Functionally, this means that an activity as routine as rising from a chair or walking a short distance on a level surface may represent physical work of a level of exertion equated with moderate- to high-intensity exercise. Because of the reduction in maximal attainable HR with age, older adults may be working close to their VO_2max range even in usual activities of daily living.[76,77]

Because HR essentially signals the work of the heart, with each beat representing ventricular contraction, increased HR relates closely to increased heart work and increased oxygen consumption by the myocardium.[75] Given that afterload on the heart increases with age, the overall work of the heart for each beat is likely greater as well.[11,22,24,25] A more representative way to estimate the work of the heart during activity for older adults is the rate pressure product (RPP),[79-81] using HR and SBP as follows:

$$RPP = HR \times SBP$$

The linear relationship between VO_2max and HR for younger adults actually levels off for older adults.[82] Because of this, HR alone cannot accurately reflect the physiological work that the older patient experiences; the RPP provides a clearer impression of relative work.[81] For older individuals with HR reserve limited by age, adjusting activity to keep the rise in HR within the lower end of the HR reserve is wise, especially for those with known coronary artery compromise.

Blood Pressure as a Warning Sign

An older person's blood pressure (BP) must also be considered. Hypertension, particularly increased SBP, is common in older adults. SBP also provides a relative indication of the level of afterload on the heart.[25,83,84] Resting BP can be used to indicate whether an older person can safely tolerate increased physiological work. Persons with resting BPs of more than 180/95 mm Hg may have difficulty with increased activity. A conservative estimate of the safe range of exercise suggests that exercise should be stopped if and when BP exceeds 220/110 mm Hg, although some consider 220 mm Hg too conservative a limit for older adults.[75] SBP should rise with increasing activity or exercise.[78]

The older adult with limited HR reserve must increase SV to achieve the required CO.[22,24,49] SBP rises as SV increases and blood volume in the peripheral vasculature rises.[25] If SBP fails to rise or actually decreases during activity, this is a significant concern.[75] The drop or lack of change in SBP indicates that the heart is an ineffective pump, unable to contract and force a reasonable volume of blood out of the left ventricle. Continuing exercise or activity in the presence of a dropping SBP returns more blood to a heart that is incapable of pumping it back out to the body. Elevated diastolic blood pressure suggests that the left ventricle is maintaining a higher pressure during the filling period.[24,25,68] Early diastolic filling during preload will be compromised,[6,25,45] and the heart will be unable to capitalize on the Frank-Starling mechanism to enhance the force of ventricular contraction.[22,49]

Respiratory Warning Signs

Dyspnea, or shortness of breath, is an important warning sign as well. Age-related changes in the pulmonary system increase the work of breathing, and breathing becomes less efficient as work increases.[72] Because an older person is prone to shortness of breath, recovering from shortness of breath during exercise may be difficult. Breathing more deeply requires a disproportionately greater amount of respiratory muscle work, which further increases the cost of ventilation.[55,73,74] The use of supplemental oxygen by nasal cannula for the postoperative or medically ill older adult who is beginning rehabilitation may be quite beneficial.

Oxygen supplementation may prevent or minimize shortness of breath, enabling an older person to tolerate increased activity better and to participate in rehabilitation more fully. During this oxygen-assisted time, any conditioning exercise to improve muscular performance (especially if combined with nutritional support) delivers blood to the working tissues and improves tissue oxygenation, ultimately aiding pulmonary function. Improved muscular conditioning and cardiovascular function may prevent or delay onset of lactic acidemia and the resultant increased desire to breathe that would trigger shortness of breath.[72,85]

Optimizing Cardiopulmonary Performance

For most older adults, conditioning or training is an effective way to improve function, although some may need a longer training period to accomplish their desired level of physical performance as compared with younger adults.[86-90] Physical conditioning, in situations of acute and chronic illness, enables the older person to do more work and better accomplish desired tasks or activities.

Older adults, including those who are quite debilitated, experience improvement in physical performance as a result of conditioning exercise[88] (Figure 4-5). For some, significant gains are made as work capacity increases from an initial state below the threshold necessary for function, such that an older person appears to make greater gains than a younger individual in similar circumstances.[91,92] In many cases the cardiopulmonary system efficiency gained through conditioning means the difference between independence and dependency; functional recovery and minimal improvement; life without extraordinary means and life support; and, for some older individuals, life and death.

The physiological mechanisms for achieving the conditioned responses of the old may vary slightly from those of the young. With increasing activity or exercise in the submaximal range, older adults demonstrate greater increases

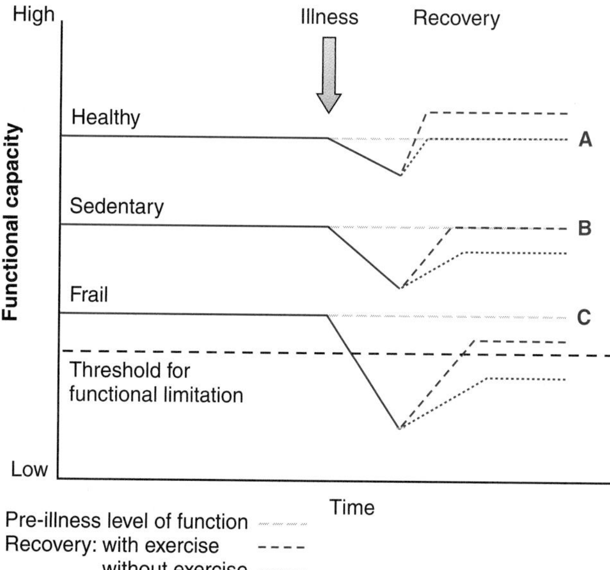

Figure 4-5

Comparison of the impact of illness or prolonged inactivity, or both, on functional status and of exercise on recovery of premorbid functional levels of healthy, sedentary, and frail older adults. Each individual's functional reserve is represented by the distance between the threshold for functional limitation and their functional capacity. A, *Healthy older adults have the most functional reserve and may recover preillness functional capacity without conditioning exercise but often show improvement above baseline with exercise.* B, *Sedentary older adults may not resume preillness functional capacity without the benefit of conditioning exercise.* C, *Frail older adults have the least functional reserve, often fall below threshold for function when illness occurs, and tend to remain below this threshold without conditioning exercise. However, even frail older adults can regain functional status with conditioning exercise.*

in SV and less rise in HR than do young adults.[22,25,45,49,75] This increase in SV is accomplished with an increased EDV, usually without change in the ESV.[22,25,45] Increasing the EDV enhances the force of ventricular contraction by the Frank-Starling mechanism, which, in turn, increases CO despite the age-related impairment of the cardioacceleratory responses, which limits the rise in HR.[22,24,25,45,49] An increased preload, which improves CO, is the usual outcome of training at any age because improved conditioning of the peripheral musculature prevents distal pooling of blood and increased resting tension of the muscles assists blood return.[75]

Preparation for Activity and Exercise

Simple lower extremity exercise as a warm-up before any functional activity or training session enhances the preload of the heart. Any gentle, repetitive, active lower extremity motions (e.g., ankle "pumps" in dorsiflexion/plantar flexion, knee flexion/extension, or cycling movements of the legs) before transfer or ambulation activities, before upper trunk and upper extremity activities, or as part of the warm-up portion of an aerobic or strength training exercise effectively improve the EDV. This increased EDV compensates in part for age-related preload problems, which might otherwise compromise work capacity.

Additionally, the muscular work of preliminary lower extremity exercise initiates the electrolyte and hormonal changes that promote the metabolic changes and vasodilation in peripheral tissues necessary to support aerobic metabolism for meeting energy demands of the task.[75,88] Peripheral oxygen exchange improves as much as 16% with regular exercise training.[22] The peripheral vasodilation associated with exercise helps to check the rise in afterload on the heart and also minimizes the development of lactic acidemia and the resulting drive to breathe more rapidly.[73,74]

As submaximal levels of exercise increase toward maximal exercise, SV continues to increase, maintaining CO.[22,45,49] When cardiopulmonary disease is present in addition to aging, however, this continued increase in SV is likely to be blunted.[24,75] Under these circumstances, the reduced sensitivity of the heart to sympathetic stimulation limits the force of contraction of the ventricle so that the ejection fraction decreases and the ESV rises slightly.[25]

Monitoring the Cardiorespiratory Response to Exercise

Consistent monitoring of the cardiopulmonary response is an essential component of rehabilitation interventions aimed at optimizing endurance or fitness of older frail or deconditioned individuals.[76,93,94] The positive effects of training only occur when the older person is appropriately challenged by the exercise or activity. According to the principle of overload, functional improvements occur only when the body is asked to do more than the customary workload for that individual.[5] For an individual who has been on prolonged bed rest and is quite deconditioned, simple lower extremity exercises while sitting upright may be as challenging as training for a marathon in a healthy young adult. The level of physiological exertion is relative to the individual's customary work. Providing the physiological overload necessary to produce improvements in performance, while avoiding a decline in performance because of exercise-induced fatigue or exhaustion, requires that the therapist monitor an individual's level of exertion.

Heart Rate and Blood Pressure

Maximum oxygen consumption (VO_2max) is the most accurate and sensitive measure of the individual workload, but the special equipment and technology necessary to determine VO_2max are not typically available in routine clinical practice.[75,76] Although the linear relationship between HR and VO_2max plateaus so that HR becomes an inaccurate reflection of the workload for older adults, HR does partially indicate the work of the heart.[75,79,82] For a rapid clinical impression of the physiological burden of an activity or exercise, HR is helpful as long as the clinician recognizes its limitations when using the measure with elders. Preexercise or activity BP provides some indication of likely afterload against which the heart will be working.[25,75,78] Continuing to monitor BP during the activity helps the clinician to recognize if the exercising cardiovascular system can meet the requirements of an increasing workload.[75] Calculation of the RPP (HR × BP) may be a more accurate estimate of cardiac workload for older adults.[78-81]

Perceived Exertion

Ratings of perceived exertion are also effective indicators of the level of physiological exertion experienced by patients who are exercising or involved in a strenuous physical activity[75,95,96] (Table 4-4).

These scales ask individuals to assess subjectively how much effort they are expending during an exercise session or activity, with higher ratings indicating greater effort. Similar scales have been developed to assess breathlessness, fatigue, and discomfort or pain during exercise (Table 4-5). In the clinical use of these ratings of perceived exertion, many older persons using ratings of perceived exertion tend to overestimate their true physiological stress, as indicated by their HR during exercise sessions.[75,95] Clinicians who appropriately, but bravely, recommend exercise for older adults relying on perceived exertion to limit the activity safely may find this phenomenon comforting.

Exercise Testing Protocols

Standard exercise testing protocols are appropriate for assessment of the status of conditioning of the cardiovascular system and exercise tolerance of older adults.[76,97] The "gold standard" treadmill test, a cycle ergometer, or a step test can be used in assessing cardiovascular performance of the older person, unless the specific clinical setting or associated musculoskeletal dysfunction (e.g., balance problems, arthritic joints, or lower extremity muscle weakness) precludes this type of testing.[76] Alternatives for individuals who can walk distances include the One-Mile Walk Test[98] and the Six-Minute Walk Test.[99,100] A brief step test performed while sitting in a chair has been developed for individuals who cannot otherwise be safely tested on a treadmill, with an ergometer, or by distance walked.[75,101]

Careful monitoring of HR and BP before the sitting step test, at predetermined points during testing, at the completion of a brief bout of exercise, and a short while into recovery from the exercise bout provides a comprehensive picture of cardiovascular function of any given older patient. This information often proves important in clinical decision making and program planning. Similarly, careful monitoring of HR and BP before, during, and after a bout of exercise during rehabilitation allows the clinician to compare the

Table 4-4
Borg Scales: Ratings of Perceived Exertion

Linear Scale		*Ratio Scale*	
Value	*Description*	*Value*	*Description*
6	No exertion	0	No effort at all
7–8	Extremely light effort	1	Very little (very weak) effort
9–10	Very light effort	2	Light (weak) effort
11–12	Light effort	3	Moderate effort
13–14	Somewhat hard effort	4	Somewhat strong effort
15–16	Heavy or hard	5–6	Strong effort
17–18	Very hard effort	7–8	Very strong effort
19	Extremely hard effort	9	Extremely strong effort
20	Maximum exertion	10	Maximal exertion

Modified from Borg G, Ottoson D. *The Perception of Exertion in Physical Work.* London: Macmillan, 1986.

Table 4-5
Ratio Scales of Perceived Breathlessness, Fatigue, or Discomfort during Exercise

Value	*Breathlessness/Dyspnea*	*Fatigue*	*Discomfort or Pain*
0	No breathlessness at all	No fatigue at all	No pain or discomfort
1	Very light breathlessness	Very light fatigue	Very little (weak) pain
2	Light breathlessness	Light fatigue	Little (weak) discomfort
3	Moderate breathlessness	Moderate fatigue	Moderate discomfort
4	Somewhat hard to breathe	Somewhat hard	Somewhat strong discomfort
5–6	Heavy breathing	Heavy work/fatigue	Strong discomfort or pain
7–8	Very heavy breathing	Very heavy fatigue	Very heavy discomfort
9	Very, very breathless	Very, very fatigued	Very, very hard discomfort
10	Maximum breathlessness	Maximally fatigued	Maximal discomfort or pain

Modified from Dean E. Mobilization and exercise. In Frownfelten D, Dean E (eds), *Principles and Practice of Cardiopulmonary Physical Therapy*, 3rd ed. St. Louis: Mosby, 1996, p. 282.

pattern of responses with the expected pattern for conditioned adults.[102] Normal exercise-induced cardiovascular responses include a slow rate of rise of HR, a rise in SBP, and minimal (if any) rise in diastolic BP during the exercise bout. For the conditioned older adult, HR and SBP should return toward preexercise values during the immediate postexercise recovery period on the order of 50% of the changes during exercise. The pattern of change in the RPP for the exercise bout and recovery period may be an even more descriptive measure of the cardiovascular response.

Expecting individuals who are significantly deconditioned, can barely tolerate sitting for 30 minutes, are short of breath after 10 repetitions of simple lower extremity exercises while sitting, or are fatigued after 5 minutes of a sitting step test to be fully able to participate in gait and balance training is unreasonable. How can older individuals who are working at 90% or more of their maximum target HR be truly concerned with much more than delivering oxygen to the working tissues? Deconditioned individuals who are working at a high intensity in simple, well-known tasks have seriously restricted energy reserves; they are likely to have difficulty with focus and attention, processing, and the therapist's directions and supporting muscle activity—all necessary components for motor learning in performing a new skill such as gait training with a prosthetic device. Under these circumstances emphasis must first be placed on improving cardiovascular conditioning, to improve energy reserves so that subsequent functional training with an orthosis or prosthesis has greater likelihood of a successful outcome.

Physical Performance Training

The same principles of training that are used with young adult athletes can be adapted and applied to frail or deconditioned older adults who are recovering from amputation in prosthetic rehabilitation or a neuromuscular or musculoskeletal event that necessitates use of an orthosis. The primary goals of conditioning for frail individuals are: (1) to develop enough aerobic capacity to do work and (2) to ensure efficient muscle function to produce work.[75,76,103] These concepts can guide any single rehabilitation session, as well as the progression of the rehabilitation program over time. An understanding of exercise for improving fitness and of the few physiological age-related changes in cardiopulmonary function provide a foundation for exercise prescription, which then is individualized on the basis of current exercise tolerance of a specific older patient. This strategy can likely optimize the performance and recovery of older adults in rehabilitation.

An effective strategy to improve cardiopulmonary response to exercise and activity for older patients who are deconditioned by bed rest, acute illness, or sedentary lifestyle begins with a warm-up of continuous alternating movements using large muscle groups, particularly of the lower extremities. The goal of such activity is facilitation of the preload and SV; any increase in SV realized through this training regimen helps an older patient to maximize cardiovascular function despite age-associated limitations in HR, cardioacceleratory responses, and baroreceptor sensitivity.

For healthy young adults the recommended regimen for aerobic conditioning and endurance training involves at least three sessions per week of 30 to 60 minutes' duration in activities that use large muscles (running, cycling, swimming, brisk walking) and keep HR in a target range between 60% and 80% of the individual's maximal attainable HR.[104] This may be unreasonable for an older adult who is recovering from an acute illness, habitually sedentary, or coping with age- or pathology-related impairments of cardiac or pulmonary function. Evidence suggests that, for older adults who are deconditioned, slower but significant improvement in work capacity can occur at exercise intensities as low as 30% to 45% of maximal HR.[87,105-107] Although high-frequency, high-intensity exercise can maximize increase in work capacity (VO_2max), high-intensity exercise performed less frequently and low-intensity exercise performed more frequently can also yield positive endurance training effects.[107] Evidence is also growing of improvement in oxygen extraction and muscle function when elders are involved in regular endurance training.[90]

In addition to aerobic conditioning, the rehabilitation program might include exercises that focus on flexibility. One goal of stretching and flexibility exercise for older adults is to preserve or restore any limited joint mobility that would otherwise compromise essential functions.[108] As flexibility of the trunk and thorax improves, a more effective alignment of the diaphragm and improved elastic recoil of the chest wall will have a positive impact on VC and inspiratory reserve volume and minimize RV, reducing the work of breathing and improving ventilation. Availability of essential range of motion is especially important for energy-efficient gait with lower limb orthoses or prostheses: Contracture of the hip, knee, or ankle has an impact on the alignment of orthotic and prosthetic components and often leads to greater sway and smaller stride length during gait, significantly increasing the energy cost or workload of walking.

Muscle strengthening can begin as soon as the aerobic conditioning appears adequate to oxygenate the peripheral muscular tissue sufficiently. Assessment of the adequacy of peripheral oxygenation might include monitoring the coloring of the distal extremities before and during exercise and noting whether cramping or claudication occurs during exercise. One of the most sensitive indicators of appropriate intensity and duration of exercise is whether the activity can be increased without a marked rise in respiratory rate or onset of shortness of breath; a potent stimulus for frequency of breathing is the pH of the exercising tissues, with decreases as lactic acid builds up during anaerobic exercise.[73,74]

Two factors should be considered when including strengthening exercises in a rehabilitation program.[94] First, is there adequate muscle strength for consistent and safe performance of the motor tasks needed for functional independence (including the use of assistive devices)? Second, is the muscle mass large enough to support a VO_2max that allows activities of daily living to represent a light to modest work intensity level? For many older people who have lost muscle mass (whether as a result of disuse and sedentary lifestyle or because of recent health problems that limit activity), development of more muscle mass increases lean body mass and improves the basal metabolic rate, improving overall health, fitness, and functional status.[109,110]

ENERGY COST OF WALKING

The human body is designed to be energy efficient during upright bipedal gait. Muscles of the trunk and extremities are activated by the CNS in a precise rhythmic cycle to move the body forward while maintaining dynamic stability, adapting stride length and gait speed to the constraints and demands of the task, the force of gravity, and the characteristics of the environment in which walking is occurring.[111,112] The advancing foot is lifted just enough to clear the surface in swing, and muscle activity at the stance-side hip and lower torso keeps the pelvis fairly level and the trunk erect, minimizing vertical displacement of the body's center of mass.[113] Normal arthrokinematic and osteokinematic relationships between body segments ensure a narrow base of support in quiet stance and relaxed walking, and reciprocal arm swing counterbalances the dynamic pendular motion of the lower extremities, ensuring that the center of mass progresses forward with minimal mediolateral sway.[113-116] Much of the energy cost of walking is related to the muscular work performed to keep the center of mass moving forward with a minimum of vertical and mediolateral displacement.[117]

Any musculoskeletal or neuromuscular pathology that interferes with alignment of body segments, the carefully controlled sequential activation of muscles, or the effectiveness of muscle contraction increases the energy cost of walking. As vertical displacement and mediolateral sway increase and gait deviations occur, muscles must work harder to keep the center of mass moving forward despite extraneous displacing moments. As muscle work increases, the cardiopulmonary system responds to this physiological demand with increased HR, SV, and respiratory rate. Any orthosis or prosthesis that adds mass to or alters movement of the lower extremity potentially increases the work of walking. However, in individuals with amputation or neuromuscular dysfunction, walking with an appropriate prosthesis or orthosis may actually require less energy than walking without it.[117-119]

Measuring Energy Costs of Walking

Measurement of physiological energy expenditure by direct calorimetry is not realistic in all but the most sophisticated research laboratory settings. Instead, several indirect indicators have been found to be reliable estimates of the energy cost and the efficiency of gait in research and clinical applications. These include calculation of oxygen consumption (VO_2max) and oxygen cost while walking, monitoring blood lactate levels, calculating the physiological cost index (PCI) of walking, and monitoring heart and respiratory rates during activity.

Oxygen Rate and Oxygen Cost

The most precise indirect measurements of energy and gait efficiency use special equipment (e.g., a portable spirometer or a Douglas bag) to monitor ventilatory volumes and to measure how much oxygen is taken in and carbon dioxide exhaled during physical activity. This type of testing is usually done while the subject or patient walks, runs on a treadmill or track, or cycles on a stationary bicycle. The rate of *oxygen consumption* (O_2 rate), measured as volume of oxygen consumed per unit of body weight in 1 minute (ml/kg/min), provides an index of intensity of physical work at any given time.[115,120] VO_2max is the highest rate of oxygen uptake possible and is determined by progressing the exercise test to the point of voluntary exhaustion, when the age-adjusted maximum attainable HR is approached or reached.[121,122]

If oxygen consumption during gait is low, an individual is likely to be able to walk long distances. If it is high, however, the distance of functional gait is likely to be limited. The *oxygen cost* of walking is determined by dividing the rate of oxygen consumption by the speed of walking. Oxygen cost is a precise indicator of efficiency of gait, the amount of energy expended to walk over a standard distance (ml/kg/m).[115] Most of what researchers currently understand about energy expenditure when using a prosthesis or orthosis is based on studies that have measured oxygen rate and oxygen cost of walking.

Serum Lactate

The energy efficiency of walking is also assessed by evaluation of serum carbon dioxide and lactate levels as indicators of anaerobic energy production. The energy (adenosine triphosphate [ATP]) required for muscle contraction during gait can be derived from a combination of aerobic oxidative and anaerobic glycolytic pathways.[123] The aerobic oxidative pathway, which depends on oxygen delivery to active muscle cells, is the most efficient source of energy, producing almost 19 times as much ATP as the anaerobic pathway. In healthy, fit individuals, this aerobic pathway is more than able to meet energy requirements of relaxed walking. If energy demands of an exercise or activity are met by aerobic oxidation, the activity can be sustained for long periods with relatively low levels of fatigue. As activity becomes strenuous (i.e., as gait speed or surface incline increases) and the need for energy begins to exceed the availability of oxygen for aerobic oxidation, additional energy is accessed through anaerobic metabolism.[124] This transition to anaerobic metabolism is reported to begin at work levels of 55% of VO_2max in healthy, untrained individuals but may begin at 80% of VO_2max in highly trained athletes.[125]

When the ability to deliver oxygen is compromised by the physical deconditioning of a sedentary lifestyle or by cardiac, pulmonary, or musculoskeletal pathology, anaerobic glycolysis becomes a primary source of energy at lower levels of work.[126] Whenever the anaerobic pathway is the major source of energy, blood levels of lactate and carbon dioxide rise, lowering blood pH and increasing the respiratory exchange ratio (CO_2 production/O_2 consumption).[127] Under these conditions, the ability to sustain activity is limited, with an earlier onset of fatigue as workload increases. Serum lactate levels are most often used in studies of assisted ambulation using hybrid orthotic/functional electrical stimulation systems for those with spinal cord injury.

Heart Rate and Physiological Cost Index

High correlations between HR and oxygen consumption during gait have been reported for children and for healthy young adults at a variety of gait speeds.[128,129] Although this suggests that HR monitoring may be a reliable substitute for oxygen rate determination, it should be used with caution in older adults because of the age-related changes in cardiopulmonary function discussed earlier in this chapter. This is especially true for older adults with heart disease who are being managed with medications that further blunt HR response.[130-131] The RPP or the PCI may be more appropriate indicators of the energy cost of walking in these circumstances. The Physiological Cost Index (PCI) is calculated as follows[132]:

$$\text{PCI} = (\text{HR walking} - \text{HR resting}) \div \text{gait speed}$$

Measured in beats per meter, the PCI reflects the effort of walking; low values suggest energy-efficient gait. The PCI was originally used to assess gait restrictions in adults with rheumatoid arthritis and similar inflammatory joint disease.[132] For children between 3 and 12 years of age, the mean PCI at self-selected or preferred gait speed has been reported to be between 0.38 and 0.40 beats per meter.[133] Typical PCI values for adolescents and young adults at usual gait speeds ranged from .3 to .4 beats per meter.[134] In a study of healthy adults older than the age of 65, the mean PCI value when walking on a flat 10-m track was .43 + .13 beats per meter; when calculated while walking on a treadmill, mean PCI increased to .60 + .26 beats per meter.[135]

The PCI has been used to assess the effect of different assistive devices on the effort of walking,[136] evaluate the short- and long-term impact on neuromuscular stimulation on the ability to walk and run in older adults and in children with hemiplegia,[137-141] assess outcomes of orthopedic surgery in children with cerebral palsy,[142] and evaluate the efficacy of reciprocal gait orthosis/functional electrical stimulation systems for individuals with spinal cord injury.[143-145] High correlation among the PCI, percent maximum HR, and oxygen rate ($r = 0.91$, $p > .005$) in able-bodied children and children with transtibial amputation supports its validity as an indicator of energy cost for children.[146] A similar study of energy cost of walking in young adults using a microprocessor-controlled transfemoral prosthesis suggests that PCI is comparable with oxygen uptake as an indicator of the energy cost of walking.[147] The PCI has also been used to compare energy cost of walking in different types of transfemoral prosthetic sockets[148] and assess efficacy of a stance control knee orthosis.[149]

Studies of variability in PCI values on repeated measures have raised questions about its accuracy and sensitivity to change in energy cost of gait, as compared with monitoring of oxygen consumption and oxygen cost.[150-152] Although the relationship between PCI and the "gold standards" of oxygen consumption and oxygen cost may not be strong enough for researchers, it remains an important tool for clinicians who lack the technology necessary to monitor oxygen consumption and cost yet want to estimate the energy cost of walking and assess the impact of orthotic or prosthetic rehabilitation over time.

Energy Expenditure in Normal Gait

The energy requirements of walking vary with age and gait speed.[154-158] Oxygen consumption is highest in childhood and decreases to approximately 12 ml/kg/min in healthy adults and elders.[155] When oxygen consumption during walking is expressed as a percent of VO_2max, a slightly different picture emerges. For a healthy, untrained young adult, oxygen consumption at a comfortable walking speed may be 32% of VO_2max, whereas for an older adult walking at a similar speed, oxygen consumption may be as much as 48% of VO_2max.[113,159] For functional gait, if walking is to cover large distances or is to be sustained over long periods of time, oxygen consumption must be less than 50% of that individual's VO_2max so that aerobic oxidation will be used as the primary source of energy.[5] At comfortable gait speeds, older adults are working nearer the threshold for transition to anaerobic metabolism than are younger adults. If some form of gait dysfunction is superimposed, increasing the energy cost of gait, the work of walking will transition to anaerobic glycolysis unless a cardiovascular conditioning program is included in the rehabilitation program.[160]

For individuals without neuromuscular or musculoskeletal impairment, the relationship between the energy cost of walking and gait speed is nearly linear[155,161] (Figure 4-6). Gait is most efficient, as indicated by oxygen cost (O_2 rate/velocity), at an individual's self-selected or customary walking speed; energy requirements increase whenever gait speed is much slower or much faster.[162-164] The customary walking speed of most individuals with neuromuscular or musculoskeletal impairments is often much slower, a strategy that minimizes the rate of energy used during walking. As a result of slower speed, however, it takes longer to cover any

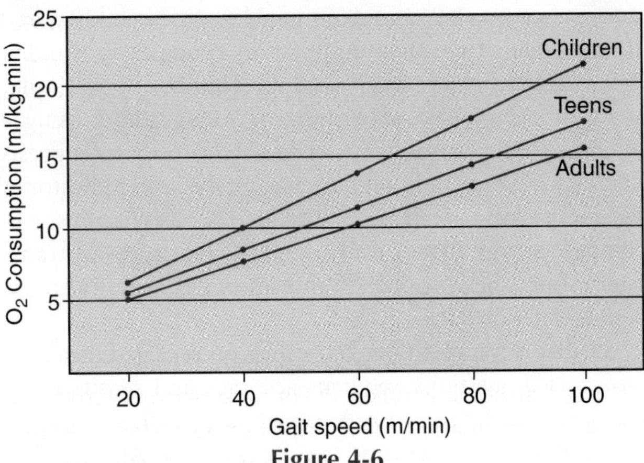

Figure 4-6

Relationship between gait speed and oxygen consumption (O_2 rate). The differences in O_2 rate between children and adults (20 to 80 years) are attributed, in part, to differences in body composition. (From gait-velocity regression formulas reported by RL Waters. Energy expenditure. In Perry J [ed], Gait Analysis: Normal and Pathological Function. *Thorofare, NJ: Slack, 1992. pp. 443-489.)*

given distance. Any impairment that reduces gait speed leads to increased oxygen cost, even if oxygen consumption remains close to normal.[165-170]

The weight and design of the prosthesis or orthosis are also determinants of energy cost of gait. The impact of added mass on the energy cost of gait depends on where the load is placed: Extra weight loaded on the trunk (such as a heavy backpack) changes oxygen rate during walking less than would a smaller load placed around the ankle.[171] This highlights the importance of minimizing weight of lower extremity orthoses and prostheses to keep the energy cost of walking within an individual's aerobic capacity.[172]

Work of Walking with an Orthosis

When discussing the energy cost of walking with an orthosis, it is important to remember that, for those with significant neuromuscular or musculoskeletal impairment, the energy cost of walking without the orthosis is typically higher than walking with an appropriate orthosis.[173-175] One of the determinants of energy cost when walking with a cast or an orthosis is the degree of immobility that the orthosis imposes on the ankle, knee, and hip and the associated change in gait speed.[170,176] For individuals with restriction of knee motion because of a cast or orthosis, the energy cost of gait can be reduced by placing a shoe lift on the contralateral limb to improve swing limb clearance.[177]

For individuals with spinal cord injury, regardless of age, the potential for functional ambulation appears to be determined by four conditions: the ability to use a reciprocal gait pattern, the adequacy of trunk stability, at least fair hip flexor strength bilaterally, and fair quadriceps strength of at least one limb.[178-179] This corresponds to an ambulatory motor index (AMI) score of 18 of 30 possible points, or 60% of "good" lower extremity strength.[179] In this instance, gait may be possible with bilateral ankle-foot orthoses (AFOs) or an AFO and knee-ankle-foot orthosis combination. Those with spinal cord injury at mid to low thoracic levels with AMI scores of less than 60% often require bilateral knee-ankle-foot orthoses, with Lofstrand or axillary crutches in a swing-through gait pattern to ambulate. Waters[117] reports a near linear positive relationship between AMI scores and gait velocity, as well as a somewhat curvilinear inverse relationship between AMI score and oxygen rate (% above normal), and oxygen cost. For persons with spinal cord injury who have the potential for functional ambulation, continued cardiovascular conditioning after discharge from rehabilitation improves the efficiency of walking, as reflected in lower oxygen cost and improvement in gait speed.[179-181] The development of reciprocal gait orthoses and "parawalkers," at times augmented by functional electrical stimulation, has also made modified ambulation possible for those with injury at mid and upper thoracic levels.[182-190] The high energy cost of the intense upper extremity work using crutches to propel the body forward during swing and maintain upright position in stance, however, restricts functional ambulation as a primary means of mobility.

The movement dysfunction associated with stroke and other neuromuscular impairments tends to reduce gait speed, with the degree of slowing determined by the severity of neuromuscular impairment.[166,174,191] As abnormal movement patterns and impaired postural responses compromise the cyclic and dynamic flow of walking, the higher levels of muscle activity that are required to remain upright and to move forward increase the energy cost of gait.[192,193] Reduction of gait speed is a functional strategy to keep energy expenditure within physiological limits. Oxygen rate (consumption) of persons with stroke who walk at a reduced gait speed is close to that of elders who walk at their customary gait speed. However, oxygen cost is significantly higher.[117,166,194] When compared with unimpaired individuals who walk at similar speeds, persons with hemiplegia wearing an AFO use 52% more energy; when they walk without an orthosis, their energy cost can increase to as much as 65% more than unimpaired gait.[195]

Work of Walking with a Prosthesis

The characteristics of gait and the energy cost of walking with a prosthesis are related to the etiology and the level of amputation.[196,197] The gait speed, stride length, and cadence of persons with lower extremity amputation who walk with a prosthesis are typically lower than those of individuals without impairment, regardless of the cause of amputation,[198] although individuals with traumatic etiology tend to walk faster than those with dysvascular etiology.[199-200]

Additionally, biomechanical and energy efficiency of prosthetic gait decreases as amputation level increases: Preservation of the anatomical knee joint appears to be especially important.[198,201]

A classic study by Waters and colleagues[198] (Table 4-6) demonstrated that, for young adults with traumatic transtibial amputation, gait speed, oxygen rate, and oxygen cost were quite close to normal values reported by Perry.[113] For those with traumatic transfemoral or dysvascular amputation, diminishing gait speeds kept oxygen consumption close to that of normal adult gait; however, oxygen cost increased well beyond the normal value of 0.15 mg/kg/m.[200] Although gait speeds reported 20 years later by Torburn and colleagues[199] are much higher (most likely due to biomechanical advances in prosthetic components in the time between the studies), the difference in performance between traumatic and dysvascular groups was consistent. Other studies report oxygen costs of prosthetic gait at between 16% and 28% above normal for individuals with transtibial amputation[202-203] and between 60% and 110% above normal for individuals with transfemoral amputation.[204-206] Although the relationship between gait speed and oxygen rate (consumption) in prosthetic gait is linear, just as it is in unimpaired gait, the slope is significantly steeper[207]: the clinical implication of this relationship is that the rate of energy consumption and of cardiac work, at any gait speed, is higher for those with amputation and that the threshold for transition from aerobic to anaerobic metabolism is reached at lower gait speeds.[208]

Several explanations are possible for the differences in prosthetic gait performance after traumatic versus dysvascular amputation. Because those with dysvascular amputation are typically older than those with traumatic amputation, differences in performance may be the result of age-related changes and concurrent cardiovascular disease in the dysvascular group.[202,209,210] For many older patients with dysvascular amputation, the energy source for walking with a prosthesis may be anaerobic rather than the more efficient aerobic metabolic pathways.[199] A larger cardiac and respiratory functional reserve capacity in younger persons with traumatic transtibial amputation may permit them to meet the increased metabolic demands of prosthetic use, as proximal muscle groups work for longer periods at higher intensities to compensate for the loss of those at the ankle.[199,207,211]

Importantly, for most individuals with unilateral transtibial and transfemoral amputation, regardless of age or etiology of amputation, the energy cost of walking with a prosthesis is less than that expended when walking without it using crutches or a walker.[200] For most persons with a new transtibial amputation, the ability to ambulate before amputation is the best predictor of tolerance of the increased energy cost of walking with a prosthesis after surgery.[209] For some older individuals with transfemoral amputation and concurrent cardiovascular or respiratory disease, and for those with bilateral amputation at transfemoral/transtibial or bilateral transfemoral levels, wheelchair mobility may be preferred.[212-215]

Since the 1990s significant efforts have been made to reduce the energy cost of prosthetic gait by developing dynamic response (energy storing) prosthetic feet[216-227] and cadence-responsive and microprocessor-controlled prosthetic knee units[228-230] using lightweight but durable materials in prosthetic sockets and components and improving the fit and alignment of the prosthesis.[231,232] The flexible keels of most dynamic response prosthetic feet are designed to mimic those of normal ankle mobility, such that mechanical energy stored by compression during stance is released to enhance "push-off" in the terminal stance.[218] The impact of different prosthetic foot designs on the energy cost is not clear, however. For adults with transtibial amputation, the FlexFoot functioned more like an anatomical ankle than did four other dynamic response feet and the SACH foot, but little difference in stride, velocity, or energy cost was noted.[199,211,221,222] However, the materials and design of most dynamic response feet may enable transtibial prosthetic

Table 4-6
Gait Speed, Oxygen Consumption, and Oxygen Cost in Prosthetic Gait: Comparison of Etiology and Level of Unilateral Amputation

Etiology and Level: Parameter	*Traumatic Transtibial*	*Traumatic Transfemoral*	*Dysvascular Transtibial*	*Dysvascular Transfemoral*
Waters et al, 1976[199]				
Gait speed (m/min)	71	52	45	36
O_2 rate (ml/kg/min)	12.4	10.3	9.4	10.8
O_2 cost (ml/kg/m)	0.16	0.20	0.20	0.28
Torburn et al, 1995[198]				
Gait speed (m/min)	82.3	–	61.7	–
O_2 rate (ml/kg/min)	17.7	–	13.2	–
O_2 cost (ml/kg/m)	0.22	–	0.21	–

users to jump, run, and use a step-over step pattern in stair climbing; these activities are difficult or not possible with a traditional SACH foot.[223-227] Additionally, many individuals with transtibial amputation wear their prosthesis for longer periods during the day and report less fatigue in prolonged walking when using a prosthesis with a dynamic response foot.[209]

SUMMARY

An understanding of normal cardiopulmonary function and how it changes in aging, as a result of sedentary lifestyle or pathological conditions, provides a necessary foundation for rehabilitation professionals working with patients who require an orthosis or prosthesis to walk. This chapter has reviewed the anatomy and physiology of the cardiopulmonary system, with attention to age-related changes, energy expenditure, and principles of aerobic conditioning for older adults.

Optimal performance of the cardiopulmonary system is influenced by three interrelated factors. First, the patient must have sufficient flexibility and mobility of the trunk for efficient and uncompromised ventilation. Second, adequate mobility of the extremities and excursion of the joints must be present for efficient performance of functional tasks. Third, the individual must have enough muscle mass, strength, and endurance to support the performance of the activity and function of the heart. Immediate and ongoing interventions that functionally enhance preload by returning blood to the older heart and avoidance of conditions (e.g., isometric muscle contraction and Valsalva maneuvers) that unnecessarily increase afterload can result in marked improvement in physical performance of the older person. With these conditions, as well as compensation for the beta-adrenergic receptor-reduced sensitivity with a prolonged period of warm-up exercises, an older person is capable of physical performance that is quite similar to that of younger counterparts and essential for the process of recovery of function for the optimal outcome of rehabilitation.

The energy cost and efficiency of gait are affected by aging, deconditioning of a sedentary lifestyle, and neuromuscular and musculoskeletal impairments that alter motor control or the biomechanics of walking. Although an orthosis that restricts joint motion increases the energy cost in unimpaired individuals, the same orthosis leads to more efficient gait in those with neuromuscular impairment. Determinants of efficiency of prosthetic gait include the level and etiology of the amputation. Reduction of gait speed when using an orthosis or prosthesis helps to maintain oxygen consumption at close to normal levels; however, this tends to compromise overall efficiency of gait, as indicated by oxygen cost. Attention to the principles of cardiovascular conditioning including monitoring the response to exercise so that patients are challenged appropriately optimizes the outcomes of rehabilitation programs.

REFERENCES

1. Des Jardins TR. *Cardiopulmonary Anatomy and Physiology: Essentials for Respiratory Care.* Albany, NY: Delmar Publishers, 1998.
2. Phibbs B. *The Human Heart: a Basic Guide to Heart Disease.* Philadelphia: Lippincott-Raven Publishers, 1997.
3. Saltin B, Secher NH, Mitchel J, et al (eds). *Exercise and Circulation in Health and Disease.* Champaign, IL: Human Kinetics, 2000.
4. Ekblom B, Astrand P, Saltin B, et al. Effect of training on circulatory response to exercise. *J Appl Physiol* 1968;24(4): 518-528.
5. Astrand P, Rodahl K. *Textbook of Work Physiology: the Physiological Bases of Exercise,* 3rd ed. New York: McGraw-Hill, 1986.
6. Pugh KG, Wei JY. Clinical implications of physiological changes in the aging heart. *Drugs Aging,* 2001;18(4):263-276.
7. Rehman HU. Age and the cardiovascular system. *Hosp Med* 1999;60(9):645-650.
8. Roffe C. Ageing of the heart. *Br J Biomed Sci* 1998;55(2): 136-148.
9. Schulman SP. Cardiovascular consequences of the aging process. *Cardiol Clin* 1999;17(1):35-49.
10. Alexander NB, Dengel DR, Olson RJ, et al. Oxygen uptake (VO_2) kinetics and functional mobility performance in impaired older adults. *J Gerontol Biol Med Sci* 2003;58(8): 734-739.
11. Wei JY, Epstein FH. Age and the cardiovascular system. *N Engl J Med* 1992;327(24):1735-1739.
12. Lakatta EG, Sollott SJ. Perspectives on mammalian cardiovascular aging: humans to molecules. *Comp Biochem Physiol A Mol Integr Physiol* 2002;132(4):699-722.
13. Olivetti G, Melissari M, Capsso JM, et al. Cardiomyopathy of the aging human heart: myocyte loss and reactive cellular hypertrophy. *Circ Res* 1991;68(6):1560-1568.
14. Olivetti G, Cigola E, Maestri R, et al. Recent advances in cardiac hypertrophy. *Cardiovasc Res* 2000;45(1):68-75.
15. Kitzman DW, Scholz DG, Hagen PT, et al. Age-related changes in normal human hearts during the first ten decades. Part II (Maturity): a quantitative anatomic study of 765 specimens from subjects 70 to 99 years old. *Mayo Clin Proc* 1988;63(2):137-146.
16. Lakatta EG. Do hypertension and aging have similar effect on the myocardium? *Circulation* 1987;75(Suppl 1):69-77.
17. Smulyan H, Safar ME. Systolic blood pressure revisited. *J Am Coll Cardiol* 1997;29(7):1407-1413.
18. Roberts WC, Shirani J. Comparison of cardiac findings at necropsy in octogenarians, nonagenarians, and centenarians. *Am J Cardiol* 1998;82(5):627-631.
19. Selzer A. Changing aspects of the natural history of valvular aortic stensosis. *N Engl J Med* 1987;317(2):91-98.
20. Seals DR, Monahan KD, Bell C, et al. The aging cardiovascular system: changes in autonomic function at rest and in response to exercise. *Int J Sport Nutr Exerc Metab* 2001;11(Suppl):S189-195.
21. Davy KP, Seals DR, Tanaka H. Augmented cardiopulmonary and integrative sympathetic baroreflexes but attenuated peripheral vasoconstriction with age. *Hypertension* 1998;32(2):298-304.

22. Rodeheffer RJ, Gerstenblith G, Becker LC, et al. Exercise cardiac output is maintained with advancing age in healthy human subjects: cardiac dilation and increased stroke volume compensate for a diminished heart rate. *Circulation* 1984;69(2):203-213.
23. Ghali JK, Liao Y, Cooper RS. Left ventricular hypertrophy in the elderly. *Am J Geriatr Cardiol* 1997;6(1):38-49.
24. Kitzman DW. Aging and the heart. *Dev Cardiol* 1994;1(1):1-15.
25. Lakatta EB, Mitchell JH, Pomerance A, et al. Human aging: changes in structure and function III. Characteristics of specific cardiovascular diseases in the elderly. *J Am Coll Cardiol* 1987;10(2SupplA):42-47.
26. Paulus WJ, Vantrimpont PJ, Rousseau MF. Diastolic function of the nonfilling human left ventricle. *J Am Coll Cardiol* 1992;20(7):1524-1532.
27. Kitzman DW, Edwards WE. Age-related changes in the anatomy of the normal human heart. *J Gerontol Biol Med Sci* 1990;45(1):33-39.
28. Binder EF, Schechtman KB, Ehsani AA, et al. Effects of exercise training on frailty in community dwelling older adults: results of a randomized controlled clinical trial. *J Am Geriatr Soc* 2002;50(12):1921-1928.
29. Lakatta EG. Cardiovascular regulatory mechanism in advanced age. *Physiol Rev* 1993;73(2):413-467.
30. Shiaishi I, Takamatsu T, Minamikawa T, et al. Quantitative histological analysis of the human sinoatrial node during growth and aging. *Circulation* 1992;85(6):2176-2184.
31. Erol-Yilmaz A, Schrama TA, Tanka JS, et al. Individual optimization of pacing sensors improves exercise capacity without influencing quality of life. *Pacing Clin Electrophysiol* 2005;28(1):17-25.
32. Squires RW. *Exercise Prescription for the High Risk Cardiac Patient.* Champaign, IL: Human Kinetics, 1998.
33. Tsakiris A, Doumas M, Nearchos N, et al. Aortic calcification is associated with age and sex but not left ventricular mass in essential hypertension. *J Clin Hypertens* 2004;6(2):65-70.
34. Lindroos M, Kupari M, Valvanne J, et al. Factors associated with calcific aortic valve degeneration in the elderly. *Eur Heart J* 1994;15(7):865-870.
35. Robert L. Aging of the vascular wall and atherosclerosis. *Exp Gerontol* 1999;34(4):491-501.
36. Newman AB, Arnold AM, Burke GL, et al. Cardiovascular disease and mortality in older adults with small abdominal aortic aneurysms detected by ultrasonography: the cardiovascular health study. *Ann Intern Med* 2001;134(3):182-190.
37. Lakatta EG. Altered autonomic modulation of cardiovascular function with adult aging; perspectives from studies ranging from man to cells. In HL Stone, WB Weglicki (eds), *Pathobiology of Cardiovascular Injury.* Boston: Martinus Nijhoff, 1985. pp. 441-460.
38. Turner MJ, Mier CM, Spina RJ, et al. Effects of aging and gender on cardiovascular responses to isoproterenol. *J Gerontol* 1999;54A(9):B393-400.
39. Lakatta EG. Cardiovascular regulatory mechanisms in advanced age. *Physiol Rev* 1993;73(2):413-467.
40. Shimada K, Kitazumi T, Ogura H. Differences in age-dependent effects of blood pressure on baroreflex sensitivity between normal and hypertensive subjects. *Clin Sci* 1986;70(5):763-766.
41. Guyton AC, Hall JE. Textbook of Medical Physiology. Philadelphia: Saunders, 1996.
42. Mukai S, Lipsitz LA. Orthostatic hypotension. *Clin Geriatr Med* 2002;18(2):253-268.
43. Jansen RW, Lipsitz LA. Postprandial hypotension: epidemiology, pathophysiology, and clinical management. *Ann Intern Med* 1995;122(4):286-295.
44. Gardin JM, Arnold AM, Bild DE, et al. Left ventricular diastolic filling in the elderly: the cardiovascular health study. *Am J Cardiol* 1998;82(3):345-352.
45. Kitzman DW, Higginbotham MB, Sullivan MJ. Aging and the cardiovascular response to exercise. *Cardiol Elderly* 1993;1(6):543-550.
46. Green JS, Crouse SF. Endurance training, cardiovascular function, and the aged. *Sports Med* 1993;16(5):331-341.
47. Cheitlin MD. Cardiovascular physiology—changes with age. *Am J Geriatr Cardiol* 2003;12(1):9-13.
48. Steinberg DH. Diastolic dysfunction of the left ventricle. A review of the physiology, causes, diagnosis, treatment, and implications. *J Insur Med* 1997;29(2):12-125.
49. Port S, Cobb FR, Coleman E, et al. Effect of age on the response of the left ventricular ejection fraction to exercise. *N Engl J Med* 1980;303(20):1133-1137.
50. Nichols WW, O'Rourke MF, Avolio AP. Effects of age on ventricular-vascular coupling. *Am J Cardiol* 1985;55(9): 1179-1184.
51. Devereux RB, Roman MJ, Paranicas M, et al. A population-based assessment of left ventricular systolic dysfunction in middle-aged and older adults: the Strong Heart Study. *Am Heart J* 2001;141(3):439-446.
52. Lakatta EG. Changes in cardiovascular function with aging. *Eur Heart J* 1990;11(Suppl C):22-29.
53. Jurimae T, Jurimae J, Pihl E. Circulatory response to single circuit weight and walking training sessions of similar energy cost in middle-aged overweight females. *Clin Physiol* 2000;20(2):143-149.
54. Vaitkevicius PV, Ebersold C, Muhammad S, et al. Effects of aerobic exercise training in community-based subjects aged 80 and older: a pilot study. *J Am Geriatr Soc* 2002;50(12):2009-2013.
55. Zadia CC. Pulmonary physiology of aging: the role of rehabilitation. *Top Geriatr Rehab* 1985;1(1):49-57.
56. Amara CE, Koval JJ, Paterson DH, et al. Lung function in older humans: the contribution of body composition, physical activity, and smoking. *Ann Human Biol* 2001;28(5):522-537.
57. McRae H. Cardiovascular and pulmonary function. In Spirduso WW, Francis KL, MacRae PG (eds), *Physical Dimensions of Aging,* 2nd ed. Champaign, IL: Human Kinetics, 2005. pp. 87-106.
58. Bourgeois MC, Zadai CC. Impaired ventilation and respiration in the older adult. In Guccione AA (ed), *Geriatric Physical Therapy.* St. Louis: Mosby, 2000. pp. 226-244.
59. Wright RR. Elastic tissue of normal and emphysematous lungs. *Am J Pathol* 1961;39(3):355-367.
60. Rossi A, Ganassini A, Tantucci C, et al. Aging and the respiratory system. *Aging* 1996;8(3):143-161.
61. Zaugg M, Lucchinetti E. Respiratory function in the elderly. *Anesthes Clin North Am* 2000;18(1):47-58.

62. Neuman DA. Arthokinesiologic considerations in the aged adult. In Guccione AA (ed), *Geriatric Physical Therapy.* St. Louis: Mosby, 2000. pp. 56-77.
63. Davidson WR, Fee EC. Influence of aging on pulmonary hemodynamics in a population free of coronary artery disease. *Am J Cardiol* 1990;65(22):1454-1458.
64. Dempsey JA, Seals DR. Ageing, exercise, and cardiopulmonary function. In Giolier CV, Nadel E (eds), *Perspectives in Exercise Science and Sports Medicine,* vol 8. Carmel, IN: Cooper Publishing, 1995. pp. 237-304.
65. Babb TG. Mechanical ventilatory constraints in aging, lung disease, and obesity: perspectives and brief review. *Med Sci Sports Exercise* 1999;31(Suppl 1):12-22.
66. Tolep K, Kelsen SG. Effects of aging in respiratory skeletal muscles. *Clin Chest Med* 1993;14(3):363-378.
67. Brooks SV, Faulkner JA. Effects of aging on the structure and function of skeletal muscle. In Roussos C (ed), *The Thorax.* New York: Academic Press, 1995. pp. 295-312.
68. Sadowsky HS. Cardiovascular and respiratory physiology. In Hillegass EA, Sadowsky HS (eds), *Essentials of Cardiopulmonary Physical Therapy,* 2nd ed. Philadelphia: Saunders, 2001, pp. 48-87.
69. McClaran SR, Babcock MA, Pegelow DF, et al. Longitudinal effects of aging on lung function at rest and exercise in healthy active elderly adults. *J Appl Physiol* 1995;78(5):1957-1968.
70. Zeleznik J. Normative aging of the respiratory system. *Clin Geriatr Med* 2003;19(1):1-18.
71. Camhi SL, Enright PL. How to assess pulmonary function in older persons. *J Resp Dis* 2000;21(6):395.
72. Stulberg M, Carrieri-Kohlman V. Conceptual approach to the treatment of dyspnea: focus on the role of exercise. *Cardiopulmonary Phys Ther* 1992;3(1):9-12.
73. Wasserman K, Casaburi R. Dyspnea: physiological and pathophysiologic mechanisms. *Ann Rev Med* 1988;39: 503-515.
74. Casaburi R, Patessio A, Ioli F. Reductions in exercise lactic acidosis and ventilation as a result of exercise training in patients with obstructive lung disease. *Am Rev Respir Dis* 1991;143(1):9-18.
75. Pollock ML, Wilmore JH (eds), *Exercise in Health and Disease.* Philadelphia: Saunders, 1990.
76. Kohrt WM, Brown M. Endurance training of the older adult. In Guccione AA (ed), *Geriatric Physical Therapy,* 2nd ed. St. Louis: Mosby, 2000. pp. 245-258.
77. Host HH, Sinacore DR, Turner MJ, et al. Oxygen uptakes at preferred gait velocities of frail elderly subjects. *Phys Ther* 1996;76(4):S69.
78. Naughton J. *Exercise Testing: Physiological, Biomedical, and Clinical Principles.* Mount Kisco, NY: Futura, 1988.
79. Kitamura K, Jorgensen CR, Gobel FL, et al. Hemodynamic correlates of myocardial oxygen consumption during upright exercise. *J Appl Physiol* 1972;32(4):516-522.
80. Ellestad MH. *Stress Testing: Principles and Practice,* 3rd ed. Philadelphia: F.A. Davis, 1986.
81. DeVries HA. *Physiology of Exercise,* 4th ed. Dubuque, IA: WMC Brown, 1986.
82. Tonino RP, Driscoll PA. Reliability of maximal and submaximal parameters of treadmill testing for the measurement of physical training in older persons. *J Gerontol* 1988;42(2):M101-104.
83. Materson BJ. Isolated systolic blood pressure: new answers, more questions. *J Am Geriatr Soc* 1991;39(12):1237-1238.
84. Applegate WB, Davis BR, Black HR. Prevalence of postural hypotension at baseline in the systolic hypertension in the elderly program (SHEP) cohort. *J Am Geriatr Soc* 1991;39(11):1057-1064.
85. Cahalin L, Sadowsky HS. Pulmonary medications. In Hillegass EA, Sadowsky HS (eds), *Essentials of Cardiopulmonary Physical Therapy,* 2nd ed. Philadelphia: Saunders, 2001. pp. 587-607.
86. Shepherd RJ. The cardiovascular benefits of exercise in the elderly. *Top Geriatr Rehab* 1985;1(1):1-10.
87. Badenhop DT, Cleary PA, Schaal SF, et al. Physiological adjustments to higher- or lower-intensity exercise in elders. *Med Sci Sports Exerc* 1983;15(6):496-502.
88. Hagberg JM, Allen WK, Seals DR. A hemodynamic comparison of young and older endurance athletes during exercise. *J Appl Physiol* 1985;58(6):2041-2046.
89. Julius S, Amery A, Whitlock LS, et al. Influence of age on the hemodynamic response to exercise. *Circulation* 1967;36(2):222-230.
90. Seals DR, Hagberg JM, Hurley BF, et al. Endurance training in older men and women. 1: Cardiovascular responses to exercise. *J Appl Physiol* 1984;57(4):1024-1029.
91. Higginbotham MB, Morris KG, Williams RS. Physiologic basis for the age related decline in aerobic work capacity. *Am J Cardiol* 1986;57(4):1374-1379.
92. Yarasheski KE. Managing sarcopenia with progressive resistance exercise training. *J Nutr Health Aging* 2002;6(5):349-356.
93. Martin L. Methods of assessing exercise capacity. In Cherniack NS, Altose MD, Homma I (eds), *Rehabilitation of the Patient with Respiratory Disease.* New York: McGraw-Hill, 1999. pp. 217-232.
94. Brown M. Muscle fatigue and impaired muscle endurance in older adults. In Guccione AA (ed), *Geriatric Physical Therapy,* 2nd ed. St. Louis: Mosby, 2000. pp. 259-264.
95. Borg G. Perceived exertion as an indicator of somatic stress. *Scand J Rehabil Med* 1970;2(3):92-97.
96. Borg G, Ottoson D. *The Perception of Exertion in Physical Work.* London: Macmillan, 1986.
97. Fleg JL. Diagnostic and prognostic value of stress testing in older persons. *J Am Geriatr Soc* 1995;43(2):190-194.
98. Kline GM, Porcari JP, Hintermeister R, et al. Estimation of VO_2max from a one-mile track walk, gender, age, and body weight. *Med Sci Sports Ex* 1987;19(3):253-259.
99. Butland RJ, Pang J, Gross ER, et al. Two- , six-, and 12-minute walking tests in respiratory disease. *Br Med J* 1982;284(6329):1607-1608.
100. Guyatt GH, Sullivan MJ, Thompson PJ, et al. The 6-minute walk test: a new measure of exercise capacity in patients with chronic heart failure. *Can Med Assoc J* 1985;132(8):9919-9923.
101. Smith EL, Gilligan C. Physical activity perception for the older adult. *Phys Sports Med* 1993;11:91-101.
102. Prentice WE. *Armheim's Principles of Athletic Training: a Competency Based Approach,* 12th ed. New York: McGraw-Hill, 2005.
103. Durstine JL, Moore GE. *ACSM's Exercise Management for Persons with Chronic Diseases and Disabilities,* 2nd ed. Champaign, IL: Human Kinetics, 2003.

104. Kaminsky LA, Bonzheim KA, Garber CE, et al (eds). *ACSM's Resource Manual for Guidelines for Exercise Testing and Prescription,* 5th ed. Philadelphia: Lippincott Williams & Wilkins, 2006.
105. Yerg JE, Seals DR, Hagberg JM, et al. Effects of endurance exercise training on ventilatory function in the older individual. *J Appl Physiol* 1985;58(3):791-794.
106. Frontera WR, Evans WJ. Exercise performance and endurance training in the elderly. *Top Geriatr Rehab* 1986;2(1):17-32.
107. Seals DR, Hagberg JM, Hurley BF, et al. Effects of endurance training on glucose tolerance and plasma lipid levels in older men and women. *JAMA* 1984;252(5):645-649.
108. Lewis CB, Kellems S. Musculoskeletal changes with age: clinical implications. In Lewis CB (ed), *Aging the Health Care Challenge,* 4th ed. Philadelphia: F.A. Davis, 2002. pp. 104-126.
109. Mazzeo RS, Tanaka H. Exercise prescription for the elderly; current recommendations. *Sports Med* 2001;31(11): 809-818.
110. Hunter GR, McCarthy JP, Bamman MM. Effects of resistance training on older adults. *Sports Med* 2004;34(5):329-348.
111. Palta AF. Neurobiomechanical bases for the control of human movement. In Bronstein A, Brandt T, Woollacott M (eds), *Clinical Disorders of Balance, Posture, and Gait.* London: Arnold; 1996. pp. 19-40.
112. Bianchi L, Angelini D, Orani GP, et al. Kinematic coordination in human gait: relation to mechanical energy cost. *J Neurophysiol* 1998;79(4):2155-2170.
113. Perry J. Basic functions. In Perry J (ed), *Gait Analysis: Normal and Pathological Function.* Thorofare, NJ: Slack, 1992. pp. 19-48.
114. Olney SJ. Gait. In Levangie PK, Norkin CC (eds), *Joint Structure and Function: A Comprehensive Analysis,* 4th ed. Philadelphia: F.A. Davis, 2005. pp. 517-568.
115. Winter DA, Quanbury AO, Reimer GD. Analysis of instantaneous energy of normal gait. *J Biomech* 1976;9(4):252-257.
116. Rose J, Gamble JG. *Human Walking,* 2nd ed. Baltimore: Lippincott Williams & Wilkins, 1994.
117. Waters RL. Energy expenditure. In Perry J (ed), *Gait Analysis: Normal and Pathological Function.* Thorofare, NJ: Slack; 1992. pp. 443-489.
118. Water RL, Mulroy SJ. Energy expenditure of walking in individuals with lower limb amputation. In Smith DC, Michael JW, Bowker JH (eds), *Atlas of Amputations and Limb Deficiency: Surgical, Prosthetics and Rehabilitation Principles,* 3rd ed. Rosemont, IL: American Academy of Orthopedic Surgeons; 2004. pp. 395-408.
119. Perry J. Normal and pathological gait. In Goldberg B, Hsu JD (eds), *Atlas of Orthoses and Assistive Devices,* 3rd ed. St. Louis: Mosby, 1997. pp. 67-92.
120. Whaley MH, Brubaker PH, Otto RM (eds). *ACSM's Guidelines for Exercise Testing and Prescription,* 7th ed. Philadelphia: Lippincott Williams & Wilkins, 2006.
121. Sidney KH, Shepherd RJ. Maximum and submaximum exercise tests in men and women in the seventh, eighth and ninth decades of life. *J Appl Physiol* 1977;43(2):280.
122. Thomas SG, Cunningham DA, Rechnitzer PA, et al. Protocols and reliability of maximal oxygen uptake in the elderly. *Can J Sport Sci* 1987;12:144.
123. Leeuwenburgh C, Heinecke JW. Oxidative stress and antioxidants in exercise. *Curr Med Chem* 2001;8(7):829-838.
124. Fleg JL, Morrell CH, Bos AG, et al. Accelerated longitudinal decline of aerobic capacity in healthy older adults. *Circulation* 2005;112(5):674-682.
125. Saltin B, Blomquist G, Mitchell JH, et al. Response to submaximal and maximal exercise after bedrest and training. *Circulation* 1968;38(Suppl 7):1-78.
126. Davis JA. Anaerobic threshold: review of the concept and directions for future research. *Med Sci Sports Exerc* 1985;17(1):6-8.
127. McArdle WD, Katch FI, Katch VL. *Exercise Physiology: Energy, Nutrition, and Human Performance,* 5th ed. Philadelphia: Lippincott Williams & Wilkins, 2001.
128. Rose J, Gamble JG, Medeiros J, et al. Energy cost of walking in normal children and in those with cerebral palsy: comparison of heart rate and oxygen uptake. *J Pediatr Orthop* 1989;9(3):276-279.
129. Rose GK. Clinical gait assessment. *J Med Eng Technol* 1983;7(6):273-279.
130. Eston R, Connolly D. The use of ratings of perceived exertion for exercise prescription in patients receiving beta-blocker therapy. *Sports Med* 1996;21(3):176-190.
131. Faulhaber M, Flatz M, Burtscher M. Beta-blockers may provoke oxygen desaturation during submaximal exercise at moderate altitudes in elderly persons. *High Alt Med Biol* 2003;4(4):475-478.
132. Steven MM, Capell HA, Sturrock RD, et al. The physiological cost of gait (PCG): a new technique for evaluating non-steroidal anti-inflammatory drugs in rheumatoid arthritis. *Br J Rheumatol* 1983;22(3):141-145.
133. Butler P, Engelbrecht M, Major RE, et al. Physiological cost index of walking for normal children and its use as an indicator of physical handicap. *Dev Med Child Neurol* 1984;26(5):607-612.
134. Nene AV. Physiological cost index of walking in able-bodied adolescents and adults. *Clin Rehabil* 1993;7(4):319-326.
135. Peebles KC, Woodman-Aldridge AD, Skinner MA. The physiological cost index in elderly subjects during treadmill and floor walking. *NZ J Physiother* 2003;3(1):11-16.
136. Hamzeh MA, Bowker P, Sayeqh A, et al. The energy cost of ambulation using 2 types of walking frames. *Clin Rehabil* 1988;2:119-123.
137. Johnson CA, Burridge JH, Strike PW, et al. The effect of combined use of botulinum toxin type A and functional electrical stimulation in the treatment of spastic foot drop after stroke: a preliminary investigation. *Arch Phys Med Rehabil* 2004;85(6):902-909.
138. Kottink AI, Oostendorp LJ, Buurke JH, et al. The orthotic effect of functional electrical stimulation on the improvement of walking in stroke patients with dropped foot: a systematic review. *Artif Organs* 2004;28(6):577-586.
139. Burridge JH, Taylor PN, Hagan SA, et al. The effects of common peroneal nerve stimulation on the effort and speed of walking: a randomized controlled clinical trial with chronic hemiplegic patients. *Clin Rehabil* 1997;11(3): 201-210.
140. Burridge J, Taylor P, Hagan S, et al. Experience of clinical use of the Odstock dropped foot stimulator. *Artif Organs* 1997;21(3):254-260.

141. Carmick J. Clinical use of neuromuscular electrical stimulation for children with cerebral palsy: lower extremity. *Phys Ther* 1993;73(8):505-513.
142. Nene AV, Evans GA, Patrick JH. Simultaneous multiple operations for spastic diplegia: Outcome and functional assessment of walking in 18 patients. *J Bone Joint Surg Br* 1993;75(3):488-494.
143. Yang L, Condie DN, Granat MP, et al. Effects of joint motion constraints on normal subjects and their implications on the further development of hybrid FES orthosis for paraplegic persons. *J Biomech* 1996;29(2):217-226.
144. Nene AV, Jennings SJ. Physiological cost index of paraplegic locomotion using the ORLAU ParaWalker. *Paraplegia* 1992;30(4):246-252.
145. Stallard J, Major RE. The influence of stiffness on paraplegic ambulation and its implications for functional electrical stimulation walking systems. *Prosthet Orthot Int* 1995;19(2):108-114.
146. Engsberg JR, Herbert LM, Grimston SK, et al. Relation among indices of effort and oxygen uptake in below knee and able-bodied children. *Arch Phys Med Rehabil* 1994;75(12):1335-1341
147. Chin T, Sawamura S, Fujita H, et al. The efficacy of physiological cost index measurement of a subject walking with an intelligent prosthesis. *Prosthet Orthot Int* 1999;23(10):45-49.
148. Hachisuka K, Umezu Y, Ohmine S, et al. Subjective evaluations and objective measurements of the ischial-ramal containment prosthesis. *J UOEH* 1999;21(2):107-118.
149. Herbert JS, Liggins AB. Gait evaluations of an automatic stance control knee orthosis in a patient with post-poliomyelitis. *Arch Phys Med Rehabil* 2005;86(8):1676-1680.
150. Bowen TR, Lennon N, Castagno P, et al. Variability of energy consumption measures in children with cerebral palsy. *J Pediatr Orthop* 1998;18(6):738-742.
151. Boyd R, Fatone S, Rodda J, et al. High- or low-technology measurements of energy expenditure in clinical gait analysis? *Dev Med Child Neurol* 1999;41(10):676-682.
152. Genin JJ, Bastien GJ, Lopez N, et al. Does the physiological cost index reflect the cost of walking? *Arch Physiol Biochem* 2004;112(Suppl):73.
153. Morgan DW, Tseh W, Caputo JL, et al. Longitudinal stratification of gait economy in young boys and girls: the locomotion energy and growth study, *Eur J Appl Physiol* 2004;91(1):30-34.
154. Waters RL, Hislop HJ, Thomas L, et al. Energy cost of walking in normal children and teenagers. *Dev Med Child Neurol* 1983;25(2):184-188.
155. Waters RL, Lunsford BR, Perry J, et al. Energy-speed relationship of walking: standard tables. *J Orthop Res* 1988;6(2):215-222.
156. Waters RL, Hislop HJ, Perry J, et al. Comparative cost of walking in young and old adults. *J Orthop Res* 1983;1(1): 73-76.
157. Aoyagi Y, Togo F, Matsuki S, et al. Walking velocity measured over 5 m as a basis of exercise prescription for the elderly: preliminary data from the Nakanojo Study. *Eur J Appl Physiol* 2004;93(1-2);217-223.
158. Malatesta D, Simar D, Dauvilliers Y, et al. Aerobic determinants of the decline in preferred walking speed in healthy, active 65- and 80-year-olds. *Eur J Physiol [Pflugers Arch]* 2004;447(6):915-921.
159. Astrand A, Astrand I, Hallback I, et al. Reduction in maximal oxygen uptake with age. *J Appl Physiol* 1973;35(5):649-654.
160. Binder EF, Schechtman KB, Ehsani AA, et al. Effects of exercise training on frailty in community-dwelling older adults: results of a randomized, controlled trial. *J Am Geriatr Soc* 2002;50(12):1921-1928.
161. Corcoran PJ, Gelmanan B. Oxygen reuptake in normal and handicapped subjects in relation to the speed of walking beside a velocity controlled cart. *Arch Phys Med Rehabil* 1970;51(2):78-87.
162. Holt KG, Hamill J, Andres RO. Predicting the minimal energy cost of human walking. *Med Sci Sports Exerc* 1991;23(4):491-498.
163. Duff Raffaele M, Kerrigan DC, Corcoran PJ, et al. The proportional work of lifting the center of mass during walking. *Am J Phys Med* 1996;75(5):375-379.
164. Hanada E, Kerrigan DC. Energy consumption during level walking with arm and knee immobilized. *Arch Phys Med Rehabil* 2001;82(9):1251-1254.
165. Waters RL, Perry J, Conaty P, et al. The energy cost of walking with arthritis of the hip and knee. *Clin Orthop* 1987;2(14):278-284.
166. Detrembleur C, Dierick F, Stoquart G, et al. Energy cost, mechanical work, and efficiency of hemiparetic walking. *Gait Posture* 2003;18(2):47-55.
167. Brophy LS. Gait in cerebral palsy. *Orthop Phys Ther Clin North Am* 2001;10(1):55-76.
168. Patrick JH. The case for gait analysis as part of the management of incomplete spinal cord injury. *Spinal Cord* 2003;41(9):479-482.
169. Gussoni M, Margonato V, Ventura R, et al. Energy cost of walking with hip joint impairment. *Phys Ther* 1990;70(5):295-301.
170. Waters RL, Barnes G, Husserl T, et al. Comparable energy expenditure following arthrodesis of the hip and ankle. *J Bone Joint Surg* 1988;70(7):1032-1037.
171. Inman, VT, Ralston HJ, Todd F. *Human Walking.* Baltimore: Waverly, 1981.
172. Waters RL, Lunsford BR. Energy expenditure of normal and pathological gait: Application to orthotic prescription. In Bowker JH, Michael JW (eds). *Atlas of Orthotics,* St. Louis: Mosby, 1985. pp. 151–159.
173. Buckon CE, Thomas SS, Jakobson-Huston S, et al. Comparison of three ankle-foot orthosis configurations for children with spastic diplegia. *Dev Med Child Neurol* 2004;46(9):590-598.
174. Franceschini M, Massucci M, Ferrari L, et al. Effects of an ankle-foot orthosis on spatiotemporal parameters and energy cost of hemiparetic gait. *Clin Rehabil* 2003;17(4): 368-372.
175. Kaufman KR, Irby SE, Mathewson JW, et al. Energy-efficient knee-ankle-foot orthosis: a case study. *J Prosthet Orthot* 1996;8(3):79-85.
176. Waters RL, Campbell J, Thomas L, et al. Energy costs of walking in lower-extremity plaster casts. *J Bone Joint Surg Am* 1982;64(6):896-899.
177. Abudulhadi HM, Kerrigan DC, LaRaia PJ. Contralateral shoe-lift: effect on oxygen cost of walking with an

immobilized knee. *Arch Phys Med Rehabil* 1996;77(7): 760-762.

178. Morganti B, Scivoletto G, Ditunno P, et al. Walking index for spinal cord injury (WISCI): criterion validation. *Spinal Cord* 2005;43(1):27-33.
179. Hussey RW, Stauffer ES. Spinal cord injury: requirements for ambulation. *Arch Phys Med Rehabil* 1973;54(12):544-547.
180. Yakura JS, Waters RL, Adkins RH. Changes in ambulation parameters in spinal cord injury individuals following rehabilitation. *Paraplegia* 1990;28(6):364-370.
181. Waters RL, Yakura JS, Adkins RH. Gait performance after spinal cord injury. *Clin Orthop* 1993;March(228):87-96.
182. Johnston TE, Smith BT, Betz RR. Strengthening of partially denervated knee extensors using percutaneous electric stimulation in a young man with spinal cord injury. *Arch Phys Med Rehabil* 2005;86(5):1037-1042.
183. Johnston TE, Finson RL, Smith BT, et al. Technical perspective. Functional electrical stimulation for augmented walking in adolescents with incomplete spinal cord injury. *J Spinal Cord Med* 2003;26(4):390-400.
184. Brissot R, Gallien P, Le Bot M, et al. Clinical experience with functional electrical stimulation-assisted gait with parastep in spinal cord-injured patients. *Spine* 2000;25(4):501-508.
185. Solomonow M, Baratta R, D'Ambrosia R. Standing and walking after spinal cord injury: experience with the reciprocating gait orthosis powered by electrical muscle stimulation. *Top Spinal Cord Inj Rehabil* 2000;5(4):29-53.
186. Franceschini M, Baratta S, Zampolini M, et al. Reciprocating gait orthoses: a multicenter study of their use by spinal cord injured patients. *Arch Phys Med Rehabil* 1997;78(6):582-586.
187. Thoumie P, Le Claire G, Beillot J, et al. Restoration of functional gait in paraplegic patients with the RGO-II hybrid orthosis. A multicenter controlled study. II: Physiological evaluation. *Paraplegia* 1995;33(11):654-659.
188. Winchester P, Caroolo JJ, Habasevich R. Physiological costs of reciprocal gait in FES assisted walking. *Paraplegia* 1994;32(10):680-686.
189. Ferrarin M, Pedotti A, Boccardi S, et al. Biomechanical assessment of paraplegic locomotion with hip guidance orthosis (HGO). *Clin Rehabil* 1993;7(4):303-308.
190. Yang L, Granat MH, Paul JP, et al. Further development of hybrid functional electrical stimulation orthoses. *Artif Organs* 1997;21(3):183-187.
191. Ryerson SD. Hemiplegia. In Umphred DA (ed), *Neurological Rehabilitation,* 4th ed. St. Louis: Mosby, 2001. pp. 741-789.
192. da Cunha IT, Lim PA, Qureshy H, et al. Gait outcomes after acute stroke rehabilitation with supported treadmill ambulation training: a randomized controlled pilot study. *Arch Phys Med Rehabil* 2002;83(9);1258-1265.
193. Chen G, Patten C, Kothari DH, et al. Gait deviations associated with post-stroke hemiparesis: improvement during treadmill walking using weight support, speed, support stiffness, and handrail hold. *Gait Posture* 2005;22(1):57-62.
194. Hash D. Energetics of wheelchair propulsion and walking in stroke patients. *Orthop Clin North Am* 1978;9(2):372-374.
195. Mauritz KH, Hesse S. Neurological rehabilitation of gait and balance disorders. In Bronstein AM, Brandt T, Woollacott MH (eds), *Clinical Disorders of Balance, Posture and Gait.* London: Arnold, 1996. pp. 236-250.
196. Ward KH, Meyers MC. Exercise performance of lower extremity amputees. *Sports Med* 1995;20(4):207-214.
197. Lin-Chan S, Nielsen DH, Shurr DG, et al. Physiological responses to multiple speed treadmill walking for Syme vs. transtibial amputation—a case report. *Disabil Rehabil* 2003;25(23):1333-1338.
198. Winter DA, Sienko SE. Biomechanics of below-knee amputee gait. *J Biomech* 1988;21(5):361-367.
199. Torburn L, Powers CM, Guiterrez R, et al. Energy expenditure during ambulation in dysvascular and traumatic below-knee amputees: a comparison of five prosthetic feet. *J Rehabil Res Dev* 1995;32(2):111-119.
200. Waters RL, Perry J, Antonelli D, et al. The energy cost of walking of amputees: influence of level of amputation. *J Bone Joint Surg* 1976;58(1):42-46.
201. Esqienazi A. Geriatric amputee rehabilitation. *Clin Geriatr Med* 1993;9(5):731-743.
202. Ganguli S, Datta SR, Chatterjee B. Performance evaluation of amputee-prosthesis system in below knee amputees. *Ergonomics* 1973;16(6):797-810.
203. Gailey RS, Wenger MA, Raya M, et al. Energy expenditure of transtibial amputees during ambulation at self-selected pace. *Prosthet Orthot Int* 1994;18(2):84-91.
204. Otis JC, Lane JM, Kroll MA. Energy cost during gait in osteosarcoma patients after resection and knee replacement and after above the knee amputation. *J Bone Joint Surg* 1985;67A(4):606-611.
205. Fisher SV, Gullickson G. Energy cost of ambulation in health and disability: a literature review. *Arch Phys Med Rehabil* 1978;59(3):124-133.
206. Jaeger SM, Vos LD, Rispens P, et al. The relationship between comfortable and most metabolically efficient walking speed in persons with unilateral above knee amputations. *Arch Phys Med Rehabil* 1993;74(5):521-525.
207. Molen NH. Energy/speed relation of below knee amputees walking on a motor driven treadmill. *Int Z Angewandte Physiol* 1973;31(3):173-185.
208. Czerniecki JM. Rehabilitation of limb deficiency. 1: Gait and motion analysis. *Arch Phys Med Rehabil* 1996;77(Suppl 35):S29-37, S81-82.
209. May BJ. Lower extremity prosthetic management. In *Amputation and Prosthetics: A Case Study Approach,* 2nd ed. Philadelphia: F.A. Davis, 2002.
210. Andrews KL. Rehabilitation in limb deficiency. 3: The geriatric amputee. *Arch Phys Med Rehabil* 1996;77(3): S14-17.
211. Torburn L, Perry J, Ayyappa E, et al. Below knee amputee gait with dynamic elastic response feet: a pilot study. *J Rehabil Res Dev* 1990;27(4):369-384.
212. Dubow LL, Witt PL, Kadaba MP, et al. Oxygen consumption of elderly persons with bilateral below knee amputation: ambulation vs. wheelchair propulsion. *Arch Phys Med Rehabil* 1983;64(6):255-259.
213. Wu YJ, Chen SY, Lin MC, et al. Energy expenditure of wheeling and walking during prosthetic rehabilitation in a woman with bilateral transfemoral amputation. *Arch Phys Med Rehabil* 2001;82(2):265-259.
214. Nissen SJ, Newman WP. Factors influencing reintegration to normal living after amputation. *Arch Phys Med Rehabil* 1992;73(6):548-551.

215. Nitz JC. Rehabilitation outcomes after bilateral lower limb amputation for vascular disease. *Physiother Theory Pract* 1993;9(3):165-170.
216. Hofstad C, Van der Linde H, Van Limbeek J, et al. *Prescription of Prosthetic Ankle Foot Mechanisms after Lower Limb Amputation.* Washington, DC: Cochrane Library, 2004, 003978.
217. Hsu MJ, Nielsen DH, Yack JH, et al. Physiological measurements of walking and running in people with transtibial amputations with 3 different prostheses. *J Orthop Sports Phys Ther* 1999;29(9):526-533.
218. Gitter A, Czerniecki JM, DeGroot DM. Biomechanical analysis of the influence of prosthetic feet on below knee amputee walking. *Am J Phys Med Rehabil* 1991;70(3): 142-148.
219. Schneider K, Zernicke RF, Setoguchi Y, et al. Dynamics of below-knee child amputee gait: SACH foot versus Flex foot. *J Biomech* 1993;26(10):1191-1204.
220. Colborne GR, Naumann S, Longmuir PE, et al. Analysis of mechanical and metabolic factors in the gait of congenital below knee amputees: a comparison of SACH and Seattle feet. *Am J Phys Med Rehabil* 1992;71(5):272-278.
221. Barth DG, Shumacher L, Sienko-Thomas S. Gait analysis and energy cost of below-knee amputees wearing six different prosthetic feet. *J Prosthet Orthot* 1992;4(2):63-75.
222. McFarlane PA, Nielsen DH, Shurr DG, et al. Gait comparisons for below-knee amputees using a FlexFoot versus a conventional prosthetic foot. *J Prosthet Orthot* 1991;3(4):150-161.
223. Wirta RW, Mason R, Calvo K, et al. Effect on gait using various prosthetic ankle foot devices. *J Rehabil Res Dev* 1991;28(2):13-24.
224. Czerniecki JM, Gitter A. The impact of energy storing prosthetic feet on below knee amputation gait. *Arch Phys Med Rehabil* 1989;70(13):918.
225. Czerniecki JM, Gitter A, Murno C. Joint moment and muscle power output characteristics of below knee amputees during running: the influence of energy storing prosthetic feet. *J Biomech* 1991;24(1):63-75.
226. Casillas JM, Dulieu V, Cohen M, et al. Bioenergetic comparison of a new energy storing foot and SAHD foot in traumatic below-knee vascular amputations. *Arch Phys Med Rehabil* 1995;76(1):39-44.
227. Torburn L, Schweiger GP, Perry J, et al. Below knee amputee gait in stair climbing: a comparison of stride characteristics using five different prosthetic feet. *Clin Orthop* 1994;June(303):185-192.
228. Perry J, Burnfield JM, Newsam CJ, et al. Energy expenditures and gait characteristics of a bilateral amputee walking with C-leg prostheses compared with stubby and conventional articulating prostheses. *Arch Phys Med Rehabil* 2004;85(10):1711-1717.
229. Buckley JG, Spence WD, Solomonidis SE. Energy of walking: comparison of "intelligent prosthesis" with conventional mechanism. *Arch Phys Med Rehabil* 1997;78(3):330-333.
230. Boonstra AM, Schrama J, Fidler V, et al. Energy cost during ambulation in transfemoral amputees: a knee joint with mechanical swing phase control vs a knee joint with a pneumatic swing phase control. *Scand J Rehabil Med* 1995;27(2):77-81.
231. Gailey RS, Lawrence D, Burditt C, et al. The CAT-CAM socket and quadrilateral socket: a comparison of energy cost during ambulation. *Prosthet Orthot Int* 1993;17(2):95-100.
232. Flandry F, Beskin J, Chambers RB, et al. The effect of the CAT-CAM above knee prosthetic on functional rehabilitation. *Clin Orthop* 1989;Feb(239):249-262.

5

Motor Learning and Motor Control in Orthotic and Prosthetic Rehabilitation

DONNA M. BOWERS AND MICHELLE M. LUSARDI

LEARNING OBJECTIVES

On completion of this chapter, the reader will be able to do the following:

1. Discuss the strengths, limitations, and implementation for practice of current models of motor control.
2. Compare and contrast the tenets of current motor learning theories.
3. Apply principles of practice conditions in the design of therapeutic interventions for individuals using orthoses or prostheses.
4. Appropriately use augmented feedback in therapeutic situations with individuals using orthoses or prostheses.
5. Describe the role of mental practice and imagery on skill acquisition for individuals using orthoses or prostheses.

WHY THINK ABOUT MOTOR CONTROL AND MOTOR LEARNING?

The primary focus of rehabilitation professionals is to assist individuals with movement dysfunction to improve or adapt their ways of moving so that they are safe, efficient, and satisfied with their level of function in all the activities that they consider important for their quality of life.[1] A wide variety of impairments, across any of the physiological systems of the body, can contribute to ineffective or abnormal patterns of movement.[2,3]

Several premises influence current thinking about how people move. The first is that movement is *goal directed.* Individuals move in order to accomplish a task or activity that they want to do in their self-care, activities of daily living (ADLs), work, and leisure activities.[4] The second is that there are *many different ways* that the central nervous system can organize our muscles and bodies to accomplish any given task; there is no single "best" way of moving.[5] The third is that we tend to move in ways that are *most efficient* for our own, individual physical characteristics; although there are many possible movement strategies available, people develop preferential ways of moving.[6] Preferential movement patterns, however, are not always optimal ways of moving. Repetitive motion injuries, for example, may be the result of preferential movement patterns that are not biomechanically effective, stressing tissues until inflammation or permanent deformation occurs.[7]

When there are impairments of musculoskeletal, neuromuscular, or cardiopulmonary systems, the resources that an individual can bring to movement may be altered, limited, or restricted. Because movement is goal directed, an individual with impairments will find a way to accomplish their movement goal that "works," often using a less effective or abnormal movement strategy. These altered strategies are recognized clinically as movement dysfunction.[7] The use of ineffective or abnormal movement patterns, over time, can lead to inflammation, tissue remodeling, or even deformity.[8] In an individual recovering from stroke, for example, an "abnormal" extensor synergy of the lower extremity may provide stance stability but will impair swing limb advancement, leading to a compensatory circumduction or vaulting step.[9] Abnormal tone may contribute to habitual plantar flexion and eventually an equinus deformity.[10] Someone with a painful knee or back will alter the way he or she uses those joints, as well as the limbs or trunk, when walking and moving between sitting and standing.[11-14] Over time, the individual may develop secondary musculoskeletal problems at distal or proximal joints or become physically deconditioned, compounding his or her movement dysfunction.[15,16] An individual with shortness of breath or a sense of fatigue (whether due to disease or deconditioning) may choose to be less active to "conserve" energy and, as a result, become even more deconditioned, develop soft tissue tightness that impairs flexibility, and lose muscle mass that limits functional strength.[17-19]

Physical therapists use various types of therapeutic exercise (e.g., strengthening, endurance programs, flexibility, balance activities), as well as functional training (often with assistive devices or ambulatory aids, orthoses, and prostheses), in order to minimize movement dysfunction and to remediate or accommodate the underlying impairments.[20] To be effective in our interventions, rehabilitation professionals must understand the principles of exercise and the effect that exercise has on the human body.[21] They must know both the purpose of an orthosis, prosthesis, or assistive device and how the design of the device will enhance or constrain movement and function.[22,23] If the goal of rehabilitation professionals is to help those with movement dysfunction learn more effective ways to accomplish what is important to them, they also must be aware of the process of learning, both on a cognitive and a motor level, and integrate this understanding into the interventions they plan and implement.[24]

This chapter provides an overview of recent thought on motor control, using a dynamic systems perspective. The chapter also reviews the tenets of motor learning and considers practice, augmented feedback, and mental imagery as tools to assist development of new or adapted movement skills. The case studies at the end of the chapter are designed to help readers integrate growing understanding of the principles of motor control and of motor learning into the planning of interventions for movement dysfunction.

THEORIES OF MOTOR CONTROL

Human movement has traditionally been examined from two distinct fields of study: a neurophysiological control approach and a motor behavioral approach.[25-31] The traditional neurophysiological approach explained movement within a hierarchical system of control on the basis of the development of neural mechanisms within the central and peripheral nervous systems and the interaction of sensory and motor systems.[25-28] The motor behavioral approach examined movement performance from the perspectives largely from the field of psychology.[29-32] Only in the past few decades have the two fields of study interfaced to bring about newer theories regarding human movement that more fully explain human movement and performance.[29]

Dynamic Systems Perspectives

Rehabilitation professionals think about the human body as a complex system with many interacting elements and subsystems. These components have an infinite number of ways to work together in accomplishing a goal-directed motor act.[4] Because the human body is a dynamic, adaptive, and inherently complex biological system, motor behaviors and ways of moving become more efficient with practice and time: Our motor control systems can consistently generate simple and well-organized movement from a complex array of movement possibilities.[33] The dynamic systems perspective of motor control is founded on understanding of behaviors that physical systems of various types have in common: the ability to change over time, the ability to be adaptive yet have preference for habitual tendencies, and the context of interaction with the environment in which movement occurs.[34,35] In the human movement system, there is great "motor abundance"; each person has a wide variety of ways to accomplish an intended movement goal (i.e., solve a functional movement problem) in whatever environmental conditions or circumstances that function occurs.[36]

According to Bernstein's model of motor control, individuals have the capacity "to make a choice within a multitude of accessible trajectories . . . of a most appropriate trajectory."[37] Bernstein's model suggests that there are both opportunities and challenges presented by interaction of the environment and the individual's will to move.[37] Unlike dynamic systems that are purely physical, the human biological system is a smart, special-purpose machine able to instantaneously and efficiently work to meet the many parallel and serial functional demands.[38] In addition, biological systems such as the human body are *self-organizing*; the mutually dependent and complex processes among the body's subsystems allow this wonderfully dynamic structure to enact efficient functional movement patterns. As an inherently multi-dimensional biological system, the human body prefers to be in a state of relative *equilibrium*. This is the reason that the gait cycle at comfortable walking speeds tends to center around one cycle per second and that most individuals transition from walk to run, as gait speed increases, at nearly the same velocity.[38] The human body, as a smart and dynamic biological system, is also *intentional*; there is a purposeful, goal-directed, and task-oriented nature in most motor behaviors. Theorists with a dynamic systems perspective define an intention as a purposeful or desired act that influences (attracts) the human system to organize motor behavior toward the desired outcome, in the context of the environment in which the movement is occurring.[40] The organism and the environment are interdependent; each is defined with respect to the other.[41] The combination of resources available to the organism-environment interaction, in conjunction with the individual's intention, shapes (constrains) how task-oriented motor behavior is organized.

Motor control has been defined by Shumway-Cook and Woollacott as "the ability to regulate or direct the mechanisms essential to movement."[27] An individual possesses his or her own set of systems including neurological, musculoskeletal, sensory/perceptual, cardiorespiratory, cognitive, and biomechanical components that interact to regulate or direct movement. Human movement or motor control is a product of the interaction of the individual (with all of his or her subsystems), the characteristics of the environment, and the nature of the specific task or goal that the individual is involved in (Figure 5-1). Movement, then, is goal directed and purposeful; makes use of the innate and learned resources available to the individual; and is subject to the influences of the environment in which it is performed. By considering each of these essential contributors to functional movement, rehabilitation professionals can assess potential sources of movement dysfunction, explore alternative movement strategies, and adapt or alter the task or environment to improve movement outcomes.

Resources of the Individual

The first component to consider in this model of motor control is the individual, with his or her ability to think and reason, to sense and perceive, and to actively respond or initiate movement (Figure 5-2). An individual's *cognitive* resources include the abilities to critically think and integrate concepts, assign emotional meaning/significance (i.e., limbic system, central set), problem solve, access memory, and learn. An individual's *perceptual* resources are the products of the ability to receive and collect many different types of sensory information (i.e., data) and to integrate and interpret these data at both subcortical and cortical levels of information processing. An individual's resources for *action* include the ability to motor plan and refine motion at cortical and subcortical levels of control; pyramidal and extrapyramidal motor systems; and the neuromuscular, musculoskeletal, and cardiopulmonary/cardiovascular contributors to "effector" systems.

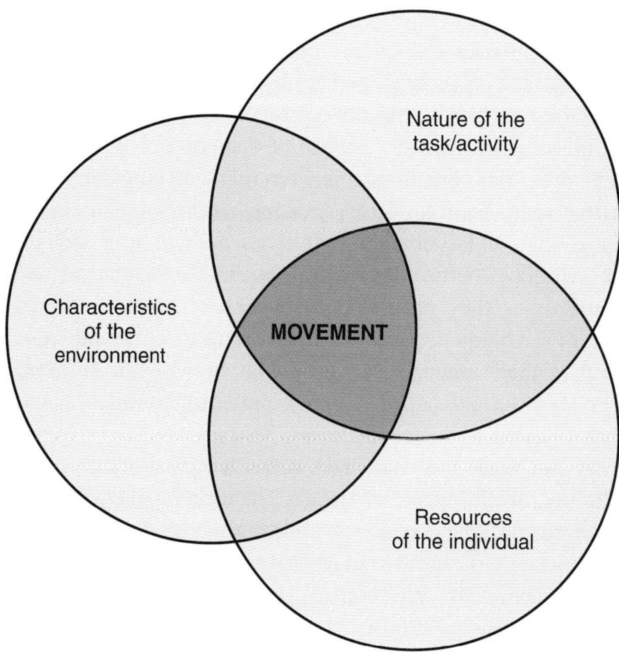

Figure 5-1
A contemporary model of motor control: movement emerges from the interaction of the individual, the environment, and the task being attempted.

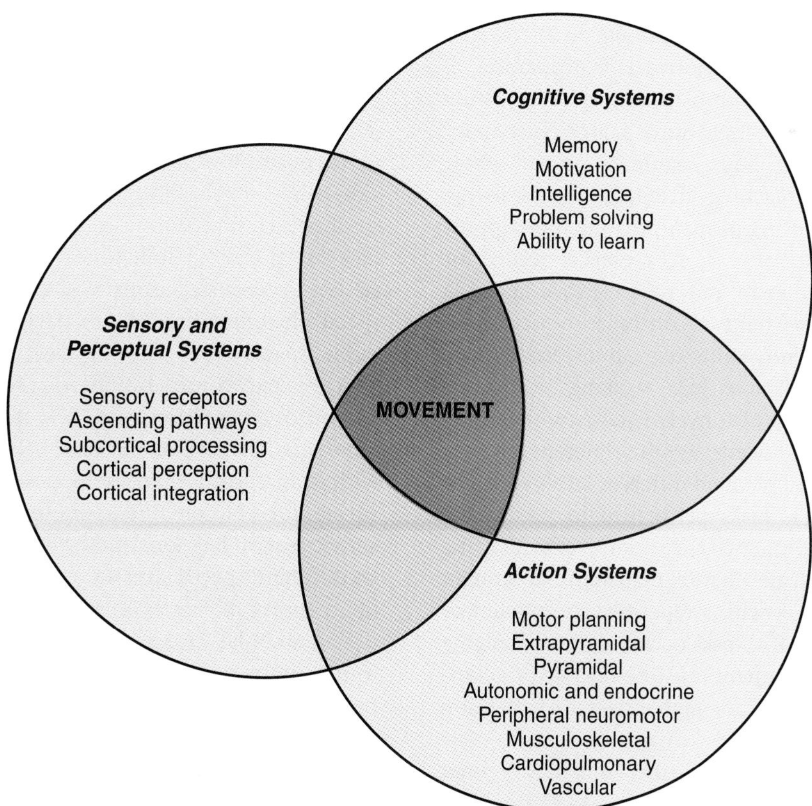

Figure 5-2
The individual resources that contribute to movement include those in the sensory/perceptual systems, the cognitive systems, and the action systems.

An example to consider is two individuals walking after a major-league baseball game across a gravel-surfaced parking area with a slightly sloped and slightly unstable support surface. One person has the typical "stocking-glove" sensory and motor impairment typical of diabetic polyneuropathy. The other has consumed a few too many servings of beer in cheering his team to victory, making his thinking and motor behavior a bit less efficient than it normally is. Both are likely to exhibit less efficient postural response and unsteady gait patterns as they return to their vehicle, but for different reasons. The quality of the sensory data that the individual with diabetic neuropathy can collect may not be sufficient for accurate perception of environmental conditions, and, complicated by distal weakness, her patterns of movement may not meet the challenges presented by the sloped and slightly movable ground surface. The individual who is tipsy has "normal" data collection ability; however, the temporary impairment in cognitive function (judgment and perception) and less efficient "error control" associated with alcohol consumption lead to motor behaviors that are not matched to environmental demands. Both baseball fans may stumble, walk with a wide base of support, or reach for the support of solid objects as they make their way toward their car, but the underlying "individual" contributors to this motor outcome are quite different.

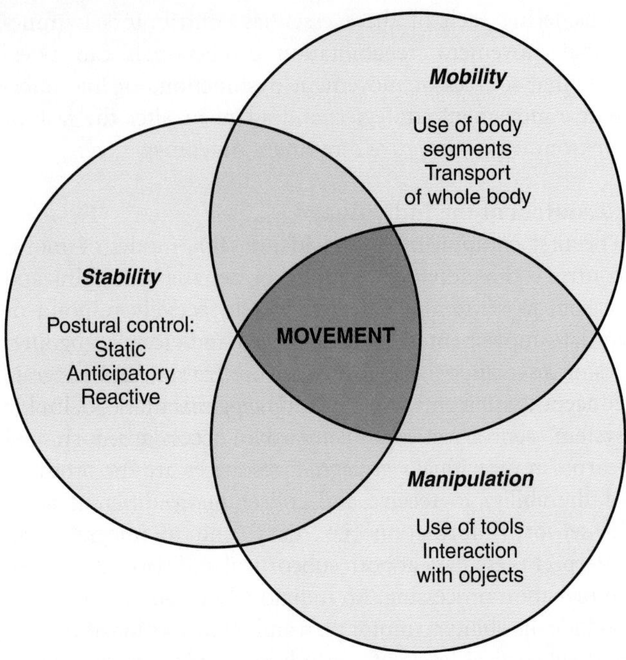

Figure 5-3
The components or nature of the task being attempted also influence the movement that emerges: The task can include or combine goals of stability, mobility, and manipulation of tools or objects.

Nature of the Task

The task is the second essential component to the overall outcome or motor behavior performed. Components of goal-directed movement include maintaining or adjusting antigravity posture (stability: static, anticipatory, reactionary postural control), moving body segments or the whole body through space (e.g., reaching, lifting, carrying, walking, hopping, running), and using or manipulating tools appropriate to the task (e.g., assistive devices, objects needed for ADLs (Figure 5-3). All tasks can be described along a number of different dimensions or continua: they can have discrete beginning and end points (e.g., transferring from bed to chair) or be continuous (e.g., walking or running over large distances). They can involve stability or require mobility, occur at various speeds, require different levels of accuracy or precision, and demand different levels of attention or focus (Box 5-1). Tasks performed in predictable (closed or fixed) environments are often executed using habitual movement strategies that require minimal thought or attention (e.g., any task with a repetitive component or that has been "overlearned"). Tasks occurring in a changing (dynamic or open) environment must be flexible or adaptable to be successful and require a higher degree of attention during performance.

One way to understand the nature of a task (either broken into components or as a whole) is to examine or classify the task using Gentile's Taxonomy of Movement Tasks (Figure 5-4).[28,30] The first component considered in the taxonomy is the movement task's outcome goals: does the task primarily focus on *stability* of the body or on *transport* (movement) of the body through space? As an example of a body stability task, consider the ability of an individual learning to use a transfemoral prosthesis to control hip and pelvic position while in single-limb stance on the prosthetic side, while slowly lifting the "intact" limb to place it on a stool or step placed in front of him or her. A body mobility task for the same individual might be to learn to use a cadence-responsive prosthetic knee unit by altering gait speed, changing direction, or navigating through a crowded public space.

The next consideration is whether the task involves use of, or interaction with, a tool or object (i.e., is *object manipulation* part of the task?). In working with persons with spinal cord injuries to develop postural control in sitting, for example, therapists often use "catching-tossing" activities with balloons and balls of various weights, thrown at different speeds and in varying directions, to provide opportunity to master this body stability skill. Learning to use an ambulatory assistive device (e.g., crutch walking in a four-point reciprocal pattern) is a prime example of a body mobility task that requires object manipulation.

The final component of the taxonomy asks us to consider the setting, environmental context, or conditions in which the task must be performed. Is the motor task occurring in an environment that is predictable (i.e., in a *closed environment*), or is there a degree of variability and possibility of change external to the individual (i.e., an *open environment*)

Box 5-1 *Descriptors of Movements Based on the Attributes/Nature of a Task*

Discrete:	The beginning or end point of movement, or both, as determined by the task itself (e.g., stepping onto a curb, donning a prosthesis, catching a ball)
Serial:	An ordered sequence of discrete movements, defined by the task itself (e.g., climbing a flight of stairs)
Continuous:	The beginning and end points of the task are determined and controlled by the individual (e.g., riding a bicycle, deciding when to start or stop)
Stability:	The primary task goal is to maintain position of body segments (often against gravity or in response to perturbation) or to keep the body's center of mass within the available base of support during functional activity (e.g., to provide a secure base in sitting or standing for subsequent skilled use of extremities)
Mobility:	The primary task goal is to move a body part, or the entire body, through physical space (e.g., rolling over in bed, coming to a sitting position from a supine position, rising to standing, walking or running, reaching for an object on a shelf or on the floor)
Manipulation continuum:	The degree to which a task requires the individual to use (manipulate) or interact with one or more external objects in order to complete the activity successfully (e.g., fastening buttons or handling clothes during dressing, donning/doffing a prosthesis or orthosis, opening doors during mobility, locking the brakes on a wheelchair)
Attention continuum:	The degree to which the task is well understood and can be carried out "automatically" or requires attention because of high task demand (level of preciseness, consequence of error) or the changing nature (variability) of the task or environmental conditions (e.g., threading a sewing needle, walking down an icy sloping walkway, catching a thrown object)

		Body Stability		Body Transport	
		No object manipulation	Object manipulation	No object manipulation	Object manipulation
Closed Environment	No variability	Stand in prostheses unsupported in the parallel bars	Stand in prostheses unsupported while putting on jacket	Walk the length of parallel bars at comfortable speed, turn around, repeat	Walk forward with crutches using 2 pt. gait pattern in empty hall
Closed Environment	Trial variability	Stand in prostheses in parallel bars, with diagonal weight shifts on command	Stand in prostheses in parallel bars, catching ball from different directions/speeds	Practice stepping in different directions and distances in parallel bars	Walk up to a closed door, opening it, and walking through while using a cane
Open Environment	No variability	Remain standing upright as people walk by at regular intervals, from similar directions	Retrieve an object repeatedly from the same spot on the floor in the corner of a busy PT gym	Practice ascending and descending a set of training stairs in the corner of a busy PT gym	Approach and ascend a full flight of stairs in a quiet hallway, using bilateral canes
Open Environment	Trial variability	Remain upright while standing in line in a busy public area	Retrieve various randomly dropped objects in an active busy PT gym	Ascend and descend stairs using the railing in a busy public space	Walk from car to supermarket door, pushing cart across parking lot

Figure 5-4

Examples of therapeutic activities for an individual learning to use bilateral transtibial prosthesis, based on Gentile's Taxonomy of Movement Tasks.

that will require the individual to monitor and respond more carefully while performing the task? When working with persons with acquired brain injury functioning at the Rancho Los Amigos cognitive continuum of 4 (confused and agitated), 5 (confused inappropriate), or 6 (confused appropriate), therapists provide a structured and predictable environment for functional and rehabilitative activities. A more complex environment may be overwhelming to the individual recovering from brain injury; the structured environment provides opportunity to complete key tasks with minimal frustration and behavioral complications. However, the complexity of the environment must be gradually increased as the individual prepares for discharge. Being able to cross the street safely at a crosswalk with real traffic is a more complex task than managing curbs and walking over a distance in the rehabilitation gym!

The taxonomy provides an organizational strategy for intervention planning by rehabilitation professions working with individuals with musculoskeletal or neuromuscular impairments and functional limitations in tasks. The primary goal of a man who has had a recent stroke may be to climb stairs so that he can return to his home, where the bedroom and bathroom are upstairs. In the early stages of rehabilitation, it may be necessary to first concentrate on static postural control and controlled weight shifting in sitting and standing on a firm support surface (body stability, no object manipulation, predictable environment). As the quality and control of these motor tasks become more consistent, intervention expands to include ambulation in the parallel bars (body mobility, no object manipulation, unvarying environment), then with an assistive device in a quiet hallway (body mobility, object manipulation, predictable environment), and finally a busy rehabilitation gym in which the individual must anticipate and react to others in the environment (body mobility, object manipulation, changing environment). As postural control becomes more efficient on level surfaces, task demand is increased by increasing speed or attempting more challenging surfaces such as stairs, inclines, and stepping over obstacles; this may initially occur in a relatively predictable environment but must eventually occur in an "open" situation in which the individual must dynamically react to or navigate around other persons and objects.

Characteristics of the Environment

The third component of the Shumway-Cook model is the environment in which the task is performed. Much like Gentile, Shumway-Cook examines (and purposefully manipulates) the environmental context in which functional movement occurs. For the therapeutic application of environmental variables, therapists can consider both macro-environmental influences (e.g., actual physical conditions that influence task demand, the therapeutic setting, or the involvement of family members), as well as micro-environmental influences (e.g., the level of visual and auditory "noise" present in the therapy room or variations in surfaces over which a client may be sitting or walking). Mastery of a motor task within a single, simple environment does not directly translate into safe performance of the same task under more complex and demanding environmental conditions. Navigating up and down a set of training steps in the physical therapy gym does not mean that the individual with stroke or paraplegic-level spinal cord injury will be functional and safe on a wet, leaf-covered, uneven brick staircase (with no railings) when entering or leaving his best friend's house or favorite neighborhood hangout!

Skill Acquisition Models

Movement has also been examined from the behavioral perspective, with a focus on quality of motor performance and acquisition of skilled behavior.[29,31,32] Researchers with this perspective are interested in the influence of cognitive-information processing and cognitive psychology on motor behavior.[25,42] They concentrate on the acquisition of skill, the learning processes associated with skills, and the refinement process of skills across applications.[25,42] Early on, studies of skill acquisition focused on orientation to the task; as the field developed and expanded, focus shifted toward understanding the process of skill development. This led to formulation of the concepts of motor memory and schema. Jack Adams' theory of feedback-based learning was a catalyst for later research, which gave rise to Schmidt's schema theory for motor learning.[25,42]

Current motor control theory has become a blending of the various bodies of study presented in this section, integrating neurophysiological, dynamic systems/ecological, and behavioral models. This shared interest gave rise to the study of motor learning, which is concerned with the adaptation and application of movement strategies to altered or novel functional, behavioral, and environmental contexts.

THEORIES OF MOTOR LEARNING

Although models of motor control focus on how the biological system organizes and adapts movement as it occurs, models of motor learning consider how the individual comes to understand and consistently perform a particular behavioral task. The outcome of effective motor learning is mastery of skilled behaviors so that the individual can function appropriately in his or her physical and social environment. Most models of motor learning are founded on four distinct notions about learning[42]:

1. Learning is a process of acquiring the capability for producing skilled actions.
2. Learning occurs as a direct result of practice or experience.
3. Learning cannot be observed directly but is inferred from observable changes in behavior.
4. Learning produces relatively permanent changes in the capability for skilled behavior.

According to Schmidt and Lee, ". . . motor learning is a set of processes associated with practice or experience leading to relatively permanent changes in the capability for movement."[42]

Rehabilitation professionals must distinguish between motor learning and motor performance. *Motor performance* is the observable action or behavior that can be measured (rated) qualitatively or quantitatively by an observer.[29] As health care professionals who focus on function, therapists are quite skilled at measuring motor performance, whether the individual is moving "normally" or is coping with some form of movement dysfunction. Physical therapists use both subjective ratings (e.g., perceived exertion[43]; poor, fair, good, normal/excellent static, and dynamic balance ability or endurance), as well as objective performance-based scales and measures (e.g., gait velocity, Timed Up and Go Test time,[44] Functional Reach distance,[45] Functional Independence Measure scores,[46] 6-minute walk test distance,[47] Gross Motor Functional Measure[48]).

In contrast, *motor learning* refers to the *process* that leads to changes in the quality, consistency, and efficiency of motor performance of a given individual. This process is not easily measured except by considering how consistency or other dimensions of performance of the task change over time. Comparisons of baseline performance and postpractice performance indicate changes in quality of performance. When an individual performs at a different level on a task after practice has occurred, over more than one practice session or intervention, it can be *inferred* that motor learning has occurred.

Evolution of Motor Learning

Initial models of motor learning were published in the early 1970s, the most prominent being Adams' closed-loop theory[49] and Schmidt's schema theory.[50] The *closed-loop theory* proposes that sensory information generated from motor performance provides a mechanism for *feedback* that will guide and refine subsequent performance of the motor task.[49] In contrast, *schema theory* suggests that an open-loop process occurs, in which a general set of rules for a particular movement is developed (schema) over time and the actual outcome of a particular movement is compared with an anticipated or predicted outcome on the basis of this schema via an error mechanism. According to schema models, *variability of practice* must occur to establish and strengthen the movement schema over time.[51] An alternative "ecological" model of motor learning (resonant with Bernstein's dynamic systems model of motor control) has been proposed by Newell, who believes that an individual uses a problem-solving approach to discover the optimal strategy to produce the task (performance) given both environmental and task influences.[52] Readers are referred to Shumway-Cook and Woollacott[53] and Schmidt[42] for a more detailed discussion of these theoretical models.

Temporal Considerations

Motor learning has also been explained through a temporal perspective in which learning occurs in stages over time. Various three- and two-stage models have been proposed to describe the process for acquisition of a skill and for adaptability or generalization/transfer of the skill (Table 5-1).

Three-stage models generally describe the earliest stage as the discovery stage, in which an understanding of the nature of a task is developed through trial and error, sometimes with guidance.[35,54,55] In this initial stage of motor learning, there is significant variability in task performance early on, with an eventual understanding or selection of the best plan for the task for that individual. Once a plan has been settled on, the second stage of motor learning focuses on refinement of the performance; variability of performance decreases while efficiency of performance increases, but attention is required and distraction is often problematic, interfering with performance. In the third and final stage of motor learning, the individual can generalize or adapt the learned skill to changing environmental demands; less attention to task is required, and the task can be performed under multiple task demands.

Two-stage models of motor learning focus on (1) acquisition of the skill and (2) adaptation or application of the skilled motor behavior.[30,31] The initial phase consolidates the first two components of the three-stage models: Acquisition and refinement of performance occur within the same stage. Variability of performance occurs through internal demands within the individual's attempts to find and select a preferred action/strategy before refinement. In the second stage performance is variable due to external demands of the environment: The person must adapt the task accordingly; this is quite similar to the final component of each of the three-stage models.

THE IMPORTANCE OF PRACTICE

Common to all models of motor learning is the concept of practice: Motor learning cannot occur unless the individual has an opportunity to gain experience through repeated attempts (both successful and unsuccessful) at accomplishing the desired movement task. Much of the research literature in the area of motor learning is devoted to exploration of practice and the optimal conditions or configurations in which it occurs. Conditions of practice can be classified or designed in several different ways. The type of practice used can influence the efficacy of motor learning that occurs, as well as its carry-over or generalizability to similar tasks or environmental conditions.

Practice Conditions

One way to describe practice is by whether it occurs in a blocked or random sequence. *Blocked practice* is characterized

Table 5-1
Comparison of Concepts in the Major Models of Motor Learning

Three-Stage Models	*Descriptive Stages/Movement Characteristics*		
Fitts and Posner[48]	COGNITIVE Early skill acquisition through trial and error; performance highly variable to find most effective strategy for task	ASSOCIATIVE Refinement of skill; performance less variable and more efficient	AUTONOMOUS Low attention necessary for task; transfer or adapting skill to other environments; performance of skill during multiple task demands
Vereijken, Whiting, and Beek[35]	NOVICE Discovery of task constraints; restriction of degrees of freedom to simplify task	ADVANCED Release of some degrees of freedom to coordinate movement; adapt tasks to environmental demands	EXPERT All degrees of freedom released; exploitation of mechanical forces to complement environmental forces
Larin[49] Refers to children	DISCOVERY Verbal-cognitive stage; physical and verbal guidance necessary	INTERMEDIATE Motor stage; independent performance, greater consistency	AUTONOMOUS Skilled performance; economy of effort; task adaptable to environment

Two-Stage Models	*Descriptive Stages/Movement Characteristics*	
Gentile[30]	EXPLICIT LEARNING Attainment of action-goal; conscious mapping of the movement's structure; rapid stabilization of performance	IMPLICIT LEARNING Dynamics of force generation; active and passive force components finely tuned unconsciously; gradual change in performance
Manoel and Connolly[31]	ACQUISITION Formulation of the action plan; understanding task and how to accomplish it; stabilization of action	ADAPTATION Task and environment interaction; task is fluid with range of options to cope with new situations; breakdown of stable task and reorganization for new action plans

by separate but subsequent repeated trials of the same task.[53,56] For blocked practice, the task is repeated under consistent environmental conditions. For the individual with transfemoral amputation working on stance control on the prosthetic limb, a blocked practice session might include stepping up onto a stool with the intact limb for 10 trials (repetitions), while standing in the parallel bars. The level of difficulty of the activity could be advanced by setting up an additional practice session, asking the individual to perform a similar task while supporting himself or herself with a straight cane to a practice curb or step outside the parallel bars. Theoretically, practice in the parallel bars would provide a model to use when performing a similar activity outside the parallel bars.

Comparatively, *random practice* (also described as *variable practice*) is characterized by separate trials of the target task randomly interspersed with trials of different tasks.[53,56] To practice stance phase stability using a random practice order, the individual with a transfemoral prosthesis would be involved in an ongoing session of gait training. As this person walked the length of the parallel bars (or across the gym), he or she might be asked to step up onto a stool or over an obstacle at a different point in the walk as he or she traversed the length of the bars or gym. The walk itself might be repeated 10 times, with a step up onto or over the stool at some point in each of the 10 trials of walking. These trials of stepping up or over do not occur in one following the other, but instead are interspersed throughout the entire ambulation event.

A third practice condition called *serial practice* can be thought of as a blending of the blocked and random practice order. Serial practice is a collection of different tasks performed sequentially, from a designated starting point to a defined ending point, always occurring in the same order, and repeated as a whole set of movement tasks.[53,56] In a serial practice session for an individual learning to use a transfemoral prosthesis, the therapist may instruct him or her to repeat a specific sequence of movements such as the following:

1. Rise from a seated position and take three steps toward an obstacle in your pathway.
2. Step over the stool (obstacle) with your intact (right) foot, bringing your prosthetic limb around the object in a small arc.
3. Complete three more gait cycles, and turn around to the right.

Box 5-2 *Summary of the Dimensions or Characteristics of Practice*

Blocked:	A single motor behavior (task) is repeated multiple times in unchanging environmental conditions. Performance improves within the practice session, but less than optimal retention across sessions.
Random (Variable):	Practice of the targeted motor task is interspersed or embedded within trials of different motor behaviors. Although performance in a single practice session is less consistent, there is better retention of skill across practice sessions and environmental conditions.
Serial:	A series of separate (related or unrelated) tasks is performed in the same sequence for multiple trials.
Massed:	Active practice time > rest time between trials
Distributed:	Active practice time ≤ rest time between trials
Part task training:	Each component of a motor behavior is practiced separately. Assists accuracy or efficiency of performance of the single-task component.
Whole task training:	The entire motor behavior is practiced as a single task. Enhances the individual's ability to problem solve and adapt task performance across practice sessions and differing environmental conditions.

4. Walk back toward the obstacle, stepping over it with the prosthesis first on the return.
5. Continue walking back to the chair, turn and sit down.
6. Rise to standing once again, and repeat the entire sequence until you have done it a total of X number of times.

The original task of stepping onto the stool with the right foot has been embedded into a series of different (but somewhat related) tasks performed in the same order over multiple trials.

Another way to classify practice is by the relative period of time spent in active practice versus rest time between practice sessions. In conditions of *massed practice* there is *more time* spent over a practice trial than there is rest time between trials. In conditions of *distributed practice*, the amount of practice time is *less than or equal to* the amount of rest time between trials.[53,56]

Part versus Whole Task Training

Another dimension of practice involves the type of training provided before the task is attempted. Part versus whole training pertains to the instruction or modeling provided to a client before task performance. *Whole task training* implies that the task as a whole is explained verbally or modeled in entirety from beginning to end. For example, a therapist may demonstrate a sit-to-stand transfer for a person with movement dysfunction, and then ask her to perform the task. *Partial task training* implies that the task is segmented into separate parts, and each part is explained or modeled as distinct or separate components of the task. In our sit-to-stand example, the therapist would demonstrate a forward lean to move center of mass from the pelvis to over the feet, and then ask the person with movement dysfunction to practice just this initial component of the whole sit-to-stand task.[57] The session might continue with modeling of the upward extension component of the task, followed by repeated trials of this component of the sit-to-stand task. After each of these components appears to be relatively mastered, the therapist might model or instruct the individual to complete the components into the sequence required for the entire task. The various dimensions of practice are summarized in Box 5-2.

Impact of Practice on Retention

The effectiveness of the various practice conditions on motor learning has been the subject of many studies in psychology, movement science, and rehabilitation. As we consider the evidence that these studies present to us (to determine their clinical relevance and possible application), it is important to note the specific outcome of practice that is being investigated; are they interested in change in quality of performance during practice trials (i.e., skill acquisition within a session) or in carryover of understanding of the task from one practice session to another (i.e., postpractice performance or retention over time)? This distinction is particularly important for rehabilitation professionals to keep in mind: Although performance over repeated trials in a practice session is often observed, it cannot be assumed this is a clear indicator that motor learning has occurred, unless the rehabilitation professional sees evidence of retention or a relatively permanent change in motor behavior across intervention sessions or differing environmental conditions.

Retention: Blocked versus Random Practice

Although blocked practice typically yields significant improvement when early performance in one practice session is compared with end-of-practice performance of the same session, there is strong evidence that blocked practice does *not* effectively assist retention of the ability to perform the practiced skill in subsequent practice sessions.[53,56,58-64] Conversely, performance is less accurate and more variable during a random practice session; however, there is much better carryover and retention of the task to later practice sessions. Therefore *improved retention of motor behavior,* better than that with blocked practice, is associated with the same random practice.[53,56,58-65] This presents a paradox when assessing efficacy of interventions. Rehabilitation professionals cannot assume that improved performance in a single session of practice (intervention) indicates that effective motor learning has occurred.

The work of key researchers in motor learning suggests that random practice enhances an individual's ability to problem solve the performance parameters of a task in the context of changing environmental demands.[63-65] If random practice requires the individual to adapt performance to meet challenges encountered with changing conditions, it may also contribute to the individual's ability to access multiple movement strategies and to self-select the most appropriate strategy for the current task and environmental demands. Conversely, blocked practice produces superior performance of a single strategy that may or may not be ideal for any given task with changing environmental demands. In studies comparing retention in situations of random and blocked practice, subjects in the blocked practice groups, who did not have experience with problem solving or self-selecting various strategies because they repeated the same task under the same conditions, demonstrated poorer performance on retention tests than those in the random practice groups.[35,42,55,56,58-65]

Retention: Part versus Whole Task Practice

A similar pattern emerges when retention after part-task training versus whole-task training is compared. The performance of subjects with and without movement dysfunction in a single part-task session was generally more consistent than in a single whole-task practice session, especially in early (acquisition) stages of motor learning; however, retention of skill over time was more consistent in those who practiced the entire task.[56,63,65] Scientists who study motor learning hypothesize that individuals who develop flexible learning strategies through whole-task training are better able to transfer learned skills, even those performed poorly, to novel situations. As clinicians this is critical for the individuals we care for, who will ultimately need to perform skills beyond the rehabilitation practice environment (rehabilitation settings), as they return to the "real world" environment of their homes and community. Keeping this in mind, rehabilitation professionals need to carefully consider and choose the practice conditions that will lead to the best possible functional outcomes for individuals for whom they care.

AUGMENTED INFORMATION

A second key concept in motor learning paradigms centers on the provision of augmented information during practice trials. If rehabilitation professionals understand the "what, when, why, and how" of augmented feedback information (and combine them with appropriately structured practice), then they can be much more effective in assisting clients' (patients') motor learning and ability to problem solve or adapt a motor skill. For each individual they are working with, rehabilitation professionals must ask themselves what type of information is most appropriate, as well as how and when they can best provide it.

As movement occurs, it generates *intrinsic* (actual) sensations (feedback) that the central nervous system (especially the cerebellum as a system interested in coordination and "error control") compares with the sensation that it "anticipates" (feedforward) will or should result from the movement. *Augmented feedback information* refers to information about the movement performance that is provided by an external source either before, during, or after the movement.[66-68] When rehabilitation professionals asks individuals what they expect will happen when performing a task, they are providing augmented feedforward information. If instead the rehabilitation professionals ask them to assess, during or after the task is completed, what they felt or experienced during the performance, they are providing augmented feedback information. Rehabilitation professionals do this, sometimes without careful thought, in each intervention encounter when they say "Good job!" or "Did that work out the way you expected?" or "What might you do differently next time you try this?" In providing augmented information, they call the person's attention to and enhance the use of intrinsically generated feedback (or sometimes, to substitute an alternative source of information in the presence of sensory impairment).

WHAT TYPE OF AUGMENTED FEEDBACK INFORMATION IS APPROPRIATE?

Augmented information can provide the individual who is learning a new motor strategy or skill with either *knowledge of results* (KR), information about the outcome of the movement, or *knowledge of performance* (KP), information about the execution of the movement.[53,66,67] Distinguishing between these two types of feedback enables the therapist to understand the "what" and "why" of augmented feedback information as a tool to assist motor learning.

Consensus exists in both basic and clinical research literature in the area of motor learning that augmented and intrinsic KP feedback information leads to better quality and consistency of performance during practice, but less accurate performance in retention tests.[64,68-73] Recent work has considered the specific use of KP during early motor performance for individuals with diminished information processing capabilities, especially as it relates to verbal and visual cueing.[74,75] Although KP may not enhance retention as much as hoped, it has been found to be both effective and necessary in the acquisition of complex motor tasks, as compared with mastery of simple motor tasks.[76,77]

The impact of KR on performance and retention of a newly learned motor task has also been extensively examined. Evidence in the literature suggests that, although KR does not necessarily lead to better performance during practice conditions, this type of augmented feedback information contributes to better task performance during retention tests.[52,64,68-73] The individual learning a new skill may benefit most by considering *if* he or she has accomplished a movement goal (KR), especially in early and mid stages of motor learning, rather than *how* accurately or efficiently the goal was attained (KP). Early on, details about quality of performance may interfere with the individual's developing understanding of the nature of the task and ability to sort through possible strategies that might be used. In later stages of motor learning, when focus shifts to refinement or improved precision of performance, KP is probably a more appropriate and powerful form of feedback information, as long as the task is consistently accomplished.

How and When Should Augmented Information Be Used?

Another thread within the motor learning research literature explores the efficacy of different frequencies and timing in the provision of augmented information. Frequent KR-focused feedback, provided on almost each trial of the task, often contributes to dependence on external guidance and ultimately degrades performance on retention tests. Summarized KR-focused feedback given at infrequent intervals (after multiple trials) appears to improve performance during practice, as well as on retention testing. Additionally, delaying the timing of KR appears to have a positive effect on performance during practice, as well as retention tests. Researchers have noted that KR, like random practice and whole training methods, better prepares individuals for adapting motor performance to changing environmental demands, hence better performance on retention tests.

What Modality for Feedback Is Appropriate?

Augmented information, whether KR or KP, can be provided in a number of ways, using the visual system (e.g., demonstration and modeling, targets, cues); the auditory system (e.g., informational verbal prompts or questions, use of tone of voice); and somatosensory-tactile systems (e.g., manual contacts, tapping/sweeping motions, compression of limb segments to cue stability response, traction/elongation of limb segments to cue mobility, appropriate resistance to guide movement).

Early in the motor learning process, therapists *judiciously* use all three modalities, keeping in mind that early stages of motor learning are periods of experimentation and trial/error as the individual becomes familiar with the nature of the task and problem solves strategies that lead to accomplishment of the task. Providing too much anticipatory prompting before initiation of the task or excessive feedback as the task proceeds and is completed can actually be detrimental to the learning process. Although it is tempting to explicitly direct and "tell" someone with movement dysfunction how to move more efficiently, prompting by using questions often can more effectively engage the individual in an active learning process.

As the individual moves into midstages of motor learning, augmented information is most effective if it helps the individual to recognize and respond to key elements of the intrinsic somatosensory and proprioceptive feedback that occurs as a result of the movement itself. Therapists must be aware of the need to "wean" the amount and frequency of augmented information as the individual moves toward becoming adept at the task. In the final stages of motor learning, augmented information becomes less and less essential or effective, as mastery of the motor task is achieved.

Mental Practice and Imagery

Another resource available to assist the process of motor learning is the incorporation of mental practice and imagery into therapeutic interventions. Growing evidence in both the human performance and rehabilitation literature indicates that mental practice and the use of imagery enhance learning effects and improves motor performance.[77-83] Imagery and mental practice appear to have a more powerful influence on improving performance during skill acquisition; their impact on retention of skills is not as well understood. This has implications for application to practice in therapeutic settings. Given high-volume patient case loads and the realities of multiple patients per therapist during sessions, mental imagery can be an effective tool for maintaining involvement of the client in the activity even when the therapist is attending to other patients.

APPLICATION: CASE EXAMPLES

The following case examples are presented as opportunities for readers to apply the information presented in this chapter. Readers are urged to take time to develop an appropriate plan of care/therapeutic intervention within the framework of the disablement model, using the interactive person-task-environment framework of motor control, Gentile's Taxonomy of Movement Tasks, and principles of practice and feedback for effective motor learning/acquisition of skill that have been discussed.

Questions to Consider

The authors suggest that readers consider the following strategies and questions to guide their planning.

Functional Considerations

- What tasks or activities are most appropriate or important to address in developing a physical therapy plan of care for the individual described in the case? (Prioritize three or four tasks to be targeted by physical therapy intervention.)

Motor Control Considerations

- What resources and impairments does this individual bring to the situation? In what ways are these helpful or constraining, given the person's neuromotor and musculoskeletal condition, cognitive and emotional status, and level of fitness?
- What is the nature of the tasks that have been selected (stability, mobility, with or without object manipulation)? What are the foundational skills necessary to perform the task? What skills or abilities may be difficult, given the impairments described in the case?
- Under what environmental conditions would this individual be best able to function at this time (closed/predictable versus open/variable)? What type of environment does this individual need to be able to eventually function in? How might you manipulate activities and environmental conditions to achieve function in the "real" environment?
- How might you organize/prioritize a sequence of activities, using Gentile's Taxonomy of Movement Tasks, to prepare/progress the individual toward safe independent function in the least restrictive environment?

Motor Learning Issues

Identify the *purpose* of the task trials that will be designed by the therapist:

- What stage of motor learning for the individual to function in is anticipated?
- Does the individual have an understanding or familiarity with the task, or is it completely novel?
- Is performance sufficient for the task to be functional? Is performance efficient or optimal?
- Can the individual use a variety of multiple motor strategies to accomplish or address this task?
- Can the person respond to changing environmental variables or task demands that warrant adaptability in performance?
- Can this task be broken into discrete parts? Would it be better to practice the task as a "whole"? Why or why not?
- Is performance of a particular part of the task problematic (mechanics of the task, fluidity between the components of the task)?
- Is performance of the task as a whole problematic (completion, speed, endurance)?

On the basis of your thoughts about the task trials, identify the best *practice conditions* for achieving the desired outcome:

- Is the primary goal of practice retention of motor behavior across practice sessions or improving performance within a practice session?
- Which practice condition or combination of practice conditions (blocked, random, or serial; massed or distributed; part- or whole-task training) would you use to assist retention of the skill? Why have you chosen these strategies?
- Which practice condition or combination of practice conditions (blocked, random, or serial; massed or distributed; part- or whole-task training) would assist improved performance? Why have you chosen these strategies?

What type of *augmented information* should be included during practice of the tasks to achieve the desired outcome?

- What modes of information should be used for this individual (visual cues and demonstration, verbal prompting, physical prompt/facilitation)? Why has this modality or combination of modalities been selected?
- What effect will the information have on the client's ability to recognize errors and self-correct motor behavior?
- What delivery scheme (KR or KP) should be used to provide augmented feedback?
- What is the anticipated effect of the selected delivery scheme (KR or KP) on retention versus performance of the motor skill being targeted?
- Can visual imagery or mental practice enhance the performance? What images would a rehabilitation professional want the client to visualize? What effect will imagery have on performance and on retention of the motor skill?
- What components can the client practice mentally? What effect will mental practice have on performance and on retention of the motor skill?

CASE EXAMPLE 1

An Adult with R Hemiparesis Who Is Learning to Use an Ankle-Foot Orthosis and Ambulatory Assistive Device

A. F. is a slightly obese, 78-year-old African American woman with a history of type 2 diabetes mellitus who had an ischemic stroke of the L middle cerebral artery 3 weeks ago. A computed tomography scan revealed a lacunar-shaped infarct from an embolic occlusion of a deep branch of the middle cerebral artery serving the internal capsule. A. F. was recently transferred to a skilled nursing facility for rehabilitation, particularly transfers and ambulation. She had just received a prefabricated solid ankle AFO before her arrival. She says that the brace is to help control her "back knee" and "lazy foot" position so that she can walk better. She has not had much opportunity to use the orthosis and is concerned that it may actually make it more difficult for her to walk. She indicates that she prefers to use a rolling walker, while her therapist in the hospital "made her" use a straight cane.

Chart review, interview, and physical therapy examination reveal the following:

Psychosocial: A. F. lives alone in a two-story, walk-up apartment. Her immediate family lives out of state. She retired 10 years ago from a position as a legal secretary and is heavily involved in the outreach ministry of her evangelical church.

Baseline vital signs: heart rate: 82, blood pressure: 132/94, respiratory rate: 16 beats per minute.

Cognitive status: alert and oriented times 3.

Communication: some slurring of words; has trouble finding the words she wants to say, but comprehension appears intact.

Vision: intact; typically wears trifocals.

Sensory system: cranial nerves intact, normal responses to light touch, pin prick, proprioception all extremities.

Neuromotor status:

Tone: moderate spasticity of right (R) upper extremity (UE) and lower extremity (LE); 1+ on the Modified Ashworth Scale

Range of motion (ROM): Passive ROM within normal limits for all extremities

Strength: L extremities 4+/5 throughout

R UE: shoulder elevation 1/5; hand grip 2/5; no other active movement present; R LE: function strength grades include ankle pf 3/5; degrees of freedom 0/5; knee extension 3/5; knee flexion 2/5; hip flexion 3/5; hip extension 3/5; hip abduction 3/5; and hip adduction 3+/5.

Postural control: able to sit upright against gravity, asymmetrical weight distribution with more weight borne on left side. Anticipatory posture changes are adequate when reaching toward right, inadequate when reaching toward left. Stands with supervision; requires verbal and tactile cues to bear weight on R LE.

Functional activities: rolls independently to both sides; supine to sit over edge of bed with supervision; transfers from bed to wheel chair with supervision.

Ambulation: uses straight cane with moderate assist, requiring both verbal cueing and physical prompt to improve loading response on right leg and to minimize genu recurvatum during forward advancement over right foot.

Design a physical therapy plan of care that will focus on development of motor skills necessary for safe and efficient locomotion using the AFO and straight cane.

CASE EXAMPLE 2

A Child with Cerebral Palsy Who Has Just Received New (Bilateral) Articulating Ankle-Foot Orthoses

T. D. is a delightful 2½-year-old-boy with cerebral palsy with moderate severity spastic diplegia. He was born prematurely at 27 weeks' gestation and remained in the neonatal intensive care unit for 10 weeks. By the time he was 18 months old, there were increasing indications of developmental delay and abnormal motor control. He currently attends an early intervention program (EIP), receives individual home visits from a physical therapist, and attends a therapeutic play group run by an educator and occupational therapist weekly.

EIP examination findings include the following:

Social: T. D. lives with both parents and an older brother in a two-story, single-family home. He interacts well with his family members and is on target for social development. He plays side by side with peers and occasionally interacts with them appropriately.

Cognition: T. D. scores age appropriately for cognitive tasks including cause and effect, object permanence, means to end, early numeration, and sorting by categories. His play with objects includes variety and imagination.

Language: T. D.'s comprehension, expression, and pragmatic use of language are on target for his age. He has an extensive vocabulary and uses language appropriately in various situations.

Fine motor/ADLs: T. D.'s reach, grasp, and release skills are within the age-expected range. Bimanual skills and object manipulation are also on target. Feeding skills are appropriate; T. D. uses utensils and drinks from a cup as expected for his age. His dressing skills are slightly below age expectations largely due to balance concerns in standing for putting on pants.

Gross motor: T. D.'s gross motor skills fall below age expectations. He has been walking independently with bilateral solid ankle-foot orthoses (AFOs) for 6 months. He can walk on multiple terrains including tile or wood floors, carpets, grass, asphalt, and woodchips. He has some difficulty with stairs requiring a railing or one hand held. Tripping and falling are issues with increasing speeds during ambulation and with attempts at running. T. D.'s mother is most concerned about his safety in ambulation at this point.

T. D. was having increasing difficulty with squatting and transitions into and out of standing from the floor. When discussing the problem, the rehabilitation team decided that articulating AFOs would increase the availability of ankle range of motion for these transitional tasks. T. D. just received bilateral articulating AFOs with a plantar flexion stop set at 10 degrees. He is currently having trouble descending stairs in the new orthoses, refusing to go down stairs unless both hands are held. He also has increased frequency of tripping outside while ambulating on the grass and rock driveway at home.

Design a physical therapy plan of care to help him master locomotion and transitional activities with the less-constraining articulating AFOs in the environments of a typical 2½-year-old.

CASE EXAMPLE 3

Child with Congenital Upper Limb Deficiency Learning to Use a Myoelectric Prosthesis

T. L. is a 3-year-old girl who has had a congenital right upper extremity limb deficiency since birth. She has an intact humerus and musculature of the upper limb with a functional elbow joint. Her forearm is incomplete with a shortened ulna, missing radius, and no wrist or hand complex. T. L. has been wearing a prosthesis with a passive terminal device since she was 6 months old and uses her prosthesis well in mobility tasks and to stabilize objects against her body or a support surface during bimanual activities. T. L. began a preschool program 2 months ago and has adjusted well to socialization. She engages in play with her peers appropriately. She has good functional use of her left upper extremity (intact limb) and uses the residual limb to assist herself in tasks, particularly for stabilizing objects.

T. L. has been working with her prosthetist and therapists to learn to use a two-channel (voluntary closing/voluntary opening) myoelectrically controlled terminal device for the past 2 weeks. When she wears the myoelectric prosthesis throughout the day, she primarily uses it as she did her previous passive prosthesis. She has not attempted to use the "hand" for play or ADLs unless prompted to by her parents or therapists. During her therapy sessions, she is intrigued with her new ability to open and close her "hand" but is inconsistent in controlling force of grasp and has difficulty initiating release. In today's session, she practiced picking up 1-inch blocks and placing them in a bowl, achieving the desired result in 2 of 5 trials. She was unsuccessful (and became rather frustrated) at picking up pegs that were much narrower than the blocks. The rehabilitation team's goals for T. L. include functional use of the prosthesis for grasp and release of household objects for feeding and self-care and school objects for play and participation in preschool activities. The team would like to increase the use of bimanual manipulation of various-sized objects.

Design an early intervention/rehabilitation plan of care to help T. L. master grasp and release of objects of various sizes and levels of durability in activities meaningful for a 3-year-old child.

CASE EXAMPLE 4

An Adolescent with Transtibial Amputation Working on Returning to Competition in Track Events

W. P. is a 16-year-old junior in high school who has been a star track athlete since he was a freshman. He currently holds his high school records in the 100-meter and 200-meter events, which he achieved during his sophomore year. He also finished third in the state championships that same year.

Three months ago, W. P. was seriously injured when the garden tractor/lawnmower he was operating rolled over and down an embankment as he was making a fast turn while mowing the lawn. He sustained deep lacerations to his right foot and lower leg from the mower's blade, as well as third-degree burns from the muffler. His injured limb was pinned under the tractor in a pile of leaves and debris. In the emergency department, trauma surgeons thought he did not meet criteria for limb salvage and performed a long, open transtibial amputation. After an intensive course of antibiotics, W. P. returned to the operating room 1 week later for closure to the standard transtibial level, with equal anterior/posterior flaps. When his residual limb healed without difficulty, W. P. was fit with a patellar tendon–bearing prosthesis, with a sleeve and pin suspension, and a Seattle Systems, Inc. dynamic response foot. He quickly mastered ambulation without an assistive device and returned to school in the fall.

W. P. is eager to return to track for his senior year. His prosthetist has fabricated a special prosthesis for him to wear in competition, with a Otto Bock Healthcare Sprinter prosthetic foot designed for track and field athletes. He has begun training for his events and is pleased that he can run again. He has two goals: to decrease his performance time (hoping to meet the records he set last year) and to become much more efficient at leaving the starting block.

Develop a prosthetic training regimen focusing on improving his performance as he prepares to return to track competition.

SUMMARY

This chapter has explored the concepts that shape one's understanding of human motor control, focusing on the dynamic and adaptive characteristics of the body as a biological system. Rehabilitation professionals use their understanding of (1) an individual's resources and characteristics, (2) environmental conditions, and (3) the nature and constraints of functional tasks to develop appropriate interventions aimed at improving or adapting individuals' abilities to move effectively, in ways that are safe and efficiently, to accomplish what is important for them to do.

The chapter also considered the process of motor learning, the ways in which individuals come to understand and approach a novel task or adapt a familiar task in differing environmental conditions or following injury or illness that changes personal resources. Using their understanding of the "stages" of motor learning, the purpose of augmented information, types and timing of feedback, and types of practice conditions, physical therapists can construct interventions that will effectively enhance retention of motor learning or refine performance for persons with movement dysfunction.

REFERENCES

1. American Physical Therapy Association. Who are physical therapists, and what do they do? In *Guide to Physical Therapist Practice,* 2nd ed. Alexandria, VA: APTA, 2001. pp. 39-50.
2. Jette AM. Physical disablement concepts for physical therapy research and practice. *Phys Ther* 1994;74(5):380-386.
3. Verbugge LM, Jette AM. The disablement process. *Soc Sci Med* 1994;38(1):1-14.
4. Austin GP. Motor control of human gait: a dynamic systems perspective. *Orthop Phys Ther Clin North Am* 2001;10(1): 17-34.
5. Kamen G. Neuromotor issues in human performance: introduction. *Res Q Exerc Sport* 2004;75(1):1-2.
6. Walter C, Lee TD. The dynamic systems approach to motor control and learning: promises, potential limitations and future directions. *Res Q Exerc Sport* 1998;69(4):316-318.
7. Sahrmann SA. *Diagnosis and Treatment of Movement Impairment Syndromes.* St. Louis: Mosby, 2002.
8. Mueller MJ, Maluf KS. Tissue adaptation to physical stress: a proposed "Physical Stress Theory" to guide physical therapist practice. *Phys Ther* 2002;82(4):383-403.
9. Olney SJ, Griffin MP, McBride ID. Multivariant examination of data from gait analysis of persons with stroke. *Phys Ther* 1998;78(8):814-828.
10. Harkless LB, Bembo GP. Stroke and its manifestations in the foot: a case report. *Clin Podiatr Med Surg* 1994;11(4): 635-645.
11. Manetta J, Franz LH, Moon C, et al. Comparison of hip and knee muscle movements in subjects with and without knee pain. *Gait Posture* 2002;16(3):249-254.
12. Sahai A, Perell KL, Fang M. Relationship between frontal and sagittal plane knee kinetics during walking in subjects with and without knee pain. *Clin Kinesiol* 2003;57(2):25-31.
13. Lee CE, Simmonds MJ, Novy DM, et al. Functional self-efficacy, perceived gait ability and perceived exertion in walking performance of individuals with low back pain. *Physiother Theory Pract* 2002;18(4):193-203.
14. Iverson MD, Katz JN. Examination findings and self-reported walking capacity in patients with lumbar spinal stenosis. *Phys Ther* 2001;81(7):1296-1306.
15. Dunlop DD, Semanik P, Song J, et al. Risk factors for functional decline in older adults with arthritis. *Arthritis Rheum* 2005;52(4):1274-1282.
16. Maire J, Tordi N, Parratte B, et al. Cardiovascular deconditioning in elderly with hip osteoarthritis and benefits of reconditioning program after total hip arthroplasty. *Science Sports* 2002;17(4):155-165.
17. Jette DU, Manago D, Medved E, et al. The disablement process in patients with pulmonary disease. *Phys Ther* 1997;77(4):385-394.
18. Gill TM, Allore H, Guo Z. Restricted activity and functional decline among community-living older adults. *Arch Intern Med* 2003;163(11):1317-1322.
19. Clark L, White P. The role of deconditioning and therapeutic exercise in chronic fatigue syndrome. *J Mental Health* 2005;14(3):237-252.
20. American Physical Therapy Association. What types of interventions do physical therapists provide? In *Guide to Physical Therapist Practice,* 2nd ed. Alexandria, VA: APTA, 2001. pp. 105-129.
21. Franklin BA, Whaley MH, Howley ET (eds). *ACSM's Guidelines for Exercise Testing and Prescription,* 6th ed. Philadelphia: Lippincott Williams & Wilkins, 2000.
22. May MJ. *Amputations and Prosthetics: a Case Study Approach,* 2nd ed. Philadelphia: F.A. Davis, 2002.
23. Edelstein JE, Bruckner J. *Orthotics: a Comprehensive Clinical Approach.* Thorofare, NJ: Slack, 2002.
24. Shepard KF, Jensen GM. *Handbook of Teaching for Physical Therapists,* 2nd ed. Boston: Butterworth Heinemann, 2002.
25. Schmidt R, Lee T. Evolution of a field of study. In *Motor Control and Learning: A Behavioral Emphasis,* 4th ed. Champaign, IL: Human Kinetics, 2005.
26. Shumway-Cook A, Woollacott M. Motor control issues and theories. In *Motor Control: Theory and Practical Applications,* 2nd ed. Baltimore: Lippincott Williams & Wilkins, 2001. pp. 1-25.
27. Shumway-Cook A, Woollacott M. A conceptual framework for clinical practice. In *Motor Control: Theory and Practical Applications,* 2nd ed. Baltimore: Lippincott Williams Wilkins, 2001. pp. 110-126.
28. Gentile A. Skill acquisition: action, movement, and neuromotor processes. In Carr J, Shepherd R, Gordon J (eds). *Movement Science: Foundation for Physical Therapy in Rehabilitation.* Rockville, MD: Aspen Systems, 1987. p. 115.
29. Lehto NK, Marley TL, Exekiel HJ, et al. Application of motor learning principles: the physiotherapy client as a problem solver. IV future directions. *Physiotherapy Canada* 2001;53(2):109-114.
30. Gentile A. Implicit and explicit processes during acquisition of functional skills. *Scand J Occ Ther* 1998;5(1):7-16.
31. Manoel E, Connolly K. Variability and the development of skilled actions. *Int J Psychophysiol* 1995;19(2):129-147.
32. Davis W, Burton A. Ecological task analysis: translating movement behavior theory into practice. *Adapted Phys Activ Q* 1991;8:154-177.
33. Berstein N. *The Co-ordination and Regulation of Movement.* London: Pergamon, 1967.
34. Gibson J. *The Ecological Approach to Visual Perception.* Mahwah, NJ: Erlbaum, 1986.
35. Vereijken B, Whiting H, Beek W. A dynamical systems approach to skill acquisition. *Q J Exp Psychol A* 1992;45(2):323-344.
36. Latash M. There is no redundancy in human movements: there is motor abundance. *Motor Control* 2000;4(3): 259-260.
37. Bernstein N. Essay II: On motor control. In Latash M, Turvey M (eds). *Dexterity and Its Development.* Mahway, NJ: Erlbaum, 1996. pp. 25-44.
38. Runeson S. On the possibility of "smart" perceptual mechanisms. *Scand J Psychol* 1977;18(3):172-179.
39. Diedrich F, Warren W. Why change gaits? Dynamics of the walk-run transition. *J Exp Psychol* 1995;21(1):183-202.
40. Lombardo T. *The Reciprocity of Perceiver and Environment: the Evolution of J Gibson's Ecological Psychology.* Hillsdale, NJ: Erlbaum, 1987.
41. Kugler P, Turvey M. *Information, Natural Law, and the Self-assembly of Rhythmical Movement.* Hillsdale, NJ: Erlbaum, 1987.

42. Schmidt R, Lee T (eds). Motor learning concepts and research methods. In *Motor Control and Learning: A Behavioral Emphasis,* 4th ed. Champaign, IL: Human Kinetics, 2005. pp. 263-283.
43. Borg G. Psychophysical scaling with applications in physical work and the perception of exertion. *Scand J Work Environ Health* 1990;16(suppl 1):55-58.
44. Podsiadlo D, Richardson S. The timed up and go: a test of functional mobility for frail elderly persons. *J Am Geriatr Soc* 1991;39(2):142-148.
45. Duncan PW, Weiner DK, Chandler J, et al. Functional reach; a new clinical measure of balance. *J Gerontol* 1990;45(6):m192-m197.
46. Granger CV, Hamilton BB, Linacre JM, et al. Performance profiles of the functional independence measure. *Am J Phys Med Rehabil* 1993;72(2):84-89.
47. Guyatt GH, Sullivan MJ, Thompson PJ, et al. The 6-minute walk: a new measure of exercise capacity in patients with chronic heart failure. *Can Med Assoc J* 1985;132(8);919-923.
48. Russell DJ, Rosenbaum PL, Avery LM, et al. *Gross Motor Functional Measure User's Manual.* London: MacKeith Press, 2002.
49. Adams JA. Closed loop theory of motor learning. *J Motor Behav* 1971;3(2):111-150.
50. Schmidt RA. A schema theory of discrete motor skill learning. *Psychol Rev* 1975;82(4):225-260.
51. Keele S, Heurer H (eds). *Handbook of Perception and Action: Motor Skills.* New York: Academic Press, 1997.
52. Newell KM. Motor skill acquisition. *Ann Rev Psychol* 1991;42(1):213-237.
53. Shumway-Cook A, Woollacott MJ (eds). Motor learning and recovery of function. In *Motor Control: Theory and Practical Applications,* 2nd ed. Philadelphia: Lippincott Williams & Wilkins, 2001. pp. 26-49.
54. Fitts PM, Posner MI. *Human Performance.* Belmont, CA: Brooks/Cole, 1967.
55. Larin H. Motor learning: a practical framework for paediatric physiotherapy. *Physiother Theory Practice* 1998;14(1):33-47.
56. Schmidt R, Lee T (eds). Conditions of practice. In *Motor Control and Learning: A Behavioral Emphasis,* 4th ed. Champaign, IL: Human Kinetics, 2005. pp. 285-320.
57. Ikeda ER, Schenkman ML, Riley PO, et al. Influence of age on dynamics of rising from a chair. *Phys Ther* 1991;71(6):473-481.
58. Lee T, Swinnen S, Serrien D. Cognitive effort and motor learning. *Quest* 1993;46(3):328-344.
59. Jamieson B, Rogers W. Age related effects of blocked and random practice schedules on learning a new technology. *J Gerontol,* 2000;55B(6):343-353.
60. Carson L, Wiegand R. Motor schema formation and retention in young children: a test of Schmidt's schema theory. *J Motor Behav* 1979;11(4):247-251.
61. Harbst K, Wilder P. Neurophysiologic, motor control, and motor learning basis of closed kinetic chain exercise. *Orthopedic Phys Ther Clin N Am* 2000;9(2):1059-1516.
62. Pringle R, Wyatt L. Effects of contextual interference on learning a kinesthetic sensitive skill. *J Chiropract Ed* 1996;10(2-3):47-52.
63. Shea C, Kohl R. Specificity and variability of practice. *Res Q Exerc Sport* 1990;61(2):169-177.
64. Schmidt R, Lee T (eds). Retention and transfer. In *Motor Control and Learning a Behavioral Emphasis,* 4th ed. Champaign, IL: Human Kinetics, 2005. pp. 385-408.
65. Ma H, Trombly C. The comparison of motor performance between part and whole tasks in elderly persons. *Am J Occup Ther* 2001;55(1):62-67.
66. Schmidt R, Lee T. Augmented feedback. In *Motor Control and Learning: A Behavioral Emphasis,* 4th ed. Champaign, IL: Human Kinetics, 2005. pp. 323-356.
67. Ezekiel HJ, Lehto NK, Marley TL, et al. Application of motor learning principles: the physiotherapy client as a problem solver III augmented feedback. *Physiother Can* 2001;53(1):40-46.
68. Barclay C, Newell K. Children's processing of information in motor skill acquisition. *J Exper Child Psychol* 1980;30(1): 98-108.
69. Gable C, Shea C, Wright D. Summary knowledge of results. *Res Q Exerc Sport* 1991;62(3):285-292.
70. Croce R, Horvat M, Roswal G. Augmented feedback for enhanced skill acquisition in individuals with traumatic brain injury. *Percep Motor Skills* 1996;82(2):507-514.
71. Wishart L, Lee T. Effects of aging and reduced relative frequency of knowledge of results on learning a motor skill. *Percep Motor Skills* 1997;84(3):1107-1122.
72. Kernodle M, Carlton L. Information feedback and learning of multiple degree of freedom activities. *J Motor Behav* 1992;24(2):187-196.
73. Porter J. Motor learning in the older adult. *Issues Aging* 1996;19(1):14-17.
74. Landin D. The role of verbal cues in skill learning. *Quest* 1994;46(3):299-313.
75. Wulf G, Horger M, Shea C. Benefits of blocked over serial feedback on complex motor skill learning. *J Motor Behav* 1999;31(1):95-103.
76. Wulf G, Hob M, Prinz W. Instructions for motor learning: differential effects of internal versus external focus of attention. *J Motor Behav* 1998;30(2):169-179.
77. Jarus T, Ratzon N. Can you imagine? The effect of mental practice on acquisition and retention of motor skill as a function of age. *Occup Ther J Res* 2000;20(3):163-178.
78. Page S. Imagery improves upper extremity motor function in chronic stroke patients: a pilot study. *Occup Ther J Res* 2000;20(3):200-215.
79. Decety J, Ingvar D. Brain structures participating in mental simulation of motor behavior: a neuropsychological interpretation. *Acta Psychologica* 1990;73(1):13-34.
80. Jacobsen E. Electrical measurements of neuromuscular states during mental activities. *Am J Physiol* 1931;96:122-125.
81. Goss S, Hall C, Buckholz E, et al. Imagery ability and acquisition and retention of movements. *Mem Cogn* 1986;14(6):469-477.
82. Burhans R, Richman C, Bewrgey D. Mental imagery training: Effects on running speed performance. *Int J Sport Psychol* 1988;19:26-37.
83. Yaguez L, Nagel D, Hoffman H, et al. A mental route to motor learning: improving trajectorial kinematics through imagery training. *Behav Brain Res* 1998;90(1):95-106.

6

An Evidence-based Approach to Orthotic and Prosthetic Rehabilitation

RITA A. WONG AND MICHELLE M. LUSARDI

LEARNING OBJECTIVES

On completion of this chapter, the reader will be able to do the following:

1. Describe the basic principles of evidence-based practice and apply these principles to orthotic and prosthetic rehabilitation.
2. Ask well-formulated, clearly defined, and clinically important questions applicable to orthotic and prosthetic rehabilitation.
3. Efficiently locate meaningful research, well targeted to orthotic and prosthetic rehabilitation.
4. Critically appraise the evidence for validity and clinical importance.
5. Use the orthotic and prosthetic research evidence to make sound clinical judgments that affect your practice.
6. Describe strategies to encourage practitioners to engage in greater use of evidence to inform practice.

WHAT IS EVIDENCE-BASED PRACTICE?

Providing effective health and rehabilitative care requires that providers be well informed about advances in assessment, medical management, technology, theory, and rehabilitation interventions. Relying on past experience or on the opinion of "experts" is not enough. An effective health care provider must also regularly update his or her knowledge base by tapping into the ever-growing information generated by clinical researchers and their basic science colleagues.[1] Providers in all health care disciplines face a number of challenges, however, in efficiently and accurately locating, appraising, and applying scientific evidence in the midst of their hectic clinical practice schedules.[2-4] Health care providers who routinely use such skills and strategies demonstrate an "evidence-based" approach to patient care. This chapter provides guidance to the practitioner in overcoming these challenges to engaging in evidence-based practice (EBP).

David Sackett, M.D., the "father" of evidence-based medicine, described this approach as the "integration of best research evidence with clinical expertise and patient values."[4] EBP is a broader concept that applies Sackett's physician-oriented concepts to a wide range of health professions.[4] Both models identify three major elements of evidence that are interactive and valuable, as well as a set of skills necessary to integrate each resource into an effective and informed clinical decision (Figure 6-1). The three major elements are the following:

1. Best available information from up-to-date, clinically relevant research
2. The skilled and experienced practitioner who can accurately perform diagnostic procedures and interventions, integrate findings to efficiently determine correct diagnosis, and engage in reflective clinical practice
3. The integration of the patient's and family's issues, concerns, and hopes into the care plan

All three elements are equally important for an effective clinical decision making process; optimal health care outcomes are grounded on integration of perspectives and priorities that each source of information brings to bear.

To make an informed clinical decision, the evidence-based rehabilitation professional must possess the skills to do the following:

1. Effectively search for and access relevant scientific evidence in the professional literature[5]
2. Assess strength and value of the scientific evidence that will support the decision that will be made[6]
3. Apply results of an accurate clinical examination, as well as the evidence from the literature, in the process of evaluating, determining prognosis, and developing an appropriate plan of care[7]
4. Assess and incorporate patient's/client's values, knowledge, preferences, and motivation into the intervention and anticipated outcomes.[8]

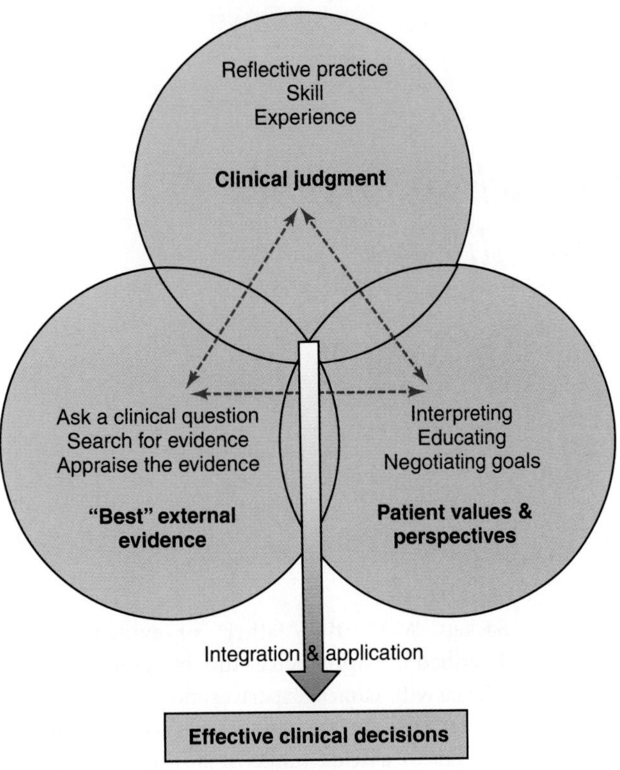

Figure 6-1

Model of three essential and interactive components necessary for effective evidence-based health care approach to guide clinical decision making, as well as the dimensions of each.

P	Patient	Patient diagnostic category or key characteristic
I	Intervention	Treatment group, or diagnostic tool, or prognostic marker
C	Comparison	Applicable if comparison is wanted between or among interventions, diagnostic tools, or prognostic markers
O	Outcome	What is the outcome of interest: presence or absence of disease? impairment? functional limitation? of disability?

Figure 6-2

The "PICO" system for formulating clinical questions includes consideration of the patient (P) *who is receiving care; the intervention* (I) *being considered; and, if available, the "gold standard" it is being compared with* (C) *and the anticipated outcomes* (O) *(positive and negative) of the intervention being considered.*

THE PROCESS OF EVIDENCE-BASED PRACTICE

EBP is, essentially, an orientation to clinical decision making that incorporates the best available sources of evidence into the process of assessment, intervention planning, and evaluation of outcomes. The skill set necessary for effective EBP develops over time, with practice and experience.

An EBP approach to the scientific literature is a systematic process with four primary steps[1,4,9]:

1. Posing a well-formulated, clinically important question
2. Locating meaningful research, well targeted to the question (developing effective and efficient search strategies)
3. Critically appraising the available evidence for validity and clinical importance
4. Using the findings to make a sound clinical judgment about changing your practice on the basis of the clinical relevance of the information applied to the needs of the individual patient

STEP 1: FORMULATING AN ANSWERABLE CLINICAL QUESTION

The questions posed by researchers and the questions posed by clinicians, while similar in many respects, are asked and answered at quite different levels. Research questions combine information from groups (samples) of individuals to develop "evidence" about relationships among characteristics, effectiveness of examination strategies, or effectiveness of intervention strategies for the group as a whole.[10] Clinical questions seek to apply this knowledge to a single person with individual characteristics.[4,5,9] They ask which examination strategy will provide the information most important for the clinical decision making process *for **THIS** particular individual*? Which intervention is likely to have the optimal outcome *for **THIS** particular individual*?

The first essential step in the EBP process is developing a well-formulated, clinically important question. Sackett identifies two categories of clinical questions: broad background questions and specifically focused foreground questions.[4] *Background questions* expand our knowledge or understanding of a disorder, impairment, or functional limitation; they are often concerned with etiology, diagnosis, prognosis, or typical clinical course. Answers to background questions expand the general knowledge base used in clinical decision making. Students and novice clinicians ask many background questions as they develop expertise in their field. Even expert clinicians routinely need to seek answers to basic background questions when they encounter an unfamiliar pathology or novel category of intervention. Answers to background questions do not, however, provide the specific evidence necessary to make individualized patient care decisions. Examples of broad background questions that might be asked by clinicians providing prosthetic and orthotic rehabilitation care include the following:

- What is the typical postsurgical rehabilitation program following a dysvascular, transtibial amputation?
- What is peripheral arterial disease (PAD) and why can it lead to limb amputation?
- What neurological functions are affected with a C7 spinal cord injury?

- What are the typical motor milestones of the first 2 years of life, and when is the achievement of these milestones considered delayed?

Foreground questions, in contrast, seek specific information to help guide care for an individual patient.[4,5,9] The most effective way to frame an answerable foreground clinical question follows the "PICO" model (Figure 6-2). It identifies the patient population of interest (P), noting specific characteristics that will link the evidence to the patient care situation prompting the question. It then identifies the examination or intervention (I) that is being considered. If appropriate, it identifies what comparisons (C) are being made, to inform choice of examination or intervention. Finally, it clearly defines the outcomes (O) that might be expected for the given patient on the basis of the best available evidence. Using the PICO model, *foreground questions* that rehabilitation professions might ask as they care for a specific individual in need of a prosthesis or orthosis include the following:

- How much does advanced age (I) affect the ability to become a functional ambulator (O) in an individual who has a dysvascular transtibial amputation (P)?
- Does supported treadmill gait training (I) improve ambulation endurance with a prosthesis (O) in older patients with dysvascular transtibial amputation (P)?
- Does the addition of functional neuromuscular stimulation (I) to a typical early rehabilitation intervention (C) enhance active muscle control (O) in individuals with incomplete spinal cord injury (P)?
- What factors (I) predict ambulation ability (O) in a young child with spastic diplegic cerebral palsy (P)?

Patient Characteristics (P)

A well-focused clinical question narrows the scope of possible *patient characteristics* to ones most applicable to a specific clinical problem or situation.[4,9] It defines the key

Table 6-1

Patient Characteristics That May Be Used to Help Focus Literature Searches for Prosthetic and Orthotic Rehabilitation

Domain	*Characteristics*	*Search Terms*
Underlying condition	Etiology	Acquired (traumatic injury, infectious process, autoimmune disease, ischemia, vascular disease, neoplasm, cancer)
		Congenital condition
		Developmental delay
		Hereditary disease
	Systems affected	Musculoskeletal
		Neuromuscular
		Cardiovascular
		Pulmonary, respiratory
		Integumentary
		Endocrine
		Systemic physiological
	Nature of condition	Chronic
		Progressive
		Degenerative
		Developmental
		Requiring remediation
		Requiring accommodation
	Comorbid conditions	Peripheral vascular disease
		Diabetes mellitus
		Systemic infections
		Cancer care, chemotherapy, radiation
		Heart disease
		Pulmonary disease
		Obesity
		Depression, anxiety
		Cognitive dysfunction
		Smoking
	Confounding factors	Alcohol use
		Other substance abuse
		Nutritional status

Continued

Table 6-1
Patient Characteristics That May Be Used to Help Focus Literature Searches for Prosthetic and Orthotic Rehabilitation—cont'd

Domain	*Characteristics*	*Search Terms*
Family and lifespan development	Age category	Infant Toddler School-age child Adolescent Young adult Midlife adult Older adult
	Family system	Roles Responsibilities Caregiver
Fitness/conditioning	Level of activity	Frail Sedentary Active Elite athlete
Mobility	Use of assistive device	None Ambulatory aid (cane, crutch, walker) Wheelchair Adaptive equipment Requiring human assistance
Environmental issues	Environment	School Home Work Leisure Accessible/inaccessible
	Living arrangements	Community dwelling (alone, independent, with caregivers or family) Assisted living setting Skilled nursing

characteristics that will best differentially guide the search for evidence. Characteristics or categories that help focus a clinical question related to orthotic or prosthetic management are summarized in Table 6-1.

Intervention (I)

The term *intervention* is used broadly in the evidence-based literature. In the EBP paradigm the intervention (I) and comparison intervention (C), described according to the PICO system, refer to the central issue for which the clinician is seeking an answer. This issue can typically revolve around an intervention, a diagnosis, or a prognosis.

a. An *intervention*: A procedure or technique (e.g., a physical modality, surgical procedure, medication) (I) that is compared with alternative procedures or techniques (C).[11,12]
b. A *diagnostic test*: A test or measure (e.g., a bone mineral density test for identification of osteoporosis; the Berg balance test for identification of falls risk) (I) that correctly differentiates patients with and without a specific condition (C).[13,14]
c. A *prognostic marker*: A specific set of characteristics or factors (I) that effectively predicts an outcome (O) for a given patient problem (P).[15]

Defining the Outcome (O)

A good clinical question focuses on the outcome that is most relevant to the patient care situation at hand. The NAGI or WHO models of disablement provide frameworks for clinicians to define the outcome they are most interested in: pathology or disease at the cellular level, impairment of a physiological system, functional limitation at the level of the individual, or disability or handicap that interferes with the normal social role[16,17] (see Figure 1-3).

CASE EXAMPLE 1

An Elderly Woman with Recent Transtibial Amputation

F. H. is an 89-year-old woman who had an "elective" transtibial amputation 4 days ago, due to PAD unrelated to diabetes. Her postoperative pain is being managed with a narcotic, and she has been mildly disoriented and distractible during rehabilitation visits. At present she requires moderate assistance in rising to standing and minimal assistance and directive cues to ambulate in a "hop to" pattern with a rolling walker. Her medical history includes mild congestive heart failure managed effectively with diuretics, hypertension managed effectively with beta-blockers, and a compression fracture (2 years ago) of the midthoracic spine secondary to osteoporosis. She recently had lens implants for cataracts. Before her hospitalization, she lived "independently" in an assisted living complex, walking long functional distances within the sprawling facility using a straight cane and eating her noon and evening meals in the communal dining room. She served as vice-chair of the Resident Council, and was the organizer of an active bridge club and book discussion group. Her nearest living relative is a granddaughter who is finishing medical residency at the hospital.

The amputation/prosthetic clinic team has been charged with developing a plan for prosthetic rehabilitation, including determining her potential for prosthetic use, the optimal setting for rehabilitation intervention, the likely duration of rehabilitative care, and preliminary prosthetic prescription.

Possible clinical questions that the team would ask in order to guide her plan of care include the following:

- Which strategies (pharmacological and nonpharmacological) for postamputation pain management (I, C) will minimize risk of delirium and assist motor and cognitive learning (O) in elderly individuals with multiple comorbidities (P)?
- Which functional and cognitive characteristics (I) provide the best indication of potential for prosthetic use (O) in elderly individuals with multiple comorbidities?
- What intrinsic and extrinsic factors (I) influence the duration of preprosthetic and prosthetic care (O) for older adults with recent transtibial amputation (P)?
- Which prosthetic foot option (nonarticulating, articulating, or dynamic response) (C, I) and suspension system (silicone suspension sleeve with pin, supracondylar cuff, waist belt, and forked-strap extension aid) (C, I) would maximize potential for safe community ambulation (O) in older patients with transtibial amputation, impaired postural control, and limited cardiovascular endurance (P)?

CASE EXAMPLE 2

A Young Adult with Incomplete Spinal Cord Injury

S. K. is a 19-year-old with incomplete C7 level spinal cord injury who has just been admitted to the rehabilitation facility, 2 weeks after injury. S. K. was a back-seat passenger injured in a driving-under-the-influence motor vehicle accident following a Thanksgiving homecoming football game victory at his high school. He was unconscious at the scene and for several hours afterward. He was given methylprednisolone in the emergency department 2 hours postinjury. Radiographs revealed an anterior wedge fracture of C6 vertebra. After intubation, he was admitted to the neurological intensive care unit; 2 days later he had surgical fusion of C4 through C8, with immobilization in a cervical halo. During the postoperative period he developed pneumonia, which has now resolved. Sensation is intact in all sacral and lumbar 3 to 5 dermatomes, and he has 2/5 strength in dorsiflexion and plantar flexion bilaterally, with hyperactive deep tendon reflex at the knee. He can tolerate sitting in a bedside recliner or high-back reclining wheelchair for approximately 45 minutes. He is anxious to know whether he will be able to walk again, and although frightened by what has occurred, appears to be motivated to begin his rehabilitation.

Before his injury, S. K. lived at home while attending a nearby state university as a biology major. His intention was to eventually apply to medical school to become an orthopedic surgeon. His parents and younger sister are involved in his care; a family member is with him for most of the day. He has a cousin, now in law school, who was born with spina bifida and uses a wheelchair for primary mobility.

Possible clinical questions that the team might ask to guide his plan of care might include the following:

- What are the most powerful indicators (I) of potential for return to functional ambulation (O) in patients with incomplete cervical spinal cord injury (P)?
- Which physical therapy interventions (I, C) will best improve functional lower extremity strength (O) in patients with incomplete cervical spinal cord injury who are immobilized in a cervical halo (P)?
- What strategies (pharmacological and nonpharmacological) (I, C) are effective in managing abnormal tone without compromising potential for strengthening (O) in patients with incomplete cervical spinal cord injury (P)?
- Will functional neuromuscular stimulation (I) reduce orthotic need and improve quality of gait (O) in patients with incomplete cervical spinal cord injury (P)?

CASE EXAMPLE 3

A Toddler with Spastic Diplegic Cerebral Palsy

E. C. is an 18-month-old with spastic diplegic cerebral palsy being cared for by an interdisciplinary early intervention team. E. C. was born prematurely at 34 weeks of gestation after her mom's high-risk first pregnancy. Her course in the neonatal intensive care unit was relatively uneventful: She did not require ventilatory assistance but did have periodic episodes of apnea and bradycardia until she reached a weight of 4 lb. She was discharged to home at 3 weeks of age and appeared to be developing fairly typically until about 8 or 9 months of age. Her parents noted increasing "stiffness" of her lower extremities when in supported standing, a tendency toward "bunny hop" rather than reciprocal creeping, and overreliance on upper extremities to pull to stand (as compared with her cousins and babies in her playgroup). Her pediatrician referred the family to a pediatric neurologist, who found mild to moderate hyperreflexia and decorticate pattern hypertonicity in her lower extremities. She has been followed in the early intervention program for 7 months; the team is charged with determining if this is an appropriate time for orthotic intervention, as she is "ready" to begin gait training. Questions that might be asked to guide her plan of care include the following:

- What are the minimal levels of muscle performance and range of motion at the hip and knee (I) necessary for effective ambulation with an articulating ankle-foot orthosis (AFO) (O) in children with spastic diplegic cerebral palsy (P)?
- Which type of therapeutic activity or approach (e.g., neurodevelopomental [NDT], sensory integration, proprioceptive neuromuscular facilitation [PNF]) (I) is most effective in assisting dynamic postural control of the lower trunk and lower extremities during transitional and locomotor tasks (O) in children with spastic diplegic cerebral palsy (P)?
- What accommodations or adaptations of her home environment (I) will best assist safety, as well as developmental progression (O), in children with spastic diplegic cerebral palsy (P)?

STEP 2: LOCATING AND ACCESSING THE BEST EVIDENCE

Once the clinical question has been clearly identified and articulated, the next step is to search the rehabilitation research literature for relevant information. Then access the full text articles that might be valuable.[18-21] Among the many ways to find citations and (hopefully) the full text of the article are the following:

- Browsing through "hard copy" of regularly received professional journals for original research articles and review articles relevant to the question at hand (which can be somewhat "hit or miss")
- Using the index in the back of up-to-date textbooks as a reliable "secondary source" of information; this can be especially useful to answer "background" questions
- Using an Internet search engine such as Google.scholar (http://scholar.google.com), which provides both unjuried and juried resources and requires the ability to carefully assess the quality of the source and of the information that has been located
- Using electronic databases of peer-reviewed journals such as PubMed/Medline/OVID or the Cumulative Index of Nursing and Allied Health Literature using appropriate key words (which can be challenging to come up with)
- Subscribing to a service that regularly updates clinicians on topic areas that they have identified as relevant to their practice

Each strategy has its "pros and cons" in terms of efficiency and availability. Health professionals who use an "evidence-based approach" to patient care develop, over time, a strategy for information seeking that will work, given their own time constraints and accessible resources.[22-24]

Sources of Evidence

Clinicians can access information from the research literature in a variety of formats and from a variety of sources. One of the most accessible formats is a journal article.[25,26] Table 6-2 provides a list of the journals particularly relevant to orthotic and prosthetic rehabilitation. These journals often contain original clinical research, reviews of the literature, and case reports focused on issues most relevant to the particular professional group.

The medical literature is divided into primary and secondary sources of information. *Primary sources* are the reports of original scientific work, commonly published as journal articles. *Secondary sources* are summary reviews of the primary literature on given topics. Secondary sources include textbooks, review articles, systematic reviews and meta-analyses, critical reviews of individual articles, clinical practice guidelines, and website summaries.

Research studies are the foundation of meaningful evidence. Academic textbooks, biomedical journals, and Internet websites aimed at health professionals and biomedical researchers are common sources of research evidence.

Textbooks

Academic textbooks can be a good starting point for locating background information, particularly for content areas that change slowly (e.g., gross anatomy or biomechanics). Evidence-based textbooks are well referenced and frequently updated. They summarize clinical studies and opinions of experts, and analyze/synthesize the impact of the research and expert opinion on the topic. Some textbooks are now available online, which provides the advantage of frequent

Table 6-2
Journals Relevant to Orthotic and Prosthetic Rehabilitation

Journal Title	*Abbreviation*
American Journal of Occupational Therapy	Am J Occ Ther
American Journal of Physical Medicine & Rehabilitation	Am J Phys Med Rehabil
American Journal of Podiatric Medicine	Am J Podiatr Med
American Journal of Surgery	Am J Surg
American Rehabilitation	Am Rehabil
Annals of Physical Medicine	Ann Phys Med
Archives of Neurology	Arch Neurol
Archives of Physical Medicine and Rehabilitation	Arch Phys Med Rehabil
Archives of Surgery	Arch Surg
Assistive Technology	Assist Tech
Athletic Training	Athletic Training
Australian Journal of Physical Therapy	Aust J Physiother
Biomechanics	Biomechanics
British Journal of Sports Medicine	Br J Sports Med
Bulletin of Prosthetic Research	Bull Prosthet Res
Canadian Journal of Occupational Therapy	Can J Occ Ther
Clinical Biomechanics	Clin Biomech
Clinics in Orthopedics and Related Research	Clin Orthoped Related Res
Clinics in Podiatric Medicine and Surgery	Clin Podiatr Med Surg
Clinics in Prosthetics and Orthotics	Clin Prosthet Orthot
Developmental Medicine & Child Neurology	Dev Med Child Neurol
Diabetes Care	Diabetes Care
Diabetic Foot	Diabetic Foot
Diabetic Medicine	Diabetic Med
Disability and Rehabilitation	Disabil Rehabil
Foot and Ankle Clinics	Foot Ankle Clin
Foot and Ankle International	Foot Ankle Int
Gait and Posture	Gait Posture
Interdisciplinary Science Reviews	Interdisc Sci Rev
International Journal of Rehabilitation Research	Int J Rehabil Res
Journal of Allied Health	J Allied Health
Journal of Applied Biomechanics	J Appl Biomech
Journal of Biomechanical Engineering	J Biomech Eng
Journal of Biomechanics	J Biomech
Journal of Bone and Joint Surgery	J Bone Joint Surg
Journal of Geriatric Physical Therapy	J Geriatric Phys Ther
Journal of Head Trauma and Rehabilitation	J Head Trauma Rehabil
Journal of Medical Engineering and Technology	J Med Eng Tech
Journal of Musculoskeletal Medicine	J Musculoskel Med
Journal of Neurologic Physical Therapy	J Neuro Phys Ther
Journal of Orthopaedic and Sports Physical Therapy	J Orthop Sports Phys Ther
Journal of Pediatric Orthopedics	J Pediatr Orthop
Journal of Prosthetics and Orthotics	J Prosthet Orthot
Journal of Rehabilitation	J Rehabil
Journal of Rehabilitation Medicine	J Rehabil Med
Journal of Rehabilitation Research and Development	J Rehabil Res Dev
Journal of Spinal Disorders	J Spinal Disord
Journal of the American Geriatrics Society	J Am Geriatr Soc
Journal of the American Medical Association	JAMA
Journal of the American Podiatry Association	J Am Podiatry Assoc
Journal of Trauma	J Trauma

Continued

Table 6-2
Journals Relevant to Orthotic and Prosthetic Rehabilitation—cont'd

Journal Title	*Abbreviation*
Medical and Biological Engineering	Med Biol Eng Comp
Orthopedic Clinics of North America	Orthop Clin North Am
Paraplegia	Paraplegia
Physiotherapy Canada	Physiother Can
Physical and Occupational Therapy in Geriatrics	Phys Occup Ther Geriatr
Physical and Occupational Therapy in Pediatrics	Phys Occup Ther Pediatr
Physical Medicine & Rehabilitation Clinics of North America	Phys Med Rehabil Clin N Am
Physical Medicine & Rehabilitation: State of the Art Reviews	Phys Med Rehabil State Art Rev
Physical Therapy	Phys Ther
Physiotherapy	Physiotherapy
Physiotherapy Research International	Physiother Res Int
Prosthetics and Orthotics International	Prosthet Orthot Int
Rehabilitation Nursing	Rehabil Nurs
Rehabilitation Psychology	Rehabil Psychol
Scandinavian Journal of Rehabilitation Medicine	Scand J Rehabil Med
Spinal Cord	Spinal Cord
Spine	Spine
Topics in Stroke Rehabilitation	Top Stroke Rehabil

Box 6-1 *Quality Indicators for Textbooks and Internet Sources of Evidence*

- Credentials of the authors
- Quality of references
- Recent/regular updating
- Endorsement by respected groups
- Peer reviewed
- Disclosure of funding source

updating of specific sections as new research evidence emerges and allows the reader to immediately hyperlink to primary research article sources. The website http://www.freebooks4doctors.com/ provides a hyperlink to most medical textbooks free of charge online. Many other online textbooks are available for purchase. Box 6-1 summarizes key quality indicators to look for in academic textbooks, both hard copy and electronic.

Primary Sources: Journal Articles

Journal articles may serve as either primary or secondary literature sources. They can be useful for both background and foreground clinical questions. *Primary research articles* are ones in which the author presents the findings of a specific original study.[27,28] It is best to use this category of evidence when dealing with rapidly evolving areas of health care (which many clinical practice questions fall into). Identifying two or three high-quality primary research articles that, in general, provide similar supporting evidence offers strong evidence on which to base a clinical decision. The time intensity required to search, critique, and synthesize primary research sources can quickly become a limitation to the ability of practitioners to use the EBP approach on a day-to-day basis.

Secondary Sources: Integrative and Systematic Review Articles

Use of high-quality *secondary source journal articles* to guide evidence-based determinations can be a time-efficient strategy for clinicians.[29,30] Quality indicators for secondary source articles include a comprehensive search of the literature to identify existing studies, an unbiased analysis of these studies, and objective conclusions and recommendations on the basis of the analysis and synthesis.[31] Secondary sources are available in a variety of formats: integrative narrative review, systematic review, meta-analysis, and clinical practice guideline (CPG). Each of these summative resources can be an effective and time-efficient method to obtain a critical assessment of a specific body of knowledge. However, there are benefits and drawbacks associated with each type of summative resource.

In an *integrative review article* the author reviews and summarizes, and sometimes analyzes or synthesizes, the work of a number of primary authors.[32] These narrative reviews are often rather broad in scope, may or may not describe how articles were chosen for inclusion in the review, and present a qualitative analysis of previous research findings. The quality (validity) of the narrative review varies with the expertise of the reviewer and requires careful assessment by the reader.

Table 6-3
Systematic Reviews Published from 2000-2005, Identified by Searching PubMed Electronic Research Database Using Search Terms "Limb Amputation AND Rehabilitation AND Systematic [Sb]"

Title	*Authors*	*Original Journal*
Type of incision for below knee amputation	Tisi PV, Callam MJ	*Cochrane Database Syst Rev* 2004(1):CD003749
Prescription of prosthetic ankle-foot mechanisms after lower limb amputation	Hofstad C, Linde H, Limbeek J, et al.	*Cochrane Database Syst Rev* 2004(1):CD003978
Spinal cord stimulation for nonreconstructable chronic critical leg ischemia	Ubbink DT, Vermeulen H	*Cochrane Database Syst Rev* 2003(3):CD004001
Postoperative dressing and management strategies for transtibial amputations: a critical review	Smith DG, McFarland LV, Sangeorzan BJ, et al.	*J Rehabil Res Dev* May-Jun 2003;40(3):213-224
Intermittent claudication: pharmacoeconomics and quality-of-life aspects of treatment	Brevetti G, Annecchini R, Bucur R	*Pharmacoeconomics* 2002;20(3):169-181
Evidence for the optimal management of acute and chronic phantom pain: a systematic review	Halbert J, Crotty M, Cameron ID	*Clin J Pain* 2002, 18(2):84092
Mobility of people with lower limb amputations: scales and questionnaires: a review	Rommers GM, Vos LD, Groothoff JW, et al.	*Clin Rehabil Feb* 2001;15(1):92-102

Systematic reviews are particularly powerful secondary sources of evidence that typically analyze and synthesize controlled clinical trials.[29,31,33] Well-done systematic reviews are valuable sources of evidence and should always be sought out when initiating a search. Box 6-2 provides key indicators of a quality systematic review. Systematic reviews are typically focused on a fairly narrow clinical question, are based on a comprehensive search of relevant literature, and use well-defined inclusion and exclusion criteria to select high-quality studies (typically randomized controlled trials) for inclusion in the review. Each study included in the review has been carefully appraised for quality and relevance to the specific clinical topic. The author attempts to identify commonalities among study methods and outcomes, as well as account for differences in approaches and findings. A good systematic review is labor intensive to prepare; thus only about 1.5% of all journal articles referenced in Medline are true systematic reviews.[34] Although the numbers are low, increasing numbers of systematic reviews are being published including ones on topics relevant to orthotics and prosthetics. For example, a PubMed search of the literature published between 2000 and 2005 using the terms "limb amputation AND rehabilitation" combined with the subject "systematic" [Sb] uncovered seven applicable systematic reviews (Table 6-3).

A *meta-analysis* is a type of systematic review that quantitatively aggregates outcome data from multiple studies to analyze treatment effects (typically using the "odds ratio" statistic) as if the data represented one large rather than multiple small samples of individuals.[29,31] The limitation to performing a meta-analysis is that, in order to combine studies, the category of patients, the interventions, and the outcome measures across the studies must all be similar. Meta-analyses can provide more powerful statements of the strength of the evidence either supporting or refuting a given treatment effect than the separate assessment of each study. Because of the difficulty in identifying studies with enough similarity to combine data, only a small subset of systematic reviews have been carried to the level of a meta-analysis. No meta-analyses were identified in PubMed on the topic of "limb amputation AND rehabilitation" during the 2000-2005 time period. Two meta-analyses were identified in PubMed on the topic of "lower limb orthotic" AND "rehabilitation" when the PubMed publication type was limited to "meta-analysis."[35,36]

Box 6-2 *Quality Indicators for Systematic Review Articles*

- Exhaustive search for evidence
- Clearly identified quality criteria for inclusion
- Multiple authors with independent judgments
- Impartial, unbiased summary
- Clearly stated conclusions: ready for clinical application
- If meta-analysis: statistical manipulation across studies

Clinical Practice Guidelines

Finally, another secondary resource for clinicians may be CPGs that have been developed for application to clinical practice on the basis of the best available current evidence.[37] Most existing CPGs have been developed for screening, diagnosis, and intervention in medical practice. CPGs are intended to direct clinical decision making about appropriate health care for specific diseases among specific populations of patients. The "best available evidence" on which CPGs are typically based combines expert consensus and review of clinical research literature.[38] Most are interpreted as "prescriptive," using algorithms to assist decision making for appropriate examination and intervention strategies for patients with given characteristics. Examples of CPGs that may be relevant to orthotic and prosthetic rehabilitation are listed in Table 6-4. The National Guidelines Clearinghouse is the most comprehensive database in the United States for CPGs (www.guidelines.gov).

Table 6-4
Examples of Clinical Practice Guidelines Available from the National Guideline Clearinghouse (www.guideline.gov)

SEARCH TERMS: ORTHOSIS OR ORTHOTIC AND REHABILITATION			
Title	*Original Source*	*NCG #*	*Sponsoring Professional Organizations*
American Academy of Orthopaedic Surgeons clinical guidelines on low back pain/sciatica, phases I and II	Rosemont, IL: American Academy of Orthopaedic Surgeons (AAOS), 2002	003672	American Academy of Orthopaedic Surgeons (AAOS). AAOS clinical guidelines on low back pain
Clinical guideline on osteoarthritis of the knee (phase II)	Rosemont, IL: American Academy of Orthopaedic Surgeons, 2003	003374	American Academy of Orthopaedic Surgeons
Diabetic foot disorders: a clinical practice guideline	Frykberg RG, Armstrong DG, Giurini J, et al. *J Foot Ankle Surg* 2000; 39(5 Suppl):S1-60	002118	American College of Foot and Ankle Surgeons
Diagnosis and treatment of pediatric flatfoot	*J Foot Ankle Surg* 2004; 43(6):341-373	004086	American College of Foot and Ankle Surgeons
Diagnosis and treatment of adult degenerative joint disease (DJD) of the knee	Bloomington, MN: Institute for Clinical Systems Improvement (ICSI), 2004 Nov	003972	Institute for Clinical Systems Improvement (ICSI)
Health professional's guide to rehabilitation of the patient with osteoporosis	Washington, DC: National Osteoporosis Foundation, 2003	003074	National Osteoporosis Foundation, American Academy of Pain Medicine, American Academy of Physical Medicine and Rehabilitation, American Association of Clinical Endocrinology, American College of Obstetrics/Gynecology, American College of Radiology, American Geriatric Society, American Medical Association, American Society for Bone and Mineral Research, International Society of Physical Medicine and Rehabilitation
Lower extremity musculoskeletal disorders; a guide to diagnosis and treatment	Boston: Brigham and Women's Hospital, 2003	003437	Brigham and Women's Hospital (Boston)
Pain in osteoarthritis, rheumatoid arthritis, and juvenile chronic arthritis	Simon LS, Lipman AG, Jacox AK, et al. 2nd ed. Glenview, IL: American Pain Society, 2002	002917	American Pain Society

Table 6-4
Examples of Clinical Practice Guidelines Available from the National Guideline Clearinghouse (www.guideline.gov)—cont'd

SEARCH TERMS: ORTHOSIS OR ORTHOTIC AND REHABILITATION			
Title	*Original Source*	*NCG #*	*Sponsoring Professional Organizations*
Physical activity and exercise recommendations for stroke survivors	Gordon NF, Gulanick M, Costa F, et al. *Circulation* 2004;Apr 27;109(16): 2031-2041	003661	American Heart Association, American Stroke Association
Use of back belts to prevent occupational low-back pain	*Can Med Assoc J* 2003;169(3):213-214	003237	Canadian Task Force on Preventive Health Care
VA/DoD clinical practice guideline for the management of stroke rehabilitation in the primary care setting	Washington, DC: Department of Veteran Affairs, 2003 Feb	003061	Veterans Health Administration, Department of Defense

SEARCH TERMS: PROSTHESIS OR AMPUTATION AND REHABILITATION			
Title	*Original Source*	*NCG #*	*Professional* Organization
Adult diabetes clinical practice guidelines	Oakland, CA: Kaiser Permanente, Care Management Institute, 2004 Mar	003597	Kaiser Permanente Care Management Institute
Assessment of function: of critical importance to acute care of older adults	Kresevic DM, Mezey M. Assessment of function, In Geriatric nursing protocols for best practice, 2nd ed. New York: Springer, 2003	002730	The John A. Hartford Foundation Institute for Geriatric Nursing—Academic Institution
Clinical guidelines for type 2 diabetes. Prevention and management of foot problems	London (UK): National Institute for Clinical Excellence (NICE), 2004 Jun	003546	National Collaborating Centre for Primary Care
Clinical practice guideline for the management of postoperative pain	Version 1.2. Washington, DC: Department of Defense, Veterans Health Administration, 2002 May	002510	Department of Defense, Veterans Health Administration
Diagnosis and treatment of diabetic foot infections	Lipsky BA, Berendt AR, Deery HG, et al. *Clin Infect Dis* 2004 Oct 1;39(7):885-910	003874	Infectious Diseases Society of America
Guideline for management of wounds in patients with lower-extremity arterial disease	Glenview, IL: Wound, Ostomy and Continence Nurses Society (WOCN), 2002 Jun	002516	Wound, Ostomy and Continence Nurses Society (WOCN)
Guideline for management of wounds in patients with lower-extremity neuropathic disease	Glenview, IL: Wound, Ostomy and Continence Nurses Society (WOCN), 2004	003898	Wound, Ostomy and Continence Nurses Society (WOCN)

Continued

Table 6-4
Examples of Clinical Practice Guidelines Available from the National Guideline Clearinghouse (www.guideline.gov)—cont'd

SEARCH TERMS: PROSTHESIS OR AMPUTATION AND REHABILITATION			
Title	*Original Source*	*NCG #*	*Sponsoring Professional Organizations*
	clinical practice guideline; no. 3)		
Initiating exercise in adults with chronic illnesses	Austin, TX: University of Texas at Austin, School of Nursing, 2004 May	003724	University of Texas at Austin, School of Nursing, Family Nurse Practitioner Program
Medical guidelines for the management of diabetes mellitus: AACE system of intensive diabetes self-management—2002 update	*Endocr Pract* 2002 Jan-Feb;8(Suppl 1):40-82	002398	American Association of Clinical Endocrinologists, American College of Endocrinology
Physical activity/exercise and diabetes	Zinman B, Ruderman N, Campaigne BN, et al. *Diabetes Care* 2004; 27(Suppl 1):S58-62	003417	American College of Sports Medicine, American Diabetes Association (ADA)
Reducing foot complications for people with diabetes	Toronto: Registered Nurses Association of Ontario (RNAO), 2004 Mar	003635	Registered Nurses Association of Ontario (RNAO)
Standards of medical care in diabetes	*Diabetes Care* 2004 Jan;27(Suppl 1):S15-35	003413	American Diabetes Association
VA/DoD clinical practice guideline for the management of diabetes mellitus	Washington, DC: Veterans Health Administration, Department of Defense, 2003	003567	Veterans Health Administration, Department of Defense

Electronic Resources and Search Strategies

A number of electronic databases can assist clinicians in quickly locating primary and secondary sources of evidence to guide clinical decision making (Table 6-5). It is often helpful, in seeking articles, to use several different databases.

Using an electronic database effectively is a two-step process. First, the searcher must locate applicable citations that provide the title of the article, author, and other key identifying information (e.g., journal, issue, year, pages). Most often, these citations also provide an abstract of the article. Sometimes the searcher can gather enough information about the applicability of the article for his or her needs purely on the basis of the information found in the title and abstract. Most often, however, the searcher must access the full-text article in order to adequately assess the findings of the study. Citations and abstracts are readily available free of charge from numerous databases. Access to the full text of articles often requires access to databases one must pay for.

Locating Citations

The National Library of Medicine, through the database PubMed, produces and maintains Medline, the largest publicly available database of English language biomedical references in the world. PubMed references more than 4600 journals including many key non-English language biomedical journals. These journals, in the aggregate, include more than 12 million individual journal article citations. This database is also a rich source of citations for quality systematic reviews. Journals indexed in PubMed must meet rigorous standards for their level of peer review and the quality of the articles published in the journal; this gives the searcher some degree of confidence in the information that he or she locates through the PubMed system. PubMed can be accessed through the National Library of Medicine's website (http://www.nlm.nih.gov/entrez/query.fcgi). OVID is another Medline resource, typically accessed via library subscription, and often has links to full text articles.

Table 6-5
Examples of Electronic Databases Used to Search for Relevant Evidence

Acronym	*Database Information*	*Access*
—	Academic Search Premier	By library access
Best Evidence	ACP Journal Club and Evidence Based Medicine (critical and systematic reviews)	http://hiru.mcmaster.ca/acpjc/acpod.htm
CCTR	Cochrane Controlled Trials Register	By subscription or library access
CDSR	Cochrane Database of Systematic Reviews	By subscription or library access
CHID	Combined Health Information Data Base (titles, abstracts, resources, program descriptions not indexed elsewhere)	www.chid.nih.gov
CINAHL	Cumulative Index of Nursing and Allied Health Literature (citations and abstracts)	By subscription or library access (www.cinahl.com)
DARE	Cochrane Database of Abstracts of Reviews of Effectiveness	By subscription or library access
EBM Online	Evidence-based Medicine for Primary Care and Internal Medicine (critical reviews and systematic reviews)	By subscription (http://www.ebm.bmjjournals.com)
Embase	Embase/Elsevier Science (Citations and abstracts)	By subscription (http://www.embase.com)
—	Hooked on Evidence/American Physical Therapy Association (citations, abstracts, annotations)	By membership in American Physical Therapy Association (http://www.apta.org)
Medline	National Library of Medicine (abstracts)	By library access
Ovid	A collection of health and medical subject databases (abstracts and full text)	By subscription or library access (http://www.gateway.ovid.com)
PEDro	The Physiotherapy Evidence Database (systematic reviews)	http://www.pedro.fhs.usyd.edu.au/index.html
PubMed	National Library of Medicine (abstracts)	http://www.ncbi.nlm.nih.gov/entrez (no charge)

The Cumulative Index of Nursing and Allied Health Literature (CINAHL) includes journal citations from a larger pool of nursing and allied health fields than found in Medline. Many of these journals have a much smaller circulation than the typical Medline cited journals, and the quality of these smaller circulation journals may not meet PubMed requirements. Thus the reader must be aware that closer scrutiny of validity and methodological quality may be necessary. However, the greater inclusion of rehabilitation-focused journals in the CINAHL database makes this an important database for rehabilitation professionals. This database is only available to paid subscribers (library or individual subscriptions).

Hooked on Evidence is a database of the American Physical Therapy Association (APTA) and is available free of charge to members of the association. Presently Hooked on Evidence consists of primary intervention studies only. Articles in Hooked on Evidence have been reviewed and abstracted by physical therapy academicians and researchers, graduate students, and clinicians. PEDro is a database of the Centre for Evidence-based Physiotherapy at the University of Sydney, Australia available to the public free of charge (http://www.pedro.fhs.usyd.edu.au/index.html). PEDro lists clinical practice guidelines, systematic reviews, and primary studies across intervention, diagnosis, and prognosis categories. Both databases focus exclusively on high-quality studies related to physical therapy. Neither database provides the full text of the articles that they reference. Their benefit is ease of identifying citations applicable to physical therapy and rehabilitation. To search either database successfully, the research question should be fairly broad, using synonyms that represent words in the title. Both databases contain only a fraction of the citations found in PubMed; all of the citations, however, are directly applicable to rehabilitation. A search of PEDro using "orthoses" only took seconds and identified one practice guideline, 11 systematic reviews, and

11 clinical trials, all relevant to physical therapy (Table 6-6). A similar search in Hooked on Evidence found 27 clinical trials, 15 of which were published since 2000 (Table 6-7).

The Cochrane Database of Systematic Reviews is widely accepted as the gold standard for systematic reviews. Groups of experts perform comprehensive analysis and synthesis of the existing research on well-focused topics and distill the findings into scientifically supported recommendations. Cochrane reviews use a standardized format and carefully follow rules to decrease bias in the choice of articles to review and in the interpretation of the evidence. Although few address physical therapy exclusively, rehabilitation procedures and approaches are a component of many of these reviews. The findings are reported in structured abstracts that summarize the key aspects of the full review including the authors' conclusions about the strength of the evidence and their recommendations. These structured abstracts are available free online. Access to full-text review articles requires a paid subscription, however.

Finding valuable secondary references on the web is increasingly possible. However, searchers must carefully scrutinize these materials as there is wide variability in accuracy and objectivity of the published information.[39] This evidence represents such varied sources as reports of original research, research reviews from trusted experts, student summaries that are non–peer reviewed, marketing advertisements (sometimes presented visually to appear to be a peer-reviewed research report), and lobbying groups' perspectives and persuasive arguments. There are many patient-focused sites and fewer practitioner-focused ones. The quality indicators identified in Table 6-2 are applicable to Internet Web sites as well as textbooks.

Executing Search Strategies

Often, the first search for citations results in one of two extremes: hundreds or thousands of citations with only a few related to the clinical question being asked, or almost no citations focused on the topic of interest.[18,40,41] Searchers should look carefully at the citations that have pulled up. In the search that is too broad, the searcher must examine closely what he or she is REALLY looking for, comparing this with the titles and key words that have resulted from the search. Often, the search is repeated, by rewording or setting limiters to narrow results and omit the previously identified unrelated citations. A searcher who uses the search term "prosthesis" may find that the results of his or her search include articles about such diverse topics as joint prostheses, dental prostheses, and skin prostheses, as well as limb prostheses. Search terms should be as applicable to the specific clinical question being posed as possible; using more precise search terms such as limb prosthesis, leg prosthesis, arm prosthesis, or artificial limb may be more effective.

Searchers should recognize that the search engine is simply matching the search words that the searcher has entered with subject headings linked to the article by the database administrator or librarian using predefined medical subject heading names or words included in the title or abstract. Searchers may need to "play" with search terms in order to find any applicable references if they exist. For example, a PubMed search of the English language literature between 1995 and 2003 using the search terms "below-knee amputation" combined with the search term "prosthetic rehabilitation" located 12 citations. The same search but with "transtibial amputation" substituted for below-knee amputation located 9 citations, with no overlap between the two sets of citations. A third search using the term "trans-tibial amputation" in place of "transtibial amputation" located five citations, only one of which was overlapped with the other two searches.

A search can be unforgiving to misspellings or, as described earlier, slight differences in search terms. If the searcher has found one citation that is on target for the topic of interest, repeating the search using words from that article's title or abstract, as well as subject headings (key words), may yield additional appropriate citations. Using a variety of synonyms when repeating the search can help the searcher be more confident that he or she is targeting the correct concepts. Searchers should always make a note of search terms that resulted in successful searches so that future searches can be most efficient. Searchers using PubMed can set up a permanent search by establishing a "cubby." This service is free and fully available via Internet connection to PubMed. Online directions help users to set up cubbies that save the search terms. Searchers can periodically check their cubbies and ask for literature updates on the topic.

In addition to the search topic, a good clinical question will often focus on one of three broad categories of clinical questions: treatment/intervention/therapy, diagnosis, or prognosis.[42] Searchers can use these terms to narrow their search as needed. Searchers must recognize that each database uses its own set of key words and may (or may not) include the title words, abstract words, or common sense clinical terms in their electronic search process. Familiarity with key headings used by the database can minimize frustration during the search process; combining words from the title or abstract (e.g., by using Boolean operators such as "AND," "OR," or "NOT"), as well as using synonyms for the clinical terms or concepts of interest, can also assist the search process. In many databases, searchers can choose to limit the search to systematic reviews addressing their topic of interest.

Searching for Interventions

Words that are likely to limit the search to studies that focus on interventions include the following[43]:

- Therapeutic use
- Clinical trials
- Therapy

Table 6-6
Results of Search Using PEDro Database

KEY WORD: ORTHOSES (LIMITED TO ARTICLES/ABSTRACTS PUBLISHED JANUARY 2000-JUNE 2005)			
Type of Study	*Title*	*Authors*	*Source*
Practice guidelines	CPG on the use of manipulation in the treatment of adults with mechanical neck disorders	Gross AR, Kay TM, Kennedy C, et al.	*Manual Ther* 2002;7(4):193-205
Systematic reviews	Therapeutic orthosis and electrical stimulation for upper extremity hemiplegia after stroke: a review of effectiveness based on evidence	Aoyagi Y, Tsubahara A	*Top Stroke Rehabil* 2004;11(3):9-15
	Interventions for treating plantar heel pain (Cochrane Review)	Crawford F, Thomson C	*The Cochrane Library* (Oxford) 2005;(3):CD000416
	Splints/orthoses in the treatment of rheumatoid arthritis (Cochrane Review)	Egan M, Brosseau L, Farmer M, et al.	*Cochrane Database Syst Rev* 2001;(1):CD 004018
	Interventions for preventing ankle ligament injuries (Cochrane Review)	Handoll HH, Rowe BH, Quinn KM, et al.	*The Cochrane Library (Oxford)* 2005;(3):CD000018
	A systematic review of physical interventions for patellofemoral pain syndrome	Crossley K	*Clin J Sport Med* 2001;11(2):103-110
	The effects of knee-ankle-foot orthoses in the treatment of Duchenne muscular dystrophy: review of the literature	Bakker JP, Groot IJ, Beckerman H, et al.	*Clin Rehabil* 2000;14(4)343-359
	Systematic review of conservative interventions for subacute low back pain	Pengel HM, Maher CG, Refshauge KM	*Clin Rehabil* 2002;16(8):811-820
	A review of efficacy of lower-limb orthoses used for cerebral palsy	Morris C	*Dev Med Child Neurol* 2002; 44(3):205-211
Clinical trials	Surgery vs. orthosis vs. watchful waiting for hallux valgus: a randomized controlled trial	Torkki M, Malmivaara A, Seitsalo S, et al.	*JAMA* 2001;285(19):2474-2480
	Can custom-made biomechanical shoe orthoses prevent problems in the back and lower extremities? A randomized, controlled intervention trial of 146 military conscripts	Larsen K, Weidich F, Leboueft-Yde C	*J Manipulative Physiol Ther* 2002;25(5):326-31
	Extracorporeal shockwave therapy (ESWT) in patients with chronic proximal plantar fasciitis	Hammer DS, Adam F, Kreutz A, et al.	*Foot Ankle Int* 2003;24(11):823-828

Table 6-7
Results of Search Using Hooked on Evidence, APTA

KEY WORD: ORTHOSES (LISTED ARTICLES/ABSTRACTS PUBLISHED JANUARY 2000-JUNE 2005)		
Title	*Authors*	*Source*
The effect of static traction and orthoses in the treatment of knee contractures in preschool children with juvenile chronic arthritis: a single-subject design	Fredriksen B, Mengshoel AM	*Arthritis Care Res* 2000;13(6):352-359
Use of orthoses lowers the O_2 cost of walking in children with spastic cerebral palsy	Maltais D, Bar-Or O, Galea V, et al.	*Med Sci Sports Exerc* 2001;33(2):320-325
The effect of foot orthoses on standing foot posture and gait of young children with Down syndrome	Selby-Silverstein L, Hillstrom HJ, Palisano RJ	*NeuroRehabilitation* 2001;16(3):183-193
A comparison of the effects of solid, articulated, and posterior leaf-spring ankle-foot orthoses and shoes alone on gait and energy expenditure in children with spastic diplegic cerebral palsy	Smiley SJ, Jacobsen FS, Mielke C, et al.	*Orthopedics* 2002;25(4):411-415
Effects of orthoses on upright functional skills of children and adolescents with cerebral palsy	Kott KM, Held SL	*Pediatr Phys Ther* 2002;14(4):199-207
Clinically prescribed orthoses demonstrate an increase in velocity of gait in children with cerebral palsy: a retrospective study	White H, Jenkins J, Neace WP, et al.	*Dev Med Child Neurol* 2002;44(4): 227-232
A randomized controlled trial of foot orthoses in rheumatoid arthritis	Woodburn J, Barker S, Helliwell PS	*J Rheumatol* 2002;29(7):1377-1383
Do static or dynamic ankle-foot-orthoses (AFOs) improve balance?	Cattaneo D, Marazzini F, Crippa A, et al	*Clin Rehabil* 2002;16(8):894-899
The effect of foot orthoses on patellofemoral pain syndrome	Saxena A, Haddad J	*J Am Podiatr Med Assoc* 2003;93(4):264-271
Nonoperative management of functional hallux limitus in a patient with rheumatoid arthritis	Shrader JA, Siegel KL	*Phys Ther* 2003;83(9):831-843
Effect of inverted orthoses on lower-extremity mechanics in runners	Williams DS, McClay-Davis I, Baitch SP	*Med Sci Sports Exerc* 2003;35(12):2060-2068
Effects of supramalleolar orthoses on postural stability in children with Down syndrome	Martin K	*Dev Med Child Neurol* 2004;46(6):406-411
A prospective study of the effect of foot orthoses composition and fabrication on comfort and the incidence of overuse injuries	Finestone A, Novack V, Farfel A, et al.	*Foot Ankle Int* 2004;25(7):462-466
Effects of foot orthoses on quality of life for individuals with patellofemoral pain syndrome	Johnston LB, Gross MT	*J Orthop Sports Phys Ther* 2004;34(8):440-448
Effect of foot orthoses on tibialis posterior activation in persons with pes planus	Kulig K, Burnfield JM, Reischl S, et al.	*Med Sci Sports Exerc* 2005;37(1):24-29

- Comparative studies
- Randomized controlled trial (to limit search to articles of highest quality, only if there are many relevant articles)
- Rehabilitation

Examples of search terms for therapeutic interventions commonly used in prosthetics and orthotics include the following:

- Prosthetic rehabilitation
- Orthotic use
- Physical therapy techniques
- Prosthetic fitting
- Prosthetic training
- Gait training
- Therapeutic exercise
- Edema management
- Balance training
- Skin care
- Strength training

Diagnosis as the Intervention

If the primary clinical question relates to making an accurate and efficacious diagnosis about some aspect of the patient's condition, or on screening patients to determine the need for more specific assessment, the health practitioner will want to search the "diagnosis" literature for relevant studies. General search terms that help limit the search to general studies focusing on diagnosis include the following[42]:

- Diagnosis (actual disease or disorder)
- Diagnostic use (tool used in diagnosis)
- Diagnosis, differential
- Sensitivity
- Specificity
- Accuracy
- Predictive value
- Construct validity

Natural History or Prognosis

Studies of the prognosis of medical pathologies and impairments are becoming increasingly available. Such studies attempt to predict who is most likely to benefit from specific treatment interventions or determine if specific characteristics of patients or their environment predict outcomes. Search terms that are likely to limit the citations to those focused on the general category of prognosis include the following[43]:

- Exp cohort studies
- Prognosis
- Prognostic factors
- Disease progression
- Recurrence
- Morbidity
- Mortality
- Incidence
- Prevalence
- Clinical course
- Outcomes

Systematic Review

Currently PubMed does not identify systematic review as a specific "publication type." When "systematic review" is used as a search term, several types of reviews are retrieved, not limited to actual systematic reviews. Articles commonly identified as review-academic, CPGs, review-tutorial, meta-analysis, guideline, and consensus development conference are all categorized in PubMed under the term *systematic review.* Search terms that are likely to limit the citations to ones focused on true systematic reviews include the following:

- Systematic review (as a title word [tw])
- Systematic (as a key word)
- Meta-analysis
- Development
- Validation
- Cochrane database of systematic reviews (as a journal name [jn])

Locating Full-Text Articles

Once appropriate citations have been found via a search of the literature, the next step is to locate the full text of articles that appear to be most closely related to the clinical question of concern. Individual journals are published and owned by publishing companies that support themselves by paid journal subscriptions. Each journal has its own mechanism for providing access to the articles it contains. If the journal is published by a specific professional organization, members of that organization typically have access to a delivered hard copy of the journal or access via the organization's website (by entering an assigned user name and password).

Libraries purchase hard copy and online access to specific journals, either bundled together as part of an intermediary company service (e.g., EBSCO or Proquest), as stand-alone subscriptions or as a publisher aggregated offering of several or all of its journals at a specified price. Libraries make the online copies of these journals available to their library patrons, either free of charge or for a specified library fee. Some journals provide full text free to the public via the Internet, either for all issues or for articles published after a certain period of time (e.g., 1 to 2 years after publication). Most journals provide full text of individual articles for a fee; this fee may be as much as $20 to $25 per article. One benefit of searching the literature on PubMed is that this database provides a link to any online access to a specific citation, both those with free access sources and those with a fee attached. The website http://www.Freejournals4docs.com lists the various biomedical journals that provide full text free, provides the hyperlink to the journal website, and identifies any limitations to free access (often time since publication). Health care practitioners should search out the availability of full-text biomedical journal articles (either hard copy or online) from the libraries to which they have regular access. Access will vary widely on the basis of the work setting and the mission of the library at the health facility or in the community.

STEP 3: CRITICALLY APPRAISING THE EVIDENCE

Once the clinician has located and screened the article to ensure that it is reasonably focused on the clinical research question of interest and applicable to the patients in his or her clinical practice, the clinician must critically appraise the methodological and analytical quality of the research process used in the study.[44] This is a skill that clinicians can develop with consistent practice, over time, and is well worth the effort involved.[22,23] Participation in study groups or journal clubs often helps development of this useful EBP skill.[45,46]

Overall Methodological Quality

The "best" quality research evidence comes from studies with a carefully articulated research question, an appropriate design and methodology, and a sample representative of the population of interest. No clinical research study or article is "perfect," and the critical appraiser of the research literature must develop skills to "weigh the evidence" that an article provides, in order to determine if the information is accurate, relevant, and clinically important for his or her patients.[44,47] Just because something is published and in print does not ensure that it provides valuable or accurate information. Whether the clinical study focuses on treatment/intervention, prognosis, or diagnosis, the overall purpose of critical appraisal is to determine the extent to which threats to internal and external validity of the study bias, and potentially invalidate, the findings of the study.[48] The clinician is interested in determining whether, and to what degree, the findings of the study truly represent the "answer" to the research question asked in the study. Box 6-3 lists a series of questions about the overall quality and applicability of primary research studies. Some questions are applicable across all categories of primary research; others are specific to certain categories. Box 6-4 identifies quality assessment questions applicable to the secondary source category of systematic review.

The Sample: Adequacy and Appropriateness

Sample size must be considered when making judgments about the methodological quality of a study. In studies with small sample sizes, a few nonrepresentative subjects can skew data substantially and lead to statistical findings that are nonrepresentative of the parent group.[49] Additionally, the natural variability between subjects may end up masking "real" differences when sample size is low. There is no absolute minimum number of subjects identified quantitatively as the "minimum" needed for a legitimate study. However, research textbooks often recommend 8 to 15 subjects per group as a minimum number to ensure that the

Box 6-3 *Questions to Consider in the Critical Appraisal of a Research or Review Article*

FOR ALL STUDIES

- What criteria were in place in the database used to find the study? (e.g., journal referenced in PubMed have met stringent quality criteria)
- How up to date (recent) is the study?
- Is the purpose of the study clearly stated? How closely does the purpose of the study address the clinical question of concern?
- How comprehensive is the review of the literature? How up to date and relevant are the references cited in the article? Does the review of the literature support the need for the study that is being reported?
- Are the outcome measurement tools used in the study described sufficiently? Are they appropriate to the clinical question of concern?
- Is evidence of the reliability and validity of each outcome measurement tool presented? Is the evidence adequate for the clinical question of concern?

FOR STUDIES OF INTERVENTIONS/ TREATMENTS/THERAPY

- Have subjects been randomly assigned to groups?
- Is there a control group (or placebo or "standard care" group) used to compare with the experimental group?
- Are the researchers collecting outcome data "blind" to subject group assignment?
- As feasible, subjects should be blinded to their group assignment?
- How similar are the experiment and control groups? Optimally, the only difference should be the intervention.
- Do confounding variables make the groups different before intervention?

FOR STUDIES CONCERNED WITH PROGNOSIS

- Are the researchers collecting outcome data "blind" to each subject's score on prognostic factors?
- Is the period of follow-up sufficiently long to ensure that the outcome of interest is captured?
- Is there evidence from repeated analysis with a second group of subjects, with similar results, to provide confirmation of the prognostic factors being investigated?

FOR STUDIES CONCERNED WITH DIAGNOSIS

- Has the new diagnostic test been compared with an accepted gold standard?
- Is the researcher performing the new diagnostic test "blind" to each subject's score on the gold standard?
- Is there evidence from repeated analysis with a second group of subjects, with similar results, to provide confirmation of the accuracy of the new diagnostic test?

Box 6-4 *Questions Used to Assess Quality of a Systematic Review*

FORMULATION OF OBJECTIVES

Is the topic (purpose of the review) well defined?

- The intervention
- The patients
- The outcomes of interest

LITERATURE SEARCH FOR STUDIES

Was the search for papers thorough?

- Use of search terms that fully capture key concepts
- Identification of databases or citation sources used
- Search methods exhaustive, international in scope
- Search methods described in enough detail to replicate
- International in scope
- Search terms that fully capture search concepts

STUDY SELECTION

Were study inclusion criteria clearly described and fairly applied?

- Explicit inclusion and exclusion criteria
- Criteria should "make sense," given the topic
- Selection criteria are applied in a manner that limits bias
- Account for studies that are rejected

ASSESSING QUALITY OF DESIGN AND METHODS

- Was study quality assessed by blinded or independent reviewers?
- Was missing information sought from the original study investigators?
- Do the included studies seem to indicate similar effects?
- Were the overall findings assessed for their "robustness"?
- Was the play of chance adequately assessed?

DATA GATHERING:

Was information from each article extracted using a standardized format?

Does the information gathered from each article include the following?

- Type of study (e.g., RCT)
- Characteristics of the intervention for experimental and control groups
- Key demographics of all subjects
- Primary outcome of importance
- An accounting for missing data

POOLING METHOD

Are selected studies similar enough to be pooled for analysis?

- In design
- In interventions
- In operational definition of outcome variable

DISCUSSION, CONCLUSIONS, RECOMMENDATIONS

- Are recommendations based firmly on the quality of the evidence presented?
- Are conclusions and recommendations justified on the basis of the analysis performed?

statistical analysis has at least a reasonable opportunity of demonstrating "real" differences or ""real" relationships if they are present.[10,50] The larger the sample size, the more likely that the sample will represent the population from which it has been drawn.

Researchers, as well as readers of research articles, can use a *power analysis* to evaluate adequacy of the sample size. A power analysis provides an objective estimate of the minimum sample size necessary to demonstrate "real" differences or relationships, between and among groups.[51-53] Inclusion of a power analysis as a standard part of the research design is a fairly new concept. Thus although the presence of a power analysis is helpful in assessing the adequacy of the sample size, lack of a specifically identified power analysis—particularly in older studies—does not necessarily indicate a weak study.

A power level (β) of .8 (80%) is generally considered acceptable in assuring that, if real group differences (or relationships) are present, the study design is sensitive enough to pick them up. A power analysis considers five factors in the determination of "power." Knowing any four of these five factors allows the reader to calculate the final factor.[52] The five factors include the following:

1. The significance level (α coefficient) set for the statistical analysis of the outcome variable
2. Anticipated variance (e.g., standard deviation) within each group of subjects related to the outcome variable
3. Sample and group size
4. The anticipated effect size for the intervention or relationship; how large a difference or a correlation does there need to be to ensure than the outcome under review is important or clinically meaningful?
5. The desired level of power (β coefficient), an estimate of the likelihood that a "real" difference between groups will be demonstrated if it exists (avoiding a type II error)

Power analysis performed in preparation for a study (i.e., before subject recruitment, data collection, or analysis) identifies the ideal number of subjects that should be in each group.[29] When a power analysis is performed after the data analysis has been completed, it is used to determine the likelihood that small sample size affected the statistical analysis when insignificant findings occurred.[54]

When a power analysis is performed before implementation of a study, most employ a significance level of α =.05 or lower and the power level of β = 0.8 or higher. The score for effect size and anticipated group variance will be study specific. Typically researchers provide references from prior research or their own pilot data to justify their choices of effect size and variance. This use of power analysis provides evidence of a rigorous research design and helps the clinician to trust the findings of the study.

The next important appraisal of the sample concerns its representativeness: to what extent are the subjects in the sample similar to (and therefore representative of) the "population" of interest and to the individual for whom the clinician is caring? The goal of all research studies is to make decisions about a general population of people on the basis of the findings of a representative sample from that population. How well a sample represents the larger group to which results will be generalized is a function of subject recruitment, selection, and retention.[55,56] In appraising an article to use as "evidence" for clinical decision making, the health professional must consider how subjects were selected and assigned to groups (hopefully randomly), what criteria were used to determine whether a possible subject was included or excluded from the study, and the reasons that subjects who started the study may have dropped out before data collection was completed. Study results will be biased if the sample used for the study is NOT representative of the underlying population. Small variations, randomly occurring across all subject groups, may be just fine. Larger variations, particularly ones that systematically affect one subject group more than others, may introduce unacceptable amounts of bias.

As a critical appraiser of the research, the evidence-based practitioner must be on the alert for sampling bias.[57,58] In the ideal world any subject in the patient population of interest should be equally likely to be chosen to be a subject in the study. Realistically, this is rarely the case. No one researcher has access to each older adult who has had a transtibial amputation, each child with cerebral palsy, or each young adult with an incomplete spinal cord lesion. The researcher should provide enough evidence in his or her discussion of the study's methodology that the reader can be reasonably comfortable that the methods implemented for choosing subjects provided access to subjects reasonably representative of the breadth of subjects with the target characteristics under investigation.

The article typically provides descriptive evidence from previous studies of the common characteristics of patients with the pathology of interest. The researcher then compares these "known" characteristics with the descriptive characteristics of subjects in their particular study. Any differences are hopefully identified and discussed in the article. The critical appraiser must use his or her own professional judgment to determine the extent to which potential biasing factors influence the methodological rigor of the study. If inequalities were detected, it is possible to add steps to the statistical analysis to "account for" the inequality. This should be reported in the study.

Attrition (subject dropout rate) also influences the researcher's ability to generalize the findings of their study to the larger population of individuals with the diagnosis or impairments. A useful rule of thumb for readers who are critically appraising an article is that if more than a 20% dropout rate has occurred, then findings of the study are likely suspect. In a strong research article, the researchers will explain why and when subjects were lost. Evidence-based practitioners want to know if subjects chose to leave the study because intervention made them worse or because the intervention was too difficult or painful to overcome its potential benefits. Another situation that may lead to attrition is based on a research design so burdensome or difficult that subjects were unable to meet participation requirements (so that only the most persistent individuals in the sample completed the study). Researchers attempt to account for dropouts either by performing an "intention-to-treat" analysis or presenting descriptive statistics that compare key characteristics of subjects who completed the study with those who did not complete the study.[59] If the researcher can confirm that both groups of subjects are not significantly different, particularly in terms of any characteristic that might bias outcomes, then a study may still be identified as having adequate methodological quality.

In an *intention-to-treat analysis,* all subjects who started a study but did not finish it are assigned the most negative outcome likely to occur with the measurement tool for the purposes of statistical analysis.[60] If a statistically significant finding still occurs in the presence of an intention-to-treat analysis, then even assuming that all dropouts had a bad outcome, the study still demonstrated significant effects.

Outcome Measures

In assessing methodological quality of a study's outcome measurement tools, three questions must be addressed:

- Are the outcome tools described well enough for the evidence-based practitioner to make an informed and realistic judgment about their appropriateness for assessing the variables of interest for this study?
- Are the outcome tools reasonably valid and reliable?
- Are the outcome tools reasonably responsive and sensitive to change?

A high-quality study describes the outcome measures in enough detail for the reader to understand exactly what was measured and to determine if the tools are appropriate to answer the research questions addressed in the study. The article should also provide sufficient detail to confirm reliability and validity of each outcome measurement tool. *Reliability* represents the consistency with which scores are reproduced given repetition of the test with the same tester or across numerous testers.[61,62] *Validity* represents the accuracy with which the measurement tool taps into the construct or characteristics that the test is purported to measure.[61,63-65] Table 6-8 lists the various aspects of reliability and validity.

If a test is reliable, it should perform consistently under similar testing situations regardless of who performs the test. Studies of reliability will usually report either correlation

Table 6-8
Validity and Reliability

DETERMINATION OF A TEST OR MEASURES RELIABILITY

Type of Reliability	*Question Being Addressed*
Intra-rater	Will the same examiner make consistent ratings of the same individual?
Test-retest	Is the measure stable/accurate over time?
Inter-rater	Will different examiners make consistent ratings of the same individual?
Internal consistency	How well do each of the items contribute or reflect what the test intends to measure (how well do the items "hang together")?
Parallel forms	Are different versions of the test or measure equivalent?

RELIABILITY COEFFICIENTS

Parametric		*Nonparametric*		
Continuous Measures	*Types of Reliability*	*Nominal Measures*	*Ordinal Measures*	*Types of Reliability*
Pearson Product Moment (Pearson's r) (association) (.0 to 1.0)	Intra-rater Test-retest Inter-rater Parallel forms	Percent agreement (includes chance agreement)	Percent agreement (includes chance agreement)	Intrarater Test-retest Interrater Parallel forms
Coefficient of Variation (SD/mean) (<10% suggests reliability)	Intra-rater Inter-rater	Kappa coefficient (agreement beyond chance)	Weighted percent agreement (magnitude of disparity) (includes chance agreement)	Intrarater Test-retest Interrater Parallel forms
Intraclass Correlation Coefficient (ICC) (association and agreement)	Intra-rater Test-retest Inter-rater Parallel forms		Weighted kappa (agreement beyond chance)	Intra-rater Test-retest Inter-rater Parallel forms
Cronbach's Alpha	Internal consistency			

DETERMINATION OF A TEST OR MEASURE'S VALIDITY

Type of Validity	*Question Being Addressed*	*Continuous Measures*
Content	How well do items on the test sample from the domain being evaluated?	Content expert review of items
Concurrent Criterion	How well does the measure reflect a particular event, characteristic, or outcome?	Correlation (with "gold standard" measure of characteristic or construct)
Predictive Criterion	How well does the measure predict a future event or outcome?	Correlation (with outcome variable, measured after a period of time)
Construct	Does the test measure a single underlying theoretical concept or construct?	Correlation (with variables theoretically related to the construct of interest)
	How many underlying constructs are included in the measure?	Confirmatory factor analysis
Construct Discriminant Divergent	How well does the test or measure differentiate between/among groups?	T-test or analysis of variance

coefficients or intraclass correlation coefficients as the statistical measure of the accuracy with which scores are reproduced.[66] There is no absolute standard of minimally acceptable reliability.[67] A score of 1 indicates a complete reliability (and is rarely achieved), and a score of 0 represents a complete lack of reliability. A general benchmark is that a score of $r = 0.9$ or better is strong evidence of reliability of that measure. Coefficients between .75 and .89 suggest that the measure has moderate risk of error but may be acceptable. Correlations of less than $r = .75$ are not typically perceived as having acceptable reliability.

The researchers who are reporting their study should provide an adequate description of the methodology of the study for the critical appraiser to determine which aspects of reliability are most important in this study (and therefore to determine if the authors provided evidence of the appropriate reliability). *Intertester reliability* should be reported if more than one tester measures the same outcome, and *intratester reliability* if the same tester measures outcomes on more than one occasion. *Test-retest reliability* provides evidence that the test performs consistently when repeated under similar conditions.

In addition, readers are interested in whether the validity of the measure has been assessed. To be considered valid, there must be sufficient evidence to demonstrate that the test or tool measures what it is purported to measure.[63-65] The researchers who have written the article must provide this evidence about the measure so that the critical appraiser can be comfortable that concerns about validity have been adequately addressed. Just because a tool is reliable (consistent in its measurement properties) does not mean that it is also valid (measures what it intends to measure). A tool cannot be valid, however, if it is not reliable in its measurement.[61] Ideally, the test or measures used in the study demonstrate great consistency with high reproducibility (i.e., reliability) and, at the same time, really measure the targeted characteristic (validity).

Evidence of validity is especially important if the test or tool measures an abstract concept (e.g., quality of life or functional independence) rather than a concrete physiological phenomenon (e.g., heart rate, range of motion). A valid test or measure contains enough items or questions related to the concept or characteristic being evaluated that the clinician can be confident that the results of testing will represent the subject's status in relationship to the construct being assessed. It is also important to note that a test or measure found to be reliable with one particular patient population is not automatically reliable with other populations.[61]

STEP 4: APPLICABILITY TO PATIENTS AND CLINICAL PRACTICE

The final component of an EBP approach to rehabilitative care is just as essential to provision of quality care as the ability to access and use available evidence and clinical expertise. Without consideration of the unique goals, expectations, values, and concerns that an individual in our care brings to the health care encounter, even the "perfect" plan of action will not be as efficacious as it might otherwise be. An individual's perspective and values are influenced by a number of factors including developmental issues and their position in the lifespan, their family system and culture, their work roles and responsibilities, their coping styles and strategies, their willingness or ability to access whatever resources might be available in their social support network, and their socioeconomic and educational resources.[68,69] To be as effective as possible in providing care, evidence-based practitioners must consider what the pathology, impairment, functional limitation, or disability means to the individual with respect to self-concept and sociocultural roles.[70]

Clinical Relevance

Assessing clinical importance of a study has both objective and subjective considerations. The clinician must look beyond the statistical significance of the findings.[71] Often this assessment is based on professional judgment about the impact of the extent of change. Does a statistically significant change in a functional test score or pain level translate into a change that the patient will perceive as important in daily life? Does long-term follow-up occur? That is, does the author examine the effectiveness of a given intervention 3 months, 6 months, or 1 year following the intervention? If the article only provides evidence of short-term benefits of the intervention, are these short-term benefits worth the time and effort in the long run? Would other interventions have had a better long-term outcome?

Making the decision to implement new approaches to care supported by the research literature requires the evidence-based practitioner to answer several questions related to his or her specific clinical environment[72]:

- How similar are the subjects used in the study to those in his or her clinical practice?
- How do the patient's values and expectations interact with or relate to effort, risks, and likely outcomes of the intervention being considered?

For studies of interventions/therapy/treatment consider the following:

- How likely is it that the patient will be willing and able to comply with intervention activities suggested in the study?

For studies of diagnosis consider the following:

- Is the diagnostic test adequately available, affordable, accurate, and precise for use in the clinician's setting?
- Is it likely that the patient will be willing and able to comply with the testing procedures?

For studies of prognosis consider the following:

- Will knowing the predictor factors make a clinically important difference in the way the clinician will care for his or her patients?

INTEGRATING CLINICAL EXPERTISE AND SKILL

Although the research literature is a valuable and important resource for evidence-based decision making, using evidence from the literature is not sufficient for effective EBP. Practitioners must also have strong examination, evaluation, and diagnostic skills and should be able to incorporate these skills into reflective past experience and current research findings.[73]

What is *clinical expertise?* In rehabilitation, it is the combination and integration of (a) a multidimensional knowledge base that is grounded in basic science, medical science, psychological/sociocultural sciences, and movement sciences; (b) effective clinical reasoning skills and an orientation toward function; (c) well-developed and efficient psychomotor skills for examination and intervention; and (d) the desire or commitment to help the individuals clinicians work with[74-76] (Figure 6-3).

The first chapter of this text explored the educational preparation, roles, and responsibilities of individual health professionals involved in orthotic and prosthetic rehabilitation. Each has a particular body of knowledge to bring to the care of individuals needing a prosthesis or orthosis, as well as shared understanding (albeit at various depths) of anatomy, kinesiology, biomechanics, gait analysis, mobility training, motor control and motor learning, and principles of exercise. The authors have established that effective interdisciplinary teaming, in which each profession's perspective interacts so that the team becomes "more than the sum of its parts," is an essential component in the provision of successful orthotic or prosthetic rehabilitative care.

The background knowledge important in orthotic and prosthetic rehabilitation that enables clinicians to ask sound clinical questions and apply evidence to patient care includes a strong foundation in the following areas:

- Anatomy and physiology of the musculoskeletal, neuromuscular, cardiovascular, and cardiopulmonary systems
- Kinesiology and biomechanics of the human body
- Properties of orthotic and prosthetic materials
- Principles of motor control and motor learning
- Lifespan development
- Exercise prescription and assessment of exercise tolerance
- Determinants of "normal" gait and methods of gait assessment

How does the clinician gain knowledge necessary for expert practice? Entry-level professional education is the baseline, while "on-the-job" experience via trial and error practice and discussion/debate/collaboration with colleagues moves clinicians from students toward novices.[74,76] They become more competent in their roles and responsibilities as their experience grows; they support and enhance their developing mastery and expertise with continuing education, participation in journal clubs and perusal of the clinical research litera-

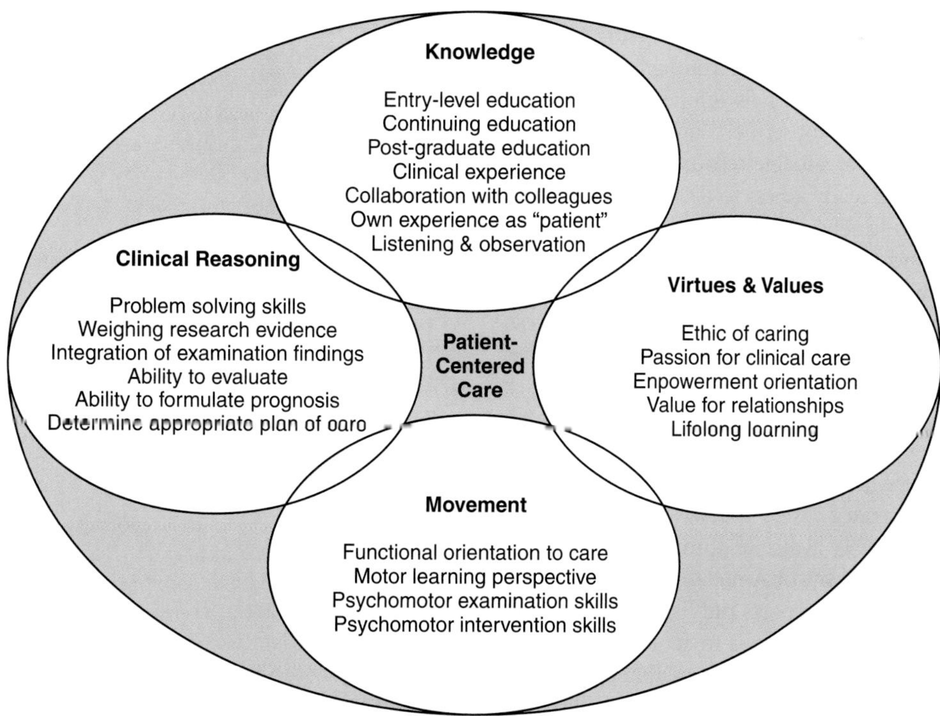

Figure 6-3
Expert "patient-centered" physical therapy practice requires integration and interaction of a provider's underlying knowledge, values, examination and intervention skills, and clinical reasoning.

ture, and postgraduate education. Another important component of increasing competence and developing expertise is the ability to actively listen to the hopes and concerns of those they work with and incorporate these into decision making and plans of care.

Clinical expertise, then, allows health care providers to quickly and efficiently identify an individual's rehabilitation diagnosis and, based on their constellation of impairments and functional limitations, select the strategies for remediation or accommodation that will assist the individual's return to a preferred lifestyle.

Staying Current with the Literature

One proactive way that a clinician can keep informed about new studies focused on his or her area of practice is to sign up for an online service that automatically sends weekly or monthly electronic updates of new articles from journals that the clinician feels are important to read or content areas that he or she wants to stay informed about. Professional organizations often offer this service as a membership benefit. Many journals allow readers to sign up for a service that electronically sends the table of contents via email whenever a new issue of the journal is released. Another valuable service (without charge) for evidence-based practitioners is available from an information management company, Amedeo (http://www.amedeo.com). When an evidence-based practitioner subscribes to Amedeo, he or she chooses from a list of topics for notification of newly published articles linked to those selected topics. Amedeo topics include rehabilitation, pain management, vascular surgery, and stroke, among many others. Amedeo routinely searches a large variety of high-quality journals for new publications on the topics selected by subscribers and sends weekly updates via email. This is a valuable resource for busy clinicians who may not have ready access to a medical library.

Two strategies, if routinely used, help health professionals to update and expand their expertise. The first is to select two or three journals (see Table 6-2) that are particularly appropriate for the clinician's area of professional interest and practice and arrange (via the journal's website) to receive an electronic copy of the table of contents of each issue. When the update arrives, it will be well worth the clinician's time and effort to scroll through the listing of articles and authors to determine which would be worth tracking down to read. The second strategy is to use whatever electronic literature update service is available through professional organizations, PubMed cubby, or Amedeo to arrange to be notified regularly of research reports published in the clinician's area of interest. The final step is to actually (and consistently) make time to read the resources that have been identified and discuss and debate them with colleagues in order to effectively integrate the new information into clinical practice.

SUMMARY

This chapter has explored the concepts underlying "evidence-based health care practice" and illustrated strategies to develop clear clinical questions, relevant to an individual patient who is receiving care. The chapter has also identified various sources of evidence available to clinicians and illustrated how electronic databases can assist the search process. The authors have suggested strategies that clinicians can use to develop critical appraisal skills and to update and expand their clinical expertise. Although much of the chapter has focused on evidence available in the research literature, it is the *integration* of the best available scientific evidence; clinical expertise and judgment; and the concerns, values, and expectations of the individual clinicians care for that determines the effectiveness of clinical decision making.

REFERENCES

1. Wong RA, Barr JO, Farina N, et al. Evidence-based practice: a resource for physical therapists. *Issues Aging* 2000;23(3):19-26.
2. Pollack N, Rochon S. Becoming an evidence based practitioner. In Law M (ed), *Evidence Based Rehabilitation: A Guide to Practice.* Thorofare, NJ: Slack, 2002. pp. 31-48.
3. Law M, Philip I. Evaluating the evidence. In Law M (ed), *Evidence Based Rehabilitation: A Guide to Practice,* Thorofare, NJ: Slack, 2002. pp. 97-108.
4. Sackett DL, Straus SE, Richardson WS, et al. *Evidence-based Medicine: How to Practice and Teach EBM,* 2nd ed. Edinburgh: Churchill Livingstone, 2000.
5. Donald A, Greenhalgh T. *A Hands-on Guide to Evidence-based Health Care: Practice and Implementation.* Oxford, UK: Blackwell Science, 2000.
6. Batavia M. *Clinical Research for Health Professionals: A User Friendly Guide.* Boston: Butterworth Heinemann, 2001.
7. Who are physical therapists, and what do they do? In American Physical Therapy Association (ed), *Guide to Physical Therapist Practice,* 2nd ed. Alexandria, VA: APTA, 2001. pp. 39-50.
8. Kassirer JP. Incorporating patient's preferences into medical decisions. *N Engl J Med* 1994;330(26):1895-1896.
9. Guyatt G, Haynes B, Jaeschke R, et al. Introduction: the philosophy of evidence-based medicine. In Guyatt G, Rennie D (eds), *Users' Guide to the Medical Literature.* Chicago: AMA Press, 2002. pp. 3-47.
10. Portney LG, Watkins MP. *Foundations of Clinical Research: Applications to Practice,* 2nd ed. Upper Saddle River, NJ: Prentice-Hall Health, 2000.
11. Greenhalgh T. Papers that report drug trials. In Greenhalgh T (ed), *How to Read a Paper: the Basics of Evidence Based Medicine,* 2nd ed. London: BMJ Books, 2001. pp. 94-104.
12. Guyatt G, Cook D, Devereaux PJ, et al. Therapy. In Guyatt G, Rennie D (eds), *Users' Guide to the Medical Literature.* Chicago: AMA Press, 2002. pp. 55-79.
13. Greenhalgh T. Papers that report diagnostic or screening tests. In Greenhalgh T, *How to Read a Paper: the Basics of Evidence Based Medicine,* 2nd ed. London: BMJ Books, 2001. pp. 105-119.

14. Fritz JM, Wainner RS. Examining diagnostic tests, an evidence-based perspective. *Phys Ther* 2001;81(9):1546-1564.
15. Randolf A, Bucher H, Richardson WS, et al. Prognosis. In Guyatt G, Rennie D (eds), *Users' Guide to the Medical Literature.* Chicago: AMA Press, 2002. pp. 55-79.
16. On what concepts is the guide based? Guide to physical therapy practice. *Phys Ther* 2001;81:27-33.
17. World Health Organization. *Toward a Common Language for Functioning, Disability, and Health.* Geneva: World Health Organization, 2002.
18. Helewa A, Walker JM. Where to look for evidence. In Helewa A, Walker JM (eds), *Critical Evaluation of Research in Physical Rehabilitation, Toward Evidence-Based Practice.* Philadelphia: Saunders; 2000. pp. 33-48.
19. Walker-Dilks C. Searching the physiotherapy evidence-based literature. *Physiother Theory Pract* 2001;17(3):137-142.
20. Maher CG, Serrington C, Elkins M, et al. Challenges for evidence-based physical therapy: accessing and interpreting high-quality evidence on therapy. *Phys Ther* 2004;84(8):644-654.
21. Greenhalgh T. Searching the literature. In Greenhalgh T (ed), *How to Read a Paper: the Basics of Evidence Based Medicine,* 2nd ed. London: BMJ Books, 2001. pp. 15-39.
22. Herbert RD, Sherrington C, Maher C, et al. Evidence-based practice—imperfect but necessary. *Physiother Theory Pract* 2001;17(3):201-211.
23. Jette DU, Bacon K, Batty C, et al. Evidence-based practice: beliefs, attitudes, knowledge, and behaviors of physical therapists. *Phys Ther* 2003;93(9):786-805.
24. Turner P. Evidence-based practice and physiotherapy in the 1990s. *Physiother Theory Pract* 2001;17(2):107-121.
25. Maher C, Moseley A, Sherrington C, et al. Core journals of evidence-based physiotherapy practice. *Physiother Theory Pract* 2001;17(3):143-151.
26. Bohannon RW. Core journals of physiotherapy. *Physiotherapy* 1999;85(6):317-321.
27. Jada A. *Randomized Controlled Clinical Trials; a User's Guide.* London: BMJ Publishing Group, 1998.
28. Helewa A, Walker JM. The nuts and bolts of research: terms, concepts, and designs. In Helewa A, Walker JM (eds), *Critical Evaluation of Research in Physical Rehabilitation: Towards Evidence-based Practice.* Philadelphia: Saunders, 2000. pp. 1-32.
29. Greenhalgh T. Papers that summarize other papers (systematic reviews and meta-analysis). In Greenhalgh T (ed), *How to Read a Paper: the Basics of Evidence Based Medicine,* 2nd ed. London: BMJ Books, 2001. pp. 120-138.
30. Cook DJ, Mulrow CD, Haynes RB. Systematic reviews: synthesis of best evidence for clinical decisions. *Ann Intern Med* 1997;126(5):376-380.
31. Montori VM, Swiontkowski MF, Cook DJ. Methodologic issues in systematic reviews and meta-analyses. *Clin Orthop Related Res* 2003;413:43-54.
32. Law M, Philip I. Systematically reviewing the evidence. In Law M (ed), *Evidence-based Rehabilitation: a Guide to Physical Therapy Practice,* Thorofare, NJ: Slack, 2002. pp. 109-126.
33. Lau J, Ionnidis JPA, Schmid CH. Quantitative synthesis in systematic reviews. *Ann Intern Med* 1997;127(9):820-826.
34. Montori VM, Wilczynski NL, Morgan D, et al. Optimal search strategies for retrieving systematic reviews from Medline: analytical survey. *BMJ* 2005;330(7482):68-71.
35. Morris C. A review of the efficacy of lower-limb orthoses used for cerebral palsy. *Dev Med Child Neurol* 2002;44(3):205-211.
36. Rome K, Handoll HH, Ashford R. Interventions for preventing and treating stress fractures and stress reactions of bone of the lower limbs in young adults. *Cochrane Database Syst Rev* 2005;(2);CD00045.
37. Nicholson D. Practice guidelines, algorithms, and clinical pathways. In Law M (ed), *Evidence-based Rehabilitation: a Guide to Physical Therapy Practice.* Thorofare, NJ: Slack, 2002. pp. 195-219.
38. Philadelphia panel evidence-based clinical practice guidelines on selected rehabilitation interventions: overview and methodology. *Phys Ther* 2001;81(10):1629-1640.
39. *A User's Guide to Finding and Evaluating Health Information on the Web.* Medical Library Association. http://www.mlanet.org/resources/userguide.html.
40. Shojania KG, Bero LA. Taking advantage of the explosion of systematic reviews: an efficient search strategy. *Eff Clin Pract* 2001;4(4):157-162.
41. O'Rourke A, Booth A. Another fine MeSH: clinical medicine meets information science. *J Info Sci* 1999;25(4):275-281.
42. Snowball R. Using the clinical question to teach search strategy: fostering transferable conceptual skills in user education by active learning. *Health Libr Rev* 1997;14(3): 167-172.
43. McKibbon KA, Richardson WS, Walker-Dilks C. EBM notebook: finding answers to well built questions. *Evid Based Med* 1999;4(6):164-167.
44. Greenhalgh T. Assessing methodological quality. In *How to Read a Paper: the Basics of Evidence-based Medicine,* 2nd ed. London: BMJ Books, 2001. pp. 59-75.
45. Fink R, Thompson CJ, Bonnes D. Overcoming barriers and promoting the use of research in practice. *J Nurs Admin* 2005;35(3):121-129.
46. Turner P, Mjolne I. Journal provision and the prevalence of journal clubs: a survey of physiotherapy departments in England and Australia. *Physiother Res Int* 2001;6(3):157-169.
47. Urschel JD. How to analyze an article. *World J Surg* 2005;29(5):557-560.
48. Crombie IK. *The Pocket Guide to Critical Appraisal.* London: BMJ Publishing Group, 1998.
49. Levangie PK. *Measurement Workshop Manual, Graduate Program in Geriatric Rehabilitation and Wellness.* Fairfield, CT: Sacred Heart University, 2003.
50. Dumholdt E. *Rehabilitation Research: Principles and Applications,* 3rd ed. Philadelphia: Saunders, 2004.
51. Archibald CP, Lee HP. Sample size estimation for clinicians. *Ann Acad Med Singapore* 1995;24(2):328-332.
52. Livingston EH, Cassidy L. Statistical power and estimation of required subjects for a study based on the t-test; a surgeons primer. *J Surg Res* 2005;126(2)149-159.
53. Chow SC, Shao J, Wang H. *Sample Size Calculation in Clinical Research,* New York: Marcel Dekker, 2003.
54. Rossi JS. Statistical power of psychological research: what have we gained in 20 years? *J Consult Clin Psychol* 1990;58(5): 646-656.
55. Daunt DJ. Ethnicity and recruitment rates in clinical research studies. *Appl Nurs Res* 2003;16(3):189-195.
56. Larson E. Exclusion of certain groups from clinical research. *Image J Nurs Scholarsh* 1994;26(3):185-190.

57. Sitthi-amorn C, Poshyachinda V. Bias. *Lancet* 1993;342(8866):286-288.
58. Morabia A. Case-control studies in clinical research: mechanism and prevention of selection bias. *Prev Med* 1997;25(5 Pt 1):674-677.
59. Mason MJ. A review of procedural and statistical methods for handling attrition and missing data in clinical research. *Measurement Eval Counsel Devel* 1999;32(2):111-118.
60. Montori VM, Guyatt GH. Intention to treat principle. *Can Med Assoc J* 2001;165(10):1339-1341.
61. Salkind NJ. Just the truth: an introduction to understanding reliability and validity. In *Statistics for People Who Think They Hate Statistics,* 2nd ed. Thousand Oaks, CA: Sage Publications, 2004. pp. 273-296.
62. Shultz KS, Whitney DJ. Classical true score theory and reliability, module 5. In *Measurement Theory in Action.* Thousand Oaks, CA: Sage Publications, 2005. pp. 69-85.
63. Shultz KS, Whitney DJ. Content validation, module 6. In *Measurement Theory in Action.* Thousand Oaks, CA: Sage Publications, 2005. pp. 87-100.
64. Shultz KS, Whitney DJ. Criterion-related validation, module 7. In *Measurement Theory in Action.* Thousand Oaks, CA: Sage Publications, 2005. pp. 101-118.
65. Shultz KS, Whitney DJ. Construct validation, module 8. In *Measurement Theory in Action.* Thousand Oaks, CA: Sage Publications, 2005. pp. 119-134.
66. Eliasziw M. Statistical methodology for the concurrent assessment of interrater and intrarater reliability: using goniometric measurements as an example. *Phys Ther* 1994;74(8):777-788.
67. Stratford PW. Getting more from the literature; estimating standard error of measurement from reliability studies. *Physiother Can* 2004;56(1):27-30.
68. Fell DW, Burnham JF. Access is key: teaching students and physical therapists to access evidence, expert opinion, and patient values for evidence based practice. *J Phys Ther Educ* 2004;18(3):12-23.
69. Lockwood S. "Evidence of me" in evidence based medicine: *BMJ* 2004;329(7473):1033-1035.
70. Spector RE. *Cultural Diversity in Health and Illness,* 6th ed. Upper Saddle River, NJ: Prentice-Hall, 2003.
71. Foster N, Barlas P, Chesterton L, et al. Critically appraised topics: one method of facilitating evidence-based practice in physiotherapy. *Physiotherapy* 2001;87(4):179-190.
72. Greenhalgh T. Implementing evidence based findings. In Greenhalgh T (ed), *How to Read a Paper: the Basics of Evidence-based Medicine,* 2nd ed. London: BMJ Books, 2001. pp. 179-199.
73. Jensen GM, Dwyer J, Shepard K, et al. Expert practice in physical therapy. *Phys Ther* 2000;80(1):28-43.
74. Hack LM. Fostering evidence-based practice in physical therapy: clinical decision making frameworks. In Wong R (ed), *Evidence-Based Healthcare Practice, Proceedings of a Consensus Conference "EBP: Where Are We Today? Where Are We Going? How Do We Get There?"* Arlington, VA: Marymount University, 2001. pp. 22-30.
75. Resnik L, Jensen GM. Using clinical outcomes to explore theory of expert practice in physical therapy. *Phys Ther* 2003;83(12):1090-1106.
76. Jensen GM, Gwyer J, Hack L, et al. *Expertise in Physical Therapy Practice.* Boston: Butterworth Heinemann, 1999.

7

Principles Influencing Orthotic and Prosthetic Design: Biomechanics, Device-User Interface, and Related Concepts

CHRISTOPHER F. HOVORKA, MARK D. GEIL, AND MICHELLE M. LUSARDI

LEARNING OBJECTIVES

On completion of this chapter, the reader will be able to do the following:

1. Describe important questions that are essential to determining the "ideal" orthosis or prosthesis for a patient.
2. Describe basic kinesiology and biomechanical principles of human joint motion, including the components of joint rotation, joint moments, and joint power.
3. Describe the design and engineering of orthoses and prostheses in distributing forces to body segments.
4. Identify interactions at the interface of the orthosis or prosthesis and the patient and distinguish among shear, friction, coefficient of friction, and pressure.
5. Describe the influence of lower limb orthoses and prostheses on the patient's gait, including factors affecting gait efficiency and physiological energy expenditure.

WHAT MAKES AN "IDEAL" ORTHOSIS?

Although no orthosis can restore "normal" function to the person with neuromuscular or musculoskeletal impairment, an effective and well-designed orthosis can enhance mobility and other functioning through various control mechanisms and improve quality of life. From the perspective of the patient with an orthosis, two important determinants of success are whether the orthosis is comfortable and the extent to which the device meets his or her needs and goals.[1] The four most important concepts the health care professional should consider when defining an "ideal" orthosis for a patient are the four *C*'s: control, comfort, cosmesis, and cost.

Control

The orthotist and therapist first ask a series of questions about how an orthosis will control function while being worn. The first question is whether (and how well) the orthosis enables the user to accomplish tasks and be involved in activities that are important to him or her without undue skin irritation, fatigue, or other orthosis-induced concerns.[2] Even the most technically advanced orthosis will remain in the user's closet or under the bed if it is too hot to wear for long periods of time or produces notable tissue breakdown.

The second question considers which body segments are being controlled by the orthosis. An ideal orthosis controls only abnormal or undesirable motions and permits motion where normal function can occur.[3] The basis for the orthosis design should be an accurate biomechanical analysis of the person who will use the device followed by selection of appropriate components and design features.

The next sets of questions to consider center on how well the orthosis achieves the intended biomechanical goals of stability or of maintenance or correction of alignment. Will the orthosis halt or limit joint motion, accommodate existing deformity, or reduce progression of deformity? Does the orthosis support or protect a joint, limb, or body segment during movement as intended? How effective is the orthosis in controlling movement in the presence of spasticity or weakness? Does the patient's functional status improve when it is worn?

Comfort

The orthotist and therapist must also assess whether the orthosis causes the user any discomfort or pain. The orthosis should accomplish its intended goals without causing secondary problems, such as skin and underlying tissue irritation or breakdown, excessive discomfort, or unnecessary stress to other joints. Patients needing orthoses are more likely to use them if they fit well by conforming to the body area, maintaining good suspension, resisting environmental factors (repetitive loading, extreme cold and heat, perspiration and other body fluids), and reliably performing desired functions. Other questions to consider are whether the the orthosis is too heavy or too cumbersome to use for more than a short period. An orthosis is more likely to be used if it is minimally cumbersome, easy to don and doff, and simple to clean and maintain.[4]

Cosmesis

Persons who wear orthoses often want them to be "cosmetic," in that they can be worn with usual clothing and not be too noticeable.[5,6] However, if an orthosis allows the wearer to accomplish a meaningful task or take part in an important activity that he or she otherwise would not be able to do, then cosmesis might not be a paramount issue.

Cost

Cost can refer to either the wearer's energy expenditure or the economic cost of the device. In terms of *energy cost*, whether an orthosis will allow the wearer to function with a reasonable (and sustainable) energy expenditure should be determined. If using the orthosis creates an excessive energy demand, the wearer often chooses not to use it. For some individuals with physiological impairments, high energy costs may actually be detrimental. Individuals with compromised cardiovascular or cardiorespiratory function or metabolic pathosis who have limited energy reserve must be carefully evaluated. Characteristics of an ideal orthosis that minimizes energy consumption or constriction of breathing include a simple and lightweight design and the ability to don and doff without difficulty. Many designs of orthoses positively affect the gait of the users and conserve physiological energy expenditure, whereas other designs may increase energy consumption in exchange for other functional controls.[7-18]

The *monetary cost* of an orthosis is determined by the materials used and the time and skill requirements for measurement, fabrication, and fitting. Orthoses that incorporate technologically sophisticated designs and components (e.g., carbon fiber lamination, microcomputer joint motion controls) usually increase the fabrication time and associated monetary costs.[19] The clinician must determine whether the patient or third-party payer can cover the fiscal cost of orthotic care and whether preauthorization procedures or other documentation are required for reimbursement when the orthosis has unique features such as polycentric joints, material reinforcements, or noncorrosive alloy coatings. Changes in health care policy have created greater demands for the provision of extensive documentation by the health care professional to the patient's funding agencies or other interested parties. As a result, the clinician needs to understand and provide documentation that details why orthotic treatment is necessary. A justification can be compelling when it shows that orthotic treatment will either reduce the monetary cost of rehabilitation or increase independence and self-care. Justification is particularly convincing when it can be stated that withholding orthotic treatment can be deleterious to a patient's health.[20]

Cost is also influenced by a number of other factors. Will the orthosis require expensive maintenance? How durable are the materials and components? Will components require frequent replacement because of excessive loading or environmental factors? Can the device consistently function and perform according to the original treatment plan?

Other Factors

The rehabilitation team must consider two other factors. One is *timing*, or the speed and efficiency with which an orthosis can be fabricated and delivered. Individuals who receive an orthosis during inpatient hospitalization usually require time for fitting and training before discharge.

The other factor is *adjustability*, the ability of the orthosis to be adjusted to accommodate growth or changes in the user's functional status. Orthoses used by children may fit optimally for a limited time or only during periods when growth is slow and progressive.[21] For others, a modular orthosis such as a knee-ankle-foot orthosis (KAFO) may provide multiple functions, such as stretching of tight hamstrings when used at night and allowing unrestricted knee movement (with the thigh section disassembled) for daily use as an ankle-foot orthosis (AFO) to enhance ambulation.[22]

The rehabilitation team is interested in the ease of fabrication and adjustment of the orthosis because these factors may affect the safe function of the device and the frequency of trips to the orthotist for repairs. Individuals with pathological conditions in which there is a period of recovery of function (e.g., upper motor neuron lesions, such as stroke) may progress from hypotonic muscle function and limited volitional control to synergistic patterns of movement and hypertonicity.[23-27] Return of movement tends to start proximally in the muscles of the limb girdle (shoulder or hip) and progress through intermediate joints (elbow or knee) toward distal limb segments (wrist/hand or ankle/foot). Distal control is often a synergistic pattern of total flexion for the upper extremity and total extension for the lower extremity.[23] Gradually, movement may come under voluntary control, but the recovery of function varies for the upper and lower extremity musculature, and the speed at which recovery takes place depends on the degree of impairment.

Individuals with spasticity and loss of voluntary motor control and joint deformity earlier in recovery may advance to lower levels of spasticity and the restoration of some "normal" residual motor strength and control and reduced joint deformity. In these cases the initial orthotic needs of the patient may be to halt motion control and limit joint deformity.[28,29] As voluntary motor control is restored, the requirements for orthotic controls change. Increasing joint motion is requisite at this stage to enhance the user's limb function in a safe and efficient fashion.[30,31] Even alteration of shapes and contours in AFO designs may provide neural feedback to improve foot alignment and possibly influence spasticity.[32-34] Optimal orthosis function is based on understanding normal joint structure and function, the kinematics of gait, the pathomechanics that result from the patient's pathological condition or impairments, the ability to conceptualize the interaction between the orthosis and the patient's body segment, and the underlying control mechanisms of the orthosis and its design.[35]

WHAT MAKES AN "IDEAL" PROSTHESIS?

Because a prosthesis replaces a missing part of the body, the ideal prosthesis should function exactly like the body part it replaces. The challenge in accomplishing this goal, assuming clinicians do not aspire to improve on anatomical function, is that the function of a body part is dynamic, complex, and often not adequately understood. As with an orthosis, the four *C*s—control, cosmesis, comfort, and cost—also play a significant role in determining the ideal features of the prosthesis. Minimizing the time the patient waits for the prosthesis and optimizing the condition of the individual's sound limb can set the stage for successful fitting of the first prosthesis.[36-38] A compromised condition of the sound limb (e.g., arthritis, intermittent claudication), long delays in prosthesis fitting and delivery, prolonged gait training, cardiac and respiratory problems, and constant residual limb pain have been shown to be significantly related to nonuse of the prosthesis.[39] Conversely, a positive result of amputation (e.g., reduced pain, feeling of well-being) is associated with increased use of the prosthesis and improved function.[40,41]

Dynamic Function

Limb segments are remarkably versatile in function. A human hand can perform tasks ranging from the precise, fine movement required to thread a needle to the rigid coupling necessary when hammering a nail. Most human body segments contain neuromotor redundancy so that the same task can be performed with different motor units or even motion paths.[42] It is challenging enough to duplicate a single task with a prosthesis; versatility and redundancy are therefore rarely included in design criteria.

Complex Function

Because human beings are able to complete so many movement tasks with so little conscious thought and direction, overlooking the complexity associated with movement is easy. A routine task such as rising from a chair involves an extraordinary range of sensory input; coordinated generation of force in agonists and antagonists; and strategies to optimize criteria related to balance, efficiency, and muscle function.[43] Prosthetists often attempt to use simplicity as a guiding design principle; however, the complexity of human movement tests this design criterion.

Poorly Understood Function

It is difficult to attempt to replace a system that is both complex and versatile. It is doubly difficult to replace a system when the function of the original body segment is poorly understood. Unfortunately, this is a common reality in human movement. For example, debate persists among students of gait about which muscles are used to advance the limb into swing phase. Although this is a fundamental and critical component of gait, no consensus exists on the role of late-stance ankle plantar flexion, with many suggesting the ankle power burst serves to propel the limb forward (push-off) and others contending that there is no ankle push-off.[44-46] Prosthesis design remains far behind this ideal, so perhaps understanding of normal human movement will continue to improve while those involved in the design of prostheses bridge the gap.

Beyond replicating movement, additional factors should be considered in the ideal prosthesis, such as suspension, socket attachment, materials, mass, and inertial properties. Prosthesis design has seen laudable progress in many of these areas, but other design criteria have been sacrificed.[47]

UNDERSTANDING HUMAN MOTION

Mechanics as a branch of engineering can be divided into *statics* and *dynamics*.[48] The application of mechanical principles to analyze the musculoskeletal system is appropriately called *biomechanics*.[48] Therefore, biomechanics includes both the study of static situations and human motion. The application of mechanical principles to study disorders of the musculoskeletal system is called *pathomechanics*.[48] Since the time of the first biomechanists such as DaVinci, Galileo, Borelli, and Newton, progress has been made in the understanding of mechanics and mathematics, with increasing application to human function. In the nineteenth and twentieth centuries, human movement analysis improved along with understanding of soft tissues and muscles. Only recently, however, has biomechanics become an independently identified discipline.[49-51] As the professions of orthopedics, physical therapy, exercise science, and orthotics and prosthetics have evolved, the study and subsequent knowledge base of biomechanics have rapidly expanded.[49,52-54]

The body of knowledge we now call orthotics and prosthetics is increasingly derived from well-established concepts in engineering, anatomy, physical and occupational therapy, orthopedics, and physical medicine. What makes the study of orthotics and prosthetics a unique body of knowledge is the combination and enrichment of these concepts. For orthotists to develop an AFO or prosthetists to develop an endoskeletal transtibial prosthesis, they must work together with the rehabilitation health care team. Health care professionals must be able to perform observational gait analysis; identify critical deviations; and understand where restraining, assisting, or resisting forces are to be applied. Orthotists and prosthetists must convert these forces into materials and components and then design, fabricate, fit, and critique the performance of the resulting AFO or the function of the endoskeletal transtibial prosthesis.[49] Ideally, the health care team then works with the patient and orthotist or prosthetist in unison to follow up the fitting process and periodically assess patient functional status and the performance of the orthotic or prosthetic device to maximize patient treatment.[55]

Because modern health care is fragmented and often interdisciplinary, a good understanding of orthosis and prosthesis design and function principles is essential for the orthotists, prosthetists, and rehabilitation team members who assess and treat the patient.[56-60] Consistency in the understanding of biomechanics and orthosis and prosthesis design criteria across health care disciplines is critical to facilitating communication and maximizing the patient's rehabilitation treatment outcome.[61-67]

Describing Motion

A line in an old children's song is "I'm all made of hinges and everything bends." Indeed, it is the "hinges," or joints, that allow the relatively rigid segments of the human body to move through space. Concerted motion of multiple joints is necessary for the majority of human motion. Consequently, an understanding of the biomechanics of human motion requires different thinking than an understanding of general motion. Human biomechanics requires a focus on joint rotation, force couples that produce joint rotation, and transfer of power through quasirigid segments by joints.

Joint Rotation

Historically, joint motion has been described by a variety of qualitative and quantitative naming conventions. Multiple standards exist to characterize mathematically the three-dimensional orientation of one body segment with respect to another, including sequential rotations (Euler/Cardan angles)[68] and screw/helical axis systems.[69] From an anatomical perspective, joint articulation might include translations such as sliding and rolling about a moving axis of rotation.[70] In fact, many prosthetic knee joints are designed to use mechanical linkages to create a polycentric joint.

Mathematical models of human joint motion usually include variable instantaneous centers so that the combination of motions is collectively calculated as joint rotation. From a clinical perspective, these mathematical descriptors of motion are characterized by more intuitive titles such as flexion, extension, and abduction. Anatomically based nomenclature is reasonably standardized and has been documented in texts in the last several decades.[71,72] The general sense of rotation in most joints is linked to three anatomical planes of motion: sagittal, transverse, and frontal (Figure 7-1).

Lower extremity motions such as hip, knee, and ankle flexion and extension are generally grouped as sagittal plane motions. Hip abduction and adduction, knee varus and valgus, and subtalar inversion and eversion are generally considered frontal plane motions. Transverse plane motions include internal and external rotation at the hip, knee, and ankle. Normal ranges of motion for these joints have been established (Table 7-1).

Although motion at the ankle/foot complex can be characterized in these separate planes, actual free motion of some joints, such as the ankle and foot, includes combinations of all three planar rotations. *Pronation* in the open kinetic chain combines motions of external rotation of the tibia and fibula, ankle dorsiflexion, and motions of the foot (subtalar eversion and forefoot abduction).[73,74] Open kinetic chain *supination* combines internal rotation of the tibia and fibula, ankle plantar flexion, and motions of the foot (subtalar inversion and forefoot adduction).[73,74]

During closed kinetic chain activities such as the stance phase of gait, motion at one joint is often coupled (has an influence on) motion at the proximal and distal joints. An example of this is the relation between pronation of the ankle/foot complex and internal (medial) rotation of proximal joints up the kinetic chain of the leg (tibia and fibula, knee, and hip) during stance phase.[75-77] The dynamics of motion vary in both the open and closed kinetic chain where the plane of motion does not always correspond with the type of motion. For example, knee flexion combined with external hip rotation means that to measure the amount of knee flexion, the perspective cannot be confined to the sagittal plane. Modern motion analysis systems use three-dimensional intersegmental angles referenced to a single global coordinate system to avoid this problem. It is more difficult to overcome when the only source of information is a two-dimensional videotape fixed in the frontal or sagittal plane.

Understanding joint rotation is essential to patient rehabilitation. Observational gait analysis methods often suggest assessment of joints in a sequential fashion from the frontal and sagittal planes to target certain joints and planes where pathologic conditions often affect locomotion. In a study of clinicians with extensive experience in observational gait analysis, subjects focused on the coronal plane of the patient under investigation, with most visual information obtained from regions around the feet, knees, and hands.[77] Instrumented gait analysis systems can provide more reliable reports of a subject's movements, containing graphs plotting the trajectory of joint angles (kinematics) sorted by planes of motion (Figure 7-2).

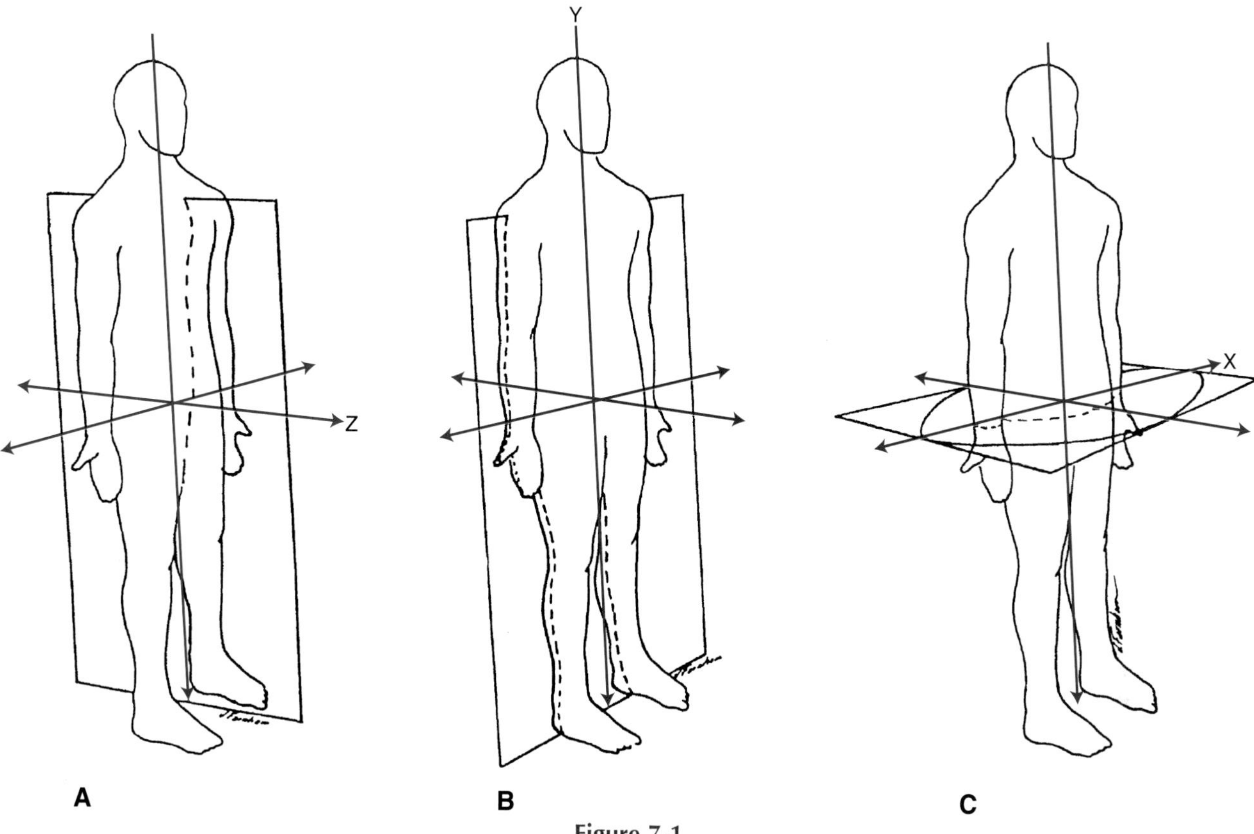

Figure 7-1

***A,** Sagittal plane motions, such as knee extension, occur around an axis of rotation in the frontal plane. **B,** Frontal plane motion, such as lateral bending of the trunk or abduction of the hip, occurs around an anteroposterior axis of rotation. **C,** Transverse plane motion, such as trunk rotation or internal rotation of the hip, occurs around a longitudinal axis of motion. (Modified from Norkin CC, Levangie PK.* Joint Structure and Function: A Comprehensive Analysis, *2nd ed, Philadelphia: F.A. Davis, 1992. p. 6.)*

Joint Moments

The importance of the forces used to generate joint rotation cannot be underestimated.[78] The human body is a complex system of muscles, levers, and joint articulations in which linear forces act at a distance from the center of a joint to cause the joint to rotate. When pairs of forces oppose one another at a distance, a force couple, or *moment,* is generated. In a joint, the moment is related to the force by the distance between the muscle's line of action and the joint center:

$$M = Fd$$

where *M* is the moment, *F* is the force, and *d* is the perpendicular distance between the force vector and the joint center, or *moment arm.* In Figure 7-3, the joint will extend if the muscle generates a force because the force acts at a distance from the joint center.

It is easier to open a door if the doorknob is placed far away from the hinges because the moment arm is greater. Following this logic, the human body attempts to use muscles as efficiently as possible by maximizing moment arms. This design is challenging within the confines of a relatively narrow arm or leg. A good example of an improved moment arm is the role of the patella in transferring quadriceps force. Quadriceps force acts by the patellar tendon with improved leverage because the patella has increased the distance of the force vector from the joint center. If Figure 7-3 represented a knee joint, the presence of a patella would increase *d,* thereby increasing the muscle moment with the same magnitude of muscle force. In the anatomical knee joint, the moment arm changes as the sagittal plane knee joint angle changes.

Joint moments can be calculated in the human body and used to analyze the biomechanics of motion. Joint moments are part of a set of information called *kinetics,* along with forces, energy, and power. The most common method used to calculate joint kinetics is called *inverse dynamics.*[79] This method combines information about the joints and the body segments they connect, such as the mass of each segment, joint kinematics (motion), and force produced by the extremity. In the case of locomotion, this force produced is measured as the ground reaction force. Joint moments are presented by motion analysis systems in the same format as joint angles: a grid of graphs with a row for each joint and a column for each plane.

Table 7-1
Normal Range of Motion of Lower Extremity Joints

Joint	*Motion*	*Magee*[138] *(active; degrees)*	*Hoppenfeld*[139] *(passive; degrees)*	*AAOS*[140] *(degrees)*	*Norkin et al*[16] *(passive; degrees)*
Hip	Flexion	110–120	120	120	120–135
	Extension	10–15	30	30	10–30
	Abduction	30–50	45–50	45	30–50
	Adduction	30	20–30	30	10–30
	External rotation	40–60	45	45	45–60
	Internal rotation	30–40	35	45	30–45
Knee	Flexion	135	135	135	130–140
	Extension	0	0–5	0	5–10
	Exterior rotation	10	10	—	40*
	Interior rotation	10	10	—	30*
Ankle	Dorsiflexion	20	20	20	20
	Plantar flexion	50	50	50	30–50
	Supination	45–60	—	—	—
	Pronation	15–30	—	—	—
	Inversion	—	—	35	—
	Eversion	—	—	15	—
	Subtalar inversion	5	5	5	—
	Subtalar eversion	5	5	5	—
Foot	Forefoot adduction	20	20	—	—
	Forefoot abduction	10	10	—	—
	Hallux MTP extension	70	70–90	70	—
	Hallux MTP flexion	45	45	45	—
	MTP extension[2–5]	—	—	40	—
	MTP flexion[2–5]	—		40	—

AAOS, American Academy of Orthopedic Surgeons; *MTP*, metatarsal-phalangeal.
*Passive external (lateral) and internal (medial) rotation of the tibia on the femur measured at 90 degrees of knee flexion.

A net joint moment provides information about the net effect of all muscle action on a joint. For example, a net moment at the knee joint can be measured in the sagittal plane. If this is an internal extensor moment, it is implied that the quadriceps are contracting to produce the moment. This does not necessarily mean that the hamstrings are not contracting, but only that the flexor moment they produce is of less magnitude than the quadriceps' extensor moment. Does an internal knee extensor moment imply that the knee is extending? Not necessarily, because muscle contractions can be concentric, eccentric, or isometric. A good example of a lengthening contraction is the biomechanics of the ankle joint during loading response in human walking (Figure 7-4).[46]

The net internal moment in the sagittal plane at the ankle joint is *dorsiflexion*, as the pretibial muscles contract to control the foot's first rocker to prevent foot slap and absorb shock during stance.[46] However, the foot is *plantar flexing* toward foot flat.

Joint Power

Joint angles describe the motion of the joints. Joint moments provide additional information about muscle forces used to rotate joints. Joint powers go one more step and add information about how quickly or slowly moments act on joints. In mechanics, work is defined as force acting to move an object over a distance. The rate at which work is done is called *power*. Calculation of joint power includes the joint moment and a measure of how quickly the joint moves. Because the focus with joints is on rotation, joint power (P) usually includes only rotational velocity (ω) and excludes linear or translational velocity:

$$P = M\omega$$

Joint power is a particularly important concept in the design of orthoses and prostheses when the devices are intended to act dynamically. Such devices use forces and leverage during human motion to redirect or augment power transfer. Examples include floor-reaction AFOs and dynamic elastic

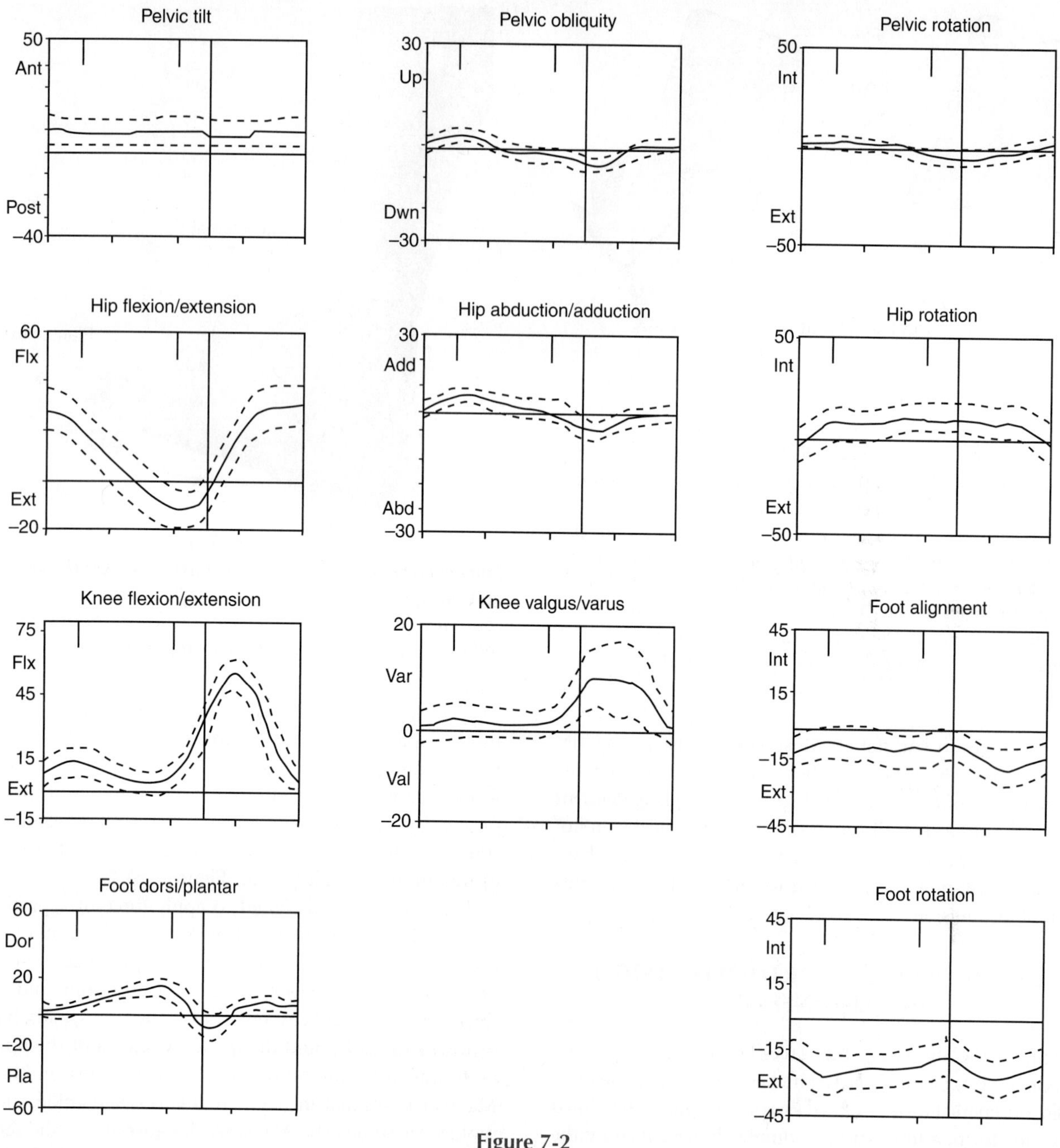

Figure 7-2

Joint kinematics presented in a typical gait report. Rows represent anatomical regions. The first column contains sagittal plane joint angles, the second contains frontal plane joint angles, and the third contains transverse joint angles, except for the foot. Often foot inversion and eversion are not reported. Each curve represents an average of several subjects. The dotted lines mark a band of plus or minus one standard deviation. (Modified from Kirtley C. CGA Normative Gait Database, http://guardian.curtin.edu.au/cga/, accessed December 2003.)

response prosthetic feet.[80] When loaded at the toeplate during midstance, the floor reaction AFO transfers loading from the toeplate to the proximal anterior pretibial section. This pushes the proximal shin in a posterior direction, resulting in a knee extension moment. The knee extension moment is particularly accentuated when the ankle portion of the AFO is aligned in slight plantar flexion, which produces an ankle plantar flexion–knee extension force coupling.[81,82] This type of orthosis design is usually indicated for individuals with ankle weakness and knee extension compromise. In addition, the fixed ankle provides swing phase foot clearance, stance ankle stability, and prevention or reduction of knee buckling.

Similarly, dynamic elastic response prosthetic feet attempt to replace the power normally generated by the ankle plantar

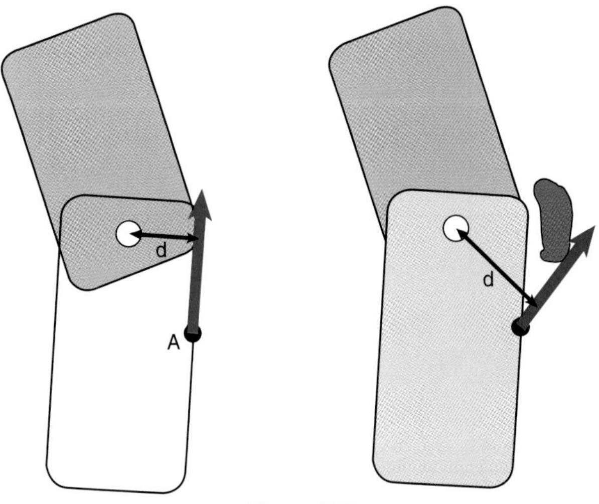

Figure 7-3

The moment a force can generate depends on its distance from the joint center. The force generated by a muscle attached at point A depends on its line of action. If the muscle acts along the line of the red vector, its moment and, consequently, its ability to rotate the joint, depends on its perpendicular distance d to the joint center (black arrow). *When considering a knee joint, for example, the moment arm d is increased by the patella, which redirects the muscle force to increase muscle moment.*

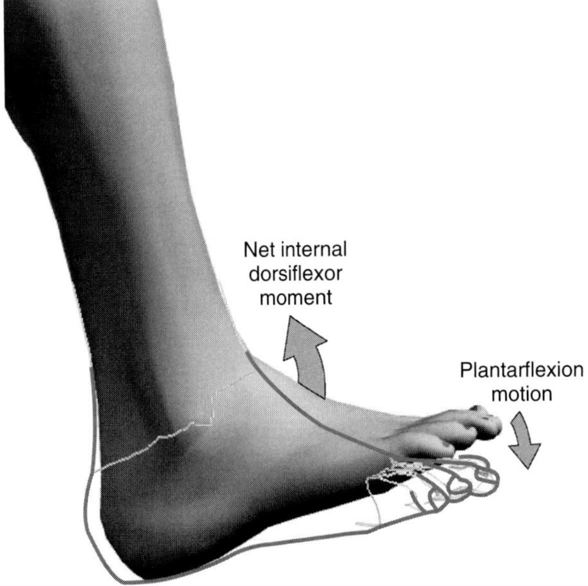

Figure 7-4

During normal loading response, the heel strikes the ground and the foot plantar flexes until foot flat. This action is controlled by the ankle dorsiflexors, which slow this natural rollover, absorbing power and reducing shock.

flexor muscles in late stance. Most varieties use a long, flat material (usually a carbon fiber composite) running the length of the foot to act as a leaf spring. The spring deforms during the equivalent of the second rocker. Near the end of stance phase, when the moment and rotational velocity have the same sign, power is returned to the proximal segments for limb propulsion.[83]

USE OF FORCES IN ORTHOSIS DESIGN AND ENGINEERING

Kinetics is the analysis of the forces that cause the motion. This analysis is based on Newton's laws of motion. Force is a basic concept that can be defined as a push or pull. Represented in vector form, a force can be completely described by the three characteristics of magnitude, direction, and point of application. The reaction force of the floor in the closed kinetic chain to the total body force (the combination of inertial forces and gravity) is the ground reaction force. Orthosis designs transfer the ground reaction force and other forces generated by the patient as part of a balanced parallel force system to control joint motion (Figure 7-5).[84]

These force systems operate, in effect, as a first-class lever system where the fulcrum lies between the two ends of the segment in which loading occurs. In a three-point loading or control system, a proximal and a distal force applied in the same direction are countered by (or balanced against) a third force applied in the opposite direction at a point somewhere in between them.[85-88] Each plane and direction of motion that the orthosis attempts to control has a three-point loading system. Some orthosis designs use additional forces, acting as balanced systems containing four, five, six, or more points, to allow better control of rotational and translational motion of the joint or provide effective control of motion in multiple planes (Figure 7-6).[84]

Each orthosis is designed to apply force of a particular magnitude at a specific point or place on the limb or body segment whether the segment is in the presence or absence of weight bearing. These forces affect the joint indirectly through the contact between orthosis (by straps, pads, bands, or total contact fit) and the tissue structures of the limb or body segment (skin, muscle, fat, fascia, tendons, and bone). Many orthoses that incorporate the foot and ankle, such as molded thermoplastic AFOs, are designed to use the shoe as a means of closure and to facilitate progression of the lower extremity during stance by applying the desired forces to the foot and ankle. The loading forces of a three- or four-point control system on a limb segment or joint may be substantial, and the interactive effect of the shoe with the proximal orthosis facilitates distribution of loading.

To examine the concept of force application between an orthosis and the patient's body segment, pressure must be defined. Pressure *(P)* is defined as the force (*F*) applied to the body segment per unit area (*A*)[49]:

$$P = F/A$$

The human body has limited tolerance for pressure. Within multiple force systems, even low pressure sustained over

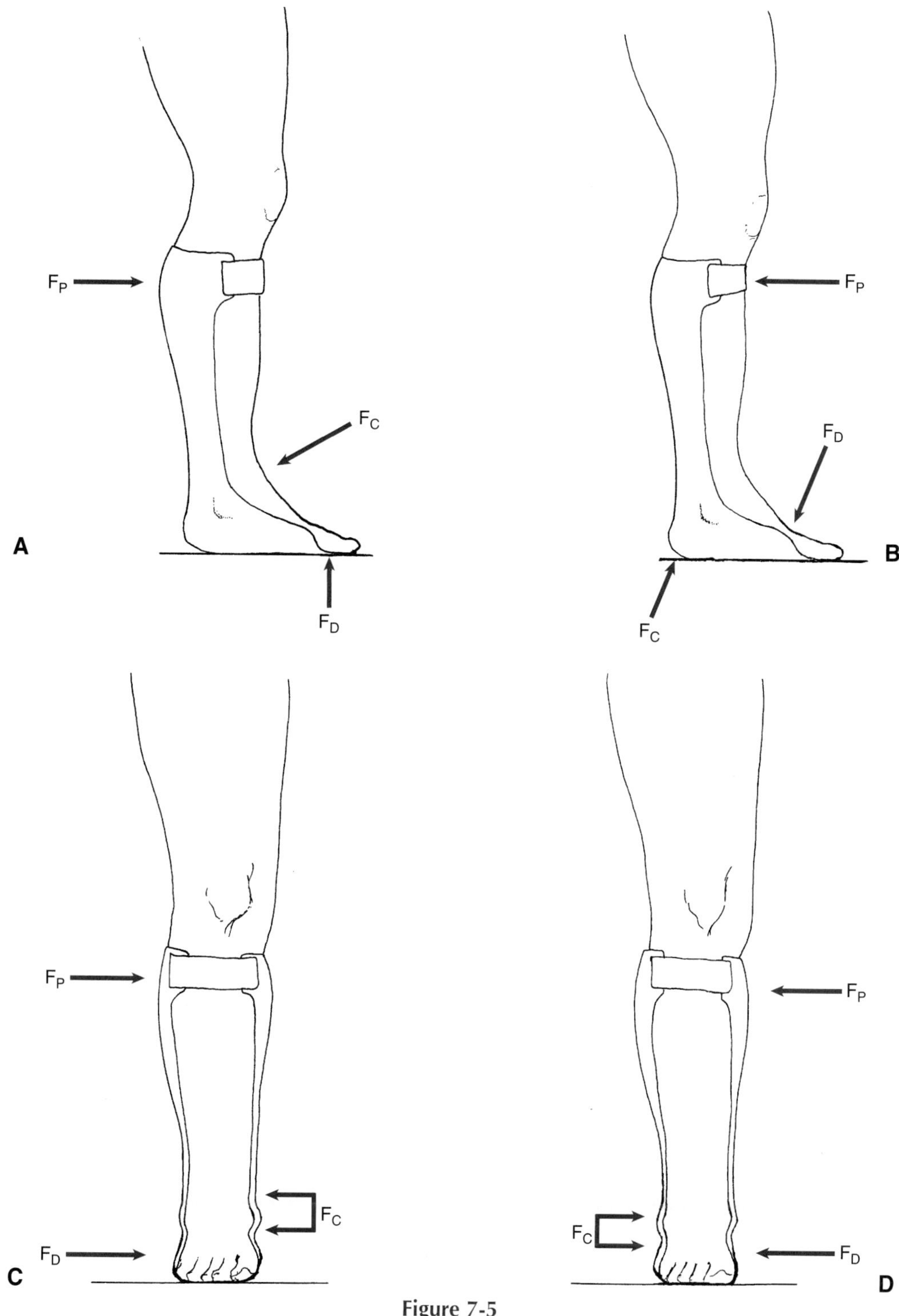

Figure 7-5

Force system in a molded thermoplastic solid-ankle AFO design. ***A,*** *Plantar flexion is controlled during swing phase by a proximal force (F_P) at the posterior calf band and a distal force at the metatarsal heads (F_D) that counters a centrally located stabilizing force (F_C) applied at the anterior ankle by shoe closure.* ***B,*** *For control of dorsiflexion during stance phase (i.e., forward progression of tibia over the foot), F_P is applied at the proximal tibia by the anterior closure, F_D at the ventral metatarsal heads by the toe box of the shoe, and counterforce F_C at the heel, snugly fit in the orthosis.* ***C,*** *The force system for eversion (valgus) locates F_D along the fifth metatarsal, F_P at the proximal lateral calf band, and F_C on either side of the medial malleolus.* ***D,*** *To control inversion (varus) of the foot and ankle, F_D is applied by the distal medial wall of the orthosis against the first metatarsal, F_P at the proximal medial calf band, and F_C at the distal lateral tibia and calcaneus/talus on either side of the lateral malleolus.*

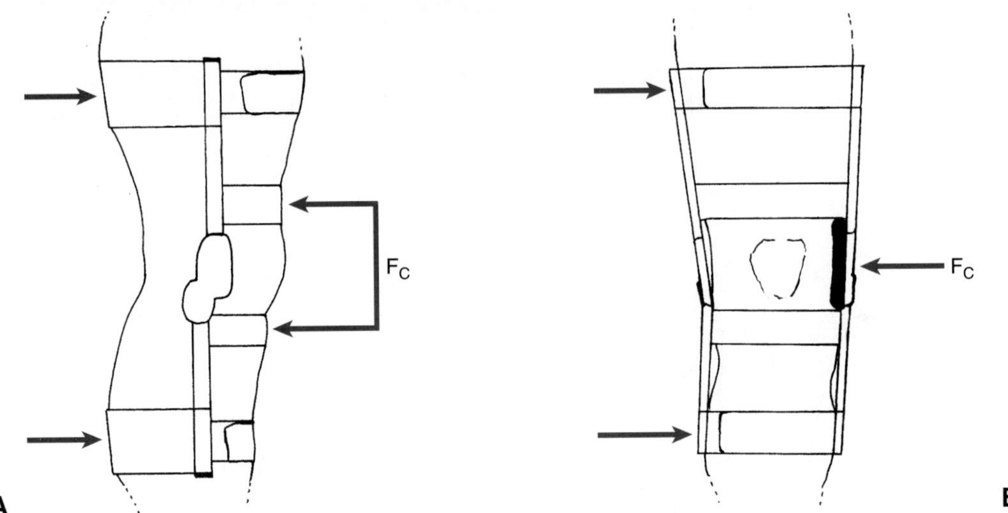

Figure 7-6

***A,** For a patient with instability of the knee, this four-point control system is designed to control sagittal plane translatory motion between the tibia and femur. Distributing the counterforce (F_c) on either side of the knee joint axis reduces shearing forces at the knee joint while simultaneously controlling knee flexion. **B,** The same orthosis controls valgus at the knee in the frontal plane with a three-point control system. Note the enlarged medial pad that is used to distribute F_C comfortably over a large area. Rotation of the tibia in the transverse plane cannot be controlled effectively by this design. To provide complete control of tibial rotation, the orthosis would have to incorporate the foot and ankle as well.*

long periods can lead to tissue deformation and breakdown through the restriction of blood and lymph flow.[86-88] For this reason, forces transferred to the body by the orthosis are often distributed over as much surface area of the limb as possible to keep pressure applied by the orthosis within levels tolerable to soft tissue and comfortable for the patient. This is especially important for patients with sensory loss, cognitive impairment, or compromised circulation, who may have increased vulnerability to tissue breakdown.

Most orthosis designs also incorporate "relief areas" where surface contours do not intimately fit over corresponding anatomical regions of bony prominence (e.g., apex or ankle malleoli in an AFO, navicular tarsal bone in a foot orthosis) or use padding or other flexible load-absorbing materials to dampen or distribute otherwise excessive forces. An example of this is the addition of rubber foam padding to the top portion of a foot orthoses to dampen repetitive loading on the plantar aspect of the foot of a long-distance runner.[89-92] The combination of durable foam materials such as cellular polyethylene foam, Spenco (Spenco Medical Corporation, Waco, Tex.), and high-temperature thermoplastic (polypropylene) can produce a rigid device resilient to impact loading and feature load-dampening capabilities when used with appropriate shoe gear. The combination of the orthosis and shoe can redistribute loading forces across the lower extremity.

As a first-class lever system, the magnitude of each of the forces in the orthotic control system is inversely related to the distance between its point of application and the axis of movement. To be in equilibrium, the forces in the system must sum to zero. Consider a knee orthosis designed to control genu recurvatum (Figure 7-7). The central force in the system is an anteriorly directed force applied at the posterior knee. The opposing paired posteriorly directed forces located above and below the central force are applied at the anterior femur and the anterior tibia. Although these forces can be applied anywhere along the shaft of the femur and tibia, the magnitude of the required force decreases as the point of application is moved upward on the femur and downward on the tibia. If the forces are in equilibrium, the central force applied at the posterior knee will be twice the magnitude of either of the other forces. The potentially negative result of this force on soft tissues of the knee is minimized by distributing the force over a large surface area. Installation of accommodative padding can also dampen forces applied from the orthosis to the body segment of the user.

Orthoses that fit over the majority of the body segment proximal and distal to the target joint provide greater leverage, which enhances the effectiveness of the design in controlling joint rotation and usually provides a more comfortable orthosis. The negative consequences of extending the length of the orthosis are compromised cosmesis and possible complications encountered by the user in donning and doffing.

Because most human movement is multiplanar, with an axis of joint motion offset from any single plane, no orthosis can perfectly match or mimic the biomechanical motion of the anatomical joint. As a result, the reactive forces that originate from the limb segment and the forces directed by

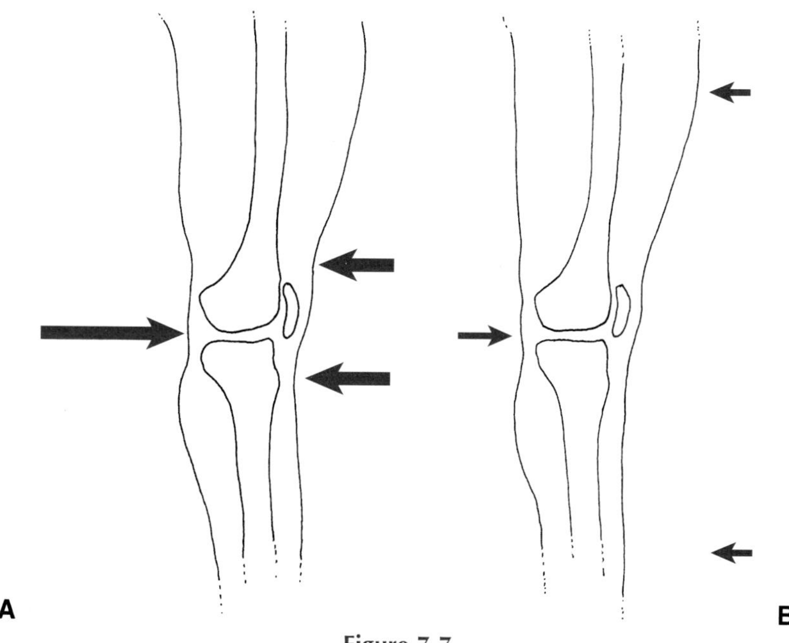

Figure 7-7

*The magnitude of forces necessary to control recurvatum decreases as the point of application is moved from close to the central force at the knee axis (**A**) to a position more proximal on the femur and distal on the tibia (**B**). Because the system is in equilibrium, moving the forces away from the joint axis also reduces the magnitude of the central force in this three-point force system.*

the orthosis will be mismatched.[93,94] Because these applied and reactive forces are, to some extent, noncollinear, any multiple-point force system applied by an orthosis to a limb in an effort to control joint motion will have a desired (corrective, controlling) and undesired (deforming) impact. These effects are best understood in terms of bending moments and shearing forces.

The bending moment, which is greatest at the point of application of the center force in a three-point system, represents the location of maximum orthosis control or correction. A separate bending moment is present in each plane of motion that the orthosis attempts to control. The efficiency of an orthosis in controlling or correcting motion is influenced by the distance between the joint axis and the point of application of each of the forces. The magnitude of the force needed if the orthosis is to achieve the desired level of correction or control decreases as the lever arm (distance from the joint axis to the point of force application) increases ($P = F/A$). The location of the point of application of the central force, where the bending moment is maximal, is also important to consider. The controlling or corrective forces are most effective (and least deforming) if the central force and the maximum bending moment coincide (are congruent) with the actual joint axis. When a discrepancy occurs, the resulting torques will have an impact on the joint and its support structures that must be taken into account.

To maximize patient comfort and compliance and minimize the long-term consequences of torque on joint and soft tissue integrity, careful placement of the straps, bands, or pads used to apply the force system becomes a priority in orthosis design.[95] Attention to width, depth, material stiffness, the intimacy of fit, and the suspension necessary to secure the orthosis and apply the desired forces plays a significant role in successful patient outcome.

When the goal of an orthosis is to control portions of joint motion rather than virtual immobilization, the congruency between the anatomical joint and orthosis mechanical joint axis is also an important consideration in orthotic design. Because most anatomical joints have a triplanar or polycentric axis and many orthotic joints are single-axis designs, incongruence occurs between the axes of the joint and the orthosis at some point in the range of motion, even in the most carefully designed orthosis.[96,97] A torque or moment subsequently results from this mismatch.

One study of four AFOs (hinged and nonhinged designs) noted that frictional/shear skin irritation may be closely related to the mechanical mismatch of the axes of rotation of the orthosis and the human ankle.[96] The greater discrepancy in orthosis hinge joint and anatomical ankle joint alignment produced greater "pistoning" (proximal and distal movement of the orthosis in relation to the anatomical leg throughout stance). The study points to the importance of the selection of polycentric joints that closely align to the anatomical joint axis in hinged AFOs and intimate fitting nonhinged AFOs with stiff mechanical properties to resist plastic "buckling" and reduce ankle dorsiflexion during the third rocker of stance phase.[96]

Knee joint technology has also advanced in that some polycentric joints are available that provide electromechanical mechanisms to lock the joint in stance phase (providing knee stability) and unlock the joint during swing phase (to provide knee flexion) and reduce the patient's need to develop alternative biomechanical strategies to achieve foot clearance.[98]

USE OF FORCES IN PROSTHESIS DESIGN AND ENGINEERING

A prosthesis design must consider force in a variety of locations and for a variety of purposes. Force and pressure are integral in prosthesis suspension and socket design. In the design of the upper extremity prosthesis with an articulating terminal device, the forces required for grasping and manipulating objects of different masses and surface characteristics must be considered.[99] A prosthetic knee joint might use friction forces or extension assists to control swing. A prosthetic foot becomes the primary lever for the realization of forward progression. Designers must consider these forces when choosing materials and their geometries.

Prosthetic Pylons

Traditionally, endoskeletal prosthetic pylons have simply transmitted force between components and to the socket (although some foot designs do not attach to pylons). To serve this purpose, pylons have been designed with inexpensive, lightweight materials and shapes but with adequate stiffness to remain relatively rigid under normal loading conditions. The hollow cylinder has served this purpose well and is usually made of aluminum or carbon fiber.

More recent pylon designs have sought to dissipate force in multiple planes. Vertical shock absorbers contain dampers to absorb power during loading response. Most shock-absorbing pylons are telescopic mechanisms that physically shorten during loading response. Gard and Konz[100] noted improved shock reduction in transtibial amputees with an Endolite Telescopic-Torsion pylon, reporting that the effect was more evident at higher walking velocities. In consideration of transverse plane motion, some prostheses incorporate a rotator along with the pylon to allow motion in the transverse plane.[101] Some rotators allow free rotation in an unweighted limb, which is useful for providing the transfemoral amputee with improved automobile ingress and egress or even simply allowing the crossing of legs while sitting. Because uninhibited motion in the transverse plane would create instability, rotators also dampen forces.

Prosthetic Knees

Modern prosthetic knees maintain stability in weight bearing over a small degree of flexion, beyond which they are free to flex. These properties make prosthetic knees stable in swing phase but still allow flexion necessary for swing phase clearance.[102,103] Despite the designed stability, individuals with transfemoral amputation often adopt locomotor strategies to maintain a ground reaction force orientation anterior to the knee. This creates a moment that extends the knee and guarantees stability. Newer prosthetic knees include designs that dynamically adjust their stiffness properties for different types of motion.[104] By increasing the stiffness of a knee, a larger moment is required to flex it. This characteristic becomes particularly beneficial when persons with transfemoral amputation attempt to descend stairs because the gravity-induced flexion moment will not collapse a stiffer knee joint.[105]

Prosthetic Feet

In general, prosthetic feet serve two important purposes in locomotion: force dissipation during loading response and force transmission for the remainder of stance phase. Most foot designs either mimic anatomical function in loading response through controlled plantar flexion or maintain a solid ankle and dissipate force with dampening foam in the heel region. For the remainder of stance phase, the majority of foot designs attempt to store and return energy. Herein lies a design challenge. Because most prosthetic feet are passive devices, they maintain constant structural properties. A foot's stiffness might be well matched for a given user's body mass and cadence, but that stiffness can become inappropriate at faster or slower walking speeds. In addition, any leaf spring will have an inherent natural frequency (Figure 7-8).[106] Its energy return will be more efficient when the cadence of gait is close to the natural frequency. Slower or faster walking velocities might hinder the function of a prosthetic foot.

Terminal Devices

The function of a terminal device such as a hook or hand is to provide the patient with a means of grasp. Hook designs emulate two-point grasp with each "finger" of the hook coming into opposition. Hands provide a rudimentary three-jaw chuck in which the thumb, index, and middle "fingers" oppose the others. The means of grasp is controlled either voluntarily through body power cable systems or through a substitute external motorized unit powered with a battery. Body-powered designs require joints proximal to the missing limb segment to transfer excursion through a cable connected to the terminal device and the prosthetic socket and harness. More distal levels of limb loss usually allow the user to access elbow and shoulder motions, which are transferred to the terminal device. Hook terminal devices usually are lightweight and require less force and cable excursion to operate, whereas prosthetic hands are heavier and require more body-powered force and cable excursion. The increased weight, bulk, and mechanical linkages create a terminal device that also requires more muscle function to operate. Body-powered systems are more readily activated because they are under the user's voluntary control.

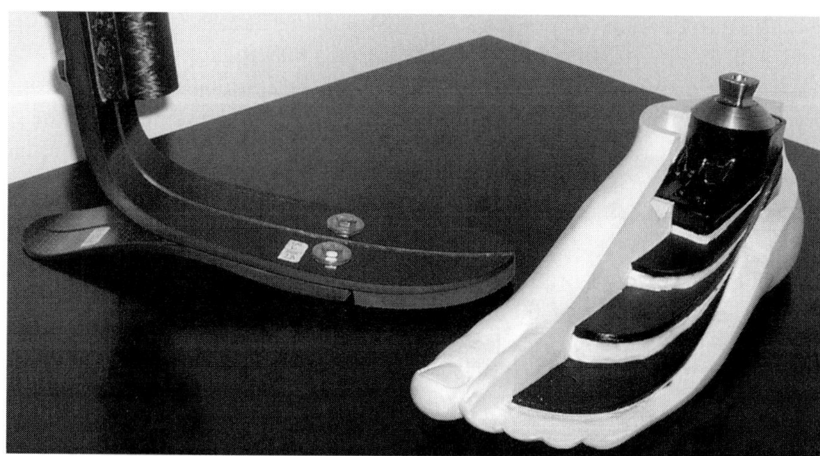

Figure 7-8

Dynamic elastic response prosthetic feet. These two models of prosthetic feet use carbon fiber as a leaf spring to store energy for use in limb propulsion in late stance.

Alternatives to body-powered systems are myoelectric designs. Myoelectric systems require greater time for activation of the terminal device and are limited by the speed of the sensor and motor that powers the prosthesis. Wrist units enhance the user's abilities to pre-position the terminal device by providing wrist flexion, extension, and rudimentary pronation and supination. As with lower extremity prosthesis components, the emphasis on reduced weight and minimal friction in movable parts means greater efficiency and less power to operate the terminal device; new design approaches in terminal devices should provide a greater range of gripping modes.[107,108]

Myoelectric Prostheses

The human hand measures temperature, pressure, and force along with many other sensory parameters that could be measured by a prosthetic hand. Microprocessor control algorithms in powered prosthetic hands have enabled the measurement of force to improve an amputee's ability to grasp and manipulate an object without damaging it. Myoelectric prostheses include sensors placed over residual muscles to enable volitional articulation of the prosthetic hand, wrist, and elbow. For example, electrodes placed on the skin over certain shoulder muscles detect the voltage output of the muscles when they contract. Contraction is mapped to specific motions in the prosthesis: grasping, rotating the wrist, and so on. In addition, muscle contraction intensity is mapped to force production in the prosthesis, usually within broad ranges such as high-, medium-, and low-intensity contractions.[109]

INTERACTIONS AT THE INTERFACE BETWEEN THE ORTHOSIS/PROSTHESIS AND PATIENT

The interface between the material of the orthosis or prosthesis and the body segment of the patient has not been well described. In light of this, the engineering challenge in orthosis and prosthesis design has been to create supporting surfaces that provide adequate mechanical stability while protecting the soft tissues from trauma and ulceration. Support surfaces of the orthosis or prosthesis must be designed so that soft tissues can tolerate the mechanical forces applied to them. Because persons with disabilities typically subject skin and underlying connective tissue to higher magnitude or longer duration of loading, the tissues are at risk for breakdown.[110] The skin of persons with pathological conditions affecting the autonomic nervous system (e.g., hereditary sensory motor neuropathies, diabetes mellitus, spinal cord injury) does not tolerate many types of stressors. Skin integrity can be compromised and weakened because it may lack elasticity or become dry or cracked from the reduced production of oils and other natural lubricants. Compromised peripheral sensation reduces the individual's ability to detect skin breakdown. As a result, the skin and underlying soft tissue envelope are vulnerable to a variety of stressors such as friction, shear, and pressure.[111]

Friction

When two surfaces are pressed together, a force parallel to the two surfaces is required to make one surface slide over the other. The resistance to this force developed at the surface of contact is termed the frictional force (F_f). The magnitude of the frictional force is directly proportional to the coefficient of friction (C_f) and the normal force (N):

$$F_f = C_f \times N$$

Therefore, if a material with high C_f value is used in an orthosis or prosthesis made from commercially available cellular polyethylene foams, such as Plastazote (Apex Foot Health Industries, Teaneck, N.J.), Pe-Lite (Fillauer Inc, Chattanooga, Tenn.), Poron (Rogers Corp., Woodstock, Conn.), Aliplast (Alimed, Dedham, Mass.), or similar materials, the frictional force will notably increase. The introduction of liquid (perspiration, other body fluids) to the interface environment also increases the value of C_f.[111] If a material with lower C_f value is used (e.g., slippery covering over the foam padding), the frictional force may be substantially reduced. Inevitably, the characteristics at the surface of materials influence whether the skin and underlying soft tissues of the patient's body segment become damaged.

The anatomical location where the orthosis or prosthesis is worn is important to consider. Some areas of the body are better suited to handle repeated high frictional force loads (sole of foot), whereas other areas are not (ankle malleoli).[111,112] As a result, planning of the material interface and the corresponding anatomical location the materials will impart forces on the body of the patient that are of paramount importance in determining the design of the device.

Shear

Shear is significant type of stress that can play a crucial role in adaptation or breakdown of the skin interface. The detrimental effects of shear forces have not been widely addressed in the scientific literature because of the lack of measurement instrumentation to quantify this aspect of load stress. What we do know is that shear represents a force couple in which forces are applied in the same plane in opposite directions. These opposing stresses that occur at the level of the surface of the orthosis or prosthesis and skin/soft tissue envelope interface also affect whether skin breakdown or other underlying tissue trauma will be induced to the body segment.

When skin is loaded under cyclic normal and shear force, the energy required to induce a blister is greater for the combination of low force and high number of cycles than for high force and low number of cycles.[113,114] Because of the great variety and characteristics of various shear-reducing materials, understanding the patient's tissue tolerances is essential to match the correct material appropriately to optimize the device design. The therapist can play a significant role in preparing the patient to be fit with an orthosis or prosthesis through conditioning of the skin and underlying soft tissue.[111,115,116]

By changing the surface characteristics of the orthosis or prosthesis and incorporating materials with a lower C_f value, interface shear can be reduced. For example, polyethylene is a smooth, uniform material with low C_f value. This is a major reason why plastic in orthosis shells or in prosthetic sockets provides an effective friction- and shear-reducing interface. As with friction, many types of padding materials can irritate the skin. Although commonly used as a lining for orthoses and prostheses, foam has a high C_f value and when notable rubbing occurs between the device and skin of a user, breakdown can occur. Covering the surface of foams with sheet materials possessing low C_f value such as ShearBan (Tamarack Habilitation Technologies, Inc., Blaine, Minn.) may reduce skin trauma.

The deleterious effects of excessive perspiration increase the C_f value of the skin, leaving the skin and soft tissue envelope vulnerable.[117] The use of interface garments (e.g., socks, shirts) may reduce skin breakdown, especially synthetic materials that provide a "wicking" effect in environments where perspiration exists.[111]

Pressure

In orthosis and prosthesis design, a great deal of attention has been focused on pressure dynamics. The assessment of pressure is important when attempting to evaluate the effect of component forces on the skin and the underlying soft tissues next to the bone where capillary gas exchange can be compromised.[49] A simple clinical method to assess the skin/soft tissue envelope reaction to pressure dynamics is capillary refill time. Patients wearing orthoses or prostheses in which excessive pressure and other force couples are imparted by the device onto the body segment have shorter capillary refill time. This indicates the tissues are possibly inflamed, and hydrostatic pressure in capillaries and interstitial tissue could be elevated. The arterial system may route additional blood to the area in response to excessive forces on the skin/soft tissue envelope. If the loading remains unchecked, the skin and underlying soft tissue may eventually break down, first becoming discolored and later forming a blister or ulcer.[111]

Typically, once breakdown occurs, a period of rest is required and the person is unable to use the orthosis or prosthesis. The occurrence of breakdown can be a serious or debilitating secondary injury that can impair mobility and be frustrating to the patient. In severe cases, the tissue does not heal and surgery to repair or remove tissue is required.[114]

Individuals with lower extremity limb loss at the transtibial level who use a prosthesis subject their residual limb to cyclic pressures and shear stresses during ambulation and often have breakdown near bony prominences intolerant to high pressure (e.g., the distal anterior tibial crest or the region of the fibular head).[118] Persons with insensate feet or poor circulation in their extremities often have foot ulcers over the heels or metatarsal heads. Although different areas of the body are affected in each of these cases, all are at risk of tissue damage. As a result of the pressure, shear stress distribution, and load duration at the body support surface, the soft tissues can respond unfavorably and break down.[119]

Some strategies exist to control or limit the potentially destructive forces at the interface between the orthosis or prosthesis and the user. Total contact at the interface between the orthosis or prosthesis and the patient's skin (soft tissue) may also reduce spiking of pressure and redistribute loads.[117,119-125] The rehabilitation professional can also play a significant role in encouraging the skin to adapt and become load tolerant to the force levels it will be subjected to by an orthosis or prosthesis.[111] Skin structure and bioprocesses are modified according to the mechanical demands placed on the skin.[85]

INFLUENCE OF LOWER EXTREMITY ORTHOSES ON GAIT

Any time a lower extremity orthosis alters anatomical joint motion, it is also likely to change progression through the gait cycle in some way. A solid-ankle AFO, which holds the ankle in a neutral position, facilitates toe clearance during swing and optimally positions the limb for heel strike at initial contact. In loading response, however, the fixed ankle cannot move into plantar flexion to reach foot flat, hampering the first rocker of gait. Instead, the rigid orthosis causes the tibia to accelerate forward quickly so that the forefoot makes contact with the ground. As a consequence, disruption of the normal shock absorption mechanism occurs with a potential disruption of postural stability in early stance.

With the progression from midstance to terminal stance, the fixed angle of the ankle in a solid-ankle AFO prevents forward progression of the tibia over the foot. Disruption of this second rocker of gait hampers forward progression of the center of mass and ultimately reduces step length of the opposite swinging limb. If the orthosis has a relatively stiff extended toe plate, the extension (dorsiflexion) of the toes necessary for continued forward progression and heel rise may be blocked as well. The stance phase trade-offs of a solid-ankle AFO can be addressed by footwear; shoes with a compressible heel and rocker sole are effective substitutes when the rockers of gait are constrained by an orthosis.

Ambulation with a KAFO with a locked knee has an impact on stance and swing phase of gait. With a knee that is prevented from flexing during loading response, the shock absorption eccentric function of the quadriceps is compromised, and impact forces are transmitted upward to the hip and low back. Stance phase stability during midstance and terminal stance is ensured by the locked knee, but the relative shortening of the limb that usually occurs as a result of knee flexion in preswing is prevented. Similarly, swing limb clearance becomes problematic in initial swing and midswing because the knee remains in extension, and the patient must use a compensatory strategy, such as circumduction or vaulting, to advance the limb successfully.

Most individuals who are fitted with lower extremity orthoses, such as a solid-ankle AFO or a KAFO with a locked knee, possess musculoskeletal-based biomechanical dysfunction or neuromuscular impairments of motor control that compromise functional ambulation. Whenever an orthosis is prescribed, the relative merits of an orthosis design are weighed carefully against the constraints imposed by the device. For this reason, orthotists and therapists strive to determine which orthosis design can maximally enhance the patient's function with the minimal possible external support or control. An orthosis that minimizes or eliminates particular joint motions may be as problematic as an orthosis that does too little to assist or improve function and likely may not be worn.

INFLUENCE OF LOWER EXTREMITY PROSTHESES ON GAIT

Assuming proper suspension, socket interface, and fit, locomotion with a lower extremity prosthesis largely depends on the function of the prosthetic foot and, when present, the prosthetic knee. Dozens of varieties of each component are available and are usually intended for specific uses and specific types of amputees. Nonetheless, generalizations can be drawn about the biomechanical effects of feet and knees when used in gait.

Role of the Prosthetic Foot

The foot/ankle complex serves two primary purposes during normal gait. First, the foot provides a stable surface for loading response while absorbing some of the tremendous impulse forces associated with the sudden cessation of the motion of the swinging limb. Second, the foot acts as a lever to maintain balance and facilitate a power burst by the ankle plantar flexors in late stance.[126]

Prosthetic feet have been designed with both purposes in mind. Shock absorption in loading response has been achieved by compressible bumpers and articulated ankles; by foam material in the heel coupled with a solid ankle; and in current designs by deformable plates, linkages, and cylinders. Most designs still incorporate the solid-ankle, cushion-heel (SACH) foot model. Normal controlled ankle plantar flexion to foot flat is replaced by deformation material such as polyurethane in the heel region. The most notable consequence is a delay in reaching foot flat because of the loss of the first ankle rocker. The first dynamic response feet were built on the SACH model but added deformation plates to the forefoot.[127] These plates are intended to act as a leaf spring, storing energy when the foot is dorsiflexed through stance and returning some of that energy. This design addresses the second major function of the foot and ankle, but instead of acting as a lever for an ankle power burst, energy is returned to the system in a spring.[128] (See Chapter 24 for more information about the design and characteristics of the different classes of prosthetic feet.)

A comparison of the power curves for the ankle during stance phase of an intact extremity and a prosthesis reveals much about the impact of these design features on gait (Figure 7-9). The normal ankle power curve reveals an extended period of energy absorption, both initially during

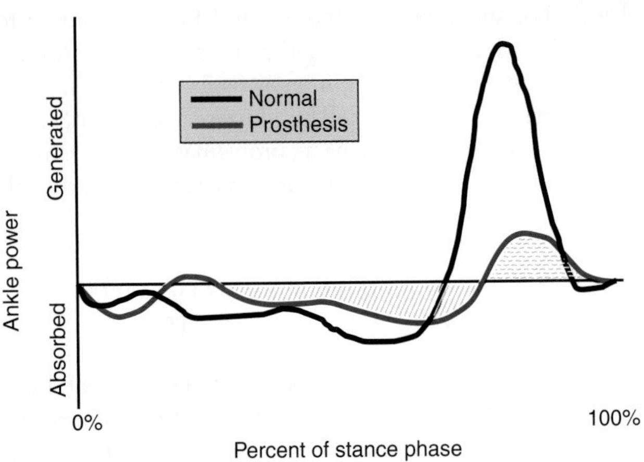

Figure 7-9

Typical ankle joint power results for normal gait and amputee gait with a prosthesis. Area under the curve represents energy either stored/dissipated or returned/produced.

loading response and then into the second rocker, followed by a power burst by the ankle plantar flexors in late stance.[129] The solid-ankle prosthesis also demonstrates power absorption during loading response and, on occasion, enough return of energy from the compressible heel to produce a period of positive power in early stance. If the forefoot of the prosthesis is capable of storing energy, the subsequent negative power is a combination of energy storage in the spring and energy dissipation (mainly in the cosmetic covering). The smaller-than-normal positive power in late stance is then returned as energy from the spring. Note that no spring can return more energy than it has stored. Energy is visualized as the area under the power curve. By association, no passive prosthetic foot/ankle power curve will have a larger area of positive late-stance power than negative midstance power.

The ratio of energy returned to energy absorbed has been called a prosthetic foot's efficiency. Varying efficiencies have been cited in the literature, ranging from 30% in a SACH foot[130] to 84% efficiency in a Flexfoot during running.[131] Efficiency and, more importantly, the overall amount of energy return depend on several factors, most obviously the stiffness of the spring material. Not to be overlooked is the natural frequency of the spring and how well that frequency is matched to the cadence of the intended user.[106]

Role of the Prosthetic Knee

For persons with amputation at or above the knee whose prosthesis includes a prosthetic knee joint, stability is a high priority. The knee is an inherently unstable joint, and the anatomical knee sees periods of agonist and antagonist co-contraction to increase joint stiffness during initial contact. Just as there are periods when stiffness is essential in the knee joint, its flexibility plays an important role in swing phase clearance (see Table 7-1). The individual with transfemoral amputation will usually demonstrate gait adaptations at two critical areas: at initial contact into loading response and in swing phase.

During loading response, stability is paramount and individuals with transfemoral amputation often demonstrate pronounced gait adaptations to guarantee full extension in the knee joint and ensure the ground reaction force remains anterior to the knee joint. These adaptations might include *dynamic limb retraction*, in which the swinging leg is brought back toward the stance leg for a brief period at the end of swing phase, producing a retrograde anteroposterior shear force. Also, anterior trunk lean may be used to shift the body's center of mass and, consequently, the center of pressure beneath the foot, forward.[132]

In swing phase, the limb acts as a double pendulum to enable knee flexion and ground clearance. This pendulum motion is controlled by the hip flexors, which advance the thigh and flex the knee, and the hip extensors, which eccentrically slow the thigh and, relying on inertia, extend the knee. A freely flexing unloaded knee joint can produce excessive flexion in early swing, as the foot kicks up behind the amputee, or a sudden and rapid stop at the end of swing phase as the knee reaches its mechanical limit of extension. This motion is controlled by friction in the joint or by hydraulic or pneumatic dampening within the knee unit.

OTHER IMPORTANT CONSIDERATIONS

The efficiency of gait and the effect on the physiological energy cost associated with the use of an orthosis or prosthesis is related to its weight as well as to the impact of the device on joint motion and gait. Weight of the orthosis or prosthesis is determined by the materials used in its fabrication and how much of the limb is encompassed by the device. Lighter-weight thermoplastics, composites, and metal alloys have replaced traditional stainless steel and leather lower extremity orthosis designs.[133] Similarly, many prostheses now incorporate thermoplastics and composites in unique combinations and shapes to reduce physiological energy expenditure during gait.[134] Consequently ambulation is a feasible goal for patients with a wider variety of diagnoses. For example, lightweight thermoplastic KAFOs may extend the age at which an individual diagnosed with muscular dystrophy may stand and ambulate.

Compared with their heavier-weight counterparts, lighter-weight prosthetic components, improved suspension techniques, and the proliferation of dynamic responsive feet and knees has resulted in reduced fatigue, improved gait mechanics, and improved physiological energy expenditure by the user. Even sprinting performance has dramatically improved in persons with lower limb loss who compete athletically at the elite level.[135]

Some of the adaptations persons with limb loss use to successfully ambulate with a prosthesis have been clarified.[136] In stance phase the prosthetic limb of persons with a transtibial amputation exhibits approximately 50% of the muscle work seen in normal individuals.[137] Persons with higher levels of limb loss exhibit increasing levels of energy expenditure as the remaining musculature compensates for lost power. Metabolic costs for an individual with ankle disarticulation are 15% higher than normal, whereas those for persons with traumatic transtibial amputation are 25% higher than normal. Individual with traumatic or dysvascular amputation at the transfemoral level correspondingly display the greatest expenditure of energy at 40% and 100% of normal, respectively.[136]

SUMMARY

As part of a rehabilitation treatment process, orthoses and prostheses serve an important role in enhancing function in persons with neuromusculoskeletal impairments or limb loss. The challenge in assessing the needs of persons with impairments and designing and creating these devices is the fact that their functional goal is to replace or augment portions of the human body. From a clinical, biomechanical, and engineering perspective, no orthosis or prosthesis can completely reproduce the full breadth of anatomical function of the human body. Therefore, orthoses and prostheses are designed as part of the patient's health care process to target certain functional goals, often at the cost of other goals. A "performance trade-off" dilemma is often encountered when provision of function has consequences of cosmesis, control, comfort, monetary cost, or physiological energy expenditure. The challenge is in optimizing the trade-offs. To accomplish this effectively, clinicians must understand the mechanical properties of both normal human function and the orthoses and prosthesis being considered as part of the rehabilitation process. Rehabilitation professionals play a significant role in influencing the outcome of this process, and through understanding the principles they can improve care they provide to the patient.

REFERENCES

1. Klasson B, Jones D. ISPO workshop on quality management in prosthetics and orthotics. *Prosthet Orthot Int* 2000;24(3):188-195.
2. Shurr DG, Michael JW. Methods, Materials, and Mechanics. In *Prosthetics and Orthotics,* 2nd ed. Norwalk, CT: Appleton & Lange, 2002. pp. 21-37.
3. McCollough NC. Biomechanical analysis systems for orthotic prescription. In Bunch WH, Keagy R, Kritter AE, et al (eds), *Atlas of Orthotics: Biomechanical Principles and Application.* 2nd ed. St. Louis: Mosby, 1985. pp. 34-75.
4. Polliack AA, Moser S. Outcomes forum. Clinical outcomes of an orthopedic ankle stabilizing boot. *J Prosthet Orthot* 1998;10(2):37-41.
5. Climent J, Sanchez J. Impact of the type of brace on the quality of life of adolescents with spine deformities. *Spine* 1999;24(10):1903-1908.
6. MacLean W, Green N, Pierre C, et al. Stress and coping with scoliosis. Psychological effects on adolescents and their families *J Ped Orthop* 1989;9(3):257-261.
7. Ryerson SD. The foot in hemiplegia. In Hunt CG (ed), *Physical Therapy of the Foot and Ankle.* New York: Churchill Livingstone, 1988. pp. 109-131.
8. Huber SR. Therapeutic application of orthotics. In Umphred DA (ed), *Neurologic Rehabilitation,* 4th ed. St. Louis: Mosby, 2001. pp. 773-789.
9. Edelstein JE. Orthotic assessment and management. In O'Sullivan SB, Schmitz TJ (eds), *Physical Rehabilitation: Assessment and Treatment.* Philadelphia: F.A. Davis, 1994.
10. Corcoran PJ, Jebsen RH, Brengelmann GL, et al. Effects of plastic and metal leg braces on speed and energy cost of hemiparetic ambulation. *Arch Phys Med Rehabil* 1970;51(2):69-77.
11. Davie JB. Use of heart rate in assessment of orthoses. *Physiotherapy* 1977;63(1):112-115.
12. Mossberg KA, Linton KA, Friske K. Ankle-foot orthoses: effect on energy expenditure of gait in spastic diplegic children. *Arch Phys Med Rehabil* 1990;71(7):490-494.
13. Stallard J, Rose GK, Tait JH, et al. Assessment of orthoses by means of speed and heart rate. *J Med Eng Tech* 1978;2:22-24.
14. Stallard J, Rose GK. Clinical decision making with the aid of ambulatory monitoring of heart rate. *Prosthet Orthot Int* 1980;4(2):91-96.
15. Guidera KJ, Smith S, Raney E, et al. Use of the reciprocating gait orthosis in myelodysplasia. *J Pediat Orthop* 1993;13(3):341-348.
16. Sykes L, Edwards J, Powell ES, et al. The reciprocating gait orthosis: long-term usage patterns. *Arch Phys Med Rehabil* 1995;76(8):779-783.
17. Franceschini M, Baratta S, Zampolini M, et al. Reciprocating gait orthoses: a multicenter study of their use by spinal cord injured patients. *Arch Phys Med Rehabil* 1997;78(6): 582-586.
18. Clinkingbeard JR, Gersten JW, Hoehn D. Energy cost of ambulation in traumatic paraplegia. *Am J Phys Med* 1964;43:157-165.
19. Muccio P, Andrews B, Marsolais B. Electronic orthoses: technology, prototypes and practices. *J Prosthet Orthot* 1989:1(1):3-17.
20. Lunsford TR, Wallace JM. The orthotic prescription. In Goldberg B, Hsu JD (eds), *Atlas of Orthoses and Assistive Devices,* 3rd ed. St. Louis: Mosby, 1997. pp. 3-14.
21. Supan TJ, Hovorka CF. A review of thermoplastic ankle foot orthoses adjustments/replacements in young cerebral palsy and spina bifida patients. *J Prosthet Orthot* 1995;7(1):15-22.
22. Supan TJ, Fisk JF. Cerebral palsy. In Goldberg B, Hsu JD (eds), *Atlas of Orthoses and Assistive Devices,* 3rd ed. St. Louis: Mosby, 1997. pp. 538-540.
23. Brunnstrom S. *Movement therapy in hemiplegia.* New York: Harper & Row, 1970.
24. Saladin L. Cerebrovascular disease: stroke. In Fredericks CM, Saladin LK (eds), *Pathophysiology of Motor Systems.* Philadelphia: F.A. Davis, 1996. pp. 486-489.
25. Twitchell T. The restoration of motor function following hemiplegia in man. *Brain* 1951;74(4):443-480.
26. Brunnstrom S. Motor testing procedures in hemiplegia based on recovery stages. *J Am Phys Ther Assoc* 1966;46(4):357-375.

27. Bobath B. *Adult Hemiplegia: Evaluation and Treatment,* 2nd ed. London: Heinemann, 1978.
28. Fishman S, Berger N, Edelstein JE, et al. Lower-limb orthoses. In *Atlas of Orthotics,* 2nd ed. St. Louis: C.V. Mosby, 1985. pp. 199-237.
29. Lehmann JF. Lower limb orthosis. In Redford JB (ed), *Orthotics Etcetera,* 3rd ed. Baltimore: Williams & Wilkins, 1986. pp. 278-351.
30. Aisen ML. *Orthotics in neurologic rehabilitation. Volume 5: Comprehensive Neurologic Rehabilitation.* New York: Demos Publications, 1992. pp. 1-23.
31. Shamp JK. Neurophysiologic orthotics designs in the treatment of central nervous system disorders. *J Prosthet Orthot* 1989;2(1):14-32.
32. Lima D. Overview of the causes, treatment, and orthotic management of lower limb spasticity. *J Prosthet Orthot* 1989;2(1):1-13.
33. Mueller K, Cornwall M, McPoil T. Effect of a tone inhibiting dynamic ankle-foot orthosis on the foot loading pattern of a hemiplegic adult: a preliminary study. *J Prosthet Orthot* 1992;4(2):86-92.
34. Hylton NM. Postural and functional impact of dynamic AFOs and FOs in a pediatric population. *J Prosthet Orthot* 1990;2:40-53.
35. Seymour R. *Prosthetics and Orthotics Lower Limb and Spinal.* Philadelphia: Lippincott Williams & Wilkins, 2002. pp. 62-74.
36. Mueller MJ. Comparison of rigid removable dressings and elastic bandages in preprosthetic management of patients with below knee amputation. *Phys Ther* 1982;62(10):1438-1441.
37. Burgess R, Romano R, Zettl J. *The Management of Lower Extremity Amputations* [CD-ROM]; Seattle: Prosthetic Research Specialists, 1998.
38. Ullendahl JE. Patient care booklet for below knee amputees. Alexandria, VA: American Academy of Orthotists and Prosthetists, 1988. pp. 6-7.
39. Gauthier-Gagnon C, Grise MC, Potvin D. Enabling factors related to prosthetic use by people with a transtibial and transfemoral amputation. *Arch Phys Med Rehabil* 1999;80(6):706-713.
40. Jones L, Hall M, Schuld W. Ability or disability? A study of the functional outcome of 65 consecutive lower limb amputees treated at the Royal South Syndey Hospital in 1988-1989. *Disabil Rehabil* 1993;15(4):184-188.
41. Boonstra AM, Rijnders LJ, Groothoff JW, et al. Children with congenital deficiencies or acquired amputations of the lower limbs: functional aspects. *Prosthet Orthot Int* 2000;24(1):19-27.
42. Carrasco DI, English AW. Mechanical actions of compartments of the cat hamstring muscle, biceps femoris. *Prog Brain Res* 1999;123:397-403.
43. Sibella F, Galli M, Romei M, et al. Biomechanical analysis of sit-to-stand movement in normal and obese subjects. *Clin Biomech* 2003;18(8):745-50.
44. Winter DA. Mechanical power in human movement: generation, absorption, and transfer. *Med Sports Sci* 1987;25:34-45.
45. Kepple TM, Siegel KL, Stanhope SJ. Relative contributions of the lower extremity joint moments to forward progression and support during gait. *Gait Posture* 1997;6(1):1-8.
46. Perry J. *Gait Analysis: Normal and Pathological Function.* Thorofare, NJ: Slack, 1992.
47. Raschke SU, Ford N. Report on key points arising from visioning process on prosthetic and orthotic education done at the British Columbia Institute of Technology. *J Prosthet Orthot* 2002(14):1:23-26.
48. Frankel VH, Nordin M. *Basic Biomechanics of the Skeletal System.* Philadelphia: Lea & Febiger, 1980.
49. Lunsford T. *Orthology Pathomechanics of Lower Limb Orthotic Design.* Alexandria, VA: American Academy of Orthotists and Prosthetists, 1998.
50. Contini R, Drillis R. Biomechanics. *Appl Mech Rev* 1954;7(2):49-52.
51. Nigg B, Herzog W. *Biomechanics of the Musculo-Skeletal System.* Chichester, England: John Wiley and Sons, 1994.
52. Rasch PJ. Notes toward a history of kinesiology, parts I, II, and III. *J Am Osteopath Assoc* 1958:58:572-574, 641-644.
53. Contini R, Drillis R. *Biomechanics in Applied Mechanics Review.* New York: Spartan Books, 1966.
54. Miller DI, Nelson RC. *Biomechanics of Sport.* Philadelphia: Lea & Febiger, 1973.
55. Cary JM, Lusskin R, Thompson RG. Prescription principles. In *Atlas of Orthotics: Biomechanical Principles and Application.* St. Louis: Mosby, 1975.
56. Lary MJ, Lavigne SE, Muma RD, et al. Breaking down barriers: multidisciplinary education model. *J Allied Health* 1997;26(2):63-69.
57. Nielsen CC. Orthotics and prosthetic in rehabilitation: the multidisciplinary approach. In Lusardi MM, Nielsen CC (eds), *Orthotics and Prosthetics in Rehabilitation.* Boston: Butterworth-Heinemann, 2000. pp. 3-9.
58. Nagi SZ. Teamwork in health care in the United States: a sociological perspective. *Milbank Q* 1975;53(3):75-91.
59. Mariano C. The case for interdisciplinary collaboration. *Nurs Outlook* 1999;37(6):285-288.
60. Hentges CJ. The team approach to the orthotic treatment of idiopathic scoliosis and Scheuermann's kyphosis. *J Prosthet Orthot* 2003;15 suppl 4:S49-S52.
61. Hovorka CF. Steel will: a multidisciplinary prosthetic care team can help patients with amputations reclaim their lives. *Advance for Directors in Rehabilitation* 2001;10(5):36-40.
62. Umbrell C. Educating tomorrow's practitioners, a practical debate. *O&P Almanac* 2001;50(2):40-45.
63. Erickson B, McHarney-Brown C, Seeger K, et al. Overcoming barriers to interprofessional health sciences education. *Education for Health* 1998;11(2):143-149.
64. Casto M. Interprofessional work in the USA: education and practice. In Leathard A (ed), *Going Interprofessional. Working Together for Health and Welfare.* London: Routledge, 1994. pp. 8-40.
65. Hall P, Weaver L. Interdisciplinary education and teamwork: a long and winding road. *Med Educ* 2001;35(9):867-875.
66. Areskog N. The need for multiprofessional health education in undergraduate studies. *Med Educ* 1988;22(4):251-252.
67. Davis R, Thurecht R. Care planning and case conferencing. Building effective multidisciplinary teams. *Aust Fam Physician* 2001;30(1):78-81.
68. Tupling SJ, Pierrynowski MR. Use of Cardan angles to locate rigid bodies in three-dimensional space. *Med Biol Eng Comp* 1987;25(5):527-532.
69. HJ Woltring. 3-D attitude representation of human joints: a standardization proposal. *J Biomech* 1994;27(12):1139-1414.

70. Levangie PK, Norkin CC. *Joint Structure and Function. A Comprehensive Analysis,* 3rd ed. Philadelphia: F.A. Davis, 2001.
71. Kapandji IA. *The Physiology of the Joints. Vol 1: Upper Limb.* Edinburgh, UK: Churchill Livingstone, 1970.
72. Shipman P, Walker A, Bichell D. *The Human Skeleton.* Cambridge, MA: Harvard University Press, 1985.
73. Sarrafian SK. *Anatomy of the Foot and Ankle.* Philadelphia: J.B. Lippincott, 1983.
74. Wright DG, DeSai SM, Henderson WH. Action of the subtalar and ankle-joint complex during the stance phase of walking. *J Bone Joint Surg* 1964;46A:361-382.
75. Oatis CA. Biomechanics of the foot and ankle under static conditions. *Phys Ther* 1988;68(12):1815-1821.
76. Rodgers MM. Dynamic foot biomechanics. *J Orthop Sports Phys Ther* 1995;21(6):306-316.
77. Ford N. *Visual Observational Gail Analysis* [dissertation]. LaTrobe University, Melbourne, Victoria, Australia. 2001;113-166.
78. Seymour R. *Prosthetics and Orthotics Lower Limb and Spinal.* Philadelphia: Lippincott Williams & Wilkins, 2002. pp. 84-86.
79. Bresler B, Frankel JB. The forces and movements in the leg during level walking. *Trans ASME* 1950;72:27-36.
80. Perry J, Shanfield S. Efficiency of dynamic elastic response prosthetic feet. *J Rehabil Res Dev* 1993;30(1):137-143.
81. Harrington E, Lin R, Gage J. Use of an anterior floor reaction orthosis in patients with cerebral palsy. *Orthot Prosthet* 1983;37(4):34-42.
82. Yang G, Chu D, Ann J, et al. Floor reaction orthosis: clinical experience. *Orthot Prosthet* 1986;40(1):33-37.
83. Geil MD. Energy loss and stiffness properties of dynamic elastic response prosthetic feet. *J Prosthet Orthot* 2001;13(3):70-73.
84. Norkin CC, Levangie PK. Basic concepts in biomechanics. In *Joint Structure and Function: A Comprehensive Analysis.* Philadelphia: F.A. Davis, 1992. pp. 1-56.
85. Trautman P. Lower limb orthoses. In Redford JB, Basmajian JV, Trautman P (eds), *Orthotics: Clinical Practice and Rehabilitation Technology.* New York: Churchill Livingstone, 1995. pp. 13-39.
86. Nawoczenski DA. Introduction to orthotics: rationale for treatment. In Nawoczenski DA, Epler ME (eds), *Orthotics in Functional Rehabilitation of the Lower Limb.* Philadelphia: Saunders, 1997. pp. 1-14.
87. Lunsford T. *Orthology Pathomechanics of Lower-Limb Orthotic Design.* Alexandria, VA: American Academy of Orthotists and Prosthetists, 1998. pp. 35-41.
88. Biomechanics and gait. In Weber D (ed), *Clinical Aspects of Lower Extremity Orthotics.* Winnipeg, Canada: Canadian Association of Orthotists and Prosthetists, 1993. pp. 61-82.
89. Brodsky RW, Kourosh S, Stills M. Objective evaluation of insert material for diabetic and athletic footwear. *Foot Ankle* 1988;9(3):111-116.
90. Eckhous D. *Comparison of Orthotic Insert Materials.* Downey, CA: Rancho Los Amigos Medical Center; 1985. pp. 6-14.
91. Lewis G, Tan T, Shive YS. Characteristics of the performance of shoe insert materials. *J Am Podiatr Med Assoc* 1991;81(8):418-424.
92. Pratt DJ, Rees PH, Rodgers C. Assessment of some shock absorbing insoles. *Prosthet Orthot Int* 1986;10(1):43-45.
93. Byars EF, Snyder RD, Plants HL. *Engineering Mechanics for Deformable Bodies,* 4th ed. New York: Harper & Row, 1983. pp. 224-237.
94. Smith EM, Juvinall RC. Mechanics of orthotics. In Redford JB (ed), *Orthotics Etcetera,* 3rd ed. Baltimore: Williams & Wilkins, 1986. pp. 26-32.
95. Trautman P. Lower limb orthotics. In Redford JB, Basmajian JV, Trautman P (eds), *Orthotics: Clinical Practice and Rehabilitation Technology.* New York: Churchill Livingstone, 1995. pp. 13-53.
96. Singerman R, Hoy DJ, Mansour JM. Design changes in ankle-foot orthosis intended to alter stiffness also alters orthosis kinematics. *J Prosthet Orthot* 1999(11):3:48-56.
97. Sumiya T, Suzuki Y, Kasahara T, et al. Instantaneous centers of rotation in dorsi/plantar flexion movements of posterior-type plastic ankle-foot orthoses. *J Rehabil Res* 1997;34(3):279-285.
98. McMillan AG, Kendrick K, Horton GW, et al. Stance control orthosis to improve functional gait. Proceedings of the American Academy of Orthotists and Prosthetists Annual Meeting, San Diego, CA, March 20-22, 2003.
99. Radocy R. A new dawn: upper extremity prosthetic technology shows promise despite daunting engineering and efficiency demands. *Advance for Directors in Rehabilitation* 2003;12(9):77-80.
100. Gard S, Konz R. The effect of a shock-absorbing pylon on the gait of persons with unilateral transtibial amputation. *J Rehab Res Dev* 2003;40(3):109-124.
101. Twiste M, Rithalia S. Transverse rotation and longitudinal translation during prosthetic gait—a literature review. *J Rehab Res Dev* 2003;40(1):9-18.
102. Michael JW. Prosthetic knee mechanisms. *Phys Med Rehabil* 1994;8(1):147-164.
103. Gard S, Childress DS, Ullendahl JE. The influence of four-bar linkage knees on prosthetic swing-phase floor clearance. *J Prosthet Orthot* 1996;8(2):34-40.
104. Breakey JW. Microprocessor C-leg: the learning curve. Proceedings of the American Academy of Orthotists and Prosthetists Annual Meeting and Scientific Symposium, San Diego, CA, March 20-23, 2003.
105. Blumentritt S, Werner Scherer H, Wellershaus U, et al. Design principles, biomechanical data and clinical experience with a polycentric knee offering controlled stance phase knee flexion: a preliminary report. *J Prosthet Orthot* 1997;9(1):18-24.
106. Lehmann JF, Price R, Boswell-Bessette D, et al. Comprehensive analysis of energy storing prosthetic feet: Flexfoot and Seattle Foot versus standard SACH foot. *Arch Phys Med Rehabil* 1993;74(11):1225-1231.
107. Lamb DW, Dick TD, Douglas WB. A new prosthesis for the upper limb. *J Bone Joint Surg [Br]* 1988;70B(1):140-144.
108. Nader M. The artificial substitution of missing hands with myoelectric prostheses. *Clin Orthop* 1990;(258):9-17.
109. Bonivento C, Davalli A, Fantuzzi C, et al. Automatic tuning of myoelectric prostheses. *J Rehabil Res Dev* 1998;35(3):294-304.
110. Norkin CC, Levangie PK. Joint structure and function. In *Joint Structure and Function: A Comprehensive Analysis.* Philadelphia: F.A. Davis, 1992. pp. 57-91.
111. Sanders JE, Goldstein BS, Leotta DF. Skin response to mechanical stress: adaptation rather than breakdown—a review of the literature. *J Rehabil Res Dev* 1995;32(3):214-226.

112. Sulzberger MB, Cortese TA, Fishman L, et al. Studies on blisters produced by friction. I. Results of linear rubbing and twisting techniques. *J Invest Dermatol* 1966;47(5):456-465.
113. Naylor PFD. Experimental friction blisters. *Brit J Dermatol* 1955;67(10):327-344.
114. Sanders JE, Silver-Thorn MB, Brienza DM. Introduction to "soft tissue interfaces in rehabilitation" [editorial]. *IEEE Trans Rehabil Eng* 1996;4(4):285-287.
115. Griffiths BH. Advances in the treatment of decubitis ulcers. *Surg Clin North Am* 1963;43:245-260.
116. Rubin L. Hyperkeratosis in response to mechanical irritation. *J Invest Dermatol* 1949;13(6):313-315.
117. Highley DR. Frictional properties of the skin. *J Invest Dermatol* 1977;69:303-305.
118. Naylor PFD. The skin surface and friction. *Br J Dermatol* 1955;67(7):239-246.
119. Wersche JJ, Frank LW, Hongsheng A, et al. Plantar pressures with total contact casting. *J Rehabil Res Dev* 1995;32(3): 205-209.
120. Burden AC, Jones GR, Jones R, et al. Use of "scotch cast boot" in treating diabetic foot ulcers. *Br Med J* 1983;286(6377):1555-1557.
121. Helm PA, Walker SC, Pullium G. Total contact casting in diabetic patients with neuropathic foot ulcerations. *Arch Phys Med Rehabil* 1984;65(11):691-693.
122. Helm PA, Walker SC, Pullium G. Recurrence of neuropathic ulceration following healing in a total contact cast. *Arch Phys Med Rehabil* 1991;72(12):967-970.
123. Bremmer MA. An ambulatory approach to the neuropathic ulceration. *J Am Podiat Assoc* 1974:64:862.
124. Mueller MJ, Diamond JE, Sinacore DR, et al. Total contact casting in treatment of diabetic plantar ulcers: controlled clinical trial. *Diabetes Care* 1989:12(6):384-388.
125. Boulton AJM, Bowker JH, Gadia M, et al. Use of plaster casts in the management of diabetic neuropathic foot ulcers. *Diabetes Care* 1986;9(2):149-152.
126. Winter DA, Sienko SE. Biomechanics of below knee amputee gait. *J Biomech* 1988;21(5):361-367.
127. Menard MR, McBride ME, Sanderson DJ, et al. Comparative biomechanical analysis of energy storing prosthetic feet. *Arch Phys Med Rehabil* 1992;73(5):451-458.
128. Michael J. Energy storing feet: a clinical comparison. *Clin Prosth Orth* 1987;11:154-168.
129. Winter DA. Energy generation and absorption at the ankle and knee during fast, natural, and slow cadences. *Clin Orthop Rel Res* 1983;175:147-154.
130. Barr AE, Siegel KL, Kanoff JV, et al. Biomechanical comparison of the energy storing capabilities of the SACH and Carbon Copy II prosthetic feet during stance phase of gait in a person with below knee amputation. *Phys Ther* 1992;72(5):344-354.
131. Czerniecki JM, Gitter A, Munro C. Joint moment and muscle power output characteristics of below knee amputees running: the influence of energy storing feet. *J Biomech* 1991;24(1):63-75.
132. Whittle M. *Gait Analysis: An Introduction,* 3rd ed. Oxford: Butterworth Heinemann, 2002.
133. Michael JW, Bowker JH. Prosthetics/orthotics research for the twenty-first century: summary of 1992 conference proceedings. *J Prosthet Orthot* 1992;6(4):100-107.
134. Phillips SL, Craelius W. Comparison of material properties of laminated prosthetic sockets. Proceedings of the American Academy of Orthotists and Prosthetists Annual Meeting and Scientific Symposium. San Diego, CA, March 20-23, 2003.
135. Martin J. Historical analysis of amputee sprinting performance. Proceedings of the American Academy of Orthotists and Prosthetists Annual Meeting and Scientific Symposium. San Diego, CA, March 20-23, 2003.
136. Czerniecki JM. Rehabilitation in limb deficiency. 1. Gait and motion analysis. *Arch Phys Med Rehabil* 1996;77(3S):S3-S8.
137. Czerniecki JM, Gitter A. Insights into amputee running: a muscle work analysis. *Am J Phys Med Rehabil* 1992;71(4):209-218.
138. Magee DJ. *Orthopedic Physical Assessment,* 3rd ed. Philadelphia: Saunders, 1997.
139. Hoppenfeld S. *Physical Examination of the Spine and Extremities,* Norwalk, Conn: Appleton & Lange, 1976.
140. American Academy of Orthopedic Surgeons: *Joint Motion: Method of Measuring and Recording.* Chicago: American Academy of Orthopedic Surgeons, 1965.
141. Norkin CC, White DJ. *Measurement of Joint Motion: A Guide to Goniometry,* 2nd ed, Philadelphia: F.A. Davis, 1995.

8

Footwear: Foundation for Lower Extremity Orthoses

JENNIFER M. BOTTOMLEY

LEARNING OBJECTIVES

On completion of this chapter, the reader will be able to do the following:

1. Determine the proper fit of standard footwear on the basis of necessary function of the foot during gait and the contour and alignment of a patient's foot.
2. Recommend appropriate footwear styles and characteristics for patients with foot deformity and for patients who wear orthoses or prostheses.
3. Describe the shoe modifications and accommodative orthoses that can be used to address musculoskeletal problems affecting the foot and lower limb.
4. Describe the effect of selected problems and deformity of the forefoot, midfoot, or rearfoot on weight bearing and efficiency of the gait cycle, and suggest appropriate footwear or orthotic interventions to reduce pain and improve function.
5. Identify special footwear needs for individuals with arthritis, gout, diabetes, peripheral vascular disease, hemiplegia, and amputation or congenital deformity of the foot and leg.

The most essential element of clothing in any person's wardrobe is the shoe. No other article of clothing is designed to fit so precisely. Continuous pressure from tight shoes can produce ulceration and deformities. Ill-fitting shoes can create shear forces that lead to skin breakdown, create and facilitate toe and foot deformities, and lead to falls.[1] Shoes perform the vital functions of transferring body weight to the floor during walking and of protecting the wearer from any hazards in the environment. A well-designed shoe is the necessary foundation for many lower extremity orthoses and for prosthetic alignment and an energy-efficient gait. This chapter discusses the components and characteristics of shoes, ensuring proper fit, and choosing appropriate footwear for patients with foot dysfunction and deformity.

COMPONENTS OF A GOOD SHOE

A suitable pair of shoes minimizes stress on all portions of the feet, provides support, and acts as a shock absorber of ground reaction forces.[2] The basic parts of a shoe are the sole, upper, heel, and last. Each of these parts is further divided into component parts or areas that are required for proper shoe design (Figure 8-1). Each component is crucial to the prescription of appropriate shoes for the person's individual needs.

Sole

The sole protects the plantar surface of the foot. The traditional sole consists of two pieces of leather sewn together with a layer of compressible cork between. An additional layer, the insole, is situated next to the foot in most shoes. A heavy thick sole protects the foot against walking surface irregularities. The rigidity or stiffness of the sole is also important. Although it needs to be durable, the sole must not be so rigid as to interfere with the toe rocker of the metatarsophalangeal (MTP) hyperextension during terminal stance and preswing phases of gait.

Various areas of the sole are identified by location. The *welt* is the inside piece of the external sole; the *outsole* is the portion that is most external. The area that lies between the heel and the ball of the shoe, the *shank,* is commonly fabricated to provide reinforcement and shape using materials such as spring steel, steel and leatherboard, or wood strips between the welt and the outsole. The purpose of the shank is to prevent collapse of the material between the heel and the ball of the foot and to provide extra support. In most athletic shoes the sole is rubber to provide maximal traction. Rubber soles absorb shock, thereby minimizing heel impact forces.

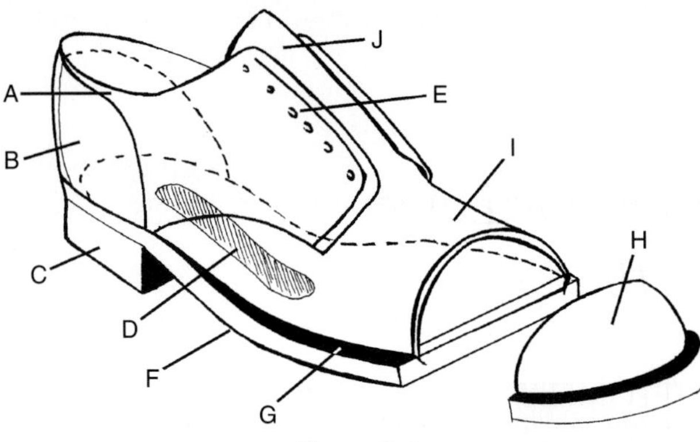

Figure 8-1

Basic parts of a shoe. The upper is made up of the quarter (A) *and its reinforcing counter* (B), *which stabilize the rearfoot within the shoe; the closure* (E) *and the tongue* (J) *across the midfoot; and the shaft* (vamp; I) *and toe box* (H), *which enclose the forefoot. The exterior outsole* (F) *is often reinforced with a steel shank* (D) *and is attached to the upper at the welt* (G). *The standard heel* (C) *is ¾-inch high.*

Upper

The upper of the shoe—divided into the *vamp, tongue,* and *rear quarters*—covers the dorsum of the foot. The vamp extends from the insole forward. The tongue is an extension of the vamp in a blucher-style closure, but in the bal-type oxford, the tongue is separate (Figure 8-2). The blucher-style closure can be opened slightly more than the bal oxford closure to allow the foot into the shoe. The toe of the vamp is often covered with a separate piece of leather called the *tip.* The rearward line of the tip may be straight or winged. The vamp is joined to the quarters, which make up the sides and back of the upper. The two quarters are joined at a back seam. The design of the shoe dictates the shape and size of the quarters. For the oxford shoe, the outside quarter is cut lower than the inside to avoid contact with the malleoli. In the bal oxford, the back edges of the vamp cover the forward edges of the quarter. The forward edges of the quarters are on the top of the vamp in the blucher style of shoe.

For individuals wearing orthoses and those with foot deformity, the blucher closure is preferable to the bal-style closure because of its construction. The blucher closure has a separation between the distal margins of the lace stays, thus offering a wide inlet and making the shoes easier to don and doff and readily adjustable in circumference. High shoes, which encase the malleoli, provide additional mediolateral stability.

Heel

The heel is located beneath the outer sole under the anatomic heel. The heel base is usually rigid rubber, plastic, or wood with a resilient plantar surface. As heel height increases, the ankle range of motion necessary to lower the forefoot to the floor increases. Weight-bearing pressures (vertical forces) on the forefoot and hallux also increase in midstance to late stance.[3] The individual with limited ankle motion may benefit from a compressible heel base to absorb shock and achieve plantar flexion during the early stance phase. A broad, low heel maximizes stability and minimizes stress on the metatarsal heads. Most lower extremity orthoses and prosthetic feet are designed for a specific heel height; efficacy of the orthosis or quality of the prosthetic gait can be significantly compromised if used with shoes that have higher or lower heels.

Reinforcements

Strategic shoe reinforcements contribute to foot protection. Toe boxing at the distal vamp shields the toes and prevents the anterior portion of the vamp from losing its shape. The toe box can also be increased in depth to protect and accommodate any toe deformities. The heel counter reinforces the quarters to help secure the shoe to the anatomic heel. The medial counter helps support the medial arch of the shoe, and the heel counter aids in controlling the rearfoot. The convex shank piece stiffens the sole between the distal border of the shoe heel and the MTP joints and aids in supporting the longitudinal arch.

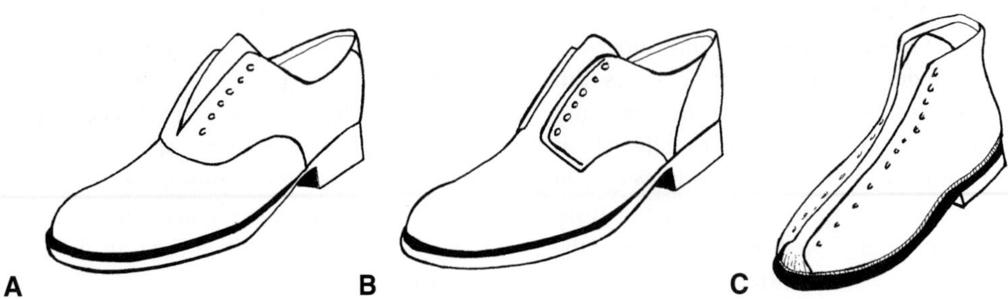

Figure 8-2

Three types of shoe closures. **A,** *In the bal oxford style, the tongue is a separate piece sewn to the vamp and anterior edges of the quarters.* **B,** *In the blucher style, the tongue is an extension of the vamp and can be opened slightly wider.* **C,** *For patients with rigid ankle orthoses, fixed deformity, or fragile neuropathic feet, the lace-to-toe (surgical) style may be necessary.*

Lasts

Shoes are constructed over a model of the foot stylized from wood, plaster, or plastic that is called a *last.* Manufacturers are now converting to computer-aided last designs. Regardless of the origin of the last, it determines the fit, walking ease, and appearance of the shoe. Commercial shoes are made over many different lasts in thousands of size combinations. Most shoes are made with a medial last, which means that the toe box is directed inward from the heel (Figure 8-3). Shoes that have a conventional last, straight last, inflared or medial last, or outflared or lateral last can also be obtained.

FASHION VERSUS FUNCTION

A revolution to create comfortable and "healthy" shoes has occurred within the shoe industry[4] in response to an epidemic of footwear-related health problems, the result of long-term wearing of improperly fitting shoes, which costs more than $3 billion annually in surgery.[5] Even the most savvy, health-conscious women sometimes buy shoes for looks, not fit. A survey of 356 women concluded that almost 90% of women wore shoes that were one to two sizes too small.[6] This trend contributes significantly to the development of bunions, hammertoes, claw toes, mallet deformities, corns and calluses, and other disabling foot problems in midlife and later life.[7]

Enhancing Function

Foot stability is critical to minimizing ankle injury, excessive pronation, and slipping of the heel during the gait cycle. A well-designed shoe provides a broad heel base, ankle collar, and close-fitting heel counter. A keystone of a good shoe is its ability to absorb shock. The construction of and materials used for the insole, midsole, and outer sole determine the amount of shock absorption that the shoe will provide.

A good shoe must be flexible and provide stability with each step. Flexible construction is especially important in the sole to enhance the toe rocker in late stance phase. The sole should also provide adequate traction as it contacts the ground, especially in early stance as body weight is transferred onto the foot. A coefficient of friction that is sufficient to minimize slips and near slips is vital. Heel height can create stress on the forefoot during gait. Heels of more than $1\frac{1}{2}$ inches exponentially increase weight-bearing forces on the metatarsal heads.[7]

The ability of a shoe to handle moisture is also an important consideration. For optimal foot health and comfort, perspiration must be wicked away and, at the same time, external moisture must be kept out.

The upper should be soft and pliable. Modern tanning techniques can create strong but supple uppers that surround the feet supportively and protectively without rubbing and chafing, while allowing the foot to breathe.

Orthotic-Related Function

A molded insole contributes to foot stability, shock absorption, and a transfer of shear forces away from problem areas. Orthoses can enhance the function of the shoes. Chapter 9 presents the principles and practices of orthotic prescription in commonly occurring conditions of the foot.

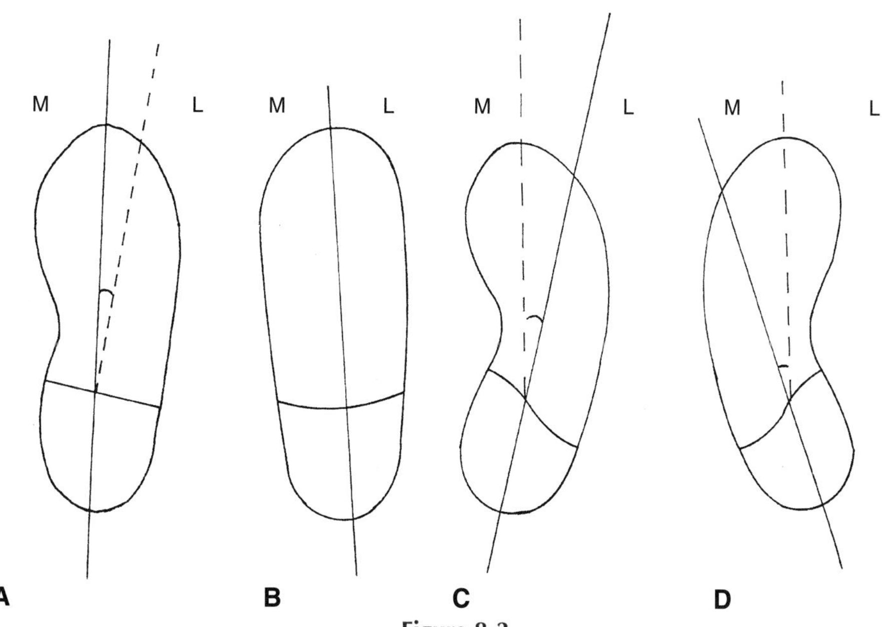

Figure 8-3

The last determines the shape of the shoe. ***A,*** *In a conventional last, the forefoot is directly slightly lateral* (L) *to the midline.* ***B,*** *A straight last is symmetric around the midline.* ***C,*** *An inflared last directs the forefoot medially, and* ***D,*** *an outflared last directs it more laterally than a conventional last.* (M, *medial.)*

PROPER FITTING OF A SHOE: "IF THE SHOE FITS"

The two primary determinants of proper shoe fit are shoe shape and shoe size. *Shoe shape* refers to the shape of the sole and the upper. Proper fit is achieved when shoe shape is matched to foot shape. *Shoe size* is determined by arch length, not by overall foot length.[9] The proper shoe size is the one that accommodates the first metatarsal joint in the widest part of the shoe. Properly fitting shoes are important in avoiding foot discomfort and deformity and are absolutely essential in individuals with arthritis, diabetes, and other foot disorders.

Great variability is found in human foot size and shape. Mass-produced shoes, however, are formed over fairly standard lasts that give a shoe its special size and shape. In the well-fit shoe, the shape determined by the last approximates the human foot. The design and construction of the shoe should allow for a roomy toe box; it should be wide enough for normal toe alignment and be ½ inch longer than the longest toe. Proper fit of the forefoot in the shoe can be a critical factor in reducing the incidence of bunions, hammertoes, and other forefoot deformities. In general, the shoe should be wide enough to accommodate the widest part of the forefoot. A tracing of the foot (standing) should fit within an outline of the shoe bottom.

Proper fit presupposes proper design, shape, and construction and is fundamentally wedded to availability in widths as well as lengths. It is important that the clinician cultivate a consumer mindset that realizes the medical importance of modifying the old cliché "if the shoe fits, wear it" to "if the shoe fits, wear it, and if it doesn't, order it in the correct size."

Determining Measurements

The average shoe salesperson does not offer to measure the foot, instead relying on the consumer to know his or her foot size. However, because foot size changes over time, periodic measurement of both feet for length and width is important. Many shoe styles that are available in retail shoe stores do not appropriately match the shape of an individual's foot. As a result, comfort and protection are compromised in the name of "style." This is especially problematic in the presence of foot deformity. Hallux valgus is a foot deformity that is aggravated by wearing shoes too narrow across the metatarsal heads and triangularly shaped in the toe box. Shoes should be wide enough to allow the material of the upper that surrounds the widest region of the forefoot (i.e., the metatarsal heads) to be compressed at least ¹⁄₁₆ inch before bony contact is made. Likewise, there should be at least a ½ inch between the tip of the longest toe and the front of the toe box in weight bearing (generally the width of the thumb).

In the United States, 12 standard shoe widths are manufactured. They range from the very narrow AAAAA to the very wide EEEE—that is, AAAAA, AAAA, AAA, AA, A, B, C, D, E, EE, EEE, EEEE. Because most retail stores stock shoes of midrange widths (A-E), patients with narrow or wide feet often have difficulty finding shoes of the optimal width.

Standard shoe sizes are available in half-size increments, from an infant's size 0 to a man's size 16 in U.S. sizes. The difference in length between half sizes is ¹⁄₁₆ inch, with concomitant adjustments in girth measurements. Standard shoe-sizing classifications are made by groups and lasts: infants' sizes 0 to 2; boys' sizes 2½ to 6; girls' sizes 2½ to 9; women's sizes 3 to 10; and men's sizes 6 to 12. Sizes larger than women's size 10 and men's size 12 must often be special ordered. A U.S. women's shoe size is usually three half sizes smaller than the corresponding men's size (e.g., women's size 9 is the same as a men's size 7½.

European and U.K. manufacturers use a different numbering system. The comparison of European and U.K. women's to men's sizes is based on centimeters (e.g., women's size 38 EUR/5 UK is the same as men's size 40 EUR/5 UK). Table 8-1 compares the standard sizes for U.S., European, and U.K. shoe manufacturers, in addition to the measures for each size).

Foot Contour

Foot contour changes throughout the life cycle. Aging, pregnancy, obesity, and everyday stresses on the foot cause it to widen. Deformities such as bunions increase the width and shape of the foot, and splaying of the metatarsal heads creates a collapse of the transverse arch, further increasing the width of the forefoot.[10] Forefoot height may increase in the presence of toe deformities. Deformities such as pes planus (flat foot) or pes cavus (high arches) change the contour of the midfoot. The shape of the foot must be considered and accommodated when an individual is measured for shoes. Often a "combined last" (where the last in the toe box is different from the rearfoot counter) is required to accommodate the contour of the foot. The relationship of the forefoot to the rearfoot is an important consideration in determining if the shoe shape, provided by the last, corresponds to the shape of the foot. Shoes with medial, straight, or lateral lasts can be ordered to best meet patient needs.

Obesity and Edema

The additional mechanical stress of carrying excess weight takes its toll on the feet, often resulting in problems such as plantar fasciitis, arthritis and bursitis, heel pain, neuroma, and gait changes.[11] Frey and associates[11] found that a weight gain of as little as 9 lb over a 5-year period increased foot size by one full size. Obesity has been shown to increase the length and the width of the foot. The Frey study also revealed that although women tended to adjust for length increases by purchasing a longer shoe, they rarely increased shoe width. The net result over the 5-year study period

Table 8-1
Comparison of Standardized Shoe Sizes

United States	*Europe*	*United Kingdom*	*Centimeters*
WOMEN'S SIZES			
3	34	1	20
3½	34.5	1.5	20.5
4	35	2	21
4½	35.5	2.5	21.5
5	36	3	22
5½	36.5	3.5	22.5
6	37	4	23
6½	37.5	4.5	23.5
7	38	5	24
7½	38.5	5.5	24.5
8	39	6	25
8½	39.5	6.5	25.5
9	40	7	26
9½	40.5	7.5	26.5
10	41	8	27
MEN'S SIZES			
6	40	5	24
6½	40.5	5.5	24.5
7	41	6	25
7½	41.5	6.5	25.5
8	42	7	26
8½	42.5	7.5	26.5
9	43	8	27
9½	43.5	8.5	27.5
10	44	9	28
10½	44.5	9.5	28.5
11	45	10	29
11½	45.5	10.5	29.5
12	46	11	30

included increased incidence of calluses, corns, bunions, hammertoes, ingrown toenails, and neuromas.

Obesity also has an impact on gait patterns. Persons with obesity demonstrate increased step width, increased ankle dorsiflexion with reduced plantar flexion, increased Q angles at the knee, increased hip abduction angles, increased abducted foot angles, greater out toeing, a tendency for flat-footed weight acceptance early in the gait cycle, increased touchdown angles, more eversion at the subtalar joint, and a faster maximum eversion velocity. These gait changes may be an attempt to increase stability during gait. The net effect, however, is an increased incidence of overuse injuries as a result of everyday activities.[11]

Proper shoe fitting is essential for preventing secondary foot problems that stem from ill-fitting shoes. Overweight individuals should be encouraged to have their feet measured regularly, particularly if they have had a significant weight gain. It is often helpful to shop for shoes at the end of the day, when feet are largest; to fit the largest foot while standing; and to ensure that ½ inch is between the end of the longest toe and the edge of the toe box. The shoes should be comfortable the moment they are worn.

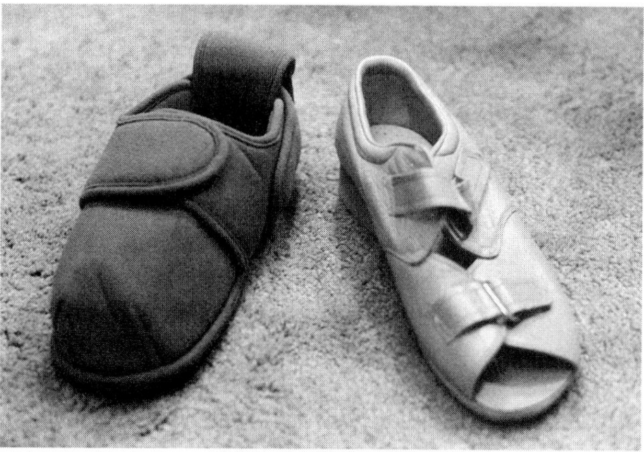

Figure 8-4
Thermold (P. W. Minor Shoes, Batavia, N.Y.) Velcro closure shoe/sandal. Adjustable Velcro closures are recommended to accommodate edematous feet and prevent tissue damage due to high pressure.

Fluctuation in foot size in individuals with edema (e.g., those with kidney dysfunction or congestive heart failure or any patient who is taking diuretic medication) creates a challenge when fitting shoes. The contour of the foot is constantly changing. For someone with severe edema, a Thermold (P. W. Minor Shoes, Batavia, N.Y.) Velcro closure shoe/sandal (Figure 8-4) is recommended to accommodate and support the foot and prevent the undue pressures imposed by a shoe that becomes too small during the course of the day.

CONSEQUENCES OF THE ILL-FITTING SHOE

The national obsession with beauty has created some not-so-beautiful sites on feet, such as bunions, hammertoes, and neuromas. These are particular problems for women, who often select poorly fitting shoes in an attempt to have the foot appear to be smaller, daintier, and narrower than it actually is. In Frey and associates' study,[6] 90% of women surveyed wore shoes that were too small by one or two width and length sizes, and 80% of these women had foot problems. Snow and associates[12] report that 90% of 795,000 surgeries for bunions, hammertoes/claw toes/mallet toes, neuromas, and Taylor bunions could be directly attributed to wearing ill-fitting shoes. Foot problems including bunions, lesser toe deformities, and neuromas are the primary consequences of wearing ill-fitting shoes. Clearly, many of these problems would be prevented by habitual use of properly fitting shoes.

SPECIAL CONSIDERATIONS

Feet come in many shapes, sizes, and conditions of health. The biomechanical and functional characteristics of feet change over an individual's lifetime and must also be reflected in shoe choice. An infant's foot must adapt to weight bearing, especially as walking becomes functional. The foot of a child continues to adapt as normal growth changes alignment of pelvis, femur, and tibia. The influence of hormones during pregnancy also affects the structure and function of the foot. Finally, the combined influence of the aging process, obesity, and diseases that are common in later life can create special footwear needs for the elderly.

Pediatric Foot

Many pediatric and lower extremity foot disorders are minimally symptomatic and do not require treatment, whereas others require more aggressive management. An understanding of the natural history of many of these disorders is important in establishing the appropriate footwear for toddlers and children as they begin to walk and run.[13-15]

In toeing is a problem caused by positional factors in utero and during sleep, muscle imbalances due to paralytic disorders, and decreased range of motion in the lower kinetic chain. It may also be due to metatarsus adductus, internal tibia torsion, or internal femoral torsion. (Note: Some of the best athletes are in-toers. The Dennis Browne bars or the counter rotation splint is used in combination with a reverse last shoe to remodel the bones during growth. Persistent severe toeing created by internal tibial torsion requires a derotational osteotomy of the tibia/fibula in the supramalleolar region.)

Metatarsus adductus is characterized by a bean-shaped foot that results from adduction of the forefoot. In most children (approximately 85%), this disorder resolves itself spontaneously.[16] If it does not improve over the first 6 to 12 weeks of life, the treatment of choice is an outflared shoe. The bones of the foot are soft and can be corrected with positioning in the outflared shoe (reverse last) or Bebax shoe (Camp Healthcare, Jackson, Mich.).

Internal tibial torsion is a twist between the knee and the ankle. Generally, this torsion disappears by 5 years of age. Torsion can be exacerbated by abnormal sitting and sleep postures with the foot turned inward.

Internal femoral torsion can also be the cause of in toeing with a twist between the knee and hip. Neither splints nor shoes are effective in treatment of torsion. Habitual sitting in the "W" position (e.g., when a child is watching television or playing games on the floor) can aggravate the problem. Children with internal femoral torsion should be encouraged to sit "X" legged as an alternative.

Out toeing occurs in children who sleep in the frog position and have soft tissue contractures around the hip. This is usually a hip or a long bone torsion problem and is not affected by footwear.

Toe walking can be the result of an in utero shortening or a congenital shortening of the Achilles tendon but can also be an early sign of cerebral palsy, muscular dystrophy, or Charcot-Marie-Tooth disease.[16] Until 4 years of age, the ability to stretch the tendon is well preserved, and conservative treatment includes stretching, casting, ankle-foot orthoses, and/or a night splint. Z-plasty lengthening is performed if conservative interventions fail. Shoe prescription objectives follow the same principles as those in the older adult with Achilles tendinitis (see the section Achilles Tendinitis, Bursitis, and Haglund's Deformity).

Flexible flatfoot appears to reflect generalized, hereditary ligamentous laxity.[17] Treatment for flatfootedness in children has changed over time. Currently, the shoe used to treat flatfoot is designed to correct heel valgus, support the arch, and pronate the forefoot in relation to the rearfoot. Forefoot pronation is achieved by using a lateral shoe wedge combined with a medial heel wedge. A scaphoid pad supports the arch, and a strong medial counter prevents medial rollover. A Thomas heel is often used to provide additional support for the arch.

Calcaneovalgus is a congenital positional deformity. The heel is in severe valgus, and the foot is dorsiflexed so much that it rests against the anterolateral aspect of the tibia. Calcaneovalgus is usually secondary to intrauterine position. Most cases correct spontaneously. Treatment of the severe cases includes stretching and serial casting. A few severe cases, if left untreated, persist into adolescence as pes planus.

An *accessory navicular bone* is a small ossicle at the medial tuberosity of the navicular. Individuals with an accessory navicular bone often complain of pressure and discomfort when wearing shoes. Often, placement of a prefabricated arch support in the shoe lifts the arch just enough to minimize rubbing on the shoe.

Hallux valgus (bunions) is most often the consequence of rearfoot valgus, leading to varus of the first metatarsal. The conservative approaches to treating this condition in children are orthoses and comfortable shoes, with a good heel counter to maintain the heel in subtalar neutral.

Curly toes involve the congenital shortening of the flexor tendons. Treated conservatively, flexors are stretched, and a rocker-like insole is used in the shoe to support the toes in extension. Shoes must have extra depth with plenty of room in the toe box.

Shoe prescription for these biomechanical problems of the foot and lower extremity in childhood is as valuable as a conservative corrective intervention. Overall, if a child's foot is developing normally and does not exhibit any signs of an abnormality, a soft-soled shoe is appropriate.[18,19] If some degree of abnormality exists, a more supportive, rigid shoe is indicated for toddlers. In general, the stiffer the heel counter, the more effective the intervention.

The most common prescription shoe for young children is a straight last shoe. This type of shoe is roomy enough to accommodate pads or wedges. In addition, a straight last shoe does not generate any abnormal forces against the child's foot.

Foot during Pregnancy

During pregnancy, women may experience problems in lower extremities, including edema, leg cramps, restless legs syndrome, joint laxity, and low back pain. As a result, foot pain is a common problem in pregnant women.[20] An important consideration is the provision of shoes with maximum shock absorption. Gel-cushioned running shoes are recommended, especially if women continue to jog or walk for exercise. Expectant mothers are also advised to exercise on soft surfaces to prevent problems caused by repetitive pounding on unforgiving surfaces.

High-heeled shoes exaggerate the lordotic curve and are inadvisable during pregnancy. Many women possess an intuitive level of common sense when it comes to wearing comfortable shoes during pregnancy. As weight distribution shifts with advancing pregnancy, especially if edema occurs, many women choose to wear shoes with laces or a Velcro closure. Athletic and walking shoes provide good support, excellent cushioning, and a solid heel counter. If a heel is desired for special occasions, a 1-inch or lower heeled shoe should be recommended. Many comfortable and attractive low-heeled dress shoes are now manufactured so that expectant mothers need not sacrifice fashion for function. Even low but tiny tapered heels cause women to wobble as they walk.

Many women find that their feet have "grown" during pregnancy; after having returned to prepregnancy weight and clothing, their shoes no longer fit. Measurements often reflect an increase in shoe length of one half to a full size. The stress of extra body weight coupled with ligamentous laxity can reduce arch height, adding length to feet. This process is a normal age-related change in foot structure, associated with wear and tear of the body over time, which is hastened during pregnancy. The hormonally induced tissue laxity of pregnancy leads to a broader forefoot as the metatarsal heads separate and the distal transverse arch flattens and to a longer foot as the longitudinal arch is less efficiently supported by soft tissue structures. For this reason, pregnant women are advised to wear a larger shoe size, with a square or deeper toe box, or both, especially if edema is also a problem.

Garbalosa and McClure[21] found that almost 80% of the general population has a forefoot varum deformity. This foot deformity displaces the center of gravity forward, which can increase stress on the back during pregnancy. Forefoot varum deformity produces instability whenever the center of gravity is moved anteriorly over the forefoot in weight bearing, forcing the foot into exaggerated pronation.[22] The net effect of the hormonal changes, pregnancy-induced forward displacement of the center of gravity, and the presence of forefoot varum is increased strain on the axial skeleton and reduced efficiency of gait. An orthosis to support the metatarsal heads and medial longitudinal arch, placed in shoes with good shock absorption ability, can help to decrease foot discomfort and prevent injury to the low back during pregnancy.

Foot in Later Life

Foot problems are one of the most common complaints of the elderly. The foot is also the most frequently neglected area of evaluation by most health care practitioners. In a study of patients who resided in a long-term care facility, 40% did not own properly fitting shoes. A subsequent survey indicated that the majority of community elders preferred to wear slippers and did not own adequate footwear.[23]

Gait disorders are a major cause of morbidity and mortality in the elderly, significantly contributing to the risk of disabling injury.[24] Gait changes, poor health, and impaired vision are the major predictors for falls.[25] Many older persons attribute their problems with walking to pain or a sense of unsteadiness, stiffness, dizziness, numbness, weakness, or impaired proprioception.[25]

Physical therapists work with patients to maximize their functional abilities and mobility. Treating foot pain and dysfunction can be a fundamental contributor to becoming functional in ambulation. As Helfand so eloquently stated, "Ambulation is many times the key or the catalyst between an individual retaining dignity and remaining in a normal living environment or being institutionalized."[26]

Gait and foot problems in the elderly are associated with diseases that are common in later life and with the aging process itself. Examples of conditions that can compromise gait and foot function include the residuals of congenital deformities, ventricular enlargement, spinal cord diseases, joint deformities, muscle contractures, peripheral nerve injuries, peripheral vascular disease, cerebrovascular accidents, trauma, ulcers, arthritis, diabetes, inactivity, and degenerative and chronic diseases.[24] The anatomical and biomechanical considerations of podogeriatrics focus on the interrelationships of the rearfoot, midfoot, and forefoot, established by osseous, muscle, and connective tissue structures. Movement of one joint influences movement of other joints in the foot and ankle. Soft tissue structures establish an interdependency of the foot and ankle to the entire lower limb. As tissues age, they become stiffer, less compliant, weaker, and more vulnerable to breakdown.

Foot contour alters with aging; the foot gets wider, and bunions and splaying occur from collapse of the transverse arch.[27] Forefoot height increases in the presence of toe deformities. Fat pads under the metatarsal joints atrophy and shift position distally, whereas the calcaneal fat pad atrophies and shifts laterally. These changes leave bony prominences that are vulnerable to breakdown.

In the diabetic patient, development of Charcot's joint (neuropathic arthropathy) is a relatively painless, progressive, and degenerative destruction of the tarsometatarsal or

MTP joints.[28-31] With the sensory losses that are common in diabetes, these joints are subjected to extreme stresses without the benefits of normal protective mechanisms. Capsular and ligamentous stretching, joint laxity, distention, subluxation, dislocation, cartilage fibrillation, osteochondral fragmentation, and fracture occur.[32,33] Hyperemia increases the blood supply, which promotes resorption of bone debris with resorption of normal bone as well. The foot often fuses in a deformed rocker bottom shape, vulnerable to pseudoarthrosis, instability, abnormal weight-bearing surfaces, ulcerations, and infections.[34,35]

The majority of foot problems in geriatric patients can be managed with proper shoe fitting and minimal shoe modifications. The most inexpensive footwear for this patient population is running or walking shoes. These are less expensive and fit within a fixed-income budget.[36] They provide good foot support and can be purchased with Velcro straps for closure if hand function or foot edema is a problem. The Thermold shoe is also a blessing for all the pathological and structural deformities with which the elderly patient must deal.

CHOOSING APPROPRIATE FOOTWEAR AND SOCKS

A vast, and somewhat bewildering, variety of "off-the-shelf" footwear is available to consumers. Many shoes are designed with certain types of activities in mind. Understanding the design and construction, as well as ensuring proper fit, enhances foot health and minimizes the risk of foot dysfunction, injury, and pain.

Athletic Shoe Gear

Many people jump into fitness activities "feet first" and develop blisters, calluses, and other foot injuries because of inappropriate footwear. A well-fit, activity-appropriate athletic shoe enhances enjoyment of the activity by protecting and supporting the foot and minimizing injury. Athletic shoes are designed for specific activities. A running shoe is designed with a high-force heel impact and forward foot movement in mind; the various shoe models have specific features that are designed for different surface conditions and distances in running. Basketball shoes do not provide as much cushioning as do running shoes but instead focus on foot support during quick lateral movement. Aerobic shoes are also designed for lateral movement but provide more cushioning for the impact anticipated on the ball of the foot. Shoe soles are also designed for the surface on which the activity is performed. Some shoes are manufactured as cross-training shoes so that they can go from the workout in the gym to jogging but are not designed for high-mileage runners.

Determining the foot type is important in prescribing the best shoe. For individuals with a flat low-arched foot, a shoe that provides maximum stability to prevent the foot from rolling in with each step is required. High-arched feet demand a shoe that is more flexible. "Normal" feet do best in a shoe that combines the last to accommodate the heel and the forefoot and that has forefoot flexibility. The size and shape of the toe box must also be considered. Enough room should be available in the toe box to prevent blisters, ulcers, and chafing of the toes. Shoes made from materials that "breathe" so that perspiration can escape are desirable. Athletic shoes are best used only for their intended activity and should be replaced at regular intervals to maximize their effectiveness.

Most athletic footwear is available in medium widths, although a few manufacturers provide shoes in several widths. Children's athletic footwear is available in narrow, medium, and wide widths. Women's athletic footwear may be available in AA, B, and D widths. Men's athletic footwear may be available in B, D, EE, and EEE widths. The key element in proper fit of athletic shoes is comfort from the moment the shoe is put on, with no break-in period needed. The shoe should also provide adequate support and shock absorption for the sport or activity that is being pursued.

Walking Shoes

A well-designed walking shoe provides stable rearfoot control, ample forefoot room, and a shock absorption heel and sole. This type of footwear may be specifically designed by an athletic footwear manufacturer or even by an orthopedic footwear manufacturer. Walking shoes are available in various widths and in several different lasts. Long medial counters, Thomas heels, and crepe soles can be used to modify this type of shoe gear to meet specific patient needs.

Dress Shoes

Despite the fashionable preference for shoes with narrow or pointed toes and slim high heels, the most foot-friendly dress shoe for women is a rounded-toe Mary Jane style with boxy heels. A good dress shoe approximates the shape of the individual's foot and provides flexibility and sufficient shock absorption. Prerequisites of a good dress shoe include a roomy toe box, low stable heel, proper width in the ball of the foot area, flexible outsole with skid-proof bottoms, and arch support.[37]

Triangular toe boxes and high heels, no matter how dainty, are best avoided because they can and do cause deformity. For a high-heeled shoe to stay on the foot, it must fit closely around the toes, resulting in no room for anything but the foot. The foot is virtually unsupported at the distal end of the shank, and extreme high pressure is present under the metatarsal heads. Heels higher than 2 inches make any kind of orthosis ineffectual.[38] Because the angle of the foot causes the heel of the orthosis to lift up, high heels can transform an orthosis into a catapult. Although orthoses can help to relieve metatarsal and heel pain and provide arch support, they cannot offer any corrective features in a shoe that is designed so unnaturally for the human foot.[12]

Socks

The sock is often overlooked when shoes of any kind are prescribed. Socks can aid in shock absorption, shield the skin from abrasion by the shoe stitching and lining, and prevent skin irritation from shoe dyes and synthetic leather materials. Additionally, clean, freshly laundered socks are integral to a sanitary foot environment. Unbleached, white cotton socks are ideal because they lack dyes, are hypoallergenic, and absorb perspiration readily. Cotton socks also provide ample toe room, unlike socks that are made from stretchable fabric, which often crowds the toes.

The size and style of socks also influence foot health. Socks that are too short crowd the toes; those that are too long wrinkle within the shoe, creating potential shear pressure points. If knee-high socks are worn, the proximal band must not be unduly restrictive; similarly, the use of circumferential garters to hold socks can impede circulation to the foot. Any holes worn into the sock also potentially create shear pressures and should be discarded. Mended holes in socks, because of the difference in thickness and materials, can irritate delicate or insensate soft tissue. An open hole at the toes pinches and constricts the digits, with excessive friction at the edges of the hole.

The Thor-lo (Thor-lo, Inc., Statesville, N.C.) sock is specially designed to support and cushion the insensitive foot or athletic/military foot that is exposed to repetitive frictional forces. Use of these specially designed socks not only reduces the frictional shearing forces but also significantly decreases vertical ground reaction pressure forces, preventing blistering and ulceration.[39-44] Extra high-density padding functions as a natural fat pad, reducing the deteriorating effects of shearing forces and the pressure and friction in the toe area. The Thor-lo concept of stockings is beneficial for patients with insensitive feet. It has also been used for individuals involved in aerobic exercise, baseball, basketball, cycling, golf, hiking, trekking and climbing, skiing, tennis, walking, and running.

PRESCRIPTION FOOTWEAR, CUSTOM-MOLDED SHOES, ACCOMMODATIVE MOLDED ORTHOSES, AND SHOE MODIFICATIONS

Alteration of foot function and alignment can be accomplished with one or more of the following strategies: foot orthoses of the appropriate materials, prescription shoes, and modifications of shoes themselves.[45-47] These strategies are used to relieve pain and improve balance and function during standing and locomotion. These alternatives are indicated when a transfer of forces from sensitive to pressure-tolerant areas is needed to reduce friction, shock, and shear forces; to modify weight transfer patterns; to correct flexible foot deformities; to accommodate for fixed foot deformities; and to limit motion in painful, inflamed, or unstable joints.

When special protective or prescription footwear is being considered, the functional objectives must be clearly stated so that the appropriate specific prescription can be developed. Careful examination of the foot helps the clinician identify pathology or mechanical factors, or both, that must be addressed and choose the appropriate materials and footwear styles to meet the patient's specific needs.

Moldable Leathers

Thermold is an example of prescription footwear that can be used to protect feet that are vulnerable due to vascular insufficiency, neuropathy, or deformity (Figure 8-5). It is a cross-linked, closed-cell polyethylene foam laminated to the leather upper of the footwear that can be heat molded directly to the foot. This makes modification for foot deformity easily managed and far less expensive than custom molding. Thermold shoes are also available in extra-depth styles, with a removable ¼-inch insole. Extra-depth shoes enable adequate room for custom-made insoles or orthoses to become an intricate adjunct to the footwear. In some instances, the Thermold can be used as an alternative to the custom-molded footwear.

Custom-Molded Shoes

Some foot problems cannot be accommodated in conventional footwear, and the best solution is custom-molded footwear. This footwear is molded directly over a plaster reproduction of the foot rather than a standard last. Special modifications, such as toe fillers, Plastazote (Zoteforms, Inc., Hackettstown, N.J.), rocker bars, and elevations, can be

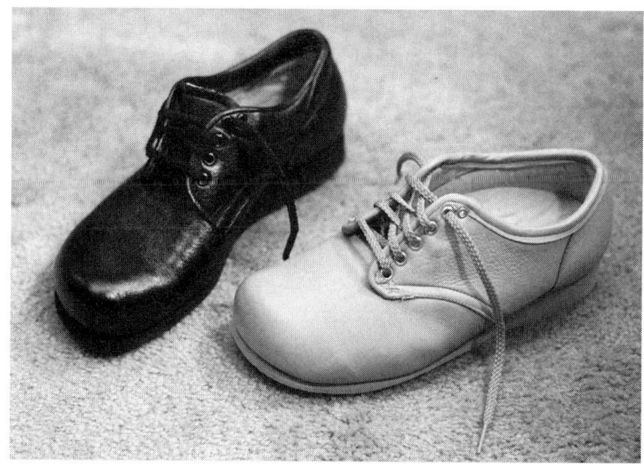

Figure 8-5
Thermold shoes (P. W. Minor Shoes, Batavia, N.Y.). These shoes allow for easy modification to accommodate foot deformities.

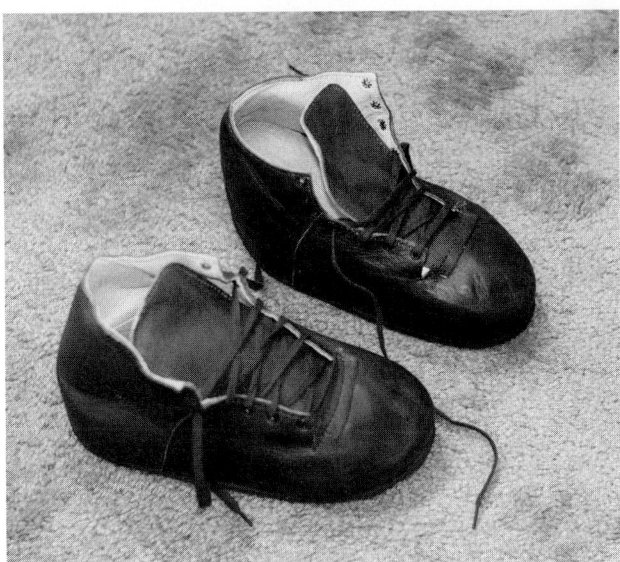

Figure 8-6
Examples of custom-molded shoes. These shoes are prescribed when foot deformities are too severe for accommodation in a conventional shoe.

added during manufacturing to meet the specific requirements of each foot. Because of this process, custom-molded shoes are made to conform to the foot shape in all respects (Figure 8-6). Custom orthopedic shoes represent the ultimate combination of function and aesthetics. Incorporating biomechanics and craftsmanship, shoes can redistribute weight, restrict joint motion, facilitate ambulation, and decrease the probability of neuropathic ulceration.[48,49]

Plastazote Shoe or Sandal

For patients with insensitive or ulcerated feet, a "healing sandal" or Plastazote shoe is often prescribed. This custom shoe is fabricated using a plaster cast of the individual's foot for construction.[50] Temporary protective footwear, such as a Plastazote boot or shoe or a healing sandal, is often used during neuropathic ulcer wound healing to allow for ambulation without pressure on the healing area, especially for patients who are unable to walk or noncompliant with non–weight-bearing ambulation.

Shoe Modifications

Various shoe modifications can be used to address functional and anatomical deformities of the foot and leg. Clearly stated objectives, based on careful evaluation, ensure that the appropriate shoe modifications are chosen.

Lifts for Leg-Length Discrepancy

For patients with leg-length discrepancy of $^3/_8$ inch or more, a full-length external lift can be mounted to the sole of the shoe on the shorter limb to equalize leg length and reduce proximal stresses at the hips and spine. If the length difference is less than $^3/_8$ inch, the discrepancy can usually be accommodated with an orthotic heel wedge worn inside the shoe. If the discrepancy is a result of a unilateral equinus deformity, a heel wedge can be attached to the external surface of the shoe. Leg length discrepancy is a common result of a hip fracture, congenital anomaly, or biomechanical imbalance such as pelvic rotation, hip anteversion or retroversion, or unilateral foot pronation. The level of the pelvis and absolute and relative measures of leg length should be part of a comprehensive gait evaluation.

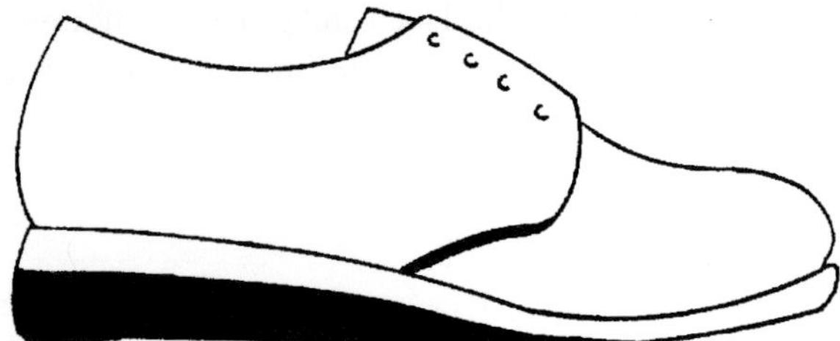

Figure 8-7
A heel wedge provides elevation of the heel for equinus deformity.

Heel Wedging

Wedging is used to alter lines of stress to facilitate a more normal gait pattern. The most effective wedges range from $^1/_8$ to $^1/_4$ inches in thickness at their apex. Larger wedges tend to cause the foot to slide away from the wedge toward the opposite side of the shoe, drastically reducing the effectiveness of the modification. Wedging is useful for children with a rotational problem, such as tibial torsion. In adults, wedges are used for accommodation in conditions such as a fixed valgus deformity of the calcaneus (Figure 8-7).

A medial heel wedge is used when flexible valgus of the calcaneus is present (Figure 8-8, *A*). As the wedge elevates the medial heel, a resultant varus tilt acts on the calcaneus, preventing excessive pronation of the foot. A lateral heel wedge is used when flexible varus of the calcaneus is present (see Figure 8-8, *B*). Elevation of the lateral heel decreases the medial drive on floor contact at heel strike, tipping the calcaneus into valgus. A full heel wedge is sometimes used in the presence of fixed or functional equinus deformity. The goal of wedging is to obtain a subtalar neutral position during the stance phase of gait.

Sole Wedging

Wedging can also be used to modify midfoot and forefoot positions. A medial sole wedge produces an inversion effect on the forefoot. This wedge is positioned along the medial aspect of the footwear, from a point just proximal of the first metatarsal head to the midline of the footwear (see Figure 8-8, *C*). Conversely, a lateral sole wedge creates an eversion effect at the forefoot. This wedge is placed proximal to

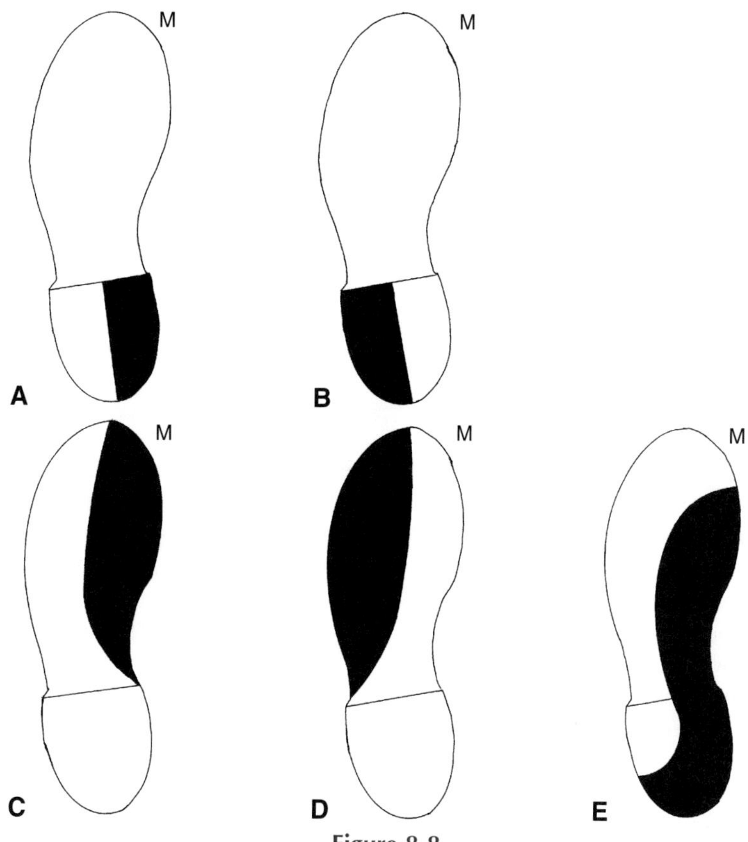

Figure 8-8

Examples of heel and sole wedge modifications. A medial (M) *heel wedge* **(A)** *is used when flexible valgus of the calcaneus is present; a lateral heel wedge* **(B)** *is used for flexible varus of the calcaneus. Medial sole wedges* **(C)** *create an inversion effect of the forefoot, whereas lateral sole wedges* **(D)** *create an eversion effect. A Barton wedge* **(E)** *supports the navicular bone and helps invert the calcaneus, shifting the body weight laterally.*

the fifth metatarsal head to the midline of the footwear. The apex of this wedge is the fifth metatarsal head (see Figure 8-8, *D*).

A Barton wedge (see Figure 8-8, *E*) is used in the presence of severe, flexible pronation deformities, such as those seen in pes planus, when control of the midfoot is the goal. The Barton wedge, usually made with $^{3}/_{16}$-inch leather, extends along the medial side of the foot to the midtarsal joint and tapers laterally just anterior to the cuboid bone. It provides support to the navicular and helps to invert the calcaneus. It is used when it is necessary to shift body weight laterally. When a Barton wedge is used, the shoe must have a firm medial counter. The Barton wedge can be incorporated in an internally placed lateral heel wedge for patients with fixed calcaneal varus or clubfoot deformity. Because an internal wedge is closer to the target deformity, it creates a positive force of greater magnitude than is possible with the external Barton wedge. Instead of tilting the footgear, the wedge tilts the calcaneus into the desired position.

Steel Spring

The steel spring, an external shoe modification, is a piece of flexible metal that is $^{1}/_{16}$ inch in depth and 1 inch in width, extending along the length of the footwear. It is usually placed between the insole and outsole of the shoe to restrict flexion of the sole. The need to enhance the strength of the shoe shank is often required to control the foot when lower extremity bracing is necessary. A steel spring is frequently helpful in assisting an individual who has hemiplegia with forward propulsion during the vertical pathway of the foot, from initial contact through midstance and into push-off/terminal stance.

Metatarsal Bars and Rocker Bottoms

A metatarsal bar is a block of material (usually stacked pieces of leather or rubber) that is attached to the sole of the shoe. Its placement proximal to the metatarsal heads significantly reduces pressure at the metatarsal heads during the push-off phase of the gait cycle.[51] The curved distal edge of the metatarsal bar is designed to follow the curve of the metatarsal heads. It is commonly used to adapt shoes worn by patients with transmetatarsal amputations, fixed arthritic deformities, diabetes, forefoot deformities such as hallux rigidus, and neuromas. The placement of a metatarsal bar or rocker facilitates push-off by simulating forward propulsion in the absence of metatarsal flexibility.

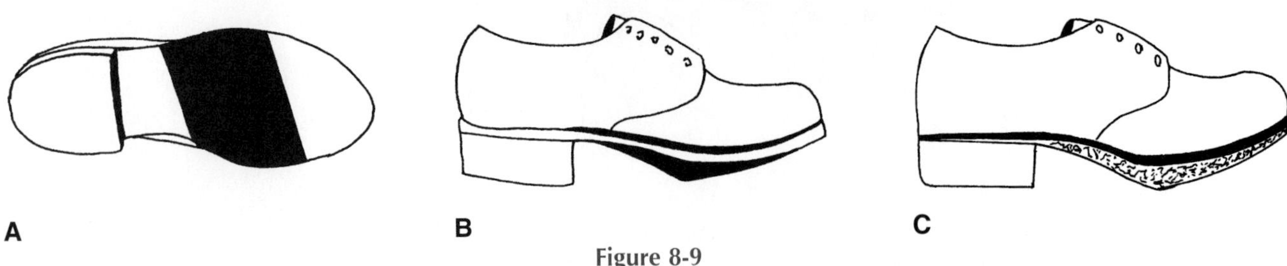

Figure 8-9

*Examples of rocker bottom soles. A metatarsal bar (**A**) prevents undue pressure at the metatarsal heads during push-off in late stance. A rigid leather rocker sole (**B**) or an extended crepe rocker bar (**C**) redistributes body weight over the entire plantar surface, facilitating a smoother and more normal gait pattern while reducing stress and trauma in the forefoot.*

Rocker bottoms are made of either lightweight crepe or leather (Figure 8-9). These modifications are flush with the heel and toe, in an arch with an apex of $\frac{1}{2}$ to $\frac{5}{8}$ inch. The rocker bar redistributes body forces over the entire plantar surface of the foot while in weight bearing. It facilitates a smooth roll during the stance phase of gait, while reducing sheer stress and trauma to the midfoot and forefoot. It is often used to modify shoes worn by patients with partial foot amputations, arthritis, and diabetes. It is also used for patients who have any lower extremity orthosis that limits forward progression of the tibia over the foot and toes during mid- and late-stance phases. For patients with diabetes, a rigid rocker sole (a steel-spring heel to toe with the toes extended and a rocking axis near the center of the foot) can be used to help distribute body weight and compel knee flexion at toe-off, reducing the length of stride and sheer stress on the metatarsal heads.

Thomas Heels

The Thomas heel is designed to improve foot balance and relieve excessive pressure on the shank portion of the footwear. Applied as either a lateral or a medial flare of the heel, its goal is to increase stability during gait by assimilating subtalar neutral. A laterally flared heel is used with a rearfoot varus to decrease the incidence of inversion injuries. A medially flared heel is used with a rearfoot valgus to decrease the incidence of eversion injuries (Figure 8-10). For instance, a medial flare from the heel to the sustentaculum tali prevents excessive pronation of the foot during gait.

Offset Heels and Shoe Counters

The offset heel is a modification used to help correct valgus or varus deformities. It offers a broad support base, especially at the superior surface of the heel, where the broad buildup against the shoe's counter provides reinforcement either medially or laterally. A heel counter is an extension along the medial or lateral borders of the shoe from the heel to the proximal border of the fifth or the first metatarsal head. This shoe modification strengthens the shank portion of the footwear for better control of the hind foot. The heel counter is often used in combination with the appropriate Thomas heel. A counter can also be placed medially or laterally in the midfoot region. A patient whose gait exhibits excessive pronation, such as is common in rheumatoid arthritis, may require a firm medial counter to prevent the shoe from collapsing medially and to assist in realigning the foot into a neutral position.

Attachments for Orthoses

For some patients with neuromuscular dysfunction (e.g., hemiplegia, paraplegia, multiple sclerosis), a traditional, metal, double-upright, lower-extremity orthosis can be prescribed. If so, the shoe must be modified: A U-shaped orthotic bracket (stirrup) is attached to the shoe by means of three copper rivets, one on the heel and two in the shank. The metal is riveted through the outsole to the insole. To accomplish this, the heel is removed and the plate of the stirrup is attached. The groove is then cut through the heel, and the heel is reattached. The appropriate orthotic ankle joint is then attached to uprights of the stirrup.

Shoe Stretching

Shoes with leather uppers can be stretched almost one full width. Although a shoe cannot be truly lengthened, it can be made to feel longer with a toe box stretcher device that looks like the shape of the foot and is inserted into the shoe to expand it (Figure 8-11). After the leather is moistened or softened, this device effectively raises and slightly rounds the toe box. Frequently, the pressure of a flat toe box on the toes is more problematic than the length of the shoe. Specific points in the shoe can be softened and expanded by placing an "expansion knob" on the toe-box stretcher or using a ball-and-socket device. Site-specific stretching is particularly helpful for patients with toe deformities such as hallux valgus, hammertoe, mallet toe, claw toe, overlapping toes, and Taylor bunion deformity.

Blowout Patches and Gussets

Patients with foot deformities who prefer conventional shoes to Thermold shoes may find temporary pain relief if a blowout patch or gusset is applied to their shoe. The shoe leather around the area of deformity is cut away and replaced with a softer blowout patch or gusset of moleskin, soft leather, or suede.

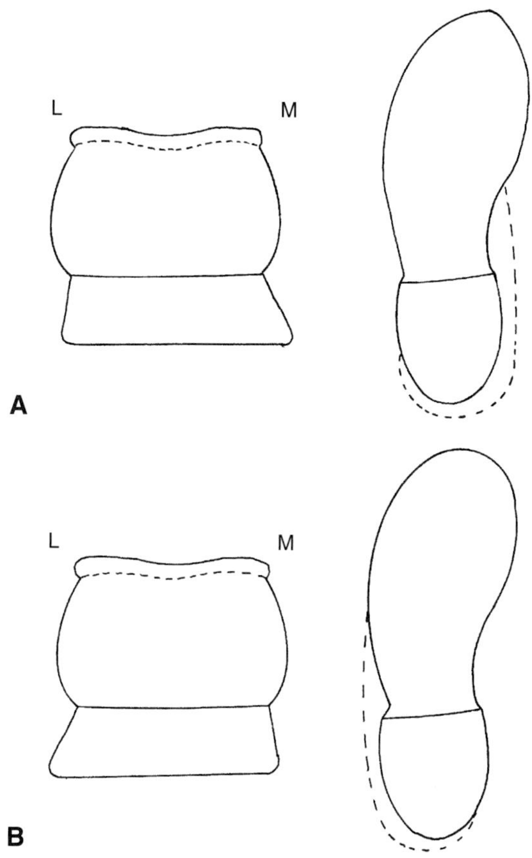

Figure 8-10
Examples of Thomas heels. ***A,*** *A medial* (M) *flared heel provides a broader base of support and prevents eversion of the ankle.* ***B,*** *A lateral* (L) *flared heel prevents inversion of the ankle.*

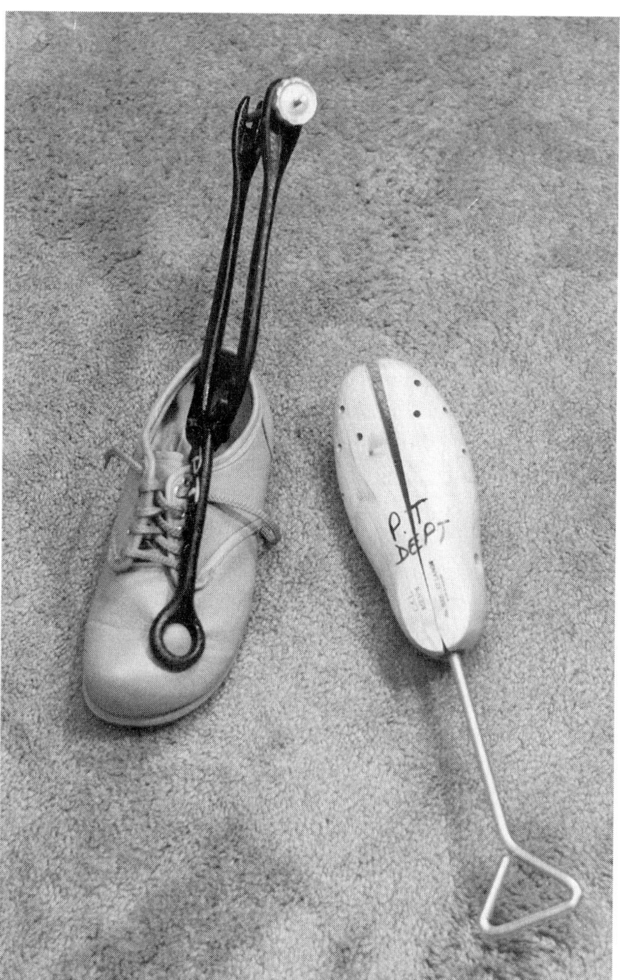

Figure 8-11
Tools that are used to stretch leather shoes. Stretching often provides adequate accommodation for deformities in conventional shoes. The toe box stretcher (right) *can increase width by one size. The ball-and-socket device* (left) *is used to stretch specific points that correspond to the forefoot and toe deformity.*

FOOTWEAR FOR COMMON FOOT DEFORMITIES AND PROBLEMS

Conservative management of common forefoot, midfoot, and rearfoot deformities often involves modification of shoes or prescription footwear, or both. Specific footwear strategies for several common foot problems are described in the following section.

Problems in the Forefoot

The most common footwear variation used for abnormalities in the forefoot is a high toe box. High toe boxes are available in various footgear, including athletic sneakers, comfort shoes, Thermolds, and prescription footwear. To accommodate forefoot deformity optimally, the maximum height of the abnormal toes must be measured in a weight-bearing position. Tables of manufactured shoes by toe box space are available to guide the clinician in recommending shoes that most closely match patient needs.[52]

Metatarsalgia

Metatarsalgia is pain around the metatarsal heads that results from compression of the plantar digital nerve as it courses between the metatarsal heads. Excessive weight bearing with atrophy of the metatarsal fat pad can result in irritation of the nerves and potentially lead to development of a neuroma. The three major objectives in shoe prescription for patients with metatarsalgia are to (1) transfer pressure from painful, sensitive areas to more pressure-tolerant areas; (2) reduce friction by stabilizing the MTP joint; and (3) stabilize the rearfoot and midfoot to reduce pressure on the metatarsal heads.[53] Characteristics of the shoe that will accomplish these goals include wide width to reduce pressure on the transverse metatarsal arch, long fitting to eliminate plantar-flexed MTP joints, cushion soles to enhance shock absorption, and a high toe box to allow forefoot flexion and extension. Additionally, the shoe should include a long medial counter to stabilize the rearfoot, a lower heel to minimize pressure at the metatarsal heads, and preferably Thermoldable leather to accommodate deformities. Shoe modifications often include a transverse metatarsal bar to redistribute pressure from metatarsal heads to metatarsal shafts and shorten stride and a rocker sole to reduce motion of painful joints.

Sesamoiditis

Sesamoiditis is an inflammation around the sesamoid bones under the first metatarsal head. It often results from a loss of soft tissue padding under the first metatarsal head and from toe deformities such as hallux valgus and hallux rigidus. The objective of shoe prescription for patients with sesamoiditis is to redistribute weight-bearing forces from the first MTP joint and its sesamoids to the long medial arch and shafts of the lesser metatarsals. A transverse metatarsal bar is used to redistribute pressure from metatarsal heads to metatarsal shafts and to shorten stride. A rocker sole can be used to reduce motion of the painful hallux joint.

Morton's Syndrome

With repetitive irritation of the plantar digital nerve between the first and second metatarsal heads, a neuroma is likely to develop.[54] This condition is known as *Morton's syndrome.* The three major objectives in shoe prescription for patients with Morton's syndrome are to (1) redistribute weight from the lesser metatarsals (especially the second and third) to the proximal phalanx of the hallux, (2) stabilize the rearfoot by maintaining subtalar joint neutral, and (3) accommodate forefoot varus as well as a possibly dorsiflexed first metatarsal. Shoe prescription includes a long medial counter for rearfoot support and stability; a straight or flared last to accommodate foot shape; a high, wide toe box to reduce compression across the transverse metatarsal arch; a large enough shoe size to accommodate the long second toe; and a Thomas heel or wedge sole to support the medial longitudinal arch. A medial heel and medial sole wedge may be necessary when symptoms are severe.

Morton's (Interdigital) Neuroma

Overstretching of the digital nerves in extreme toe extension at the proximal phalanx can also result in the development of a neuroma. Two objectives should be considered for patients with Morton's neuroma. First, the patient must obtain relief from the pain and burning, especially in the third interspace of the MTP joint. Second, compression of the digital nerve as it passes between the heads of the third and fourth metatarsals needs to be reduced. To achieve these goals, the shoe should be wide enough to eliminate transverse compression and have enough length to reduce plantar flexion of the MTP joints. A long medial counter can help to reduce pronation; a cushioned sole increases shock absorption, and a low heel unloads pressure on the metatarsals. Elastic laces may be helpful in allowing expansion of the forefoot. Shoe modifications for Morton's neuroma might include a metatarsal bar to elevate the metatarsals and redistribute weight, or a metatarsal rocker bar to immobilize the metatarsals, or a combination of both.

Metatarsalgia of the Fifth Metatarsophalangeal Joint

Like the metatarsalgia described previously, metatarsalgia of the fifth MTP joint results in plantar digital nerve irritation at the interdigital space of the fourth and fifth metatarsal heads. When metatarsalgia of the fifth MTP joint is present, the goals of intervention are to redistribute weight forces to the fifth metatarsal shaft and to provide a broad base of support along the lateral border of the foot. The optimal shoe has a last with enough lateral flare to accommodate the lateral aspect of the foot and fifth metatarsal shaft, a firm lateral counter, and a firm leather or rubber sole. Possible shoe modifications include a lateral heel and sole flare ending proximal to the fifth metatarsal head to provide a broader base of support. Lateral heel and sole wedges may be useful for patients with flexible feet.

Hallux Rigidus (Limitus)

Degenerative joint disease of the first MTP joint causes pain, loss of mobility, and eventually fusion of the joint. Osteophyte formation on the dorsal aspects of the metatarsal head and base of the proximal phalanx can be quite painful and result in a loss of extension. For patients with hallux rigidus or limitus, the goals are to limit motion of the hallux and first MTP joint and to reduce pressure on the dorsal and plantar aspects of the hallux and first MTP joint.[55] To accomplish this, the shoe should have a high and wide toe box and Thermold or soft leather uppers. When significant deformity is present, a steel shank from heel to phalanx of the hallux and a rigid rocker sole with compensating heel elevation may be necessary.

Hallux Valgus (Bunions)

A prominent bony formation on the medial aspect of the first MTP joint can result from lateral deviation of the hallux and from foot pronation.[56] This deformity is often associated with long-term wearing of shoes with a triangular toe box. Five objectives should be considered in the prescription of shoes for patients with hallux valgus: (1) to reduce friction and pressure to the first MTP joint, (2) to eliminate abnormal pressure from narrow-fitting shoes, (3) to reduce pronation of the foot from heel strike to midstance, (4) to correct eversion, and (5) to relieve posterior tibial tendon and ligamentous strain. Patients with hallux valgus benefit from shoes with high, wide toe boxes and Thermold or soft leather uppers. A combined last with increased last width in the toe box and a smaller heel for better control of the subtalar joint may also be indicated. Additionally, the choice of a shoe that is longer and wider helps to accommodate deformity; a lower heel to reduce forefoot pressure and a reinforced medial counter help to prevent pronation.

Hammertoes, Claw Toes, and Mallet Toes

Hammertoe deformity is characterized by hyperextension of the MTP joint, flexion of the proximal interphalangeal (PIP) joint, and extension of the distal interphalangeal (DIP) joint. This results in high load during weight bearing at the plantar metatarsal heads and at the plantar surface of the distal phalanx. Claw toe deformity features hyperflexion of the PIP and DIP joints, although the MTP joint can be hyperextended or hyperflexed. Mallet toe deformity results from hyperextension of the MTP joint, flexion of the PIP, and a neutral position of the DIP, so that weight bearing is on the tip of the distal phalanx. Deformities of the lesser toes can be problematic, especially for patients with compromised circulation and neuropathy. For these individuals, there are two major footwear goals: (1) to transfer pressure away from the metatarsal heads, the PIP joints, and the distal phalanx joints, and (2) to encourage flexion of the MTP joints and extension of the PIP joints.[57] Patients with lesser toe deformities should wear shoes with a high, wide toe box made of Thermold or soft leather to reduce the likelihood of microtrauma over the bony prominences. The shoe should also be long enough to allow flexion of MTP joints and extension of PIP joints rather than cramping the toes. Finally, a soft cushion outsole and low heel further reduce pressure on the metatarsal heads. Commonly used shoe modifications for lesser toe deformities include metatarsal bars to reduce pressure to metatarsal heads and shift weight bearing to metatarsal shafts and rocker bars or rocker soles to accommodate rollover on fixed deformities.

Problems in the Midfoot

Shoe prescriptions or modifications, or both, are also helpful in managing midfoot dysfunction and deformity. The most commonly encountered problems include pes planus pes equinus, pes cavus, and plantar fasciitis.

Pes Planus

Pes planus is pronation of the midfoot that results in a failure of the foot to supinate during midstance. The longitudinal arch flattens, causing a splaying of the forefoot and lateral deviation of the metatarsals. This deformity can be either flexible or fixed (rigid).

For patients with a flexible pes planus, the goals of intervention are to reduce pronation from heel strike to midstance, correct eversion, relieve tension on the posterior tibial tendonitis, and relieve ligamentous strain. To do these things, the shoe should offer a long medial heel counter, a Thomas heel (medial extension) or a firm wedge sole, and a straight last. A custom shoe is recommended for severe cases. Shoe modifications may include a medial heel wedge to correct eversion and reduce pronation or a medial heel and sole flare in extreme cases.

Because of the fixed nature of a rigid pes planus, the goals are somewhat different: to relieve ligamentous strain, to relieve arch pain, and to correct eversion of the foot. The optimal shoe should offer a broad shank (extra wide midfoot), a straight last, and a long medial counter. Additionally, a wedge sole is applied to reduce the load on the metatarsal heads, stabilize the intertarsal joint, and provide a dorsiflexion assist.

Pes Equinus

In *pes equinus,* the plantar flexor muscles and Achilles tendon are tightened, which limits dorsiflexion of the ankle and results in a plantar flexion deformity. For patients with a flexible pes equinus, the footwear prescribed attempts to reduce ankle plantar flexion, reduce the load on the metatarsal heads, and stabilize the subtalar joint. This can be accomplished in a shoe with a low heel. A rocker bottom can be applied to the sole to provide a dorsiflexion assist and further reduce load on the metatarsal heads.

When the pes equinus deformity is rigid or fixed, the goals of footwear intervention change. Instead of trying to reduce plantar flexion, a posterior platform supports the rearfoot from heel strike to midstance and mimics the dorsiflexion needed at toe-off. It is important to contain the entire foot in the shoe, reducing the load on the metatarsal heads. For patients with unilateral deformity, it is also important to equalize the relative leg length difference between the normal foot and the equinus foot through all phases of gait. Shoe prescription for patients with a fixed equinus deformity includes a Cuban (elevated) heel to provide a platform and deep quarter or high-top shoes. If modifications are necessary, they might include posterior heel elevation on the equinus side, as well as on the contralateral limb, to facilitate swing of the involved limb and reduce pelvic obliquity.

Pes Cavus

Pes cavus is an exaggerated longitudinal arch that can lead to a plantar flexed forefoot with retraction of the toes and severe weight-bearing stresses on the metatarsal heads and heel. Patients with pes cavus benefit from shoes that provide a broad platform for stability; reduce loading at the heels, lateral borders, and metatarsal heads; and accommodate the deformed foot within the shoe. The shoe should also have a firm heel counter to maintain rearfoot stability and a modified, curved last to accommodate foot shape. Custom-molded shoes are recommended in severe cases. Possible shoe modifications for patients with pes cavus include a lateral flare to provide a platform for greater stability, a cushion sole to absorb shock on the heel and metatarsal heads, and a metatarsal bar to shift weight from the metatarsal heads.

Plantar Fasciitis

Plantar fasciitis is inflammation of the plantar fascia at its insertion to the medial aspect of the calcaneus. This inflammatory process can lead to the development of calcification at that insertion, commonly referred to as a *heel spur*. Plantar fasciitis is often a consequence of loss of the longitudinal arch in conditions such as pes planus or of undo stresses created in the forefoot with tightness of the gastrocnemius and soleus muscles or an elevated longitudinal arch. To reduce the painful signs and symptoms of plantar fasciitis, the goals of intervention are to transfer weight-bearing pressure from painful to more tolerant areas, to reduce tension on the plantar fascia and Achilles tendon, to control pronation from heel strike to midstance, and to maintain the subtalar joint in a neutral position. The shoe prescribed for plantar fasciitis has a long medial heel counter to limit heel valgus, a high heel to reduce tension on the plantar fascia and Achilles tendon, and adequate length to minimize compression and promote supination from midstance to toe-off. The types of shoe modifications that may be useful include a posterior heel elevation to reduce tension on the plantar fascia and Achilles tendon.

Problems in the Rearfoot

The most common dysfunctions and deformities of the rearfoot that can be addressed by footwear prescription or modification include arthrodesis, Achilles tendinitis or bursitis, and Haglund's deformity (pump bump).

Arthrodesis

Arthrodesis is a loss of mobility at the ankle mortise, the junction of the talus with the tibia and fibula. This deformity prevents motion at the ankle in all planes and alters progression through the stance phase of gait, and it may also compromise limb clearance in swing phase. When arthrodesis of the ankle is present, the major objectives are to provide effective shock absorption and controlled lowering of the forefoot at loading response, to improve comfort and efficiency of push-off, and to accommodate any shortening or residual equinus. Shoes that address the problems of arthrodesis have a reinforced counter and may have a medial or a lateral flared heel (or a combination of both) to provide greater stability. Some patients benefit from a high-top shoe as well. Modifications that protect the foot and facilitate a more normal gait pattern include application of a cushioned heel to absorb shock and simulate plantar flexion after heel strike and a rocker sole to mimic the dorsiflexion needed in the late stance phase.

Achilles Tendinitis, Bursitis, and Haglund's Deformity

Undue stresses of the Achilles tendon, direct pressure of a too-short shoe, and/or tightness of the gastrocnemius and soleus muscles can result in tendinitis or bursitis. *Haglund's deformity* is an osseous formation at the insertion of the Achilles tendon at the calcaneus. The goals of shoe prescription for patients with Achilles tendinitis, bursitis, and/or Haglund's deformity (pump bump) are similar: (1) to reduce tension on the Achilles tendon, (2) to provide dorsiflexion assist at heel strike and at toe-off, (3) to reduce abnormal pronation, and (4) to reduce pressure and friction (shear) at the insertion of the calcaneus. Patients with these problems require a slightly higher heel to reduce dorsiflexion, a long medial counter to limit subtalar motion, a longer shoe size to reduce compression pressure, and a backless shoe to prevent irritation of the pump bump. The types of shoe modifications that may be helpful include a posterior heel elevation to reduce tension on the Achilles tendon or a foam-filled posterior heel counter.

DIAGNOSIS-RELATED CONSIDERATIONS IN SHOE PRESCRIPTION

Prescription footwear and shoe modifications are also extremely useful tools to protect joints, prevent skin problems, and enhance normal function of patients who are coping with arthritis and gout or diabetes and peripheral vascular disease. Adaptations to footwear may also be helpful for patients with hemiplegia, partial foot amputations, or congenital deformities.

Arthritis

Arthritis, whether degenerative, rheumatoid, or traumatic, leads to destruction of joints. In working with patients with foot arthritis, the goals of intervention are to prevent or limit abnormal motion, accommodate for arthritic deformities, and cushion impact loading and reduce microtrauma within the joint.[58] A reinforced counter can help to limit subtalar motion; a high-top design shoe can also help to limit ankle motion. Extra-depth shoes may be needed to accommodate deformities of the midfoot and forefoot. Thermoldable leather is preferable if deformities need further accommodation. The application of a rocker bottom helps to improve push-off by shortening the distance between the heel and the MTP joint. It also reduces the total ankle motion required for push-off. Shock-absorbing accommodative orthoses can be placed inside the shoe, and a cushion heel can be added to absorb even more force at heel strike, as well as to limit ankle and subtalar motion.[59] A flared heel can reduce medial/lateral movement at the subtalar joint.

Gout

For patients with gout, the treatment objectives are similar to those for patients with arthritis— preventing or limiting motion of painful or inflamed joints, accommodating foot deformities, and cushioning the impact of loading on the involved joints. A reinforced counter to limit subtalar motion or a high-top design to limit overall ankle motion should be considered. An extra-depth shoe of thermoldable leather is best able to accommodate deformities without creating pain and discomfort over sensitive joints. A rocker bottom can be applied to assist push-off, prevent pedal joint movement, and reduce ankle motion required for push-off.

Shock-absorbing accommodative orthoses and cushion heels provide even more comfort and protection of inflamed joints during gait.

Diabetes

The loss of protective sensation in patients with diabetic neuropathy creates significant vulnerability to injury from repetitive microtrauma. Protection of the plantar surface of the diabetic foot from microtrauma is of paramount importance. Patients with diabetic neuropathy often have significant weakness of intrinsic muscles. Forefoot deformities develop, including claw toes, which are susceptible to breakdown in areas of excessive shoe pressures. The risk of nonhealing, infection, and subsequent amputation is quite high; prevention is the most effective treatment strategy. Total-contact full-foot orthoses using soft, shock-absorbing materials helps to distribute weight-bearing pressures over the entire plantar surface of the foot away from the vulnerable bony prominences. A Thermold leather shoe is recommended for the insensitive diabetic foot. (See Chapter 21 for comprehensive management of vulnerable feet.)

Peripheral Vascular Disease

Because the ability to heal is compromised in patients with peripheral vascular disease, any irritation or ulceration exponentially increases the risk of infection and subsequent amputation. Here, too, prevention of skin breakdown and protection of the vulnerable foot are the primary goals. The ability to fit and protect the foot effectively is further challenged by fluctuating edema. A Thermold sandal with Velcro closure is often recommended for patients with peripheral vascular disease-related edema as a safe and effective alternative to standard shoes. If edema is not a problem, a soft Thermold shoe protects the plantar surface of the foot from repetitive pressures and accommodates deformities that are at risk for shoe pressure–related trauma. Because hypersensitivity is often a problem with circulatory pathologies in the lower extremities, a shoe that cushions the foot may be helpful. Elastic shoelaces allow expansion of the shoe for patients with minimal edema-related fluctuations in foot size.

Hemiplegia

The patient with hemiplegia after a cerebrovascular accident (e.g., stroke, brain attack) may have inadequate or excessive tone of the lower extremity. Many of these patients need orthotic intervention to control the foot and ankle in some or all phases of gait, to accommodate for any fixed deformities and to cushion impact loading at initial contact. Footwear is selected to enhance orthotic function or, in some instances, to directly impact mild dysfunction. A reinforced heel counter helps to limit subtalar motion and stabilize the foot on heel strike. A flared heel or high-top shoe may be recommended to enhance foot placement and stance stability. A rigid shoe shank may be required for some types of lower extremity orthoses. In the presence of an equinus deformity, a heel lift on the shoe provides total contact during weight bearing and facilitates stability. In severe deformities of the ankle, a custom-molded shoe may be the only alternative.

The most common ankle-foot orthoses used in hemiplegia tend to increase shoe length, width, and depth by a half to a whole size. Often the insole can be replaced with an insert foundation, to garner a little more room for the orthosis within the shoe. Extra-depth shoes are particularly helpful for patients who are faced with difficulty in donning their orthosis and shoe because of upper extremity dysfunction in hemiplegia.

Amputation and Congenital Deformity

The foot that is shortened surgically or is congenitally deformed is a management challenge because the weight-bearing surface is reduced or altered, increasing the likelihood of tissue breakdown with repeated loading in gait. The type of protective footwear used can range from an over-the-counter extra-depth shoe for a mild deformity to a custom-molded shoe for a severe deformity. When the feet are of unequal size, it is more difficult to fit them without buying two pairs of shoes or having custom footwear made. If the difference between the feet is no more than one size in length, the larger size can be used with toe padding for the shorter deformed or amputated foot or with an orthosis to accommodate the deformity (Figure 8-12). Frequently, the shorter foot is also wider and must be accommodated by the appropriate orthosis custom molded to the shoe. A toe filler prevents the shortened foot from sliding within the shoe

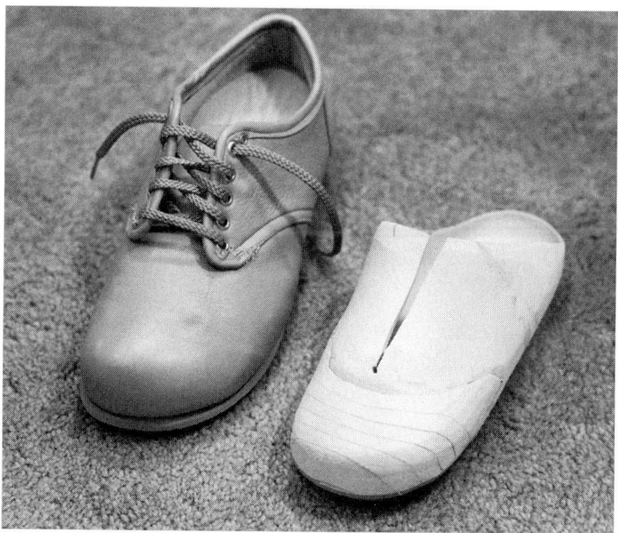

Figure 8-12
A toe filler can be used on a foot that has been shortened by amputation or congenital deformity.

during gait but also increases the risk of skin breakdown. It is crucial that the first MTP joint be aligned with the "toe break" point in the shoe. If the foot falls posterior to the toe break, stress is concentrated at the distal end of the foot, increasing the chance of pressure imposition by the "filler."

READING THE WEAR ON SHOES

For the clinician who is faced with decisions about modifying, repairing, or replacing footwear, examination of patterns of wear and erosion provides important information. Deterioration of the shoe itself impairs tactile sensibility and position sense judgment.[60] Shoes that have outlasted their purpose often create abnormal forces and shearing that increase the risk of repetitive microtrauma to the skin and joints of the foot and ankle. Analysis of the wear and erosion of the shoe is a prescriptive tool in advising, prescribing, and modifying a shoe to fit individual needs.

CASE EXAMPLE 1

A Diabetic Patient Who Is Homeless and Has a Neuropathic Ulcer

J. H. is a 71-year-old homeless, Hispanic man with a 22-year history of type 2 diabetes mellitus treated with glibenclamide 2.5 mg three times daily. He presents with a large ulcer (6.552 cm^2) of the plantar surface of the midfoot with significant arch deformity of the right foot, subsequent to an episode of Charcot arthropathy several years ago. J. H. reports that the ulcer has been present for more than 1 year. He has complications resulting from diabetes, including retinopathy, peripheral neuropathy, and history of numerous neuropathic ulcerations involving both feet. He also has a 24-year history of arterial hypertension and a documented myocardial infarct in July 1993. He is currently managed with ACE inhibitors and calcium antagonists. It is unclear how regularly he has taken his medications, although they are available at no cost through the shelter's clinic. J. H. has been homeless for 7 years.

J. H. is referred to the health clinic at the homeless shelter for diabetic and hypertensive assessment and conservative treatment of the foot ulceration. His first appointment at the clinic is on August 29, 2004.

Questions to Consider

- What tests and measures might the foot clinic team use to assess current status and changes in J. H.'s neuropathic wound, the deformity of his feet, the circulation and sensory status of his limbs, and his functional status and gait? What is the evidence of reliability and validity of these measures?
- What does the team need to understand about his current health status and diabetic control? How will they gather this information?
- What are the immediate needs, in terms of footwear, for J. H.? How might his needs change over time as his wound heals?
- Given his current health status and lifestyle, what factors will likely affect (both positively and negatively) clinical decision making about footwear, wound care, diabetic management, and follow-up care? How might the team prioritize goals and possible interventions?
- How would the team assess efficacy of their interventions?

Initial Plan of Care

Satisfactory metabolic control and blood pressure values are reached during the initial week of medical management at the shelter clinic, and J. H. is referred to Boston City Hospital (BCH) for a series of tests and measures on an outpatient basis. Although J. H. is found to have bilateral diabetic retinopathy (*fundus oculi*), there was no evidence of diabetic nephropathy. Echocardiogram evidences a left ventricular hypertrophy with a normal regional kinesis and an ejection fraction of 50%.

Electromyography shows normal conduction velocity and slight abnormalities of sensory action potentials in the nerves of both lower extremities. An elevated threshold of 40 V to biothesiometer and a partial loss of sensitivity (nine of nine areas tested are insensitive bilaterally) to Semmes-Weinstein 5.07 monofilament are recorded. The transcutaneous oxygen tension is 30 mm Hg at the dorsum of the involved foot (right) and 15 mm Hg at the perilesional site. In the ulcerated limb, the ankle-brachial index measured with Doppler technique is 0.8. Duplex scanning shows widespread atheromasic lesions in the carotids and in the lower limb arteries without hemodynamically significant stenoses and no significant alterations in the venous district of the lower limbs.

J. H.'s ulcer on the right foot appears superficial and is graded as a Wagner grade II ulcer. The ulcer is covered by a fibrinous exudate with keratotic margins. The microbiological cultures are negative. A surgical debridement is performed at BCH September 18, 2004, and the patient/client is sent back to the shelter with instructions for local treatment before and after daily sharps debridement consisting of the daily application of sterile paraffin gauze and for "evaluation and conservative treatment" by physical therapy. The wound is surgically debrided again on September 24 and October 10, 2004.

Questions to Consider

- How might the team interpret the results of the tests performed at BCH? How will this information influence or inform wound care and recommendations for footwear for this gentleman?
- What additional information will the physical therapist and foot care clinic team need to gather?

- What are the primary goals of physical therapy/foot care intervention? What is the prognosis and anticipated outcome? What is the anticipated duration of this episode of care? How frequently might J. H. receive care?
- What interventions would be most appropriate to address the goals of wound healing and prevention of future recurrence of neuropathic ulcers?

Physical Therapy Evaluation and Intervention

J. H. is evaluated at the shelter by a physical therapist on the Foot Clinic Team on September 18, 2004. He arrives at the clinic ambulating independently, without any assistive devices. The ulcer on the plantar surface of his midfoot measures 6.552 cm^2, in the Charcot joint deformity region of the right foot. The ulcer is determined to be secondary to repetitive trauma to this region in shoes that had a large hole in the midsection of the sole.

A total contact cast is applied. Selective padding of the cast includes foam padding over the toes and an ulcerated area of the foot; felt pads over the malleoli and navicular prominence; and cotton cast padding around the proximal and anterior lower leg, heel, sides, and dorsum of the foot. (Chapter 21 covers additional information about total contact casting and conservative management of neuropathic ulcers.) A rubber heel mount is applied to the cast for ambulation. Fiberglass casting material is used to decrease the effects of the elements (weather) on a plaster cast in this homeless individual who spends much time outdoors. The cast is also bifurcated to allow high galvanic electrical stimulation to be used as a local treatment modality to the wound and to provide access for daily debridement, application of dressings, and monitoring for secondary lesions. The cast is secured using Velcro strapping. The patient is allowed to walk freely and is highly compliant, wearing the cast continuously.

The ulcer responds favorably to a combination of periodic surgical debridement, local wound care and daily sharps debridement, a modified total contact casting protocol, and high galvanic electrical stimulation. By the end of December 2004, complete closure of the ulcer is achieved, with the patient remaining stable since. J. H. is subsequently fitted with a total contact foot orthosis bilaterally and provided with a pair of Reebok walking sneakers with an extra width to accommodate for the Charcot foot deformity bilaterally.

With proper intervention and attention to the patient's/client's social situation, it is determined that the prognosis for healing his wound is good and that he can be integrated into appropriate home, community, and work environments within the context of his disability. J. H. is placed in a permanent shelter-housing residence on November 13, 2004 and assumes part-time employment as a guide at the Boston Museum of Science.

Discussion

For individuals with neuropathic wounds, total contact casting allows ambulation with protection from external stress and trauma. In addition, because the cast is well molded and minimal padding is applied, pressure is distributed evenly and maintained as long as the cast is worn. This total-contact cast also counteracts lymphatic congestion, which compromises the healing process. For J. H., the cast was bifurcated to allow for daily wound care while providing consistent pressure relief and foot protection.

Once wounds are healed, the major objectives in treating the diabetic foot are to protect the plantar surface from repetitive microtrauma and accommodate deformities that could be traumatized by excessive shoe pressures resulting in ulceration and amputation. A total-contact, full-foot orthosis using soft shock-absorbing materials helps to distribute weight-bearing pressures over the entire plantar surface of the foot away from the vulnerable bony prominences. A Thermold leather shoe or good walking sneaker is recommended for the insensitive diabetic foot.

Accommodative devices are insoles that are placed in shoes to balance the feet, allowing pressures to be evenly distributed and permitting support and shock absorption of the foot. An orthosis, in contrast, supports and also controls the foot by neutralizing pronatory forces. Following wound healing, a total-contact orthosis (Plastazote with a layer of $^3/_8$-inch PPT) was fabricated for J. H. and placed in a pair of extra-depth Reebok walking shoes.

Accommodating shoe gear should be used by diabetic patients, and walking barefooted should be prohibited. The shoe's upper should be soft, so as not to irritate any prominence or developing deformity. The accommodative insole that is used should be adaptable to changes as well. A combination of an expanded polyethylene such as Plastazote, which can be heat molded to provide total contact, mounted on a shock-absorbing material such as PPT, or covered with a neoprene like Spenco that is soft and retains its shape, makes an excellent accommodative insole. This type of accommodative orthosis protects the foot from trauma to prominent areas and redistributes the forces to provide even weight bearing through total contact upon the plantar surface (Figure 8-13). When accommodative orthoses are used, the shoe must have adequate depth to accommodate it. Extra-depth shoes such as Thermold shoes or extra-depth sneakers allow not only the room needed for the accommodative insole but also modification of the upper through heat molding to accommodate lesser toe deformities. A rigid-sole rocker-bottom shoe might also be recommended to reduce pressures under the metatarsal heads during push-off. The apex of the rocker is positioned just proximal to the metatarsal heads, allowing for the shoe itself to provide forward propulsion of the foot.

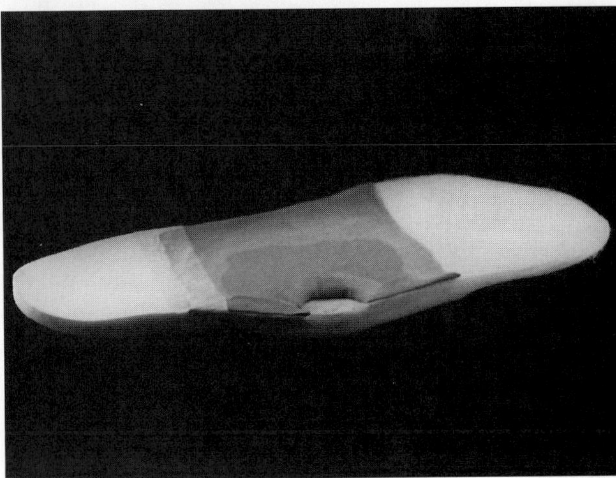

Figure 8-13
An example of an accommodative orthosis for a patient with diabetic neuropathy and Charcot deformity of the left midfoot. Note the "cut out" to reduce weight-bearing pressure on the most prominent area of bony deformity and the use of materials to "fill" space around the deformity and distribute weight-bearing pressures over the entire plantar surface of the foot.

SUMMARY

The shoe is an essential interface between the foot and the ground. It protects the foot from trauma and supports the structures of the foot as an individual walks, runs, and changes direction. Fashionable footwear, especially for women, often compromises, rather than enhances, foot function. Foot function and footwear needs have a developmental aspect as well; an understanding of how the foot changes over the life span and of the special needs of children, pregnant women, and the elderly is essential. Knowledge about the components of shoes and their variations, the criteria for proper fitting, and the relationship between shoe design and activity-related demands is an important tool for clinical practice. Physical therapists are often called on to recommend footwear for patients with special needs. A baseline knowledge of shoe characteristics and modifications for certain types of deformities or diagnoses enhances this ability.

REFERENCES

1. Finlay OE. Footwear management in the elderly care programme. *Physiotherapy* 1986;72(4):171-178.
2. Fuller EA. A review of the biomechanics of shoes. *Clin Podiatr Med Surg* 1994;11(2):241-258.
3. Mandato MG, Nester E. The effects of heel height on forefoot peak pressure. *J Am Podiatr Med Assoc* 1999;89(2):75-80.
4. Black E, Black E. Comfort shoes: the long overdue revolution. *Biomechanics* 1995;2(10):27-33.
5. Frey C. If the shoe fits . . . *Biomechanics* 1995;2(4):26-28.
6. Frey C, Thompson F, Smith J, et al. American Orthopaedic Foot and Ankle Society Women's Shoe Survey. *Foot Ankle* 1993;14(2):78-81.
7. Coughlin MJ. Lesser toe abnormalities. Oregon Health Science University, *Instructional course lectures,* 2003;52:421-444.
8. Snow RE, Williams KR. High heeled shoes: their effect on center of mass, position, posture, three-dimensional kinematics, rearfoot motion, and ground reaction forces. *Arch Phys Med Rehabil* 1994;75(5):568-576.
9. Janisse DJ. The art and science of fitting shoes. *Foot Ankle* 1992;13(5):257-262.
10. Herman HH, Bottomley JB. Anatomical and biomechanical considerations of the elder foot. *Top Geriatr Rehabil* 1992;7(3):1-13.
11. Frey C. Chan C, Carrasco N. Obesity: do weight gains lead to lower extremity pain? *Biomechanics* 1996;3(1):30-35.
12. Snow RE, Williams KR, Holmes GB. The effects of wearing high heeled shoes on pedal pressures in women. *Foot Ankle* 1992;13(2):85-92.
13. Sass P, Hassan G. Lower extremity abnormalities in children. *Am Fam Physician* 2003;68(3):417-419.
14. Charrette M. Foot care: do children need corrective footwear? *Dynamic Chiropract* 2003; 21(12):28-33.
15. Hein NM. [Inserts and shoes for foot deformities]. *Orthopade* 2003;32(2):119-1329.
16. Shapiro S. Pediatrics: a reasoned approach to common lower limb disorders. *Biomechanics* 1995;2(5):18-21.
17. Rao UB, Joseph B. The influence of footwear on the prevalence of flat foot: a survey of 2300 children. *J Bone Joint Surg* 1992;74(4):630-631.
18. Valmassy RL. Pediatric biomechanics. *Podiatry Today* 1989;May:86-92.
19. Valmassy RL. The use of gait plates for in-toed and out-toed deformities. *Clin Podiatry Med Surg* 1994;11(2):211-217.
20. Black E, Cooke Anastasi S. Pregnancy and the lower extremities. *Biomechanics* 1995;2(4):22-25, 68-69.
21. Garbalosa JC, McClure MH. The frontal plane relationship of the forefoot to the rearfoot in an asymptomatic population. *J Sports Phys Ther* 1994;20(4):200-206.
22. Rothbart BA, Hansen KH, Yerratt MK. Resolving chronic low back pain: the foot connection. *Am J Podiatry Med* 1995;5(3):84-90.
23. Karpman R. Geriatric prefab. *Biomechanics* 1995;2(5):53-58.
24. Sudarsky L, Ronthal M. Gait disorders among elderly patients. *Arch Neurol* 1993;40(2):740-743.
25. Hough JC, McHenry MP, Kammer LM. Gait disorders in the elderly. *Assoc Prescription Footwear* 1987;35(6):191-196.
26. Helfand AE. Common foot problems in the aged and rehabilitative management. In Williams TF (ed), *Rehabilitation in the Aging.* New York: Raven, 1984. pp. 291-303.
27. Edelstein JE. Foot care for the aging. *Phys Ther* 1988;68(12):1882-1886.
28. Pinzur MS. Charcot's foot. *Foot Ankle Clin* 2000;5(4):897-912.
29. Pinzur MS, Shields N, Trepman E, et al. Current practice patterns in the treatment of Charcot foot. *Foot Ankle Int* 2000;21(11):916-920.
30. Frykberg RG, Kozak GP. The diabetic Charcot foot. In Kozak GP, Hoar CS, Rowbotham JL, et al. (eds), *Management of Diabetic Foot Problems.* Philadelphia: Saunders, 1984. pp. 103-112.

31. Frykerg RG. Podiatric problems in diabetes. In Kozak GP, Hoar CS, Rowbotham JL, et al. (eds), *Management of Diabetic Foot Problems.* Philadelphia: Saunders, 1984. pp. 45-67.
32. Prior T, Gardiner A, Thomas A, Maitland P. Footwear requirements of patients with diabetes mellitus. *Diabet Foot* 2000;3(1):24-28.
33. Ramuglia VJ, Palmarozzo PM, Rzonca EC. Biomechanical concepts in the treatment of ulcers in the diabetic foot. *Clin Podiatr Med Surg* 1988;5(3):613-626.
34. Bailey TS, Yu HM, Rayfield EJ. Patterns of foot examination in a diabetes clinic. *Am J Med* 1985;78(3):371-374.
35. Pinzur MS. Benchmark analysis of diabetic patients with neuropathic (Charcot) foot deformity. *Foot Ankle Int* 1999;20(9):564-567.
36. Bottomley JB, Herman H. Making simple, inexpensive changes for the management of foot problems in the aged. *Top Geriatr Rehabil* 1992;7(3):62-77.
37. Seale KS. Women and their shoes: unrealistic expectations? American College of Podiatry, Instructional course lectures, 1995;44:379-384.
38. Corrigan JP, Moore DP, Stephens MM. Effect of heel height on forefoot loading. *Foot Ankle* 1993;14(3):148-152.
39. Herring KM, Richie DH. Friction blisters and sock fiber composition: a double-blind study. *J Am Podiatry Med Assoc* 1990;80(2):3-7.
40. Richie DH, Herring KM. Friction blisters and sock construction. Presented at the annual meeting of the American Academy of Podiatric Sports Medicine, Miami, May 29, 1990.
41. Herring KM, Richie DH. Friction blisters and sock fiber composition: a single-blind study. Part 2. Presented at 75th annual meeting of the American Podiatric Medical Association, Las Vegas, August 15, 1990.
42. Murray HJ, Veves A, Young MJ, et al. Role of experimental socks in the care of the high-risk diabetic foot. *Diabetes Care* 1993;16(8):1190-1192.
43. Veves A, Masson E, Fernando D, Boulton AJM. Use of experimental padded hosiery to reduce abnormal foot pressures in diabetic neuropathy. *Diabetes Care* 1989;12(9):16-19.
44. Veves A, Masson E, Fernando D, Boulton AJM. Studies of experimental hosiery in diabetic neuropathic patients with high foot pressures. *Diabet Med* 1990;7(3):324-326.
45. Lord M, Hosein R. Pressure redistribution by molded inserts in diabetic footwear. *J Rehabil Res Devel* 1994;31(3):214-222.
46. Shrader JA. Nonsurgical management of the fool and ankle affected by rheumatoid arthritis. *J Orthop Sports Phys Ther* 1999;29(12):703-717.
47. Egan M, Brosseau L, Farmer M, et al. Splints and orthosis for treating rheumatoid arthritis. *Cochrane Database Syst Rev* 2003, (1)(CD004018).
48. White J. Custom shoe therapy. Current concepts, designs, and special considerations. *Clin Podiatr Med Surg* 1994; 11(2):259-270.
49. Reiber GE, Smith DG, Wallace C, et al. Effect of therapeutic footwear on foot reulceration in patients with diabetes: a randomized controlled trial. *JAMA* 2002;287(19):2552-2558.
50. Breuer U. Diabetic patient's compliance with bespoke footwear after healing of neuropathic foot ulcers. *Diabetes Metab* 1994;20(4):415-419.
51. Brown D, Wertsch JJ, Harris GF, et al. The effect of rocker soles on plantar pressure. *Arch Phys Med Rehabil* 2004;85(1):81-86.
52. Kaye RA. The extra-depth toe box: a rational approach. *Foot Ankle Int* 1994;15(3):146-150.
53. Kelly A, Winson I. Use of ready made insoles in the treatment of lesser metatarsalgia: a prospective randomized controlled clinical trial. *Foot Ankle Int* 1998;19(4):217-220.
54. Childs SG. Diagnosis and treatment of interdigital perineuronal fibroma (a.k.a Morton's syndrome). *Orthop Nurs* 2002;21(6):32-24.
55. Shrader JA, Siegel KL. Non-operative management of functional hallux limitus in a patient with rheumatoid arthritis. *Phys Ther* 2003;83(10):831-844.
56. Caselli MA. Foot deformities: biomechanical and pathomechanical changes associated with aging. *Clin Podiatr Med Surg* 2003;20(3):487-509.
57. Hurwitz S. Hammer toe in adults: recognition and clinical management. *J Musculoskel Med* 1999;16(8):460-465.
58. Michelson J, Easley M, Wigley FM, Hellmann D. Foot and ankle problems in rheumatoid arthritis. *Foot Ankle Int* 1994;15(11):608-613.
59. Li CY, Imaishi K, Shiba SJ, et al. Biomechanical evaluation of foot pressure and loading force during gait in rheumatoid arthritic patients with and without foot orthosis. *Kurume Med J* 2000;47(3):211-217.
60. Robbins S, Waked E, McClaran J. Proprioception and stability: foot position awareness as a function of age and footwear. *Age Ageing* 1995;24(1):67-72.

II

Orthotics in Rehabilitation

9

Functional Foot Orthoses

ROBERTA NOLE, DONALD S. KOWALSKY, AND
JUAN C. GARBALOSA

LEARNING OBJECTIVES

On completion of this chapter, the reader will be able to do the following:

1. Describe the major anatomical structures of the foot as well as the basic biomechanical principles associated with these structures.
2. Describe effects of extrinsic and intrinsic deformities and of abnormal pronation on the function of the foot during the various phases of gait.
3. Understand strategies used to examine and evaluate intrinsic foot deformities.
4. Describe abnormal pronation and the pathological conditions that contribute to abnormal pronation in gait.
5. Describe components of a foot orthosis, goals of orthotic intervention, and specific purposes of the most common orthotic interventions.
6. Discuss controversy related to traditional orthotic theory.
7. Understand current literature related to the effect of foot types on lower extremity biomechanics and injury occurrence.
8. Understand current literature related to the biomechanical effects of foot orthoses.
9. Understand current literature related to the efficacy of foot orthoses.

HISTORY OF THE FUNCTIONAL FOOT ORTHOSIS

The use of foot orthoses as an effective treatment tool for biomechanical dysfunction of the feet has evolved during the twentieth century. Early on, foot orthoses were used to redistribute plantar foot forces to alleviate discomfort in pressure-sensitive areas of the foot. Little consideration was given to the specific foot abnormality that led to the pathological condition.[1] In the early 1900s metal foot braces began to be used to control motion at specific joints of the foot and prevent pathological conditions.[2] These devices, although functional, were often not well tolerated because of the rigidity of the materials and the mismatch between brace design and foot pathokinesiology. In 1948, Schreber and Weineman first identified forefoot invertus (varus) and evertus (valgus) as primary foot deformities that required correction by an orthosis.[3] In the 1960s, Merton Root developed neutral impression casting techniques, positive cast modifications, and posting (mechanical correction) techniques. The standards he established have enhanced orthotic comfort and function.[3] During the past few decades, functional foot orthosis use has increased considerably as theories linking the mechanics of the foot and ankle and the causes of musculoskeletal disorders have evolved.[4]

TRIPLANAR STRUCTURE OF THE FOOT

The foot is a complex of bones interconnected by a series of multiplanar articulations supported by soft tissue structures. It is subdivided into three functional components: the rearfoot, the midfoot, and the forefoot.

Several important articulations of the foot (talocrural, subtalar, midtarsal, first and fifth rays) are *triplanar*; the axis of rotation in these joints is not perpendicular to any of the cardinal planes (sagittal, horizontal, frontal) of the human body. As a result, motion about triplanar joints leads to simultaneous movement in all three of these cardinal planes.[5] The amount of motion evident in any single plane is related to the pitch (inclination) of the triplanar axis from the respective cardinal plane.[6] Triplanar motion occurs in three-dimensional space; the breakdown of triplanar motion into its three constituent cardinal plane movements is artificial.

Because motion about a triplanar axis is three dimensional, motion occurs simultaneously in the three cardinal planes. Blocking any one component of triplanar motion in a single cardinal plane prevents movement in the other two planes as well. This "all or nothing" rule is the premise for orthotic posting or wedging.[5] Theoretically, the addition of a post or wedge to an orthosis blocks the frontal plane component of triplanar motion, which in turn blocks or limits the triplanar motion of pronation. The design principles of foot orthoses are founded on knowledge of the functional anatomy of the foot.

Talocrural Joint

The talocrural joint (TCJ) (articulation between tibia, fibula, and talus, connecting the foot to the lower leg) has a triplanar axis of rotation. In neutral position, the TCJ axis passes through the tips of the medial and lateral malleoli, pitched 10 degrees from the transverse plane and 20 to 30 degrees from the frontal plane (Figure 9-1).[7-10] Although sagittal plane plantar flexion and dorsiflexion are primary motions at this joint, the slight inclination of the TCJ axis of rotation leads to concomitant transverse and frontal plane motion. During plantar flexion, the foot adducts and inverts; with dorsiflexion it abducts and everts.[11] Normal range of motion (ROM) of the TCJ is between 12 and 20 degrees of dorsiflexion and 50 and 56 degrees of plantar flexion.[12,13] The medial (deltoid) and lateral collateral ligaments stabilize and limit motion that occurs at the TCJ.[14]

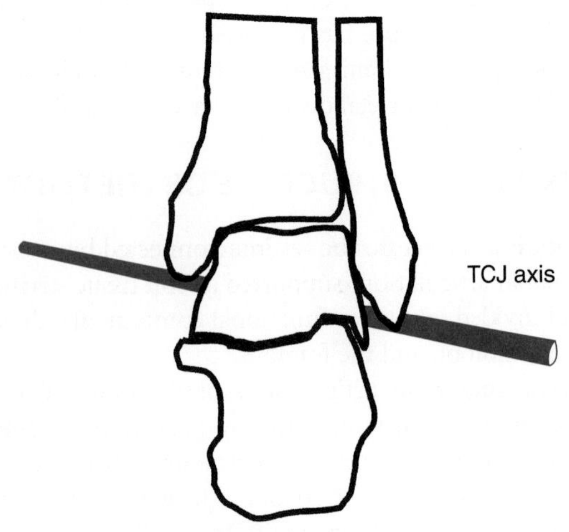

Figure 9-1
Posterior view of the osseous components and axis of the talocrural joint. The osseous components of the talocrural joint are the tibia medially and superiorly, the fibula laterally, and the talus inferiorly. The axis of the joint passes in a posterolateral to anteromedial direction through the tips of the lateral and medial malleoli. (Courtesy Juan C. Garbalosa, University of Hartford, West Hartford, Conn.)

Rearfoot

The osseous structures of the rearfoot are the calcaneus (inferior) and the talus (superior) (Figure 9-2). The articulation between the calcaneus and talus is the subtalar joint (STJ). Three joint surfaces are present in this articulation: posterior, anterior, and middle. The posterior joint surface has a concave talar and convex calcaneal portion, whereas the anterior and middle joint surfaces have convex talar and concave calcaneal arrangements. This structurally based articular geometry, along with the interosseous talocalcaneal ligament, limits the amount and type of motion occurring at the STJ.[11,15] The medial and lateral collateral ligaments and the posterior and lateral talocalcaneal ligaments also offer support to the STJ.[16]

At the STJ, the triplanar axis of rotation is oriented in an anterosuperior to posteroinferior direction, pitched approximately 42 degrees from the transverse plane, 48 degrees from the frontal plane, and 16 degrees from the sagittal plane (see Figure 9-2). The location of the STJ axis in the human foot varies greatly. Manter[17] reported that the inclination from the transverse and sagittal planes varies from 29 degrees to 47 degrees and 8 degrees to 24 degrees, respectively.

The triplanar motions at the STJ are supination and pronation. Supination of the weight-bearing foot leads to dorsiflexion and abduction of the talus with simultaneous inversion of the calcaneus. Pronation of the weight-bearing foot results in plantar flexion and adduction of the talus and eversion of the calcaneus.[5] Because of the variability in location of the axis of rotation of the STJ, the component motions of supination and pronation vary as well. As the axis becomes more perpendicular to a particular cardinal plane, the motion occurring in that plane becomes more pronounced, whereas the other motions become less prominent.[18,19] This variability affects coupled motion between the joints of the foot and the lower leg. During pronation and supination of the rearfoot, the tibia and fibula rotate internally and externally in the transverse plane.[5,20,21] An increase in the frontal plane motion of the rearfoot could cause a simultaneous increase in the transverse plane motion of the lower leg.

Midfoot

The midfoot is composed of two bones: the cuboid and the navicular. The talonavicular and calcaneocuboid articulations between the midfoot and rearfoot form an important composite joint: the midtarsal joint (MTJ) or transverse tarsal joint. The articular surfaces of the talonavicular joint are convex-concave, whereas the surfaces of the calcaneocuboid joint are sellar shaped.[8,17] MTJ movement is supported and restricted by the bifurcate, short and long plantar, and plantar calcaneonavicular (spring) ligaments. The short and long plantar ligaments and the plantar calcaneonavicular ligaments also support the longitudinal and transverse plantar arches of the foot.[22]

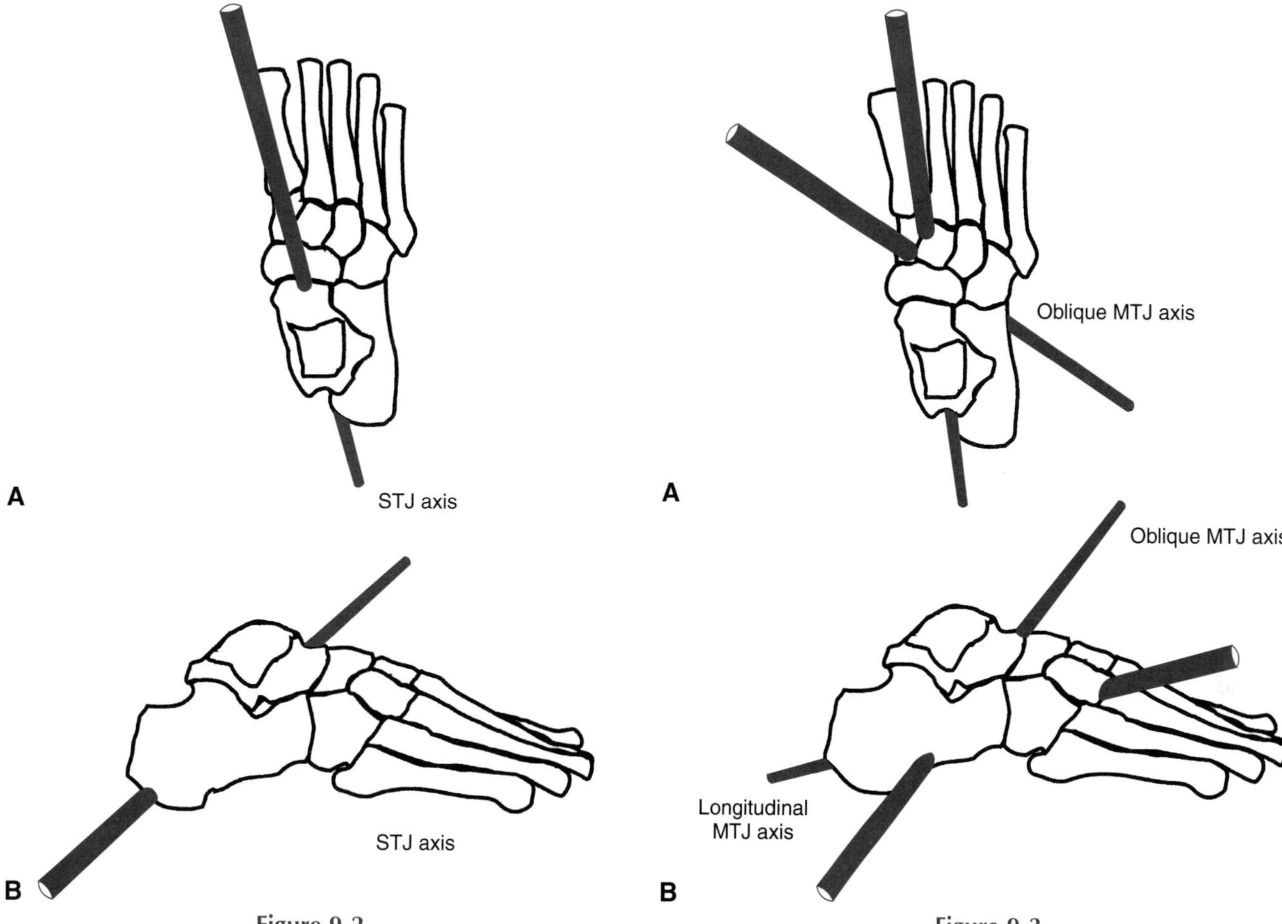

Figure 9-2

*Superior (**A**) and lateral (**B**) views of the osseous structures in the rearfoot: the superior talus and inferior calcaneus. Also pictured is the triplanar axis of the subtalar joint. Note the inclination of the axis from all three cardinal planes of the body. (Courtesy Juan C. Garbalosa, University of Hartford, West Hartford, Conn.)*

Figure 9-3

*A superior (**A**) and lateral (**B**) view of the osseous components of the midtarsal joint (MTJ). The anterior portion of the MTJ is composed of the navicular and cuboid bones, whereas the posterior portion is composed of the calcaneus and talus. The two axes of the MTJ, the oblique and longitudinal axes, are also depicted. Like the STJ, both axes of the MTJ are triplanar. (Courtesy Juan C. Garbalosa, University of Hartford, West Hartford, Conn.)*

Because the MTJ is a composite joint, motion occurs about two separate triplanar joint axes: a longitudinal and an oblique axis (Figure 9-3). Movement of the forefoot about each joint axis can occur independently of the other. Manter[17] reported that the longitudinal axis is inclined superiorly 15 degrees from the transverse plane and medially 9 degrees from the sagittal plane, whereas the oblique axis is pitched superiorly 52 degrees from the transverse plane and medially 57 degrees from the sagittal plane. The predominant motion about the longitudinal axis is frontal plane inversion and eversion. Because of the slight deviation of the longitudinal axis from the three cardinal planes, small amounts of forefoot plantar flexion and dorsiflexion and adduction and abduction occur during inversion and eversion. Plantar flexion and dorsiflexion and abduction and adduction are the predominant movements around the oblique MTJ axis, with little concomitant inversion and eversion.[5,15]

These two joint axes produce the combined motion of supination and pronation of the MTJ. During supination and pronation, the forefoot inverts and everts about the longitudinal axis. The motion around the oblique axis is plantar flexion with adduction and dorsiflexion with abduction. The amount of motion possible at these MTJ axes is determined by the position of the STJ. In STJ supination, the two joint axes are nearly perpendicular so that MTJ mobility is restricted. This mechanism helps convert the forefoot into a rigid structure for propulsion during the push-off phase of gait (from heel rise through toe-off).[17,23] When the STJ is pronated the joint axes are more parallel, allowing a greater degree of MTJ mobility.

Forefoot

The forefoot includes all structures distal to the navicular and cuboid bones; it is subdivided into five rays and toes.

The first through third rays consist of a cuneiform and its associated metatarsal bone; the fourth and fifth rays consist only of a metatarsal. The tarsometatarsal joints, the primary joints of the ray complexes, have two opposing planar surfaces.[5,22] The hallux, or first toe, has two bones (a proximal and distal phalanx) and two corresponding joints (metatarsophalangeal [MTP] and interphalangeal [IP]). The lesser toes have three bones (proximal, middle, and distal phalanges) and three associated joints. The proximal articular surfaces of the MTP and IP joints are convex, and the distal articular surface is concave.[5] Numerous soft tissue structures support these joints.[24,25]

Although each ray has its own axis of motion, the first and fifth rays are of particular interest. The triplanar axes of rotation of these two joints are nearly perpendicular. The axis of the first ray is pitched at a 45-degree angle from the sagittal and frontal planes; the primary motions possible are plantar flexion with eversion and dorsiflexion with inversion. Because the axis of the first ray is minimally pitched from the transverse plane, insignificant transverse motion occurs.[5] In contrast, the axis of rotation of the fifth ray is oriented at a 20-degree angle from the transverse plane and a 35-degree angle from the sagittal plane. The resulting motions combine inversion with plantar flexion and eversion with dorsiflexion. Less motion is present about the axis of rotation of the fifth ray than of the first ray.[5] MTP joints have two separate axes of rotation: the vertical axis (abduction and adduction) and the transverse axis (plantar flexion and dorsiflexion).[5,8,22] Little frontal plane motion at MTP joints is normal; frontal plane motion leads to subluxation.[5]

Plantar Fascia and Arches of the Foot

The plantar aponeurosis, one of the most functionally important soft tissue structures of the foot, is a sheath of fascia spanning most of the foot's plantar surface. Arising from the medial process of the calcanean tuberosity, it passes distally along the plantar aspect of the foot, then divides into five slips for its distal attachment at the base of the proximal phalanges by the plantar pads.[26] This fascial sheath plays an extremely important role in providing the stability needed by the foot during the toe-off phase of stance during gait and in supporting the longitudinal arch of the foot.

The medial longitudinal and transverse arches are formed by the ligamentous and osseous structures of a "normal" foot.[27] The medial longitudinal arch (MLA) extends from the calcaneus (posterior) to the first metatarsal head (anterior) and is supported by the plantar aponeurosis, short and long plantar ligaments, and the spring ligament. During weight bearing the height of the arch is reduced as the supporting ligamentous structures are elongated. The transverse arch reaches across the foot from medial to lateral borders. The height of the arch varies along the length of the foot: Its maximum height occurs at the cuboid-cuneiform bones of the midfoot, and its lowest point is at the metatarsal heads.

FUNCTION OF THE FOOT IN GAIT

The foot and ankle complex has three major functions in the gait cycle: attenuating the impact forces, maintaining equilibrium, and transmitting propulsive forces. For optimal biomechanical and energy-efficient performance, the joints of the foot and ankle must work in harmony. In early stance, the foot-ankle complex absorbs energy generated at initial contact and decreases forces transmitted to proximal structures during loading. The foot and ankle must also adapt to surface conditions encountered by the foot as stance begins. In late stance, the foot and lower leg transmit propulsive forces generated by muscles of the lower extremity onto the ground. The ability of the foot and lower leg to accomplish these functions depends on the integrity of the various structures of the foot. Gait abnormalities occur when the foot and ankle complex is unable to compensate for deficits in motion or structure.

The kinematic, kinetic, and neuromuscular events of the normal human gait cycle have been described in many ways.[5,28,29] Most focus on five distinct events: initial contact (IC) or heel strike, loading response (LR) or foot flat, midstance (MSt), terminal stance (TSt) or heel off, and preswing (PSw) or toe off. See Chapter 3 for a more detailed description of the gait cycle.

Shock Absorption

Musculoskeletal structures of the lower limb act from IC to MSt to attenuate impact forces.[5,28,30] Force plate recording of ground reaction forces (GRFs) estimates the foot's ability to absorb energy and decelerate the lower leg. The push of the foot against the floor creates a GRF with three components: vertical, medial and lateral, and fore and aft forces. The vertical component of a typical GRF record has a bimodal shape (Figure 9-4). The brief first peak results from the impact of the heel with the ground. Some of the vertical GRF is attributed to acceleration of the centers of mass of the foot and shank of the leg.

In early stance, from IC to LR, the STJ moves into pronation as the TCJ is plantarflexing.[5,28,31,32] The fibula and tibia internally rotate with respect to the foot.[20,21] Pronation of the STJ is controlled by eccentric contraction of the tibialis anterior, posterior tibialis, flexor hallucis longus, and flexor digitorum longus muscles.[5,28,33] Plantar flexion of the foot is controlled primarily by eccentric action of the tibialis anterior.[5,32] The combined muscle activity decelerates plantar flexion and pronation motion of the TCJ, STJ, and MTJ, slowing vertical and anterior movement of the center of mass of the foot and shank and decreasing impact forces encountered at IC.

The viscoelastic plantar fat pad absorbs some of the energy generated between IC and LR.[34] Pronation of the STJ flattens the arches of the foot, elongating plantar connective tissue structures. Because these tissues are viscoelastic, they also absorb some of the energy generated from IC to LR.

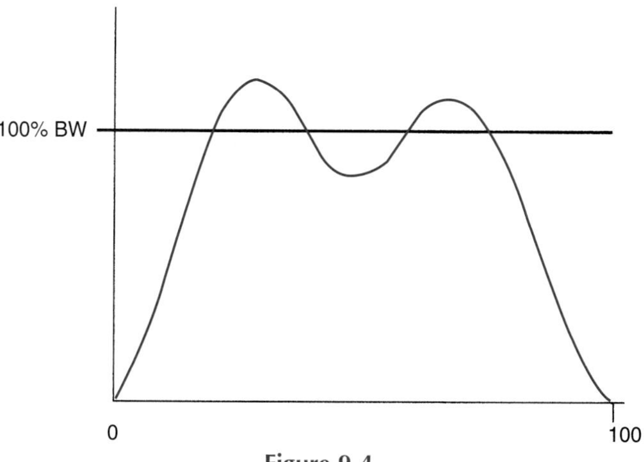

Figure 9-4
Typical vertical ground reaction pattern during walking. Note the bimodal shape of the ground reaction force. The first peak occurs at initial contact, and the second peak occurs during the toe-off phase of gait. The recorded ground reaction force represents the whole body center of mass acceleration. BW, *Body weight. (From Valiant GA. Transmission and attenuation of heelstrike accelerations. In Cavanagh PR (ed),* Biomechanics of Distance Running, *Champaign, Ill: Human Kinetics, 1990. pp. 225-249.)*

Adaptation to Surfaces

In everyday walking, the foot must be able to adapt quickly to many types of terrains and uneven surfaces. The key contributor to surface adaptation is STJ pronation, which unlocks the MTJ, permitting the joints of the foot to function in loose-packed positions and enabling the osseous elements to shift their relative positions.

At IC, the forefoot is in a supinatory twist (inverted) about the longitudinal MTJ axis. Eccentric action of the anterior tibialis decelerates plantar flexion of the forefoot, lowering it to the ground. The MTJ becomes fully supinated at LR, as a result of eversion of the STJ and GRFs acting upward on the foot's medial border. Contraction of the extensor digitorum longus and peroneus tertius abducts and dorsiflexes (pronates) the forefoot, locking it about the oblique MTJ axis and preparing the forefoot to receive the loading forces encountered at MSt.[5]

Propulsion

During MSt (LR to PSw), the STJ is maximally pronated and begins to resupinate. At this time, the GRF maintains the MTJ in a pronated position about its oblique axis. At the same time, a pronatory twist is initiated at the longitudinal axis by concentric action of the peroneals. The MTJ locks in a fully pronated position around the longitudinal axis just before heel rise, as the STJ reaches its neutral position. The MTJ must remain locked in this position throughout propulsion, as the peroneals contract to lift the lateral side of the foot from the ground and transfer weight medially to the other foot. As the heel is raised from the ground, the rearfoot continues to supinate (talus abducts and dorsiflexes) as the lower limb rotates externally. This coupled motion necessitates supination of the MTJ about the oblique axis to maximize joint stability and convert the foot into a rigid lever for propulsion.

Supination of the STJ occurs with concentric action of the tibialis posterior, flexor hallucis longus, and flexor digitorum longus and soleus, as well as the antagonistic functioning of the peroneus brevis.[5,28] The concentric activity of the gastrocnemius and soleus muscles causes vertical acceleration of the foot and lower leg. Propulsive forces generated by the foot and lower leg are transmitted to the floor.[5,28,32] The second peak of a GRF curve corresponds to propulsion in late stance phase (see Figure 9-4).

Supination of the STJ and locking of the MTJ about the longitudinal axis place the foot in a closed-packed position, transforming the foot into a rigid lever.[5,10,20,28] This transformation is aided by the action of the plantar aponeurosis as it wraps around the metatarsal heads. During TSt, the MTP joints extend (dorsiflex), creating a "windlass effect." This action compresses joints of the midfoot and forefoot, facilitating the transition from flexibility to rigidity required for effective push-off.[10,15,20,26,27]

BIOMECHANICAL EXAMINATION

The biomechanical examination of the foot and ankle has three components: a non–weight-bearing assessment, a static weight-bearing assessment, and a dynamic gait analysis (Figure 9-5). Five common intrinsic foot deformities are identified in the biomechanical examination: rearfoot varus, forefoot varus, forefoot valgus, equinus deformity, and plantar flexed first ray.

The theoretical model of biomechanical foot and ankle examination is based on the work of Root and colleagues.[5] Debate continues about the validity of Root's criteria for normalcy and the assumption that the STJ is in neutral position from MSt to TSt of the gait cycle. Reliability of the measurement techniques used to determine STJ neutral position has also been questioned.[35-37] Although controversial, Root's theory and his biomechanical evaluation and treatment techniques are used by many clinicians.

Root describes deviations from normal foot alignment as "intrinsic" foot deformities, which can lead to aberrant lower extremity function and musculoskeletal pathological conditions.[5,38] To prescribe an appropriate biomechanical foot orthosis, the source of the pathological condition or deformity must be determined by a detailed patient history and a comprehensive biomechanical examination.[39] This helps the clinician identify resultant pathomechanical abnormalities and determine the benefits of orthotic intervention.

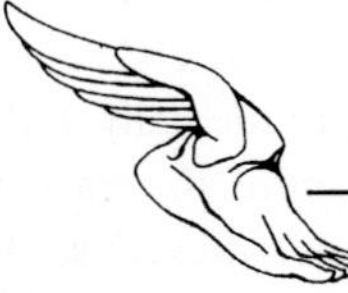

STRIDE, Inc.

Physical Therapy and Pedorthic Services
530 Middlebury Road • Suite 102 • Middlebury, CT 06762
TEL.: (203) 598-0070 • FAX: (203) 598-0075

BIOMECHANICAL FOOT EVALUATION

Patient: ______________________ Phone: __________

Address: ______________________

Age: ________ Height: ________ Weight: ________ Shoe size: ________ Shoe Style: ______

Occupation: __________ Activity level: ________ Sports: __________

Referring Practitioner: ______________________ Date of Evaluation: ________

Diagnosis: ______________________

I. NON-WEIGHTBEARING EVALUATION

	Left	Right
Rearfoot:		
STN position	________ varus	________ varus
calcaneal inversion	________ degrees	________ degrees
calcaneal eversion	________ degrees	________ degrees
rearfoot dorsiflexion	________ degrees	________ degrees
Forefoot:		
STN position	________ varus/valgus	________ varus/valgus
locking mechanism	poor — fair — normal — rigid	poor — fair — normal — rigid
MTJ dorsiflexion	________ degrees	________ degrees
First Ray:		
STN position and mobility		
hallux dorsiflexion	________ degrees	________ degrees
Arch Position:	low — med — high	low — med — high
Toe Position/Deformities:	________	________

Lesions/Shoe Wear:

R L

L R

Calluses:

L R

Figure 9-5

Biomechanical examination form outlining components of the non–weight-bearing and weight-bearing assessment. Ante, *Femoral anteversion;* ASIS, *anterior superior iliac spine;* DLS, *double-limb stance;* Gastroc, *gastrocnemius;* G.T., *greater trochanter;* ITB, *iliotibial band;* M.M., *medial malleolus;* PSIS, *posterior inferior iliac spine;* Retro, *femoral retroversion;* SLS, *single-limb stance;* T.T., *tibial tubercle;* VAR, *varus;* VAL, *valgus. (Courtesy Stride, Inc., Middlebury, Conn.)*

II. Weightbearing Evaluation

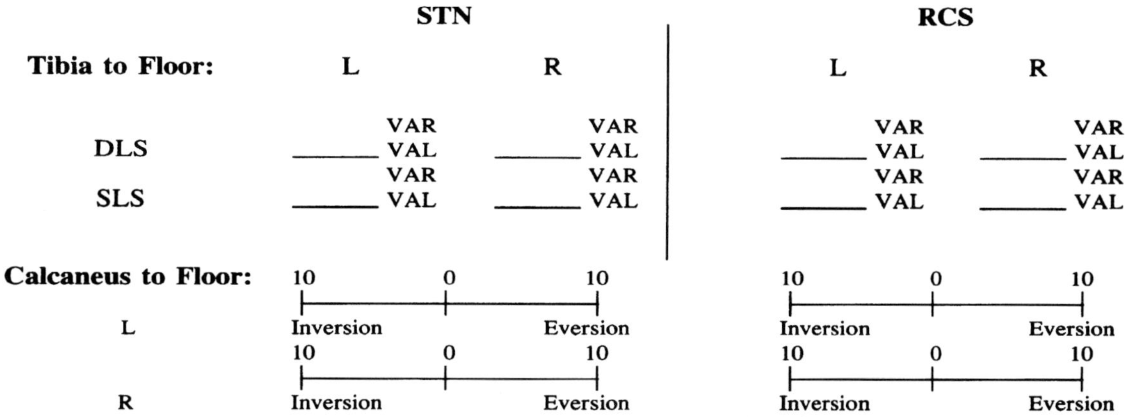

	STN		RCS	
Tibia to Floor:	L	R	L	R
DLS	______ VAR / VAL	______ VAR / VAL	______ VAR / VAL	______ VAR / VAL
SLS	______ VAR / VAL	______ VAR / VAL	______ VAR / VAL	______ VAR / VAL

Calcaneus to Floor:

	STN	RCS
L	10 (Inversion) — 0 — 10 (Eversion)	10 (Inversion) — 0 — 10 (Eversion)
R	10 (Inversion) — 0 — 10 (Eversion)	10 (Inversion) — 0 — 10 (Eversion)

III. Soft Tissue Restrictions

	L	R
Iliopsoas	______	______
Rectus Femoris	______	______
ITB	______	______
Hamstring	______	______
Gastroc	______	______
Soleus	______	______

	L	R
Hip Rotation (Hips 90°, Knees 90°)		
Internal	______	______
External	______	______
Hip Rotation (Hips 0°, Knees 90°)		
Internal	______	______
External	______	______

IV. Postural Observations

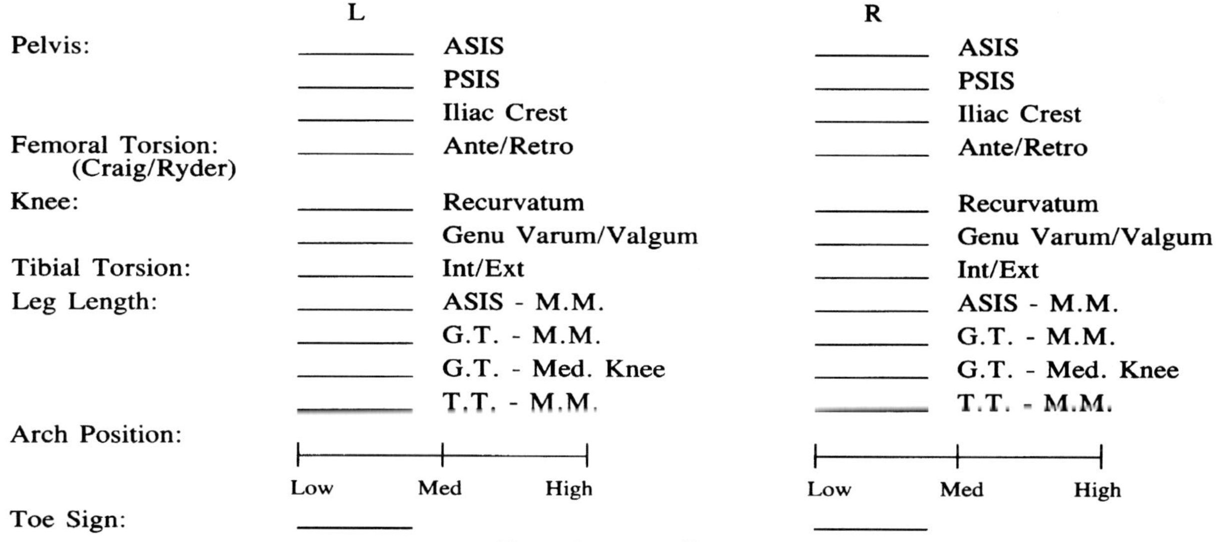

	L		R	
Pelvis:	______	ASIS	______	ASIS
	______	PSIS	______	PSIS
	______	Iliac Crest	______	Iliac Crest
Femoral Torsion: (Craig/Ryder)	______	Ante/Retro	______	Ante/Retro
Knee:	______	Recurvatum	______	Recurvatum
	______	Genu Varum/Valgum	______	Genu Varum/Valgum
Tibial Torsion:	______	Int/Ext	______	Int/Ext
Leg Length:	______	ASIS - M.M.	______	ASIS - M.M.
	______	G.T. - M.M.	______	G.T. - M.M.
	______	G.T. - Med. Knee	______	G.T. - Med. Knee
	______	T.T. - M.M.	______	T.T. - M.M.
Arch Position:	Low — Med — High		Low — Med — High	
Toe Sign:	______		______	

Figure 9-5—cont'd

Biomechanical examination form outlining components of the weight-bearing assessment.

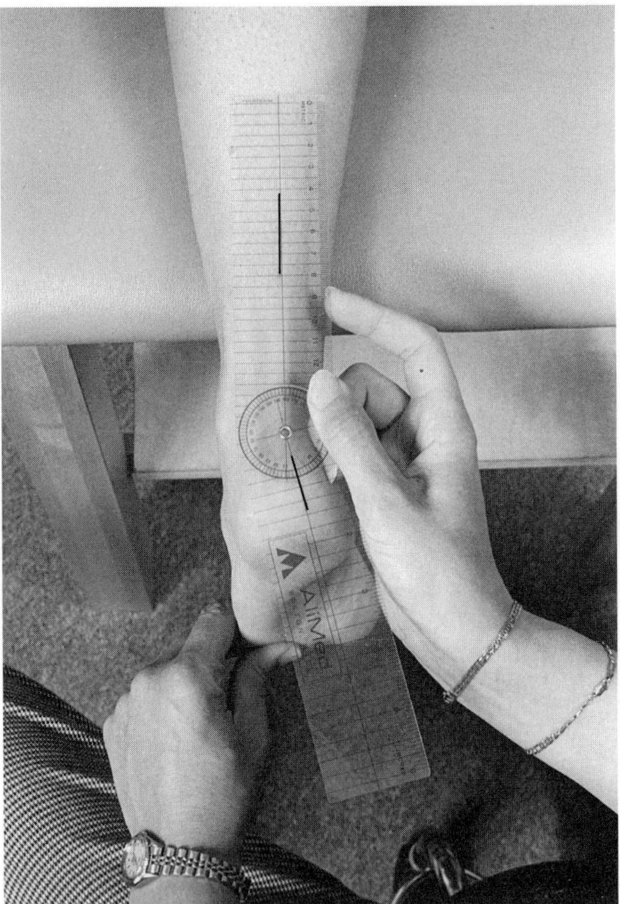

Figure 9-6
Non–weight-bearing goniometric technique. A loading force applied by the examiner over the fourth and fifth metatarsal heads locks the forefoot on the rearfoot while the examiner's opposite hand operates the goniometer to measure subtalar neutral position and calcaneal range of motion. The examiner is seated at the distal end of the treatment table, with chair height adjusted to position the patient's foot at chest level.

NON–WEIGHT-BEARING, OPEN CHAIN EXAMINATION

During the non–weight-bearing, open chain examination, the basic architecture of the foot and ankle is assessed. Any bony deformities or prominence of the joints, rays (toes), and callosities are noted. The examiner uses a goniometer to locate the subtalar neutral (STN) position and identify any intrinsic foot deformities.

The non–weight-bearing goniometric examination is performed with the patient in the prone position, with the targeted lower extremity positioned with extended knee, and the foot 6 to 8 inches off the treatment table. Placing the contralateral lower extremity in a figure-of-four position orients the ipsilateral lower extremity in the frontal plane, reducing the influence of proximal rotational limb disorders on measurement.[40]

Examination of the Rearfoot

Goniometric measurements of the non–weight-bearing examination assess the rearfoot with respect to STN position, as well as STJ mobility, based on calcaneal positioning in the frontal plane. Calcaneal frontal plane motion is the most readily examined component of triplanar STJ motion. To perform the examination, the stationary arm of a goniometer is aligned with an imagined bisection of the lower third of the limb (tibiofibular complex), the mobile arm is aligned with an imaginary bisection of the posterior surface of the calcaneus, and the axis of the goniometer is aligned at the STJ axis, just above the superior border of the calcaneus but beneath the level of the medial and lateral malleoli (Figure 9-6).[40,41]

Subtalar Neutral Position

STN position can be manually estimated by palpation or by using a mathematical model developed by Root. If using palpation, the examiner identifies the anteromedial and anterolateral aspects of the talar head with the thumb and index fingers of the hand closest to the patient's midline, placing the thumb just proximal to the navicular tuberosity, approximately 1 inch below and 1 inch distal to the medial malleolus (Figure 9-7). In STJ pronation, the anteromedial talar head is most prominent beneath the thumb, and an anterolateral sulcus (the sinus tarsi) is apparent. The index finger is placed in this sulcus, where the talar head is found to protrude when the foot is fully supinated. The thumb and index finger of the other hand grasp the fourth and fifth metatarsal heads, moving the foot in an arc of adduction and inversion (supination) and abduction and eversion (pronation). STN is the point where the talar head is equally prominent anteromedially and anterolaterally.[38,40,41] The examiner then "loads" the foot by applying a dorsally directed pressure against the fourth and fifth metatarsal heads until slight resistance is felt. The loading procedure locks the MTJ against the rearfoot, mimicking GRFs of MSt.[5,42] The angular relation between the bisection of the calcaneus and the bisection of the lower third of the leg is measured with a goniometer (see Figure 9-6), recorded on the evaluation form as rearfoot STN position.

Root's mathematical model for determining STN position uses a quantitative goniometric formula.[5,38] First, end ROM calcaneal inversion and eversion are determined by goniometric measurement. Total calcaneal ROM is the sum of the inversion and eversion values. The STN position is determined as the calcaneus is moved into inversion at one third of the total calcaneal ROM. If end-range calcaneal inversion is 25 degrees and end-range calcaneal eversion is +5 degrees, total calcaneal ROM would be 30 degrees. STN position is calculated to be at 5 degrees calcaneal inversion, one third of the distance from its fully everted position.

Reliability and clinical validity of both models have been debated.[37,38,40,43-45] Diamond and colleagues[46] reported that although acceptable reliability is possible, it is influenced by examiner experience. Palpation to determine STN position is efficient in terms of time but requires more advanced manual skills and experience than the mathematical model. The mathematical model may be more reliable for the entry-level practitioner.

Calcaneal Range of Motion

Calcaneal inversion and eversion occur primarily at the STJ, with lesser contributions from the TCJ. Calcaneal ROM is assessed with the patient in the prone position with the same anatomical landmarks and lines of bisection as for STN assessment. The examiner grasps the calcaneus in one hand, fully inverts it in the frontal plane until end ROM is achieved, and then takes a goniometric measurement.[45] The procedure is repeated for calcaneal eversion. The TCJ must be maintained in a neutral to slightly dorsiflexed position while measuring to lock it in a closed-packed position and better isolate STJ motion.[47] Normative values of 20 degrees for calcaneal inversion and 10 degrees beyond vertical for eversion have been reported.[5]

Because values of calcaneal eversion are larger when assessed in a full weight-bearing position, some clinicians suggest that this position is more clinically valid.[35,45] Assessment of calcaneal eversion in the weight-bearing position represents a total "functional" pronation and eversion that is the summation of motion occurring at the STJ and compensatory motion occurring extrinsic to the STJ (e.g., TCJ, MTJ). Passive assessment of calcaneal eversion in non–weight bearing remains the most accurate method to determine the degree of composite pronation acquired from the STJ itself.

Talocrural Joint Range of Motion

In normal walking, the TCJ is maximally dorsiflexed just before heel rise, when the knee is fully extended and the STJ is in a nearly neutral position.[5,48] When and whether an actual STN position ever occurs during gait is disputed.[35] The use of a standard position of knee extension and STN, however, offers a consistent point of reference when assessing TCJ dorsiflexion. According to most sources, a minimum of 10 degrees TCJ dorsiflexion is required for normal gait; anything less is classified as an equinus deformity.[5,48-51] A minimum of 20 degrees of plantar flexion is also required for normal gait.[5]

Ankle dorsiflexion is measured in a non–weight-bearing position with the STJ held in the neutral position and the knee extended. The examiner forcefully dorsiflexes the ankle with active assistance from the patient. Active assistance encourages reciprocal inhibition of the calf muscle group and is essential for accurate measurement.[48] The proximal arm of the goniometer is positioned along the lateral aspect of the fibula, the distal arm along the lateral border of the fifth metatarsal, and the axis distal to the lateral malleolus.[53] An alternative placement of the distal arm of the goniometer

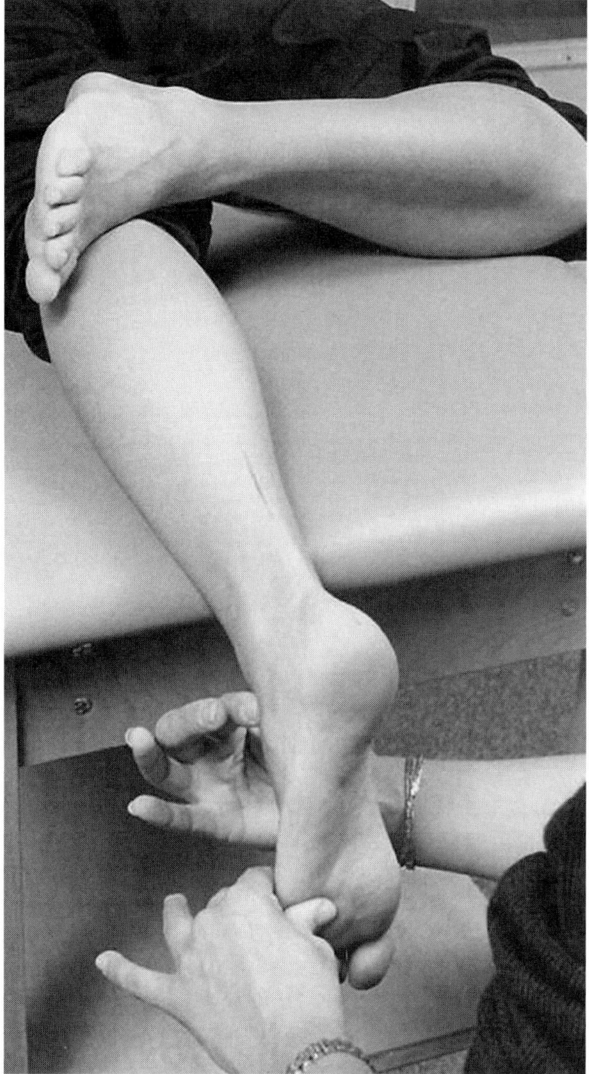

Figure 9-7
To determine subtalar neutral position, the examiner moves the forefoot slowly between supination and pronation until the anteromedial and anterolateral surfaces of the head of the talus are equally prominent.

along the inferolateral border of the calcaneus may more effectively isolate true TCJ dorsiflexion (Figure 9-8). This value is recorded as rearfoot dorsiflexion. Forefoot dorsiflexion is measured by repositioning the distal arm along the lateral aspect of the fifth metatarsal. This method allows the examiner to identify contributions or restrictions in sagittal plane motion from the oblique axis of the MTJ.

If ankle dorsiflexion is less than 10 degrees when measured with the knee extended, remeasurement with the knee flexed may rule out soft tissue restriction of the gastrocnemius-soleus complex.[5,48] If dorsiflexion values are consistent in both positions, the limitation is likely a result of osseous equinus formation of the ankle.

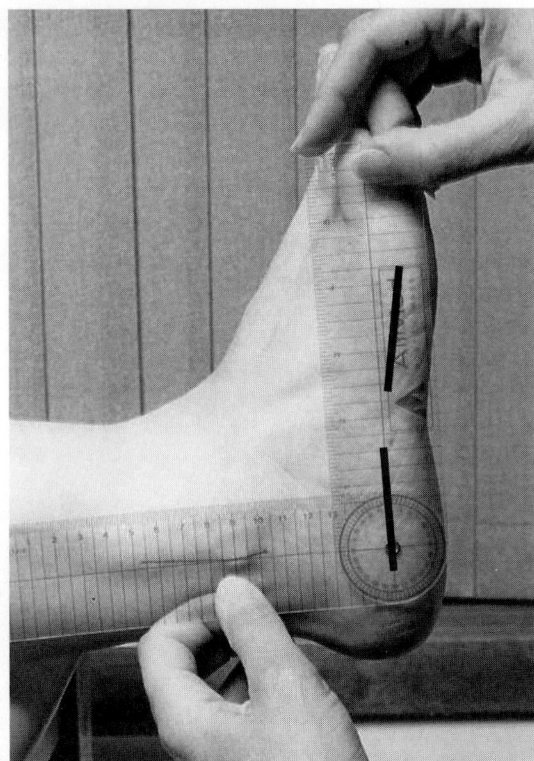

Figure 9-8
Alignment of the distal arm of the goniometer along the inferior-lateral border of the calcaneus may provide a more accurate measure of talocrural joint dorsiflexion than the traditional alignment along the shaft of the fifth metatarsal used to measure overall ankle dorsiflexion.

During gait, ankle dorsiflexion occurs in a closed kinetic chain as the tibia and fibula rotate forward over a fixed foot. On the basis of this, some have suggested that assessing ankle dorsiflexion may be more accurate with the patient in a weight-bearing position.[35,49] The weight-bearing technique measures the angle between the tibia and the floor as the patient leans forward with the foot flat on the floor. Unwanted compensations are often difficult to control during weight bearing and may mask true TCJ limitations. The non–weight-bearing technique allows the examiner to assess end feel and joint play, as well as mechanical blocks or joint laxity, providing additional information not accessible in the weight-bearing examination.

Rearfoot Deformities

Normal rearfoot position is one in which STN is 1 to 4 degrees of varus.[36,37,44,45] Values of more than 4 degrees are described as a *rearfoot varus deformity*. This deformity may be the result of ontogenetic failure of the calcaneus to derotate sufficiently during early childhood development.[5,42,54] Because this deformity is a torsional structural malalignment of the calcaneus, not a joint-related problem, the TCJ and STJ lines remain congruent when observed in the non–weight-bearing STN position. As a structural deformity, it cannot be corrected or reduced by joint mobilization or a strengthening program. Instead, it is managed with a functional foot orthosis that partially supports the calcaneus in its inverted alignment while preventing excessive STJ pronation.

Assessment of calcaneal ROM predicts quality of motion and the integrity of the STJ. Measuring calcaneal motion into eversion allows the examiner to determine whether a rearfoot deformity is compensated or uncompensated (Figure 9-9).

In a *compensated* rearfoot varus deformity, the calcaneus fully everts to vertical or beyond in weight bearing because the STJ possesses an adequate amount of pronatory motion to compensate for the deformity. A compensated rearfoot varus deformity of 10 degrees (STN position) requires that the STJ pronate or evert at least 10 degrees to enable the medial condyle of the calcaneus to achieve ground contact in weight bearing. Such excessive pronatory motion causes medial gapping and lateral constriction at the STJ line and a medial bulge of the talus as it moves into adduction and plantar flexion.

In an *uncompensated* rearfoot varus deformity, the calcaneus remains fixed in its inverted STN position with no eversion motion at the STJ. A *partially compensated* rearfoot varus deformity allows for partial STJ eversion so that the medial condyle of the calcaneus does not make complete contact with the ground on weight bearing. Alternative compensatory motion, extrinsic to the STJ, is necessary to achieve weight bearing on the medial aspect of the foot. One of the common compensations is an acquired soft tissue (valgus) deformity of the forefoot caused by a plantar flexed first ray. Other sources of compensatory motion can occur at the MTJ or proximally at the knee, hip, or sacroiliac joints.

An *equinus deformity* occurs when fewer than 10 degrees of ankle dorsiflexion are available as a result of osseous or muscular problems.[49,51,55,56] Clubfoot (talipes equinovarus) is a congenital osseous deformity that includes varus deformity of both rearfoot and forefoot, rearfoot equinus, and an inverted and adducted forefoot.[57,58] The angular relation between the body and the head and neck of the talus is decreased, and the navicular is shifted medially. Muscular forms of equinus include congenital or acquired soft tissue shortening or muscle spasm.[51] Tissue contracture or shortening occurs in both contractile tissues (gastrocnemius, soleus, and plantaris) and noncontractile tissues (teno Achilles and plantar fascia).[49,51]

Compensation for an equinus deformity occurs at the foot through pronation, perpetuating soft tissue contractures. The STJ is forced to pronate maximally to gain as much sagittal plane dorsiflexion as possible. Although foot pronation allows some dorsiflexion from the STJ, the amount is often inadequate. Pronation of the STJ unlocks the MTJ, creating an unstable midfoot while allowing further dorsiflexion and forefoot abduction from the oblique axis of the MTJ.[51] Other compensatory strategies for equinus deformity include knee flexion (especially in individuals with cerebral palsy), early heel rise, toe walking, shortened stride length of the contralateral lower limb, and toe-out walking.[28,38,51] Clinical consequences of long-term ankle equinus include many conditions normally associated with the excessively pronated foot: plantar fasciitis, heel spurs, bunions, and capsulitis.[51]

Examination of the Forefoot

Forefoot position is assessed with the STJ in neutral position. Because the first and fifth rays have independent axes of motion, forefoot orientation is defined by the planar relation of the second, third, and fourth rays to the bisection line of the calcaneus.

Neutral Forefoot Position

If the forefoot is properly balanced, the plane of the three central metatarsals is perpendicular to the bisection of the calcaneus when in STN (Figure 9-10). In a forefoot varus deformity, the forefoot is excessively supinated or inverted, whereas in a forefoot valgus the forefoot is excessively pronated or everted.

Mobility Testing: Locking Mechanism

To isolate STN position in the non–weight-bearing examination, the examiner attempts to lock the MTJ by applying a dorsally directed loading pressure with the thumb and index fingers over the fourth and fifth metatarsal heads of the patient's foot (see Figures 9-6 and 9-7). Loading force must be gently applied over the fourth and fifth metatarsal heads until tissue slack is taken up from the normally plantar flexed resting position of the ankle.[5,52] Overload of the forefoot leads to dorsiflexion and abduction of the foot, placing the forefoot in an excessively pronated position and giving a false valgus orientation.

Although many forefoot measurement devices are available, forefoot orientation can be accurately assessed with a standard goniometer.[44] To assess the forefoot to rearfoot relation, the proximal arm of the goniometer is aligned along the bisection of the calcaneus, with the axis just below its distal border. The distal arm is positioned in the plane of the three central metatarsal heads (Figure 9-11). The angular displacement is recorded on the evaluation form under STN position for the forefoot assessment (see Figure 9-5).

In normal walking, the MTJ locks as heel rise begins so that the foot is converted into a rigid lever for propulsion. This lock requires that the STJ be in the neutral position. Clinical assessment of MTJ mobility and the locking mechanism is an advanced manual skill. Observations made during weight-bearing assessment (e.g., toe sign, navicular drop test, talar bulge) provide an elementary method to identify an MTJ unable to lock.

An ineffective locking mechanism at the MTJ is often more clinically significant than the absolute degree of forefoot deformity. For example, a forefoot varus deformity of

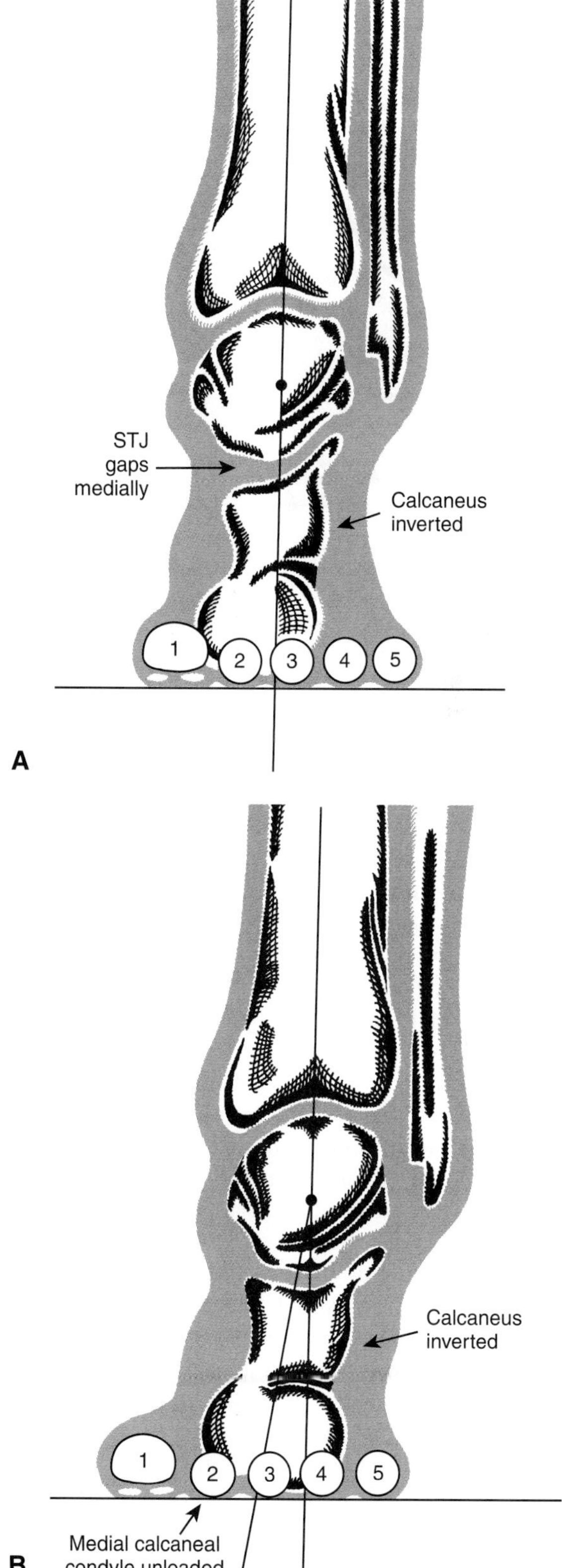

Figure 9-9

A, *In relaxed calcaneal stance, compensation for a rearfoot varus is normally subtalar joint pronation.* ***B,*** *In an uncompensated rearfoot varus, the subtalar joint cannot pronate and instead may develop compensatory midtarsal joint pronation about the longitudinal joint axis. (Courtesy Stride, Inc., Middlebury, Conn.)*

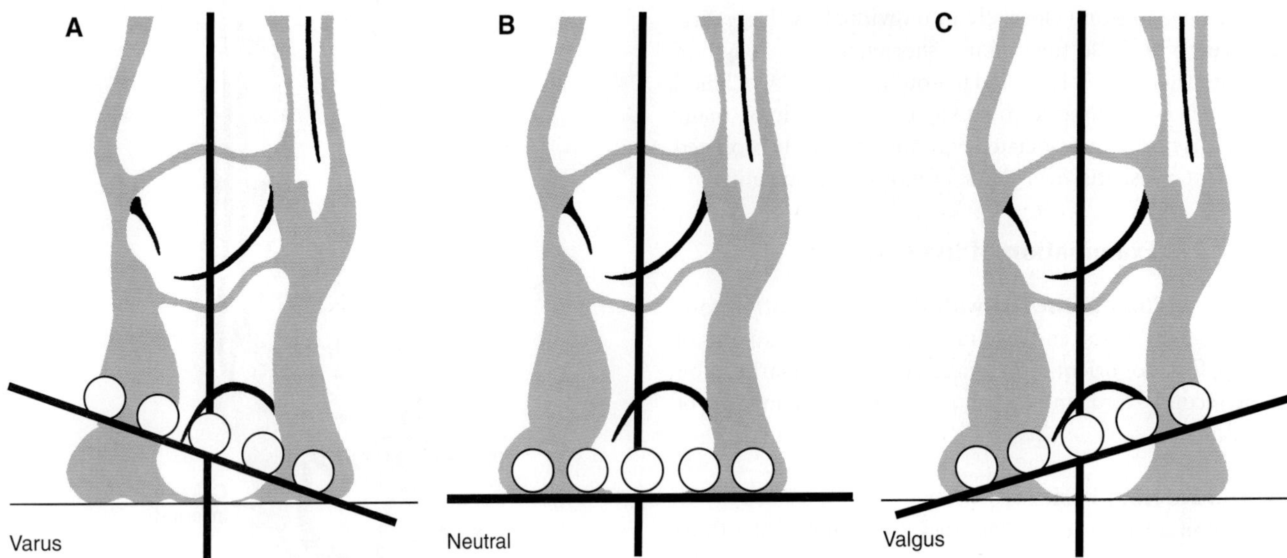

Figure 9-10
*In subtalar neutral position, the normal orientation of the forefoot to the calcaneus (**B**) is perpendicular. Excessive supination and inversion of the forefoot in subtalar neutral position indicates a forefoot varus (**A**), whereas excessive pronation and eversion of the forefoot indicates a forefoot valgus (**C**). (Courtesy Stride, Inc., Middlebury, Conn.)*

3 degrees with a poor MTJ locking mechanism may be symptomatic, whereas an 8-degree forefoot varus deformity with a normal MTJ locking mechanism may not be.

Identifying Forefoot Deformities

Although the prevalence of forefoot deformity, with or without symptoms, is well documented, less agreement exists regarding which types of deformity are most common.[44,59] If an individual has bilateral forefoot deformity, the deformities may not be of the same severity or type. MTJ deformities change the location of the lock of the forefoot against the rearfoot.[5] Although these osseous frontal plane deformities alter the direction of motion, they do not limit the total ROM of the MTJ.[5] In forefoot varus, locking of the forefoot occurs in an inverted position relative to the rearfoot.[5] Forefoot varus results from ontogenetic failure of the normal valgus rotation of the head and neck of the talus in relation to its body during early childhood development.[5,42,54]

Compensations for foot deformities are viewed in a relaxed weight-bearing position referred to as *relaxed calcaneal stance* (RCS). When excessive pronation of the STJ compensates for the deformity on weight bearing, the condition is called a *compensated forefoot varus* (Figure 9-12, *A*). When the STJ cannot adequately pronate to accommodate an inverted forefoot, an *uncompensated forefoot varus* is present.[5] The medial forefoot does not make contact with the ground, and the lateral forefoot is subjected to excessive pressure. Thick callus develops beneath the head of the fifth metatarsal, and the risk of stress fracture is increased. Plantar flexion of the first ray and pronation at the MTJ are common compensations that allow the medial forefoot to make contact with the ground (Figure 9-12, *B*). Persistent MTJ stress may lead to joint damage and excessive forefoot abduction and eversion.

Forefoot valgus occurs in the frontal plane deformity, locking the forefoot in eversion relative to the rearfoot.[5] Root suggests this deformity results from ontogenetic overrotation of the talar head and neck in relation to its body during early childhood development.[5,42,54] Forefoot valgus can be a rigid or flexible deformity. In rigid forefoot valgus, the compensatory weight-bearing mechanism occurs at the STJ as excessive supination or calcaneal inversion. It is a result of excessive premature GRFs at the first metatarsal head, causing rapid STJ inversion and increasing loading forces beneath the fifth metatarsal head. Thick callosities are often present beneath the first and fifth metatarsal heads. In contrast, flexible forefoot valgus is usually an acquired soft tissue condition. It most often occurs as a consequence of uncompensated rearfoot varus as an attempt to increase weight bearing along the medial foot. Because this deformity is flexible, no compensatory mechanism is necessary. Contact force beneath the first metatarsal head simply pushes it up out of the way, and the foot functions as if this condition were not present.

The First Ray

Assessment of first ray position is also carried out in STN position. Ideally, the first ray lies within the common transverse plane of the lesser metatarsal heads. To examine mobility of the first ray, the examiner holds the first metatarsal head between the thumb and index finger and performs a dorsal and plantar glide while stabilizing the lesser metatarsal heads with the other hand. Normally, first ray movement is at least one thumb width above and below the plane of the other metatarsal heads.[5]

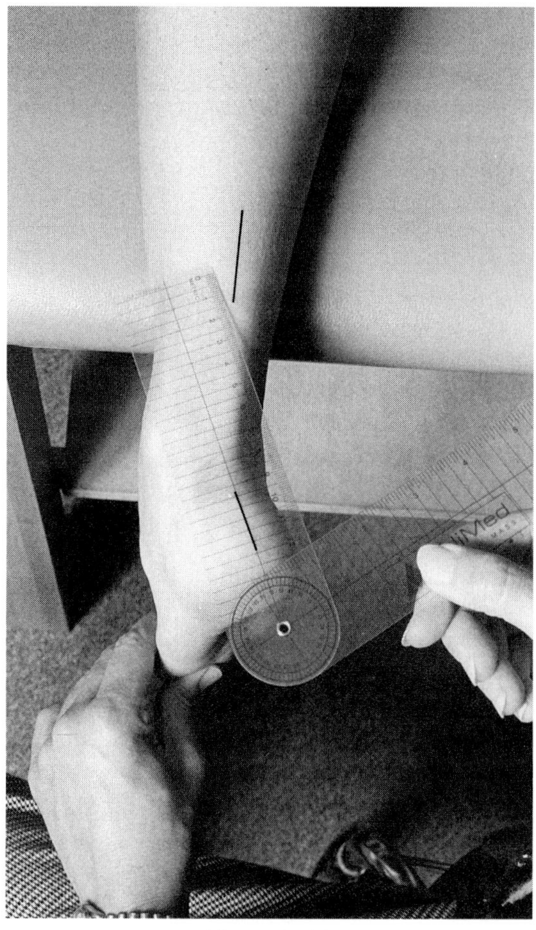

Figure 9-11
Measurement of forefoot orientation in subtalar neutral position with a standard goniometer. The proximal arm of the goniometer is aligned with the bisection of the posterior surface of the calcaneus, and the distal arm parallels the plane of the metatarsal heads. The axis lies beneath the distal aspect of the calcaneus.

As stance phase is completed, activity of the peroneus longus creates a pronatory twist of the forefoot, stabilizing the medial column of the foot on the ground, locking the MTJ about its longitudinal axis, and converting the foot to a rigid lever for propulsion. Adequate plantar flexion of the first ray must be present for conversion from flexible forefoot to a rigid lever. How much first ray plantar flexion must occur is determined by three factors: amount of inversion of the foot at propulsion, width of the foot, and length of the second metatarsal.[5] The more the foot inverts during propulsion, the further the first ray must plantarflex to make ground contact. Elevation of the medial forefoot is related to foot width; wide feet require more first ray plantar flexion. An excessively long second metatarsal also increases the distance that the first ray must plantarflex to make ground contact.

In some instances, the first ray is inappropriately dorsiflexed above the plane of the other metatarsals, resulting in

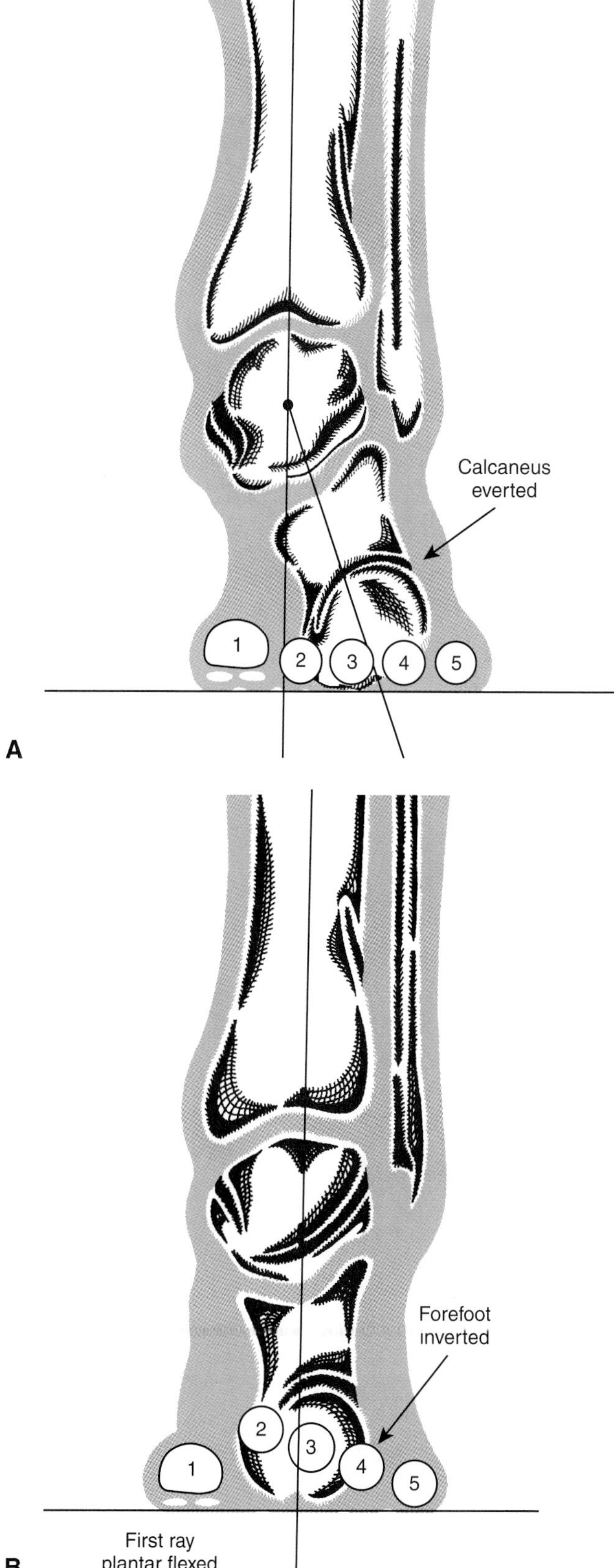

Figure 9-12
***A,** In relaxed calcaneal stance, compensation for a forefoot varus deformity is normally subtalar joint pronation, resulting in an everted calcaneus. **B,** In an uncompensated forefoot varus, the subtalar joint is unable to compensate. Instead, the first ray plantarflexes to achieve weight bearing medially on the foot. (Courtesy Stride, Inc., Middlebury, Conn.)*

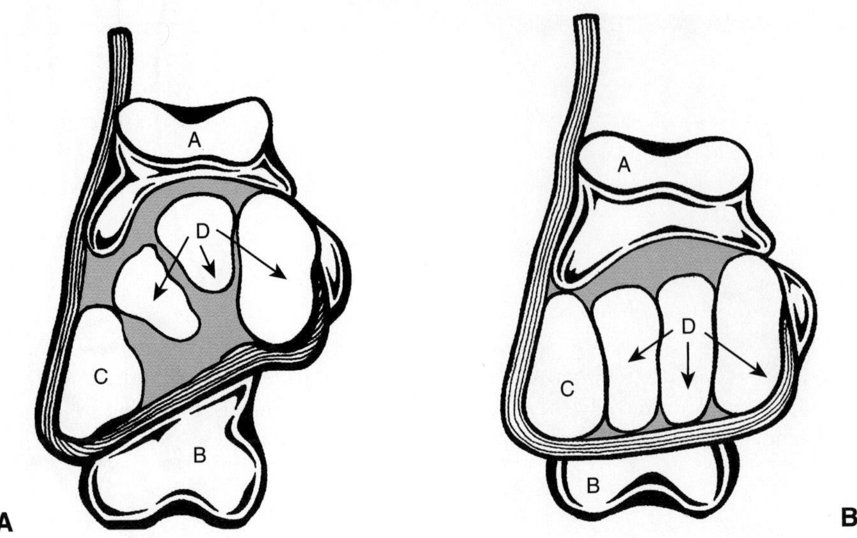

Figure 9-13

***A,** Cuboid pulley mechanism in a normal foot. **B,** In an abnormally pronated foot, the mechanical advantage of the peroneals is impaired.* A, *Talus;* B, *calcaneus;* C, *cuboid;* D, *the cuneiforms. (Courtesy Stride, Inc., Middlebury, Conn.)*

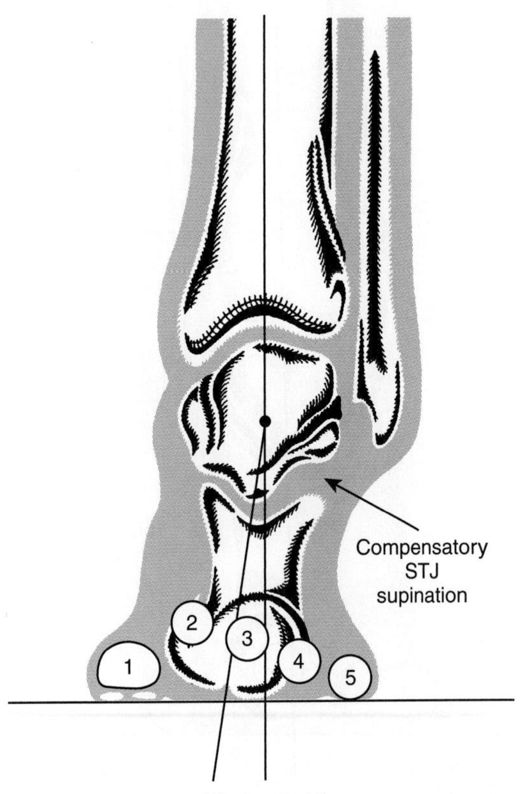

Figure 9-14

Plantarflexed first ray deformity in relaxed calcaneal stance. Compensation occurs at the subtalar joint, with lateral gapping and medial compression. (Courtesy Stride, Inc., Middlebury, Conn.)

restriction of plantar flexion and impeding normal propulsion. The first ray may also be plantar flexed below the plane of the other metatarsals. In uncompensated rearfoot varus, for example, the eversion motion of the calcaneus is insufficient, the medial condyle fails to make contact with the ground, and excessive weight bearing is present on the lateral border of the foot. The peroneus longus contracts to pull the first metatarsal head toward the ground in an attempt to load the medial side of the foot. This action is possible because of the cuboid pulley system (Figure 9-13).[5] When the STJ remains abnormally pronated in late stance phase, orientation of the cuboid tunnel is altered and the mechanical advantage of the peroneus longus is lost. The MTJ cannot lock, and the foot is unstable throughout propulsion.

The presence of a rigid plantar flexed first ray sometimes results in a functional forefoot valgus (Figure 9-14). The compensatory mechanism for this condition is similar to that for rigid forefoot valgus: STJ supination or calcaneal inversion on weight bearing to lower the lateral aspect of the foot to the ground.

The Hallux

In normal gait, dorsiflexion of the hallux occurs during the late propulsive phase as the body moves forward over the foot. Sagittal plane motion of the hallux is assessed as passive ROM. The stabile arm of the goniometer is positioned along the medial first metatarsal and the mobile arm along the medial proximal phalanx of the hallux. The axis is medial to the first MTP joint.[53] Sufficient force is applied to bring the hallux to its end ROM. Normal range of hallux dorsiflexion is between 70 and 90 degrees.[5,53]

In *hallux limitus* deformity, pathomechanical functioning of the first MTP joint prevents the hallux from moving through its full range of dorsiflexion during propulsion.

Repetitive trauma to the first MTP joint can lead to ankylosis, or *hallux rigidus*. Functional hallux limitus is a condition in which full first MTP ROM is present when non–weight bearing, but a functional restriction of hallux dorsiflexion occurs during gait. Functional hallux limitus disrupts the normal windlass mechanism previously described.[60,61]

Limitation of hallux dorsiflexion prohibits the normal progression of the foot and interferes with propulsion of the body over the hallux. Several gait compensations can overcome this limitation.[60,61] An abducted or toe-out gait pattern shifts propulsion to the medial border of the hallux. A pinched callus then develops from friction between the hallux and shoe during propulsion. Alternatively, the IP joint of the hallux may hyperextend, causing a callus in the sulcus of the IP joint.

Hallux abductovalgus (HAV) is a progressive, acquired deformity of the first MTP joint that eventually results in a valgus subluxation of the hallux.[5,42] This deformity is caused by abnormal STJ pronation with hypermobility of the first ray.[5] A common misconception is that HAV is hereditary. Although the congenital osseous abnormalities that lead to aberrant STJ pronation are hereditary, HAV occurs to compensate for these other deformities. Another misconception is that HAV is caused by restrictive footwear. Although inappropriate or restrictive footwear can accentuate or speed the progression of HAV deformity when present, the deformity is frequently observed in populations that do not typically wear shoes.[5,42]

Additional Observations

Several other important observations are made as the non–weight-bearing examination is completed. Non–weight-bearing arch height is observed for later comparison to weight-bearing arch height as a composite estimate of foot pronation. Toes are inspected for positional deformities such as hammertoe, claw toe, crossover deformity, and the presence of bunions or bunionettes. The plantar foot is checked for callus, plantar warts, or other signs of excessive pressure. The shoes are inspected for excessive or uneven wear patterns.

STATIC WEIGHT-BEARING, CLOSED KINETIC CHAIN EXAMINATION

The open chain kinetic motion evaluated in the non–weight-bearing examination is dramatically different from the functional sequence of events in the closed kinetic chain of standing and walking. Open kinetic chain pronation (calcaneal dorsiflexion, eversion, and abduction) and supination (calcaneal plantar flexion, inversion, and adduction) are triplanar motions around the STJ.[5,8,26] During closed kinetic chain pronation, internal rotation of the leg is coupled with talar adduction and calcaneal plantar flexion and eversion. Closed kinetic chain supination couples external rotation of the leg with talar abduction and calcaneal dorsiflexion and inversion. In the open kinetic chain, movement is initiated in the distal segment (the foot). In the closed kinetic chain, motion is initiated proximally (at the tibia and talus). A thorough closed kinetic chain examination includes static postural observations, dynamic motion testing, and gait assessment.

Compensatory mechanisms that result from intrinsic deformities are assessed as the foot is subjected to GRFs during the static weight-bearing examination. This provides valuable insight regarding how the body compensates for the intrinsic foot deformities or impairments of normal foot joint function identified in the non–weight-bearing examination. Improper foot functioning can lead to a complex series of compensations that influence the mobility patterns of the foot and lower leg, as well as the knee, hip, pelvis, and spine.

The patient stands in a relaxed, weight-bearing posture (RCS). The examiner observes the patient's preferred stance, noting postural alignment and foot placement angle. The patient then adjusts the stance position, if necessary, to assume equal weight-bearing double-limb support, with feet 5 to 10 cm apart and oriented in neutral toe-in and toe-out foot placement angle. This adjusted posture, with neutral foot placement angle, offers a better frame of reference for assessing planar alignment and enhances the reliability and consistency of the measurement.[38] Postural alignment or body symmetry of the patient is evaluated in the frontal, sagittal, and transverse planes.

Frontal Plane

Static weight-bearing examination in the frontal plane focuses on the angular relation of the calcaneus and the tibia and fibula with respect to the floor and the relation between the pelvis and the lower leg.

Calcaneal Alignment to the Floor

With the patient in double-limb stance posture, a line bisecting the posterior surface of the calcaneus is visualized and the angular relation between the line and the floor taken. Because the infracalcaneal fat pad often migrates (related to prolonged weight bearing), care must be taken to avoid errors in visual assessment (Figure 9-15). Palpation of the osseous medial, lateral, and inferior borders of the calcaneus helps factor out fat pad migration and improve measurement accuracy. Calcaneal alignment can also be quantified with a protractor to measure the degree of calcaneal tilt relative to vertical.[62]

The key question to answer is whether the calcaneus is inverted, vertical, or everted relative to the floor during stance; the actual angular degree is not as important as the relative orientation of the calcaneus. This component of the examination assesses the ability of the STJ to provide enough pronation to compensate for its neutral position. In the normal closed chain STN position, the calcaneus is in 1 to 4 degrees of varus (inversion). The STJ must have an equal amount of compensatory pronation to lower the medial condyle to the ground for a vertical calcaneus. If a patient has uncompensated rearfoot varus of 10 degrees in STN as well as restricted calcaneal motion (–4 degrees) eversion, the STJ would not be able to achieve sufficient pronation or eversion in stance for normal calcaneal alignment. Instead the calcaneus would be in an inverted alignment relative to the floor. Inverted calcaneal position also occurs when a rigid forefoot valgus or rigid plantarflexed first ray deformity is present. STJ supination is a compensatory mechanism for both deformities.

In contrast, forefoot varus deformity requires excessive compensatory STJ pronation; calcaneal eversion occurs in weight bearing. The position of the calcaneus with respect to the floor provides insight into the type of STJ compensation present and can be correlated with the biomechanical findings of the non–weight-bearing examination. If the STJ is unable to pronate enough to compensate completely for a deformity, additional pronatory motion occurs at the MTJ or by eversion tilting of the talus within the ankle mortise.[5,38,45] The functional rearfoot unit (calcaneus and talus) may assume a valgus (everted) position relative to the floor, even if calcaneal eversion is restricted.

Tibiofibular Alignment

Proximal structural malalignments, such as tibial varum or valgum, contribute to abnormal foot pronation and overuse injuries. In osseous congenital tibial varum, the distal third of the tibia is angled medially in the frontal plane, whereas in tibial valgum the distal tibia inclines away from the midline.[38]

Tibial alignment can be measured with either a standard goniometer (Figure 9-16) or a bubble inclinometer; both assess, the angular relation between the bisection of the distal third of the lower leg relative to the supporting surface.[38,63] Radiographic measurement of lower leg position is better correlated with clinically assessed tibiofibular position values than with isolated tibial position. Radiographic measure-

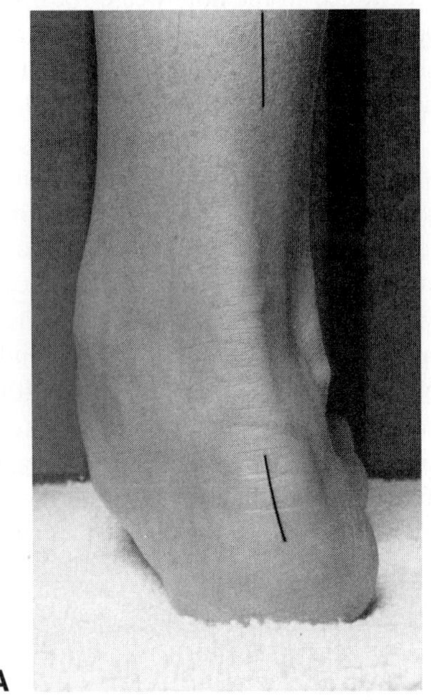

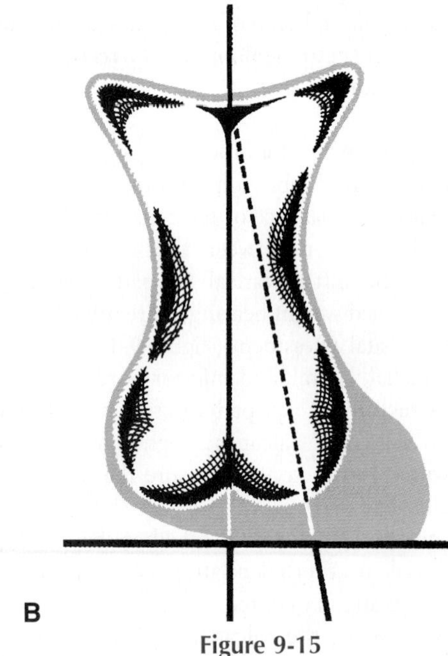

Figure 9-15
A, Calcaneal alignment to floor. B, Lateral migration of the infracalcaneal fat pad can give the illusion of an everted calcaneal to floor alignment. (Courtesy Stride, Inc., Middlebury, Conn.)

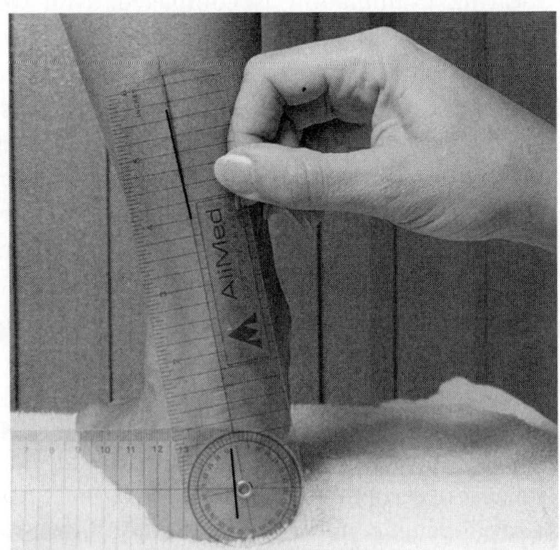

Figure 9-16
Goniometric assessment of tibiofibular varum. The proximal arm of the goniometer is aligned with the bisection of the distal third of the tibiofibular complex, and the distal arm is level with the floor. The axis of measurement shifts with the degree of varum or valgum deformity and may not always fall directly behind the calcaneus.

ment may be the most accurate method to isolate true tibial varum.[64]

Test position is critical because variation in STJ alignment greatly influences tibiofibular varum measurement values. Tibiofibular varum values are larger in RCS than in the STN position because of the combined effects of osseous malalignment and varus leg alignment associated with compensatory STJ pronation in stance.[63-65] The incidence of tibiofibular varum appears to be high, although no clear normative values have been established.

The alignment of the distal third of the leg relative to the floor more accurately represents tibiofibular position than tibial position. Values assessed in STN reflect neutral tibiofibular alignment, whereas values assessed in RCS represent compensatory tibiofibular repositioning in response to STJ and MTJ pronation. High tibiofibular varum values measured in STN elevate the medial foot from the supporting surface, requiring excessive compensatory foot pronation during gait. High tibiofibular varum values in RCS suggest excessive foot pronation, although the source of that pronation cannot be isolated.

Alignment of the Pelvis and Lower Leg

The final component of the frontal plane assessment evaluates symmetry of the anterior superior iliac spines, iliac crests, greater trochanters, gluteal folds, popliteal creases, genu varum or valgum deformities, fibular heads, patellae, and malleolar levels. Asymmetry often indicates sacroiliac joint dysfunction or leg-length discrepancy, influencing foot position and function in the closed kinetic chain.

Sagittal Plane

The second component of the weight-bearing examination considers function in the sagittal plane. The examiner looks for evidence of genu recurvatum or excessive knee flexion, navicular drop, talar bulge, and inadequate or excessive height of the longitudinal arch.

Knee Position

Viewing the patient's stance from the side, the examiner observes the verticality of the tibia. In genu recurvatum the proximal tibia is aligned behind the axis of the TCJ, resulting in hyperextension of the knee and plantar flexion of the TCJ with relative shortening of the limb. Genu recurvatum also occurs as a compensation for equinus deformity at the ankle. When true leg-length discrepancy is present, two types of compensation are possible. If limb length difference is small, genu recurvatum may adequately shorten the longer limb. For larger limb length differences, knee flexion of the longer limb is often used to minimize asymmetry.

Navicular Drop

The position of the navicular is examined by using the navicular drop test, a composite measure of foot pronation focusing on displacement of the navicular tuberosity as a patient moves from closed kinetic chain STN to RCS position.[66] Excessive navicular displacement is associated with collapse of the MLA and may be correlated with midfoot pain or other symptoms of excessive foot pronation.[38] Subotnick[67] established an interdependency between MTJ and STJ function based on articulation of the navicular and cuboid with the talus and calcaneus. Brody[66] suggested that the navicular drop test is a valid assessment of STJ function in the closed kinetic chain. Although navicular drop occurs with STJ pronation that stems from intrinsic foot deformity, it can also be the result of muscle insufficiency or ligamentous laxity.[38]

To measure navicular drop, an index card is held perpendicular to the medial foot, the level of the navicular tuberosity is marked in STN position and RCS, and the distance between the marks is calculated.[36] Normative studies report a mean navicular drop of between 7.3 and 9.0 mm.[36,68] A navicular drop of more than 10 mm is considered abnormal.[68]

Talar Bulge and Arch Height

When excessive STJ pronation is present in stance, the talus moves into adduction and plantar flexion. Displacement of the talar head causes an observable medial bulge in the region of the talonavicular joint.[69] The height of the MLA normally decreases moderately in weight bearing as a result of normal STJ pronation. Pes planus deformity (flatfootedness) is characterized by excessive collapse of the MLA. In hereditary rigid flatfoot, the MLA is low or absent in non–weight-bearing and weight-bearing positions. In flexible flatfoot, the height of the MLA is normal in non–weight bearing but drops excessively in weight bearing because of abnormal STJ pronation. In normal foot alignment, the medial malleolus, navicular tuberosity, and first metatarsal head fall along the Feiss line.[69] In a severely pronated foot, the navicular tuberosity lies below the Feiss line. In extreme cases the tuberosity may even rest on the floor.[69,70]

Transverse Plane

The final component of the static weight-bearing examination considers foot function in the transverse plane. The examiner looks for signs of excessive pronation or forefoot adduction and torsional deformities of the lower extremities.

Toe Sign

A positive toe sign indicates excessive pronation or abduction of the foot in the transverse plane (Figure 9-17). The sign is determined by the number of toes that can be seen, in a posterior view, when the patient is standing in RCS with a neutral foot placement angle.[58] Normally no more than 1.5 toes are visible beyond the lateral border of the foot. If more toes can be seen, abnormal pronation may be present, causing excessive transverse plane motion or abduction of the foot. A false-positive toe sign can occur in the presence of a relative toe-out foot placement angle associated with lateral rotational deformities (e.g., femoral retroversion) or muscle imbalances that limit internal rotation of the hip (e.g., tight piriformis). Ensuring that the patient's patellae are oriented in the frontal plane before assessing toe sign reduces the risk of false-positive findings.

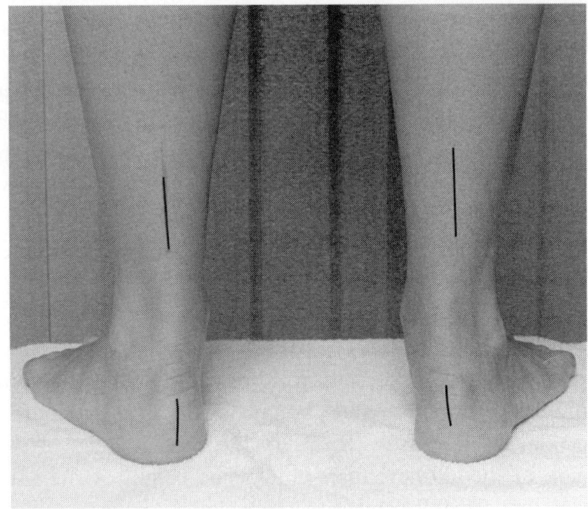

Figure 9-17
Toe sign, demonstrating excessive transverse plane motion as evidenced by the abducted position of the forefoot.

Torsional Deformities

Transverse plane abnormalities of the femur and tibia also adversely affect normal foot functioning. The femoral shaft normally has 12 degrees of medial rotation relative to the femoral head and neck (Figure 9-18). In femoral anteversion more than 12 degrees of rotation are present, whereas in retroversion fewer than the expected 12 degrees of medial rotation are present.[69] In normal transverse plane tibial alignment, the fibular malleolus is situated posterior to the tibial malleolus, for 20 to 30 degrees of lateral rotation.[69] Internal tibial torsion or femoral anteversion increase medial rotational forces, leading to abnormal foot pronation. Excessive external tibial rotation or femoral retroversion increases lateral rotational forces, leading to abnormal foot supination.

To assess femoral torsion, the patient lies in the prone position with the knee in 90 degrees of flexion.[38] The examiner palpates the greater trochanter as the lower limb is passively moved laterally (representing hip internal rotation) and medially (representing hip external rotation). Femoral torsion is measured at the point where the greater trochanter is most prominent (Figure 9-19). When there is "normal" anteversion of 12 degrees, tibial position will indicate slight internal rotation of the hip. A vertical tibia indicates femoral retroversion.

Tibial torsion is assessed with the patient in the supine position, with 90 degrees of ankle dorsiflexion and the leg placed neutrally in the frontal plane (Figure 9-20). The examiner holds the stationary arm of the goniometer parallel to the table surface while the mobile arm is aligned with the TCJ axis as it passes through the medial and lateral malleoli. This angular displacement represents tibial torsion. Normally 20 degrees of external tibial torsion are present.

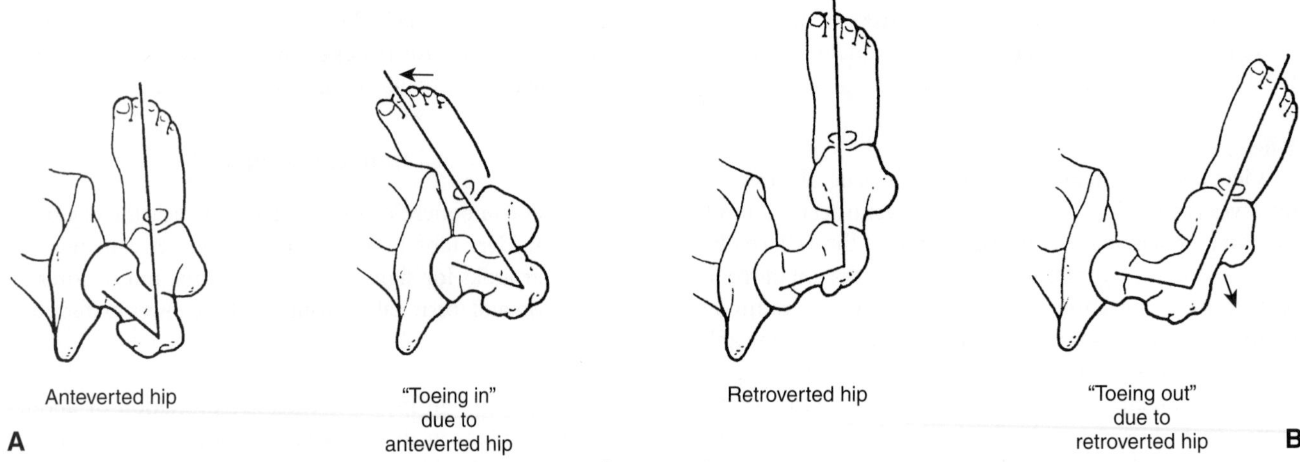

Figure 9-18
A, *With excessive femoral anteversion, the limb appears to be internally rotated when the head of the femur is well seated in the acetabulum.* ***B,*** *With femoral retroversion, the limb appears to be externally rotated when the femur is well seated in the acetabulum. (From Magee DJ.* Orthopedic Physical Assessment, *3rd ed. Philadelphia: Saunders, 1997. p. 475.)*

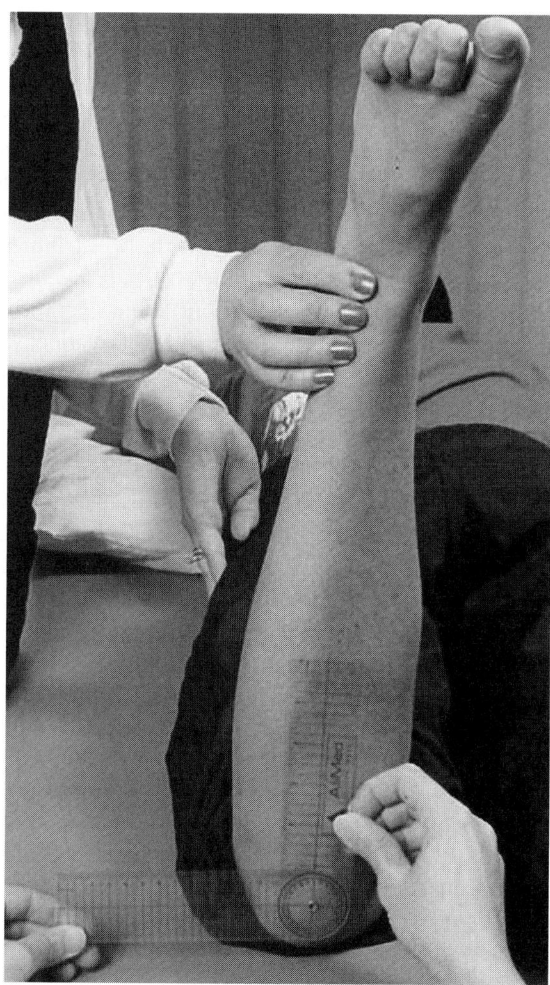

Figure 9-19
Assessment of femoral torsion in prone position with a standard goniometer. The examiner palpates the greater trochanter and rotates the lower leg. Femoral torsion is measured at the point of greatest prominence of the greater trochanter.

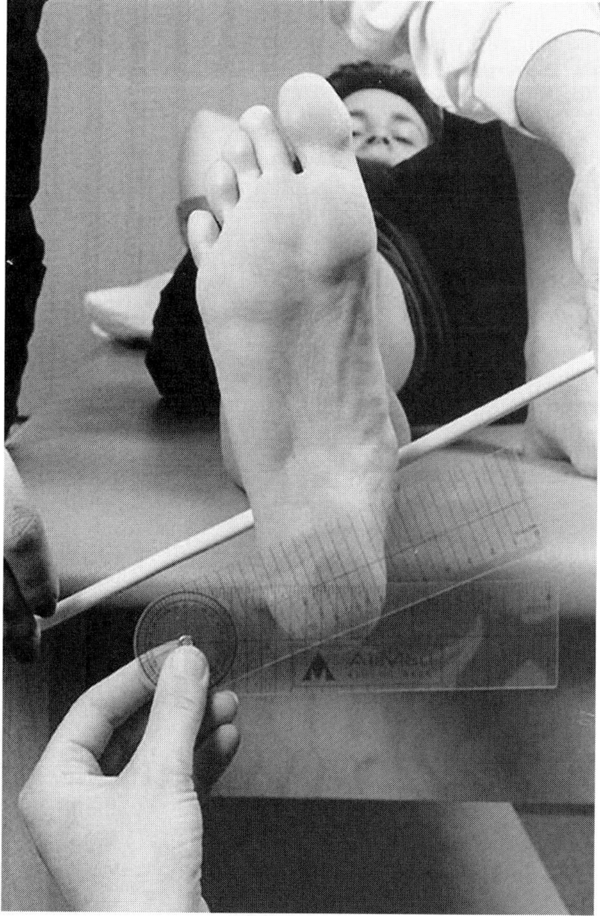

Figure 9-20
Tibial torsion is measured as the angle between horizontal and the plane of the axis of the talocrural joint.

DYNAMIC GAIT ASSESSMENT

The final component of the clinical evaluation is observation of foot function during walking. During the dynamic gait assessment, extrinsic factors that affect foot function (e.g., muscle imbalances or weaknesses, proximal structural deformities, kinesthetic or proprioceptive losses) are observed. Videotaping the individual while he or she is walking on a runway or treadmill may enhance the accuracy of the assessment. The function of the rearfoot, midfoot, and forefoot is examined at each of the subphases of the gait cycle, with special attention to compensatory gait mechanisms. See Chapter 3 for more information on dynamic gait assessment.

CASE EXAMPLE 1A

An Individual with Rearfoot and Forefoot Dysfunction

M. L. is an active 50-year-old woman who recently began to train for a local 10-km race. She is referred by her family physician for evaluation and intervention because of thickened and painful plantar callus under the second and fourth metatarsal heads and on the lateral surface of the hallux in both feet. The discomfort has increased to a point that she is unable to complete the distances she needs to run to prepare for the upcoming race.

M. L. is 5 feet, 5 inches tall and weights 132 lbs. In relaxed standing no leg-length discrepancy is apparent, although both patellae are rotated inward, slight hyperextension and recurvatum at the knee is present (left more than right), and both feet are markedly pronated.

The following values are recorded in the non-weight-bearing and weight-bearing examinations:

Non–Weight-Bearing Examination Component	*Left*	*Right*
Rearfoot STN position	6 degrees varus	7 degrees varus
Calcaneus inversion	18 degrees	22 degrees
Calcaneus eversion	12 degrees	14 degrees
Ankle dorsiflexion	9 degrees	7 degrees
Rearfoot dorsiflexion	2 degrees	0 degrees
Forefoot STN position	Mild valgus	Moderate valgus
Locking mechanism	Fair	Poor
First ray	Slightly plantar flexed	Slightly plantar flexed
Hallux dorsiflexion	75 degrees	80 degrees
Medial longitudinal arch	Medium height	Medium height

Weight-Bearing Examination Component	*Left*	*Right*
Calcaneal/floor alignment	Eversion	Eversion
Tibiofibular position	40 degrees	37 degrees
Navicular drop (STN to relaxed calcaneal stance)	10 mm	12 mm
Navicular position (Feiss)	Slightly below	Moderately below
Toe sign	2.5 toes visible	3 toes visible
Femoral torsion	14 degrees	16 degrees
Tibial torsion	25 degrees	27 degrees

Questions to Consider

- What are the normative values for non–weight-bearing range of motion in the rearfoot (STN position, calcaneal inversion and eversion, dorsiflexion) and forefoot (STN position, midtarsal joint dorsiflexion, first ray position, and mobility)?
- What rearfoot and forefoot deformities do M. L.'s examination findings suggest?
- What are normal findings for the closed chain, static weight-bearing examination?
- How should the findings for M. L.'s weight-bearing examination be interpreted?
- How do the findings of M. L.'s non–weighting-bearing and weight-bearing examinations relate to each other? What deformities are compensated versus uncompensated?

FUNCTIONAL FOOT ORTHOSES

Although 4 to 6 degrees of triplanar STJ pronation are necessary to provide adequate shock absorption and accommodation to uneven ground terrain, persistent or recurrent abnormal pronation disrupts normal temporal sequencing of the gait cycle.[5,8,31,71] This disruption creates an unstable osseous and arthrokinematic situation that contributes to pathological musculoskeletal conditions.[5,38]

Compensatory motion occurs in the primary plane of a given deformity. In frontal plane deformities (e.g., rearfoot varus or forefoot varus), the typical compensatory motion is eversion at the STJ. In transverse plane deformities (e.g., torsional deformities of the hip, femur, or tibia), the typical compensatory motion is adduction at the STJ. In sagittal plane deformities (e.g., ankle equinus), the typical compensatory motion is dorsiflexion at the STJ. Root's model suggests that single-plane compensatory motion is beneficial, allowing adequate accommodation for a deformity.[5] Because the STJ is a triplanar structure, however, movement in one plane leads to movement in the others as well. The associated motion of the other planes has the potential to become dysfunctional and destructive.[5]

A *functional foot orthosis* is an orthopedic device designed to promote structural integrity of the joints of the foot and lower limb by resisting the GRFs that cause abnormal skeletal motion during the stance phase of gait.[42] A functional foot orthosis attempts to control abnormal foot functioning during stance by controlling excessive STJ and MTJ motion, decelerating pronation, and allowing the STJ to function closer to its neutral position at MSt.[72-74] In contrast, an accommodative foot orthosis is used to distribute pressures over the plantar surface for individuals with fixed deformity or vulnerable neuropathic feet. (See Chapter 21 for more information on accommodative foot orthoses.)

Criteria for Abnormal Pronation

Five criteria are used to determine if pronation is abnormal. Pronation is considered an abnormal mechanical condition when the following conditions are present:

1. STJ pronation is more than the normal 4 to 6 degrees.[5,8,31,71]
2. The foot pronates at the wrong time, disrupting the normal sequencing of events during closed kinetic chain motion.
3. Pronation is recurrent, with each step contributing to repetitive microtrauma to musculoskeletal structures.
4. Pronation happens at a location other than the STJ (e.g., when MTJ pronation compensates for limited STJ motion).
5. Unnecessary destructive compensatory motion occurs in the other planes of motion of the STJ.[5]

Causes of Abnormal Foot Mechanics

Three pathological situations contribute to abnormal foot mechanics: structural malalignment, muscle weakness or imbalance, and loss of structural integrity.

Structural Malalignment

Structural malalignment can be intrinsic or extrinsic to the foot or caused by abnormal mechanical forces.[5] Rearfoot and forefoot varus and valgus, ankle equinus, and deformities of the rays are examples of intrinsic deformities. Congenital and developmental conditions, such as tibial varum or valgum, torsional deformities of the tibia or femur, and other conditions that occur above the foot and ankle are extrinsic deformities. The types of abnormal mechanical forces that might contribute to pathomechanical foot function include obesity, leg length discrepancies, and genu valgum or varum. Orthotic management for structural malalignment is preventive; control of aberrant or excessive STJ and MTJ motion forestalls the sequence of mechanical events associated with abnormal pronation or supination, minimizing the consequences of painful foot conditions.

Muscle Weakness or Imbalance

A variety of upper and lower motor neuron diseases result in muscular weakness, abnormal muscle tone, or paralysis of the foot, with resultant instability of foot structure and reduced mechanical efficiency during gait.[39] In Charcot-Marie-Tooth disease (hereditary sensory motor neuropathy), for example, weakness of intrinsic, peroneal, and anterior tibial muscles contributes to development of a "cavus" foot, with claw toes, metatarsus adductus, or other deformities of the rays.[39] When muscle weakness or imbalance is present, the examiner must identify its origin and extent, the specific soft tissue structures involved, the resultant mechanical foot deformities, and the potential to reduce them. An effective foot orthosis for a patient with muscular weakness deters the pathomechanical sequelae that result from such induced structural foot deformities.

Compromised Joint Integrity

Compromised joint integrity and mechanical instability can also be caused by pathological musculoskeletal conditions of the foot or ankle, including arthritis, acute trauma, or chronic repetitive injury. In rheumatoid arthritis, for example, joint deformity results from synovitis and pannus formation. Autodestruction of connective tissue weakens tendons, contributes to muscle spasm and shortening, and erodes cartilaginous surfaces. Eventually, joint dislocations occur.[75]

The loss of protective sensation associated with peripheral neuropathy also contributes to compromised joint integrity. Patients with diabetes mellitus, chronic alcoholism, or Hansen's disease (leprosy) are particularly vulnerable. Inability to perceive microtrauma because of sensory compromise, weakness of intrinsic muscles of the foot, compromised autonomic control of the distal blood flow, and the poor nutritional and metabolic state of soft tissues combine to increase the risk of plantar foot ulceration. If neuropathic osteoarthropathy (Charcot-Marie-Tooth disease) occurs, significant bone and joint destruction, collapse of the midfoot, and a fixed rocker bottom deformity can result.[76] Plantar ulceration at the apex of the collapsed cuneiforms or cuboid is common.[77] Whenever mechanical instability is present, normal joint orientation is altered, and gait compensation shifts weight-bearing forces. A foot orthosis can be used to reduce pain, reduce weight-bearing stresses, control abnormal or excessive joint motion, or compensate for restricted motion.

GOALS OF ORTHOTIC INTERVENTION

A functional foot orthosis attempts to improve foot mechanics during walking, regardless of the cause of foot dysfunction, by the following actions:

- Controlling velocity of pronation
- Redistributing plantar pressures
- Supporting abnormal structural forefoot positions that lead to abnormal rearfoot function in stance
- Supporting abnormal rearfoot deformities that lead to excessive STJ pronation
- Resisting extrinsic forces of the leg that lead to aberrant pronation and supination of the foot
- Improving calcaneal positioning at IC
- Repositioning the STJ in neutral position just before heel rise
- Fully pronating the MTJ, when the STJ is in the neutral position, to lock and stabilize the foot, converting it into a rigid lever for propulsion
- Allowing normal plantar flexion of the first ray and stabilizing the forefoot in response to the retrograde GRFs sustained during propulsion
- Providing a normal degree of shock absorption during LR

A functional foot orthosis does not support the MLA of the foot; STJ pronation is controlled by the pressure of the rearfoot post on the calcaneus at the sustentaculum tali. The ultimate goal is to stop, reduce, or slow abnormal compensatory motion of the joints of the foot as the foot and leg interact with the GRFs.

MEASUREMENT AND FABRICATION

The information gathered in the non–weight-bearing and static weight-bearing examinations and in gait analysis provides direction for orthotic prescription. A simple plaster cast is used to make an accurate negative impression of the patient's foot in the STN position. A positive model based on this impression is then prepared. Thermoplastic materials are heat molded over the model to form an orthotic shell. Accommodative padding, soft tissue supplements, and covering materials are added to address the patient's functional foot problem. The orthosis is fitted to the patient, and its effect on foot function during gait is evaluated. An early wearing schedule is devised, and an appointment for a recheck visit is scheduled.

Negative Impression

If a foot orthosis is to control abnormal pronation and supination effectively and minimize painful symptoms in

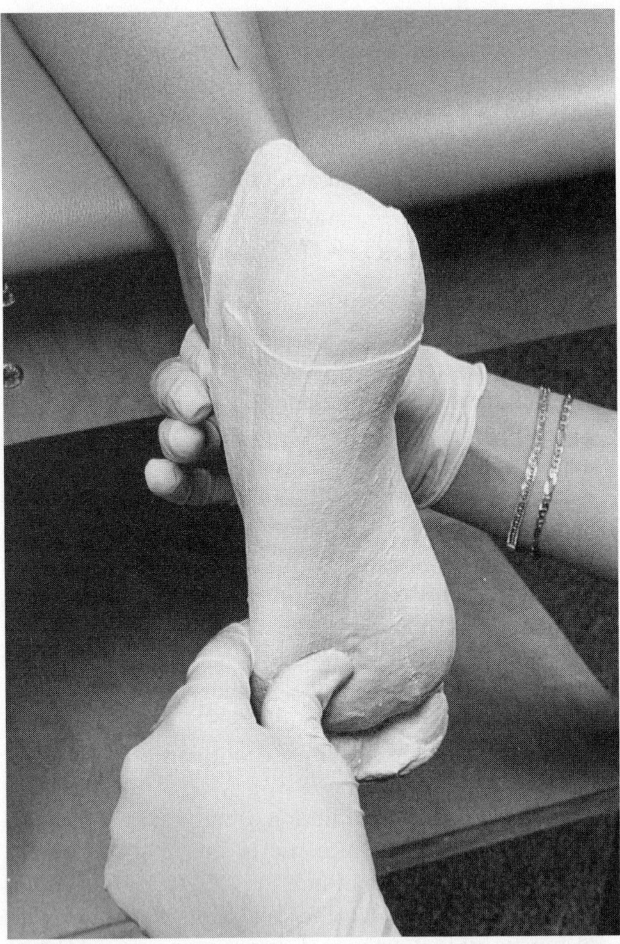

Figure 9-21
Negative cast impression by the direct pressure technique. The foot is maintained in STN position while the plaster hardens.

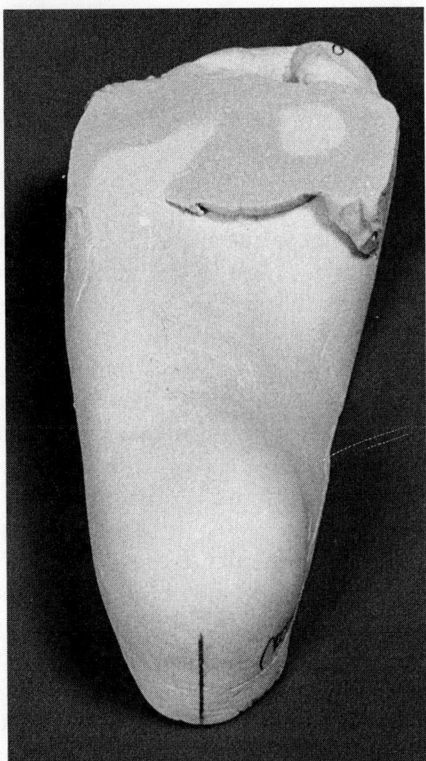

Figure 9-22
The modification process of forefront position on a positive cast.

gait, the negative foot impression must precisely duplicate the existing foot structure, including any intrinsic deformities. The goal of the foot impression is to capture the patient's STN position during the MSt phase of the gait cycle. Multiple strategies can be used to take negative impressions, including suspension techniques, modified suspension techniques, direct pressure techniques, foam impression systems, semi–weight bearing, and in-shoe vacuum casts. Because maintenance of the STN position and correct loading of the forefoot are difficult to control in weight-bearing impression techniques, suspension and direct pressure non–weight-bearing techniques appear to be the most reliable methods for making accurate negative impressions. The direct pressure technique, one of the easiest procedures to learn, captures the STN position by loading the fourth and fifth metatarsal heads to mimic GRFs during MSt (Figure 9-21). Alternative casting procedures are also available.[78,79]

Direct Pressure Impression Technique

The patient is placed in the prone position, in the figure-of-four position used for goniometric measurement. Two double-layer thickness wraps of 5-inch plaster bandage are used to make the negative cast. The first wrap is cut to surround the foot from just distal to the fifth metatarsal head, around the posterior heel, to just beyond the first metatarsal head. The second wrap is cut so that, when draped over the plantar surface of the forefoot, it overlaps the first wrap at the metatarsals.

The first wrap is thoroughly moistened with tepid water and any wrinkles in the mesh are smoothed. The top edge of the plaster splint is folded 0.5 inch, providing reinforcement to prevent distortion when the cast is later removed. The first wrap is draped over the heel, just below the malleoli, and along the borders of the foot to just beyond the first and fifth metatarsal heads. Because total contact with the sole of the foot is essential, the plaster is carefully smoothed along the sides of the foot, across its plantar surface, and around the curves of the malleoli. The second wrap is moistened and draped around the forefoot, overlapping the distal edges of the first layer. Any excess bandage is folded into the sulcus of the toes. This layer should also have a wrinkle-free total contact with the foot and toes.

Once both wraps are in place, the foot is positioned in the STN position by maintaining appropriate forefoot loading pressure at the fourth and fifth metatarsal heads. The plaster splint is sufficiently hardened when an audible click is produced when it is tapped. The negative cast is then carefully

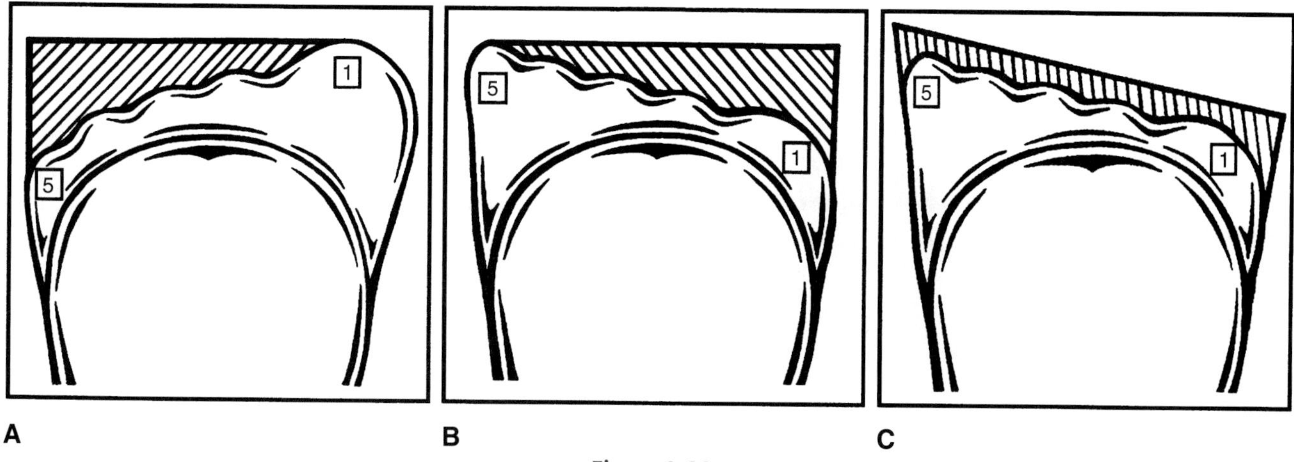

Figure 9-23

Cross section at the level of the metatarsophalangeal joints, with first and fifth metatarsals labeled, demonstrating intrinsic modifications to the positive mold. ***A,*** *A lateral platform corrects forefoot valgus.* ***B,*** *A medial platform corrects forefoot varus.* ***C,*** *A neutral balancing platform maintains forefoot alignment and serves as a base for extrinsic posts. (Courtesy Stride, Inc., Middlebury, Conn.)*

removed. The skin is gently pulled around the reinforced top edge to loosen contact from the cast. A downward force over the superior border of the heel cup is exerted to free the heel from the cast. A gentle forward force is then provided to free the forefoot and remove the cast from the foot.

Errors in Negative Casting

Accuracy in the negative impression is the key to an effective orthotic. Although the casting procedure is simple, three types of errors during the process can compromise the efficacy of orthotic design.

First, the foot may be inadvertently supinated at the longitudinal MTJ axis as a result of contraction of the anterior tibialis while the patient "helps" hold the foot still. Alternatively, the loading force may be applied too far medially at the forefoot, creating a false forefoot varus. An orthosis manufactured from such a cast can cause excessive pressure plantar to the distal aspect of the first metatarsal shaft. It can also lead to lateral ankle instability or the development of a functional hallux limitus or HAV deformities.[80]

The second common casting error occurs when the foot is excessively supinated at the oblique MTJ axis. Improper loading at the fourth and fifth metatarsal heads results in insufficient dorsiflexion of the forefoot. When this happens, transverse skin folds can be seen inside the negative cast at the MTJ. An orthosis manufactured from this cast creates an excessive sagittal plane angulation plantar to the calcaneocuboid joint (lateral longitudinal arch), with pain and irritation on weight bearing.[80]

The third error occurs when the STJ is excessively pronated during casting, placing the foot in a false forefoot valgus position. An orthosis manufactured from this cast does not capture the STN position and is ineffective in controlling the symptoms of abnormal pronation.[80]

Positive Cast Modifications

Once a satisfactory negative impression of the patient's foot has been obtained, a positive cast is made and then modified. The hardened negative impression is filled with liquid plaster and allowed to dry. The negative cast is peeled away, leaving a positive mold of the foot (Figure 9-22). Modifications to the positive cast ensure an effective correction in foot alignment and function by redirecting forces through the foot. Those made to enhance comfort include plaster additions to relieve pressure-sensitive regions of the forefoot and MLA. Because the negative cast is taken in a non–weight-bearing position, it is also modified to allow for the elongation of the foot and expansion of the soft tissues in weight bearing. The cast is also modified to allow for normal plantar flexion of the first metatarsal during propulsion.[42,81] Intrinsic or extrinsic posts can be added for further correction of forefoot or rearfoot deformities.

Forefoot Posting

Two techniques can be used to provide orthotic correction for forefoot deformity. Both are based on modification of the positive cast impression. The first, a traditional Root functional orthosis, uses an intrinsic correction. A plaster platform is applied to the positive cast at the level of the MTP joints to balance the abnormal forefoot to rearfoot relation (Figure 9-23). A lateral platform corrects forefoot valgus, and a medial platform corrects forefoot varus.[42] When the shell is pressed over the modified positive mold, it creates a convexity at the distal anterior border of the orthosis. This posting technique achieves correction by effectively realigning the skeletal structure of the foot.[81] The intrinsic posting technique is often selected when shoe volume is limited, as in some women's footwear.

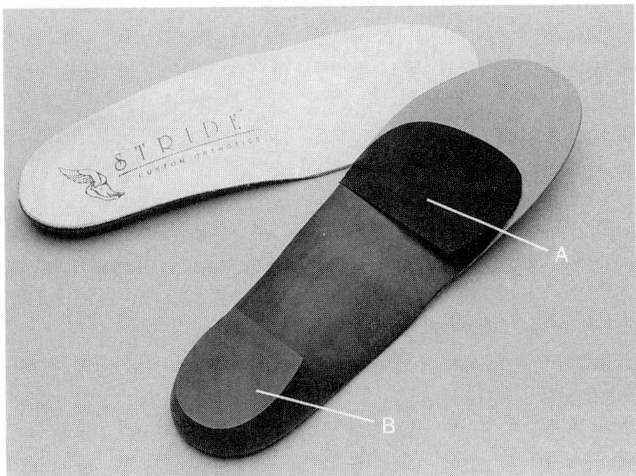

Figure 9-24
Standard biomechanical orthosis with an extrinsic forefoot post (A) *and an extrinsic rearfoot post* (B).

A second forefoot posting technique involves a variation of Root's original design, referred to as a *standard biomechanical orthosis.* In this technique a neutral platform is formed on the positive mold, but the existing valgus or varus position of the forefoot is maintained. An extrinsic forefoot post or wedge is attached to the bottom of the orthotic shell to support the forefoot in its position of deformity. Unwanted compensatory motion is prevented by stabilizing the distal border of the orthosis (Figure 9-24). Although an orthosis with an extrinsic correction takes up more space inside the shoe than an intrinsically corrected orthosis, it can more easily be modified if the individual has difficulty tolerating the original posting prescription.

Rearfoot Posting

As the foot makes contact with the ground and moves through stance during gait, GRFs act on the joints of the foot. An orthosis acts as an interface between the ground and the foot, creating its own orthosis reactive force. In a foot that pronates excessively, the foot orthosis is designed to decrease STJ pronation during weight bearing by creating a supination moment acting medial to the STJ axis.[2] This can be accomplished by adding an extrinsic rearfoot post or wedge to the inferior surface of the heel cup or by modifying the plaster mold to incorporate an intrinsic rearfoot post to the heel cup of the orthosis. A rearfoot post effectively reduces rearfoot pronation (eversion) during the contact phase of gait as well as the angular velocity of eversion.[2,82,83]

Extrinsic rearfoot posts are attached to the bottom of the orthosis shell beneath the heel (see Figure 9-24, *B*). A medial wedge or rearfoot post increases orthosis reactive forces at the sustentaculum tali (medial to the STJ axis) to reduce abnormal STJ pronation. It also promotes stability of the heel by increasing the contact surface of the orthosis beneath the heel.[82,83] An intrinsic rearfoot post can be made with a medial heel skive technique. A plaster modification is performed on the medial aspect of the heel of the positive mold to increase the amount of varus (medial) sloping within the heel cup of the orthosis in an effort to control pronation.[2] An intrinsic rearfoot post reduces overall bulk of the orthosis for optimal fit within a shoe. A combination of intrinsic and extrinsic rearfoot posting permits more correction than possible with either method independently.

The Orthotic Shell

To be effective, a functional orthosis must be made on the basis of a neutral position model of the patient's foot. Prefabricated foot supports do not offer adequate control of foot motion or resistance to GRFs and cannot fulfill all criteria of functional foot orthoses. A custom orthosis, made of rigid or semirigid materials, can offer maximal resistance to weight-bearing forces and optimal realignment of foot structure. Accommodative orthoses, made of softer materials, support the arches of the foot and provide relief to pressure-sensitive areas while offering minimal control of STJ motion.[84,85] A semifunctional orthosis is a hybrid of functional and accommodative orthoses that combines the motion effectiveness of a semirigid shell with soft posting and accommodative material to cushion the foot.

Many studies have evaluated the effectiveness of the different types of orthotic materials in controlling rearfoot mechanics and clinical symptoms.[84-88] Some suggest that orthotic materials be classified by degree of rigidity (soft, semi-rigid, rigid), but standards for the classification of materials are not well established.[1]

A rigid orthosis achieves maximal motion control and biomechanical correction of a foot deformity, is lightweight, and takes up the least space within the shoe. Some clinicians are concerned that orthoses made of rigid materials are uncomfortable to the wearer. Anthony[42] suggested, however, that those "who propose rigid devices to be patient intolerant are generally less acquainted with the theory of podiatric biomechanics and the correct diagnostics and prescription formularies that are critical for the provision of a truly functional foot orthosis."

Semirigid materials, such as polypropylene and TL-2100 (Performance Materials Corp., Camarillo, Calif.), are attractive alternatives to rigid orthotic shells. Polypropylene is a flexible olefin polymer that resists breakage. TL-2100 is a thermoplastic composite of resin and fiber that is harder and more rigid than polypropylene.[1]

Soft orthoses are often made of closed-cell foams manufactured from heat-expanded polyethylene. Examples of such foams include Aliplast and Nickleplast (Alimed, Inc., Dedham, Mass.) and Plastazote (Bakelite Xylonite Ltd, Croydon, United Kingdom), cross-linked polyethylene expanded foams available in many densities. Pelite (Fillauer,

Table 9-1
Accommodative Padding and Soft Tissue Supplements for Functional Foot Orthotics

Supplement	*Description*
Metatarsal mound	A dome-shaped addition in the form of a teardrop positioned with the apex just proximal to the metatarsal heads to support a collapsed transverse metatarsal arch. Often used to control symptoms of neuroma by reducing shearing of the metatarsals during contact phase. Reduction of the shearing eliminates irritation to the interdigital nerves of the forefoot.
2-5 bar	A pad of uniform thickness placed beneath the second through fifth metatarsal heads relieves pressure beneath the first metatarsal head during propulsion. Used when a rigid plantar flexed first ray is present.
Metatarsal head cutout	A U-shaped pad positioned beneath a rigid plantar flexed metatarsal head to relieve pressure from a painful callosity. Often used for hammertoe deformity.
Morton's extension	An extension of the plastic shell, or the addition of an inlay made of dense material, beneath the shaft of the first metatarsal to the sulcus of the hallux. Often used for a dorsiflexed first ray or Morton's toe.
Heel cushion	Placed in the heel cup of the orthosis to enhance heel cushioning and shock absorption. Often made of the soft tissue–supplementing material Poron (Rodgers Co., Rogers, Conn.) or a viscoelastic polymer. Used when irritation or atrophy of the infracalcaneal fat pad is present or for calcaneal stress fracture.
Forefoot extension	A soft tissue–supplementing material such as Poron is added to the distal end of the orthotic shell to cushion the metatarsal heads or as a base for other forefoot inlays.
Scaphoid pad	A material of soft to medium density placed beneath the medial longitudinal arch to decelerate pronatory forces.

Inc., Chattanooga, Tenn.) is a cross-linked, closed-cell foam that can be heat molded in the fabrication of semiflexible foot orthoses. Various rubberized or thermoplastic cork materials are also used.[1] Lightweight and available in different densities, these materials are effective in orthotics for which accommodation and shock absorption are desirable. These same features limit the durability and the useful life of the orthosis, however, because these materials are prone to rapid and permanent shape deformation.[1]

For some individuals, extrinsic accommodative modifications are necessary to address a particular deformity. Examples of accommodative supplements are listed in Table 9-1.

Covering Materials

Once appropriate posts and supportive materials are attached to the shell of the orthosis, a covering material is applied to provide an interface with the skin of the foot. Vinyl is a commonly used orthosis-covering material. Spenco (Spenco Medical Corporation, Waco, Tex.) and various other fabric-covered neoprene materials are resistant to shearing and enhance shock absorption. They are often chosen as covering materials for certain sport orthoses when shear forces are expected to be high or for occupational situations that demand prolonged standing on hard surfaces.

MANAGING REARFOOT DEFORMITY

In a well-aligned foot, 4 to 6 degrees of STJ pronation occur during the stance phase of gait. In rearfoot varus, more than 6 degrees of STJ pronation are present. A fully compensated rearfoot varus deformity of 10 degrees pronates at the STJ 10 degrees during gait to lower the medial condyle of the calcaneus to the ground, but only 6 degrees of this pronation are considered excessive.

The appropriate orthotic design for rearfoot varus is a *medial post* or *medial wedge*. Complete orthotic correction is difficult to achieve and quite uncomfortable for the individual wearing the orthosis. Because of this, the initial goal is often to create an orthosis that provides 50% correction of a rearfoot deformity. To correct the excessive 6 degrees of pronation, for example, a medial rearfoot post or wedge of 3 degrees would be applied to the orthosis.

If an individual with a rearfoot varus deformity of 10 degrees is uncompensated to –5 degrees of calcaneal eversion, a medial or varus wedge of 3 degrees is not effective because the STJ would reach its end-range eversion motion (–5 degrees) before the orthosis provided support. To manage uncompensated rearfoot deformity effectively, the varus wedge must be large enough to prevent the STJ from reaching its end ROM. In this example, a larger medial rearfoot varus post or wedge of at least 5 degrees is necessary. When the rearfoot is aggressively posted (more than 3 or 4 degrees of varus posting), the distal medial aspect of the orthosis shell loses contact with the ground, as if a forefoot varus deformity were present. In these circumstances, a medial forefoot post is used to counteract the induced apparent forefoot varus.

MANAGING FOREFOOT DEFORMITY

For forefoot varus deformities, a medial (varus) wedge or post is indicated. For forefoot valgus deformities, lateral (valgus) posts or wedges are used. Forefoot deformities can be corrected through intrinsic plaster modifications or extrinsic posting. For an orthosis to be accurately balanced so that it does not wobble, a forefoot deformity must be corrected to its fullest extent (e.g., an 8-degree forefoot varus deformity requires an 8-degree medial wedge or post).

The addition of a large extrinsic post to the distal end of the orthotic shell often creates problems with shoe fit. One possible solution is to correct large forefoot deformities with a combination of intrinsic and extrinsic techniques. In this example, a 4-degree medial intrinsic plaster platform and a 4-degree extrinsic medial forefoot post or wedge would provide the desired correction without bulkiness. For individuals with a forefoot varus deformity of 10 degrees or more, a semipronated or pronated negative cast can reduce the forefoot deformity to a more manageable degree.[78]

Plantar flexion of the first ray is managed according to the level of flexibility of the deformity. A fully flexible plantar flexed first ray deformity does not require orthotic intervention. A semirigid or rigid plantar flexed first ray deformity requires the addition of a metatarsal (second through fifth) bar inlay. The thickness of the inlay is determined by how far below the first metatarsal head lies relative to the plane of the remaining metatarsal heads. The orthotic intervention for patients with a rigid plantar flexed first ray and forefoot varus is an extended medial forefoot wedge. The forefoot post is modified with a cutout to accommodate the dropped first metatarsal head position. In some cases, a small forefoot varus deformity combined with a large, rigidly plantar flexed first ray deformity results in a functional forefoot valgus (see Figure 9-14).

ORTHOTIC CHECKOUT AND TROUBLESHOOTING

Delivery of an orthosis includes evaluation of its fit, comfort, and mechanical alignment. The orthotic shell should end just proximal to the metatarsal heads. The width is evaluated to ensure that normal first ray plantar flexion and propulsion are not compromised. The position of the orthosis within the shoe is also evaluated; its volume, impact on heel height, points of excessive pressure, and tendency to cause pistoning during gait are considered. On initial fitting, many individuals report that the orthosis feels slightly strange or unusual. The orthosis should not, however, cause undue discomfort. Fit and mechanical functioning of the orthosis are evaluated in standing and walking.

Patient education in appropriate break-in protocols and wearing schedules is an important component of orthotic delivery. A new orthosis is usually worn for 2 hours on day 1, 4 hours on day 2, 6 hours on day 3, and so forth, until the individual is able to wear the orthosis comfortably all day. A follow-up visit is scheduled after the orthosis has been worn for at least 2 weeks. By this time the patient should feel comfortable with the orthosis for normal activities of daily living. Thereafter, progressively increased use of the orthosis for all activities, including sport and occupational use, should be well tolerated. Adjustments are occasionally necessary to optimize patient comfort and mechanical alignment.

CASE EXAMPLE 1B

An Individual with Rearfoot and Forefoot Dysfunction

M. L. wants to continue training for her upcoming race without increasing her pain and further damaging soft tissue in her feet. An appropriate prescription is being created for M. L. on the basis of the findings of her examination and the principles of orthotic design.

Examination Findings

Relaxed standing: no apparent leg-length discrepancy, both patella rotated inward, slight hyperextension and recurvatum at the knee (left more than right), marked pronation of both feet.

Non–Weight-Bearing Examination Component	*Left*	*Right*
Rearfoot STN position	6 degrees varus	7 degrees varus
Calcaneus inversion	18 degrees	22 degrees
Calcaneus eversion	12 degrees	14 degrees
Ankle dorsiflexion	9 degrees	7 degrees
Rearfoot dorsiflexion	2 degrees	0 degrees
Forefoot STN position	Mild valgus	Moderate valgus
Locking mechanism	Fair	Poor
First ray	Slightly plantar flexed	Slightly plantar flexed
Hallux dorsiflexion	75 degrees	80 degrees
Medial longitudinal arch	Medium height	Medium height

Weight-Bearing Examination Component	*Left*	*Right*
Calcaneal/floor alignment	Eversion	Eversion
Tibiofibular position	40 degrees	37 degrees
Navicular drop (STN to relaxed calcaneal stance)	10 mm	12 mm
Navicular position (Feiss)	Slightly below	Moderately below
Toe sign	2.5 toes visible	3 toes visible
Femoral torsion	14 degrees	16 degrees
Tibial torsion	25 degrees	27 degrees

Questions to Consider

- What are the primary short-term and long-term goals of orthotic intervention for M. L.? Are the therapeutic goals for orthotic intervention similar to or different from M. L.'s goals? How quickly will the orthosis have an impact on level of pain and function?
- What options should be considered in addressing her forefoot deformity in each foot? What type of posting (intrinsic versus extrinsic, medial versus lateral) is most appropriate? How much of a wedge or post should be recommended? Why? How might the recommendations for each foot be similar or different?
- What options should be considered in addressing the rearfoot deformity in each foot? What type of posting (intrinsic versus extrinsic, medial versus lateral) would be most appropriate? How much of a wedge or post should be recommended? Why? How might the recommendations for each foot be similar or different?
- What type of materials would be most appropriate to use in her orthosis? Why?
- Is fabricating orthoses for both her running shoes and her usual daily footwear advisable? Why or why not?
- What type of wearing schedule should be recommended? Should she alter her training schedule or expectations about participating in the upcoming race? Why or why not?
- How frequently should M. L. be followed up during this episode of care? How should the outcomes of orthotic intervention be assessed?

CONTROVERSY WITH ROOT'S PARADIGM

Much discussion on the basic components of Root's theory has occurred in the past decade.[48,89-96] Payne and Bird[96] suggested that "no other aspect of podiatric medical practice is undergoing such a far-reaching theoretical and scientific debate as podiatric biomechanics and the use of functional foot orthoses."

Root's theory is founded on "normal" foot structure and the concept of the STN position: the point of maximal congruence in the articulation of the talus and navicular.[5,8,26,52] STN position supposedly (1) minimizes stress to the surrounding joints and ligaments, (2) is the most efficient position regarding muscle function and attenuation of the impact forces at IC, and (3) represents the point at which the foot converts from a mobile adapter to a rigid lever.[5,38,52] According to Root's traditional theory, normal foot alignment occurs just before TSt during gait, when the STJ is in the neutral position and the MTJ is fully locked.[5]

The major criticisms of Root's paradigm raise concerns about reliability of measurement of the STN position, the position of STN position during the gait cycle, and criteria for "normal" foot alignment.[35,89,91,95]

Reliability of Measurement

When considering available evidence about reliability of foot measurements and the STN position, although acceptable levels of intrarater reliability exist,[36,37,43,45,46,97,98] interrater reliability of foot measurements and the STN position is low.[35,89,91,95] Diamond and colleagues[46] and Cook and colleagues[98] found that interrater reliability can be improved with training. McPoil and Hunt[35] noted that considerable confusion exists regarding the definition and measurement of STN position. They suggested that Root's STN position may misinterpret the of work by Wright and colleagues,[99] who referenced relaxed standing position, not STN neutral, as the basis of their work. To further add to the confusion, the definition of STN position used in some reliability studies was not identical to Root's methods.[95] Based on the review of reliability studies, McPoil and Hunt[35] suggested that physical therapists are not able to agree on position and motion of the STJ.

Subtalar Position in Stance

According to Root, ideal foot alignment occurs just before TSt during gait, when the STJ is in the neutral position and the MTJ is fully locked.[5,100] In a study of rearfoot motion of 50 healthy adults, McPoil and Cornwall[101] marked patients' lower leg and calcaneus with bisection lines and then filmed relative calcaneal and lower leg position while walking, while standing in a double-support relaxed standing, and while in STN position. Their findings did not support Root's paradigm. They found that (1) the rearfoot is slightly inverted before IC, (2) maximal rearfoot pronation was reached at the 37.9% point of stance phase, and (3) the neutral position of the rearfoot for the typical pattern of rearfoot motion should be the resting standing foot posture rather than STN position.[101] As a result, they suggested that the relaxed standing foot position rather than the STN position should be used during casting.[101]

Pierrynowski and Smith[102] used three-dimensional analysis and six experienced raters to study the pattern of rearfoot motion throughout the gait cycle relative to the STN position. The right lower extremities of nine patients were evaluated by each rater six to seven times, and the STN position was recorded. Patients then walked on a treadmill and were recorded for 30 seconds to allow the capture of approximately 25 walking cycles. For most patients, the rearfoot was everted throughout stance, with maximal eversion occurring at 44% of the gait cycle.[102] They found that STN position occurs at 64% and 74% of the gait cycle, with the rearfoot inverted between these points. The rearfoot was everting from 0% to 44%, inverting from 44% to 70%, everting from 70% to 90%, and inverting from 90% to 100% of the gait cycle.[102] The authors concluded that the manufacture of foot orthoses should not be associated with the STN position.[102]

Criteria for Normal Alignment

Root described deviations from normal foot alignment as intrinsic foot deformities, which can lead to aberrant lower extremity function and musculoskeletal pathological conditions.[5,52] Root and colleagues[100] defined three criteria for normal foot and ankle alignment in the loaded STN position: (1) a bisection of the lower leg being in parallel to the bisection of the calcaneus, (2) the plane of the metatarsal heads being perpendicular to the bisection of the calcaneus, and (3) the distal third of the lower leg being perpendicular to the floor. McPoil and colleagues[35,89] examined 116 feet in 58 asymptomatic individuals, finding 8.6% with forefoot varus, 44.8% with forefoot valgus, 14.7% with a plantar flexed first ray, 83.6% with subtalar varus, and 98.3% with tibiofibular varum. Only 17% (116 feet) of the 58 individuals evaluated demonstrated normal criteria.[35] In an examination of forefoot to rearfoot relations of 120 healthy asymptomatic individuals, Garbalosa and colleagues[44] found that only 4.58% of the 234 feet studied exhibited normal criteria, 86.67% had forefoot varus, and 7.75% had forefoot valgus. Astrom and Arvidson[103] performed standardized clinical assessments on 121 healthy individuals, finding that none demonstrated an ideal foot position; most had a valgus position in the STN position (mean, 2 degrees), forefoot in varus (mean, 6 degrees), calcaneal valgus in stance valgus (mean, 7 degrees), and 6 degrees of tibial varus with respect to vertical. The evidence from these studies suggests that an "ideal" foot may be based on a questionable theoretical concept.

FOOT TYPE AND LOWER EXTREMITY BIOMECHANICS

A question that has been the focus of recent research focuses on the relation between various foot types and the amount of pronation during gait. Recent reviews of the literature suggest this question might not have a simple answer. According to Razeghi and Batt,[104] foot type alone cannot explain ankle and foot kinematics because of the interrelated function of the subtalar, talocrural, and knee joints. Their findings may explain why several studies have failed to demonstrate relations between several static and dynamic measures of the foot and lower extremity.[105-107] Ball and Afheldt[95] suggested that attempts to justify static classification of foot type schemes as a means of predicting dynamic joint function have had mixed results.

FOOT TYPE AND LOWER EXTREMITY OVERUSE INJURIES

Many researchers have reported an association between abnormal alignment of the foot and lower extremity and occurrence of lower extremity injuries. Dahle and colleagues[108] studied the relation between foot type (classified in standing as supinated, pronated, or neutral) and occurrence of ankle sprain and knee pain in 55 athletes during the football and cross country seasons. Although the relation between foot type and subsequent ankle sprain was not supported, foot type was strongly related to knee pain; 48% of those with pronated feet and 50% of those with supinated feet had significant knee pain compared with 21% of those classified with neutral alignment. In a study of 20 individuals with unilateral overuse injuries, Tomaro[63] reported that the injured extremity demonstrated more tibiofibular varum compared with the uninjured extremity. This may be explained by the need for more pronation related to increased subtalar compensation to place the foot flat on the floor. Powers and colleagues[109] compared prone STN rearfoot position of 15 patients diagnosed with patellofemoral pain with 15 control subjects, reporting a statistically significant difference in rearfoot varus found in the patellofemoral group (8.9%) compared with control subjects (6.8%). In a retrospective study of the relation between foot posture and incidence of medial tibial stress syndrome, Sommer and Vallentyne[110] measured foot angle in 14 standing limbs with medial tibial stress syndrome (MTSS) and 36 control limbs. They reported mean foot angle of 137 degrees in symptomatic limbs compared with 145 degrees in asymptomatic limbs. They also reported that a standing foot angle of less than140 degrees and a varus alignment of the rearfoot or forefoot, measured qualitatively in STN position, were predictive of a previous history of MTSS.

Some reports do not support the relation between foot type and lower extremity injury. Donatelli and colleagues[111] reported no statistically significant relations among static or dynamic foot posture and injury status in professional baseball players. Razeghi and Batt[104] suggested that arch height may not influence injury occurrence. Similarly, Cowan and colleagues[112,113] found that individuals in the U.S. Army with low arches might be less likely to have lower extremity injury. Considering the variety of reports in the literature,

Razeghi and Batt[104] surmised that "the effect of foot type on the occurrence of lower extremity injuries has not been the subject of well-controlled studies and few, if any, causal correlations have been demonstrated."

ORTHOSES AND LOWER EXTREMITY FUNCTION

Overpronation has been implicated as a cause of many overuse injuries. Traditionally a foot orthosis is used to help control abnormal foot functioning during the stance phase by controlling excessive STJ motion, decelerating pronation, and allowing the STJ to function closer to its neutral position during stance.[72-74] Literature about efficacy of foot orthoses in controlling lower extremity and foot biomechanics is growing.

Effect on Rearfoot Biomechanics

The use of foot orthoses is based on the premise that control of frontal plane rearfoot motion in stance provides a means of controlling pronation of the foot. Novick and Kelley[114] investigated the effects of medially posted rigid orthoses in 20 asymptomatic individuals during the LR phase of the gait cycle. They report a significant decrease in calcaneal angle (angle between the sagittal plane and bisected posterior tubercle of the calcaneus), calcaneal eversion angle (mathematical sum of the tibia vara angle plus the calcaneal angle), angular velocities and angular accelerations, as well as a shift medially in the center of pressure relative to the ankle joint. These findings that an orthosis is able to reposition the rearfoot concur with earlier studies examining the effects of orthoses on rearfoot mechanics.[85,88,115,116] McCulloch and colleagues[117] examined 10 orthotic wearers with and without their orthoses, finding significant decrease in overall pronation (measured as the degree of calcaneal eversion) during the stance phase when orthoses were worn but no reduction in velocity of pronation during early stance. They suggested that orthoses can be effective in controlling abnormal pronation during walking and running.

Johanson and colleagues[118] examined the effects of three different orthotic posting methods on subtalar pronation during ambulation in 22 individuals with a forefoot varus deformity of at least 8 degrees. Individuals ambulated in running shoes with (1) unposted prefabricated shells with a polyurethane arch support and (2) individualized shells posted at the rearfoot, (3) at the forefoot, and (4) at both the rearfoot and forefoot. Forefoot posts were approximately 50% of the measured forefoot varus deformity, and the rearfoot posts were 80% of the forefoot post. Running shoes without shells were used as the control. Measurements of calf to calcaneus and calcaneus to vertical were recorded for each situation. Shells with and without posting decreased calcaneal angles compared with running shoes alone. Concurrent posts of rearfoot and forefoot decreased calcaneal angles similar to rearfoot posting alone; both decreased the angle more than forefoot posting alone. Similarly, Genova and Gross[119] found significant reduction in calcaneal eversion during static stance with shoes alone and shoes with orthoses, compared with the barefoot condition, in 13 individuals with barefoot standing calcaneal eversion angles of at least 10 degrees. The condition of the shoes and the orthoses was not statistically different in controlling eversion in static standing. Individuals demonstrated lower angles for maximal calcaneal eversion during stance and for calcaneal eversion at heel rise for the shoe with an orthosis compared with the shoe alone during fast walking on a treadmill. Branthwaite and colleagues[120] investigated the biomechanical effects of simple orthotic designs at rearfoot in 9 individuals with varus deformities of the feet by using biplanar orthoses (medial wedging at the heel) or cobra pads (medial wedging and an arch support). A decrease in calcaneal eversion occurred with the biplanar orthosis compared with no insole, but no difference occurred with cobra insoles. Neither condition produced significant changes in the maximal eversion velocity.

The difficulty in predicting the biomechanical effects of orthoses on the rearfoot was demonstrated by Brown and colleagues,[121] who compared shoes only, over-the-counter arch supports, and custom-made semirigid orthoses to control rearfoot pronation in 24 patients with a forefoot varus deformity. Custom-made orthoses were posted at both the rearfoot and forefoot, with forefoot posts at 60% of the forefoot deformity and rearfoot posts at 50% of the forefoot deformity. Although a difference was found in the total pronation among the three groups, the authors suggest additional research is warranted to identify orthotic factors responsible for the biomechanical effects associated with the clinical successes of foot orthotics. Butler and colleagues[122] found that rigid or soft orthoses posted 6 degrees at rearfoot were unable to control calcaneal eversion excursion, peak eversion, and eversion velocity during running in individuals with normal foot alignment.

Miller and colleagues[123] suggested that mechanisms by which orthoses control rearfoot motions are not as clear as might be expected. The examination of GRFs during ambulation of 25 individuals with pes planus with or without a rearfoot device found no significant change in the mediolateral GRFs during the stance phase of gait. Significant differences were found, however, in the vertical and anterior posterior GRFs during various percentages of the stance phase.

Several variables that must considered in interpreting these disparate findings, including the materials used, whether individuals are running or walking, foot alignment and biomechanics, and posting methods. Although rearfoot mechanics appear to be altered by foot orthoses, further investigation into the mechanisms responsible for these effects is needed.

Effect on Lower Limb Biomechanics

Foot orthoses influence lower extremity kinematics and kinetics as well as rearfoot mechanics. Eng and Pierrynowski[87] examined the three-dimensional effects of soft foot orthoses during the contact, MSt, and propulsion phases of walking and running on the talocrural and subtalar joints and knee joints in 10 women with a history of patellofemoral joint pain and forefoot varus or calcaneal valgus greater than 6 degrees. Soft orthoses produced a modest decrease in frontal and transverse plane motion in the talocrural and subtalar joints and knee joint during walking and running. Knee joint motion in the frontal plane decreased during the early and MSt phases of walking but increased during the contact and MSt phases of running. This work demonstrates the complex coupling of lower extremity kinematics with motions of the STJ; reductions in subtalar motion in the frontal plane have an impact on knee function in both the frontal and transverse planes during walking. Lafortune and colleagues[124] used three-dimensional analysis to examine the effects of pronation and supination on the knee. Intracortical pins were surgically placed into the tibia and femur of five unaffected individuals who then ambulated with regular shoes or with 10-degree varus and 10-degree valgus wedged shoes designed to produce supination and pronation. Subtle changes occurred with the modified shoe wear, with a 4-degree increase in tibial internal rotation with the valgus (pronation-inducing) wedging. The authors attribute the minimal impact on angular and translatory patterns of the tibiofemoral joint to unaffected individuals' ability to resolve rotational changes at the hip joint with the integrity of knee ligaments and musculature. The authors propose that the combination of ligament laxities and prolonged pronation, along with the increased stresses of running, might produce greater changes than were seen in this cross-sectional study.

Nawoczenski and colleagues[125] clarified the effects of orthoses on lower extremity axial rotations by examining the effects of semirigid orthoses on 20 recreational runners with lower extremity symptoms. Individuals were characterized as having either a high (pes cavus) or low (pes planus) foot profile on the basis of radiographs. No differences in total range of tibial internal and external rotation or tibial abduction and adduction were found between the groups, with or without orthoses. Orthoses did decrease total tibial rotation from heel contact to maximal tibial rotation in both groups by 2 degrees: a 31% decrease in the low-profile group and a 22% reduction in the high-profile group. The orthoses did not affect frontal plane movement. The authors proposed that benefits of orthoses result from alterations of tibial rotation during early stance rather than alterations in calcaneal eversion.

McPoil and Cornwall[126] also studied the effects of soft and rigid orthoses on tibial rotation. Ten individuals with documented rearfoot or forefoot deformity ambulated with unposted, premolded, soft orthoses and rigid polyethylene orthoses posted according to the individual's deformity. Both orthoses decreased the rate and amount of tibial internal rotation during walking. Stacoff and colleagues[127] observed the effects of medially posted cork orthoses on calcaneal and tibial motions in 5 runners. Three-dimensional tibiocalcaneal rotations were assessed after inserting intracortical bone pins into the calcaneus and tibia. Although the effects on eversion and tibial rotation were small and variable, a statistically significant orthotic effect was present for total tibial rotation. The authors, noting that the differences were unsystematic across conditions and were specific to each individual, speculated that the effects of orthoses might be proprioceptive as well as mechanical.

Tillman and colleagues[128] evaluated the impact of orthotic posting on the tibial rotation induced by jumping from a 43-cm-high platform in seven women without foot malalignments by using three conditions (shoes only, shoes with orthoses posted 8 degrees medially, and shoes with orthoses posted 8 degrees laterally). Tibial internal rotation increased by 2.6 degrees with laterally posted inserts and decreased by 3.1 degrees with medially posted inserts. Nester and colleagues[129] examined the effects of medially and laterally wedged orthoses on the kinematics of the rearfoot, knee, hip, and pelvis during walking, reporting main effects on the rearfoot, with minimal effects at knee, hip, or pelvis. Laterally wedged orthoses increased pronation and decreased laterally directed ground forces, whereas medially wedged orthoses decreased pronation and increased the laterally directed ground forces.

Williams and colleagues[130] examined the effects of graphite "inverted" orthoses (orthoses used to provide more aggressive control of pronation by using an inverted position as opposed to a more vertical orientation), standard graphite orthoses posted with a 4-degree medial wedge, or shoes alone in 11 runners who had been initially fitted with the standard orthoses for various lower extremity injuries. Surprisingly, the three conditions produced no significant differences in the peak rearfoot eversion or rearfoot eversion excursion.

A significant decrease in the rearfoot inversion moment and work with the inverted orthosis suggests this orthotic design might decrease demand on the structures controlling eversion. However, increased internal tibial rotation as well as an adduction moment at the knee occurred with the inverted orthosis, raising concern that potential for lateral stress increases with this aggressive orthotic approach.

Stackhouse and colleagues[131] studied biomechanics during running in 15 individuals with normal alignment. Individuals ran with both rearfoot and forefoot strike patterns and with and without semirigid orthoses with 6 degrees of rearfoot posting. The orthoses did not change rearfoot motion in either strike pattern but did reduce internal rotation and genu valgum by approximately 2 degrees through most of the stance phase. Although no statistically significant

reduction occurred in the inversion moment and inversion work, the authors believed that the reductions they found were clinically relevant and might explain the reduction of injuries seen when orthoses are used.

Although evidence supports the fact that foot orthoses can and do influence lower extremity kinematics and kinetics, the variability of individual responses makes it difficult to determine exactly which biomechanical effects will occur. This variability also makes it difficult to forecast who is likely to benefit from orthotic intervention. Efficacy of foot orthoses is not solely the result of altered rearfoot kinematics, as proposed by Root. The contribution of the neuromuscular system to the effect of orthotic intervention is now being considered.

Effect of the Neuromuscular System

Nigg and colleagues,[132] citing problems in previous studies (e.g., small skeletal changes produced by orthotic use, minimal decrease in impact forces, and nonsystematic effects caused by individual variability), proposed that mechanisms involving the neuromuscular system contribute to the way that foot orthoses alter lower extremity function. They were especially interested in sensitivity of the foot and pressure distribution on the foot surface, noting that (1) the foot has many sensory receptors to detect forces and deformations acting on it, (2) the sensors detected input signals into the foot with patient-specific thresholds, and (3) individuals with similar sensitivity thresholds seem to respond to their movement patterns in a similar way.[132] They suggested that force signals from the floor were filtered by the shoe, the orthosis, and finally by the plantar surface of the foot, which then transferred the filtered information to the central nervous system. The central nervous system, in turn, prompted dynamic responses in the lower extremity on the basis of patient-specific conditions. Comfort of the orthosis is an important consideration; a comfortable orthosis is likely to minimize muscular work during walking. According to Nigg and colleagues,[132] an optimal orthosis would reduce muscle activity, feel comfortable, and improve musculoskeletal and neuromuscular performance in walking.

Based on his analysis of the role of impact forces on foot function in gait, Nigg[133] proposed a new paradigm focusing on locomotor systems and strategies for impact and movement control. The dynamical systems model of motor control suggests that locomotor systems keep general kinematic and kinetic situations similar for any given task. Nigg suggests that a muscle tuning reaction occurs to cause forces that affect muscle activation before ground contact, and that muscle adaptation (to ensure constant joint movement pattern) affects muscle activation during ground contact. The interplay of realignment of the skeleton and locomotor system muscle tuning affects joint and tendon loading and, in turn, fatigue, comfort, work, and performance.[133]

Electromyographic Evidence

Several recent studies have suggested that the neuromuscular mechanisms proposed by Nigg and colleagues[132,133] are affected by orthoses. Mundermann and colleagues[134] studied 21 recreational runners who used a flat shoe insert, posting alone, custom-molded orthoses, and custom-molded orthoses and posting. They analyzed the effects of each condition on lower extremity kinematics, kinetics, and electromyographic data as well as comfort during use. Thirty-five percent of differences in comfort were explained by changes in 15 kinematic, kinetic, and electromyographic variables, and these 15 variables correctly classified the corresponding orthotic condition in 75% of cases. Mundermann and colleagues[134] suggested that comfort not only reflected subjective perceptions but was also related to biomechanical variables. In an extension of their work, Mundermann and colleagues[135] observed that the effects of molding were more important than posting on change in kinematic and kinetic variables.

Nawoczenski and Ludewig[136] examined electromyographic activity of lower extremity muscles of 12 symptomatic recreational runners during the first 50% of the stance phase, comparing electromyographic signals in two conditions: when using custom-molded, semirigid orthoses and shoes without orthoses. Surface electromyographic activity data of the tibialis anterior, medial gastrocnemius, vastus medialis, vastus lateralis, and biceps femoris were collected while the patients ran on a treadmill. Although electromyographic activity was not different in the medial gastrocnemius, vastus medialis, or vastus lateralis with orthotic use, a decrease in biceps femoris activity and an increase in tibialis anterior activity occurred with orthotic use. The activity for patients was concluded to be highly individualized.

Bird and colleagues[137] considered electromyographic activity of lumbar erector spinae and gluteus medius muscles with prefabricated foot wedges (a 5-degree lateral wedge, a 5-degree medial wedge, or a 2-cm heel wedge). Although no change in amplitude of electromyographic signal occurred, wedging at the heel and lateral forefoot led to earlier electromyographic activity of the erector spinae. Gluteus muscle activity was delayed with bilateral heel wedges, as was ipsilateral gluteus activity when a unilateral heel wedge was used. Although changes of onset for the erector spinae and gluteus medius averaged only 4% and 2% of the gait cycle, respectively, the researchers suggested that these changes are likely to be clinically significant over the course of a day.

Vanicek and colleagues[138] considered how foot orthoses affected the ability of six healthy alpine skiers to hold a skier's squat position and on the duration of fatigue of the vastus lateralis. Individuals were examined under three conditions: no orthoses, high-volume orthoses, and low-volume orthoses (based on the amount of foam incorporated into the orthosis). A decrease in median firing frequencies toward the end of contraction suggested that high-volume orthoses reduced

myoelectric fatigue. However, no significant differences in the ability to sustain a squat occurred under the three conditions.

Postural Control

If neuromuscular systems play a role in the effectiveness of orthoses, changes in balance and posture control would be anticipated with their use. Guskiewicz and Perrin[139] examined the effects of custom orthoses in 13 patients with acute ankle inversion sprains and in 12 noninjured patients. As anticipated, orthoses reduced postural sway in the medial and lateral and inversion and eversion directions, with a larger effect in patients who had the injury. The researchers propose that, by restricting undesirable motions, the orthoses enhanced the ability of joint mechanoreceptors to detect movement. In contrast, Hertel and colleagues[140] found that six different orthotic interventions (shoe only; molded Aquaplast orthoses [Aquaplast Thermoplastics, Wyckoff, NJ]; orthoses in the neutral, medially posted, and laterally posted positions; and a prefabricated, rigid, laterally posted heel wedge) did not influence postural sway in 15 patients with unilateral ankle sprains while they performed unilateral standing. None of the orthotic conditions decreased frontal or sagittal postural sway compared with shoes alone. Hertel and colleagues[141] also studied 15 healthy patients with normally aligned feet under the same six conditions, focusing on center of pressure length and velocity in both the frontal and sagittal planes during unilateral stance. In this study, sagittal plane motion was not different among the various conditions; however, medially posted orthoses reduced frontal plane motion more than the other conditions. Frontal plane center of pressure excursion increased with a prefabricated, rigid, laterally posted heel wedge compared with medially and neutrally posted conditions. Frontal plane velocity was lower with medial posting compared with a prefabricated, rigid, laterally posted heel wedge and neutral orthoses. The prefabricated, rigid, laterally posted heel wedge, however, produced significantly greater frontal plane velocities than the medially or laterally posted conditions.

Percy and Menz[142] found that orthoses did not affect postural stability in 30 professional soccer players in bipedal, dominant leg, and tandem stance. Sway was assessed under four conditions: barefoot, soccer shoes only, soccer shoes with soft insoles, and soccer shoes with rigid orthoses. The researchers concluded that orthoses had no beneficial or detrimental effects in the elite athletes studied. In contrast, Olmsted and Hertel[143] found that foot orthoses differentially benefit those with various foot types. They assessed static and dynamic postural control in 30 patients grouped by rectus, planus, or cavus foot type. Patients wore custom-molded, semirigid foot orthoses for 2 weeks between baseline and posttest measurement. Improvement in reach occurred in three of eight directions on the Star Excursion Balance Test in those with cavus foot type. Patients with cavus foot type also demonstrated a decreased center of pressure velocity in static stance.

Rome and Brown[144] examined postural sway in 50 patients identified as pronators (per the Foot Posture Index) in a randomized clinical trial. Patients were assigned either to a control or orthotic group. The orthotic group wore prefabricated, high-density ethyl vinyl acetate orthoses with low-density ethyl vinyl acetate rearfoot wedging for 4 weeks. At 4 weeks, medial-lateral sway decreased in the orthotic group; however, no differences in anterior-posterior sway or mean balance occurred between the groups.

Collectively, these studies suggest that orthoses do affect electromyographic activity, balance, and postural control. Health professionals may be better able to identify those most likely to benefit from orthotic intervention if measures of postural control and neuromuscular function are incorporated along with the assessment of lower extremity and foot skeletal alignment.

MANAGEMENT OF OVERUSE INJURIES

Although the specific biomechanical and neurological effects of foot orthoses on walking and running are not completely understood, orthoses can and do reduce symptoms and improve function. Although current evidence does not include many randomized, controlled clinical trials, the available evidence does support efficacy of orthotic intervention in the management of lower extremity injuries.

Pain Associated with Foot Deformity

Riegler[145] surveyed 235 individuals provided with molded thermoplastic orthoses for a variety of lower extremity injuries. In 176 returned surveys (75% return rate), 20.5% demonstrated complete improvement in symptoms, 29.5% reported a 75% improvement, 29.5% reported 50% improvement, 13.6% reported 25% improvement, and 6.8% reported no improvement. D'Ambrosia[146] reported on 200 individuals who had used orthoses to manage a variety of running injuries, including posterior tibial syndrome, pes planovalgum, metatarsalgia, plantar fasciitis, and iliotibial band tendonitis. Almost all had severe pronation with forefoot varus before prescription of an orthosis. Rates of reported improvement were quite high: 73% in posterior tibial syndrome, 90% in pes planovalgum, 86% in metatarsalgia, 82% in plantar fasciitis, and 66% in iliotibial band syndrome. Of those with cavus foot type, only 25% showed improvement with orthotic use.

Donatelli and colleagues[147] received follow-up surveys from 53 (65%) of 81 individuals who had previously been fitted with custom-molded, semirigid orthoses for pes planus and chondromalacia, with 95% having a forefoot varus deformity. All respondents had a 6- to 8-week trial of temporary orthoses modified according to alterations in pain before receiving custom-molded, semirigid orthoses. Respondents were asked to describe or rate pain relief with orthoses, orthotic satisfaction, continued use of orthoses,

and ability to return to previous level of activity. Ninety-six percent of respondents reported pain relief, 91% were satisfied with their orthoses, 94% were still wearing their orthoses (length of time with orthoses varied from 3 months to 2 years from time surveyed), and 70% were able to return to their previous level of activity.

Moraros and Hodge[148] surveyed 525 individuals who used custom-fitted orthoses provided by podiatric physicians to determine effectiveness and patient satisfaction. Of the 453 records completed in useable form (89% response rate), the chief symptom was fully resolved in 62.5%, partially resolved in 32.8%, and unresolved in 4.7%. Overall satisfaction for fit and quality was 83.1%. Although limitations are inherent in survey research, the relatively high response rate and sample support the usefulness of orthoses in relieving painful foot symptoms.

Patellofemoral Pain Syndrome

The effect of foot orthoses on patellofemoral joint pain has been the subject of several studies. Tiberio[48] presented a model in which excessive pronation and associated lower extremity rotation explain abnormal lateral articular compression at the knee. Compensatory internal rotation of the femur in response to increased internal rotation of the tibia produced by excessive subtalar pronation is a potential cause of dysfunction. Based on evidence about orthotic effects on lower extremity biomechanics, this explanation is plausible.

Eng and Pierrynowski[87] evaluated the effect of soft foot orthotics on patellofemoral pain syndrome (PFPS) of at least 6 weeks' duration in 20 adolescent women with excessive pronation. A control group performed exercise (stretching of quadriceps and hamstrings, isometric quadriceps exercise, isotonic hamstring strengthening).[10] An experimental group participated in exercise and wore soft orthoses with medial posts at the forefoot and rearfoot (to position the STJ closer to neutral position).[10] Over an 8-week period, patients rated their pain during various activities by using a visual analog scale. Although both groups reported less pain over time, the total reduction in pain was greater in the orthotic group at weeks 4, 6, and 8.

In a single subject design, Way[149] investigated the use of a custom-molded thermoplastic foot orthosis on PFPS in a 19-year-old collegiate softball player with a mild forefoot varus bilaterally and increased midfoot pronation during MSt and TSt. Intervention included pain-free stretching and strengthening exercise, modalities, and nonsteroidal anti-inflammatory medication. The study design involved a 13-day baseline phase, a 17-day intervention phase (after which the patient removed orthoses for an 11-day withdrawal phase), and a second intervention phase in which orthoses were reintroduced for the last 32 days of the study. Pain was rated by a visual analog scale, and function was evaluated with the Functional Index Questionnaire. Pain decreased in each consecutive phase; function improved between phases for seven of the nine functional activities assessed in the Functional Index Questionnaire. On the basis of these findings, Way[149] suggested that orthotic intervention is appropriate for PFPS.

Saxena and Haddad[150] retrospectively reviewed 102 outcomes of interventions in individuals with chondromalacia patella, retropatellar dysplasia, or PFPS. Multiple interventions were noted, including semiflexible orthotics. Overall, 76.5% of patients demonstrated a reduction in pain and improved function, and 2% were asymptomatic after a 2- to 4-week intervention period.

Sutlive and colleagues[151] sought to identify characteristics of patients with PFPS likely to improve with a combination of orthoses and modified activity. They examined 50 patients in active military duty who had symptoms of PFPS during a partial squat or when ascending stairs. Measures included (1) rearfoot alignment in STN, (2) forefoot to rearfoot alignment, (3) navicular drop, (4) RCS, (5) Q angle, (6) tibial varum or valgum, (7) tibial torsion, (8) leg length, and (9) standard goniometric and postural test positions to determine ROM and tissue tightness. Patients wore unposted, premolded, full-length insoles with full arch support and heel cushioning for 21 days while concurrently limiting various activities. All completed a visual analog scale and a Global Rating of Change Questionnaire at baseline and at the end of the intervention period. Thirty-three of 50 patients completed the study, with a total of 78 knees with PFPS (many had bilateral symptoms). Data from 27 patients who demonstrated 50% or more improvement in visual analog scale scores were examined to determine which patient characteristics could predict orthotic success. Likehood ratios identified several predictors of successful outcome: forefoot valgus of 2 degrees or more, great toe extension of 78 degrees or less, and navicular drop of 3 mm or less. Of those with PFPS, the patients with these three characteristics were more likely to respond to orthotic intervention.

In a systematic review of the literature on the theoretical and research basis for the use of foot orthoses in PFPS, Gross and Foxworth[152] concluded that "taken together, the studies . . . suggest that foot orthoses may improve symptoms of pain and ratings of physical function for patients with patellofemoral pain who demonstrate excessive foot pronation." They emphasized the need for additional randomized trials with reliable outcome measures and careful definition of patient inclusion criteria.

Plantar Fasciitis

The use of foot orthoses in the management of plantar fasciitis has also been examined. A multicenter study by Pfeffer and colleagues[153] compared the effectiveness of prefabricated and custom orthoses on acute plantar fasciitis pain in 200 of 236 patients receiving care. All patients performed end Achilles and plantar fascia stretching exercises for 10 minutes twice a day. Patients were randomly assigned to one of five

intervention groups: (1) stretching only, (2) silicon heel pad, (3) felt heel insert, (4) rubber heel cup, and (5) a custom-made polypropylene neutral orthosis. All were examined and completed questionnaires and the pain subscale of the Foot Function Index at baseline and after 8 weeks of intervention. Reduction in pain after intervention was 95% for the silicon insert group, 88% for the rubber insert group, 81% for the felt insert group, 72% for the stretching only group, and 68% for the custom orthoses group. When prefabricated groups were combined, the rate of improvement was higher than stretching alone, and those who stretched alone were significantly improved compared with the custom-made orthoses group. In interpreting study results, several limitations must be considered; patients were not grouped by foot type, and all custom orthoses were made in neutral position without posting.

Gross and colleagues[154] studied 15 individuals with plantar fasciitis for at least 1 month. Eight patients had excessively pronated feet, and seven had a cavus foot type. Eleven of 15 had unsuccessfully used noncustom arch supports before enrollment in the study. At baseline, patients completed the pain and disability index of the Foot Function Index, were timed during a 100-m walk, and rated pain experienced during the walk with the visual analog scale. They received custom-fabricated, posted, multilayer orthoses with a thermoplastic core and were reevaluated after 12 to 17 days of orthotic use. Although no differences in preintervention and postintervention walk times occurred, visual analog scale pain ratings after the walk were lower than baseline, with only one patient demonstrating increased pain after the walk test. The scores on the subsections of the Foot Function Index also improved after orthotic use, with improvement of 66% in the pain subscale and 75% in the disability subscale. All patients continued to wear their orthoses at a follow-up phone call made 2 to 6 months after testing.

Seligman and Dawson[155] retrospectively evaluated 10 older individuals (mean age, 71 years) with heel pain from plantar fasciitis who used a heel pad made of Sorbothane (Sorbothane, Inc., Kent, Ohio) attached to a custom-molded, medium-density Plastazote insert reinforced with cork in the medial longitudinal arch. Duration of pain ranged from 6 months to several years; 5 of 10 patients previously tried other interventions. Pain was rated by a 10-point Likert pain rating scale. A significant difference occurred between baseline pain ratings (5.7/10) and postintervention pain ratings (1.85/10). The authors suggested that this orthosis, costing approximately $25 to fabricate, is an effective first-line intervention for painful plantar fasciitis in older adults.

Morton's Neuroma

Kilmartin and Wallace[156] found that orthotic intervention did not improve symptoms of Morton's neuroma. Twenty-three individuals with pain of the third and fourth intermetatarsal space, aggravated by exercise and relieved by rest, were randomly assigned to two groups, with no consideration of foot type. Those in the supination group wore a Cobra orthosis with a thicker medial heel and arch filler. Those in the pronation group wore a reverse Cobra orthosis with a thicker lateral heel. Pain was measured by a visual analog scale. Sensory impairment and pain were objectively measured by tests that elicit neuroma pain. Function was assessed with the McMaster-Toronto Arthritis Patient Function Preference Questionnaire patient-specific measure of maximal function. No differences in pain or function occurred between the supination and pronation groups. Neither orthosis produced additional symptoms in the lower extremity.

The authors suggested that prescribing a custom orthosis based on foot type would have provided greater relief of symptoms.

Low Back Pain

Dananberg and Guiliano[157] examined the effects of orthotic intervention in 32 patients with chronic low pain. Patients completed the Quebec Back Pain Disability Scale at baseline, after wearing foot orthoses for 1 month, and after wearing orthoses for at least 6 months. The Quebec Scale provided a back pain score and a disability score. Permanent orthoses were fabricated on the basis of the results of temporary orthoses with modifications specific to each patient, in-shoe pressure analysis, gait video analysis, and clinical examination. At 1 month, significant reduction was observed in the mean pain and disability scores. Twenty-three of the original 32 patients were contacted at 6-month follow-up and reported significant improvement in function and reduction in pain. In comparing their outcomes to previous work by Kopec and colleagues,[158] who used the Quebec Back Pain Disability Scale to evaluate improvement in 178 patients undergoing standard back care interventions, the authors suggested that the use of foot orthoses enhanced outcomes over traditional back care. Of note, the protocol for evaluating patients for permanent orthoses was extensive.[157]

Although few randomized, controlled clinical studies have been undertaken, and most have been done with a small sample size in specific patient populations, current evidence supports that foot orthoses reduce symptoms of pain and improve function in individuals with overuse injury. Foot structure and type, orthotic materials, posting methods, and fabrication methods must be considered in determining who is likely to respond to orthotic intervention and comparing the effectiveness of various orthotic interventions.

SUMMARY

Although many components of Root's theory have been questioned, little doubt is present concerning the importance of his work in the field of foot biomechanics and orthotic intervention. Root's work provides a foundation for most of

the research performed to gain a better understanding of the influence of the foot on lower extremity biomechanics and overuse injuries. Although research has provided some answers about mechanisms underlying efficacy of orthotic intervention, many more questions have also been raised. Additional research is necessary before clinicians will be able to prescribe orthoses confidently based on likely outcomes.

The effectiveness of biomechanical foot orthoses depends on a number of factors. An understanding of causes and effects of aberrant foot motion on pathological conditions of the foot is essential in determining the appropriate orthosis prescription and plan of care. Clinicians who do not carefully consider biomechanical principles and other factors that contribute to clinical signs and symptoms are likely to prescribe an ineffective or inappropriate orthosis. Information gathered from all three components of the biomechanical examination (non–weight-bearing, static weight-bearing, and dynamic gait assessment) is critical for orthotic design and prescription.

Historically, the principles and design of the Root functional orthosis and the biomechanical foot orthosis have had consistently effective clinical results. Root's model demands a keen understanding of foot biomechanics, careful prescription, and advanced fabrication skills. With this understanding and attention to detail, the end result may be a lightweight, durable, cost-effective foot orthosis that substantially reduces the detrimental effects of aberrant foot motion.

REFERENCES

1. Olson WR. Orthotic materials. In Valmassy RL (ed), *Clinical Biomechanics of the Lower Extremities,* St. Louis: Mosby–Year Book, 1996. pp. 307-326.
2. Kirby KA. The medial heel skive technique. Improving pronation control in foot orthoses. *J Am Podiatry Med Assoc* 1992;82(4):177-188.
3. Shuster RO. A history of orthopaedics in podiatry. *J Am Podiatry Assoc* 1974;64(5):322.
4. Rossi WA. Orthotics: the miracle cure-all? *Footwear News* 1995;22.
5. Root ML, Orien WP, Weed JH. *Normal and Abnormal Function of the Foot,* vol 2, Los Angeles: Clinical Biomechanics Corporation, 1977.
6. Burns ML. Biomechanics. In McGlamry ED (ed), *Fundamentals of Foot Surgery,* Baltimore: Williams & Wilkins, 1987. pp. 111-135.
7. Barnett CH, Napier JR. The axis of rotation at the ankle joint in man. Its influence upon the form of the talus and the mobility of the fibula. *J Anat (Lond)* 1952;86:1-9.
8. Hicks JH. The mechanics of the foot. Part I: the joints. *J Anat* 1953;87:345-347.
9. Isman RE, Inman VT. Anthropometric studies of the human foot and ankle. *Bull Prosthet Res* 1969;10-11:97-129.
10. Morris JM. Biomechanics of the foot and ankle. *Clin Orthop* 1977;122(1):10-17.
11. Norkin CC, Levangie PK. The ankle foot complex. In Levangie PK, Edd CC, Norkin PT (eds), *Joint Structure and Function: A Comprehensive Analysis,* 2nd ed. Philadelphia: F.A. Davis, 1992. pp. 379-419.
12. American Orthopedics Association. *Manual of Orthopedic Surgery,* Chicago: American Orthopedics Association, 1972.
13. Boone DC, Azen SP. Normal range of motion of joints in male subjects. *J Bone Joint Surg* 1979;61A(5):756-759.
14. Rasmussen O, Tovberg-Jevsen I. Mobility of the ankle joint. *Acta Orthop Scand* 1982;53(1):155-160.
15. Lapidius PW. Kinesiology and mechanics of the tarsal joints. *Clin Orthop* 1963;30:20-35.
16. Kjaergaard-Andersen P, Wethelund J, Nielsen S. Lateral talocalcaneal instability following section of the calcaneofibular ligament: a kinesiologic study. *Foot Ankle* 1987;7(6):355-361.
17. Manter JT. Movements of the subtalar and transverse tarsal joints. *Anat Rec* 1941;80:397-410.
18. Phillips RD, Christeck R, Phillips RL. Clinical measurement of the axis of the subtalar joint. *J Am Podiatry Assoc* 1985;75(3):119-131.
19. Green DR, Carol A. Planal dominance. *J Am Podiatry Med Assoc* 1984;74(2):98-103.
20. Perry J. Anatomy and biomechanics of the hindfoot. *Clin Orthop* 1983;177(1):9-15.
21. Olerud C, Rosendahl Y. Torsion-transmitting properties of the hindfoot. *Clin Orthop* 1987;Jan(214):285-294.
22. Warwick R, Williams PL (eds). *Gray's Anatomy,* 35th ed. Philadelphia: Saunders, 1973. pp. 373-385, 460-471, 571-585.
23. Elftman H. The transverse tarsal joint and its control. *Clin Orthop* 1960;16:41-45.
24. Sarrafian SK. *Anatomy of the Foot and Ankle: Descriptive, Topographic, and Functional,* Philadelphia: J.B. Lippincott, 1983.
25. Moore KL. *Clinically Oriented Anatomy,* Baltimore: Williams & Wilkins, 1980.
26. Hicks JH. The mechanics of the foot. Part II: the plantar aponeurosis and the arch. *J Anat* 1954;88:25-31.
27. Sarafian SK. Functional characteristics of the foot and plantar aponeurosis under tibiotalar loading. *Foot Ankle* 1987;8(1):1-4.
28. Perry J. *Gait Analysis: Normal and Pathological Function,* Thorofare, NJ: Slack, 1992. pp. 69-85.
29. Vaughn CL, Davis DL, O'Connor JC. *Dynamics of Human Gait,* Champaign, Ill: Human Kinetics, 1992. pp. 7-14.
30. James SL, Jones DC. Biomechanical aspects of distance running injuries. In Cavanagh PR (ed), *Biomechanics of Distance Running,* Champaign, Ill: Human Kinetics, 1990. pp. 249-271.
31. Wright DG, Desai M, Henderson WH. Action of the subtalar and ankle-joint complex during the stance phase of walking. *J Bone Joint Surg* 1964;46A(2):361-382.
32. Perry J, Hislop HJ. *Principles of Lower Extremity Bracing,* Washington, DC: American Physical Therapy Association, 1967. pp. 9-32.
33. Close JR, Todd FN. The phasic activity of the muscles of the lower extremity and the effect of tendon transfer. *J Bone Joint Surg* 1959;41A(2):189-208.
34. Valiant GA. Transmission and attenuation of heelstrike accelerations. In Cavanagh PR (ed), *Biomechanics of Distance Running,* Champaign, IL: Human Kinetics, 1990. pp. 225-249.

35. McPoil TG, Hunt GC. Evaluation and management of foot and ankle disorders. Present problems and future directions. *J Occup Sports Phys Ther* 1995;21(6):381-388.
36. Picciano AM, Rowlands MS, Worrell T. Reliability of open and closed kinetic chain subtalar joint neutral positions and navicular drop test. *J Occup Sports Phys Ther* 1993;18(4): 553-558.
37. Smith-Oricchio K, Harris BE. Interrater reliability of subtalar neutral, calcaneal inversion and eversion. *J Occup Sports Phys Ther* 1990;12(1):10-15.
38. Gross MT. Lower quarter screening for skeletal malalignment. Suggestions for orthotics and shoewear. *J Occup Sports Phys Ther* 1995;21(6):389-405.
39. Pratt D, Tollafield D, Johnson G, et al. Foot orthoses. In Wallace WA (ed), *Biomechanical Basis of Orthotic Management,* Oxford: Butterworth-Heinemann, 1993. pp. 70-98.
40. Wooden MJ. Biomechanical evaluation for functional orthotics. In Donatelli RA (ed), *The Biomechanics of the Foot and Ankle,* 2nd ed. Philadelphia: F.A. Davis, 1996. pp. 168-183.
41. McPoil TG, Brocato RS. The foot and ankle. In Gould JA, Davis GJ (eds), *Orthopaedics and Sports Physical Therapy,* St. Louis: Mosby, 1985. pp. 322-325.
42. Anthony RJ. *The Manufacture and Use of the Functional Foot Orthosis,* Basel, Switzerland: Karger, 1991. pp. 1-178.
43. Elveru RA, Rothstein JM, Lamb RC. Goniometric reliability in a clinical setting. Subtalar and ankle joint measurements. *Phys Ther* 1988;68(5):672-677.
44. Garbalosa JC, McClure MH, Catlin PA, et al. The frontal plane relationship of the forefoot to the rearfoot in an asymptomatic population. *J Occup Sports Phys Ther* 1994;20(4):200-206.
45. Lattanza L, Gray GW, Kantner RM. Closed versus open kinematic chain measurements of subtalar joint eversion. Implications for clinical practice. *J Occup Sports Phys Ther* 1988;9(9):310-314.
46. Diamond JE, Mueller MJ, Delitto A, et al. Reliability of a diabetic foot evaluation. *Phys Ther* 1989;69:797-802.
47. Vitasalo JT, Kvist M. Some biomechanical aspects of the foot and ankle in athletes with and without shin splints. *Am J Sports Med* 1983;2(3):125-130.
48. Tiberio D. Evaluation of functional ankle dorsiflexion using subtalar neutral position. *Phys Ther* 1987;67(6):955-957.
49. Baggett BD, Young G. Ankle joint dorsiflexion. Establishment of a normal range. *J Am Podiatry Med Assoc* 1993;83(5): 251-254.
50. Hillstrom HJ, Perlberg G, Sieglers S, et al. Objective identification of ankle equinus deformity and resulting contracture. *J Am Podiatry Med Assoc* 1991;81(10):519-524.
51. Hill RS. Ankle equinus: prevalence and linkage to common foot pathology. *J Am Podiatry Assoc* 1995;85(6):295-300.
52. D'Ambrosia RD. Orthotic devices in running injuries. *Clin Sports Med* 1985;4(4):611-619.
53. Hoppenfeld S. *Physical Examination of the Spine and Extremities,* Norwalk, Conn: Appleton-Century-Crofts, 1976. pp. 197-235.
54. Tachdjian MO. *The Child's Foot,* Philadelphia: Saunders, 1985.
55. McGlamry ED, Kitting RW. Equinus foot. An analysis of the etiology, pathology, and treatment techniques. *J Am Podiatry Assoc* 1973;63:165.
56. Whitney AK, Green DR. Pseudo equinus. *J Am Podiatry Assoc* 1982;72:365.
57. Davidson RS. Deformities of the child's foot. In Sammarco JG (ed), *Foot and Ankle Manual,* Philadelphia: Lea & Febiger, 1991. p. 296.
58. Donatelli RA. Abnormal biomechanics. In Donatelli RA (ed), *The Biomechanics of the Foot and Ankle,* Philadelphia: F.A. Davis, 1990. pp. 32-65.
59. McPoil TG, Knecht HG, Schuit D. A survey of foot types in normal females between the ages of 18 and 30 years. *J Occup Sports Phys Ther* 1988;9(12):346-349.
60. Dananberg HJ. Gait style as an etiology to chronic postural pain. Part I: functional hallux limitus. *J Am Podiatry Med Assoc* 1993;83(8):433-441.
61. Dananberg HJ. Gait style as an etiology to chronic postural pain. Part II: postural compensatory process. *J Am Podiatry Med Assoc* 1993;83(11):615-624.
62. Gastwirth BW. Biomechanical examination of the foot and lower extremity. In Valmassy RL (ed), *Clinical Biomechanics of the Lower Extremities,* St. Louis: Mosby–Year Book, 1996. pp. 132-147.
63. Tomaro J. Measurement of tibiofibular varum in subjects with unilateral overuse symptoms. *J Occup Sports Phys Ther* 1995;21(2):86-89.
64. McPoil TG, Schuit D, Knecht HG. A comparison of three positions used to evaluate tibial varum. *J Am Podiatry Med Assoc* 1988;78(1):22-28.
65. Lohmann KN, Rayhel HE, Schneiderwind P, et al. Static measurement of tibial vara. Reliability and effect of lower extremity position. *Phys Ther* 1987;67(2):196-200.
66. Brody D. Techniques in evaluation and treatment of the injured runner. *Orthop Clin North Am* 1982;13(3): 541-558.
67. Subotnick SI. Biomechanics of the subtalar and midtarsal joints. *J Am Podiatry Assoc* 1975;65(8):756-764.
68. Mueller MJ, Host JV, Norton BJ. Navicular drop as a composite measure of excessive pronation. *J Am Podiatry Med Assoc* 1993;83(4):198-202.
69. Norkin C, Levangie P. *Joint Structure and Function: A Comprehensive Analysis,* Philadelphia: F.A. Davis, 1983. pp. 261-387.
70. Dahle LK, Mueller M, Delitto A, et al. Visual assessment of foot type and relationship of foot type to lower extremity injury. *J Occup Sports Phys Ther* 1991;14(2):70-74.
71. Close JR, Inman VT, Poor PM, et al. The function of the subtalar joint. *Clin Orthop* 1967;50(1-2):159-179.
72. Donatelli R, Hurlbert C, Conaway D, et al. Biomechanical foot orthotics. A retrospective study. *J Occup Sports Phys Ther* 1988;10(6):205-212.
73. Inman VT, Rolston HJ, Todd F. *Human Walking,* Baltimore: Williams & Wilkins, 1981.
74. Johnson MA, Donatelli R, Wooden M, et al. Effects of three different posting methods on controlling abnormal subtalar pronation. *Phys Ther* 1994;74(2):149-161.
75. Schumacher HR. *Primer of the Rheumatoid Diseases,* 10th ed. Atlanta: The Arthritis Foundation, 1993.

76. Harper MC. Failed treatment and residual deformity of the midfoot and hindfoot. In Sammarco JG (ed), *Foot and Ankle Manual,* Philadelphia: Lea & Febiger, 1991. pp. 212-213.
77. Boulton A. Diabetic neuropathy. In Frykberg RG (ed), *The High Risk Foot in Diabetes Mellitus,* New York: Churchill Livingstone, 1991. pp. 49-59.
78. Valmassy RL. Advantages and disadvantages of various casting techniques. *J Am Podiatry Assoc* 1979;69(12):707-712.
79. McPoil TG, Schuit D, Knecht HG. Comparison of three methods used to obtain a neutral plaster foot impression. *Phys Ther* 1989;69(6):448-450.
80. Kirby KA. Troubleshooting functional foot orthoses. In Valmassy RL (ed), *Clinical Biomechanics of the Lower Extremities,* St. Louis: Mosby–Year Book, 1996. pp. 327-348.
81. Philps JW. *The Functional Foot Orthosis,* Edinburgh: Churchill Livingstone, 1995. pp. 39-53.
82. Blake RL, Ferguson H. Extrinsic rearfoot posts. *J Am Podiatry Med Assoc* 1992;82(4):202-207.
83. Blake RL, Ferguson HJ. Effect of extrinsic rearfoot posts on rearfoot position. *J Am Podiatry Med Assoc* 1993;83(8):202.
84. Brown GP, Donatelli R, Catlin PA, et al. The effects of two types of foot orthoses on rearfoot mechanics. *J Occup Sports Phys Ther* 1995;21(5):258-267.
85. Smith LS, Clarke TE, Hamill CL, et al. The effects of soft and semi-rigid orthoses upon movement in running. *J Am Podiatry Med Assoc* 1986;76(4):227-233.
86. Eng JJ, Pierrynowski MR. The effects of soft foot orthotics on three-dimensional lower-limb kinematics during walking and running. *Phys Ther* 1994;74(9):836-844.
87. Eng JJ, Pierrynowski MR. Evaluation of soft foot orthotics in the treatment of patellofemoral pain syndrome. *Phys Ther* 1993;73(2):62-70.
88. Rodgers MM, Leveau BF. Effectiveness of foot orthotic devices used to modify pronation in runners. *J Occup Sports Phys Ther* 1982;4(2):86-90.
89. McPoil TG, Hunt GC. *An Evaluation and Treatment Paradigm for the Future in Physical Therapy of the Foot and Ankle,* 2nd ed. Philadelphia: Churchill Livingstone, 1995. pp. 1-10.
90. Sobel E, Levitz SJ. Reappraisal of the negative impression cast and the subtalar joint neutral position. *J Am Podiatr Med Assoc* 1997;8(1):32-33.
91. Payne CB. The past present and future of podiatric biomechanics. *J Am Podiatr Med Assoc* 1998;88(2):53-63.
92. Payne C, Chuter V. The clash between theory and science of the kinematic effectiveness of foot orthoses. *Clin Podiatr Med Surg* 2001;18(4):705-713.
93. Lee WE, Podiatric biomechanics. An historical appraisal and discussion of the Root model as a clinical system of approach in the present context of theoretical uncertainty. *Clin Podiatr Med Surg* 2001;18(4):555-684.
94. Ball KA, Afheldt MJ. Evolution of foot orthotics-part 1: coherent theory or coherent practice. *J Manipulative Physiol Ther* 2002;25(2):116-124.
95. Ball KA, Afheldt MJ. Evolution of foot orthotics-part 2: research reshapes long-standing theory. *J Manipulative Physiol Ther* 2002;25(2):125-134.
96. Payne CB, Bird AR. Teaching clinical biomechanics in the context of uncertainty. *J Am Podiatr Med Assoc* 1999;89(10):525-530.
97. Pierrynowski MR, Smith SB, Mlynarczyk JH. Proficiency of foot care specialists to place the rearfoot at subtalar neutral. *J Am Podiatr Med Assoc* 1996;86:217-223.
98. Cook A, Gorman I, Morris J. Evaluation of the neutral position of the subtalar joint. *J Am Podiatr Med Assoc* 1988;78:449-451.
99. Wright DG, Desai SM, Henderson WH. Action of the subtalar joint and ankle joint complex during the stance phase of walking. *J Bone Joint Surg (Am)* 1964;46A:361-382.
100. Root ML, Orien WP, Weed JH, et al. *Biomechanical Examination of the Foot,* vol 1. Los Angeles: Clinical Biomechanics, 1971.
101. McPoil TG, Cornwall MW. Relationship between neutral subtalar joint position and pattern of rearfoot motion during walking. *Foot Ankle Int* 1996;15:141-145.
102. Pierrynowski MR, Smith SB. Rear foot inversion/eversion during gait relative to the subtalar joint neutral position. *Foot Ankle Int* 1996;17(7):406-412.
103. Astrom M, Arvidson T. Alignment and joint motion in the normal foot. *J Orthop Sports Phys Ther* 1995;22(5):216-222.
104. Razeghi M, Batt ME. Biomechanical analysis of the effect of orthotic shoe inserts; review of the literature. *Sports Med* 2000;29(6):425-438.
105. Hamill J, Bates BT, Knutzen KM, et al. Relationship between selected static and dynamic lower extremity measures. *Clin Biomech* 1989;4:217-225.
106. Knutzen KM, Price A. Lower extremity static and dynamic relationships with rearfoot motion in gait. *J Am Podiatr Med Assoc* 1994;84:171-80.
107. McPoil TG, Comwall MW. The relationship between static lower extremity measurements and rearfoot motion during walking. *J Orthop Sports Phys Ther* 1996;24(5):304-314.
108. Dahle LK, Mueller M, Delitto A, et al. Visual assessment of foot types and relationship of foot type to lower extremity injury. *J Orthop Sports Phys Ther* 1991;14(2):70-74.
109. Powers CM, Maffucci R, Hampton S. Rearfoot posture in subjects with patellofemoral pain. *J Orthop Sports Phys Ther* 1995;22(4):155-160.
110. Sommer HM, Vallentyne SW. Effect of foot posture on the incidence of medial tibial stress syndrome. *Med Sci Sports Exerc* 1995;27(6):800-804.
111. Donatelli R, Wooden M, Ekedahl SR, et al. Relationship between static and dynamic foot postures in professional baseball players. *J Orthop Sports Phys Ther* 1999;29(6):316-330.
112. Cowan DN, Jones BH, Robinson JR. Medial longitudinal arch height and risk of training-associated injury. *Med Sci Sports Exerc* 1989;21(suppl):S60.
113. Cowan DN, Jones BH, Robinson JR. Foot morphology and alignment and risk of exercise-related injury in runners. *Arch Fam Med* 1993;2:273-277.
114. Novick A, Kelley D. Position and movement changes of the foot with orthotic intervention during the loading response of gait. *J Orthop Sports Phys Ther* 1990;11(7):301-312.
115. Bates BT, Osternig LR, Mason B, et al. Foot orthotic devices to modify selected aspects of lower extremity mechanics. *Am J Sports Med* 1979;7:338-342.
116. Clark TE, Fredrick EC, Hlavac HF. Effects of a soft orthotic device on rearfoot movements in running. *Pod Sports Med* 1983;1(1):26-33.

117. McCulloch MU, Brunt D, Vanderlinden D, The effect of foot orthotics and gait velocity on lower limb kinematics and temporal events of stance. *J Orthop Sports Phys Ther* 1993;17(1):2-10.
118. Johanson MA, Donatelli R, Woodon MJ, et al. Effects of three different posting methods on controlling abnormal subtalar pronation. *Phys Ther* 1994;74(2):149-161.
119. Genova JM, Gross MT. Effect of foot orthotics on calcaneal eversion during standing and treadmill walking for subjects with abnormal pronation. *J Orthop Sports Phys Ther* 2000;30(11):664-675.
120. Branthwaite HR, Payton CJ, Chockalingam N. The effect of simple insoles on three-dimensional foot motion during normal walking. *Clin Biomech* 2004;19(9):972-977.
121. Brown GP, Donatelli R, Catlin PA, et al. The effect of two types of foot orthoses on rearfoot mechanics. *J Orthop Sports Phys Ther* 1995;21(5):258-267.
122. Butler RJ, Davis IM, Laughton CM, et al. Dual-function foot orthosis: effect on shock and control of rearfoot motion. *Foot Ankle Int* 2003;24(5):410-414.
123. Miller CD, Laskowski ER, Suman VJ. Effect of corrective rearfoot orthotic devices on ground reaction forces during ambulation. *Mayo Clin Proc* 1996;71(8):757-762.
124. Lafortune MA, Cavanagh PR, Sommer HJ, et al. Foot inversion-eversion and knee kinematics during walking. *J Orthop Res* 1994;12:412-420.
125. Nawoczenski DA, Cook TM, Saltzman CL. The effect of foot orthotics on three-dimensional kinematics of the leg and rearfoot during running. *J Orthop Sports Phys Ther* 1995;21(6):317-327.
126. McPoil TG, Cornwall MW. The effect of foot orthoses on transverse tibial rotation during walking. *J Am Podiatr Med Assoc* 2000;90(1):2-11.
127. Stacoff A, Reinschmidt C, Nigg BM, et al. Effects of foot orthotics on skeletal motion during running. *Clin Biomech* 2000;15:54-64.
128. Tillman MD, Chiumento AB, Trimble MH, et al. Tibiofemoral rotation in landing: the influence of medially and laterally posted orthotics. *Phys Ther Sport* 2003;4(1):34-39.
129. Nester CJ, van der Linden ML, Bowker P. Effect of foot orthoses on the kinematics and kinetics of normal walking gait. *Gait Posture* 2003;17(2):180-187.
130. Williams DS, Davis IM, Baitch SP. Effect of inverted orthosis on lower extremity mechanics in runners. *Med Sci Sports Exerc* 2003;35(12):2060-2968.
131. Stackhouse CL, Davis IM, Hamill J. Orthotic intervention in forefoot and rearfoot strike running patterns. *Clin Biomech* 2004;19(1):64-70.
132. Nigg BM, Nurse MA, Stefanyshyn DJ. Shoe inserts and orthotics for sport and physical activities. *Med Sci Sports Exerc* 1999;31(7 suppl):S421-S428.
133. Nigg BM. The role of impact forces and foot pronation: a new paradigm. *Clin J Sport Med* 2001;11(1):2-9.
134. Mundermann A, Nigg BM, Humble RN, et al. Orthotic comfort is related to kinematics, kinetics, and EMG in recreational runners. *Med Sci Sports Exerc* 2003;35(10):1710-1719.
135. Mundermann A, Nigg BM, Humble RN, et al. Foot orthotics affect lower extremity kinematics and kinetics during running. *Clin Biomech* 2003;18(3):254-262.
136. Nawoczenski DA, Ludewig PM. Electromyographic effects of foot orthotics on selected lower extremity muscles during running. *Arch Phys Med Rehabil* 1999;80(5):540-544.
137. Bird AR, Bendrups AP, Payne CB. The effect of foot wedging on electromyographic activity in the erector spinae and gluteus medius muscles during walking. *Gait Posture* 2003;18(2):81-91.
138. Vanicek KN, Kingman J, Hencken C. The effect of foot orthotics on myoelectric fatigue in the vastus lateralis during a simulated skiers squat. *J Electromyography Kinesiology* 2004;14(6):693-698.
139. Guskiewicz KM, Perrin DH. Effect of orthotics on postural sway following inversion ankle sprain. *J Orthop Sports Phys Ther* 1996;23(5):326-331.
140. Hertel J, Denegar CR, Buckley WE, et al. Effect of rearfoot orthotics on postural sway after lateral ankle sprain. *Arch Phys Med Rehabil* 2001;82(7):1000-1003.
141. Hertel J, Denegar CR, Buckley WE, et al. Effect of rearfoot orthotics on postural control in healthy subjects. *J Sports Rehabil* 2001;100:36-47.
142. Percy ML, Menz HB. Effects of prefabricated foot orthoses and soft insoles on postural stability in professional soccer players. *J Am Podiatr Med Assoc* 2001;91(4):194-202.
143. Olmsted LC, Hertel J. Influence of foot type and orthotics on static and dynamic postural control. *J Sports Rehabil* 2004;13(1):54-66.
144. Rome K, Brown CL. Randomized clinical trial into the impact of rigid foot orthoses on balance parameters in excessively pronated feet. *Clin Rehabil* 2004;18(6):624-630.
145. Riegler HF. Orthotic devices for the foot. *Orthop Rev* 1987;16(5)27-37.
146. D'Ambrosia RD. Orthotic devices in running injuries. *Clin Sports Med* 1985;4(4):611-619.
147. Donatelli R, Hulbert C, Conaway D, et al. Biomechanical foot orthotics: a retrospective study. *J Orthop Sports Phys Ther* 1988;10(6):205-212.
148. Moraros J, Hodge W. Orthotic survey preliminary results. *J Am Podiatr Med Assoc* 1993;83(3):139-148.
149. Way MC. Effects of a thermoplastic foot orthosis on patellofemoral pain in a collegiate athlete: a single subject design. *J Orthop Sports Phys Ther* 1999;29(6):331-338.
150. Saxena A, Haddad J. The effect of foot orthoses on patellofemoral pain syndrome. *J Am Podiatr Med Assoc* 2003;93(4):264-271.
151. Sutlive TG, Mitchell SD, Maxfield SN, et al. Identification of individuals with patellofemoral pain whose symptoms improved after a combined program of foot orthosis use and modified activity: a preliminary investigation. *Phys Ther* 2004;84(1):49-61.
152. Gross MT, Foxworth JL. The role of foot orthoses as an intervention for patellofemoral pain. *J Orthop Sports Phys Ther* 2003;33(11):661-670.
153. Pfeffer G, Bacchetti P, Deland J, et al. Comparison of custom and prefabricated orthosis in the initial treatment of proximal plantar fasciitis. *Foot Ankle Int* 1999;20(4):214-221.
154. Gross MT, Byers JM, Krafft JL, et al. The impact of custom semirigid foot orthotics on pain and disability for individuals with plantar fasciitis. *J Orthop Sports Phys Ther* 2002;32(4):149-157.

155. Seligman DA, Dawson DR. Customized heel pads and soft orthotics to treat heel pain and plantar fasciitis. *Arch Phys Med Rehabil* 2003;84(10):1564-1567.
156. Kilmartin TE, Wallace WA. Effect of pronation and supination orthosis on Morton's neuroma and lower extremity function. *Foot Ankle Int* 1994;15(5):256-262.
157. Dananberg HJ, Guiliano M. Chronic low-back pain and its response to custom made foot orthoses. *J Am Podiatr Med Assoc* 1999;89(3):109-117.
158. Kopec JA, Esdaile JM, Abrahamowicz M, et al. The Quebec Back Pain Disability Scale: measurement properties. *Spine* 1995;20(3):341-352.

10

Ankle-Foot Orthoses

ROBERT S. LIN

LEARNING OBJECTIVES

On completion of this chapter, the reader will be able to do the following:

1. Describe how an ankle-foot orthosis (AFO) is designed to enhance achievement of stance stability, swing clearance, limb prepositioning, adequate step length, and efficiency of gait.
2. Describe the biomechanical forces systems use in the most common AFO designs.
3. Compare and contrast the indications and limitations of prefabricated, custom-fit, and custom-molded AFOs.
4. Describe how each commonly prescribed AFO design affects transition through the rockers of stance and on the swing phase of gait.
5. Compare and contrast the clinical indications for static or dynamic AFO designs.
6. Apply knowledge of normal and pathological gaits, assessment of impairment, and functional potential in the selection of appropriate AFOs for patients with neuromuscular impairments.

AFOs can be prescribed for patients with musculoskeletal or neuromuscular dysfunction to accomplish various goals. For patients with unstable ankles, whether from injury or muscular imbalance, AFOs can be used to support the feet and ankles, maintain optimal functional alignment during activity, or limit motion to protect healing structures. For patients with neuromotor dysfunction, the AFO can substitute for inadequate muscle function during key points in the gait cycle, optimize alignment and help to manage abnormal tone, or minimize the risk of deformity (e.g., equinovarus) associated with long-term hypertonicity. In this chapter, we focus on the AFO as a means of improving gait in children and adults with neuromuscular dysfunction, such as in cerebral palsy or after stroke. For a discussion of orthotic management of common musculoskeletal injuries of the ankle, the reader is referred to Epler.[1]

The development of a prescription for an AFO usually involves an interdisciplinary team (orthotist, therapist, physician, patient, and primary caregiver). The combined knowledge and skills of the team ensure that the prescription will best match orthotic design to the patient's functional needs. To create an optimal prescription, the team must consider a number of important issues. First, the biomechanical and neuromotor aspects of normal human locomotion must be thoroughly understood. With this foundation, team members can recognize primary gait pathologies and their most common compensations and select appropriate components or design from among the many options. Second, an understanding of the specific disease or disorder is also essential; this includes the natural history and likely prognosis and the types of secondary musculoskeletal problems commonly encountered, as well as any cognitive or other multisystem involvement that may be associated with the disease.[2] Practical issues, such as who will be responsible for applying (donning) or removing (doffing) the device and the ease with which this can be accomplished must also be considered if the optimal orthotic outcome is to be achieved.

PREREQUISITES OF FUNCTIONAL GAIT

Five fundamental prerequisites are necessary for safe, energy-efficient walking.[3] First, the lower limb must be stable enough to accept and support body weight during the stance phase, especially during single-limb support. Second, foot clearance must be adequate during the swing phase. Third, the foot must be properly prepositioned in preparation for initial contact and loading response in the early stance. Fourth, at the same time, reasonable control and adequate motion must be present at the foot, ankle, knee, and hip if step length is to be efficient and adequate. Fifth, if any component is compromised, the energy cost of walking increases significantly, and efficiency of upright mobility is negatively affected. For some patients whose neuromuscular dysfunction substantially interferes with these prerequisites, functional ambulation may be an unrealistic goal unless an appropriate orthosis is provided.

Stability in Stance

When the support limb is in stance phase, it must respond with substantial stability to the biomechanical forces that act on the body. In the presence of neuromotor or musculoskeletal dysfunction, an orthosis can effectively augment function by supporting anatomical structures that are prone to angulation and/or weakness during loading.[4] The application of an AFO's three-point force mechanism can moderate dynamic (nonfixed) functional deformities, such as ankle varus, by optimally positioning the limb and providing an external support for effective single-limb stance. A dynamic ankle varus deformity, which is commonly encountered in spastic cerebral palsy or after stroke, can be effectively controlled with the application of key forces with the orthosis. For example, the distal lateral force serves as a fulcrum for forces applied at the proximal-medial tibia and distal medial foot (Figure 10-1). An additional force system controls dorsiflexion/plantar flexion position in the sagittal plane: the fulcrum is at the anterior ankle, and the counterforces are applied at the plantar surface of the foot and the posterior proximal calf.

Clearance in Swing

In normal gait, synergistic hip and knee flexion combined with dorsiflexion of the ankle (to a neutral position) during midswing provides just enough elevation for effective clearance of the foot. The ability to clear the foot without dragging or catching the toes is often compromised in patients with neuromuscular or musculoskeletal impairment. Both weakness of dorsiflexor muscles and an abnormal extensor synergy pattern of the lower extremity can, singly or in combination, effectively "lengthen" the swing limb such that toe clearance cannot be achieved. An AFO of appropriate design and strength can position the foot and ankle to enhance clearance. An AFO cannot, however, compensate for inadequate knee or hip flexion.

Swing Phase Prepositioning

Preparation for initial contact, as swing phase ends, is similar in many ways to that of an airplane just before landing: The plane's nose is held slightly upward, its wings are level, and its tail is slightly down. At the end of swing phase, while the extremity is "airborne," the ankle-foot complex is preparing to accept forces imposed during loading in early stance: the toes are up as a result of knee extension and ankle dorsiflexion to neutral, the foot is level without excessive inversion or eversion, and the heel is positioned to make first contact with the ground. Optimal alignment of the foot-ankle complex is essential for successful prepositioning in preparation for stance.

Adequate Step Length

Step length is determined by two things: appropriately timed activity of proximal musculature and the pendulum effect of the lower limb below the knee during swing. Sagittal plane stability at the talocrural joint in terminal stance and preswing also contributes to step length. As a first-class lever, a stable talocrural joint facilitates effective forward propulsion of the limb in swing. When this stability is compromised, propulsion is less effective and step length is curtailed.

Energy Conservation

Sustained functional ambulation requires careful timing, strength, balance, and coordination of the contributing lower extremity segments. If the synergistic patterns of these segments are disrupted or exaggerated, ambulation may occur at much too high an energy cost. This fifth prerequisite of gait relates to the reasonable amount of energy consumed during ambulation so that walking can be an efficient primary means of mobility. By guiding and controlling ankle and knee joint position and motion during the stance and swing phases of gait, an AFO may reduce energy cost associated with pathological gait patterns in patients with neuromuscular impairment, making ambulation a functional possibility.[5]

ROCKERS OF STANCE PHASE IN GAIT

Three transitional periods (rockers) occur during stance phase as the body progresses forward over the foot (Figure 10-2).[3] The first rocker (*heel rocker*) begins at initial contact and ends when the foot-flat position is achieved in loading response. During the first rocker, a controlled deceleration of the foot toward the floor occurs, as well as an acceptance of body weight as the limb is loaded. In individuals with normal neuromuscular function, eccentric contraction of the quadriceps and anterior tibialis prevents "foot slap" and protects the knee as ground reaction forces are translated upward toward the knee.

During the second rocker (*ankle rocker*) the tibia advances over the ankle-foot complex, from approximately 10 degrees of plantar flexion at the end of loading response to 10 degrees of dorsiflexion at the end of midstance. The gastrocnemius-soleus complex contracts eccentrically to control the speed (deceleration) of forward tibial progression.

The third and final rocker (*toe rocker*) begins as the heel rises off the ground surface, and body weight rolls over the

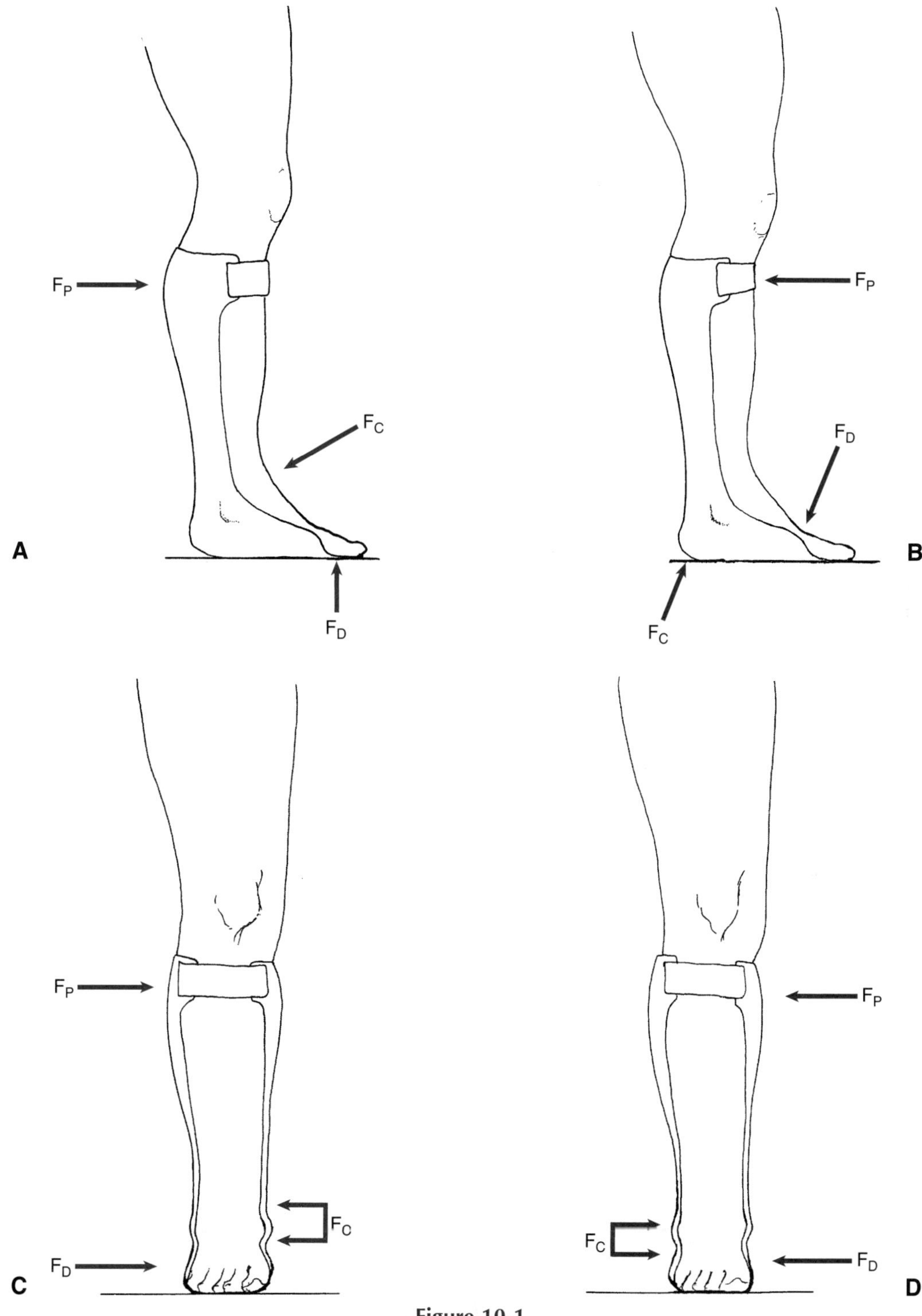

Figure 10-1

The four force systems in a molded, thermoplastic, solid-ankle ankle-foot orthosis design. ***A,*** *Plantar flexion is controlled during swing phase by a proximal force* (F_p) *at the posterior calf band and a distal force at the metatarsal heads* (F_d) *that counter a centrally located stabilizing force* (F_c) *applied at the ankle by shoe closure.* ***B,*** *For control of dorsiflexion during stance phase (i.e., forward progression of the tibia over the foot),* F_p *is applied at the proximal tibia by the anterior closure,* F_d *at the ventral metatarsal heads by the toe box of the shoe, and counterforce* F_c *at the heel, snuggly fit in the orthosis.* ***C,*** *The force system for eversion (valgus) locates* F_d *along the fifth metatarsal,* F_p *at the proximal lateral calf band, and* F_c *on either side of the malleolus.* ***D,*** *To control inversion (varus) of the foot and ankle,* F_d *is applied by the distal medial wall of the orthosis against the first metatarsal,* F_p *at the proximal medial calf band, and* F_c *at the distal lateral tibia and calcaneus/talus, on either side of the lateral malleolus.*

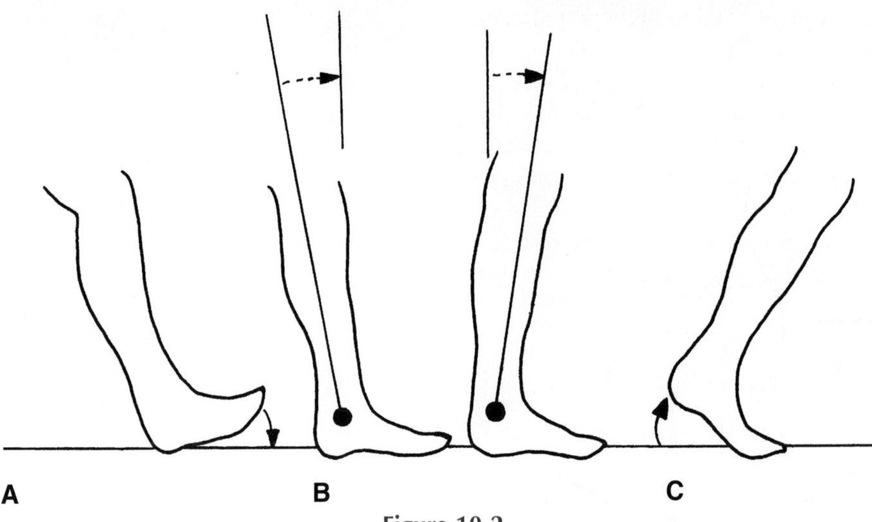

Figure 10-2

Three transitional rocker periods occur as the body moves forward over the foot during stance. ***A,*** *During first rocker, the transition from swing into early stance, controlled lowering of the forefoot occurs, with a fulcrum at the heel.* ***B,*** *During second rocker, controlled forward progression of the tibia over the foot occurs, with motion of the talocrural joint of the ankle.* ***C,*** *In the third rocker, transition from stance toward swing occurs as the heel rises, with dorsiflexion of the metatarsophalangeal joints.*

first metatarsophalangeal joint through push-off in terminal stance. During fast walking, acceleration, rather than deceleration, actually occurs as active contraction of the gastrocnemius-soleus complex propels the foot and leg into swing phase.

Because most lower-extremity orthoses provide external stability, they necessarily have an impact on the smooth transition through one or more of the stance phase rockers. Any disruption of forward progression compromises the mobility parameters of gait, such as step length, cadence, and single support time. An effective orthotic intervention attempts to balance the patient's need for external stability with the orthosis's potentially deleterious effects on mobility. The goal is to provide the minimal amount of stability necessary so that the greatest amount of mobility is possible.

For patients with dorsiflexion weakness, three gait problems must be addressed:

1. Swing clearance
2. Prepositioning for initial contact
3. Controlled lowering of the foot in early stance

The optimal orthotic design addresses these issues without restricting forward progression of the tibia in the second rocker or rolling over the forefoot in the third rocker. A patient with significant extensor hypertonicity and equinovarus, however, may have a greater need to control foot and ankle position throughout stance, such that all three rockers of gait may be compromised. Shoe modifications, such as rocker bottom soles, can compensate for some of this compromise in mobility.

The rehabilitation team weighs the impact of stability provided by an orthosis on progression through stance with its impact on a patient's functional status. At times compromise is unavoidable if the patient's functional deficits are to be addressed effectively.

BIOMECHANICAL PRINCIPLES OF ANKLE-FOOT ORTHOSES

To understand the biomechanical principles of AFOs, one must understand the functional anatomy of the ankle-foot complex itself. Dorsiflexion and plantar flexion of the ankle occur as the talus rotates through the mortise of the ankle. The interior of the mortise is formed from the syndesmosis (fibrous articulation) between the distal tibia and the distal fibula. The medial malleolus is the downward extension of the tibia. The corresponding lateral malleolus of the fibula is slightly longer and located more posteriorly. The shape of the articular surfaces of the talus and mortise, combined with spatial orientation of the malleoli, results in a joint axis that is slightly oblique. Because the axis of motion runs in an anteromedial to posterolateral direction, motion occurs in more than one plane. Dorsiflexion is associated with forefoot pronation with abduction and hindfoot valgus, whereas plantar flexion is accompanied by forefoot supination with adduction and hindfoot varus.

If a lower extremity orthosis includes mechanical ankle joints, it is essential that the joints' axis be aligned, as closely as possible, to the obliquely oriented anatomical axis of motion (Figure 10-3). Although no mechanical ankle joints can model the multiplanar motion of the anatomical ankle exactly, approximating this axis reduces the likelihood of abnormal torque and shearing between the orthosis and limb during gait. Typically, a pair of mechanical joints is incorporated into the medial and lateral aspects of the orthosis. The distal border (tip) of the medial malleolus is used as a reference point for placement of the mechanical joint in the coronal plane. A horizontal line that bisects the medial and lateral malleolus at the same height from the ground is used to position the lateral joint. In the transverse plane, the mechanical joint axes should be parallel to each other, to follow the line of progression and degree of external rotation dictated by the patient's tibial torsion. The specific mechanical joint heads are placed at approximately midline of the malleoli in the sagittal plane. If significant incongruency is present between the anatomical and mechanical axes, excessive motion of the extremity within the orthoses and a limitation of motion and efficiency of the mechanical joint often occur.

MATERIALS AND METHODOLOGIES

The development of thermoplastic materials has had a profound impact on the design and manufacture of lower extremity orthoses. Although AFOs can be constructed of various materials including metals, leathers, and thermosetting materials, the many advantages of thermoplastic have made it the material of choice for most patients requiring AFOs. AFOs can be (1) prefabricated ("off-the-shelf") devices; (2) custom fit to the patient, with preshaped "blanks" or component parts adapted to meet the patient's needs; or (3) individually custom molded to exactly fit a patient's limb. When compared with the metal double-upright AFO designs of the polio era, today's thermoplastic AFOs have significantly lighter weight, are much more cosmetic and comfortable to wear, and can be worn in more than one pair of shoes (Figure 10-4).

A custom-molded thermoplastic AFO is heat formed over a positive model of the patient's own limb. The resulting intimate fit provides more effective control of the extremity than is possible with a traditional double-upright AFO, with which control is limited by the structural integrity and fit of the patient's shoe. The closely fitting molded AFO effectively distributes forces exerted on the limb more broadly over the limb's surface area, reducing the potential of high pressure and skin breakdown.[6] This is especially beneficial for patients with sensory impairment, who would not recognize discomfort and skin irritation from friction or high or prolonged pressure within a shoe.[7-9]

Thermosetting materials have also been used in the fabrication of AFOs (Figure 10-5). Manufacture of a thermoset AFO is a time- and labor-intensive process: multiple layers of material, often reinforced with glass or carbon fibers, must be laminated together. Thermosetting materials are used when a high degree of stiffness is desired. It is important to note, however, that thermoset materials cannot be heat molded to adjust fit. These materials also tend to fail at points of high stress. In virtually all instances, a thermoplastic version can be fabricated more quickly and cheaply than other materials. Continued development of new manufacturing techniques and the introduction of composite reinforcements clearly make thermoplastic the material of choice for most AFOs.

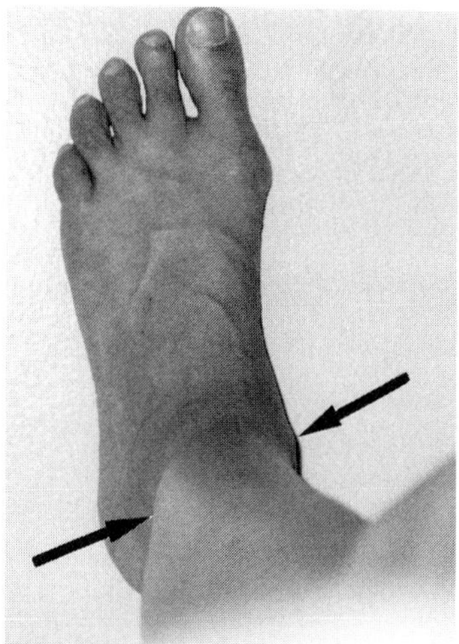

Figure 10-3
Alignment of the mechanical ankle joint axes must reflect the degree of external rotation/tibial torsion that is present in the transverse plane.

Prefabricated Orthoses

Prefabricated orthoses are mass-produced in various "typical" sizes and in various materials. Most have generous contouring, although the degree to which they can be modified or adjusted to fit an individual patient varies. Although they are much less expensive than custom-molded AFOs, their ability to achieve desired control of motion, as well as their durability, can be compromised by the quality of material used and the lack of intimate fit to a given patient's limb. Prefabricated orthoses are often used by therapists as an evaluative tool to determine which orthotic design might best meet a patient's needs, as an interim device while a custom orthotic is being prepared, or when the condition warranting use of an AFO is temporary or of short duration.

Custom-Fit Orthoses

Some manufacturers provide an orthotic "blank" that can be custom fit for a given patient using various heating or relieving techniques, or application of additional materials, to obtain as close a fit as possible. Although custom-fit devices provide better orthotic control than do most prefabricated versions, they often do not achieve the same accuracy of fit and degree of function that a custom-molded orthosis can provide. This option may be considered when change in functional status (either improvement or deterioration) is anticipated, and the orthosis must be replaced relatively frequently.

Custom-Molded Orthoses

Custom-molded orthoses provide optimal control of the limb and are especially important for patients with impaired

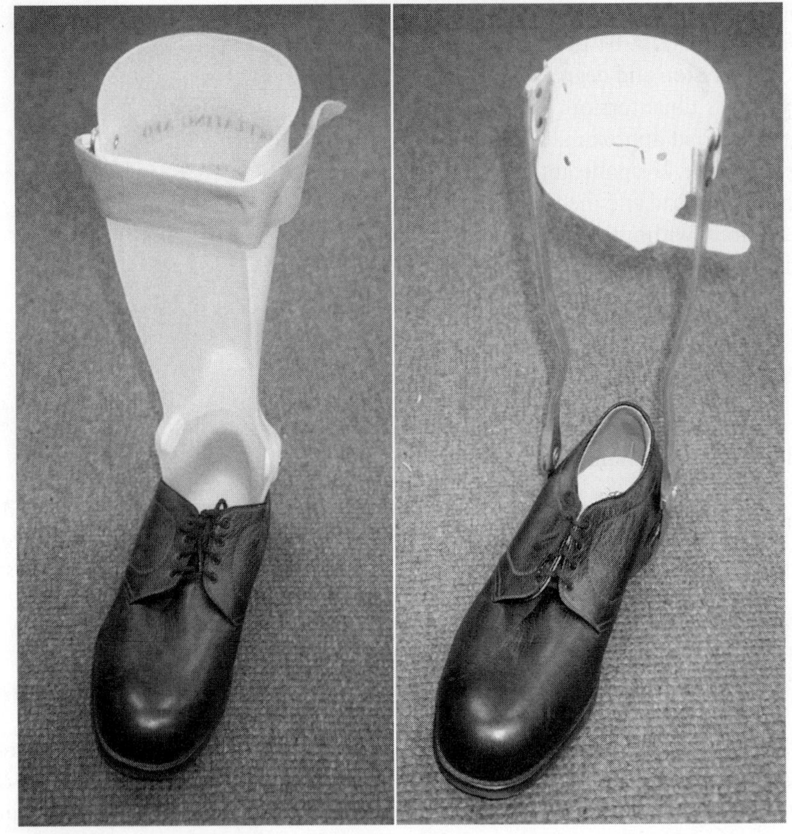

Figure 10-4

***A,** A custom-molded, thermoplastic, hinged-ankle, ankle-foot orthosis closely follows the contours of the limb, with its intimate fit providing excellent motion control. **B,** A conventional double-upright, hinged-ankle, ankle-foot orthosis with shoe stirrup and calf band may be appropriate when limb volume fluctuates significantly.*

sensation or significant hypertonicity or who are at risk of progressive deformity associated with their condition.

Custom-molded orthoses require *casting* of the affected body part to obtain a *negative mold* in the desired alignment. Once the cast is set and removed, it is filled with plaster of Paris to obtain a *positive model* of the patient's extremity. This positive model is *rectified,* or modified, to provide pressure relief in intolerant areas (e.g., around a bony prominence) or to apply corrective or stabilizing forces as dictated by the design of the orthosis. This modification sequence is the most critical design step in the application of biomechanical forces and orthotic fit and function.

The first step in the manufacture of a custom-molded AFO is casting for an accurate negative mold of the patient's limb. One or two rolls of plaster gauze wrap are smoothed over the limb, and then the limb is held in optimal alignment until the cast is set. The flexible tubing along the anterior leg is used as a guide for cast removal (see Figure 2-2).

The only true contraindication of a custom-molded thermoplastic design is significantly fluctuating limb size, associated with edema of the braced extremity. When the limb is at its lowest volume, the intimacy of fit can be lost so that excessive movement of the limb within the orthosis occurs. When the limb is significantly edematous, the intimate fit of the AFO may be too constricting, leading to pressure-related problems. In this instance, the total contact of a molded design may be inappropriate, and a conventional double-upright system should be considered.

Many factors influence the decision to choose a prefabricated, custom-fit, or custom-molded orthosis. The patient's functional needs are paramount but must be tempered by access to an orthotist for fit, education, and service; the rate of growth and need for ongoing adjustments; anticipated length of time that the orthosis will be required; likelihood of progression of dysfunction or evolution of deformity as it relates to preciseness of orthotic control; and, of course, cost of the orthosis. Many current health insurance plans have limitations in coverage for orthoses, leaving patients with proportional out-of-pocket expenses.

NAMING ANKLE-FOOT ORTHOSES

Acronyms used to name lower extremity orthoses describe joints that the orthoses encompass, not necessarily all the joints in which functions are affected by the orthoses.[10]

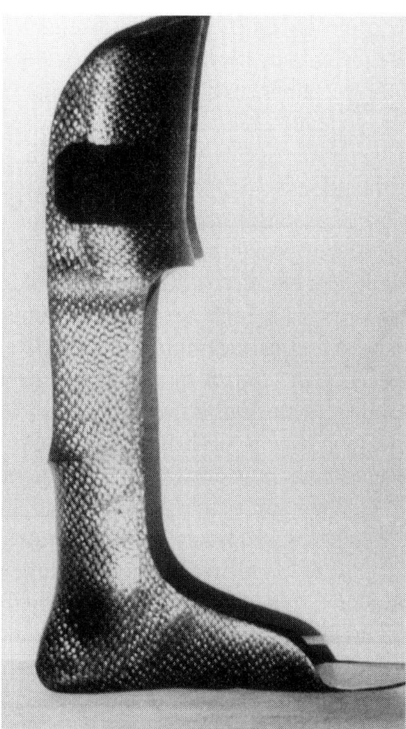

Figure 10-5
This floor reaction ankle-foot orthosis was fabricated using carbon graphite and fiberglass in a thermosetting process because of the desire to provide maximum stiffness. The combination of a solid-ankle design and an anterior wall produces a knee extension moment at midstance and enhances stance phase stability.

The foot orthosis category includes arch supports, biomechanical foot orthoses, University of California Biomechanics Laboratory (UCBL) orthoses, and heel cups. A supramalleolar orthosis (SMO) encompasses the ankle-foot complex but terminates just above the proximal border of the medial malleolus.

AFO designs are the most frequently fabricated orthoses for children and adults with neuromuscular disorders. An AFO typically includes a toe plate that extends under the phalanges or a footplate that extends to just behind the metatarsal heads, a heel cup that holds the subtalar joint in neutral, a mechanical ankle joint with a plantar flexion stop, and a proximal upright with a trimline reaching a level just distal to the tibial tubercle on the anterior surface and an inch below the apex of the fibular head laterally. In addition to affecting function of the foot-ankle complex, AFOs also have a biomechanical impact at the knee and hip.

Despite numerous variations in design details, most AFOs can be classified either as *static orthoses* (prohibiting motion at the ankle) or *dynamic orthoses* (permitting ankle motion, primarily in the sagittal plane). The solid-ankle AFO, the anterior floor reaction brace, and the patellar tendon-bearing (PTB) AFO are examples of static AFOs.

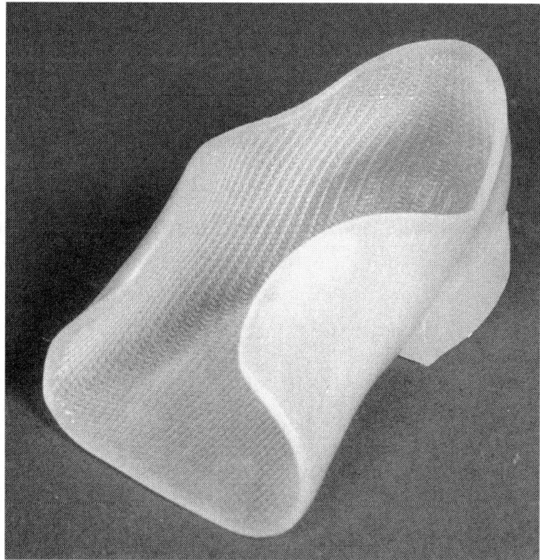

Figure 10-6
The University of California Biomechanics Laboratory orthosis is designed to position the calcaneus optimally for effective subtalar joint function. The deep heel cup, with its high medial and lateral trimlines, snugly holds the calcaneus. The orthosis also encompasses the joints of the midfoot, providing support for the longitudinal arch. In this example, a medial post (Gillette modification) has been added.

Those in the dynamic group include posterior leaf spring and hinged-ankle (articulating) AFO designs.

University of California Biomechanics Laboratory Orthosis

Subtalar instability is a functional problem that can be effectively addressed by orthotic intervention. In the 1970s, researchers at UCBL developed a custom-molded shoe insert, now known as the *UCBL orthosis* or simply *UCBL* (Figure 10-6).[11] The UCBL effectively controls flexible calcaneal deformities (rearfoot valgus or varus), as well as transverse plane deformities of the midtarsal joints (forefoot abduction or adduction).[12]

The UCBL differs from the biomechanical foot orthosis described in the previous chapter in its intimate rearfoot fit, which "grabs" the calcaneus, and its hold on the midfoot with high medial and lateral trimlines. The UCBL is based on the premise that the calcaneus is the key structure for subtalar joint orientation. The orthosis realigns the calcaneus, improving the angle of pull of the Achilles tendon, and proves a more stable foundation for the articular surfaces of the talus, navicular, and cuboids.

The UCBL can also restore and support a supple longitudinal arch deformity. The *Gillette modification*, an external post positioned either on the medial or lateral border of the heel cup, can be used to apply additional rotatory moments to the calcaneus during weight bearing.

As with other custom orthoses, the UCBL begins with the patient's limb casted in a subtalar neutral position to provide a negative mold and create a positive model of the foot. Once the positive model is appropriately rectified and modified, thermoplastic material is heat molded, cooled, and trimmed to form the UCBL orthosis.

The UCBL orthosis is most commonly used for dynamic control of coronal plane deformities at the subtalar joint. This type of orthosis is not effective for sagittal plane problems of the ankle and foot or when a patient has difficulty with swing phase clearance. In these cases, an orthosis with trimline above the ankle joint is necessary.

Supramalleolar and Dynamic Ankle-Foot Orthoses

The SMO and dynamic ankle-foot orthosis (DAFO) are relatively new orthotic designs that have evolved from the UCBL in an effort to address sagittal plane problems and to facilitate foot clearance in swing. One design variant consists of a UCBL-like shoe insert modified with medial and lateral extensions. The medial and lateral extensions represent an attempt to improve control of subtalar valgus or varus by lengthening the proximal lever arm upward. A number of SMO designs are currently being used in clinical practice. Some versions include a mechanical ankle joint (Figure 10-7). One version, also called a *dynamic AFO*, attempts to inhibit hypertonicity and dynamic equinovarus deformity by supporting normal triplanar motion of the ankle joint through stabilization of ankle position with nonjointed medial and lateral extensions (Figure 10-8).[13] Early evidence suggests that this version enhances biomechanical function of the foot during gait; however, its impact on abnormal tone is not as well supported.[14-18] The proximal trimlines of an SMO or dynamic AFO can be positioned anywhere between the superior aspects of the malleoli and just below the belly of the soleus.

The design of an SMO mimics the effect of a high-top sneaker or shoe but provides more intimate control of the ankle-foot complex because of its custom-molded fabrication. For children with mild to moderate neuromuscular impairment who are just beginning to ambulate, the SMO may provide enough control of coronal plane motion to enhance stability as the gait pattern matures, without the restrictions imposed by a full-height solid-ankle orthosis.[19] Older children can be transitioned from an articulating AFO into an SMO if their gait pattern has matured and become stable. The SMO may be chosen for children with cerebral palsy who have had corrective orthopedic surgery and no longer require the external stability provided by their preoperative solid-ankle AFO. The SMO may also be indicated for patients with chronic inversion instability at the subtalar joint secondary to trauma, arthritic changes, peripheral neuropathy, or muscle disease.

Controversy as to the effectiveness of the SMO centers on its impact on sagittal plane motion. The position of the ankle joint axis in an adult of average height is approximately 7 cm above the ground surface. If the SMO transverses this level with a definitive closure, it will limit sagittal plane motion of the ankle, and its impact on the rockers of gait may be profound. An additional concern is the patient's tolerance of forces applied at the proximal closure as the

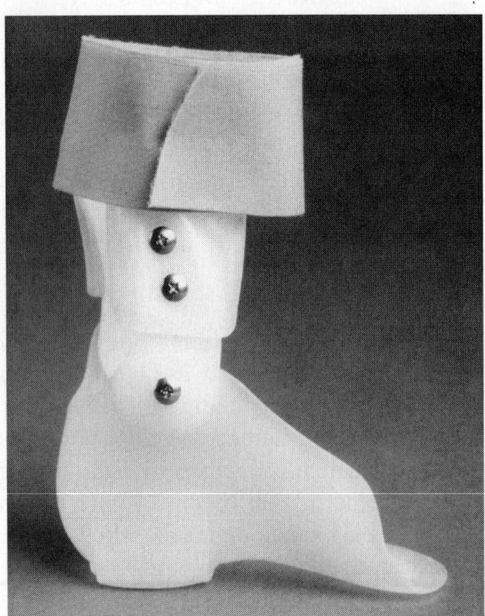

Figure 10-7
A low-profile supramalleolar orthosis with a mechanical ankle joint. Note the University of California Biomechanics Laboratory–style foot orthosis with a medial post. Note also the relatively short lever arm of the proximal closure in controlling forward progression of the tibia through the period of midstance.

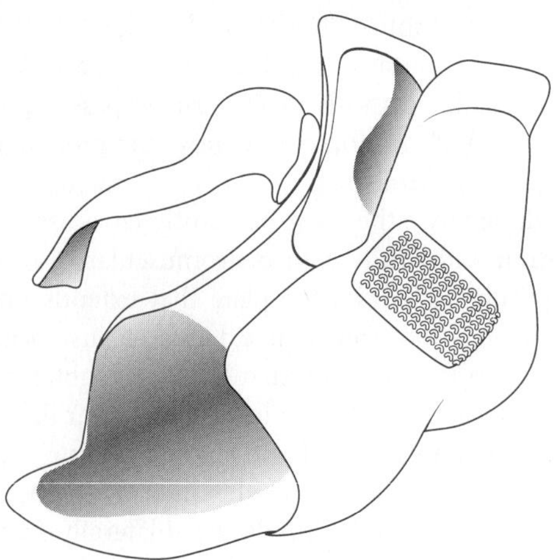

Figure 10-8
The dynamic ankle-foot orthosis (DAFO) is a flexible polypropylene brace designed to optimize subtalar joint alignment through its supramalleolar design. (From Zablotny CM. Use of orthoses for the adult with neurological involvement. In DA Nawoczenski, ME Epler (eds). Orthotics in Functional Rehabilitation of the Lower Limb. *Philadelphia: Saunders, 1997. p. 229.)*

SMO controls forward progression of the tibia; the force on the anterior aspect of the tibia increases exponentially as the height of the proximal closure decreases (Figure 10-9). An SMO design that incorporates an elastic closure or a set of articulating mechanical ankle joints may enable tibial advancement over the foot. If control of tibial advancement in stance is a primary orthotic goal, a standard AFO, with a proximal trimline placed 1 to 1½ inches below the apex of the fibular head, may be a more biomechanically effective and comfortable choice.

Static Ankle-Foot Orthoses

The three orthoses in the static category hold the ankle in a fixed position, as close to neutral ankle, subtalar, and forefoot alignment as the patient is able to tolerate. These orthoses are able to assist swing clearance, effectively preposition the foot for initial contact, and provide external stability for the ankle and knee during stance. The design of static orthoses, however, also compromises the first, second, and, to a lesser extent, third rocker of gait.

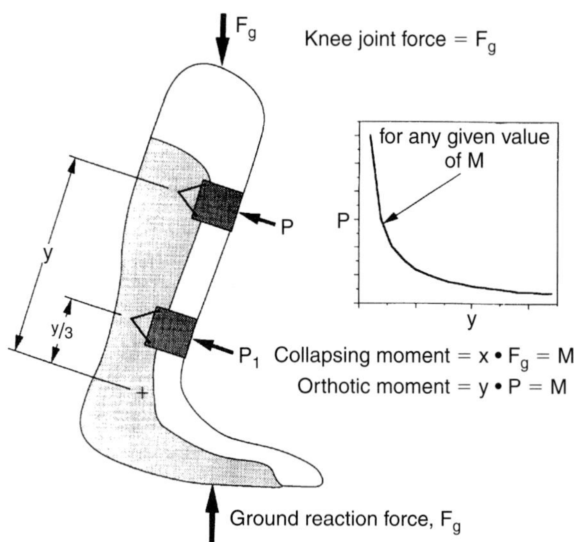

Figure 10-9
Comparison of anterior forces at the proximal closure of a standard ankle-foot orthosis (AFO) ***(P)*** *and supramalleolar orthosis* (P_1) *in controlling forward advancement of the tibia during stance. The distance from the ankle axis* (+) *to the proximal closure of the supramalleolar orthosis* (y/3) *is one-third that of the standard AFO* (y). *To counteract the collapsing moment that results from the force of gravity* (F_g), *the anterior force of the supramalleolar orthosis* (P_1) *must be nine times greater than the anterior force of the AFO* (P). *The graph illustrates the exponential relationship between the anterior force* (P) *and lever arm (distance between the joint axis and the proximal closure,* y*).*

Solid-Ankle Ankle-Foot Orthosis

The solid-ankle AFO is designed to provide maximum immobilization of the ankle-foot complex in all three planes of motion. This AFO, usually fabricated from thermoplastic materials, encompasses as much of the lower leg and foot as possible, without making it too difficult to don the orthosis. The anterior/posterior trimline of the solid-ankle AFO is usually placed at or near the midline of the medial and lateral malleolus (Figure 10-10). The proximal border is usually trimmed at 1½ inches below the apex of the head of the fibula.

For children with cerebral palsy, the *footplate* can extend distally under the toes to reduce the likelihood of abnormal toe grasp reflex. For adults, the footplate is usually trimmed just proximally to the metatarsal heads to facilitate the fit and donning of shoes. The ankle is held in a neutral 90-degree position, and the heel is well seated to control the position of the calcaneus and subtalar joint. For adults with hemiplegia

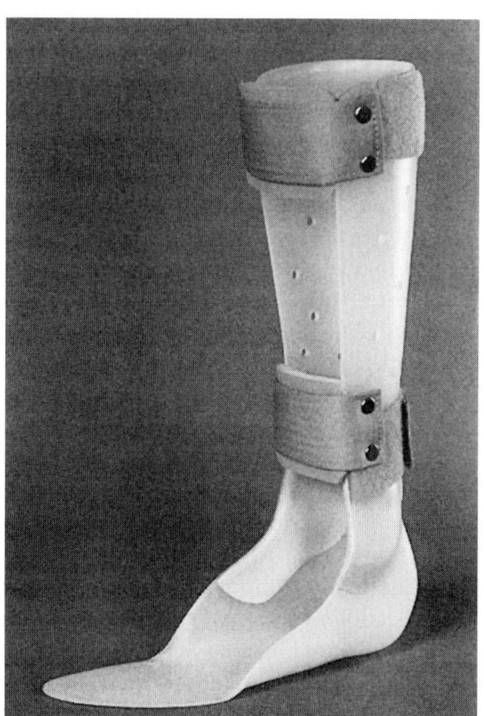

Figure 10-10
Custom-molded, solid-ankle ankle-foot orthosis holds the ankle in as close to optimal static alignment as possible for a given patient. Mediolateral ankle stability is a result of trimlines at the midline of the malleoli. Note the high medial border at the foot and the slight flaring just proximal to the medial malleolus. This strategy is used to counteract an abnormal, flexible subtalar valgus. The crossed Velcro strap anterior to the ankle helps to position the rearfoot appropriately within the heel section of the orthosis. (From Zablotny CM: Use of orthoses for the adult with neurological involvement. In Nawoczenski DA, Epler ME, (eds), Orthotics in Functional Rehabilitation of the Lower Limb. *Philadelphia: Saunders, 1997. p. 223.)*

and significant hypertonicity secondary to tonic toe flexion reflex, an extended toeplate and the addition of a tone-inhibiting bar appears to improve gait speed as well as stride length.[20]

The solid-ankle AFO design incorporates four force systems to control the ankle (see Figure 10-1).[21] The force system that provides resistance to plantar flexion in swing has a fulcrum at the anterior ankle, with an upward counterforce on the plantar surface of the foot and anteriorly directed counterforce at the proximal posterior aspect of the orthosis. The foot section is designed to control excessive angular forces at the subtalar joints during stance.[22] The fulcrum of the varus/inversion control system is a medially directed force applied to the distal fibula and calcaneus across the lateral malleolus, with two laterally directed counterforces applied at the proximal medial tibia and the medial foot. The fulcrum of the valgus/eversion control system is a laterally directed force applied to the distal tibia and calcaneus just proximal to the medial malleolus. Two medially directed counterforces are applied just below the fibular head proximally and at the lateral foot distally. Control in the transverse plane is also determined by the trimlines of the foot section. Midtarsal joint deformity and the resultant forefoot abduction or adduction can be effectively countered with trimlines that strategically encompass the shafts of the first and fifth metatarsals. If excessive subtalar valgus is present, the foot section incorporates a high medial wall and a flange just proximal to the medial malleolus. This strategy provides a greater surface area for distribution of the fulcrum of corrective forces applied by the orthosis so that the patient is comfortable with the external stability provided by the orthosis.

The fourth force system controls dorsiflexion during stance phase (and consequently facilitates knee extension in stance). There is a compressive force on the ankle section of the orthosis, an upward force of the sole of the foot, and a posteriorly directed force on the anterior proximal tibia.

A solid-ankle AFO is appropriate for patients who require total immobilization of the ankle-foot complex to be stable or functional in standing and during gait. The solid-ankle AFO effectively provides mediolateral stability at the ankle, prevents foot drop in swing by resisting plantar flexion, controls hyperextension of the knee (if set in a few degrees of dorsiflexion at the ankle), controls hyperflexion of the knee (if set in a few degrees of plantar flexion), and assists terminal stance by preventing a collapse into dorsiflexion at the end of stance. This orthosis is often prescribed for patients with neuromotor problems such as moderate to severe hypertonicity (spasticity), unpredictable fluctuating tone (athetosis), or postural instability and ataxia.[22,23] The solid-ankle AFO may also be appropriate for patients with low tone or generalized weakness who must rely on an external device to substitute for the stability that their own muscle activity cannot effectively provide. This design has also been used to protect the ankles and midfeet in patients who are recovering from Charcot's arthropathy, to provide stabilization after foot or ankle surgery, and in patients who have ankle instability and pain secondary to rheumatoid arthritis.[24]

The calf component of the orthosis can be modified with a varus or valgus door or a padded tab for ambulatory patients with strong displacement of the subtalar joint on weight bearing. A Gillette modification can be added to the outer medial or lateral surface of the heel cup to influence valgus or varus attitude at the knee joint. A medial or lateral post (similar to those used in a biomechanical foot orthosis) can be incorporated into the foot section to equalize forefoot to rearfoot relationships or to enhance biomechanical effects on the knee.

The solid-ankle AFO has a deleterious impact on all three rockers of gait. The ankle is held in a neutral position, at approximately 90 degrees, throughout all of the stance phase. This effectively prevents the controlled lowering of the foot toward the floor during loading response; instead, a rapid knee flexion may occur to achieve a foot-flat position quickly. If the orthosis is set in slight dorsiflexion in an effort to prevent recurvatum in early stance, the patient must have at least fair eccentric strength of the quadriceps to control the rapid knee flexion moment in loading response. The proximal closure, combined with the fixed ankle position, prevents forward progression of the tibia during midstance. If the distal trimlines extend beyond the metatarsal heads and the orthosis has a stiff toe plate, the third/toe rocker of the foot will be limited. To counteract these limitations and improve the quality of gait, the patient's shoe can be modified with a cushion heel to simulate the first rocker, and/or a rocker bottom sole to substitute for orthosis-induced limitation of forward progression of the tibia in the second rocker, and impaired rollover of the forefoot in the third rocker.

CASE EXAMPLE 1

A Child with Spastic Diplegia/Cerebral Palsy

P. M. is a 7-year-old child with a primary diagnosis of spastic diplegic cerebral palsy. He tries to keep up with his nonimpaired peers at school, but his mild "crouch" gait (despite using Lofstrand crutches as assistive devices) limits his mobility and endurance. He is referred by his neurologist for evaluation in the interdisciplinary "brace clinic" at the local children's medical center.

On physical examination, P. M. is found to have moderate tightness and soft tissue shortening of his plantar flexors, distal hamstrings, adductors, and hip flexors. While he exhibits moderate flexor-pattern spasticity in both lower extremities, sagittal and coronal plane motions of his hip, knee, and ankle are within 10 degrees of normal. Structurally, he exhibits 25 degrees of femoral anteversion and 15 degrees of internal tibial torsion. Upon barefoot weight bearing, however, his foot progression angles appear to be normal, at approximately 10 degrees external (outward) angle.

Questions to Consider

- What are the most likely gait problems, in each subphase of gait, that might be effectively addressed by an AFO?
- What musculoskeletal (alignment and flexibility) and neuromuscular (control) impairments or characteristics, as well as developmental issues, should be considered by the team as they sort through orthotic options for this child?
- Which of the orthotic options (static vs. dynamic) might you choose for this child? What are the possible benefits and trade-offs of each?
- How might you assess if the orthosis chosen is accomplishing the desired outcomes?

Recommendations of the Team

Given the finding of dynamic pes planovalgus deformity and his propensity to "crouch" during stance, the team recommends that bilateral polypropylene solid-ankle AFOs be custom molded for P. M. When he receives his AFOs, he attends several sessions of outpatient gait training. His gait pattern demonstrates improved plantar flexion–knee extension couples, with virtually all pre-orthosis knee persistent knee flexion eliminated. Subtalar joint alignment is also improved, with an effective support of the medial longitudinal arch.

Follow-up Care

Three weeks after the initial visit, the patient's mother schedules a follow-up visit because she observes "the AFO is causing P. M.'s feet to turn in." On this return visit, observational gait assessment reveals an apparent 30-degree internal (inward) foot progression, bilaterally. This is causing difficulty with clearance of the advancing limb during swing phase. Examination of the fit and alignment of the AFOs reveal appropriate design and fit, with an effective subtalar neutral position.

The team recommends computerized gait analysis be performed to determine the underlying factors leading to this significant change in foot progression angle despite an appropriately fitted and designed solid-ankle AFO. The team suspects that this altered foot progression angle is most likely the result of underlying musculoskeletal deformities (tibial torsion and femoral anteversion) "unmasked" when compensatory motion of the subtalar and midtarsal joints during stance is restricted by the AFOs. In effect, when foot alignment is well supported by the AFO, the effects of excessive tibial torsion and femoral anteversion during gait become more evident.

It is not possible for an AFO to effectively address or control gait problems arising from existing underlying transverse plane (rotational) deformity. The team and family begin to consider the possibility of femoral/tibial derotation osteotomy as a solution to the gait problems that have emerged.

Anterior Floor Reaction Ankle-Foot Orthosis

All AFO designs inherently use moments that result from the ground reaction force to provide some stability in stance. An anterior floor reaction AFO (also known as a *floor reaction orthosis, FRO*) is specifically designed to harness the ground (floor) reaction moment as a primary source of sagittal plane stability for the knee joint during stance.[25,26] The FRO relies on the plantar flexion–knee extension couple where a fixed, slightly plantar-flexed ankle creates an extension moment at the knee (Figure 10-11; see Figure 10-5). The force systems that control foot and ankle position are the same as those described previously for a solid-ankle AFO.

The plantar-flexion angle and the length and rigidity of the toe plate help to determine the magnitude of the resulting knee-extension moment. When an FRO is set in neutral or a few degrees of plantar flexion, the tibia is restrained from advancing over the foot in the second rocker of gait, and the ground reaction force passes anteriorly to the knee earlier in stance phase. Additionally, as the length and stiffness of the toe plate increase, the third rocker of gait is also limited, and additional extension forces are brought to bear on the knee into extension in the latter half of stance phase. The anterior shell and mediolateral trimlines are padded at the proximal prepatellar areas so that the extra extension force being transmitted to the knee in stance is more tolerable (Figure 10-12). The FRO can be fabricated as a single solid unit (which may be difficult to don) or as a solid-ankle AFO with an additional anterior shell that is snugly strapped in place. The latter variation may be appropriate if improvement is anticipated. The anterior shell can be removed, and the orthosis used as a traditional solid-ankle orthosis.

For this orthotic design to be effective in stabilizing the knee, the vector of the ground reaction force must pass anterior to the knee axis. However, this may be problematic for patients with fixed flexion contracture of more than 10 degrees at the distal hamstring.[25] In this case, the FRO resists additional dorsiflexion and knee flexion but does not create a true extension moment. The FRO is also inappropriate for patients who exhibit recurvatum or have structural instability of the knee joint. Because the FRO design limits ankle mobility and knee flexion, it may have a negative impact on balance reactions; if patients do not have effective postural control, an assistive ambulation device (e.g., a cane) may be required, especially if FROs are worn bilaterally.

As a result of the biomechanical advantages of FRO design, a patient with little quadriceps function can be stable in stance, while fully bearing weight, without knee instability. This design has been successful in improving the quality and safety of gait for patients with poliomyelitis,

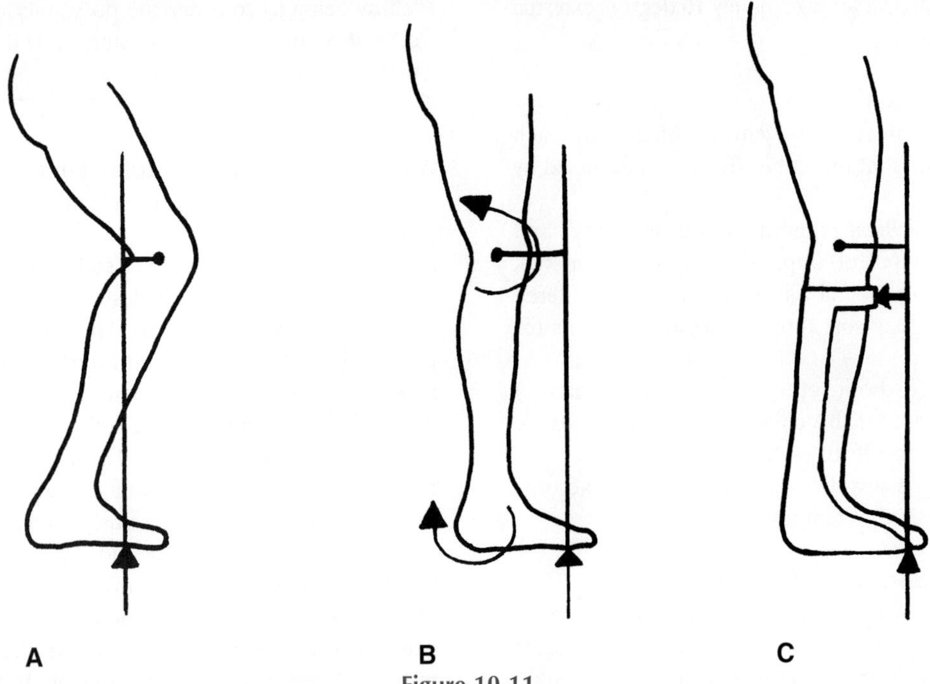

Figure 10-11

***A,** In normal gait, knee stability at midstance is assisted by a ground reaction moment as the body moves over the foot, and the ground reaction force vector passes anterior to the knee. **B,** When a patient walks in a "crouch gait" pattern, the ground reaction force vector passes behind the knee at midstance, creating a flexion moment at the knee, which must be counteracted to maintain upright position. **C,** The solid-ankle ankle-foot orthosis and the floor reaction orthotic designs use a fixed-ankle position to "harness" the ground reaction force, creating a large extension moment at the knee.*

peripheral neuropathy, and myopathy, as well as those with crouch gait from neuromuscular problems, as long as sufficient knee range of motion is possible.

Patellar Tendon–Bearing, Ankle-Foot Orthoses

The PTB AFO is a modification of the solid-ankle design, with an additional anterior shell that incorporates the weight-bearing principles of a PTB socket for a transtibial prosthesis.[27] The anterior shell of the PTB AFO is modified to include a "shelf" to support the medial tibial flare and a patellar tendon bar.

The primary goal of the PTB AFO design is to reduce axial loading of the distal limb during gait. The orthosis is oriented in approximately 10 degrees of knee flexion (with respect to vertical) so that a portion of body weight is loaded on the anterior shell of the AFO at the medial tibial flare and patellar tendon bar during stance. A portion of the axial loading forces is then transmitted down the metal uprights incorporated into the medial and lateral walls of the orthosis, reducing loading of the tibia, fibula, and bones of the foot.[28]

This design has been used for patients with Charcot's ankles, neuropathic ulcers on the plantar surface of the foot, slowly healing or nonunion fractures of the foot and ankle, ankle instability and pain associated with arthritis, and other conditions that require reduced weight bearing through the foot-ankle complex. For this design to be effective, however, the anatomical knee must have structural and skin integrity to tolerate the extra loading forces applied by the PTB design. It is also important that the patient have adequate quadriceps strength for knee stability in early stance.

Dynamic Ankle-Foot Orthoses

The family of dynamic AFOs includes thermoplastic and conventional double-upright orthotic designs. What distinguishes dynamic from static AFOs is that they allow, or have the potential to allow, sagittal plane motion at the ankle. This is accomplished by incorporation of a mechanical ankle joint or, in the case of a posterior leaf spring orthosis (PLS), strategically minimized thermoplastic trimlines.

Thermoplastic Posterior Leaf Spring Ankle-Foot Orthoses

The PLS is a thermoplastic AFO with medial and lateral trimlines placed well posteriorly to the midline of the malleoli (Figure 10-13). This design feature results in flexibility of the orthosis at the anatomical ankle joint. The degree of flexibility is determined by the thickness of the thermoplastic material used to construct the orthosis and the arc of the radius at the distal third of the AFO.

During loading response, in the first rocker of early stance, the PLS substitutes for eccentric contraction of the muscles of the anterior compartment (primarily the tibialis anterior), providing a controlled lowering of the foot toward

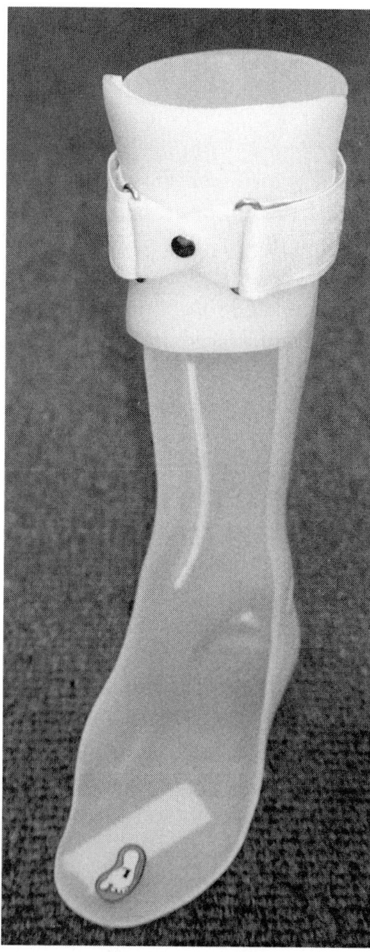

Figure 10-12
This floor reaction orthosis has a posterior shell similar to that of a solid-ankle ankle-foot orthosis (AFO). The combination of slight plantar flexion at the ankle and a stiff, long toe plate creates a plantar flexion-knee extension couple that acts in mid to late stance. The addition of a padded anterior shell more comfortably captures the resultant extension moment, stabilizing the knee. Note also the corrugation incorporated in the medial and lateral walls of the AFO to provide additional rigidity to the orthosis.

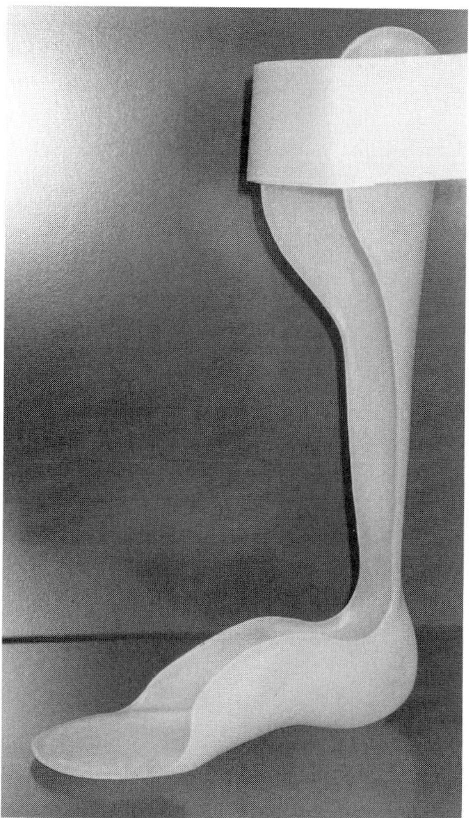

Figure 10-13
The posterior position and arc of the trimlines at the ankle, as well as the thickness of thermoplastic material used, determine the degree of flexibility of the posterior leaf spring ankle-foot orthosis. This design approximates the first and second rockers of stance phase and assists clearance and prepositioning of the foot during swing.

the ground. In the second rocker, the flexibility of the PLS allows the dorsiflexion necessary for tibial advancement over the foot during midstance. Once the limb is elevated and the swing phase begins, the PLS holds the ankle at 90 degrees, assisting clearance and appropriately positioning the foot for the subsequent initial contact.[29,30]

Because of its posterior trimlines and flexibility at the ankle, the PLS cannot "contain" the calcaneus as well as a solid-ankle design. As a result, the PLS may not be as effective in controlling mediolateral foot position and may not be appropriate for patients with flexible deformities of the rear-feet, midfeet, or forefeet.[31]

If a patient requires some external mediolateral stability at the ankle but not the rigid control of a solid-ankle AFO, the trimlines can be placed somewhere between those of a solid-ankle AFO and a PLS design. This design, known as a *semisolid AFO* or a *modified PLS orthosis,* has some of the functional characteristics of the solid-ankle and PLS AFOs. Although somewhat less flexible at the ankle than a PLS in loading response, this modified PLS design can provide some control of knee position during stance.[32]

CASE EXAMPLE 2

A Child with Idiopathic "Toe Walking," Developmental Delay, and Genu Recurvatum

G. M. is an 8-year-old child with chronically tight heel cords. He has a diagnosis of idiopathic toe walking and developmental delay. He is referred for evaluation for possible orthotic intervention because of increasing knee pain secondary to genu recurvatum at midstance.

On examination, G. M. exhibits a normal first rocker (initial contract to loading response/foot flat position) in both feet. There is a delay in the second rocker, however, complicated by 20 degrees of recurvatum after midstance. He has normal lower-extremity range of motion, and there is no evidence of spasticity or clonus. Particularly noteworthy is that he can be positioned in 10 degrees of ankle dorsiflexion when his knees are extended. On manual muscle testing, strength of the quadriceps is 4+, bilaterally.

Questions to Consider

- What are the most likely gait problems, in each subphase of gait, that you want to address by provision of an AFO?
- What musculoskeletal (alignment, flexibility) and neuromuscular (control) impairments or characteristics, as well as developmental issues, must be considered by the team as they sort through orthotic options for this child?
- Which of the orthotic options (static vs. dynamic) might you choose for this child? What are the possible benefits and tradeoffs of each? What modifications of orthotic design might be necessary to meet the orthotic goals for this child?
- How might you assess if the orthosis chosen is accomplishing the desired outcomes?

Recommendations of the Team

The team's orthotist recommends that a pair of custom-molded thermoplastic AFOs be provided. Anteroposterior trimlines around the ankle are placed for a modified (semi-solid) AFO in order to allow moderate sagittal plane motion. The foot is positioned in 5 degrees of dorsiflexion to address excessive extension forces at the knee around midstance. These design modifications are recommended because they (1) minimally limit G. M.'s ability to move through the first rocker of gait and (2) accelerate his limb through second rocker, such that the length of time the ground reaction force is anterior to the knee is minimized. This, in turn, reduces the forceful plantar flexion–knee extension couple around midstance that has been contributing to excessive recurvatum.

Follow-up Care

When G. M. returns to the clinic 3 months after receiving his orthoses for reassessment, he and his family report that his knee pain has "disappeared." He uses the AFOs during the entire school day and at home until bedtime most evenings (taking them off when he plays on the floor with his younger siblings and puppy for more than a few minutes). Observational gait analysis reveals a smooth progression through the rockers of gait, with no observable hyperextension during ambulation or in quiet stance. The team determines the semisolid AFOs with 5 degrees of dorsiflexion, by allowing some ankle joint motion yet controlling tibial position in early to mid stance, have successfully addressed G. M.'s previous gait dysfunction.

Conventional Dorsiflexion-Assist Ankle-Foot Orthosis

The conventional double-upright counterpart to the PLS uses a spring mechanism incorporated into the mechanical ankle joint to assist dorsiflexion in swing, as well as to provide a smooth transition from heel strike/initial contact to foot flat at the end of loading response. The most commonly used conventional dorsiflexion-assist joint is the Klenzak (Figures 10-14 and 10-15). The uprights are connected to the distal stirrup at the mechanical ankle joint. The stirrup is fixed between the heel and sole of the shoe. A coil spring and small ball bearing are placed in a channel in the distal uprights that runs toward the posterior edge of the stirrup. When the spring is compressed at initial contact and early loading response, it resists plantar flexion, allowing a controlled lowering of the foot to the floor. Recoil of the spring when the foot is unloaded in preswing and initial swing assists dorsiflexion for swing-phase toe clearance.[31] The amount of dorsiflexion assist provided is determined by adjustment of a screw placed in the top of the channel to compress or decompress the spring further.

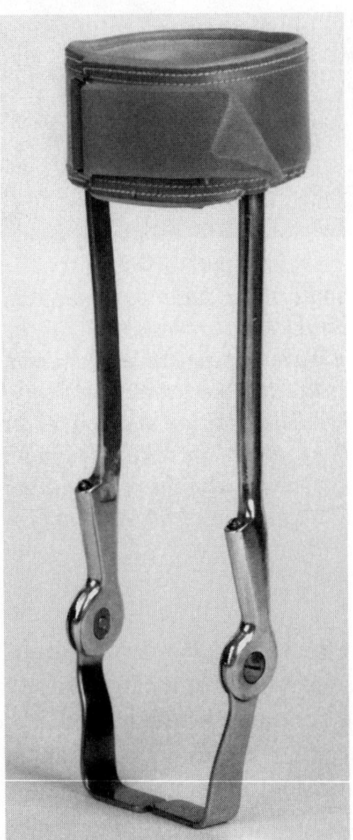

Figure 10-14

Conventional double-upright dorsiflexion-assist ankle-foot orthosis (AFO), with a single-channel Klenzak joint. Tightening the screw at the top of the channel compresses a spring to increase the amount of dorsiflexion assistance provided. This split stirrup would be fit into a shoe plate positioned between the sole and heel, making it possible for the patient to use the AFO with more than one shoe.

The PLS or dorsiflexion-assist conventional AFO is chosen when the primary problem is weakness of dorsiflexion. Patients with peroneal nerve palsy, Charcot-Marie-Tooth disease, and various peripheral neuropathies are appropriate candidates for the PLS or dorsiflexion-assist AFO. Patients with hypertonicity and neuromotor equinovarus, however, are better served by other orthotic designs: The flexible PLS is easily overpowered and rendered ineffective by abnormal tone. The PLS and dorsiflexion-assist conventional AFO are equally effective substitutes for anterior compartment muscles. The choice of orthosis is determined by factors that include weight of the orthotic, functional strength of the proximal musculature, the need for total contact to protect the foot, the ability to interchange shoes, and the wearer's desire for cosmesis.

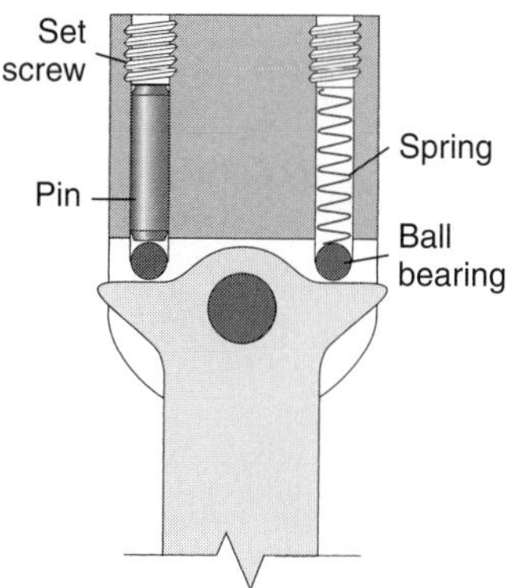

Figure 10-15

The internal anatomy of the double-adjustable ankle joint. Ankle-joint mobility restrictions (e.g., plantar flexion stop) result from the locations of the pins in the anterior and posterior channels of the orthotic joint. A spring may occupy one of the channels, as depicted here, to assist motion (e.g., dorsiflexion assistance). The ball bearings allow the brace uprights to pivot with ease over the brace stirrup. The set screw can be adjusted to change the relative positions of the rods in each of the channels. (From Zablotny CM: Use of orthoses for the adult with neurological involvement. In Nawoczenski DA, Epler ME [eds], Orthotics in Functional Rehabilitation of the Lower Limb. *Philadelphia: Saunders, 1997. p. 227.)*

Articulating Thermoplastic Ankle-Foot Orthosis

The articulating, or hinged-ankle, AFO is a thermoplastic orthotic design that incorporates a mechanical ankle joint placed between the foot and calf sections of the orthosis. Various mechanical ankle joints are commercially available (Figure 10-16). Some require an overlap of the foot and calf, whereas others do not. Those with true articulations, such as the Oklahoma joint, have a single axis of motion that should be aligned as closely as possible to the anatomical ankle joint. Other orthotic joints, such as the Gillette joint, are flexible, nonarticulating, and axisless.[21]

The configurations of the foot and calf sections of an articulating AFO are essentially the same as those of the solid-ankle AFO. The width of the orthosis at the ankle is usually slightly greater than a solid-ankle AFO because of the mechanical ankle joint. Most mechanical ankle joints allow dorsiflexion and plantar flexion (sagittal plane) motion.

For this orthosis to function effectively, the patient must have at least 5 degrees of true ankle dorsiflexion, accomplished without compromise of subtalar or midtarsal joint position.[10] Because of the need for normal subtalar and midfoot arthrokinematics in the second rocker of gait, an articulating AFO is not usually appropriate in the presence of severe spasticity that limits ankle motion or if severe instability or malalignment of the midfoot is present.[33] A 90-degree plantar flexion stop mechanism can be incorporated into the articulating AFO if prevention of plantar flexion is desired (e.g., if spastic equinovarus is a concern). This is usually accomplished by an overlapping lip or pin stop mechanism (Figure 10-17). The hinged AFO allows progression through the first rocker of gait, while controlling knee hyperextension in and around midstance, improving mobility and energy efficiency for children and adults with hemiplegia.[34]

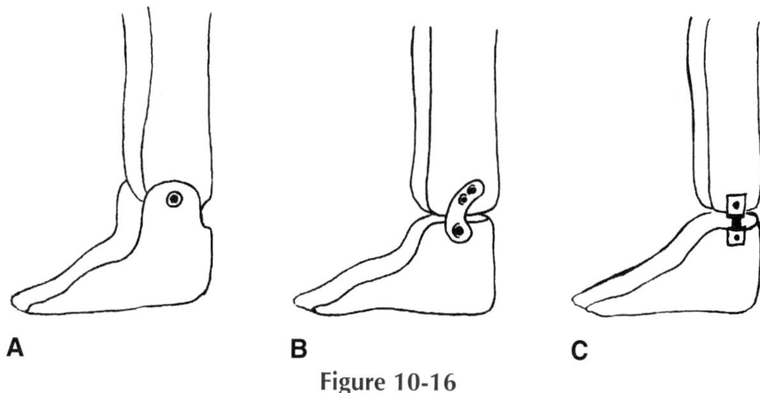

Figure 10-16

*Examples of mechanical ankle joints used in articulating ankle-foot orthoses. The overlap joint **(A)** and Oklahoma joint **(B)** are true single-axis joints, whereas the flexible Gillette mechanism **(C)** allows movement into dorsiflexion and plantar flexion without an actual articulation.*

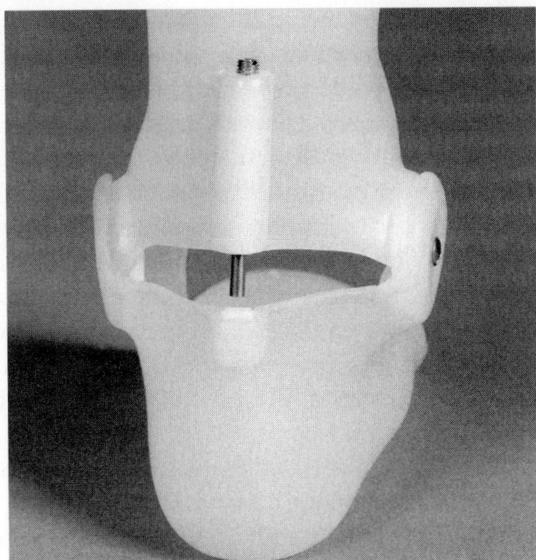

Figure 10-17
When control of plantar flexion is necessary, a posterior plantar flexion stop is incorporated into the articulating ankle-foot orthosis. In this example, a pin stop is used to limit plantar flexion, whereas the overlap mechanical ankle allows the dorsiflexion needed for an efficient second rocker of gait. The amount of plantar flexion motion is adjusted by how far the pin is screwed into the posterior channel.

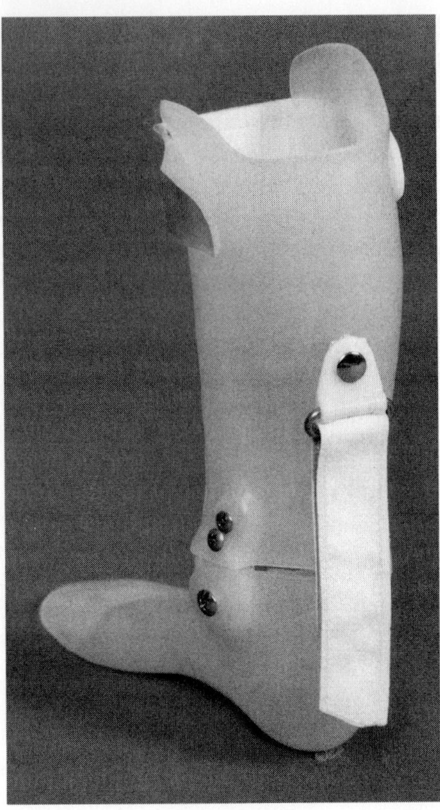

Figure 10-18
An articulating ankle-foot orthosis with Oklahoma joints and a Velcro closing posterior check strap. The mechanical ankle joint would permit free dorsiflexion and plantar flexion motion in the sagittal plane; however, plantar flexion is limited as the calf and foot components make contact. The amount of dorsiflexion possible can be adjusted as the patient progresses through gait training by loosening or elasticizing the check strap closure.

Another version of the articulating AFO uses an adjustable posterior check strap to limit the excursion into dorsiflexion (Figure 10-18). If the check strap is maximally tightened, the orthosis functions much like a solid-ankle AFO. The check strap can be loosened, lengthened, or elasticized as neuromotor control improves, allowing only as much forward progression of the tibia in the second rocker as is safe and functional for the patient.[33] This adaptation makes the articulating AFO the most versatile of all thermoplastic designs. It is often prescribed for patients in the early stages of recovery from stroke, for children with cerebral palsy after orthopedic surgery to correct deformities, or for any other patient with a rapidly changing clinical picture in whom return of function is anticipated.

Hybrid Plastic-Metal and Conventional Articulating Ankle-Foot Orthosis

The bichannel, adjustable ankle-locking joint (also referred to as a *double-action ankle joint* or a *double Klenzak joint*) used in conventional double-upright AFOs has also been adapted for use in thermoplastic designs (Figure 10-19).[22,35] The double-action mechanical joint has anterior and posterior channels. If motion assistance is desired, a coil spring is placed in the channel and a screw is used to adjust compression until the desired level of assistance is achieved. If motion is to be blocked, a solid steel pin is inserted instead of the spring, to stop motion beyond a particular point in the range of motion.

This mechanical ankle joint can be adjusted to meet individual patient needs, stopping plantar flexion and allowing or assisting dorsiflexion as neuromotor control dictates. The double-action joint can also be set to block dorsiflexion (e.g., to limit weight bearing on the anterior portion of the foot) or assist plantar flexion (for a patient with weakness of plantar flexors), should it be necessary. Because of its versatility and adjustability, the double-action ankle joint is often chosen when change in a patient's functional status (improvement or deterioration) is anticipated.

Various other mechanical ankle joints are available for patients who require a conventional double-upright AFO.[31] A simple single-axis joint can be used to provide mediolateral stability for the ankle while allowing free dorsiflexion and plantar flexion. Motion can be limited by adding a stop to the orthotic ankle joint to block either plantar flexion or dorsiflexion. Some orthotic ankle joints, such as the Friddle joint, can be adjusted to limit excursion between dorsiflexion and plantar flexion motion in increments of 7 to 9

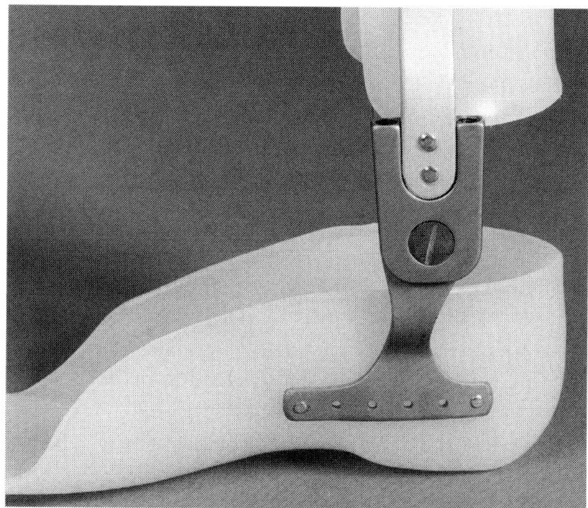

Figure 10-19
The double-action joint can be used in a conventional, double-upright, metal ankle-foot orthosis (AFO) and a thermoplastic-metal, hybrid AFO. Motion is assisted if a spring is compressed within the channel or can be blocked by placement of a steel pin within the channel.

degrees. A leather T-strap can be used in an attempt to position the rearfoot more optimally within the shoe. Proximally, the conventional double-upright AFO has a calf band and anterior closure, positioned approximately $1\frac{1}{2}$ inches from the apex of the fibular head.

SUMMARY

Several characteristics are common to all effective AFOs, regardless of their specific design or the materials and methods used in their fabrication. First, the efficacy of the orthosis is directly related to the intimacy and consistency of its fit. For some patients, an additional figure-eight ankle strap or other form of augmented closure (in addition to an appropriately closed or tied shoe) may be necessary to keep the calcaneus well seated in the orthosis during all phases of gait. Even a minimal amount of pistoning or heel elevation within the orthosis during gait can lead to skin irritation, ulceration, or an increase of underlying extensor hypertonicity.

Second, although thermoplastic AFOs are effective in controlling wide-ranging orthopedic deformities, their efficacy is dependent on a total contact, intimate fit in all three planes of motion. This is best achieved in custom-molded designs.

Finally, the ability of an AFO to achieve maximum benefit is greatly influenced by the type and condition of the shoe.[36] This point is often overlooked by patients, caregivers, and health care providers. Many patients need to increase their shoe size one half to a whole size to accommodate the orthosis. Although one of the benefits of thermoplastic AFOs is the ability to wear various shoes, changing heel heights can dramatically alter the biomechanical function of the orthosis. A PLS, articulating, or solid-ankle AFO designed to be worn with an athletic or oxford shoe that closes near the ankle is not as effective in a loafer or sandal with a more distal (or absent) closure.

Modification of a shoe's sole can counteract the limitations imposed by AFOs that restrict ankle motion. The addition of a cushion heel (similar to that used in prosthetic feet) can mimic the controlled lowering of the foot during first rocker. A rocker bar or rocker bottom placed at midfoot can simulate the second rocker, enhancing forward progression during the second half of stance phase. The orthotist and therapist share the responsibility for educating the patient and family about appropriate footwear, monitoring the condition of shoes, and evaluating the continuing efficacy of the orthosis in meeting the patient's functional needs over time.

An appropriately designed and fitted AFO can have a significant positive impact on a patient's mobility and functional status. Although thermoplastic designs are most often used, in some circumstances a conventional metal AFO may be more appropriate. The primary goal is to prescribe an orthosis that provides the appropriate external support for stability in stance and clearance in swing, with minimal compromise of the first (heel), second (ankle), and third (toe) rockers of gait. Factors that help to determine the appropriate design include the presence and degree of musculoskeletal impairment or deformity, the extent of impairment of motor control and hypertonicity, and the prognosis of the condition (growth, progression of the disease process, or likelihood of improvement). Thoughtful consideration of these factors results in a positive orthotic outcome for the patient and for members of the health care team.

REFERENCES

1. Epler ME. Orthoses for the ankle. In Nawoczenksi DA, Epler ME (eds), *Orthotics in Functional Rehabilitation of the Lower Limb.* Philadelphia: Saunders, 1997. pp. 77-114.
2. Hanna D, Harvey RL. Review of preorthotic biomechanical considerations. *Top Stroke Rehabil* 2001;7(4):29-37.
3. Perry J. *Gait Analysis: Normal and Pathological Function.* Thorofare, NJ: Slack, 1992.
4. McHugh B. Analysis of body-device interface forces in the sagittal plane for patients wearing ankle-foot orthoses. *Prosthet Orthot Int* 1999;23(1):75-81.
5. Franceschini M, Massucci M, Ferrari L, et al. Effects of an ankle foot orthosis on spatiotemporal parameters and energy cost of human gait. *Clin Rehabil* 2003;17:368-372.
6. Nowak MD, Abu-Hasaballah KS, Cooper PS. Design enhancement of a solid ankle-foot orthosis: real-time contact pressures evaluation. *J Rehabil Res Dev* 2000;37(3): 273-281.
7. Shah MK, Hugghins SY. Charcot's joint: an overlooked diagnosis. *J La State Med Soc* 2002; 154(5):246-250.
8. Inlow S, Kalla TP, Rahman J. Downloading plantar foot pressures in the diabetic patient. *Ostomy Wound Manage* 1999;45(10):28-34.

9. Landsman AS, Sage R. Off-loading neuropathic wounds associated with diabetes using an ankle-foot orthosis. *J Am Podiatr Med Assoc* 1997;87(8):349-357.
10. Bunch WH, Keagy RD, Kritter AE, et al. *Atlas of Orthotics: Biomechanical Principles and Application,* 2nd ed. St Louis: Mosby, 1985.
11. Carlson J, Berglund C. An effective orthotic design for controlling the unstable subtalar joint. *Orthot Prosthet* 1979;33(1):39-49.
12. Inman VT. Dual axis ankle control systems and the UCBL shoe insert: biomechanical considerations. *Bull Prosthet Res* 1969;Spring(10-11):130-146.
13. Knutson LM, Clark DE. Orthotic devices for ambulation in children with cerebral palsy and myelomeningocele. *Phys Ther* 1991;71(12):947-960.
14. Diamond MF, Ottenbacher KJ. Effect of a tone-inhibiting dynamic ankle-foot orthosis on stride characteristics of an adult with hemiparesis. *Phys Ther* 1990;70(7):423-430.
15. Hylton NM. Postural and functional impact of dynamic AFOs and FO in a pediatric population. *J Prosthet Orthot* 1989;2(1):40-53.
16. Mueller K, Cornwall M, McPoil T, et al. Effect of a tone-inhibiting dynamic ankle-foot orthosis on the foot loading pattern of a hemiplegic adult. *J Prosthet Orthot* 1992;4(2): 86-92.
17. Romkes J, Brunner R. Comparison of a dynamic and a hinged ankle-foot orthosis by gait analysis in patients with hemiplegic cerebral palsy. *Gait Posture* 2002;15(1):18-24.
18. Carlson WE, Vaughan CL, Damiano DL, Able MF. Orthotic management of gait in spastic diplegia. *Am J Phys Med Rehabil* 1997;76(3):219-225.
19. Bill M, McIntosh R, Myers P. A series of case studies on the effect of a midfoot control ankle foot orthosis in the prevention of unresolved pressure areas in children with cerebral palsy. *Prosthet Orthot Int* 2001;25(3):246-250.
20. Iwata M, Kondo I, Sato Y, et al. An ankle-foot orthosis with inhibitor bar: effect on hemiplegic gait. *Arch Phys Med Rehabil* 2003;84(6):924-927.
21. Trautman P. Lower limb orthotics. In JB Redford, JV Basmajian, P Trautman (eds), *Orthotics: Clinical Practice and Rehabilitation Technology.* New York: Churchill Livingstone, 1995. pp. 13-53.
22. Waters RL, Garland DE, Montgomery J. Orthotic prescription for stroke and head injury. In *American Academy of Orthopedic Surgeons, Atlas of Orthotics, Biomechanical Principles and Application.* St. Louis: Mosby, 1985. pp. 270-286.
23. Montgomery J. Orthotic management of the lower limb in head injured adults. *J Head Trauma Rehabil* 1987;2(2):57-61.
24. Carlson JM, Berglund C. An effective orthotic design for controlling the unstable subtalar joint. *J Orthot Prosthet* 1979;33(1):39-49.
25. Harrington E, Lin R, Gage J. Use of an anterior floor reaction orthosis in patients with cerebral palsy. *Orthot Prosthet* 1983;37(4):34-42.
26. Yang G, Chu D, Ahn J, et al. Floor reaction orthosis: clinical experience. *Orthot Prosthet* 1986;40(1):33-37.
27. McIlmurray WJ, Greenbaum W. A below knee weight bearing brace. *Orthop Prosthet Appl J* 1958;12(2):81-82.
28. Lehman JF. Lower limb orthotics. In JB Redford (ed), *Orthotics Etcetera,* 3rd ed. Baltimore: Williams & Wilkins, 1975. p. 317.
29. Waters RL, Garland DE, Montgomery J. Passive drop foot, clinical illustration: trauma. In *Rancho Los Amigos Medical Center Prosthetics and Orthotics Course Syllabus, Critical Decisions in Patient Management.* Downey, CA: Professional Staff Association, 1985. pp. 6:10-12.
30. Lehman JF, Esselmen PC, Ko MJ. Plastic ankle foot orthosis: evaluation of function. *Arch Phys Med Rehabil* 1983;64(9):402-407.
31. Berger N, Edelstein JE, Fishman S, et al. *Lower Limb Orthotics. Prosthetics and Orthotics.* New York: NYU Postgraduate Medical School, 1986. pp. 129-163.
32. Sumiya T, Suzuki Y, Kasahara T. Stiffness control in posterior-type plastic ankle-foot orthoses: effect of ankle trimline. Part 2: Orthosis characteristics and orthosis/patient matching. *Prosthet Orthot Int* 1996;20(2):132-137.
33. Weber D. *Clinical Aspects of Lower Extremity Orthotics.* Oakville, Ontario: Elgan, 1990.
34. Buckon CE, Thomas SS, Jakobson-Huston S, et al. Comparison of three ankle-foot orthosis configurations for children with spastic hemiplegia. *Dev Med Child Neurol* 2001;43(6):371-378.
35. Shurr DG, Cook TM, editors. Lower limb orthotics. In *Prosthetics and Orthotics.* Norwalk, CT: Appleton & Lange, 1990. pp. 123-149.
36. Churchill AJG, Halligan PW, Wake DT. Relative contribution of footwear to the efficacy of ankle foot orthoses. *Clin Rehabil* 2003;17:553-557.

11

Knee-Ankle-Foot and Hip-Knee-Ankle-Foot Orthoses

THOMAS V. DIBELLO AND JAMES H. CAMPBELL

LEARNING OBJECTIVES

On completion of this chapter, the reader will be able to do the following:

1. Delineate the functional objectives that can be addressed by the various knee-ankle-foot orthosis (KAFO) and hip-knee-ankle-foot orthosis (HKAFO) designs.
2. Explain the evaluative process used to determine appropriate prescriptions for individuals requiring KAFOs or HKAFOs.
3. Describe how typical KAFO and HKAFO designs provide stability in stance and affect mobility or gait.
4. Compare and contrast the benefits and trade-offs of comparable KAFO and HKAFO designs.
5. Identify effective strategies for donning and doffing orthoses, gait and mobility training, and orthotic maintenance for children and adults using KAFOs and HKAFOs.

For patients with neuromuscular or musculoskeletal impairments of the lower extremities who may require an orthosis to enhance functional mobility (gait or transfers, or both), decisions about orthotic prescription are best made in the context of an interdisciplinary team framework. This team comprises the patient with impairment and his or her family or caregivers; any physicians involved in the patient's care (e.g., a neurologist, orthopedist, or physiatrist); the physical and occupational therapists who are likely to be involved in functional training; and the orthotist who will design, fabricate, deliver, and maintain the orthosis. Recommendations about orthotic options are based on four types of information:

1. An understanding of the individual's diagnosis and prognosis.
2. A thorough assessment of gait, muscle function and motor control, range of motion, and alignment of the limb.
3. An understanding of the patient's general medical condition and level of fitness.
4. Discussion of the patient's typical or desired vocational and leisure activities. A clear goal or set of goals for orthotic intervention is formulated on the basis of these findings. This chapter specifically focuses on decision making for the prescription of KAFOs and HKAFOs.

The team approach allows consideration of various important influences on the eventual outcome of orthotic intervention, ranging from the specifics of the patient's diagnosis to the patient's preferred lifestyle and leisure activities. The importance of this discussion, which must include the patient with impairment, cannot be overstated. The use of an orthosis, a mechanical device that can enhance as well as constrain lower limb function, requires considerable adjustment on the part of the patient. Acceptance and consistent use of the orthosis depend, to a large extent, on how well the device meets the patient's specific needs or goals and how much use of the device is inconvenient or disruptive to the patient's lifestyle.

An important component of orthotic intervention is assessment of the patient's preconception or expectation about the outcome of orthotic intervention. A patient who expects that the success of an orthosis depends on a return to "normalcy" in walking is certain to be disappointed with the intervention and frustrated with the device. Patient education and discussion about the likely functional outcomes of KAFO or HKAFO use are especially important when expectations and reality are mismatched. Failure to discuss and define anticipated functional status and trade-offs of orthotic use early in the process often leads to difficulties with or rejection of the orthosis.

The clinical decision to provide any age of patient with a KAFO or HKAFO is based on careful consideration of the relative advantages and disadvantages of such an orthosis with respect to its impact on function, mobility, and energy cost. Although there are established decision pathways for bracing the lower extremity with KAFOs, clear indications for bracing the hip and trunk for those with significant neuromuscular or musculoskeletal impairments have not been as well documented.[1]

It is also important for the team to consider carefully the diagnosis that makes prescription of an orthosis necessary, including its etiology and prognosis. Is the patient's musculoskeletal or neuromuscular status stable and likely to remain the same over time? Does the patient's disease typically have a progressive course, such that decline in function is anticipated over time, or, as in the case of traumatic injury, will the patient's condition and functional ability improve with time as healing occurs? Diagnosis also helps the team to define what might be expected in terms of muscle function and strength, range of motion and joint function, and functional mobility and gait. The orthotic design must account for all of these factors.

This chapter describes the most commonly used components and designs of KAFOs and HKAFOs and explores their use in the management of mobility dysfunction for persons with neuromuscular impairments. It begins with a discussion of contemporary KAFO components and design, continues with an overview of traditional HKAFOs, investigates the clinical use of the parapodium and standing frames, and, finally, explores orthotic options for reciprocal gait for individuals with significant neuromuscular disease or disability.

WHAT IS THE DIFFERENCE BETWEEN A KAFO AND AN HKAFO?

The systematic approach used to prescribe orthoses defines an orthotic device by the anatomical segments or principal joints that it encompasses. A KAFO is defined as encompassing the knee joint and ankle joint, while an HKAFO, in addition to controlling the knee and ankle, extends proximally above one or both hip joints.

WHEN IS A KAFO INDICATED?

An effective assessment of the lower limb function is based on a thorough understanding of the intricacies of normal stance and swing-phase biomechanics.[2] Assessment of gait includes quantitative kinematic measures (e.g., gait speed, stride and step length, cadence, double support time) and an observational gait analysis that assists the team in identifying primary problems in the context of the gait cycle, as well as possible compensatory strategies.[2-4] For patients with complex gait problems, videotaping or computerized gait analysis may be a valuable tool for the team in appreciating what is happening during stance and swing. Clear definition and quantification of gait deviations assist the team in determining the level of orthotic intervention necessary to achieve specified goals.

KAFOs are considered when excessive movement occurs at the knee during stance phase that cannot be effectively controlled by an ankle-foot orthosis (AFO).[1] If a patient is unable to control flexion movement in early stance, stability is compromised. The patient may have hyperextension or recurvatum that jeopardizes the structural integrity of the joint and, if unchecked, will threaten stance phase stability. Abnormal or excessive varus or valgus angulation may be present when the limb is loaded in stance, which compromises joint function and structure and can further alter biomechanical function over time to compromise the patient's ability to walk in the future.

Assessment of knee function should never occur in isolation but instead be evaluated in the context of a closed chain or system: Position of and muscular action around the ankle and the hip affect knee function throughout stance and swing phases. Ankle position affects the position of the knee in relation to the ground reaction forces.

In normal gait, as loading response transitions toward midstance, the foot has moved into a foot-flat position so that the ankle is in slight plantar flexion. Concurrently, knee flexion is controlled by eccentric contraction of the quadriceps muscles to approximately 15 degrees to "absorb shock" as the limb is loaded; this is quickly followed by knee extension. The hip is supported in 30 degrees of flexion and begins to extend with forward progression, and the hip abductors work to keep the pelvis level. In this early-stance period, the ground reaction force passes through the ankle, behind the knee, and through the hip, creating an external flexion movement at the knee (Figure 11-1). To counteract this ground reaction force–derived external flexion movement, the quadriceps must contract to prevent the knee from collapsing into further flexion. In addition, the hamstrings contract to stabilize hip position, and the gastrocnemius begins to contract eccentrically to control forward progression of the tibia. This combination of muscle activity provides an internally generated knee extension movement that balances the external flexion movement at the knee generated by the ground reaction force.

If position or muscle function at the hip, knee, or ankle is altered or disturbed in any way, the system is thrown out of equilibrium, and gait will be less efficient or compromised.[5] If ankle position changes, the relative position of the ground reaction force will also change, altering the magnitude of the movement generated at the knee. If the strength or motor control of any of the involved musculature is impaired, the patient's ability to generate the appropriate internal extension movement to balance the external flexion movement may be compromised. When significant hypertonicity (spasticity) is present, excessive muscle activity that overpowers the external moment or alters the sequencing of muscle action often occurs.[6] The magnitude of disruption of the equilibrium between externally and internally generated movements determines whether the patient will recover from or compensate for the imbalance. The magnitude of disruption and the resultant impact on gait also determine the level of orthotic intervention that is necessary to achieve the specified goal. When the evaluation of lower extremity

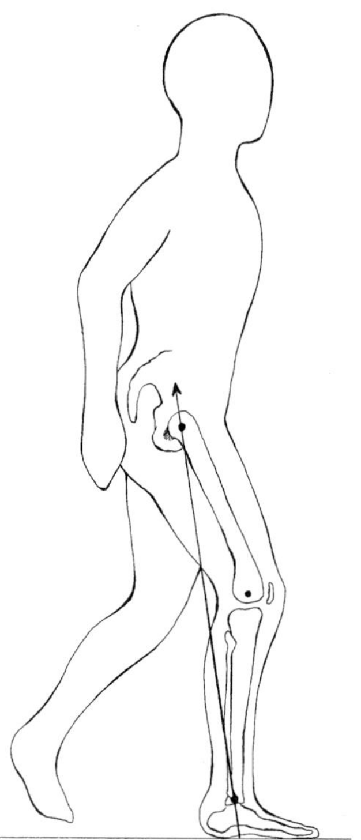

Figure 11-1
The ground reaction force passes through the ankle, behind the knee, and through the hip as loading response moves toward midstance, creating an external flexion movement at the knee. To achieve stability, muscle activity of the quadriceps, hamstrings, and gastrocnemius/soleus combine to create an internal extension movement to counterbalance the flexion movement of the ground reaction force.

function indicates that an AFO cannot effectively influence the position of the ground reaction force as it crosses the knee, a KAFO is likely to be the appropriate orthosis.

An orthosis of any kind does three things: It protects the joints of the limb that it crosses, it provides stance phase stability when structural integrity or motor control is impaired, and it affects the patient's ability to function (i.e., functionality). The relationship between functionality and stability/protection in lower extremity orthoses is somewhat inverse; any orthosis that provides stance phase stability for patients with lower limb weakness due to a neuromuscular disorder, or protection for a patient who is in rehabilitation after traumatic injury, affects mobility in swing and limb movement during other functional activities. Improved function does not imply normalcy. The goals of stability and protection are to provide patients improved function as compared with ambulation without an orthosis, but gait cannot be restored to normal.

When protection or stability of the knee is the primary goal of treatment, an AFO may not be sufficient, and a KAFO may be indicated.[7] Currently, an orthotist can choose from three classes of orthotic knee joints. When the desired control is for reduction of knee joint hyperextension or mild to moderate varus or valgus angulation is present, the KAFO can be built with a *nonlocking knee joint*. When hyperflexion (the tendency to "buckle" under body weight) or severe varus or valgus angulation is present, a *locking orthotic knee joint* is incorporated into the KAFO. When an orthosis locks the limb in extension, stance phase stability is enhanced, but swing phase clearance is compromised. A new group of *stance control orthotic knee joints* that have become available for patients with quadriceps weakness. These provide stance control without having to keep the knee locked in extension during swing phase.[8] This group of stance-and-swing-phase–influencing orthotic knee joints represents the first major change in knee joint mechanics in possibly 150 years. All these designs and their proper use and application are discussed in greater detail later in the chapter.

The decision to use a nonlocking, locking, or a swing-or-stance-phase–influencing orthotic knee joint is based on each patient's available range of motion, muscle strength, and motor control. A KAFO can be used to support one impaired limb, for example, after trauma injury or after stroke. Bilateral KAFOs are often prescribed for patients with paraplegia or with traumatic injury of both lower extremities. A patient with bilateral locked-knee KAFOs most often requires an assistive device (crutches or a walker) for external support during ambulation. The most efficient gait pattern is determined by hip function: Most patients who use bilateral KAFOs develop a swing-to or swing-through gait pattern. Some may be able to use a reciprocal pattern if sufficient muscle function is present at the hip (minimally, volitional control of hip flexion).[9]

KAFO EVALUATION AND PRESCRIPTION

The evaluation process includes assessment of the patient's height and weight, the status of circulation and sensation in the affected lower extremity, the condition and integrity of the patient's skin, soft tissue density and bony prominences, and the patient's living or working environment. Specific measurements of range of motion and fixed contractures, muscle strength and tone, and leg length and limb girth are also made. This information, when combined with functional assessment of gait and mobility tasks, helps the team to define the appropriate orthosis. Several critical decisions regarding specific aspects of the orthotic design must be made about materials and components. The orthotist must first select the appropriate type and gauge of plastic or metal to use. Decisions must be made about whether reinforcing materials will be necessary, which to choose, and where to place the reinforcements. The extent of contact that the orthosis will make with the patient's body must also be carefully considered; although intimate fit provides optimal control, one must protect areas that are vulnerable to pressure and account for potential variations in limb volume. The choices made in this planning stage ultimately define the success or failure of a particular orthosis.[7] The orthotist's knowledge and understanding of material characteristics guide the selection of appropriate materials and the decision about the most effective way to implement them. Blending combinations of plastic, metal, and composite materials permits the orthotist to provide an orthosis that is flexible where needed but rigid and stiff in other areas. In this way, a skilled clinician can maximize control while minimizing the orthosis' impact on function.

The most critical component of assessment and orthotic prescription is a clear understanding of the sequential deviations in the patient's gait pattern. This knowledge enables the orthotist to provide the maximum amount of correction without causing discomfort. While measuring the limb (for a conventional metal, double-upright orthosis) or taking an impression by casting the limb (to make a positive model for a thermoplastic orthosis), the orthotist must position the limb in optimal alignment, given that individual's neuromuscular or musculoskeletal impairments and functional limitations. The orthotist uses a series of overlapping three-point force systems, beginning at the foot and moving proximally, to achieve this optimal alignment in the design of the orthosis.[10] The orthotist must assess range of motion at each joint and then design the orthosis to reduce or eliminate each deviation in sequence through the application of appropriate three-point force systems.

Consider a patient who presents with hyperextension at the right knee while transitioning from initial contact to loading response, excessive pronation of the midfoot during midstance, and hyperextension with valgus at the knee throughout the stance phase. For this patient, one force system will control knee hyperextension throughout stance, another will address valgus, and a third will target midfoot control to minimize the abnormal pronation. The impact of each on the others as the stance phase progresses must also be considered.

KAFO DESIGN OPTIONS

Two KAFO designs are being used in contemporary clinical practice. A conventional (metal and leather) KAFO is attached to the patient's shoe by a stirrup and can be worn either under or external to clothing. A molded thermoplastic KAFO fits within the patient's shoe and is designed to have an intimate fit so that it can be worn under clothing. Any orthosis, as an external device applied to the patient's limb, in some ways facilitates and in others inhibits function. What is advantageous for one patient may be disadvantageous to another.[1] A design that is effective in meeting the needs of one patient may be contraindicated for patients with different physical characteristics or medical conditions.

In choosing materials, components, and orthotic design, the orthotist must consider many factors: durability and weight of the materials, the precise control that is possible across all planes of motion, the ease of donning and doffing the device, the ease of adjustability and maintenance, and the overall cosmesis of the finished orthosis. The decision to prescribe a conventional or thermoplastic KAFO is founded on the needs and characteristics of the individual patient.

Conventional KAFOs

A conventional KAFO has a metal frame (double uprights) that is attached to a shoe by a stirrup system and leather coverings over the calf and thigh bands (Figure 11-2). Typically, a pair of orthotic ankle joints is used to connect the stirrup to the distal (lower) metal uprights, and a pair of orthotic knee joints connects the distal (lower) and proximal (upper) metal uprights, as determined by the patient's specific needs. The uprights are most often stainless steel or aluminum. The length and contour or the uprights are based on a tracing (delineation) of the limb and on girth measurements. The uprights and joints form a rigid structure or cage around the limb. The orthosis contacts the patient's limb at leather-covered posterior bands and the anterior straps that are used to hold the limb within the orthosis. An anterior kneepad can be added as an additional contact point.

A three-point pressure system stabilizes the knee in the sagittal plane to control flexion/extension: Two anteriorly directed forces (applied by the posterior thigh band proximally and the shoe and posterior calf band distally) are opposed by a single posteriorly directed force (applied by the anterior kneepad or by anterior thigh and calf straps).[11] Theoretically, additional force systems (a pair of proximal/distal forces

Box 11-1 *Comparison of Advantages and Disadvantages of Conventional Knee-Ankle-Foot Orthoses*

ADVANTAGES
- Strong
- Most durable
- Easily adjusted

DISADVANTAGES
- Heavy
- Must be attached to shoe or shoe insert
- Less cosmetic
- Fewer contact points reduce control

INDICATIONS
- When maximum strength and durability are needed
- For individuals with significant obesity
- For individuals with uncontrolled or fluctuating edema (e.g., congestive heart failure, dialysis)

CONTRAINDICATIONS
- When issues of energy expenditure make weight of the orthosis a factor
- When control of transverse plane motion is important

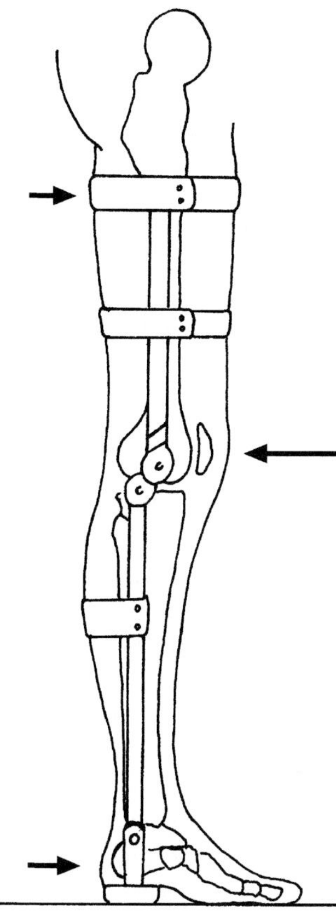

Figure 11-2

Schematic diagram of the components and sagittal plane force system acting at the knee in a conventional knee-ankle-foot orthosis.

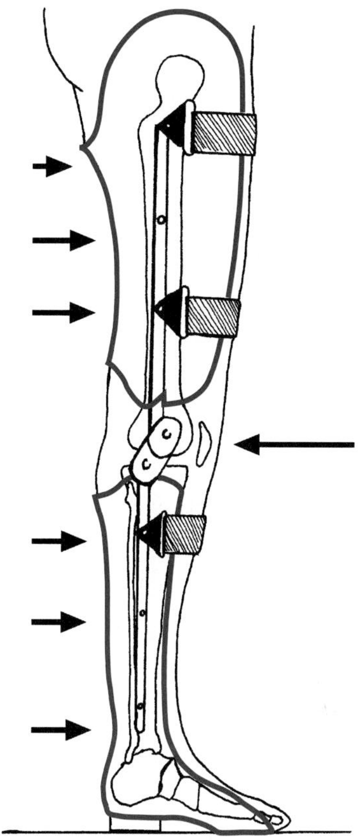

Figure 11-3

Schematic diagram of the components and sagittal plane force systems that are necessary to control knee flexion/extension. Because the point of force application is distributed over the entire posterior surface of the intimately fitting orthotic shell, more precise and more comfortable control of the limb is possible.

opposing a central force) act in the frontal plane to control varus and valgus at the knee. The less-than-intimate fit of this orthosis reduces the efficacy of varus/valgus control systems.

Although conventional KAFOs are quite durable and easily adjusted, they tend to be heavier and less cosmetically pleasing than thermoplastic versions. The advantages and disadvantages and the indications and contraindications of conventional KAFOs are summarized in Box 11-1.

Thermoplastic KAFOs

To create the thermoplastic KAFO (Figure 11-3) a shell is vacuum-formed over a positive model of the patient's limb. The distal shell, which fits intimately over the foot, ankle, and lower leg, is basically an AFO with a proximal anterior strap (usually Velcro) closure. Depending on the patient's needs, this distal component may be either a solid-ankle or articulating design. The proximal shell encases the thigh from the greater trochanter to just above the femoral condyles and typically has a pair of anterior straps (again, usually Velcro) for closure. Metal knee joints and sidebars (made of stainless steel, aluminum, or titanium) connect the proximal and distal shells. The type of plastic chosen for the shell determines the rigidity of the orthosis. An alternative custom KAFO design, using an anterior thigh shell and an anterior proximal tibial shell instead of a posterior thigh cuff and AFO, has been described as more comfortable to wear and somewhat easier to don,[12] although evidence is limited.

The key feature of this orthosis is its intimate total contact fit and resultant potential to control the limb. Covering and encompassing a large surface area with the plastic reduces the force per unit area that is required for stabilization or control of the limb, diminishing the likelihood of discomfort or skin irritation, which is associated with high or excessive pressure. On the other hand, if the fit is less than optimal such that pistoning occurs within the orthosis during gait or tissue is excessively compressed where the fit is too tight, patients will complain of discomfort, and skin problems are likely to occur.

In this design, a series of overlapping three-point force systems is possible. The force system for control of flexion and extension in the sagittal plane is essentially the same as that of a conventional KAFO, although the posterior force is distributed over a wider surface area. As a result of the total

Box 11-2 *Comparison of Advantages and Disadvantages of Thermoplastic Knee-Ankle-Foot Orthoses*

ADVANTAGES
- Lightweight
- Interchangeability of shoes
- Greater cosmesis worn under clothing

DISADVANTAGES
- Can be hot to wear

INDICATIONS
- Intimate/total contact fit makes maximum limb control possible
- When energy expenditure makes weight of the orthosis an issue
- When control of transverse plane motion is needed
- Contraindications
- Intimacy of fit is difficult when the individual is significantly obese
- Intimacy of fit is compromised when the individual has uncontrolled or fluctuating edema

contact design of the shells, a more precise control of the limb is possible, in both the frontal and transverse planes; this is particularly important when dealing with segmental deviations secondary to transverse plane rotational problems.[13] Because of the multiplanar characteristics of the knee joint, varus or valgus deviations at the knee typically include a rotatory component. Controlling this is more easily accomplished with the total contact design of the thermoplastic KAFO than with the double-upright system of a conventional KAFO. The intimate fit of the thermoplastic KAFO may be problematic, however, for patients with fluctuating limb volume secondary to edema or cyclical weight gain or loss. Many thermoplastic KAFO patients enjoy wearing a variety of shoes (as long as heel height is the same) and the cosmesis afforded by wearing the thermoplastic orthosis under their clothing. As lightweight as this orthosis is, the large contact area may make it difficult to dissipate body heat so that the orthosis is uncomfortably warm for patients who are active or live in hot climates. Advantages and disadvantages of a custom-molded thermoplastic KAFO are summarized in Box 11-2.

Controlling the Ankle

The ankle joints used in KAFOs are the same as those available for ankle-foot orthoses (AFOs). The orthotist can choose among three types of orthotic ankle joints: (1) a *nonarticulating,* or fixed-ankle, design (as in a solid-ankle AFO); (2) a *single-axis articulating* design that allows dorsiflexion (for forward progression of the tibia over the foot in stance) but blocks plantar flexion or provides dorsiflexion assistance (to enhance swing phase clearance); or (3) a *"free" single-axis articulating* design that allows dorsiflexion and plantar flexion within a specific range of motion. What is important to consider, however, is how the ankle configuration and ground reaction force influence knee function and forward progression during gait.

If a patient's condition requires a KAFO with a locked knee joint, the impact of the ground reaction force on the knee is negated.[3,14] Using an ankle joint that permits movement of the ankle through a specific range of motion is beneficial in improving the patient's level of function when the knee is locked, enhancing forward progression of the body over the foot during stance. Ambulation with both a locked knee and a locked ankle becomes difficult. Locking the ankle precludes progression through the stance phase rockers found in normal gait; forward progression over the foot in stance is significantly compromised. Additionally, clearance in swing is compromised by the locked knee. Patients walking with locked knee and ankle must use compensatory strategies for functional gait: They may have uneven stride length and stance times because of difficulty with forward progression and may vault or circumduct to enhance swing clearance of the limb in the orthosis.

When motion at the ankle must be eliminated to protect the joint or control the impact of abnormal tone and the knee joint must remained locked for stance phase stability, the orthotist often places a *rocker sole* on the patient's shoe.[15] This rocker sole simulates the normal rockers of gait, enhancing forward progression by reducing the toe lever of the orthosis, improving the smoothness of the patient's gait and reducing the likelihood of compensatory gait deviations.

Ideally, if a patient's condition or level of function requires that the orthotic knee joint remains locked during ambulation, the orthotist can use an articulating ankle joint so that some ankle motion is possible. The ability to move into plantar flexion enhances the transition from initial contact to loading response (although the locked knee may compromise the shock absorption function of loading response). The ability to move into dorsiflexion enhances the forward progression of the limb over the fixed foot, especially in the transition from midstance toward terminal stance. The design characteristics of the orthotic ankle joint (whether metal or plastic, allowing free or limited motion) must be consistent with the overall design of the KAFO. In those instances in which ankle control is not particularly influenced by the desired knee control, the type of ankle joint and ankle position is determined by the patient's particular musculoskeletal and neuromuscular function or needs at the ankle.

Controlling the Knee

A wide variety of orthotic knee joints are available for use in KAFOs in current clinical practice. In this chapter, we discuss the designs that are most often encountered by rehabilitation professionals involved in functional gait training. When a patient has a special need, the orthotist uses knowledge of mechanics and product availability to tailor a joint to the specific needs of that patient.

Single-Axis Knee Joints

The single-axis knee, also known as a *straight knee joint without drop lock* or a *free knee,* permits unrestricted flexion and extension to 180 degrees in the sagittal plane (most designs prevent hyperextension) while providing mediolateral stability (Figure 11-4, *A*). The joint is designed to pivot around a single point or axis, like a simple hinge. The orthotist positions the axis of this orthotic joint medially along the midline of the extended leg at a point approximately one half of the distance between the adductor tubercle and the medial tibial plateau. The lateral joint is also positioned at the approximate axis of the anatomical knee joint. Although some degree of torque is created by the mismatch between the single-axis orthotic knee joint and the polycentric anatomical knee joint, for most patients this is not problematic. The free, single-axis knee is appropriate for those who have enough muscle function to ensure knee stability in stance but who tend to move into recurvatum, have significant structural (mediolateral) instability of the knee joint, or fall into excessive varum or valgus in stance.[16,17]

Single-Axis Locking Knee

With the addition of a locking mechanism, such as a ring or drop lock, the single-axis or locked knee provides rigid stability to the knee in all planes (see Figure 11-4, *B*). Its alignment is the same as that of the single-axis free knee. Although a drop (ring) lock is the most commonly used locking mechanism, various other locking mechanisms are also available, depending on the patient's functional requirements. This type of orthotic knee joint is appropriate for patients who are unable to control the knee effectively during stance phase, requiring additional external stability to prevent or restrain excessive knee flexion as body weight is transferred onto the limb.[18]

Offset Knee Joint

The offset knee joint is also known as a *posteriorly offset, free knee* (see Figure 11-4, *C*). This design is aligned with its axis of rotation behind the midline of the leg, posterior to the axis of the anatomical knee. In early stance, during the period of double support, the ground reaction passes closer to the center of the axis of the orthotic joint, reducing the magnitude of the external flexion moment that is acting to flex the limb. With continued forward progression, the ground reaction force quickly moves anterior to the orthotic joint, creating an extensor force that mechanically augments stance phase stability during single-limb support.[19,20] When used properly, this joint permits the orthotist to design a device that allows stability in the knee from initial contact

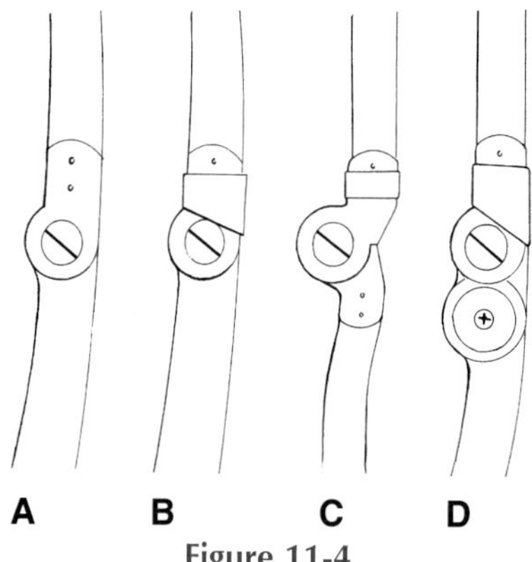

Figure 11-4

Conventional orthotic knee joints most often used in knee-ankle-foot orthoses. ***A,*** *A single-axis, or free, knee allows full flexion and extension while providing mediolateral stability to the knee joint.* ***B,*** *A locked knee is typically locked while the patient is standing, providing stability in all planes, and unlocked to permit knee flexion in sitting.* ***C,*** *The axis of the offset orthotic knee joint is positioned behind the anatomical knee axis, increasing the biomechanical stability of the orthosis. It is available with and without a locking mechanism.* ***D,*** *A variable position, or adjustable, orthotic knee joint permits the orthotist to accommodate for changing range of motion or for fixed contracture at the knee.*

through midstance; however, alignment of the knee and ankle must be precise if it is to be effective. A drop lock or other locking mechanism can be added to stabilize the knee in an extended position when the patient will be standing for long periods of time or when additional stability is advisable (e.g., when the patient is walking on uneven ground). This option is valuable for patients with limited knee control due to lower motor neuron disease, such as polio, or low thoracic–upper lumbar spinal cord injury.

Variable Position Orthotic Knee Joint

The variable position locking orthotic knee joint is also known as a *dial lock* or as an *adjustable locking knee joint* (see Figure 11-4, *D*). This design is intended for patients who are unable to achieve full extension due to knee flexion contracture. With flexion contracture, the position of the ground reaction force stays posterior to the anatomical knee joint; it may be difficult or impossible for the patient with weakness or motor control impairment to develop or maintain the necessary counteractive muscle force for stance stability. Instead, the variable position orthotic knee joint is locked in the most extended position possible, providing an external mechanical stability.[10,18] In addition to being used to accommodate a fixed knee flexion contracture, the variable position joint can be gradually adjusted into extension to assist elongation of soft tissue contracture as a patient's function improves and range of motion increases.[21] The angle of flexion is adjusted by removing the cover of the serrated disc and its matching serrated ring. Movement of one serration affects the locked angle by approximately 6 degrees.

Locking Mechanisms

The most commonly used locking mechanism is the ring or drop lock (see Figure 11-4, *B*). This simple design "captures" the male and female halves of the orthotic joint when it is fully extended, blocking subsequent movement into flexion or hyperextension. A small ball bearing incorporated into the upright ensures that the drop lock stays in the desired position until the patient purposefully unlocks or locks the orthosis. Although this mechanism is simple, durable, strong, and safe, the knee must be fully extended for the lock to be engaged or disengaged. Most KAFOs have a medial and a lateral upright. For optimal safety, a drop or ring lock should be engaged on both uprights. Having to manage drop locks on both sides of the orthosis simultaneously to engage or disengage the lock mechanism may be challenging for patients with limited hand function, significant lower extremity spasticity or contracture, or difficulty in balancing on one crutch while using a hand to work the locking mechanism.[21]

For patients who have difficulty managing drop locks, an alternative mechanism may be a spring-loaded bail lock (Figure 11-5). This is essentially a lever system, which connects the medial and lateral locks of a KAFO, permitting them to be engaged or disengaged simultaneously. Other locking mechanisms that use lever systems to manage the lock include pawl locks, cam locks, or Swiss locks.[10,21] To use a bail lock, the patient backs up against the edge of the seating surface (e.g., wheelchair, mat table, kitchen chair, desk chair); pressure against the posterior bar activates the bail's mechanism to disengage the lock, and the patient can sit with knee flexion. Although theoretically convenient and easy to use, this type of lock mechanism is most appropriate for patients with enough upper body strength and coordination to control the descent into sitting or for those who have previous experience with its use. If the exposed bail passing behind the knee is inadvertently bumped, the locks may disengage unexpectedly and the person may fall. Although the posterior edge of a properly contoured bail is angled downward to reduce the likelihood of unexpected unlocking, an upwardly directed force would still unlock these joints.

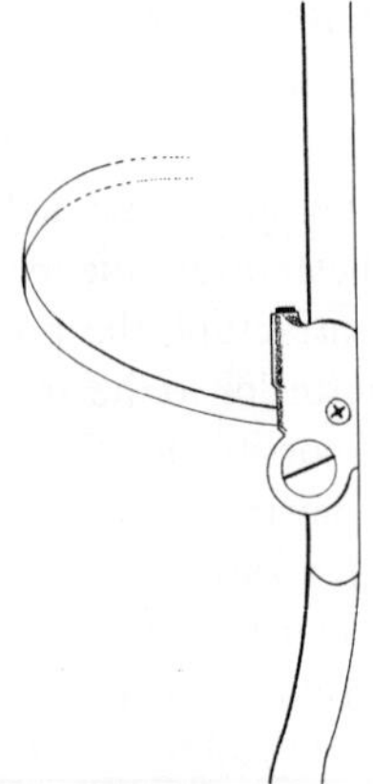

Figure 11-5
A bail-locking mechanism allows the medial and lateral knee locks to be disengaged at the same time by a posterior pressure, as against the edge of a seating surface. This mechanism is often used for patients with paraplegia who must maintain bilateral upper extremity support via crutches for stability in standing.

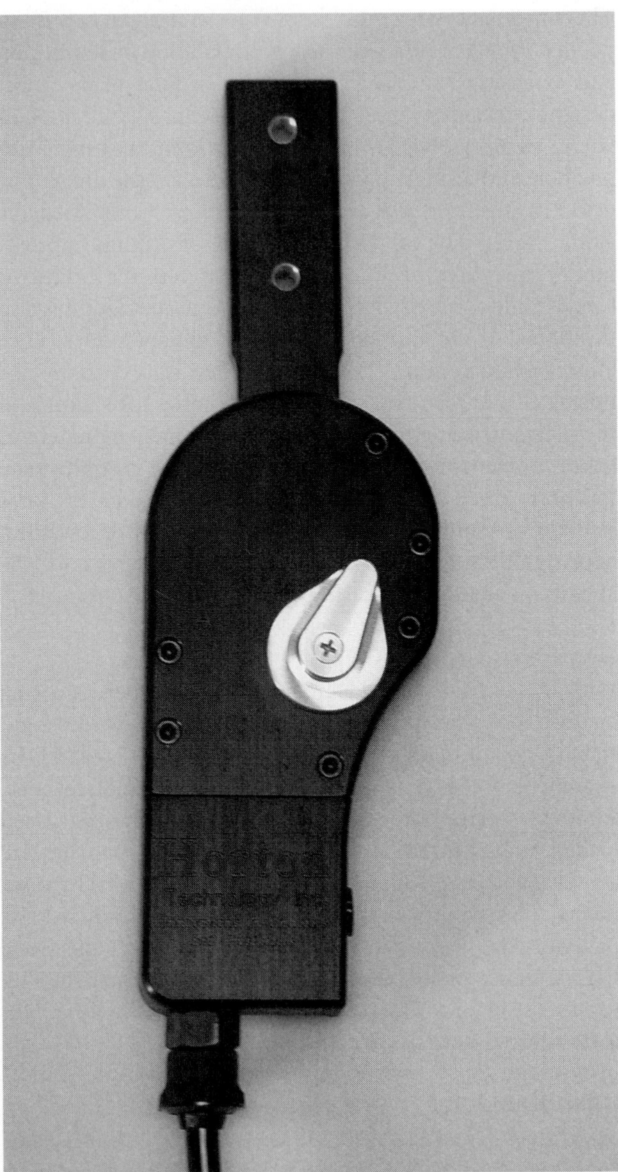

Figure 11-6
The stance control orthotic knee joint has an internal cam lock that engages the upper head assembly when slight pressure is transmitted upward through a push rod at initial contact/loading response. This blocks knee flexion during stance. As the cam is unloaded in late stance, the lock disengages, allowing knee flexion for limb clearance in swing. Depending on the patient's ability, the environment, and the nature of the task (walking versus prolonged standing), this orthotic knee can be set into any of three modes: automatic stance control, unlocked, or always locked. (Courtesy Horton's Orthotic Lab, Little Rock, Ark.)

Stance- and Swing Phase–Influencing Orthotic Knee Joints

Patients with quadriceps weakness present with a complex and varied set of problems that require the use of stance- and swing phase–influencing orthotic knee joints. Successful clinical application of these joints requires an understanding of the technical features of each joint as well as an understanding of the biomechanical deficit that is being replaced.[22] Accurate individual selection protocols have been developed and should be followed.[23,24] Designed specifically for patients with quadriceps weakness, this new family of orthotic joints allows the orthotic knee joint to lock at a point approximating initial contact (the beginning of first rocker) and unlock at a point approximating heel off (the beginning of third rocker). This arrangement permits the patient with lower limb paralysis to more closely mimic normal gait than ever before.

The advantages of the stance phase knee stability and swing phase freedom afforded by these joints is easily appreciated. Unlocking the knee at the beginning of third rocker decreases the need for a compensatory strategy such as hip hiking or circumduction to clear the foot, as would occur in swing phase in a traditional locked-knee KAFO. This reduced circumduction reduces the energy expenditure of walking[25] and provides a reasonable option for those with single-limb paralysis to compensate for absent musculature without having to use awkward mechanical movements. The reduction of hip movement in the coronal plane resulting from diminished hip hiking significantly lessens the stress and strain applied to the patient's lower back while walking.

If an orthotist is considering using an orthotic knee joint with these dynamic load–triggered locking and unlocking characteristics, every aspect of the evaluation process must be carefully performed. Special attention must be paid to the patient's ability to be trained to use this technology, as well as his or her cognitive ability to understand and apply it. Physical and possibly occupational therapy programs should be considered after fitting in order to achieve an optimal outcome.

Following is a summary of the key design features and the biomechanical rational for each component design.

Stance Control Orthotic Knee Joint

The Stance Control Orthotic Knee Joint (SCOKJ), developed by Horton Orthopedic Lab (Little Rock, AR), is a more traditional double sidebar arrangement with a push rod running from the knee joint to the ankle joint or to the heel of the orthosis.[22,27] It differs from traditional KAFO knee joints because it has a *tri-mode* (automatic, unlock, and lock) selection switch (Figure 11-6). In the automatic stance control mode, at initial contact, when the heel contacts the ground or the plantar flexion stop is engaged, the push rod causes a cam in the knee joint to block the movement of the joint, thereby preventing knee flexion but permitting knee extension. At heel off, the pressure is removed from the push rod and a

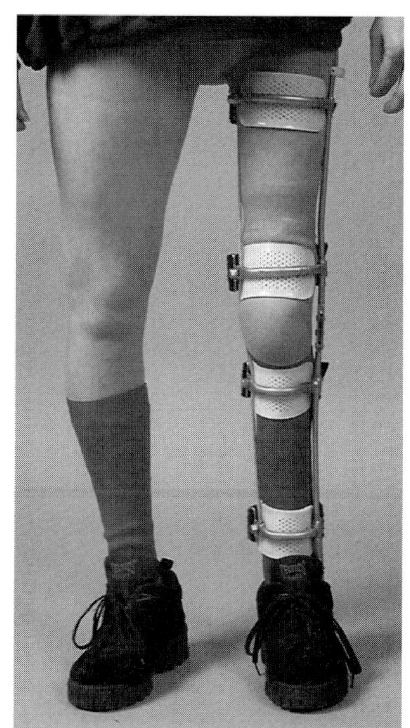
A

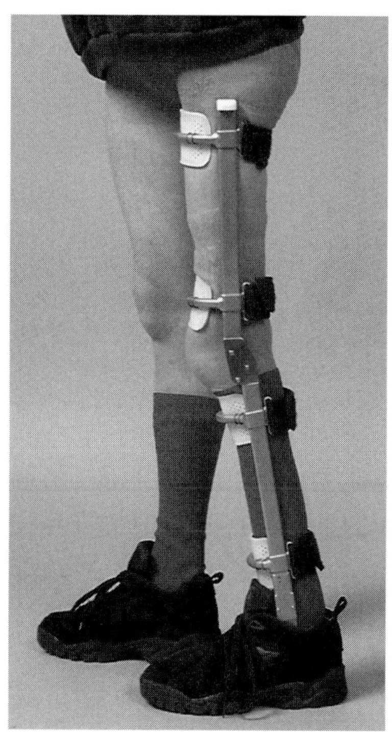
B

Figure 11-7

*An anterior (**A**) and lateral (**B**) view of the UTX Swing KAFO. This orthosis uses a lightweight lateral upright, a medial cable, anterior padded cuffs with Velcro-closing posterior straps, and an orthotic knee joint that resists flexion during stance but allows flexion during swing. (Courtesy Becker Orthopedic, Troy, Mich.)*

spring pushes the cam away from the central joint hub. When a knee extension movement is applied, the joint will unlock to facilitate swing phase. The joint is intended for patients with quadriceps absence or weakness—it is contraindicated for patients with significant or fixed knee deformity.

UTX Swing and Free Walk Joints

Based on original research and development work conducted at the University of Twente in the Netherlands by Dr. Nils van Leerdam, the UTX swing and free walk joints maintain sagittal plane stability while allowing knee flexion during swing phase for select patients with quadriceps weakness (Figure 11-7).[23,28] Both designs use a tubular steel construction to create an open-frame, lightweight design with a lateral upright. These systems have an upper weight limit of 265 pounds and are intended for patients with quadriceps weakness. They have been successfully used in clinical conditions including multiple sclerosis, polio, and incomplete lesions of the spinal cord. A strict and detailed physical assessment of each potential user should be conducted to determine the appropriateness of this prescription. Weakness of the hip musculature and angular deformity of the lower limb would be considered contraindications.

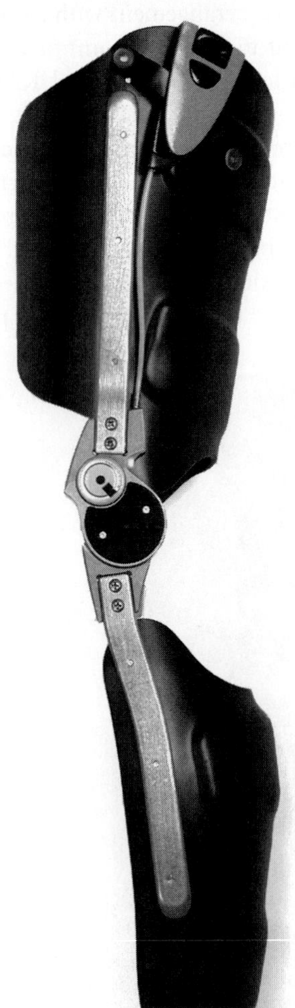

Figure 11-8
An example of the swing phase lock system developed by Basko Healthcare in the Netherlands, marketed by Fillauer, Inc. An internal mechanism of the laterally placed orthotic knee joint triggers locking before initial contract when the knee is fully extended and unlocking at the end of stance phase. A medially placed orthotic knee joint that further resists flexion during stance can also be used. (Courtesy Fillauer, Inc., Chattanooga, Tenn.)

Swing Phase Lock Orthotic Knee Joint

The Swing Phase Lock (SPL) orthotic knee joint was developed by Basko Healthcare in the Netherlands and uses a simple internal pendulum mechanism, which is designed to lock and unlock the knee depending upon the angle of the knee joint in the sagittal plane (Figure 11-8).[29] During walking, this orthotic joint locks at the end of swing phase, before initial contact, and unlocks at heel off. The locking/unlocking mechanism is therefore position dependent and could be described as gait, rather than weight, activated. Contraindications include knee or hip flexion contracture, involvement or weakness of the hip musculature, poor balance, or coordination.

Load Response Joint

The loading response phase of gait is highly demanding as the limb is destabilized by the heel rocker and then supported by a strong extensor muscle response. In normal gait, controlled stance phase knee flexion provides shock absorption for more proximal joints as weight is loaded onto the limb. The load-response orthotic knee joint has been engineered to facilitate knee flexion and provide shock absorption during stance phase.[30] It can be considered for patients with significant quadriceps weakness, as well as for those who also have weakness of hip musculature.

G Knee

In the intact lower extremity, the quadriceps restrain knee flexion in stance phase. They also act to extend the knee joint in terminal swing as the limb approaches initial contact. The G knee joint component is intended to allow passive knee flexion during swing phase and includes a gas spring that will aid knee extension and establish a stable limb and geometric stability of the knee at initial contact.[31]

E Knee

The E knee is a foot force–activated, computer-controlled, electromechanical, orthotic knee joint system that was developed by Jonathan Naft.[32] The E knee is an attempt to improve existing KAFO design by combining electronic foot force sensing, microcontroller signal processing, and control with a novel electromechanical knee actuator. Configured with a passive lock, during stance phase this joint permits knee extension while blocking knee flexion. As pressure is removed from a footplate inside the shoe, a ratcheting knee joint disengages, permitting free knee flexion and extension during swing phase.

CASE EXAMPLE 1

A Patient with Poliomyelitis-Related Impairment

M. L. is a 59-year-old woman who survived acute poliomyelitis as a 7-year-old and has been living with longstanding atrophy and weakness of her left lower extremity since that time. Until recently, she wore a conventional KAFO with drop lock to maintain full knee extension for stance phase stability. When walking with the KAFO, she used a combination of circumduction of the left (swing) limb and vaulting on the right (stance) limb to ensure clearance of the left lower extremity in midswing. Inside, on level surfaces, she can ambulate without assistive devices. Outside, and for long distances, she uses either a straight cane or a forearm (Lofstrand) crutch on the right for added stability. She recently read about the development of stance control knee joints that allow knee flexion during swing phase and has returned to the orthotic clinic to determine if this option would be appropriate for her.

Examination reveals a fairly fit and active woman with marked atrophy of thigh and calf muscles. Passive range of motion of the left hip and knee are within functional limits required for gait, although ankle dorsiflexion (0 to 7 degrees) and plantar flexion (0 to 10 degrees) are limited by long-standing soft tissue tightness. While all knee ligaments are intact, there is a mild valgus alignment, and the knee can be hyperextended 5 degrees. No rotational or torsional deformities are noted.

Left lower extremity muscle strength is as follows:

- Hip flexion and rotations, 3+
- Hip extension (gluteals) and abduction, 4
- Quadriceps (knee extension) 2, hamstring (knee flexion), 4
- Dorsiflexion, 3+
- Plantar flexion, 2+

Exteroception and kinesthesia/vibration sensation appear to be intact.

Questions to Consider

- What are the major benefits and tradeoffs associated with a conventional locked-knee KAFO versus a KAFO with a stance control orthotic knee joint?
- What are the minimal requirements for strength, range of motion, and alignment that an individual must have to use the various stance-and-swing–control orthotic knee joints currently available?
- Is M. L. a suitable candidate for a stance-control KAFO? Why or why not? Which of the stance-control joints would be appropriate for her? Why would you recommend this particular orthotic option?

Special KAFO Designs

Conventional and thermoplastic KAFO designs have been adapted or modified to meet the needs of groups of patients with special needs. For growing children with muscular dystrophy, a modular system that allows the orthotist to adjust the length of the uprights and quickly replace outgrown thigh or calf supports has been developed.[33] A pair of lightweight long-leg calipers with no knee joint have traditionally been used to facilitate function in standing for adults with spinal cord injury; however, calipers are currently being replaced by a standing frame.[20]

A Craig-Scott orthosis, also known as a *double-bar hip-stabilizing orthosis* (Figure 11-9), is a lightweight variation of a traditional KAFO that was designed for patients with

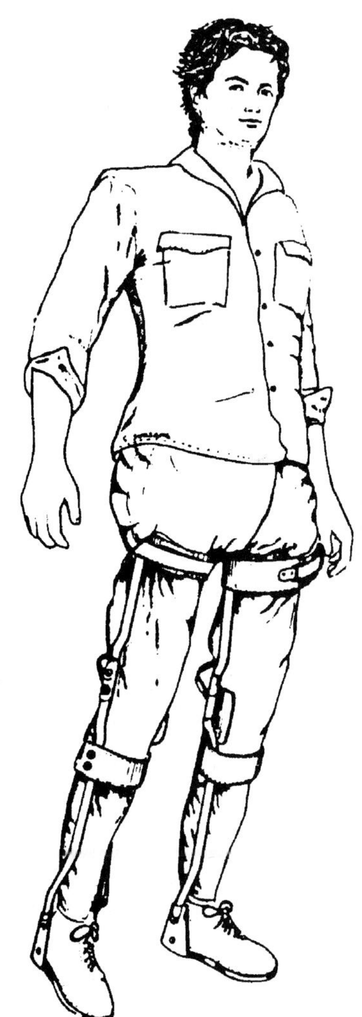

Figure 11-9
The Craig-Scott orthosis is a modified version of a conventional knee-ankle-foot orthosis, designed to be as lightweight as possible and to capitalize on alignment stability to enhance ambulation and upright activities in patients with low-thoracic and lumbar spinal cord injury. (From DG Shurr, TM Cook. Prosthetics and Orthotics. *Norwalk, CT: Appleton & Lange, 1990. p. 141.)*

paraplegia.[34] This orthosis is designed to maximize stability in stance with a minimal amount of bracing. A single thigh band and anterior strap are positioned just below the ischial tuberosity at the level of the greater trochanter; a single calf band and support are positioned just below the knee. Patients without active hip control are biomechanically stable in standing, assisted by the orthosis's dorsiassist ankle joints and offset locking knee joints when in a position of hip hyperextension and exaggerated lumbar lordosis. With this combination of orthosis and posture, the ground reaction force passes just anterior to the knee and posterior to the hip so that little or no muscular counterforce is necessary.

Conventional KAFOs are also being used in conjunction with functional electrical stimulation protocols for ambulation in patients with spinal cord injury. Various braking orthotic knee joints have been developed to augment stance stability when muscle fatigue from repeated electrical stimulation is problematic.[35] For patients with spinal cord injury, an alternative to current HKAFO designs, such as the Walkabout orthosis (WO) or the Mooring Medial Linkage Orthosis (MLO), may be an option.[36-38] These orthoses link two thermoplastic KAFOs by means of a single-axis hinge joint attached to the medial uprights of each.

CASE EXAMPLE 2

A Patient with L1 Traumatic Spinal Cord Injury

K. G. is a 19-year-old who sustained traumatic spinal cord injury in a motor vehicle accident 3 months ago. He had surgical fusion of T10-L3 spinal levels and wore a thoracolumbosacral orthosis (TLSO) for 8 weeks. He has completed his inpatient rehabilitation, is now out of his TLSO, and functions independently indoors and with minimal assistance on ramps and curbs outdoors while using a solid-frame wheelchair. His rehabilitation continues on an outpatient basis, and he wants to "give walking a try." He is referred to the Gait/Orthotic (GO) clinic at the rehabilitation center for evaluation.

At present, he presents with F- hip flexion on the right and P hip flexion on the left. Reflexes at knee and ankle are "0," with flaccid paralysis and complete sensory loss below the L1 neurological level. He has hip and knee flexion contractures of 10 degrees bilaterally. Skin is intact at the moment, although a sacral decubitus ulcer has recently healed. Upper extremity and upper body strength and flexibility are sufficient for ambulation with an appropriate assistive device.

Questions to Consider

- What additional information is important for the clinic team to gather as they prepare to make recommendations about orthotic options for K. G.? What additional tests and measures might be important to use?
- Given his current level of function, as well as his lower motor neuron spinal cord injury, what orthotic option is the team likely to consider: KAFO or HKAFO?
- If the team opts for a KAFO, which design would you recommend using: conventional leather or thermoplastic KAFOs with or without FES, a stance control KAFO, a pair of Craig Scott orthoses, a standing frame, or a set of "linked" orthoses such as the Walkabout? What are the benefits and tradeoffs of each? Why have you chosen the one you are recommending?
- In addition to learning to ambulate with the orthoses, what other motor tasks will K. G. have to master in order to use them functionally?
- How will the team evaluate the effectiveness and efficiency of the orthoses as K. G. becomes more adept at using them?

CHOOSING THE APPROPRIATE KAFO

The choice of a specific orthotic design and of a particular orthotic knee joint is based on a careful assessment of the patient's neuromuscular and musculoskeletal impairments, present and potential level of function, and a clear definition of key goals. The orthotist, after discussion with the patient and the clinic team, designs an orthosis that can most effectively achieve the desired goals. A set of general guidelines for choosing the orthotic knee joints that can best achieve desired knee control is presented in Table 11-1. This frame-

Box 11-3 *Guiding Questions for Delivering and Fitting a Knee-Ankle-Foot Orthosis*

- Is the orthosis consistent with the design criteria or prescription?
- Is the craftsmanship acceptable?
- Is the general appearance of the orthosis acceptable?
- Are the mechanisms for closure (Velcro straps or buckles) of adequate length and in the appropriate position to stabilize the limb in the orthosis?
- Will the patient be able to don/doff the orthosis independently (after functional training)?
- Is clearance or pressure relief sufficient around bony prominences or areas of fragile skin and soft tissue?
- Are the mechanical knee and ankle joints properly aligned with respect to the axis of the anatomical joints?
- Do all the mechanical parts (joints and locks) function smoothly?
- If the orthosis is of conventional design, are the uprights and cuffs the proper length and in an optimal position for the desired degree of control?
- If the orthosis is thermoplastic, is the total contact and surface area appropriate for distribution of force and the desired control of the knee and limb segments?

Table 11-1
Indications and Contraindications for Orthotic Knee Joint Designs

	Orthotic Knee Design				
Desired Knee Control	*Single Axis Unlocked*	*Single Axis Locked*	*Offset Unlocked*	*Offset Locked*	*Variable Position Locked*
Stabilization of flail knee with knee extension moment and free knee joint motion	Contraindicated	Contraindicated	**Indicated**	Contraindicated	Contraindicated
Stabilization of flail knee without use of knee extension moment and free knee joint motion	Contraindicated	**Indicated**	Contraindicated	**Indicated**	Unnecessary
Control of genu recurvatum	Contraindicated	**Indicated** if orthosis will only be locked when ambulating	**Indicated**	**Indicated** when individual will lock knee intermittently	Contraindicated
Reduction of knee flexion contracture	Contraindicated	Lacks adjustability	Contraindicated	Lacks adjustability	**Indicated**
Control of genu valgum	**Indicated**	**Indicated** Use of lock optional	**Indicated**	**Indicated** Use of lock optional	Unnecessary
Control of genu varum	**Indicated**	**Indicated** Use of lock optional	**Indicated**	**Indicated** Use of lock optional	Unnecessary

Modified from *Short course in Orthotics and Prosthetics—Course Manual.* Dallas, TX: University of Texas, Southwestern Medical Center, 1993. pp. 8–22.

work may need to be modified to meet specific or unique patient characteristics or circumstances.

DELIVERY AND FUNCTIONAL TRAINING

After the orthosis has been fabricated, the orthotist inspects the device to ensure that components work properly and that the thigh and calf bands or thermoplastic shells have been contoured appropriately, plastic edges have been smoothed and rounded, and metal surfaces have been buffed or coated. The orthotist then examines the fit of the orthosis to the patient's limb, in the intended functional, weight-bearing position (Box 11-3). The contours of cuffs or shells are reassessed in this position of function, with particular attention to vulnerable areas of skin or soft tissue. The overall length of the uprights and positions of the cuffs and shells and of the orthotic joints are inspected. Alignment of the components of the KAFO is also carefully evaluated. Ideally, the patient is able to stand comfortably, without skin irritation or pain. If minor problems with fit are identified, simple adjustments of fit and alignment can be made to address them. The orthotist and other members of the team then assess the effectiveness of the orthosis in meeting the defined functional goals, observing the degree of correction that is possible in quiet standing and during gait.

The orthotist carefully assesses any corrections that the orthosis can achieve, comparing posture and alignment to preorthotic assessment findings. Consider a patient who initially presented with 20 degrees of genu valgum in weight bearing that was correctable to 10 degrees when unweighted. The orthotist would reassess the amount of genu valgum that is present in standing, anticipating that the limb will be supported in the corrected 10-degree position.

If the orthosis fits appropriately and achieves its intended goals of protection, stability, or mobility, the patient must learn how to use the device. The patient and caregivers must understand how to don and doff the orthosis, including the way in which the limb is best positioned within the orthosis and the appropriate adjustment of stabilizing straps. They must learn about the locking mechanism at the knee, practicing the mechanics of locking and unlocking the joint several times. The patient and caregivers must be instructed in the care and maintenance of the orthosis, including keeping it clean and routinely inspecting components for wear and tear. An orthosis, as a mechanical device with moving parts, requires regular cleaning and occasional lubrication of its mechanical parts.

In most cases, especially if a patient is new to the use of an orthosis, a wearing schedule is developed, tailored to the person's specific needs and physical condition, in which the time in orthosis gradually increases to full-time wear.

Gait training begins once any adjustments to alignment or fit have been completed. Initial gait-training activities might begin with weight shifting from the intact toward the involved limb (for patients with unilateral deficits) and progress to controlled stance on the orthosis while the intact limb is in swing. Training may initially occur in the stable environment of the parallel bars but must progress to functional ambulation with the assistive device and gait pattern that are most appropriate for the individual patient, within the confines of stability necessary for safe ambulation. Often, once a patient has developed a comfortable pattern of ambulation, the orthotist reevaluates the fit and function of the orthosis to fine-tune alignment so that the most biomechanically sound and energy-efficient gait pattern is possible. Advanced gait-training activities include ambulation on uneven terrain, ramps, and stairs. It is also important to assist patients in developing strategies to manage unexpected falls; patients with sufficient upper extremity function and motor control may benefit from practicing getting up and down from the floor.

The decision to prescribe a KAFO for a patient with musculoskeletal or neuromuscular impairments is often made when knee instability cannot be adequately managed by an AFO design, as long as hip control is adequate for stable stance. A KAFO is often chosen when genu valgum or varum is problematic or when structural instability of ligaments of the knee is present. The orthotist, therapist, and other members of the team involved in the patient's care choose the most appropriate orthotic design and components on the basis of clearly defined functional goals, after careful evaluation of the patient's limb condition, motor control, and gait.

WHEN IS HKAFO INDICATED?

Clear indications for bracing the hip and trunk have not been as well documented as for the KAFO. The clinical decision to provide any individual, child or adult, with a HKAFO is typically taken after careful consideration of the relative advantages and disadvantages.[39] An HKAFO is typically a cumbersome device, and donning and doffing the orthosis can be quite challenging for both the patient and the caregivers. The additional control of joint motion that can be achieved by going above the hips must be balanced against the practical challenges that the individual patient will undoubtedly face.

The prescription of an HKAFO is based upon biomechanical deficits and neuromuscular impairments that are independent of specific conditions. Appropriate design and ultimately individual acceptance and compliance will, however, demand a thorough understanding of specific pathoses and individual requirements. The next sections describe the most commonly used HKAFO design and components and provide examples of common clinical application.

Traditional/Conventional HKAFOs

The traditional or conventional HKAFOs that were commonly prescribed for patients with polio, spinal cord injury, myelomeningocele, or spastic quadriplegic cerebral palsy before the 1980s were typically manufactured from a combination of metal and leather materials (Figure 11-10, *A*). Most often, they were applied bilaterally; occasionally, a single HKAFO was used to control the motion of just one extremity. The high energy cost of gait associated with these orthoses often limited their functional use.[39] However, just as thermoplastic materials and lighter but durable metals have become materials of choice for AFOs and KAFOs, they have been incorporated into the manufacture of HKAFOs (see Figure 11-10, *B*). Today, custom-fit and custom-fabricated thermoplastic HKAFOs are much lighter in weight. Because of the intimacy of their fit on the lower extremity, thermoplastic HKAFOs may also provide better biomechanical control of the limb.

Controlling the Hip

An orthotist can choose from various commercially available orthotic hip joints to control hip joint motion (Figure 11-11). Most designs have a single mechanical axis; some allow free flexion/extension when unlocked, and others can be set to allow motion only within a desired, more limited range. Single-axis hip joints inherently restrict motions of abduction and adduction and of rotation. Although dual-axis hip joints with separate mechanical control systems for flexion and extension and for abduction and adduction are also available, the single-axis joint provides the desired control for the majority of patients who require HKAFO systems for standing and mobility.

The orthotist selects the appropriate joint after considering the patient's functional disability, the treatment objectives, and the specific joint control that is desired. He or she can choose a joint that is designed to allow free motion, to assist or resist motion, to stop motion at a particular point in the range of motion, or to hold or eliminate all motion in the prescribed plane. The mechanical joint that best meets the patient's needs is attached proximally to a pelvic band, positioned between the trochanter and iliac crest (Figure 11-12). The center of the mechanical joint (axis of motion) is positioned just proximal and anterior to the greater trochanter. Distal stabilization is achieved by the attachment of the distal arm of the joint to the thigh cuff/upright.

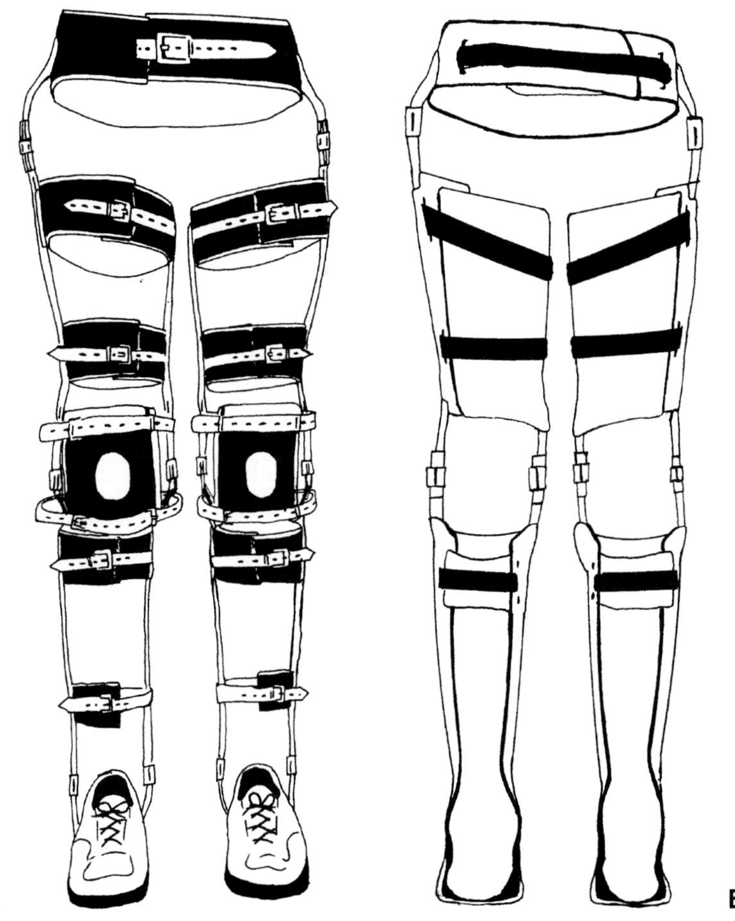

Figure 11-10

*A, Example of a traditional metal and leather hip-knee-ankle-foot orthosis (HKAFO), with its pelvic band, orthotic hip joints and locks, proximal and distal thigh bands, orthotic knee joints and stabilization pads, proximal and distal calf bands, ankle joints, and stirrups. **B,** Thermoplastic HKAFOs, typically lighter in weight than conventional HKAFOs, also have a pelvic band and orthotic hip and knee joints. Because they distribute forces over a wider thigh and calf band, an anterior knee stabilization pad may not be necessary. Many incorporate a solid-ankle or articulating ankle design of the ankle-foot orthosis, fitting inside the shoe rather than in an external stirrup.*

Traditional HKAFOs for Adults with Spinal Cord Injury

Most adults with paraplegia after lower thoracic or lumbar spinal cord injury have the potential to use bilateral KAFOs to provide the external stabilization of the knee and ankle that is required for upright activities and swing-through gait with crutches.[39,40] This is possible despite weakness of the hips and trunk by standing with an exaggerated lumbar lordosis (see Figure 11-9). In this position, the center of gravity (weight line) falls posterior to the hip joint, creating an extension movement at the hip, achieving stability by alignment. Although, theoretically, HKAFOs (which add hip joints and pelvic band, with or without thoracic extensions) would provide stability for patients with high thoracic spinal cord injury, little evidence has been found that the addition of hip joints and pelvic band is functionally beneficial.[9,39]

Traditional HKAFOs for Children with Myelomeningocele

The primary goal of rehabilitation for children with myelomeningocele (spina bifida) is to facilitate the developmental process (motor and cognitive), striving for as close to "normal" development as the child's neuromuscular and musculoskeletal impairments allow.[40] To achieve this goal, orthopedic and orthotic management of the child's spine and lower limbs focuses on achieving a stable upright posture.[41] This can only be accomplished, however, if the child's lower extremities can be positioned in hip and knee extension; prevention of flexion contracture or deformity of the hips and knees is paramount.[42] The level of motor and sensory impairment in the child's lower extremities is an important consideration in the process of orthotic prescription and fitting. Rehabilitation interventions are designed to

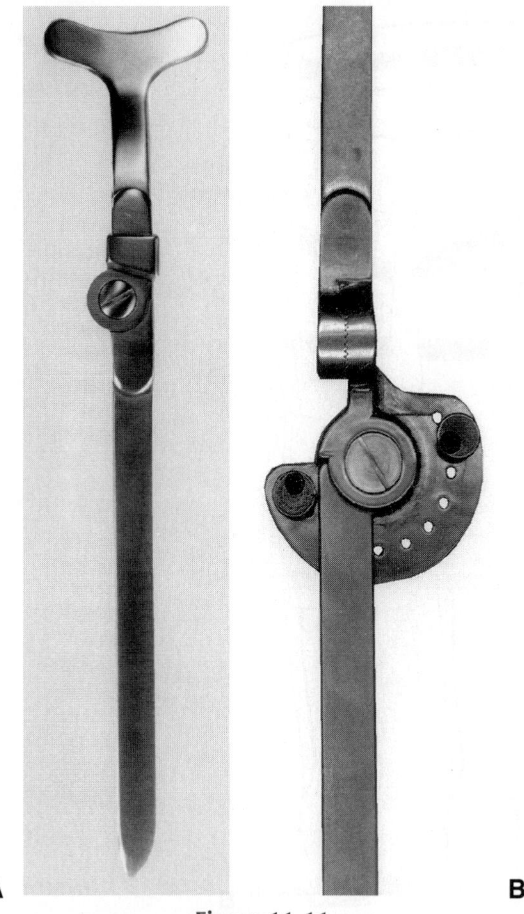

Figure 11-11
A, Examples of a single-axis hip joint. A drop lock holds the hip in extension in standing but allows free hip flexion for sitting when disengaged. B, Another type of hip joint allows controlled flexion and extension within a limited range of motion while limiting abduction/adduction and rotation.

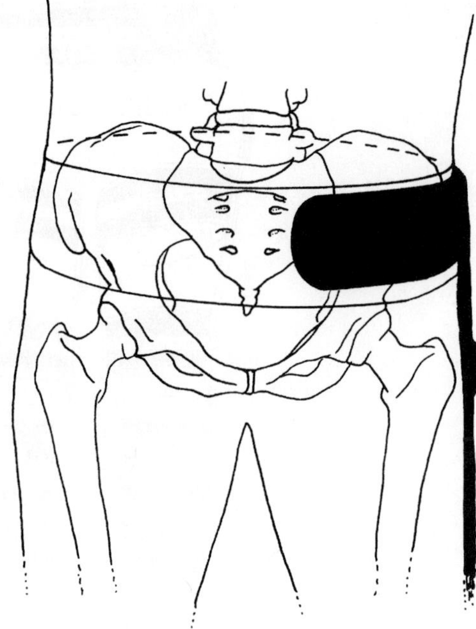

Figure 11-12
For effective control of hip motion, the pelvic band is positioned between the greater trochanter of the femur and the crest of the ilium. The orthotic hip joint is placed slightly proximal and anterior to the greater trochanter of the femur.

simulate or approximate normal developmental activities. Achieving trunk control in sitting is often the therapeutic focus for infants between 6 and 8 months of age; supported standing and locomotion activities are encouraged for children between 1 and 2 years of age.[40] The relationship between motor and cognitive development has been clearly established; orthopedic, surgical, and orthotic management support rehabilitation interventions that target age- and neurosegmental level–appropriate activities for the child.[40,42-44]

If children with myelomeningocele also develop hydrocephalus, the potential to become independent in locomotion is further challenged.[40] Any additional postural instability and intellectual impairment associated with hydrocephalus may make it more difficult for the child to learn to use the limbs or an orthosis effectively. Some children with myelomeningocele have bony deformity (such as malformation of vertebrae) that, along with their paralysis, places them at risk for development of secondary musculoskeletal impairments. Some of the most commonly encountered musculoskeletal problems include scoliosis and kyphosis, abnormalities of the rib cage, hip dislocation, osteoporosis and risk of fracture, and development of contracture or fixed limb deformities, or both, especially of the ankle and knee.[41]

Orthopedic and surgical management of children with myelomeningocele has three goals[45,46]:

1. To correct the primary deformity, maintain the correction, prevent its recurrence, and avoid the production of secondary deformities or musculoskeletal impairments
2. To obtain the best possible locomotor function
3. To prevent or minimize the effects of sensorimotor deficiency

It is critically important that orthotic management work toward these same goals.

Orthotists often become active members of the interdisciplinary rehabilitation team when a child is ready to begin standing activities, usually between 12 and 18 months of age.[40,47] In the 1960s and 1970s, conventional HKAFOs were the primary orthotic options for these children. Currently, there is considerable controversy and difference of opinion with regard to the advantages of fitting such children with this orthotic design. Providing for stability of the pelvis and hip has been problematic for children who have an imbalance of muscle power around the hip joint.[48,49] Many children with myelomeningocele may have some ability to activate hip flexor muscles (innervated by L2 and L3 nerve roots) but little or no power in hip extensors (innervated below L3 root levels). This imbalance of muscle tone and power often results in an exaggerated anterior pelvic tilt and lumbar lordosis and the development of significant hip flexor tightness or contracture.[49]

Although some clinicians argue that conventional HKAFOs provide stability and reduce the potential for hip flexion contracture, others question their ability to prevent lumbar lordosis and flexor tightness. In the authors' experience, a pelvic band can provide mediolateral hip stability but is not successful in controlling anterior pelvic tilt.[50]

Until reciprocating gait orthoses became available in the 1980s, conventional HKAFOs were routinely prescribed for children with myelomeningocele. Wearing the HKAFO, children were taught to ambulate using walkers or crutches in a pivot or swing-through gait pattern.[51,52] Most of these early HKAFOs had single-axis hip joints with drop locks, which attempted to stabilize a weak hip in an extended position and to prevent the hips from falling into a flexed position while the individual was standing. Although the HKAFO design does stabilize the lower extremities for stable stance, most have been unable to effectively control the position of the lumbar spine and pelvis biomechanically. Orthotists sought alternative strategies to control trunk and pelvic stability more effectively while allowing enough hip motion for a functional step.[53]

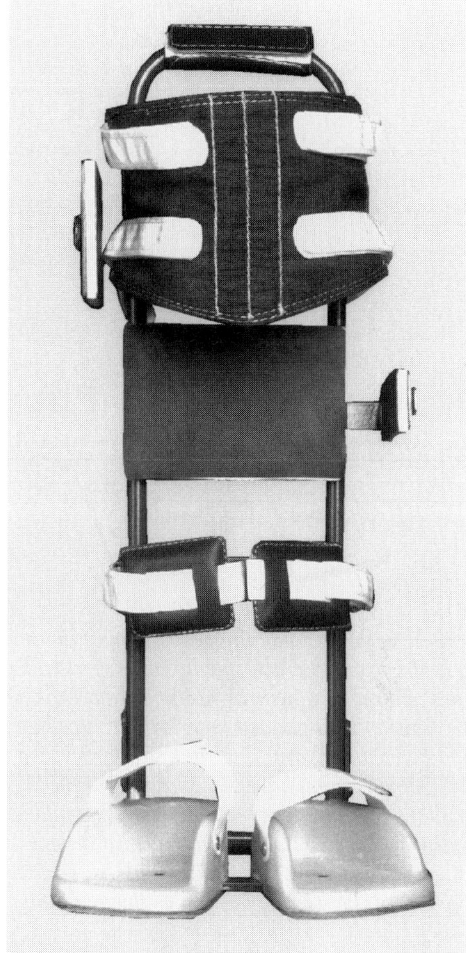

Figure 11-13
Standing frame orthosis developed at Gillette Children's Hospital, now known as Gillette Children's Specialty Healthcare, in St. Paul, Minn. Note that the tubular frame has no hip, knee, or ankle joints. The fulcrum of the three-force system used to ensure hip extension is the broad posterior pelvic pad (at the center, without Velcro straps), with counterforces delivered by the anterior thoracic corset and the anterior kneepads.

Traditional HKAFOs for Children with Cerebral Palsy

Few areas of orthotic management have attracted as much attention during the past several decades as the orthotic management of cerebral palsy. The routine practice of prescribing and fitting conventional HKAFOs for children with spastic quadriplegia or diplegia has been supplanted by more effective and less expensive forms of orthotic management. The current approach to the management of children with cerebral palsy better integrates therapeutic, orthotic, and surgical interventions based on the severity of the child's neuromuscular deficit, potential for functional mobility, and current motor and cognitive developmental status.[54] Custom-molded AFOs of various designs have been found to be effective in providing just enough external sagittal plane stability for effective upright posture in children who have the potential to become functional ambulators. It must be noted that AFOs do not influence hip position or motion in the frontal or transverse planes. HKAFOs or hip orthoses are sometimes used to protect or maintain hip position after orthopedic surgery to correct bony deformity (e.g., correction of femoral anteversion or derotation osteotomy) or after lengthening procedures of hip adductors or hamstrings.

PARAPODIUMS, STANDING FRAMES, AND SWIVEL WALKERS

Attempts to improve orthotic options for children with lower extremity neuromotor dysfunction have led to the commercial development of various parapodiums, standing frames, and swivel walkers. Although most of these orthoses include proximal components to control the thoracic and lumbar spine (and can most accurately be defined as thoracolumbar HKAFOs), they are usually classified within the HKAFO family.

These orthotic options were developed with the goal of improving function and encouraging independence for patients whose needs could not be adequately addressed by conventional HKAFOs.[45,51] Most allow the child (or adult) who is using them to function in standing and in limited ambulation with significantly less energy cost. Most can be used without a walker or crutches, leaving the hands free for functional activities. Because most designs are available in a kit form, the cost of fabrication and fitting is significantly less than that for conventional HKAFOs.

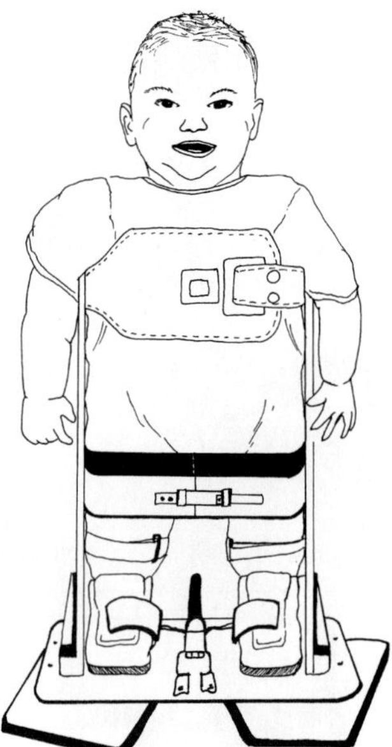

Figure 11-14
A young child with myelomeningocele, upright in an Orthotic Research and Locomotor Assessment Unit swivel walker. The ankles are stabilized in a neutral position against the foot plate, knees in extension by a padded anterior bar, hips in extension by a broad pelvic band, and the trunk supported by a broad chest strap. Some versions have orthotic joints at the knees and hips that allow the child to sit but lock when the child is assisted into standing. The child learns to use reciprocal movement of the arms to shift weight from side to side, alternately advancing one of the swivel pads under the foot plate.

All of these orthoses provide stability in standing, and some allow limited mobility as well. The earliest versions (Figure 11-13) were designed to facilitate the ability to stand; however, they did not always meet the stability needs of timid or apprehensive children who were fearful of falling. Active patients discovered that a frame's structural strength, although sufficient for quiet standing, was compromised or failed during more adventurous activities such as swing-through gait with crutches or independent transfers. Standing frames and similar orthoses are useful in the classroom, where the ability to stand at the same eye level as one's peers and to function with the hands free enhances participation and empowers students with disability to participate more fully in academic and social activities. Although many therapists acknowledge the advantages of these orthoses, others complain about the difficulty of donning and doffing the device and of the child's inability to move to and from the floor while wearing it.

The parapodium designed at Ontario Crippled Children's Center in Toronto[51] and the swivel walker (Figure 11-14) designed at the Orthotic Research and Locomotor Assessment Unit in Oswestry, England[55] are valuable orthotic options to consider when managing the child who has significant neuromuscular or skeletal deficit. Standing frames and swivel walkers are also available in adult sizes but are not used as often for adults as they are for children. They hold the same advantages for adults with paraplegia and other neuromuscular disorders who are required to sustain a hands-free upright posture for vocational, therapeutic, or practical purposes.

CASE EXAMPLE 3

A Young Child with Myelomeningocele

J. B. is an 18-month-old girl with myelomeningocele at the L1 level. Her defect was surgically closed the day after her birth, and a ventriculoperitoneal shunt was placed to control hydrocephalus when she was 2 months old. She has been attended at the spina bifida clinic at a regional children's hospital, 2 hours by car from her home, as well as a local home-based "birth to 3" program.

Currently, there is no active contraction of muscles in either lower extremity and no response to painful stimuli at or below the L1 dermatome. J. B. has consistently worn "night splints" to prevent plantar flexion contractures at the ankle. At 14 months of age, she sustained a mid-femoral fracture while playing on the floor with her older brothers and was immobilized in a Spica cast for 6 weeks. She has developed soft tissue tightness such that her lower extremities are in a somewhat abducted and externally rotated position at the hip. Knee range of motion is within functional limits for sitting and supported standing.

J. B.'s primary means of moving are by an upper extremity–powered commando crawl when playing with her brothers and similar-age cousins and by a stroller propelled by a family member. Recently, her behavior suggests she is frustrated by her inability to pull into a standing position and her limited mobility. Her family and therapists have returned to the spina bifida clinic for evaluation of her readiness for orthotic intervention that would allow J. B. to stand and to walk.

Questions to Consider

- What additional information would be important for the clinic team to gather as they prepare to make recommendations about orthotic options for J. B.? What additional tests and measures might be important to use?
- Given her current level of function and her lower motor neuron deficit, what orthotic option is the team likely to consider: KAFO or HKAFO? Why?
- If the team opts for an HKAFO, which design would you recommend: a thermoplastic HKAFO, a standing frame, a parapodium, a swivel walker, or a HKAFO that allows reciprocal gait? What are the benefits and trade-offs of each? Why have you chosen the one you are recommending?

- In addition to learning to stand and perhaps to ambulate with her HKAFO, what other motor tasks will J. B. and her family have to master in order to use them functionally?
- How will the team evaluate the effectiveness and efficiency of the orthoses as J. B. becomes more adept at using them?

HKAFOS DESIGNED FOR RECIPROCAL GAIT

Two additional lumbosacral-HKAFO systems have been developed for persons with paraplegia; both use a simple lateral weight shift from one limb to the other as the basis for orthotic-assisted reciprocal gait. The hip guidance orthosis (HGO, or parawalker) was developed at the Orthotic Research and Locomotor Assessment Unit,[43,53,56,57] and the reciprocal gait orthosis (RGO) was developed at Louisiana State University (LSU).[58-61] Both systems were designed for patients with high-level spinal cord dysfunction (congenital or traumatic) who would not otherwise be candidates for ambulation. The similarities and differences in the design and use of these orthoses have been the focus of intense research in the past decade.

Hip Guidance Orthosis

Whittle and Cochrane[62] suggest that the most important design aspect of the HGO is its rigidity in single limb support, which enhances the patient's ability to clear the contralateral limb as it advances in swing (Figure 11-15). The work of Jefferson and Whittle[63] demonstrates that in an HGO the lower limbs remain essentially parallel in the coronal plane, providing for better ground clearance of the limb in swing.

The HGO enables patients with paraplegia to walk independently with a reciprocal gait pattern.[64] Theoretically, this orthosis also reduces the energy cost of walking because the patient does not have to lift body weight off the ground, as is necessary with a swing-through gait using conventional HKAFOs and crutches. Studies that compared the physiological cost of walking in the HGO and conventional HKAFOs in children with myelomeningocele demonstrated an 87% increase in gait speed and a reduction in heart rate of 10 beats a minute when using the HGO.[57] Watkins and colleagues[64] report, on the basis of approximately 200 fittings of the orthosis, that the HGO works effectively to enable patients with complete thoracic level spinal cord injury to undertake therapeutic walking. The HGO system has also been successful in adult patients with complete spinal cord lesions ranging from C-8 to T-12 levels, with more than 85% of those fitted with an HGO continuing to use their orthosis on a regular basis at the 20-month follow-up interview.[65] Many patients who learn to use HGOs achieve independent use of their orthoses and low-energy ambulation indoors and outdoors and on various floor or ground surfaces.

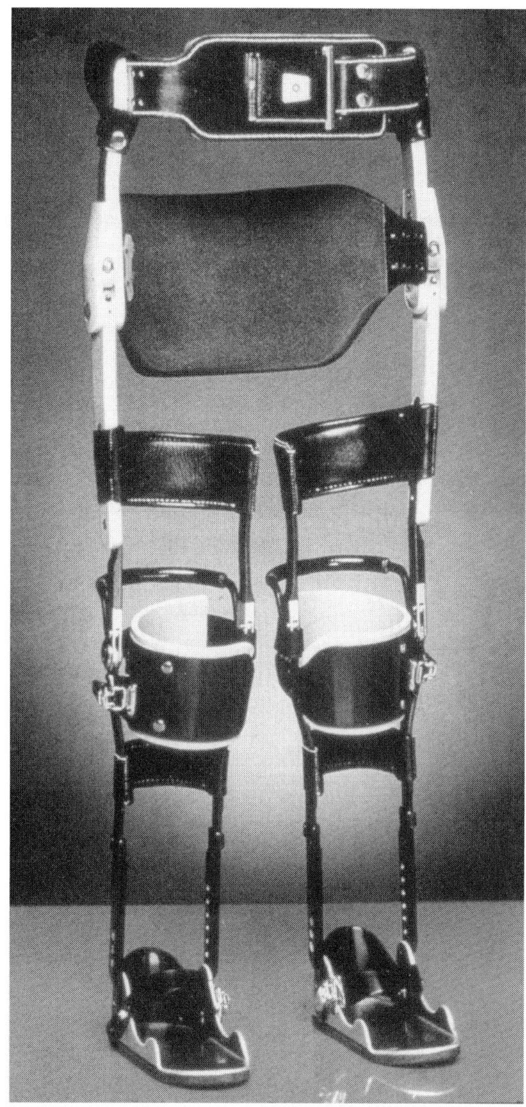

Figure 11-15
The hip guidance orthosis, usually worn over clothing, provides a rigid support system for the stance limb. Advancement of the swing limb occurs with its unweighting when the patient leans or shifts laterally onto the stable stance limb.

The HGO was originally developed for children with myelomeningocele.[64] The goal of the HGO is to provide the opportunity for functional independent ambulation. Rose and colleagues[57] define three criteria for independent orthosis-supported ambulation for these children. First, energy cost must be low at a reasonable speed of ambulation (30% to 60% of normal speed for the child's age-matched peers). Second, the child must be able to transfer independently from sitting (chair) to walking and vice versa. Third, the child must be able to don and doff the orthosis independently, within a reasonable amount of time without unreasonable effort. Researchers at the Orthotic Research

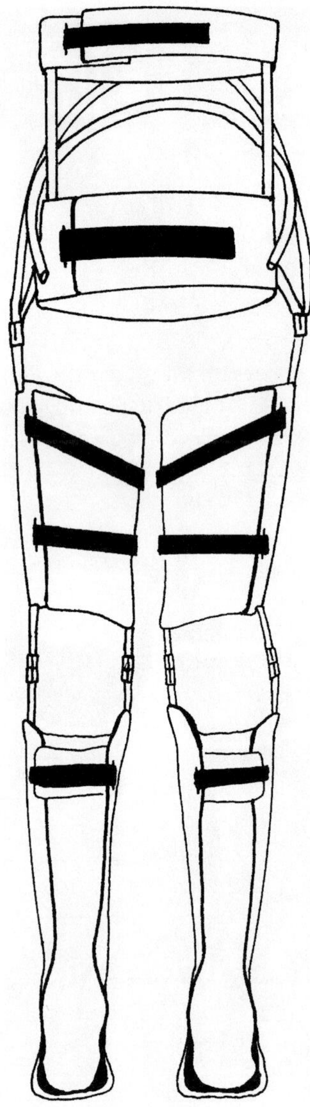

Figure 11-16
The reciprocal gait orthosis uses a dual cable system to couple flexion of one hip with extension of the other. This coupling assists forward progression of the swing limb while ensuring stability of the stance limb.

and Locomotor Assessment Unit tracked 27 children who had used the HGO for at least 6 months to evaluate the outcomes of its use. Their work has identified stability of the trunk (the ability to sit with the arms raised above the head for a prolonged period without support) as an important predictor of HGO success.[57] The HGO can provide, at low energy cost, reciprocal ambulation for children with low-thoracic and high-level lumbar lesions. Twenty-five of 27 children had been upright in another orthosis before using an HGO. Only 2 of 27 (7.6%) children developed scoliosis while using the HGO.[66] Further work is required to investigate how this extraordinarily low incidence of scoliosis is related to the use of an HGO or a conventional HKAFO.

Table 11-2
Diagnoses of Patients Who Successfully Used an RGO

Patient Diagnosis	*Number of Patients Fitted with an RGO*
Myelomeningocele	95
Traumatic paraplegia	18
Muscular dystrophy	15
Cerebral palsy	8
Multiple sclerosis	1
Sacral agenesis	1

Modified from Douglas R, Larson PF, D'Ambrosia R, et al. The LSU reciprocation gait orthosis. *Orthopedics* 6:834–839, 1983.
RGO, Reciprocal gait orthosis.

The HGO has been used mostly for school-aged children, adolescents, and adults with myelodysplasia (congenital) or acquired spinal cord injury.[67,68] Stallard and colleagues[69,70] report the development of a parawalker for young children who have a more rigid body brace and a smaller orthotic hip joint.

Reciprocal Gait Orthoses

Douglas and colleagues[58] describe the LSU RGO as a lightweight bracing system that gives structural stance phase support to the lower trunk and lower limbs of the individual with lower extremity paralysis (Figure 11-16); it uses a cable-coupling system to provide hip joint motion for swing phase. In the RGO, by means of its cable system, flexion of one hip (in swing) results in extension of the other hip (concurrently in stance). The hip joints of the orthosis are coupled together with two Bowden cables to transmit the necessary forces. (Although the original design used a single cable, functional problems and subsequent revisions evolved into the use of a second cable.) This reciprocal coupling has the added benefit of eliminating simultaneous hip flexion and reducing the risk of "jackknifing" during ambulation. Douglas and colleagues[58] have used the RGO for patients with various neuromuscular disorders (Table 11-2) and report that long-term bracing with RGO, as well as the early ambulation this makes possible, decreases the potential for development of secondary deformity. In a group of 100 adults with paraplegia fitted with an RGO, 7 were able to ambulate 100 feet with no more than two 30-second rest periods. For many patients, up to 45 hours of training were necessary to achieve functional gait with an RGO. Although the RGO has clearly been shown to be an effective intervention for reciprocal gait in adults and children with paraplegia, some extravagant claims about its success have resulted in uncertainty about prescription criteria.[71]

The RGO was initially designed to afford an upright posture and reciprocal gait pattern for children with myelomeningocele and has been used routinely for such individuals during the past 20 years.[50] Little has been published, however, to substantiate its effectiveness for this group; it is reasonable to suggest that considerably more attention has been given to its suitability for the adult paraplegic population than to the group for whom it was designed.

Yngve and colleagues[59] analyzed the effectiveness of the RGO in children with myelomeningocele who had absence or weakness of the hip extensor mechanism. Patients ranged in age from 18 months to 15 years. The function and potential benefit of three configurations of the reciprocating mechanism were evaluated. In the first configuration, ambulation was tested with the reciprocating mechanism engaged to allow hip flexion with contralateral hip extension. The first configuration represents the normal settings for the RGO. In the second configuration, the reciprocating mechanism was released to provide free flexion and extension at the hips, representing a conventional HKAFO with unlocked hip joints. In the third configuration, the hip joints were locked to eliminate hip motion, representing a conventional HKAFO with restricted hip motion.

Each child ambulated at his or her maximum velocity for 15 to 31 meters in each of the three configurations. The distance that the child walked was determined by individual strength and ability. Yngve and colleagues recorded the number of steps taken and the time to complete their distance and calculated velocity and step length. Although 17 children were included in the study sample, gait characteristics of only 8 children were analyzed. In five of these eight children, gait speed was significantly faster in the RGO than in the other configurations. Of the children in the sample, 75% had motor function at the L-3 level and only 18% had complete paralysis of hip musculature. The authors also did not provide information about how and why data from a subsample were used in the analysis. Given these concerns, it is impossible to draw any meaningful conclusions about function and neurosegmental level while a patient is wearing an RGO.

McCall and colleagues[60] fit a group of 29 children with neurological deficiencies (age range, 1 to 16 years) with the RGO at Shriners Hospital, Shreveport Unit, between 1981 and 1982. They report that the RGO offered improved standing and ambulatory potential in these neurologically deficient children while preventing development of deformity and increasing individual independence. Mazur and colleagues[72] further investigated differences in functional characteristics of reciprocal gait and swing-through gait using the technology of a gait laboratory. In a sample of three children with thoracic-level myelomeningocele, reciprocal gait with an RGO was modestly more efficient than a conventional HKAFO.

A retrospective review by Guidera and colleagues[73] evaluated the long-term usage pattern of patients fitted with reciprocating gait orthoses at the Shriners Hospital for Crippled Children in Tampa, Fla. Twenty-one children (13 boys, 8 girls; mean age, 8.75 years) were reevaluated 2 years after receiving their RGO. Nine of the children had thoracic-level lesions with no active hip flexion; 12 children had lumbar-level lesions. All of the children had required surgical correction of lower limb or spinal deformities before or during the bracing period, and 17 exhibited residual contracture. Eleven individuals required additional orthotic support of the spine. When questioned about their use of the RGO, all patients reported problems with donning and doffing, wear and tear on clothing, heat, multiple repairs, and down time. Almost half of the children were still using the RGO, but only four were community ambulators. The RGO was typically used at school rather than at home. The authors examined energy efficiency of three patients who used the RGO consistently. All were more energy efficient, and two were faster with a swing-through gait pattern as compared with the reciprocating pattern. Despite this, patient preference was to reciprocate.

Guidera and colleagues[73] then evaluated various factors that may contribute to the long-term success or failure of the RGO. Discontinuance occurred more often in children with a thoracic-level lesion, in the presence of obesity, when there was a lack of patient or family support, and if the patient had spinal deformity, mental retardation, knee flexion contracture of more than 30 degrees, or hip flexion contracture of more than 45 degrees. Other negative factors included spasticity, trunk and upper extremity weakness, asymmetric hip dislocation or motor function, and lack of prior standing or walking in a parapodium or other type of orthosis. These factors, especially in combination, have an adverse impact on long-term use and effective ambulation in an RGO.

Rogowski and colleagues[74] at Newington Children's Hospital evaluated the outcomes of RGO fittings for children with thoracic and high lumbar level of paralysis. They were especially interested in the criteria or indicators for fitting with an RGO, as well as the use and acceptance of the orthosis, using data from 48 consecutive cases fit between 1982 and 1991. The average time spent in the orthosis for their sample was 6.3 hours a day. Many of the children in the Newington study discontinued brace use between the ages of 7.5 and 11.5 years. In this study of children with paraplegia, the most important determinants of RGO use were age and level of paralysis.

Cuddeford has compared energy cost (ml/kg/min) and velocity (m/sec) of 15 children with myelomeningocele using RGOs and 11 children with myelomeningocele using traditional HKAFOs.[75] There is a trade-off between gait pattern and energy cost—the children wearing HKAFOs who used a swing-through gait pattern had a relative reduction in the energy cost of walking compared with children walking more slowly in RGOs.[75]

A version of the RGO design has been used for adults with acquired (traumatic) spinal cord injury, although there are conflicting data factors influencing continued use or rejection of the orthosis.[76-78] One modified version, the RGO II, has a ratchet locking mechanism in the orthotic knee and hip joint to provide stance stability in the presence of flexion contractures, as well as the addition of surface electrodes for functional electrical stimulation (FES) for individuals with upper motor neuron lesions of lower-cervical (C7) to low-thoracic (T10) levels of injury.[79,80] Solomonow and colleagues[81] followed 70 patients with spinal cord injury who attempted to use the RGO II during outpatient rehabilitation. Predischarge factors influencing successful RGO II use included higher levels of injury, depression, and low motivation and complications of spinal cord injury, including skin breakdown and fracture. Forty-one patients were discharged to use the device independently at home. On follow-up (6 months to 3 years after discharge), nearly 80% continued to use the orthosis at least once a week for exercise or for functional activities. Those most likely to continue to use the RGO II had lesions from mid- to low-thoracic levels, were highly motivated, and felt the RGO II contributed to health and quality of life.[82]

CASE EXAMPLE 4

An Adult with Acquired T-9 Spinal Cord Injury

L. F. is a 20-year-old who sustained multiple gunshot wounds to his abdomen and back during an armed robbery of the convenience store where he worked. He was airlifted to a regional level-1 trauma center for initial care. He underwent several surgeries to repair internal organs and remove his spleen, as well as a fusion to stabilize burst fractures of T-9 to T-11 vertebral bodies. Once stable, L. F. was transferred to a rehabilitation center, wearing a TLSO, for a 5-week stay. He is now living at home, and the TLSO has been discontinued. L. F. has continued his rehabilitation on an outpatient basis for the past 3 months. He is independent in wheelchair mobility on level surfaces, ramps, and curbs. He has been actively involved in a functional electric stimulation (FES) program using the ERGYS cycle ergometer for the past 2 months. He has expressed interest in "walking" for cardiovascular fitness exercise, perhaps combining an orthosis with FES.

At present, there is no apparent neuromotor or sensory function below the level of T-9. Deep tendon reflexes are +3 at knee and +4 at ankle, with occasional extensor spasms of lower extremities noted, typically as a sign of skin breakdown or bladder infection. Range of motion is within functional limits at knee and ankle, with 10-degree hip flexion contracture noted bilaterally.

Questions to Consider

- What additional information would be important for the clinic team to gather as they prepare to make recommendations about orthotic options for L. F.? What additional tests and measures might be important to use?
- Given his current level of function and his upper motor neuron deficit, what orthotic option is the team likely to consider: KAFO or HKAFO? Why?
- If the team opts for an HKAFO, which design would you recommend that they use: a "traditional" thermoplastic HKAFO, a reciprocal gait orthosis, or a parawalker/hip guidance orthosis? What are the benefits and trade-offs of each? Why have you chosen the one you are recommending?
- In addition to learning to stand and perhaps to ambulate with his HKAFO, what other motor tasks must L. F. master in order to use it functionally?
- How will the team evaluate the effectiveness and efficiency of the orthoses as L. F. becomes more adept at using them?

Comparison of the HGO and the RGO

The HGO and the RGO enable patients with paraplegia that results from traumatic or congenital spinal cord dysfunction to ambulate using a reciprocal gait pattern. Studies have begun to compare these orthoses in terms of energy expenditure.

Banta and colleagues[82] determined relative oxygen cost (ml/kg/m) of gait with an HGO and an RGO in five individuals (four adults and one child) with paraplegia. An oxylog was used to record oxygen consumption while the subjects ambulated during steady state. Although all of the subjects trained and used the orthoses for varying amounts of time, the data suggest that the HGO enables a more energy-efficient gait; on average, the oxygen cost while using the parawalker was 27% less than that of the RGO, with reductions of between 12% and 42%. Subjects also ambulated faster with the HGO, with a mean increase in gait speed of 33%. These preliminary results indicate that the HGO may be a more efficient orthosis for level ambulation for individuals with paraplegia.

In 1989 the Department of Health and Social Security in the United Kingdom commissioned an extensive comparative trial of both orthoses.[35,48] Twenty-two patients with paraplegia from the Nuffield Orthopedic Centre in Oxford, England (18 men, 4 women) used each orthosis for 4 months in a crossover study.[83] Clinical, ergonomic, biomechanical, psychological, and economic assessments were repeated over the course of the study. Of the individuals in the sample, 15 were able to use both orthoses, 5 were unable to use either of the orthoses, and 2 were able to use the HGO but not the RGO. At the conclusion of the trial, 12 subjects chose to keep the RGO, 4 preferred the HGO, and 6 discontinued use of both orthoses. Those who chose the RGO preferred its appearance. Those who chose the HGO appreciated how quickly the orthosis could be donned and doffed. Although Jefferson and Whittle[63] found that intersubject differences were much larger than interorthosis differences, biomechanical assessment demonstrated that the patterns of movement were not identical in the two orthoses. One limitation of the study was the composition of the sample: No children were included, although both systems were designed for the pediatric patient with paraplegia. As a result, no conclusions about the benefits or drawbacks for children with paraplegia can be drawn.

In a single-case design study that involved a 33-year-old with complete traumatic paraplegia at the T-5 level who was a proficient user of HGO and RGO systems, few differences in general gait characteristics were identified.[39] The study results were based on measurements taken from videotape and the Vicon gait analysis system (Oxford Metrics Ltd., Oxford, United Kingdom) data. Although stride length was similar with both orthoses, a smaller range of pelvic motion, as well as a more fluent gait, occurred with the HGO. In the sagittal plane, less hip extension was noted when the patient ambulated with the HGO compared with the RGO. In the coronal plane, more hip abduction occurred with the HGO than the RGO. This important difference is attributed to lower extremities that remain essentially parallel during walking, which leads to a more efficient toe clearance during swing. The major contribution of this study is a clearer understanding of the biomechanics of movement (based on objective measurement) of these two orthoses when used by an adult with paraplegia who is free of existing deformity or contracture. One of the limitations of a single-case design is the ability to apply these results to the population of those with paraplegia: In children with tightness of hip flexors, contracture has a considerable influence on pelvic measurements and stride length.

OTHER TYPES OF RECIPROCAL GAIT ORTHOSES

The advanced reciprocating gait orthosis, developed by Hugh Steeper Limited of London, is best described as a modified LSU RGO. A single push-pull cable links the mechanical hip joints. The most appreciated improvement reported by investigators who have examined this design is the ease it confers on rising from a sitting position and on sitting down again after standing. This improvement is the result of a cable link between orthotic hip and knee joints and the addition of pneumatic struts to assist knee extension. The arrangement assists patients in standing directly from a sitting position in which the knees are typically flexed, without prior manual straightening and locking of the knees.

The isocentric reciprocating gait orthosis is a further modification of the LSU RGO. In this variant, the two crossed Bowden cables are replaced by a centrally pivoting bar and tie rod arrangement.

SUMMARY

KAFOs provide an external stabilization to counteract the flexion movement that is created when the ground reaction force passes posteriorly to the knee in early stance. Conventional and thermoplastic KAFOs use a three-point force system to control the knee motion in sagittal, frontal, and transverse planes. The intimately fitting thigh and distal shells of thermoplastic KAFOs can better control forces in the transverse plane than conventional designs. Although any of the ankle joint or AFO designs can be incorporated into a KAFO, an articulating orthotic ankle joint, which allows dorsiflexion, enhances forward progression over the foot during the stance phase of gait. A number of options for orthotic knee joints are available, including free motion, static locking mechanisms, and dynamic mechanisms that lock at initial contact and unlock as swing phase begins. The choice of orthotic knee joint is determined by how well the patient can control motion actively at the knee.

After the KAFO has been fabricated, its fit and function are carefully evaluated by the orthotist, therapist, and other team members. The orthosis must be comfortable to wear and effectively achieve its functional goals if the patient is to accept and use the device. Once any necessary adjustments to alignment and fit have been made, an initial wearing schedule is developed to gradually bring "time in brace" up to full-time use. A period of gait training, including instruction and practice with the appropriate assistive device and ambulation on level and uneven surfaces, ramps, and stairs, is begun. The patient and caregivers also need to understand how to clean and maintain the orthosis; regularly scheduled rechecks with the orthotist ensure continued effectiveness of and satisfaction with the orthosis.

For children and adults with paraplegia resulting from more significant neuromuscular system impairment, evidence suggests that the HGO, or parawalker, provides better ground clearance and a smoother gait pattern than conventional KAFOs and HKAFOs. These benefits are possible because of the mechanical rigidity of the orthosis; however, they are achieved only with significant cosmetic deficit. In many instances, the improved cosmesis of the RGO is much preferred by patients. The mechanical reliability of the RGO, however, has been questioned in the literature. In more recent developments, an advanced reciprocating gait orthosis design enhances the patient's ability to rise to standing up and to sitting down without having to lock or unlock orthotic knee joints. The isocentric reciprocating gait orthosis attempts to combine the mechanical advantages of the HGO with the cosmetic and therapeutic advantages of other RGOs. Perhaps the most important finding across most of the studies comparing RGOs and HGOs relates to general gait parameters: Functional differences among the contemporary orthotic options are small.

Despite the considerable activity and associated expense within this subject area, research and clinical experience indicate that most individuals with paraplegia opt for wheelchair mobility after discharge to the community because this provides a faster, safer, and more practical means of mobility with considerably less energy expenditure.

The ability to walk remains an important objective for many children (and their parents) with congenital paraplegia and for adults with acquired paraplegia following spinal cord injury or other neurological event. The ability to reach the goal of functional ambulation depends on many factors, including the cause of the paraplegia, the level of the neuromuscular lesion, the presence of hydrocephalus, the strength of the upper limbs, the availability and effectiveness of parental support, and the child's own coordination and motivation. The ability to ambulate also depends on the prescription and fitting of an appropriate orthosis. The literature indicates that contemporary forms of orthotic management, specifically the HGO and the RGO, improve function for many children with paraplegia.[30]

What remains unclear, however, is the influence of these accepted HKAFO designs on the development of joint contracture and the progression of deformity. The problem of progressive deformity in children with paraplegia is significant. Often a spinal deformity appears within the first decade and progresses to skeletal maturity; the most common deformity is an increased lumbar lordosis. For children with a neurological level of lesion at T-12 or higher, the incidence of spinal deformity is almost 100%. The impact of fitting of an HKAFO, especially of the HGO and RGO, on the prevention of spinal deformity requires much more scholarly attention and study.

REFERENCES

1. Merritt JL. Knee-ankle foot orthoses: indications and practical applications of long leg braces. *Phys Med Rehabil State Art Rev* 2000;14(3):395-422.
2. Inman VT, Ralston HJ, Todd F. *Human Walking.* Baltimore: Williams & Wilkins, 1981.
3. Perry J. *Gait Analysis: Normal and Pathological Function.* Thorofare, NJ: Slack, 1992.
4. Los Amigos Research and Education Institute. *Rancho Los Amigos Observational Gait Handbook.* Downey, CA: Rancho Los Amigos Medical Center, 1989.
5. Smith LK, Weiss EL, Lehmjuhl DL. *Brunnstrom's Clinical Kinesiology,* 5th ed. Philadelphia: F.A. Davis, 1996.
6. Gage JR. *Gait Analysis in Cerebral Palsy.* London: Mackeiht, 1991. pp. 61-130, 177-182.
7. Cary JM, Lusskin R, Thompson RG. Prescription principles. In WH Bunch (ed), *Atlas of Orthotics: Biomechanical Principles and Application.* St Louis: Mosby, 1985. pp. 3-6.
8. Kupperman C. Stance control technology gains momentum. *Biomechanics* Feb 2004;59-69.
9. Somers MF. *Spinal Cord Injury: Functional Rehabilitation.* Norwalk, CT: Appleton & Lange, 1992.
10. Trautman P. Lower limb orthoses. In JB Redford, JV Basmajian, P Trautman (eds), *Orthotics: Clinical Practice and Rehabilitation Technology.* New York: Churchill Livingstone, 1995. pp. 13-55.
11. Perry J, Hislop HJ (eds). *Principles of Lower Extremity Bracing.* Alexandria, VA: American Physical Therapy Association, 1967.
12. Peethambaran A. The relationship between performance, satisfaction, and well being for individuals using anterior and posterior design knee-ankle-foot-orthosis. *J Prosthet Orthot* 2000;12(1):33-40.
13. Moore TJ. Lower limb orthoses. In B Goldberg, JD Haus (eds), *Atlas of Orthoses and Assistive Devices,* 3rd ed. St Louis: Mosby, 1997. pp. 377-463.
14. Fishman S. Lower limb orthoses. In WH Bunch (ed), *Atlas of Orthotics: Biomechanical Principles and Application.* St Louis: Mosby, 1985. pp. 199-237.
15. Shoe modifications and foot orthoses. In Berger N, Edelstein JE, Fishman S, et al (eds), *Lower Limb Orthotics.* New York: New York University Medical Center, Post Graduate Medical School, Prosthetics and Orthotics, 1986. pp. 110-128.
16. Edelstein JE. Orthotic assessment and management. In O'Sullivan SB, Schmitz TJ (eds), *Physical Rehabilitation: Assessment and Treatment,* 3rd ed. Philadelphia: F.A. Davis, 1994. pp. 655-684.
17. Lunsford T. Orthotic principles. In *Rancho Los Amigos Medical Center Prosthetics and Orthotics Course Syllabus: Critical Decisions in Individual Management.* Downey, CA: Professional Staff Association, 1985.
18. Zablotny CM. Use of orthoses for the adult with neurological involvement. In DA Nawoczenski, ME Eppler (eds), *Orthotics in Functional Rehabilitation of the Lower Limb.* Philadelphia: Saunders, 1997. pp. 205-243.
19. Clark D. Knee-ankle-foot orthosis design for polio. In *Rancho Los Amigos Medical Center Prosthetics and Orthotics Course Syllabus: Critical Decisions in Individual Management.* Downey, CA: Professional Staff Association, 1985.
20. Hahn HR. Lower extremity bracing in paraplegics with usage follow-up. *Paraplegia* 1970;8(3):147-153.
21. Ankle, knee, and hip orthoses. In Berger N, Edelstein JE, Fishman S, et al (eds), *Lower Limb Orthotics.* New York: New York University Medical Center, Post Graduate Medical School, Prosthetics and Orthotics, 1986. pp. 129-164.
22. Michael JW, McMillan AG, Kendrick K. Stance control orthoses: history, overview, and case example of improved KAFO function. *Alignment,* 2003:60-70.
23. Operating instructions for the free walk orthosis, Ottobock, Germany. Retrieved November 15, 2005 from *http://www.healthcare.ottobock.de/technische orthopaedei/orthosen/pdf/647H351Freewalk.pdf.*
24. Horton Orthotics and Prosthetics. Individual criteria sheet. Retrieved November 15, 2005 from *http://www.stancecontrol.com/individual_criteria_sheet.htm.*
25. Kauffman KR, Irby SE, Mathewson JW, et al. Energy efficient knee ankle foot orthosis: a case study. *J Prosthet Orthot* 1996;8(3)79-85.
26. Mattsson E, Broostrom LA. The increase in energy cost of walking with an immobilized knee or unstable ankle. *J Scand Rehab Med* 1990;22(1):51-53.
27. McMillan AG, Dendrick K, Michael JW, et al. Preliminary evidence for effectiveness of a stance control orthosis. *J Prosthet Orthot* 2004;16(1):6-13.
28. Becker Orthopedic introduces the original URX® to North America. Retrieved November 15, 2005 from *http://www.beckerorthopedic.com/utx/utx.htm.*
29. Fillauer to offer innovative orthotic technology: SPL orthotic knee joint. Retrieved November 15, 2005 from http://www.oandp.com/edge/issues/articles/2002-07_14.asp.
30. The LR-9002 load response knee joint. Retrieved November 15, 2005 from *http://www.beckerorthopedic.com/knee/ load_response.htm.*

31. Model 9003 G-knee. Retrieved November 15, 2005 from *http://www.beckerorthopedic.com/knee/g_knee.htm.*
32. Step into the future: Foot force activated, computer controlled, electromechanical orthotic knee joint, from Retrieved November 15, 2005 from *http://www.beckerorthopedic.com/knee/9001.htm.*
33. Taktak DM, Bowker P. Lightweight modular knee-ankle-foot orthosis for Duchenne muscular dystrophy: design, development, and evaluation. *Arch Phys Med Rehabil* 1995;76(12):1156-1162.
34. Hawran S, Biering-Sorensen F. The use of long leg calipers for paraplegic individuals: a follow up study of individuals discharged 1973-1982. *Spinal Cord* 1996;34(11):666-668.
35. Goldfarb M, Durfee WK. Design of a controlled brake orthosis for FES aided gait. *IEEE Trans Rehabil Eng* 1996;4(1):13-24.
36. Middleton JW, Yeo JD, Lanch L, et al. Clinical evaluation of a new orthosis, the 'Walkabout' for restoration of functional standing and short distance mobility in spinal paralyzed individuals. *Spinal Cord* 1997;35(9):574-579.
37. Middleton JW. A medial linkage orthosis to assist ambulation after spinal cord injury. *Prosthet Orthot Int* 1998;22(3): 258-265.
38. Harvey LA, Newton-John T, Davis GM, et al. A comparison of the attitude of paraplegic individuals to the walkabout orthosis and the isocentric reciprocal gait orthosis. *Spinal Cord* 1997;35(9):580-584.
39. Goldberg B, Hsu JD. *Atlas of Orthoses and Assistive Devices. American Academy of Orthopaedic Surgeons.* St Louis: Mosby, 1997. pp. 391-399.
40. Tappit-Emas E. Spina bifida. In Tecklin JS (ed), *Pediatric Physical Therapy,* 3rd ed. Philadelphia: Lippincott, 1999. pp. 163-222.
41. Menelaus MB. *The Orthopaedic Management of Spina Bifida Cystica.* Edinburgh: Churchill Livingstone, 1980. pp.
42. Williams NW, Broughton NS, Menelaus MB. Age related walking in children with spina bifida. *Dev Med Child Neurol* 1999;41:446-449.
43. Roussos N, Patrick JH, Hodnett C, Stallard J. A long term review of severely disabled spina bifida individuals using a reciprocal walking system. *Disabil Rehabil* 2001;23(6): 239-244.
44. McCall RE, Douglas R, Rightor N. Surgical treatment in individuals with myelodysplasia before using the LSU reciprocation gait system. *Orthopedics* 1983;6:843-848.
45. Rose GK. Orthoses for the severely handicapped; rational or empirical choice. *Physiotherapy* 1980;66(3):76 81.
46. Sharrard WJW. Long-term follow-up of posterior iliopsoas transplantation for paralytic dislocation of the hip. *Dev Med Child Neurol* 1969;(Suppl 1):96.
47. Pollack AA, Elliot S, Caves C, et al. Lower extremity orthoses for children with myelomeningocele: user and orthotist perspectives. *J Prosthet Orthot* 2001;13(4):123-129.
48. Glancy J. Dynamics and the L3 through L5 myelomeningocele child. *Clin Prosthet Orthot* 1984;8(3):15-23.
49. Lehneis HR. Orthotic pelvis control in spina bifida. *Clin Prosthet Orthot* 1984;8(3):26-28.
50. Campbell JH. *The Orthotic Management of the Paraplegic Child; Clinical and Biomechanical Analysis.* PhD thesis, University of Strathclyde, Glasgow, Scotland, 1996.
51. Motlock W. The parapodium: an orthotic device for neuromuscular disorders. *Artif Limbs* 1971;15:37-47.
52. Rose GK. Splintage for severe spina bifida cystica. *J Bone Joint Surg* 1970;52(1):178-179.
53. Rose GK. The principles and practice of hip guidance articulations. *Prosthet Orthot Int* 1979;3(1):37-43.
54. Styer-Acevado J. Physical therapy for the child with cerebral palsy. In Tecklin JS (ed), *Pediatric Physical Therapy,* 3rd ed. Philadelphia: J.B. Lippincott 1999;107-162.
55. Rose GK, Henshaw JT. Swivel walkers for paraplegics—considerations and problems in their design and application. *Bull Prosthet Res* 1973;10(20):62-74.
56. Major RE, Stallard J, Rose GK. The dynamics of walking using the hip guidance orthosis (HGO) with crutches. *Prosthet Orthot Int* 1981;5(1):19-22.
57. Rose GK, Stallard J, Sankarankutty M. Clinical evaluation of spina bifida patients using hip guidance orthosis. *Dev Med Child Neurol* 1981;23(1):30-40.
58. Douglas R, Larson PF, D'Ambrosia R, McCall RE. The LSU reciprocation gait orthosis. *Orthopedics* 1983;6:834-839.
59. Yngve D, Douglas R, Roberts JM. The reciprocating gait orthosis in myelomeningocele. *J Pediatr Orthop* 1984;4(3):304-310.
60. McCall RE, Schmidt We. Clinical experience with the reciprocal gait orthosis in myelodysplasia. *J Pediatr Orthop* 1986;6:157-161.
61. Guidera KJ, Smith S, Raney E, et al. Use of the reciprocating gait orthosis in myelodysplasia. *J Pediatr Orthop* 1993;13(3): 341-348.
62. Whittle MW, Cochrane GM. *A Comparative Evaluation of the Hip Guidance Orthosis (HGO) and the Reciprocating Gait Orthosis (RGO). Health Equipment Information No.192.* London: National Health Service Procurement Directorate, 1989.
63. Jefferson RJ, Whittle MW. Performance of three walking orthoses for the paralyzed: a case study using gait analysis. *Prosthet Orthot Int* 1990;14(3):103-110.
64. Watkins EM, Edwards DE, Patrick JH. Parawalker paraplegic walking. *Physiotherapy* 1987;73(2):99-100.
65. Summers BN, McClelland MR, Masri WS. A clinical review of the adult hip guidance orthosis (parawalker) in traumatic paraplegics. *Paraplegia* 1988;26(1):19-26.
66. Rose GK, Sankarankutty M, Stallard J. A clinical review of the orthotic treatment of myelomeningocele patients. *J Bone Joint Surg* 1983;65(3):242-246.
67. Major RE, Stallard J, Farmer SE. A review of 42 patients of 16 years and older using the ORLAU Parawalker. *Prosthet Orthot Int* 1997;21:147-152.
68. Moore P, Stallard RE. A clinical review of adult paraplegic patients with complete lesions using the ORLAU Parawalker. *Paraplegia* 1991;29:191-196.
69. Stallard J, Woolman PJ, Miller K, et al. An infant reciprocal walking orthosis: engineering development. *Proc Inst Mech Eng [H]* 2001;215:599-604.
70. Woolman PJ, Lomas B, Stallard J. A reciprocal walking orthosis hip joint for young pediatric patients with a variety of pathological conditions. *Prosthet Orthot Int* 2001;25(1): 47-52.
71. Patrick JH. Developmental research in paraplegic walking. *Br Med J* 1986;292(6523):788.
72. Mazur JM, Sienko-Thomas S, Wright N, Cummings U. Swing-through vs reciprocating gait patterns in patients with thoracic level spina bifida. *Z Kinderchir* 1990;45(Suppl 1): 23-25.

73. Guidera KJ, Raney E, Ogden JA, et al. The use of reciprocating gait orthosis in myelodysplasia (abstract). *J Pediatr Orthop* 1993;13(3):341-348.
74. Rogowski EM, Fezio JM, Banta W. Long term clinical experience with the reciprocating gait orthotic system. *J Assoc Child Prosthet Orthot Clin* 1992;27:54.
75. Cuddeford TJ. Energy consumption in children with myelomeningocele; a comparison between reciprocating gait orthosis and hip-knee-ankle-foot orthosis ambulators. *Dev Med Child Neurol* 1997;39(4):239-242.
76. Jaspers P, Peeraer L, VanPetegem W, Van der Perre G. The use of an advanced reciprocating gait orthosis by paraplegic patients: a follow-up study. *Spinal Cord* 1997;35:585-589.
77. Sykes L, Edwards J, Powell ES, Ross ERS. The reciprocating gait orthosis: long term usage patterns. *Arch Phys Med Rehabil* 1995;76:779-783.
78. Scivoletto G, Petreilli A, Di Lucente L, et al. One-year follow-up of spinal cord injury individuals using reciprocating gait orthosis: a preliminary report. *Spinal Cord* 2000;38:555-558.
79. Solomonow M, Baratta RV, Hirokawa S, et al. The RGO Generation II: muscle stimulations powered orthosis as a practical walking system for thoracic paraplegics. *Orthopedics* 1989;12:1309-1315.
80. Hirokawa S, Grimm M, Le T, et al. Energy consumption in paraplegic ambulation using the reciprocating gait orthosis and electrical stimulation. *Arch Phys Med Rehabil* 1990;71:687-694.
81. Solomonow M, Aguilar E, Reisen E, et al. Reciprocating gait orthosis powered with electrical muscle stimulation (RGO II): Part I: Performance evaluation of 70 paraplegic individuals. *Orthopedics* 1997;20(4):315-324.
82. Banta JV, Bell KJ, Muik EA, Fezio JM. Parawalker: energy cost of walking. *Eur J Pediatr Surg* 1991;1(Suppl 1):7-10.
83. Whittle MW, Cochrane GM, Chase AP, et al. A comparative trial of two walking systems for paralyzed people. *Paraplegia* 1991;29(2):97-102.

12

Orthotics in the Management of Neuromuscular Impairment

MICHELLE M. LUSARDI AND DONNA M. BOWERS

LEARNING OBJECTIVES

On completion of this chapter, the reader will be able to do the following:

1. Explain clinical signs and symptoms of neuromuscular pathologies on the basis of an understanding of structure and function of the central and peripheral nervous system.
2. Describe and differentiate the types of abnormal tone seen in persons with neuromuscular pathologies.
3. Select an appropriate strategy to examine and document abnormalities of muscle tone and muscle performance.
4. Describe the contributions of various central nervous system (CNS) components to, and key determinants of, effective postural control.
5. Describe the contributions of various CNS components to, and key determinants of, mobility and coordination during functional activity.
6. Discuss the roles of orthopedic and neurosurgical procedures, central and peripherally acting pharmacological agents, and various orthotic options for the management of hypertonicity.
7. Describe strategies used by rehabilitation professionals to reduce the risk of developing secondary musculoskeletal impairments in persons with hypertonicity.
8. Describe a strategy for clinical decision making in the selection of an appropriate orthosis for individuals with neurological and neuromuscular pathologies.

MOVEMENT IMPAIRMENT IN NEUROMUSCULAR DISORDERS

Pathologies of the neuromuscular system manifest in a sometimes confusing array of clinical signs and symptoms. To select the most appropriate therapeutic intervention, be it functional training or the use of various orthoses and assistive devices to accommodate for an impairment, the clinician must develop a strategy to "classify" the movement disorder that has produced the observed impairments and functional limitations.[1] The clinician must understand the medical prognosis and potential progression of the disease process, as well as the risk factors that might contribute to secondary impairments that limit function over time (even if the disease is "nonprogressive") and their impact on the individual's growth and development.[1,2]

Health professionals use a number of organizational strategies as frameworks for decision making during rehabilitation of individuals with pathologies leading to neuromuscular dysfunction. Many neurologists use a medical differential diagnosis process to locate the "lesion" as being within the CNS or involving structures of the peripheral nervous system or the muscle itself.[3] They do this by "triangulating" evidence gathered by examining tone and deep tendon reflexes, observing patterns of movement and postural control, and looking for specific types of involuntary movement.[4] They may also interpret results of special tests such as nerve conduction studies, electromyography (EMG), computed tomography (CT), and magnetic resonance imaging (MRI). These tests might pinpoint areas of denervation, ischemia, or demyelinization and help the health professionals arrive at a medical diagnosis.[5,6]

Rehabilitation professionals are most interested in the functional consequences associated with the various neuromotor conditions. They examine the ways in which abnormal tone (hypertonicity–excessive tone; hypotonicity–insufficient tone; or flaccidity–absence of tone) affects mobility and locomotion, postural control, motor planning and motor control during movement, coordination ("error control"), and muscle performance during functional activities.[7,8] Rehabilitation professionals are not only concerned about function at the present time but also consider the long-term impact of neuromotor impairment on the person's joints and posture, especially in children who are growing with abnormal tone and postures.[9]

This chapter first relates neuroanatomical structures to their functions, considering both location of lesion (per the medical model) and functional consequences of the disease process (per the disablement model used in rehabilitation). Then it examines in greater detail the roles, interactions, and goals of orthoses and adaptive equipment, pharmaceutical interventions, and surgeries in the management of persons with neuromuscular disorders. The authors specifically consider management of hypertonicity (spasticity), hypotonicity (low tone), fluctuating tone (athetosis, chorea), and flaccidity (no tone) integrating issues of postural control, coordination, and muscle performance into case studies to illustrate options for individuals with "typical" neuromuscular diseases.

Differential Diagnosis: Where Is the Problem?

Neurological and neuromuscular diseases can be classified as affecting either the CNS or the peripheral nervous system (PNS).[3,4,10] Only a few diseases such as amyotrophic lateral sclerosis affect both systems. Although both types of disease may cause motor or sensory impairment, or both, there are patterns and characteristics of dysfunction that are unique to each. Selection of the appropriate orthosis, seating/wheelchair system, or assistive devices is easiest if the therapist, orthotist, members of the rehabilitation team, patient, and patient's family understand the normal function and the consequences of the disease process of the neurological subsystem that is affected.

The Central Nervous System

The CNS is a complex of dynamic and interactive "subsystems" that mediates purposeful movement and postural control, vital autonomic "vegetative" and physiological functions, and learning of all types.[11] Readers are referred to Figure 12-1 and Table 12-1 to refresh their understanding of the functions located in specific regions of the cerebral cortex and to Figure 12-2 and Table 12-2 to review "deep" forebrain structures. Functional areas of the brainstem are illustrated and summarized in Figure 12-3 and Table 12-3, while functional areas of the spinal cord are diagrammed and discussed in Figure 12-4 and Table 12-4.

Some diseases affect a single CNS system or center (e.g., Parkinson's disease affects the basal ganglia; a "lacunar" stroke in the internal capsule may interrupt transmission only within the pyramidal/corticospinal pathway), leading to a specific array of signs/symptoms characteristic of that system or center. Other pathologies disrupt function across several systems: a thromboembolic stroke in the proximal left middle cerebral artery may disrupt volitional movement and sensation of the right side of the body, as well as communication and vision. Several exacerbations of multiple sclerosis (MS), over time, may lead to plaque formation in the cerebral peduncles/pyramidal system, superior cerebellar peduncle/error control system, restiform body/balance system, and fasciculus gracilis/lower extremity sensation; in this case it can be challenging but imperative to sort through the various types of impairments that may result in order to select the most appropriate therapeutic or orthotic intervention for the individual. Readers are referred to Table 12-5 for a summary of the most common neurological/neuromuscular disorders, the systems they affect, and the impact each has on tone, postural control, and mobility.

The *pyramidal system* is responsible for initiation of volitional movement and plays a major role in the development of skilled and manipulative activities. The cell bodies of pyramidal neurons are located in the postcentral gyrus/primary motor cortex. The motor cortex in the left cerebral hemisphere influences primarily the right side of the body (face, trunk, and extremities); the right cortex influences the left body. The axons of pyramidal neurons form the corticobulbar and corticospinal tracts, projecting toward alpha motor neurons in cranial nerve nuclei and anterior horn of the spinal cord. To reach their destination, these axons descend through the genu and posterior limb of the internal capsule, the cerebral peduncles, the basilar pons, the pyramids of the medulla, and finally the opposite lateral funiculus of the spinal cord. A lesion at any point in the pyramidal system has the potential to disrupt volitional movement. The degree of disruption varies with the extent and functional salience of the structures that are damaged, manifest on a continuum from mild weakness (paresis) to the inability to voluntarily initiate and direct movement (paralysis).

Immediately following insult or injury of the pyramidal system, during a period of "neurogenic shock," there may be substantially diminished muscle tone and sluggish or absent deep tendon reflexes.[12] As inflammation from the initial insult subsides, severely damaged neurons degenerate and are resorbed, while minimally damaged neurons may repair themselves and resume function.[13] The more neurons that are destroyed, the greater the likelihood that hypertonicity will develop over time due to the altered "balance" of descending input of pyramidal and extrapyramidal systems. As the recovery period continues, individuals may begin to move in "abnormal synergy" patterns whenever volitional movement is attempted.[14,15] When the damage to the system is less extensive, individuals may eventually recover some or all volitional motor control; the more extensive the damage to the system, the more likely there will be residual motor impairment.[15]

The *extrapyramidal* system is made up of several subcortical subsystems that influence muscle tone, organize patterns of movement from among the many possible movement strategies, and make both feedforward adjustments (in anticipation of movement) and refining feedback adjustments (in response to sensations generated as movement occurs) during performance of functional tasks.[16] The *motor*

Text continued on page 272.

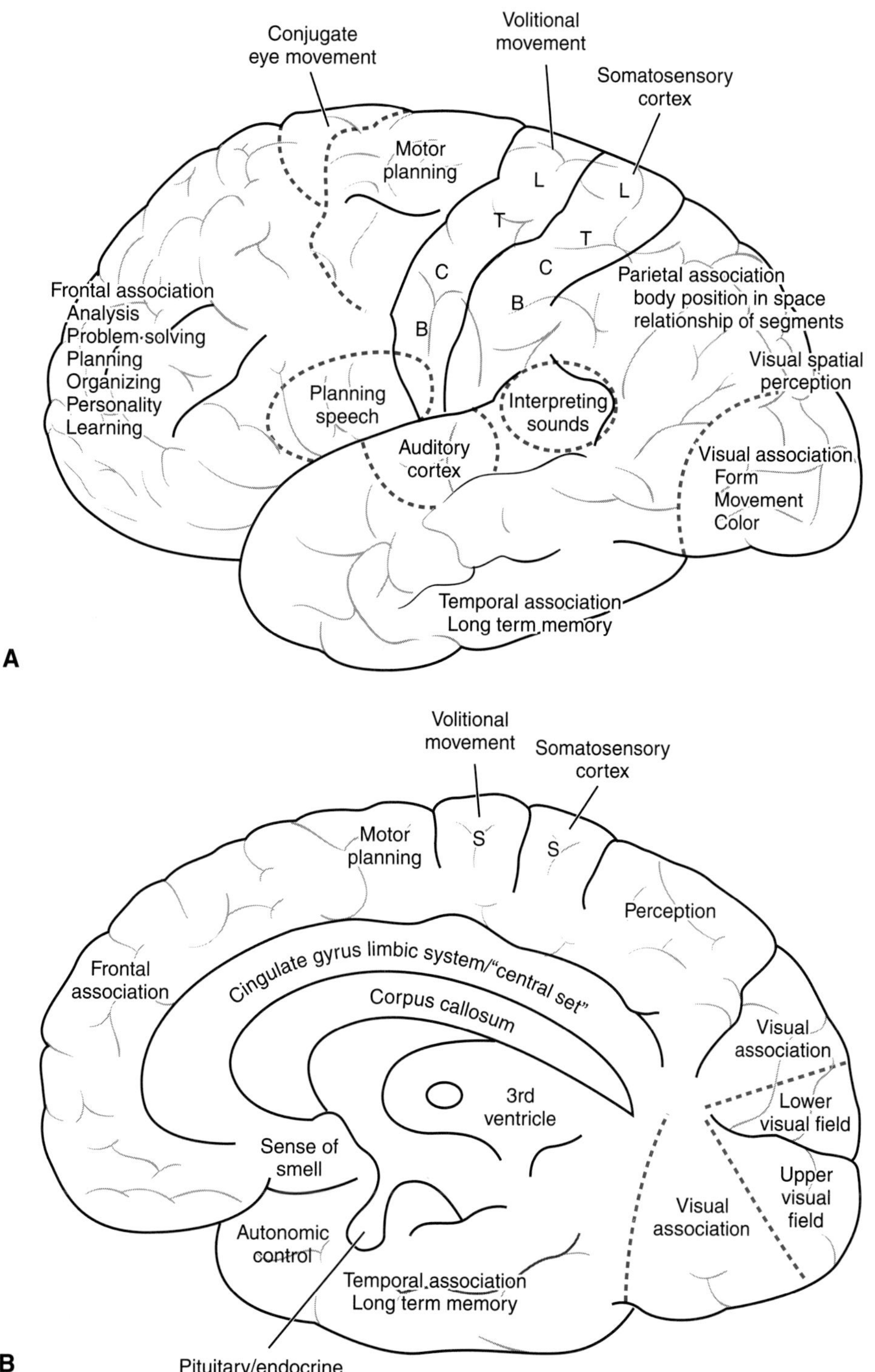

Figure 12-1

*Lateral (**A**) view of the surface of the left hemisphere and midsagittal (**B**) view of the surface of the right hemisphere, noting functional areas within each lobe of forebrain.* S, *Sacral;* L, *lumbar,* T, *thoracic;* C, *cervical;* B, *bulbar.*

Table 12-1
Functional Areas of the Cerebral Cortex

Anatomical Structure		*Function*	*Comments*
Cortex in the frontal lobe	Frontal association cortex (Brodmann's 9-12)	Intellectual ability, learning, problem solving, personality, "higher" executive function, short-term memory	Left hemisphere: analytical, sequential aspects of thought/behavior Right hemisphere: intuitive "big-picture" aspects of thought/behavior
	Frontal eye fields (Brodmann's 8)	Conjugate eye movement, visual tracking, papillary reactions	Projections to medial longitudinal fasciculus to influence oculomotor, trochlear, and abducens cranial nerve nuclei
	Primary and secondary motor planning areas (Brodmann's 6)	Planning and preparing for volitional movement (speed, direction, force)	Interacts with subcortical basal ganglia system, influences primary motor cortex
	Primary motor cortex precentral gyrus (Brodmann's 4)	Initiation of volitional, purposeful movement during functional tasks	Left hemisphere: influences right side of body Right hemisphere: influences left side of body
	Broca's association area (Brodmann's 44, 45)	Motor planning for speech, formulation of what is to be said	Left hemisphere: language function Right hemisphere: affective components of language, automatic/overused phrases
Cortex in the parietal lobe	Somatosensory cortex, postcentral gyrus (Brodmann's 3, 1, 2)	"Receiving" area for conscious exteroceptive and proprioceptive sensations	Left hemisphere: receives input from right side of body Right hemisphere: receives input from left side of body
	Parietal association areas (Brodmann's 5, 7)	Interpretation and integration of somatic sensation: kinesthetic perception, body image, understanding relationships of body segments	Perceptual function tends to be "specialized" in right hemisphere
	Wernicke's association area (Brodmann's 40, 42)	Interpretation and integration of sounds	Left hemisphere: understanding words/phrases: sequential communication sounds Right hemisphere: understanding affective aspects on spoken language and other sounds
	Angular gyrus (Brodmann's 39)	Integrative association cortex, linking somatic sensation, what is heard, what is seen	Specialized in the left hemisphere; gives meaning to sequential symbols; connects vision, hearing, speech

Table 12-1
Functional Areas of the Cerebral Cortex—cont'd

Anatomical Structure		*Function*	*Comments*
Cortex of the occipital lobe	Calcarine cortex; primary visual cortex (Brodmann's 17)	Receiving area for visual information	Left visual field represented on right calcarine cortex; right visual field represented on left calcarine cortex Upper visual field represented on lower calcarine cortex; lower visual field represented on upper calcarine cortex
	Visual association areas (Brodmann's 18, 19)	Interpretation of visual information	Left hemisphere: primarily concerned with sequential images, as in communication or symbolic materials Right hemisphere: concerned with form, shape, direction of movement of objects in the environment
Temporal cortex	Primary auditory cortex, superior temporal gyrus (Brodmann's 41)	Receiving area of all types of sound, from both ears	Determines what sounds are "communication" to be sent/interpreted to left Wernicke's area versus general sounds that will be sent/interpreted by right Wernicke's area
	Temporal association areas (multiple Brodmann's areas)	All other cortical surfaces of the temporal lobe; multiple dimensions of long-term memory	Left temporal hemisphere: tends to "store" memories that are overall impressions and affective dimensions of memory Right hemisphere: tends to "store" memories that are concerned with sequence, or order, such as language and "progression" of learned motor activity
Limbic cortex	Uncus/hippocampus (located on medial underside of temporal lobe)	Major component of limbic system, acts as channel into/out of long-term memory systems	Interacts with hypothalamus to interconnect limbic and autonomic function
	Cingulate cortex	Limbic system association area, involved with motivation, emotional/ affective aspects of behavior	Receives input from, and sends output to, most other cortical areas, as well as brainstem centers
Insular cortex	Association cortex, located deep within lateral fissure	Involved with interpretation of taste and smell	Receives input from solitary nucleus and tract, relayed through the ventral posterior medial nucleus of the thalamus

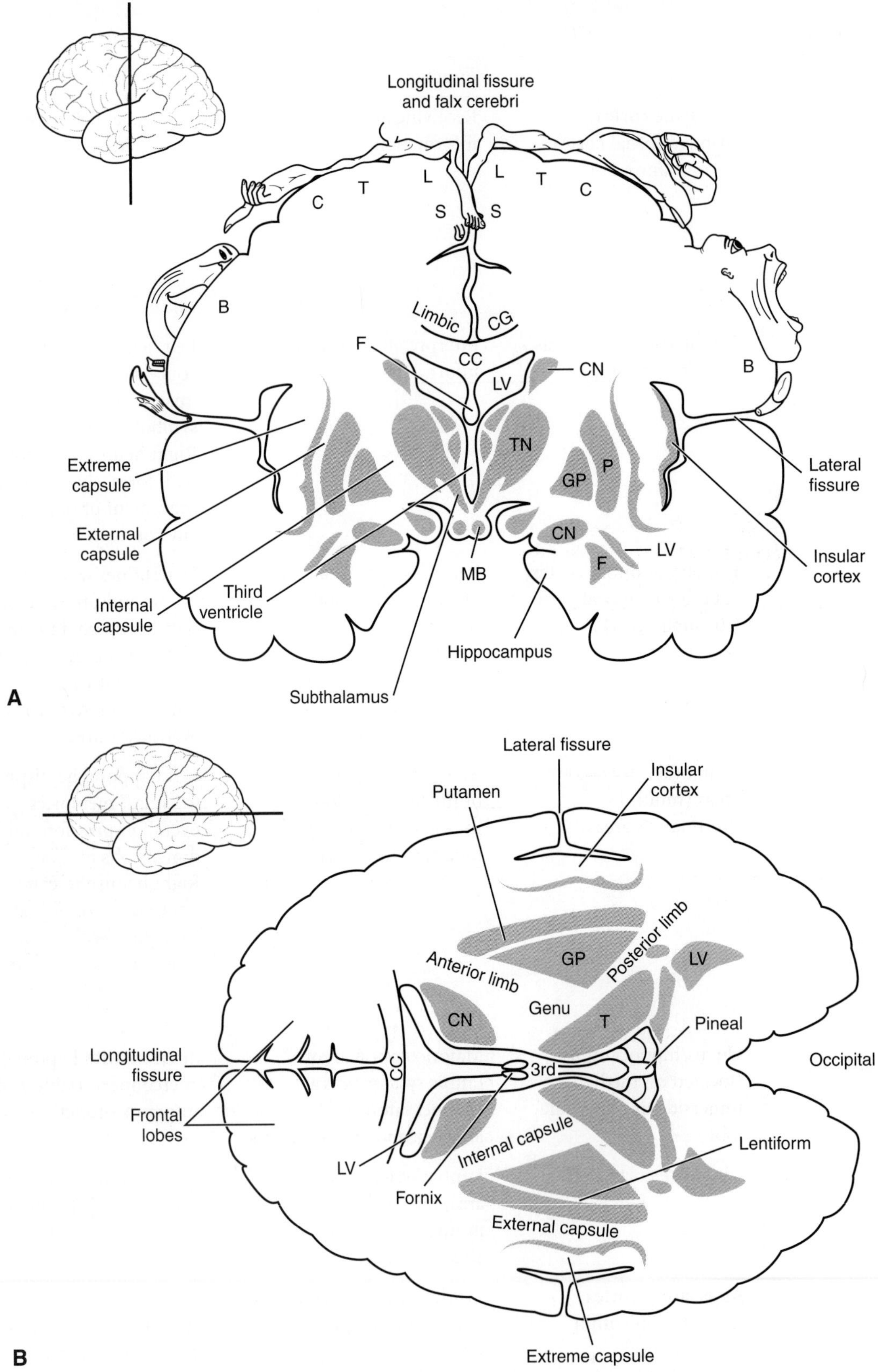

Figure 12-2

*Frontal (**A**) and horizontal (**B**) sections through the telencephalon and diencephalon, with key anatomical/functional areas labeled.* S, *Sacral;* L, *lumbar,* T, *thoracic;* C, *cervical;* B, *bulbar;* CG, *cingulate gyrus;* CC, *corpus callosum;* F, *fornix;* CN, *caudate nucleus;* P, *pulvinar;* GB, *globus pallidus;* TN, *thalamic nucleus;* LV, *lateral ventricle.*

Table 12-2
Structures within the Telencephalon and Diencephalon (Listed from Midline to Lateral Surface)

Level of Neuraxis	*Structure*	*Function*	*Comments*
Telencephalon	Corpus callosum	Major white matter interconnection containing commissural fibers traveling among all areas of cortex in left and right hemispheres	Integrates left and right brain "specialized" functions
	Fornix	White matter tract interconnecting hippocampus and mammillary bodies, part of the limbic system	Involved in Papez circuit of emotion/rage
	Lateral ventricle	C-shaped ventricle running through center of telencephalon; contains choroid plexus, which manufactures cerebrospinal fluid	Anterior horn in frontal through parietal lobes (separated by septum pellucidum), posterior horn extending into occipital lobes, inferior horn into temporal lobes
	Caudate nucleus	Component of primary and secondary subcortical "motor planning loop," corpus striatum Significant interaction with substantia nigra in mesencephalon Primary role in modulation of underlying muscle tone	Transmitter: GABA C-shaped nucleus traveling lateral to the lateral ventricle: head of caudate in frontal lobe, body through parietal lobes, tail into temporal lobes Involved in learning of many types, especially novel situations
	Amygdala nucleus	Component of limbic system, involved with physiological memory, drive states, and instincts	Located in the temporal lobe, at the anterior tip of the caudate nucleus
	Internal capsule corona radiata	Major white matter interconnection between all areas of cerebral cortex with the brainstem and spinal cord	Anterior limb: interconnections between frontal lobe and brainstem/spinal cord Genu contains primarily corticobulbar projections Posterior limb: corticospinal projections, interconnections between parietal/occipital/temporal lobes and brainstem/spinal cord
	Globus pallidus nucleus	Component of subcortical "motor planning loop," corpus striatum, and lentiform nucleus Major role in dampening all but most essential muscle activity of agonist/antagonist for functional movement	Transmitter: GABA Separated from thalamic nuclei by the internal capsule
	Putamen nucleus	Component of primary and secondary subcortical "motor planning loops," corpus striatum, and lentiform nucleus Primary role in modulation of underlying muscle tone	Transmitter: GABA
	External capsule	Secondary white matter structure interconnecting cerebral cortex with brainstem/spinal cord	

Continued

Table 12-2
Structures within the Telencephalon and Diencephalon (Listed from Midline to Lateral Surface)—cont'd

Level of Neuraxis	*Structure*	*Function*	*Comments*
	Claustrum nucleus	Small button-shaped nucleus, classified as part of anatomical basal ganglia	Function/contribution to motor behaviors not well understood
	Extreme capsule	Secondary white matter structure interconnecting cerebral cortex with brainstem/spinal cord	
	Insular cortex	Component of cerebral cortex "buried" deep within lateral fissure	Thought to be involved in interpretation/perception of taste and smell
Diencephalon	Third ventricle	At midline, contains choroid plexus	Interventricular foramen drains lateral ventricles into third ventricle, cerebral aqueduct interconnects third and fourth ventricles within brainstem
	Thalamic nuclei	MGB: relay in auditory pathway LGB: relay in visual pathway Ventral posterior lateral nucleus: relay in somatosensory pathways from spinal cord Ventral posterior medial nucleus: relay in somatosensory pathways from brainstem/cranial nerve sensory nuclei Ventral lateral nucleus: relay in "error control" system, connecting red nucleus and cerebellum to primary motor cortex Ventral anterior nucleus: relay in subcortical motor planning systems Anterior nucleus: relay in limbic system (emotion, motivation, memory) Dorsal/medial nuclear and lateral groups: interpretation/integration of physiological state with emotional state Pulvinar nucleus: integration/subcortical interpretation of visual, auditory, and somatosensory modalities Intralaminar nuclei have three functions: modulation of pain, consciousness as part of the reticular activating system, and involvement with motor planning system	Subcortical processing, interpretation, and integration of all sensory modalities (except olfaction), integration of sensory systems, motor planning and control systems, limbic/motivational systems

Table 12-2
Structures within the Telencephalon and Diencephalon (Listed from Midline to Lateral Surface)—cont'd

Level of Neuraxis	*Structure*	*Function*	*Comments*
	Epithalamus	Pineal gland (circadian rhythm, melatonic production) Habenular nucleus (limbic system structure, involved with interpretation of pleasurable sensations) Posterior commissure (white matter structure linking posterior cortical areas of occipital and temporal lobes)	
	Hypothalamic nuclei	Collection of small functional areas/regions; functions include regulation of endocrine activity (via projections to pituitary), control of autonomic nervous systems (projections to parasympathetic nuclei in brainstem, sympathetic centers in thoracic spinal cord, parasympathetic centers in lumbosacral spinal cord), integration of physiological state with emotional state (via interconnections with hippocampus, amygdala of the limbic system)	Integration of CNS systems that influence physiological function
	Subthalamus	Component of subcortical basal ganglia "motor planning" system	Thought to be involved with force production/modulation, especially of ballistic movements
	Optic nerve	White matter structure carrying information from retina to the LGB of the thalamus	Information in right ON from right eye Information in left ON from left eye If lesion : blindness of ipsilateral eye
	Optic chiasm	"Plexus" where information from nasal retina (lateral visual field) crosses midline	Reorganizes visual information so that information from one visual field is delivered to opposite hemisphere
	Optic tract	White matter structure carrying information from retina to the LGB of the thalamus	Information from right visual field (from both eyes) carried in left optic tract Information from left visual field (from both eyes) carried in right optic tract If lesion: homonymous hemianopsia (loss of some or all of a visual field)

Continued

Table 12-2
Structures within the Telencephalon and Diencephalon (Listed from Midline to Lateral Surface)—cont'd

Level of Neuraxis	*Structure*	*Function*	*Comments*
	Pituitary gland	Infundibulum or "stalk" contains axons of hypothalamic neurons projecting to neurohypophysis, as well as portal vessels to adenohypophysis Neurohypophysis/posterior lobe: produces hormones vasopressin and oxytocin Adenohypophysis/anterior lobe: produces follicle stimulating hormone, luteinizing hormone, prolactin, thyroid stimulating hormone, adrenocorticotrophic hormone, growth hormone, and somatotropic hormone	"Master" endocrine gland, influences function of other major endocrine structures
	Mammillary bodies	Relay nucleus interconnecting hippocampus to anterior and lateral nuclei of the thalamus	

CNS, Central nervous system; *GABA,* gamma-aminobutyric acid; *LGB,* lateral geniculate body; *MGB,* medial geniculate body; *ON,* optic nerve.

planning subsystem is a series of neural loops interconnecting the premotor and accessory motor cortices in the frontal lobes, the nuclei of the functional basal ganglia (caudate, putamen, globus pallidus, substantia nigra, subthalamus) and several nuclei of the thalamus. Damage to the premotor and accessory motor cortex leads to apraxia, the inability to effectively sequence components of a functional task and to understand the nature of a task and the way to use a "tool" in performance of the task.[17] If there is damage to the caudate and putamen (also called the *corpus striatum*), underlying muscle tone may fluctuate unpredictably (athetosis) and involuntary dancelike movements (chorea) are likely to occur.[18,19] Damage to the subthalamic nuclei can lead to forceful, often disruptive, involuntary movement of the extremities (ballism) that interrupts purposeful activity.[19,20] Damage to the substantia nigra characteristically leads to resting tremor, rigidity of axial and appendicular musculature (hypertonicity in all directions), and bradykinesia (difficulty initiating movement, slow movement with limited excursion during functional tasks), which are most commonly seen in persons with Parkinson's disease.[21] Motor impairments resulting from damage to the ventral anterior nucleus and related thalamic nuclei are less well understood but may contribute to less efficient motor planning, especially when the individual is learning or performing novel tasks.

Extrapyramidal structures influence muscle tone and readiness to move via a network of interconnections among motor centers in the brainstem. The reticulospinal tracts, originating in the lower pons and medulla, are thought to influence tone by acting on gamma motor neurons and their associated muscle spindles. They play a major role in balancing the "stiffness" required for antigravity position and the "flexibility" necessary for movement of the limbs through space during functional activity and are likely the "effectors" for tonic hindbrain reflexes.[16,22] The vestibulospinal tracts, also originating from the pons and medulla, influence anticipatory postural adjustment in preparation for movement and reactionary postural adjustments as movement occurs. These tracts are thought to be the "effectors" for postural control and balance.[16,22] The tectospinal tracts, originating in the collicular nuclei of the dorsal midbrain, influence linkages between the head and extremities (especially arms and hands) so that the visual and auditory systems can be used effectively to orient the head and body during tasks that require visual (eye-hand) and auditory (ear-hand) guidance.[16,22]

The "error control" or *coordination subsystem* has several interactive components.[23,24] Feedforward information (how movement is likely to occur) from the forebrain's motor cortex is relayed through the thalamus to the deep nuclei of the cerebellum via the middle cerebellar peduncle (brachium pontis). Feedback information generated by movement travels from the muscle spindle and anterior horn of the spinal cord via the inferior cerebellar peduncle (restiform body), as does sensory information from static

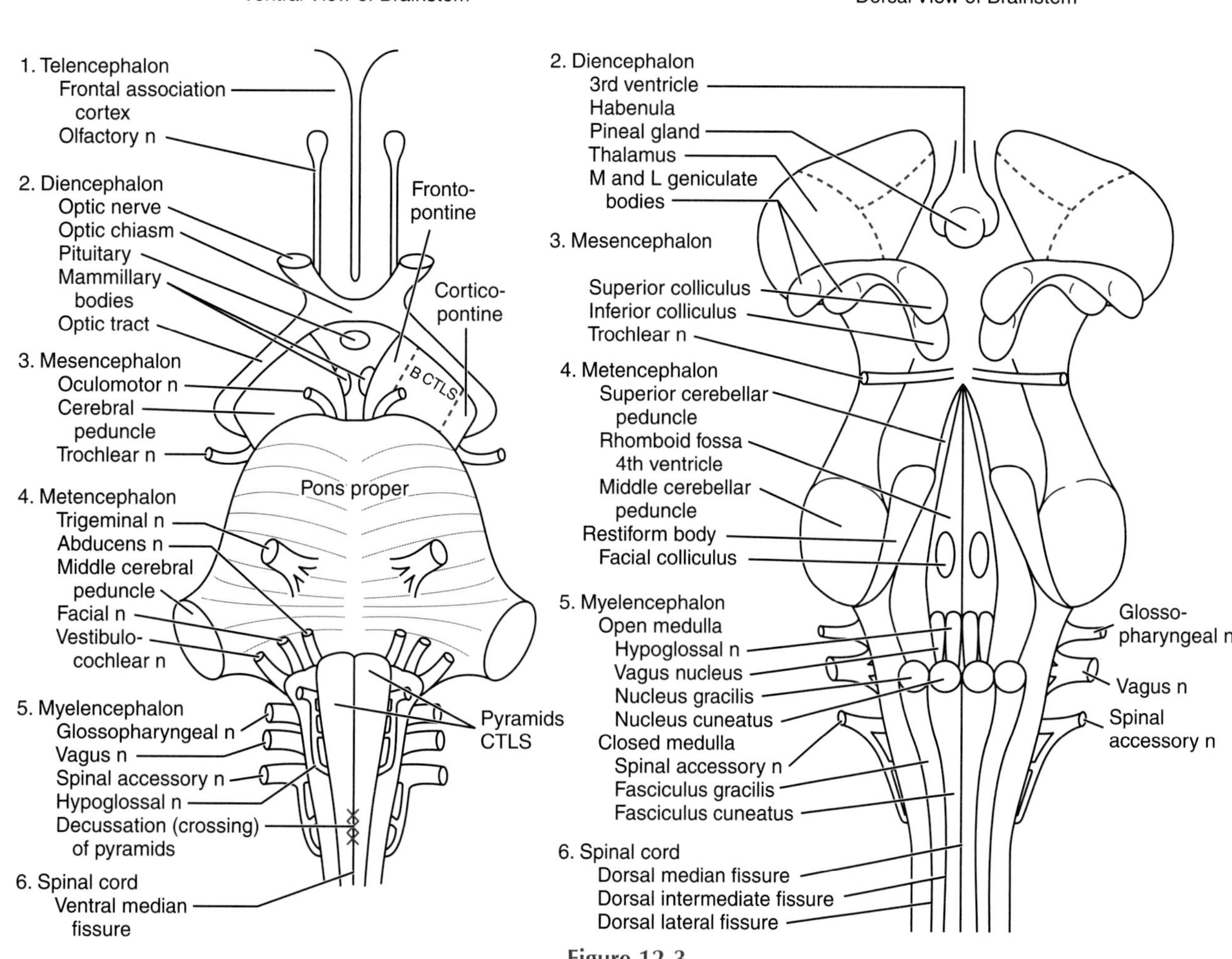

Figure 12-3

A, Ventral and dorsal views of the brainstem, with key anatomical structures labeled.

and dynamic vestibular receptors (head position and movement in space) and the vestibular nuclei in the brainstem. Through interaction of Purkinje cells in the cerebellar cortex and neurons in the deep cerebellar nuclei, the cerebellum judges how "in sync" these various types of information are (essentially asking the questions, "Did the movement occur as planned? Was the outcome of the movement as intended?") and suggests refinements for more precise and coordinated movement. These adjustments are relayed to the red nucleus in the midbrain via the superior cerebellar peduncle (brachium conjunctiva) and are forwarded back to the thalamus and the motor cortex, as well as to the spinal cord via the rubrospinal tract. The rubrospinal tract is thought to be essential for refinement and correction of direction and control of movement as it occurs.

The *somatosensory* system is composed of a set of ascending pathways, each carrying a specific sensory modality from the spinal cord and brainstem to the thalamus and postcentral gyrus of the cerebral cortex, reticular formation, or cerebellum. The anterior-lateral (spinothalamic) system carries exteroceptive information from mechanoreceptors that monitor "protective" senses (e.g., pain, temperature, irritation to skin and soft tissue).[25] This tract originates in the dorsal horn (substantia gelatinosa) of the spinal cord and the spinal trigeminal nucleus, crosses the midline of the neuraxis to ascend in the lateral funiculus of the spinal cord to the contralateral ventral posterior thalamus, and then continues to the postcentral gyrus. The dorsal column/medial lemniscus carries information from encapsulated receptors that serve as "internal monitors" of body condition and motion.[26] This tract ascends from the spinal cord to reach the nuclei gracilis and cuneatus in the medulla of the brainstem, then crosses midline to ascend to the contralateral ventral posterior thalamus and on to the posterior central gyrus. The postcentral gyrus (somatosensory cortex) is organized as a "homunculus," with each region of the body represented in a specific area (see Figure 12-2). Sensation from the lower extremities (lumbosacral spinal cord) is located at the top of the gyrus near the sagittal fissure. Moving downward toward the lateral fissure, the next area represented is the trunk (tho-

Text continued on page 297.

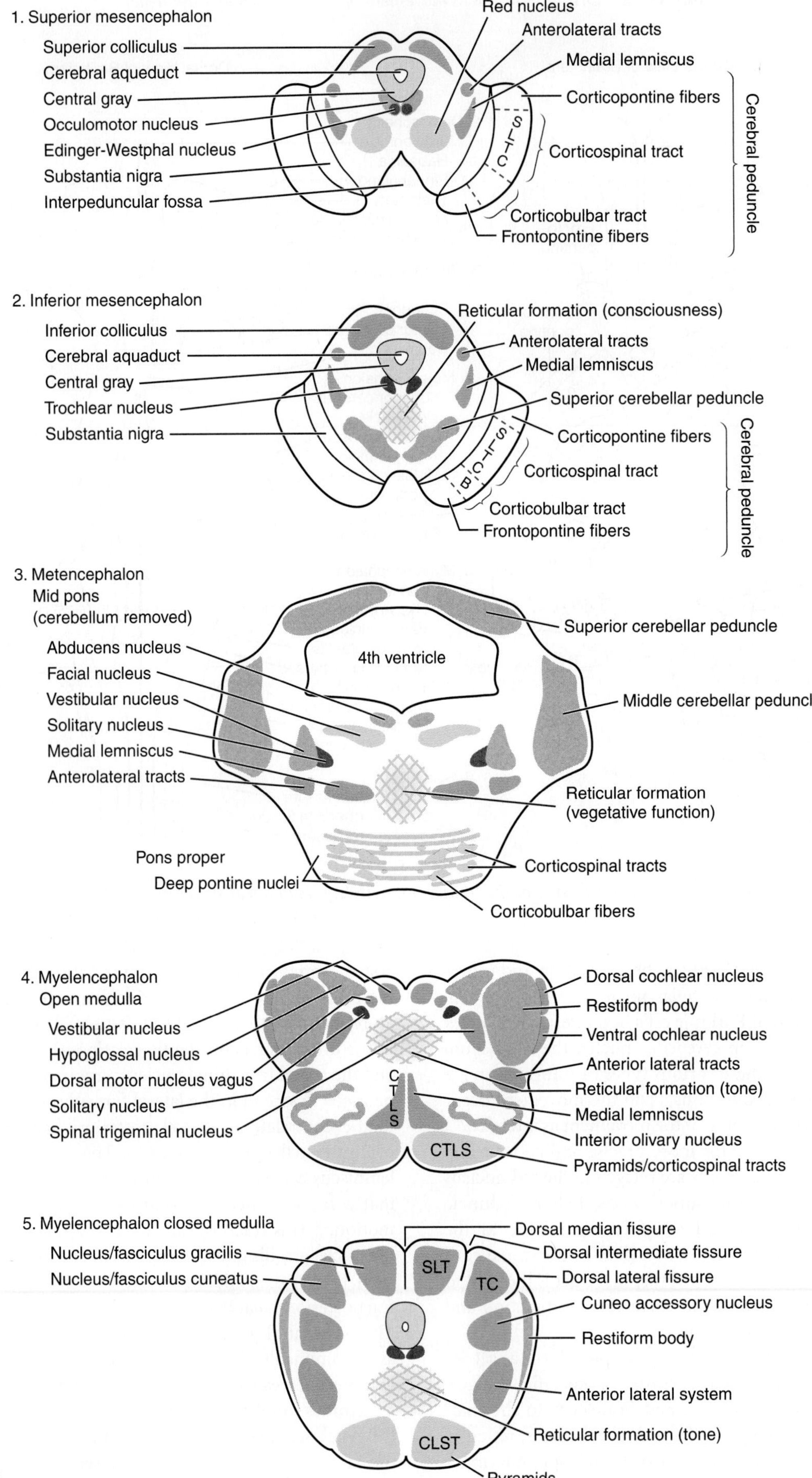
1. Superior mesencephalon
Superior colliculus
Cerebral aqueduct
Central gray
Occulomotor nucleus
Edinger-Westphal nucleus
Substantia nigra
Interpeduncular fossa
Red nucleus
Anterolateral tracts
Medial lemniscus
Corticopontine fibers
Corticospinal tract
Corticobulbar tract
Frontopontine fibers
Cerebral peduncle
S
L
T
C
2. Inferior mesencephalon
Inferior colliculus
Cerebral aquaduct
Central gray
Trochlear nucleus
Substantia nigra
Reticular formation (consciousness)
Anterolateral tracts
Medial lemniscus
Superior cerebellar peduncle
Corticopontine fibers
Corticospinal tract
Corticobulbar tract
Frontopontine fibers
Cerebral peduncle
S
L
T
C
B
3. Metencephalon
Mid pons
(cerebellum removed)
Abducens nucleus
Facial nucleus
Vestibular nucleus
Solitary nucleus
Medial lemniscus
Anterolateral tracts
4th ventricle
Superior cerebellar peduncle
Middle cerebellar peduncle
Reticular formation
(vegetative function)
Pons proper
Deep pontine nuclei
Corticospinal tracts
Corticobulbar fibers
4. Myelencephalon
Open medulla
Vestibular nucleus
Hypoglossal nucleus
Dorsal motor nucleus vagus
Solitary nucleus
Spinal trigeminal nucleus
Dorsal cochlear nucleus
Restiform body
Ventral cochlear nucleus
Anterior lateral tracts
Reticular formation (tone)
Medial lemniscus
Interior olivary nucleus
Pyramids/corticospinal tracts
C
T
L
S
CTLS
5. Myelencephalon closed medulla
Nucleus/fasciculus gracilis
Nucleus/fasciculus cuneatus
Dorsal median fissure
Dorsal intermediate fissure
Dorsal lateral fissure
Cuneo accessory nucleus
Restiform body
Anterior lateral system
Reticular formation (tone)
Pyramids
SLT
TC
CLST
B

Figure 12-3, cont'd

B, Horizontal sections taken at five representative levels of forebrain, with key tracts and nuclei labeled.

Table 12-3
Structures within the Brainstem (listed from superior to inferior)

Level of Neuraxis	*Structure*	*Function*	*Comments*
Superior mesencephalon	Superior colliculus	Links eyes/head orientation to moving objects within visual field	Relay in neural circuit for pupillary light reflexes
	Central gray	Subcortical perception/ modulation of pain	
	Cerebral aqueduct	Ventricular system link between third and fourth ventricles	
	Oculomotor nucleus	Innervation for medial, superior, and inferior rectus muscles, as well as inferior oblique	Axons form oculomotor nerve
	Edinger-Westphal nucleus	Parasympathetic nucleus involved in pupillary light reflexes	Axons form oculomotor nerve
	Anterior-lateral system (tract)	Ascending pathway carrying exteroceptive information from spinal cord to thalamus	Also known as the spinothalamic system
	Medial lemniscus	Ascending pathway carrying conscious proprioception and discriminatory sensation from spinal cord and brainstem to thalamus	Moderately myelinated pathway
	Red nucleus	Relay in cerebellum to thalamus to cortex feedback system; involved in "error control/ coordination" of voluntary movement	Original of rubrospinal (extrapyramidal) tract
	Substantia nigra	Basal ganglia nucleus with reciprocal connections to the corpus striatum (caudate and putamen nucleus) in the telencephalon Modulation of agonist/antagonist tone/activity	Transmitters: nigrostriate fibers: dopamine striatonigral fibers: GABA
	Cerebral peduncle	Frontopontine fibers (feedforward to cerebellum) Corticobulbar fibers/pyramidal system Corticospinal fibers/pyramidal system Corticopontine fibers (feedforward to brainstem and cerebellum)	Highly myelinated motor fibers, organized in a "homunculus" (bulbar medially, sacral laterally)
Inferior mesencephalon	Inferior colliculus	Links of eye and orientation to sounds with in the auditory environment	Relay in auditory pathway

Continued

Table 12-3
Structures within the Brainstem (listed from superior to inferior)—cont'd

Level of Neuraxis	*Structure*	*Function*	*Comments*
	Central gray	Subcortical perception/ modulation of pain	
	Cerebral aqueduct	Ventricular system link between third and fourth ventricles	
	Trochlear nucleus	Contains alpha and gamma motor neurons, which innervate superior oblique muscle	Involved in alignment of eyes for accommodation between close and distant vision
	Anterior-lateral system (tract)	Ascending pathway carrying exteroceptive information from the opposite side of the body projecting from spinal cord and brainstem to thalamus	Also known as the spinothalamic system
	Medial lemniscus	Ascending pathway carrying conscious proprioception and discriminatory sensation from the opposite side of the body, projecting from spinal cord and brainstem to thalamus	Moderately myelinated pathway
	Mesencephalic reticular formation	Component of the reticular activating system, involved with consciousness, attention, habituation to repetitive stimuli	Influenced by projections from prefrontal cortex, limbic system, anterior-lateral sensory system Output diverges to influence all areas of neuraxis
	Superior cerebellar peduncle	White matter connection between cerebellum/dentate nucleus and red nucleus	Component of "error control" and coordination systems
	Substantia nigra	Basal ganglia nucleus with reciprocal connections to the corpus striatum (caudate and putamen nucleus) in the telencephalon Modulation of agonist/antagonist tone/activity	Transmitters: nigrostriatal fibers: dopamine striatonigral fibers: GABA
	Cerebral peduncle	Frontopontine fibers (feedforward to cerebellum) Corticobulbar fibers/pyramidal system Corticospinal fibers/pyramidal system Corticopontine fibers (feedforward to brainstem and cerebellum)	Highly myelinated motor fibers, organized in a "homunculus" (bulbar medially, sacral laterally)

Table 12-3
Structures within the Brainstem (listed from superior to inferior)—cont'd

Level of Neuraxis	*Structure*	*Function*	*Comments*
Metencephalon (pons)	Cerebellum and its deep nuclei	Receives feedforward information about intended movement from forebrain via pontocerebellar and olivocerebellar interconnections, receives feedback information about state of body from vestibulocerebellar and spinocerebellar interconnections Provides feedback to motor cortex for more precise motor control via projections to red nucleus and thalamus	Plays major subcortical (unconscious, automatic) role in righting and equilibrium responses, in setting appropriate baseline postural tone, and in "error correction" (coordination) for skilled movement during functional activities
	Superior cerebellar peduncle	One of three structures connecting cerebellum to brainstem; carries of most of the "efferent" output from cerebellum upward to red nucleus and thalamus	Highly myelinated neurons
	Fourth ventricle with rhomboid fossa	Large diamond-shaped ventricle in the metencephalon, extending into the open medulla. Also contains choroid plexus for CSF production; location of foramina that allow CSF to enter into subarachnoid space	
	Abducens nucleus	Location of α and γ motor neurons that will innervate lateral rectus muscle of the eye	Axons form the sixth cranial nerve (abducens)
	Facial nucleus	Location of α and γ motor neurons that will innervate all muscles of facial expression	Axons form the seventh cranial nerve (facial)
	Solitary nucleus and tract	Location of first nucleus in the taste sensation pathway, surrounded by axons ascending to higher centers in forebrain	Receives input from trigeminal and other different cranial nerves
	Pontine reticular formation	Location of many "centers" that modulate vegetative function Lower pons is location of extrapyramidal motor center concerned with antigravity muscle tone, which gives rise to the medial reticulospinal tract	
	Medial lemniscus	Ascending pathway carrying information about conscious proprioception from the opposite side of the body and face	Moderately myelinated neurons

Continued

Table 12-3
Structures within the Brainstem (listed from superior to inferior)—cont'd

Level of Neuraxis	*Structure*	*Function*	*Comments*
	Anterolateral tracts	Ascending pathway carrying information about exteroception from the opposite side of the body and face	Also known as spinothalamic tract
	Middle cerebellar peduncle	Major point of entry of feedforward information from cortex and brainstem into the cerebellum, via pontocerebellar projections	Highly and moderately myelinated neurons
	Corticobulbar bundles	Descending pyramidal tract controlling voluntary movement of face (formerly traveling in the genu of the internal capsule and medial cerebral peduncle) projecting to α motor neurons in somatic motor cranial nerve nuclei	Highly myelinated neurons
	Corticospinal bundles	Descending pyramidal tract controlling voluntary movement of the body (formerly found in the posterior internal capsule and mid to lateral cerebral peduncle) projecting to motor neurons in the anterior horn of spinal cord	Highly myelinated neurons
	Deep pontine nuclei	Site of synaptic connection between frontopontine and other corticopontine fibers and pontocerebellar fibers carrying feedforward information about intended motor plan to cerebellum. Pontocerebellar fibers cross midline to enter contralateral cerebellum via middle cerebellum	
Open medulla (superior myelencephalon)	Fourth ventricle with rhomboid fossa	Large "diamond-shaped ventricle in the metencephalon, extending into the open medulla. Also contains choroid plexus for CSF production; location of foramina that allow CSF to enter into subarachnoid space	
	Nucleus ambiguous	Location of α and γ motor neurons that will innervate muscles of the soft palate, larynx, and pharynx	Axons will form glossopharyngeal (ninth) and part of vagus (tenth) cranial nerves

Table 12-3
Structures within the Brainstem (listed from superior to inferior)—cont'd

Level of Neuraxis	*Structure*	*Function*	*Comments*
	Hypoglossal nucleus	Location of α and γ motor neurons that will innervate muscles of the tongue	Axons will form hypoglossal (twelfth) cranial nerve
	Dorsal motor nucleus of the vagus	Major parasympathetic nucleus of the brainstem; influences visceral systems to maintain homeostasis; receives input from hypothalamus via dorsal longitudinal fasciculus	Axons will form vagus (tenth) and a part of spinal accessory (eleventh) cranial nerves; project to parasympathetic ganglion near target organs
	Vestibular nuclei	Set of four nuclei clustered from lower pons to closed medulla; receives input from dynamic (semicircular canals) and static (saccule and utricle) vestibular receptors via the vestibulocochlear eighth cranial nerve; major output reaches cerebellum via restiform body and brainstem somatic motor cranial nerve nuclei and spinal cord via medial longitudinal fasciculus/medial vestibulospinal tracts and lateral vestibulospinal tracts	Origin of extrapyramidal vestibulospinal tracts; key player in righting and equilibrium responses, key player in vestibulo-ocular reflexes
	Solitary nucleus and tract	Location of first nucleus in the taste sensation pathway, surrounded by axons ascending to higher centers in forebrain	Receives input for trigeminal and other afferent cranial nerves
	Spinal trigeminal nucleus and tract	First nucleus in pathway carrying exteroceptive information from face and mouth Analogous to the substantia gelatinosa lamina 1-4 in spinal cord	Receives input from trigeminal nerve, as well as other afferent cranial nerves
	Inferior cerebellar peduncle (restiform body)	Major interconnection between spinal cord and cerebellum (via spinocerebellar tracts) Also carries information from vestibular nerve and nuclei and climbing fibers projecting from the inferior olivary nucleus	Highly myelinated neurons entering cerebellum

Continued

Table 12-3
Structures within the Brainstem (listed from superior to inferior)—cont'd

Level of Neuraxis	*Structure*	*Function*	*Comments*
	Dorsal and ventral cochlear nucleus	First nucleus in auditory pathway Input from receptors in cochlea delivered bilaterally via cochlear division of eighth cranial nerve Projections, bilaterally, ascend to other nuclei in the auditory pathway (superior olive, inferior colliculus, medial geniculate body) on the way to primary auditory cortex	Multisynaptic pathway allows localization of sound in space
	Reticular formation	Location of extrapyramidal tone center that gives rise to the lateral reticulospinal tract	Together with the medial reticulospinal tract influences "hindbrain" level reflexes during development and following brain injury
	Medial lemniscus	Ascending pathway carrying information about conscious proprioception from the opposite side of the body and face	Moderately myelinated neurons
	Inferior olivary nucleus	Major projections from this nucleus into cerebellum as climbing fibers via restiform body	
	Anterolateral system	Ascending pathway carrying information about exteroception from the opposite side of the body and face	Also known as spinothalamic tract
	Pyramids	Continuation of corticospinal fibers that originated in ipsilateral primary motor cortex, descended through internal capsule, cerebral peduncle, and metencephalon (pons)	
Closed medulla (inferior myelencephalon)	Fasciculus/nucleus gracilis	In lower medulla, column of afferent fibers carrying conscious proprioception definitive from dermatomes <T6 level from ipsilateral lower extremities and lower trunk. More proximally located nucleus is location of synapse in dorsal column/medial lemniscal pathway	After synapse, second order neurons in pathway cross midline in internal arcuate fibers to ascend toward ventral posterior lateral nucleus of the thalamus

Table 12-3
Structures within the Brainstem (listed from superior to inferior)—cont'd

Level of Neuraxis	*Structure*	*Function*	*Comments*
	Fasciculus/nucleus cuneatus	In lower medulla, column of afferent fibers carrying conscious proprioception definitive from dermatomes >T6 level from ipsilateral upper trunk and upper extremities. More proximally located nucleus is location of synapse in dorsal column/medial lemniscal pathway	After synapse, second order neurons in pathway cross midline in internal arcuate fibers to ascend toward ventral posterior lateral nucleus of the thalamus
	Cuneoaccessory nucleus	Location of synapse of unconscious proprioceptive information (collected by muscle spindle and Golgi tendon organ) from ipsilateral upper extremity; surrounded by dorsal spinocerebellar tract	Enters cerebellum via restiform body
	Central canal	Ventricular component of inferior myelencephalon, continues into spinal cord	
	Central gray	Integrative/processing area surrounding central canal, continuous with lamina 10 in spinal cord	
	Reticular formation	Continuation of extrapyramidal tone center that gives rise to the lateral reticulospinal tract	Together with the medial reticulospinal tract, influences "hindbrain" level reflexes during development and following brain injury
	Hypoglossal nucleus	Location of alpha and gamma motor neurons that will innervate muscles of the tongue	Axons will form hypoglossal (twelfth) cranial nerve
	Anterolateral system	Ascending pathway carrying information about exteroception from the opposite side of the body and face	Also known as spinothalamic tract
	Pyramids	Continuation of corticospinal fibers that originated in ipsilateral primary motor cortex, descended through internal capsule, cerebral peduncle, and metencephalon (pons)	Pathway crosses midline at transition from medulla to spinal cord, into lateral funiculus

CSF, Cerebrospinal fluid.

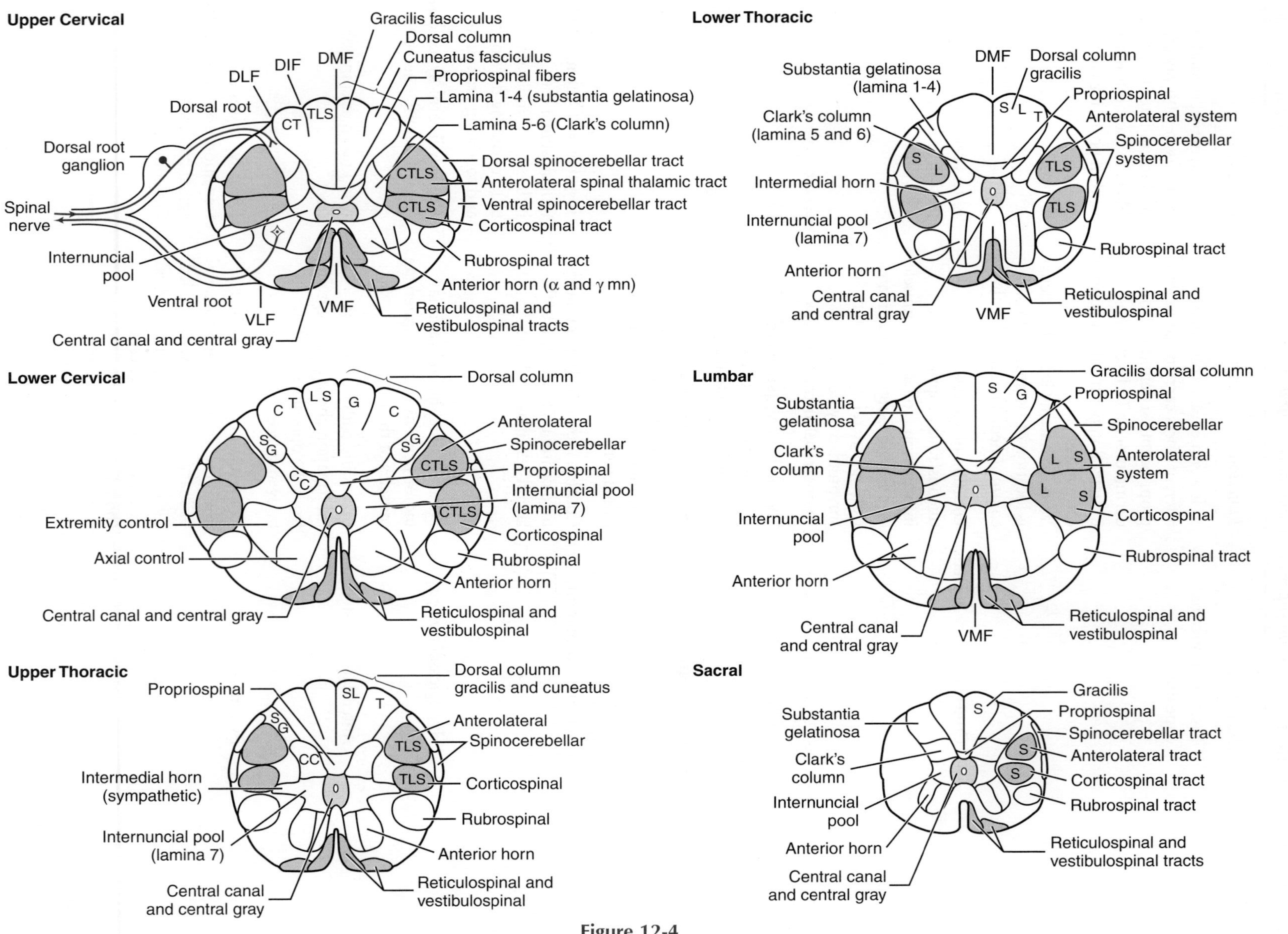

Figure 12-4
Horizontal sections taken at representative levels of the spinal cord, with key tracts in each fasciculus, and functional areas of gray matter labeled.

Table 12-4
Structures of the Spinal Cord (as they would appear dorsal to ventral on a cross section)

Location	*Structure*	*Location/Function*	*Comments*
Dorsal column (white matter)	Dorsal median fissure	At midline, divides dorsal column into left and right sides	
	Fasciculus gracilis	White matter tract carrying information from ipsilateral lower extremities and lower trunk (<T6 dermatomes) upward to nucleus gracilis in the medulla	Moderately myelinated neurons
	Dorsal intermediate fissure	Landmark dividing dorsal column into two fasciculi	Present from mid-thoracic cord through closed medulla
	Fasciculus cuneatus	White matter tract carrying information from ipsilateral upper trunk and upper extremities (>T6 dermatomes) upward to nucleus cuneatus in the medulla	Moderately myelinated neurons Present from midthoracic cord through closed medulla
Dorsal horn (gray matter)	Substantia gelatinosa	Location of synapse of exteroceptive afferent information carried in the anterolateral system After synapse, axons cross midline to ascend in the contralateral lateral column to the inferior and superior reticular formation on the way to the ventral posterior lateral nucleus of the thalamus	Also known as Rexed's laminae 1-4
	Clark's column	Not well developed in cervical spinal cord; analogous to cuneoaccessory nucleus in the closed medulla In sacral through thoracic cord, location of synapse of unconscious proprioceptive information collected by muscle spindle and Golgi tendon organ	Part of dorsal spinocerebellar system
Midgray area	Internuncial pool	Major integrative nucleus of spinal cord; site of synapse for multisynaptic spinal cord reflexes	Also known as Rexed's lamina 7
	Intermedial horn	Sympathetic center in the thoracic and upper lumbar spinal cord	Receives descending input from hypothalamus via dorsal lateral fasciculus; axons project into sympathetic chain, which runs parallel to spinal cord
	Central canal	Ventricular component of spinal cord (more of a potential than actual space in the adult spinal cord)	
	Central gray	Central integrative center within spinal cord, contributes to spinocerebellar pathways	Also known as Rexed's lamina 10

Continued

Table 12-4
Structures of the Spinal Cord (as they would appear dorsal to ventral on a cross section)—cont'd

Location	*Structure*	*Location/Function*	*Comments*
Anterior horn	Motor pools	Location of α and γ motor neurons that will innervate muscles of the axial muscles (medially) and extremities (laterally)	Also known as Rexed's laminae 8 and 9. Receives input from pyramidal system, extrapyramidical system, limbic system, and afferent/sensory systems (reciprocal innervation)
Lateral column	Dorsal and ventral spinocerebellar tracts	Afferent pathways at the edge of the lateral column carrying information about state of muscles and activity within anterior horn to cerebellum	Continues into restiform body
	Anterolateral system	Major afferent pathway, located dorsally within lateral funiculus carrying exteroceptive information from substantia gelatinosa to reticular formation and ventral posterolateral nucleus of the thalamus	Also known as spinothalamic tract
	Corticospinal tract	Major pyramidal (descending) motor pathway carrying information from contralateral primary motor cortex to α motor neurons in the anterior horn of spinal cord	Continuation of axons previously found in pyramids, cerebral peduncle, and motor fibers in posterior limb of internal capsule
	Rubrospinal tract	Extrapyramidal pathway involved in coordination and error control, arising from red nucleus in the superior mesencephalon Axons project to α and γ motor neurons in the anterior horn	Means by which cerebellum influences motor behavior at level of spinal cord
Anterior/ventral column	Reticulospinal tracts	Major extrapyramidal pathways involved in setting and adjusting postural tone, balancing readiness of agonist/antagonist muscles for contraction/activity during functional activities; originates in pontine and medullary reticular formation; influences γ motor neuron activity	Thought to be network that influences developmental reflexes of hindbrain, decorticate pattern of spasticity (following pyramidal system impairment)
	Vestibulospinal tracts	Major extrapyramidal pathways involved in righting responses and equilibrium reactions. Originates in vestibular nuclei of pons and open medulla; influences γ motor neuron activity	

Table 12-5
Structures Involved, Disease Processes, and Movement Dysfunction of Common Neuromuscular Disorders

Medical Pathology	*Etiology*	*Risk Factors*	*Structures Involved*	*Prognosis*	*Impact on Tone*	*Impact on Postural Control*	*Impact on Functional Mobility*
Stroke, brain attack, CVA	Thrombosis	Hypertension Hypercholesterolemia Diabetes Obesity Smoking	MCA lesion most common; depending on which vessel involved, may lead to impairment of some/all of the following: 1. Pyramidal motor system (hemiparesis/plegia) 2. Sensory systems 3. Perceptual systems (especially if right CVA) 4. Communication systems (especially if left CVA) 5. Visual system (homonymous hemianopsia) 6. Limbic system (emotion, learning, memory)	Static event, with evolving symptoms in weeks/months following initial damage due to initial inflammatory response and subsequent tissue remodeling/healing Severity of impairment related to degree of damage, especially to gray matter structures	Initial hypotonus (sometimes appearing to be flaccid) due to neurogenic shock Some individuals remain hypotonic, most develop various levels of hypertonus in weeks/months following event. Hyperactive deep tendon reflexes evolve over time	Frequently impaired, especially if lesion is in right hemisphere, gray matter with perceptual dysfunction	Asymmetry in ability to use trunk, limbs during functional activity; tendency to move in abnormal "synergy" (flexion UE, extension LE) Frequently require AFO and ambulatory device
	Embolus	Atrial fibrillation Arteriosclerosis in carotid/vertebral arterial systems					
	Intracranial hemorrhage	Uncontrolled hypertension, aneurysm					

Continued

Table 12-5
Structures Involved, Disease Processes, and Movement Dysfunction of Common Neuromuscular Disorders—cont'd

Medical Pathology	*Etiology*	*Risk Factors*	*Structures Involved*	*Prognosis*	*Impact on Tone*	*Impact on Postural Control*	*Impact on Functional Mobility*
Spastic cerebral palsy	Unknown	Prematurity High-risk pregnancy Low birth weight Neonatal respiratory distress/anoxia Mother's substance abuse while pregnant	Quadriplegia/tetraplegia: global impact on both gray and white matter structures in forebrain Some individuals have concomitant cognitive impairment and seizure disorders Diplegia: usually due to damage of white matter of internal capsule/corona radiata, affecting motor and sensory systems more than perceptual Hemiplegia: may be due to intercerebral hemorrhage or ischemia affecting one hemisphere	Static event occurring at or around the time of birth Signs and symptoms become apparent over first 2 years of life as developmental delay High risk of secondary musculoskeletal deformity due to impact of abnormal tone during periods of growth Level of disability often becomes more pronounced as child moves into middle childhood, adolescence, and young adulthood due to increasing body size and weight	Initial hypotonus in premature and low-birth-weight infants common Hypertonus develops over time; severity of hypertonus varies depending on extent of CNS damage Hypertonus may increase in times of growth, or in times of excitement/stress Hyperactive deep tendon reflexes, as well as abnormal tonic developmental reflexes	Often impaired due to influence of persistent tonic reflexes, and less efficient development of righting and equilibrium responses	Frequently employ movement strategies based on abnormal patterns/synergies; over time may develop rotational deformity of LE as well as joint contracture due to combination of preferred abnormal positions/patterns of movement and hypertonus Often require AFO, assistive devices, or wheelchair for locomotion Those with significant trunk and UE involvement may require adaptive equipment for feeding, communication, and ADLs Orthoses or resting splints may be used as a means of managing abnormal tone, or after orthopedic surgery to correct deformity

Table 12-5
Structures Involved, Disease Processes, and Movement Dysfunction of Common Neuromuscular Disorders—cont'd

Medical Pathology	*Etiology*	*Risk Factors*	*Structures Involved*	*Prognosis*	*Impact on Tone*	*Impact on Postural Control*	*Impact on Functional Mobility*
Choreoathetoid cerebral palsy	Unknown	Bilirubin toxicity	Basal ganglia (especially caudate nucleus)	Static event occurring at or around the time of birth Impairments and functional limitations become more obvious during development in the first years of life Level of disability may be more pronounced with growth in middle childhood and adolescence	Unpredictable fluctuation of muscle tone (from low tone to significant hypertonus), affecting muscles of limbs, axial skeleton, respiration, and phonation Often appears as writhing motions of trunk and extremity Response to tendon reflexes varies due to changing tone	May be significantly impaired; fluctuating tone challenges ability to attain and hold positions, or move dynamically through space	Often depend on external support for stability during functional tasks and locomotion May benefit from use of ambulatory device, adaptive equipment, seating systems, or UE and LE orthoses

Continued

Table 12-5
Structures Involved, Disease Processes, and Movement Dysfunction of Common Neuromuscular Disorders—cont'd

Medical Pathology	*Etiology*	*Risk Factors*	*Structures Involved*	*Prognosis*	*Impact on Tone*	*Impact on Postural Control*	*Impact on Functional Mobility*
Cerebellar cerebral palsy	Unknown	Unknown	Gray matter (cortical and deep nuclei) and white matter (cerebellar peduncles) structures of the cerebellum	Static event occurring at or around the time of birth Impairments and functional limitations become more obvious after the first year of life, when walking is delayed	Frequently hypotonic with hyperflexible joints in both appendicular and axial skeleton At risk for secondary "overuse" injury with habitual and long-term hyperflexibility during movement and in static postures Often pendular deep tendon reflexes	Sitting and standing postures tend to be "floppy," as child relies on soft tissue structures of the musculoskeletal system to support upright position because of inadequate antigravity postural control	Depending on severity of impairment, may have difficulty with trunk stability during functional tasks using UE (ADLs) and LE (walking) May use AFO to provide external support/positioning during functional tasks

Table 12-5
Structures Involved, Disease Processes, and Movement Dysfunction of Common Neuromuscular Disorders—cont'd

Medical Pathology	*Etiology*	*Risk Factors*	*Structures Involved*	*Prognosis*	*Impact on Tone*	*Impact on Postural Control*	*Impact on Functional Mobility*
Parkinson's disease	Unknown	In some instances may be familial; more common with repeated low-grade head injury (e.g., in boxers) In some individuals may be associated with use of illegal, neurotoxic substances NOTE: Elderly adults with multisystem sensory impairment appear to move like those with Parkinson's disease, but with no resting tremor or rigidity at rest	Deterioration, degeneration, or damage of the substantia nigra nucleus in the midbrain, resulting in imbalance in dopamine-cholinergic axis for motor control	Progressive decline in function characterized by tremor at rest (especially of fingers/hands), bradykinesia with limited range of active motion, masklike faces Higher incidence of cognitive impairment in those with Parkinson's disease than in general older adult population	Rigidity (hypertonicity of all muscles) but often with normal deep tendon reflex Severity of rigidity may vary, related to medication dosage and timing Some individuals may exhibit choreoathetosis as adverse effect of medications used to manage rigidity	Tendency to assume slighty flexed, somewhat asymmetrical upright posture in sitting and standing Over time, significant impairment of postural responses with increased likelihood of falling due to inefficient postural responses	Festinating or retropulsive gait Difficulty navigating through narrow spaces Difficulty with rolling, transitions into sitting from supine, and upright May into standing benefit from ambulatory assistive device; rarely require LE orthosis
Multiple sclerosis	Unknown	May be exposure to slow virus, environmental toxin; possible autoimmune component; risk higher among siblings	Unpredictable exacerbations result from inflammation and destruction of myelin around pathways within the CNS	Variable course with many types of impairment accruing over time with repeated exacerbations	Varies depending on location and size of residual plaque. Some individuals may exhibit normal tone	Postural control and equilibrium responses may be impaired due to a combination of pyramidal and/or	Mobility and locomotion may be impaired, along with postural control, depending on location of lesion Some individuals with impaired

Continued

Table 12-5

Structures Involved, Disease Processes, and Movement Dysfunction of Common Neuromuscular Disorders—cont'd

Medical Pathology	*Etiology*	*Risk Factors*	*Structures Involved*	*Prognosis*	*Impact on Tone*	*Impact on Postural Control*	*Impact on Functional Mobility*
			Residual impairments are the consequence of slowed transmission of neural impulses across "plaques" interrupting connections between CNS structures May affect any subsystem within CNS (voluntary motor, postural control, coordination, memory, perception, sensation) Diagnosis made if there have been at least 2 different episodes of impairment, involving 2 different neurological subsystems, affecting 2 different parts of the body	Typically onset of initial symptoms in young and mid adulthood Often diagnosis by exclusion; when neurological signs/ symptoms cannot be attributed to other disease processes	and deep tendon reflexes, in the presence of perceptual, postural, or coordination impairment Others may demonstrate hypertonus and hyperactive reflexes in various muscles Others may have hypotonus and impaired muscle performance	extrapyramidal motor system impairment, sensory impairment, or somatosensory, spinocerebellar, or visual pathways, or damage of major integrative white matter structures such as the corpus callosum or medial longitudinal fasciculus	muscle performance benefit from AFOs (for support and positioning of LE in gait) associated with weakness or hypertonicity Many choose to use ambulatory aids and assistive devices for function and safety Some with significantr multisystem impairment benefit from seating and wheeled mobility systems

Table 12-5
Structures Involved, Disease Processes, and Movement Dysfunction of Common Neuromuscular Disorders—cont'd

Medical Pathology	*Etiology*	*Risk Factors*	*Structures Involved*	*Prognosis*	*Impact on Tone*	*Impact on Postural Control*	*Impact on Functional Mobility*
Spina bifida myelomeningocele	Unknown	Not well understood	Incomplete closure of neural tube soon after conception; leading to flaccid paralysis and total sensory impairment of all structures innervated at and below level of lesion May be concurrent with hydrocephalus, often managed by ventriculo-peritoneal shunt	Static, nonprogressive condition; however, level of disability often becomes more pronounced as child moves into middle childhood, adolescence, and young adulthood due to increasing body size and weight High risk of secondary musculoskeletal deformity (e.g., osteoporosis, fracture, contracture) due to combination of motor and sensory impairment Depending on level of lesion, voluntary bladder and bowel control may also be impaired or absent	Typically flaccid paralysis with absent deep tendon reflexes May have spotty hypertonicity of muscle innervated by nerve roots proximal to level of lesion	Normal righting reactions and equilibrium responses above level of lesion; with absence of righting and equilibrium responses in trunk and limbs below level of lesion Postural control in sitting influenced by how much of trunk and pelvis is innervated At risk of developing hypermobility of spinal column around level of lesion	Impairment and functional limitation proportional to levelof lesion Those with sacral or low lumbar level lesions may be able to ambulate with AFO, with or without assistive devices Those with mid to high lumbar lesions may use KAFO or HKAFO for limited mobility Many individuals with lumbar and higher levels opt, over time, to use seating and wheelchair systems for functional mobility Orthoses and splints may be used after orthopedic surgeries to repair fracture or correct deformity

Continued

Table 12-5
Structures Involved, Disease Processes, and Movement Dysfunction of Common Neuromuscular Disorders—cont'd

Medical Pathology	*Etiology*	*Risk Factors*	*Structures Involved*	*Prognosis*	*Impact on Tone*	*Impact on Postural Control*	*Impact on Functional Mobility*
Spinal cord injury UMN	Traumatic, sometimes infectious (e.g., transverse myelitis)	Quadriplegia (cervical cord injury) or paraplegia (thoracic cord injury) with spastic paralysis	Consequence of compression or contusion of spinal cord as a result of dislocation or fracture of vertebrae, often sustained in fall, collision, diving, gunshot wound, or other high-speed/high-impact event; complicated by inflammatory process	Improved emergency and acute medical management often results in incomplete lesion, with varying combinations of return of function and spastic paralysis	Initial hypotonicity during period of neurogenic shock Many develop significant hypertonicity in the months postinjury; some may have muscle spasm needing pharmacological intervention Sudden increase in resting tone may signal unrecognized skin irritation, bladder distention or infection, or bowel impaction At risk of secondary musculoskeletal deformity (contracture) due to long-standing abnormal tone and limited mobility	"Disconnection" of lower motor neuron pool below level of lesion results in loss of volitional movement, as well as automatic postural responses, despite hypertonus Deep tendon reflexes often brisk, sometimes resulting in sustained clonus	May temporarily use spinal orthosis until surgical stabilization of damaged vertebrae is well healed Often require seating and wheelchair systems for mobility. May require UE splints and adaptive equipment for ADLs May require resting splints or orthoses to manage abnormal tone and prevent contracture

Table 12-5
Structures Involved, Disease Processes, and Movement Dysfunction of Common Neuromuscular Disorders—cont'd

Medical Pathology	*Etiology*	*Risk Factors*	*Structures Involved*	*Prognosis*	*Impact on Tone*	*Impact on Postural Control*	*Impact on Functional Mobility*
Spinal cord injury LMN	Usually traumatic, sometimes ischemic (complication of AAA repair)	Paraplegia (with lumbosacral cord injury)	Consequence of compression, contusion of lumbosacral nerve roots (cauda equina) within the lower spinal canal	Considered a LMN lesion with flaccid paralysis and absence of deep tendon reflexes at and below level of lesion		Postural control of trunk intact, however, flaccid paralysis of lower extremities limit stability in standing without external support of orthoses	May temporarily use TLSO until surgical stabilization of damaged vertebrae is well healed Depending on extent of impairment, may use AFO, KAFO, or HKAFO and aid for ambulation Often require seating and wheelchair systems for mobility May use resting splint or orthosis to maintain optimal ankle position
Peripheral neuropathy	Metabolic	Diabetes, kidney disease	Gradual, often insidious, onset of symptoms; typically in a "stocking glove" pattern; may include sensory impairment (e.g., loss of protective sensation), motor impairment (intrinsic weakness), and autonomic impairment (skin health, vascular regulation)	Metabolic neuropathies tend to be progressive, worsening over time	Impaired muscle performance (especially weakness) and gradual loss of deep tendon reflex as disease process advances	Impaired distal equilibrium responses increase risk of falls	May benefit from accommodative or protective orthoses to preserve functional foot position and decrease risk of secondary deformity May use ambulatory aid, such as cane, to reduce risk of falls

Continued

Table 12-5

Structures Involved, Disease Processes, and Movement Dysfunction of Common Neuromuscular Disorders—cont'd

Medical Pathology	*Etiology*	*Risk Factors*	*Structures Involved*	*Prognosis*	*Impact on Tone*	*Impact on Postural Control*	*Impact on Functional Mobility*
	Toxic	Chronic alcoholism, exposure to other toxins		Severity of toxic neuropathies related to intensity and duration of exposure Long-term impairment varies	Severity of impairment of muscle performance and deep tendon reflex response varies by toxic agent and exposure	If toxin has systemic impact, may have less efficient postural control of trunk and/or extremities in sitting and standing	If significant or permanent impairment of muscle performance, may use AFO and ambulatory device for mobility, and adaptive equipment for ADLs
	Compression or traumatic	Obesity, overuse injury, entrapment syndromes, nerve root compression due to intervertebral disk herniation or osteophyte	Sometimes resulting from acute injury to extremity or to nerve root; often gradual onset as consequence of prolonged faulty posture or positioning leading to cumulative trauma	Severity of compression and traumatic neuropathies related to duration and degree of compression or damaging force	Severity of impairment of muscle performance and deep tendon reflex response varies with extent of nerve damage	May have temporarily or permanently impaired postural responses with impaired LE muscle performance	May use ambulatory device, AFO, spinal orthosis, or UE splint or orthosis as primary intervention during acute period, or following surgical repair or reconstruction

Table 12-5
Structures Involved, Disease Processes, and Movement Dysfunction of Common Neuromuscular Disorders—cont'd

Medical Pathology	*Etiology*	*Risk Factors*	*Structures Involved*	*Prognosis*	*Impact on Tone*	*Impact on Postural Control*	*Impact on Functional Mobility*
	Infectious	Poliomyelitis, postpolio syndrome	Acute inflammation and destruction of anterior horn cell (poliomyelitis) May be "spotty" in distribution Weakness and fatigue may recur years following initial infection as postpolio syndrome	Anterior horn cell destruction leads to permanent denervation of corresponding motor units	In mild cases, diminished deep tendon reflex with weakness In more severe cases, absent deep tendon reflexes with flaccid paralysis	Extent of difficulty with postural control determined by where in the body and how many muscles lose innervation	Individuals with LE weakness and paralysis may require AFO, KO, or KAFO for mobility Those with UE muscle loss may require splint or orthosis for functional activities Those with significant involvement of trunk and limbs may require seating and wheelchair systems
		Guillain-Barré	inflammation/ destruction or myelin sheath of peripheral nerves (GB). Progresses in a fairly symmetrical distal toward proximal pattern of weakness	With resolution of inflammatory process in GB, remyelinization of peripheral nerves occurs over a period of weeks/ months	During acute phase, absent deep tendon reflexes and flaccid paralysis With recovery, return of deep tendon reflexes with paresis that usually resolves over time	Extent of difficulty with postural control determined by how many spinal nerves are affected during the acute phase of the disease	Often require AFO or KAFO, and functional UE orthoses or splints in early rehabilitation May initially require seating/wheelchair systems, or ambulatory assistive devices for mobility Often able to discontinue use of orthoses as recovery progresses

Continued

Table 12-5
Structures Involved, Disease Processes, and Movement Dysfunction of Common Neuromuscular Disorders—cont'd

Medical Pathology	*Etiology*	*Risk Factors*	*Structures Involved*	*Prognosis*	*Impact on Tone*	*Impact on Postural Control*	*Impact on Functional Mobility*
ABI	Traumatic injury involving head in MVA, fall, assault, gunshot wound, near drowning, prolonged resuscitation following cardiac arrest or electrocution	Primary injury: coup and contracoup injury to brain substance, diffuse axonal injury, secondary injury due to physiological response to injury with increasing intracranial pressure, prolonged anoxia	May cause focal damage to cerebral cortex, deep nuclei, or tracts, as well as global ischemia/anoxia affecting both brain and brainstem May also damage cranial nerve nuclei and/or nerves Can result in hemiplegic or quadriplegic movement dysfunction with abnormal tone, sensory or perceptual impairment, or both, and cognitive impairment	Severity of residual impairment related to degree of direct damage to cerebral cortex and brainstem, as well as degree and duration of ischemia, intracranial pressure, or anoxia	May observe decorticate or decerebrate posturing, with hypertonicity and hyperactive deep tendon reflexes During rehabilitation, there may be evidence of abnormal synergy patterns when persons with ABI attempt volitional movement	Postural control often compromised by re-emergence of primitive tonic reflexes and/or sensory-perceptual impairment, as well as complicated if there is also apraxia, agnosia, impulsiveness, and impaired judgment	May require AFO or KAFO for locomotion. May require resting or dynamic splints to address hypertonicity and joint contracture In cases of multiple trauma, may require fracture orthoses until bone healing is adequate

ABI, Acquired brain injury; *ADLs,* activities of daily living; *AFO,* ankle-foot orthosis; *CNS,* central nervous system; *CVA,* cerebrovascular accident; *GB,* Guillain Barre; *LE,* lower extremity; *LMN,* lower motor neuron, anterior horn cell; *MCA,* middle cerebral artery; *MVA,* motor vehicle accident; *TLSO,* thoraco-lumbo-sacral orthosis; *UE,* upper extremity; *UMN,* upper motor neuron, within the central nervous system, *KAFO,* knee-ankle-foot orthosis; *HKAFO,* hip-knee-ankle-foot orthosis; *KO,* knee orthosis; *AAA,* abdominal aortic aneurysm.

racic spinal cord), followed by upper extremities and head (cervical spinal cord), and finally face, mouth, and esophagus (trigeminal nuclei) just above the lateral fissure. A lesion such as an MS plaque in one of the ascending pathways may result in a discrete area of loss of exteroception or of conscious proprioception in one area of the body; a lesion on the somatosensory cortex can lead to a more profound, multimodality impairment on the opposite side of the body.

Although sensory information is "logged in" at the postcentral gyrus, the location of the somatosensory cortex, interpretation and integration of this information occurs in the *somatoperceptual system* in the parietal association areas, with specialization in the right hemisphere.[27] These association areas give meaning to the sensations that are generated as people move and function in their environments. This is where people understand the relationships among their various extremities and trunk (body schema), as well as their relationship to and position within our physical environment. Damage to the parietal lobes leads to problems ranging from left-right confusion to the inability to recognize and monitor the condition of a body part (neglect, agnosia), depending how much of the association area is involved.[28,29]

The *visual system* begins with processing of information gathered by the rods and cones in the multiple layers of specialized neurons in the retina, located in the posterior chamber of the eye. Axons from retinal ganglion cells are gathered into the optic nerve, which carries information from that eye toward the brain. At the optic chiasm there is reorganization of visual information, such that all information from the left visual field (from both eyes) continues in the right optic tract and that from the right field continues in the left tract. This information is relayed, through the lateral geniculate body of the thalamus, via the optic radiations, to the primary visual cortex on either side of the calcarine fissure of the midsagittal occipital lobe.[30,31] Damage to the retina or optic nerve results in loss of vision from that eye. Damage to the optic chiasm typically leads to a narrowing of the peripheral visual field (bitemporal hemianopsia); a lesion of one of the optic tracts or radiations leads to loss of part or all of the opposite visual field (homonymous hemianopsia). Damage to the visual cortex can result in cortical blindness, in which visual reflexes may be intact but vision is impaired.[32]

Visual information is interpreted in the visual association areas in the remainder of the occipital lobe.[32] The visual association areas in the left hemisphere are particularly important to interpretation of symbolic and communication information, while spatial relationships are of more interest in the right hemisphere. Specific details about the environment, especially about speed and direction of moving objects with respect to the self and of the individual with respect to a relatively stationary environment, are important contributors to functional movement and to the development of skilled abilities.[33] Interconnections between the parietal and occipital association areas serve to integrate visual and somatic/kinesthetic perception and provide important input to motor planning and motor learning systems.[34]

Effective visual information processing is founded on three interactive dimensions: visual spatial orientation, visual analysis skills, and visual motor skills.[35] Developmentally, visual spatial orientation includes spatial concepts used to understand the environment, the body, and the interaction between the body and environment that are part of functional activity (e.g., determining location or direction with respect to self, as well as respect to other objects or persons encountered as people act in their environment). Visual analysis skills allow people to discriminate and analyze visually presented information, identify and focus on key characteristics or features of what people see, use mental imagery and visual recall, and respond or perceive a "whole" when presented with representative parts. The visual motor system links what is seen to how the eyes, head, and body move, allowing one to use visual information processing skills during skilled, purposeful activities. This also provides the foundation for fine manipulative skills requiring eye-hand coordination.

The ability to problem solve, consider alternatives, plan and organize, understand conceptual relationships, multitask, and possess the initial components of learning are functions of the frontal association areas of the forebrain.[36,37] These dimensions of cognitive function are often described by the phrase *"higher executive function."* Quantitative and other analytical skills are thought to be primarily housed in the frontal association areas of the left hemisphere, while intuitive understanding and creativity may be more concentrated in the right hemisphere. Most people tap the resources available in both hemispheres (via interconnections through the corpus callosum) during daily life, although some may fall toward one end or another of the analytical-intuitive continuum. Individuals with acquired brain injury involving frontal lobes often exhibit subtle deficits that have a significant impact on their ability to function in complex environments, as well as under conditions of high task demand; difficulty in these areas certainly compromises functional efficiency and quality of life.[38]

The neuroanatomical structures that contribute to the *motivational system* include the nuclei and tracts of the limbic system, prefrontal cortex, and temporal lobes; all play major roles in managing emotions, concentration, learning, and memory. The motivational system not only has an important impact on emotional aspects of behavior but also influences autonomic/physiological function, efficacy of learning, interpretation of sensations, and preparation for movement[39-42] (Figure 12-5). Dimensions of limbic function that influence motivation and the ability to manage challenges and frustration include body image, self-concept, and self-worth as related to social roles and expectations, as well as the perceived relevance or importance (based on reward or on threat) of an activity or situation. "Central set" is a

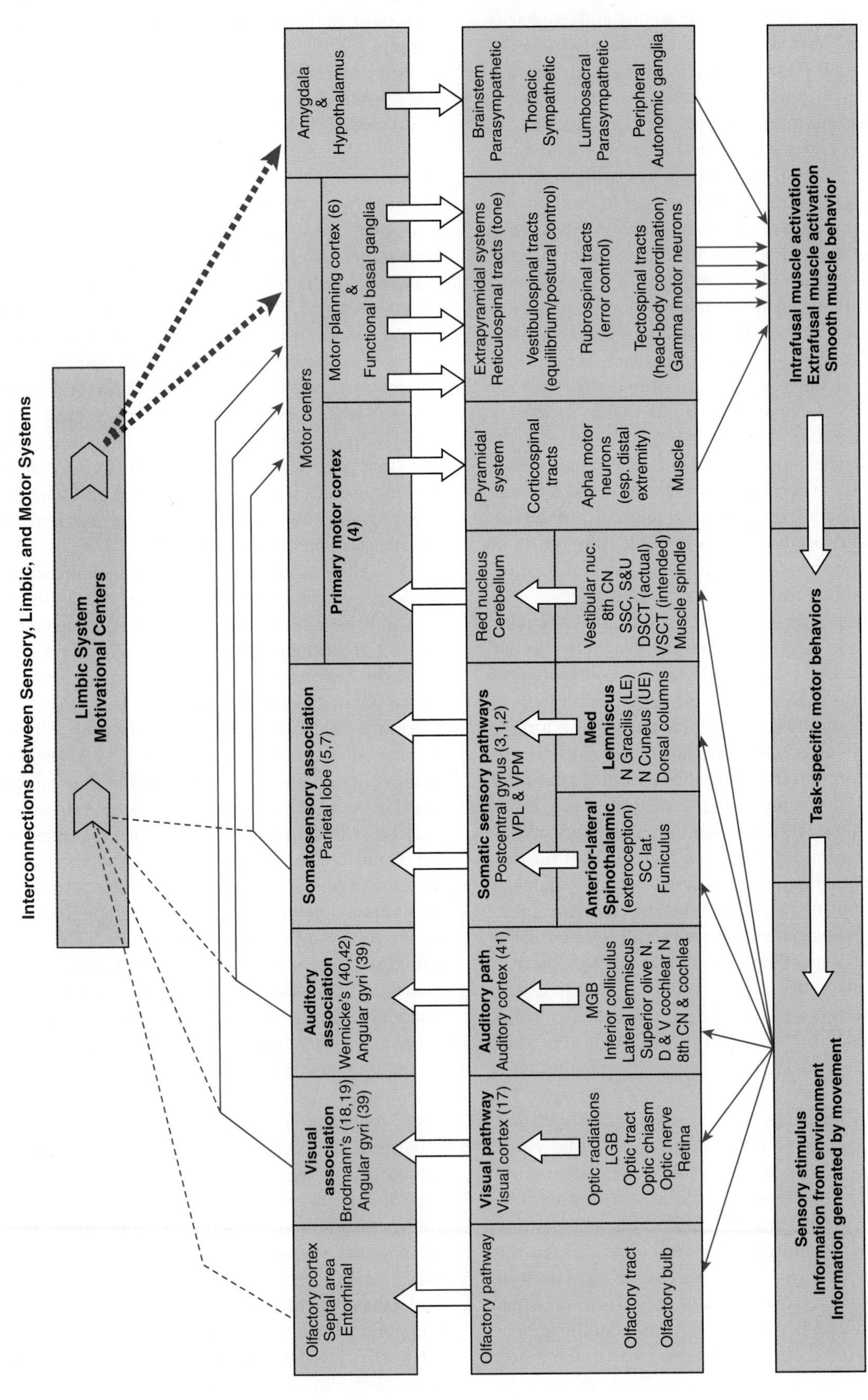

Figure 12-5

A conceptual model of the interactions and interconnections among sensory, limbic, and motor systems that influence functional movement.

phrase used to describe the limbic system's role as a motivator and repository of memory on readiness to move or act. Central set helps people to "predict" movement needs relevant to a given situation or circumstance (considering both the physical and affective dimensions of the environment in which they are acting) from past experience.[43]

The ability to be alert and oriented when functioning in a complex environment is the purview of the *consciousness system* and is a function of interaction of the brainstem's reticular formation, the filtering system of thalamic nuclei, and the thought and problem solving that occur in the association areas of the telencephalon, especially in the frontal lobes.[44,45] The reticular activating system, found in the inferior mesencephalon and upper pons of the brainstem, is the locus of sleep-wake and level of alertness. The thalamus and the reticular formation help people habituate to repetitive sensory stimuli while they focus on the type of sensory information that is most germane to the task at hand. The frontal association areas add "content" to one's consciousness: the ability to reason and to adapt to challenges encountered as one moves through daily life. Alteration in quality and level of consciousness and behavior are indicators of evolving problems within the CNS. Increasing intracranial pressure, the result of an expanding mass or inflammatory response following trauma or ischemia, may be initially manifest by confusion or agitation; progression into a state of lethargy, stupor, or unresponsiveness (coma) indicates deteriorating compromise of the CNS structures.[46]

Homeostasis and the ability to respond to physiological stressors are functions of the components of the *autonomic system*. The nuclei of the hypothalamus serve as the command center for parasympathetic and sympathetic nervous system activity via projections to cranial nerve nuclei in the brainstem and the intermedial horn in the thoracic spinal cord.[47] The hypothalamus has extensive interconnections with the limbic system, bridging physiological and emotional/psychological aspects of behavior and activity.[39] The hypothalamus also integrates neural-endocrine function through interconnections with the pituitary gland.[48]

Peripheral Nervous System

The PNS serves two primary functions: to collect information about bodies and the environment and to activate muscles during functional activities. *Afferent neurons* collect "data" from the various sensory receptors distributed throughout the body and transport this information to the spinal cord and brainstem (sensory cranial nerves) for initial interpretation and distribution to CNS centers and structures that use sensory information in the performance of their various specialized roles.[28] The interpretation process can have a direct impact on motor behavior at the spinal cord level (e.g., deep tendon reflex) or along any synapse point in the subsequent ascending pathway (e.g., righting and equilibrium responses) as sensory information is transported toward its "final" destination within the CNS. *Efferent neurons* (also described as *lower motor neurons* or, more specifically, alpha/α and gamma/γ motor neurons) carry signals from the pyramidal (voluntary motor) and extrapyramidal (supportive motor) systems to extrafusal/striated and intrafusal (within muscle spindle) muscle fibers that direct functional movement by enacting the CNS's motor plan.[22,26]

The cell bodies of these α and γ motor neurons "live" in the anterior horn of the spinal cord and in cranial nerve somatic motor nuclei. In the spinal cord, α and γ axons project through the ventral root, are gathered into the motor component of a spinal nerve, and (in cervical and lumbosacral segments) are reorganized in a plexus before continuing toward the targeted muscle as part of a peripheral nerve. In the brainstem, α and γ axons project to target muscles via motor cranial nerves (oculomotor/III, trochlear/IV, motor trigeminal/V, abducens/VI, facial/VII, glossopharyngeal/IX, spinal accessory/XI, and hypoglossal/XII. When α and γ axons reach their target set of muscle fibers (motor unit), a specialized synapse—the neuromuscular junction—triggers muscular contraction.[49]

Pathologies of the PNS can be classified by considering two factors: the modalities affected (only sensory, only motor, or a combination of both), as well as where the problem is located (at the level of the sensory receptor, along the neuron itself, in the dorsal root ganglion, in the anterior horn, at the neuromuscular junction, or in the muscle itself).[50,51] Poliomyelitis is the classic example of an anterior horn cell disease; Guillain-Barré syndrome is a demyelinating infectious-autoimmune neuropathy that impairs transmission of electrical impulses over the length of motor and sensory nerves. The polyneuropathy of diabetes (affecting motor, sensory, and autonomic fibers) is the classic example of a metabolic neuropathy. Radiculopathies (e.g., sciatica) result from compression or irritation at the level of the nerve root, while entrapment syndromes (e.g., carpal tunnel) are examples of compression neuropathies over the more distal peripheral nerve. Myasthenia gravis, tetanus, and botulism alter function at the level of the neuromuscular junction. Myopathies and muscular dystrophies are examples of primary muscle diseases.

What Is "Functional" versus "Abnormal" Tone?

Ideally the CNS can set the neuromotor system to be "stiff enough" to align and support the body in functional antigravity positions (e.g., provide sufficient baseline postural tone) but "flexible enough" in the limbs and trunk to carry out smooth and coordinated functional movement and effectively respond to changing environmental conditions or demands as daily tasks are carried out.[52] Postural tone can be conceptualized as a curvilinear continuum of "readiness" to move or respond, anchored on one end by insufficient tone and at the other by excessive tone (Figure 12-6). Among individuals, postural tone varies with level of consciousness,

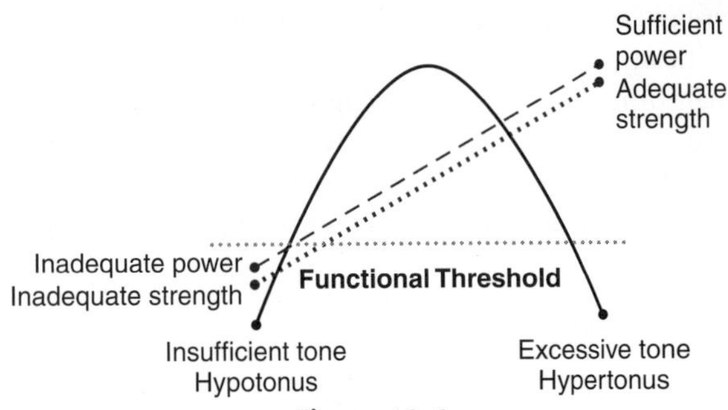

Figure 12-6

A conceptual model of the relationship between muscle tone (postural tone), and two dimensions of muscle performance (strength and power) to functional abilities. Once strength and power cross a theoretical "threshold" for functional performance, efficacy of movement increases. In contrast, both insufficient and excessive tone can contribute to functional limitation, increasing energy cost and decreasing effectiveness of movement.

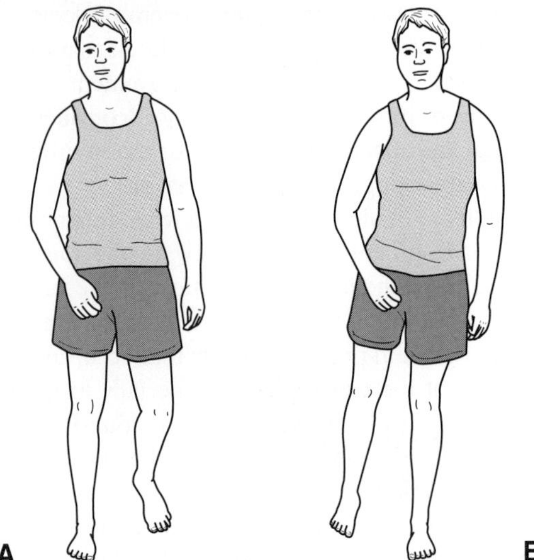

Figure 12-7

Decorticate pattern hypertonicity following cerebrovascular accident. ***A,*** *The affected upper extremity is held in a flexed posture, while the extensor bias in the lower extremity provides stability at midstance and permits swing limb advancement of the less-involved extremity.* ***B,*** *The extensor pattern hypertonus in the affected lower extremity precludes swing-limb shortening normally accomplished by hip and knee flexion; instead, the individual uses an "abnormal" strategy such as pelvic retraction and hip hiking to advance the involved limb.*

level of energy or fatigue, and perceived importance (salience) of the tasks they are involved with. Importantly, at either end of the tone continuum, function can be compromised. Also of importance is that strength (absolute force generated by the muscle) and power (the rate at which a muscle can generate force), two additional determinants of muscle performance and functional ability, are related to, but not the same as, underlying tone. Strength and power can be represented as positively sloped, perhaps parallel lines that interfere with function only on the "inadequate" side of their continua. Although it is difficult to achieve adequate strength or power when underlying tone is low, individuals with hypertonus often demonstrate weakness or inadequate power during manual muscle testing or performance of functional tasks.

Hypertonus

Hypertonus is a term used to describe muscles that are influenced to be too "stiff" or are excessively biased toward supporting antigravity function. *Spasticity* is a type of hypertonus that typically occurs when there is damage to one or more CNS structures of the pyramidal motor system and is encountered as a component of many neuromuscular pathologies.[53-56] Decrements in underlying tone and muscle performance, in bipedal humans with impairment of the pyramidal system, most often occurs in a "decorticate" pattern: the upper extremity is typically biased toward flexion (can be easily moved into flexion but not into extension), while the lower extremity is biased toward extension (when it is difficult to move into flexion) (Figure 12-7). In persons with severe acquired brain injury the entire body may be biased toward extension, a condition or posture described as "decerebrate" pattern spasticity (Sherrington originally described this phenomenon as *decerebrate rigidity*). Both decorticate and decerebrate conditions are unidirectional in nature; there is an increased stiffness and resistance to passive elongation in one group of muscles (agonists) with relatively normal functioning of opposing muscle groups (antagonists).

Spasticity is a velocity-dependent phenomenon: Under conditions of rapid passive elongation, spastic muscle groups "fight back" with increased stiffness, a result of a hypersensitive deep tendon reflex loop (Figure 12-8). This has been described as *clasp-knife spasticity,* in which the spastic limb "gives" after an initial period of resisting passive movement in the way that a pocket knife initially resists opening when near its initially closed position but then becomes more compliant once moved past a "threshold" position as it is opened. Growing evidence indicates that the stiffness encountered during passive movement has both neurological (spasticity) and musculoskeletal (changes in muscle and associated soft tissue) components that combine to increase the risk of contracture development.[57]

Given the unidirectional nature of severe hypertonus, it is common for persons with severe hypertonus to develop chronic dystonic postures. The limb or body segment assumes an end-range position that the limb would not normally be able to assume[58,59] (e.g., extreme equinovarus with

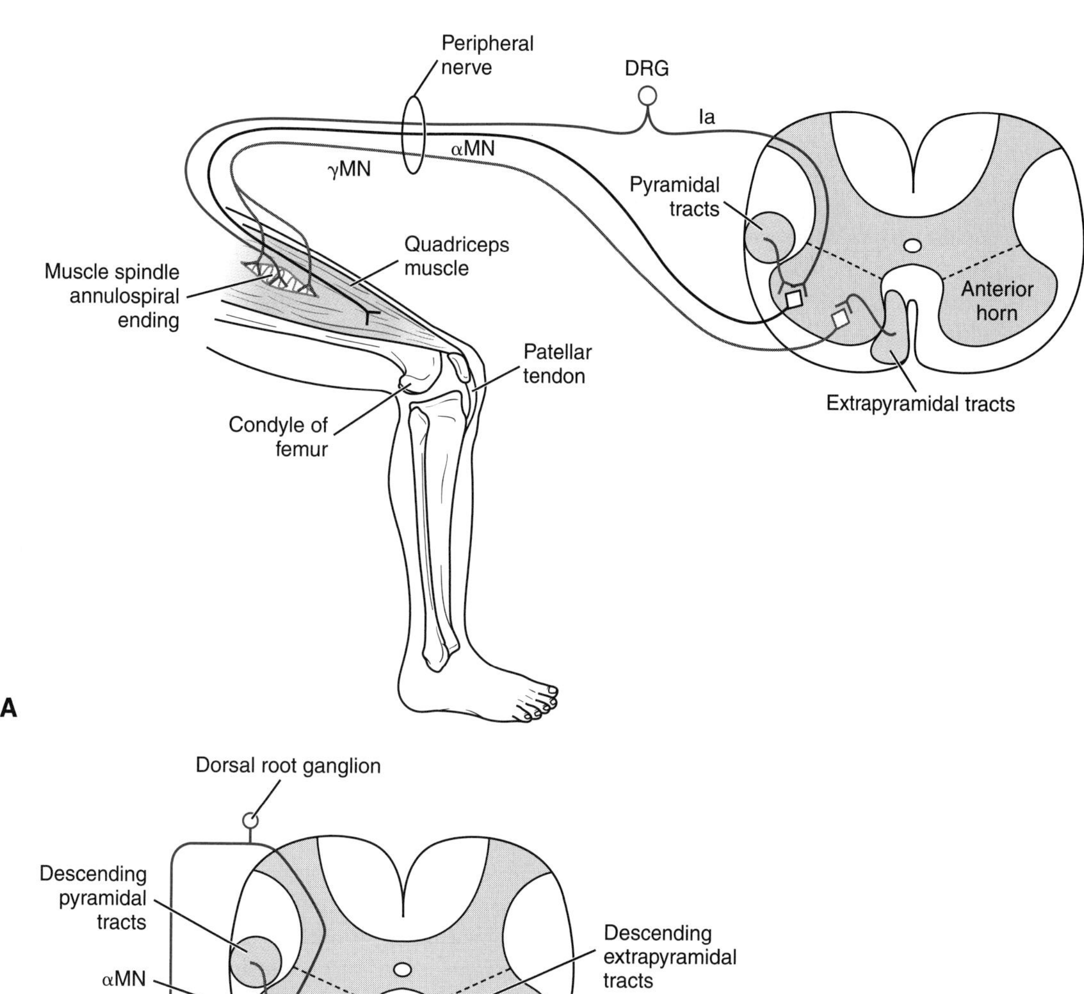

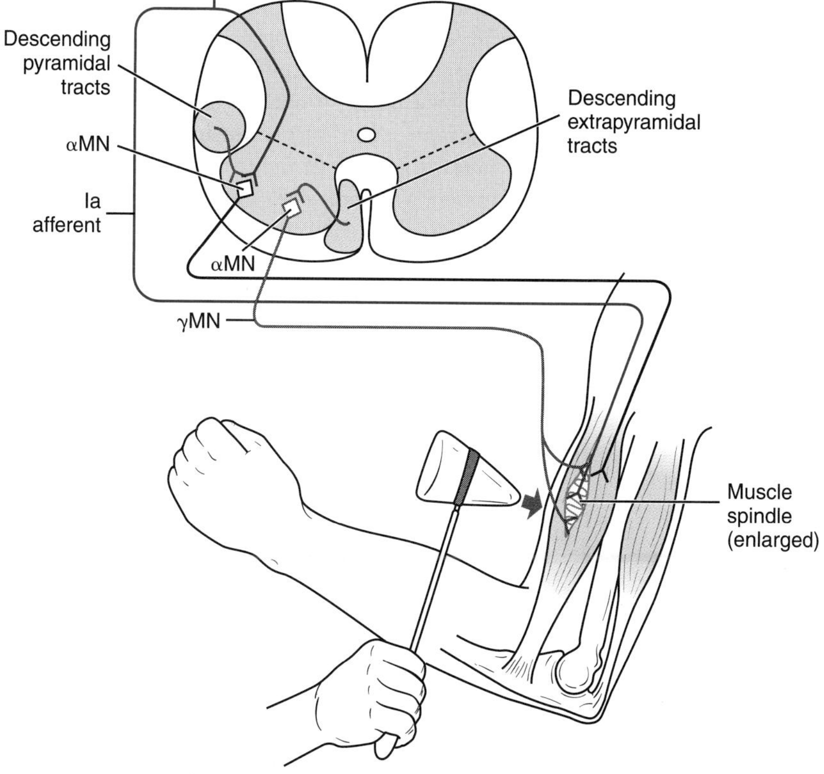

Figure 12-8

Diagram of the deep tendon reflex loop: stimulation of the annulospiral receptor within muscle spindle of the quadriceps (A) and biceps brachii (B) (via "tap" on the patellar tendon with a reflex hammer) activates 1a afferent neurons, which in turn assist motor neurons in the anterior horn of the spinal cord. These motor neurons project to extrafusal muscle fibers in the quadriceps, which contract, predictably, as a reflex response. Sensitivity of muscle spindle (threshold for stimulation) is influenced by extrapyramidal input reaching γ motor neurons in the anterior horn, which project to intrafusal muscle fibers within the muscle spindle itself.

marked supination in an individual with severe acquired brain injury, equinovalgus with marked pronation in a child with cerebral palsy [CP]). If persistent, these fixed postures are associated with a significant likelihood of secondary contracture development. Hypertonicity is also associated with deficits in muscle performance, most notably diminished strength, diminished ability to produce power (generate force quickly), diminished ability to effectively isolate limb and body segments, diminished excursions of movements within joints (i.e., moving within a limited range of motion [ROM]), and inefficiency with altering force production or timing of contractions to meet changing (fluid) demands of tasks.[60] Muscle performance deficits can contribute to an imbalance of forces around a joint that leads to habitual, "abnormal" patterns of movement. These habitual patterns are often biomechanically inefficient and, over time, contribute to the development of secondary musculoskeletal impairments such as adaptive shortening or lengthening of muscles and malalignment of joints.[57]

Individuals with Parkinson's disease and related neurological disorders often demonstrate varying levels of *rigidity*: a bidirectional, cocontracting hypertonicity in which there is resistance to passive movement of both agonistic and antagonistic muscle groups.[61,62] Cocontraction of flexor and extensor muscles of the limbs and trunk creates a bidirectional stiffness that interferes with functional movement. Rigidity is often accompanied by slowness in initiating movement (bradykinesia), decreased excursion of active ROM, and altered resting postures of the limbs and trunk (Figure 12-9). The rigidity of Parkinson's disease can be overridden under certain environmental conditions: persons with moderate to severe disease can suddenly run reciprocally if they perceive danger to themselves or a loved one; once this initial "limbic" response has dissipated, they will resume a stooped and rigid posture, with difficulty initiating voluntary movement, limited active ROM, and bradykinesia.

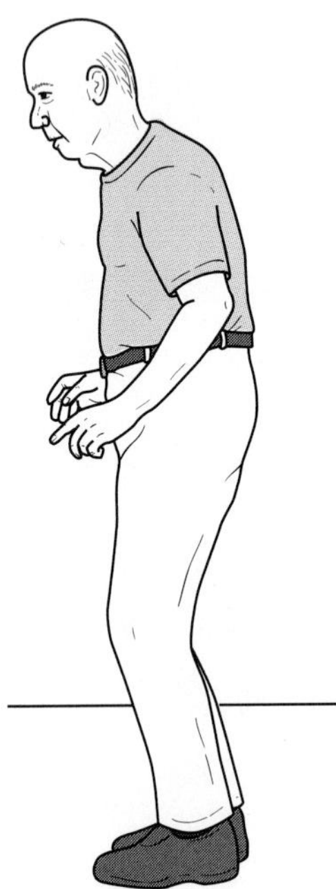

Figure 12-9

Typical standing posture in individuals with Parkinson's disease, with a forward head, kyphotic and forward flexed trunk, and flexion at hip and knees. Upper extremities are often held in protracted and flexed position. The altered position of the body's center of mass, when combined with rigidity and bradykinesia, significantly decreases the efficacy of anticipatory postural responses during ambulation, as well a response to perturbation.

Hypotonus

Hypotonus is the word used to describe the state of "readiness" of muscles that are influenced by descending extrapyramidal motor pathways and other inputs to the anterior horn to be more compliant than they are stiff.[63] As a result, hypotonic muscles are less "ready" to support upright posture against gravity or to generate force during contraction.[64] Hypotonic muscles are considerably more pliable on rapid passive elongation (i.e., less resistant to passive stretch) than muscles with typical tone, as well as those with hypertonus/spasticity. Because their postural muscles are "less ready" to be active, individuals with hypotonicity often have difficulty when assuming and sustaining antigravity positions. To compensate for their reduced postural tone, persons with hypotonicity may maintain postural alignment by holding positions at the extreme ends of the ROM (extreme extension) and using ligamentous tautness to sustain the posture[65] (Figure 12-10). With overreliance on ligaments in extreme ends of range, further degradation to joint structures often occurs.

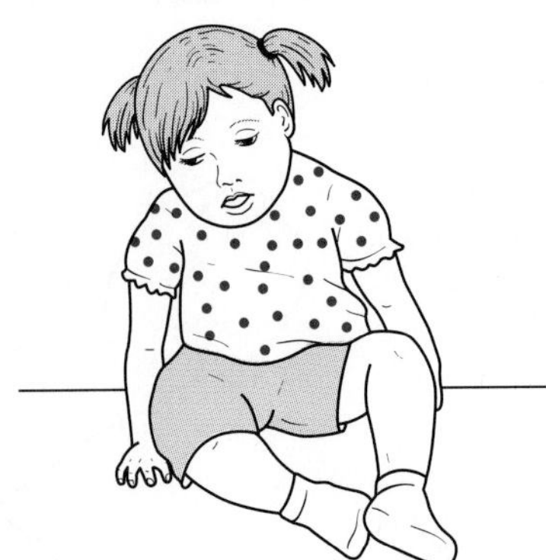

Figure 12-10

Postural control is often inefficient in children (and adults) with hypotonicity or low tone. This 10-month-old child has insufficient muscle tone to maintain her head and trunk in an upright position and use her upper extremities to reach or manipulate, visually track objects in her environment, or safely transition into and out of a sitting position. (Modified from Stokes M. Physical Management in Neurological Rehabilitation. *Edinburgh: Elsevier Mosby, 2004. p. 322.)*

In addition to postural control dysfunction, individuals with hypotonia often have difficulty with coordination of movements. This may be due to the decreased efficacy of afferent information collected by a "lax" muscle spindle during movement execution.[66] Children with hypotonia often have impaired control of movements at midrange of muscle length, suggesting that kinesthetic information is not being used efficiently to guide movement or that the ability to regulate force production throughout movements is compromised. In either case, muscle performance is notably less efficient, especially in activities that require eccentric control (e.g., controlled lowering of the body from a standing position to sitting on the floor). Individuals with hypotonia have difficulty regulating force production and may appear to use the "all or nothing" principle, in which muscles are either active or inactive and collaboration between agonists and antagonists is not well coordinated.

Immediately following an acute CNS insult or injury there is often a period of neurogenic shock in which the motor system appears to "shut down" temporarily, with apparent loss of voluntary movement (paralysis) and markedly diminished or absent deep tendon reflex responses.[67-68] This phenomenon is observed following cervical or thoracic spinal cord injury and early on following significant stroke. During this period, individuals with extreme levels of hypotonus are sometimes (erroneously) described as having flaccid paralysis. Most individuals with acute CNS dysfunction will, within days to weeks, begin to show some evidence of returning muscle tone; over time, many will develop hyperactive responses to deep tendon reflex testing and other signs of hypertonicity.[15] If they continue to have difficulty activating muscles voluntarily for efficient functional movement, these individuals are described as demonstrating spastic paralysis.

Flaccidity

The term *flaccidity* is best used to describe muscles that cannot be activated because of interruption of transmission or connection between lower motor neurons and the muscles they innervate.[69] True flaccidity is accompanied by significant atrophy of muscle tissue, well beyond the loss of muscle mass associated with inactivity; this is the result of loss of tonic influence of lower motor neurons on which muscle health is based. The flaccid paralysis seen in persons with myelomeningocele (spina bifida) occurs because incomplete closure of the neural tube during the early embryonic period (soon after conception) prevents interconnection between the primitive spinal cord and neighboring somites that will eventually develop into muscles of the extremities.[70] The flaccid paralysis observed in persons with cauda-equina level spinal cord injury is the result of damage to axons of α and γ motor neurons as they travel together as ventral roots to their respective spinal foramina to exit the spinal column as a spinal nerve.[71] After acute poliomyelitis, the loss of a portion of a muscle's lower motor neurons will lead to marked weakness; the loss of the majority of a muscle's lower motor neurons will lead to flaccid paralysis.[72] In Guillain-Barré syndrome the increasing weakness and flaccid paralysis seen in the early stages of the disease are the result of demyelination of the neuron's axons as they travel toward the muscle in a peripheral nerve.[73] After injection with botulinum toxin, muscle tone and strength are compromised because of the toxin's interference with transmitter release from the presynaptic component of the neuromuscular junction.[74]

Fluctuating Tone: Athetosis

Athetosis is the descriptor used when an individual's underlying muscle tone fluctuates unpredictably.[75] Athetosis is characterized by unpredictable changes in postural tone, with variations from hypertonus to hypotonus. Athetosis, although less common than spastic CP, can have as significant (and often more pronounced) an impact on daily function. Although etiology of athetosis is not well understood, it is most frequently described as a type of basal ganglia or thalamic dysfunction associated with bilirubin toxicity or significant perinatal anoxia.[76] Persons with athetosis typically demonstrate truncal hypotonia, with fluctuating levels of hypertonus in antigravity musculature and the extremities. In some individuals movements appear to have a writhing dancelike quality (choreoathetosis) in addition to the tonal influences. Others may compensate for postural instability by assuming end-range positions, relying on mechanical stability of joints during functional activity. Although persons with athetosis are less likely to develop joint contracture than those with long-standing hypertonicity, they are more likely to develop secondary musculoskeletal complications that compromise stability of joints, a result of extreme posturing, imbalance of forces across joint structures, and the need to stabilize in habitual postural alignment patterns for function.[77]

Dimensions of Motor Control

In considering what type of intervention would be most appropriate for persons with neuromuscular system impairment, rehabilitation professionals focus on two fundamental dimensions of motor control. The first is postural control: an individual's ability to function while maintaining his or her center of mass within the limits of stability/base of support. The second is the individual's ability to move within his or her environment in a smooth, efficient, and coordinated fashion.

Postural Control

Postural control has three key dimensions: (1) Static postural control is defined as the ability to hold antigravity postures at rest; (2) dynamic anticipatory postural control is the ability to sustain a posture during movement tasks that shift (internally perturb) the center of mass; and (3) dynamic reactionary postural control is the ability to be able to withstand or recover from externally derived perturbations without loss of balance.[78] One has functional postural control if center of mass (COM) can be maintained within one's base of support (BOS) under a wide range of task demands and environmental conditions. This requires some measure of ability across the triad of static, anticipatory, and reactionary control.

The key interactive CNS systems involved in postural control include extrapyramidal and pyramidal motor systems, visual and visual-perceptual systems, conscious (dorsal column/medial lemniscal) and unconscious (spinocerebellar) somatosensory systems, the vestibular system, and the cerebellar feedback/feedforward systems.[79,80] Clinical measures used to assess efficacy of static postural control include timing of sitting or standing activities[81] and measures of center of pressure excursion in quiet standing.[82] The sensory organization test developed by Nashner[83] and modified by Horak and Woollacott[84,85] sorts out the contribution of visual, vestibular, and proprioceptive systems' contribution to balance, as well as the individual's ability to select the most relevant sensory input when there is conflicting information collected among these systems.

Measures of anticipatory postural control such as functional reach tasks consider how far the individual is willing to shift his or her center of mass toward the edge of his or her "sway envelope."[86-88] Measures of dynamic reactionary postural control consider the individual's response to unexpected perturbations (e.g., when pushed or displaced by an external force, when tripping/slipping in conditions of high environmental demand).[89,90] Although these three dimensions of postural control are interrelated, competence in one does not necessarily ensure effective responses in the others.[91]

Many individuals with neuromuscular disorders demonstrate inefficiency or disruption of one or more of the CNS subsystems necessary for effective postural control and balance.[92] An individual with mild to moderate hypertonicity or spasticity often has difficulty with anticipatory and reactionary postural control, especially in high task demand situations within a complex or unpredictable "open" environment. Difficulty with muscle performance such as impairment of control of force production or the imbalance of forces acting across a joint might constrain anticipatory postural control in preparation for functional tasks such as reaching or stepping. Impairment of the ability to "segment" trunk from limb or to individually control joints within a limb may affect the individual's ability to react to perturbations in a timely or consistent manner.

Persons with hypotonicity, on the other hand, often have difficulty with sustaining effective postural alignment in antigravity positions such as sitting and standing. They are likely to demonstrate patterns of postural malalignment such as excessive lumbar lordosis and thoracic kyphosis. Because of difficulty with muscle force production (especially in midrange of movement), individuals with hypotonia also have difficulty with anticipatory postural control. A lack of "on demand" motor control contributes to difficulty with moving within one's postural sway envelope; this may be observed as a tendency to stay in one posture for long periods of time, with infrequent alterations in position during tasks. Reactionary control may also be altered, particularly with respect to the use of equilibrium reactions and the reliability of protective responses. Individuals with hypotonia have difficulty when a task requires them to absorb small-amplitude perturbations; they must use equilibrium or balance strategies more frequently than persons with adequate muscle tone. Additionally, a lack of stability in joints, from both tonal and ligamentous laxity, contributes to an inability to safely stop an accelerating body part as it comes into contact with a surface during a loss of balance episode.

Movement and Coordination

Many functional activities require us to move or transport the entire body (e.g., mobility or locomotion) or a segment of the body (e.g., using one's upper extremity to bring a cup toward the mouth to take a drink) through space.[93,94] The locomotion task that receives much attention in rehabilitation settings is bipedal ambulation—the ability to walk. For full functional ability, individuals must be able to manage a variety of additional locomotion tasks: running, skipping, jumping, and hopping.[95] To fully understand an individual's functional ability, therapists and orthotists must also consider the environmental context in which ambulation is occurring. What are the physical characteristics of the surface on which the individual needs to be able to walk or traverse? Is it level, unpredictably uneven, slippery or frictional, or structurally unstable? Is the ambulation task occurring where lighting is adequate for visual "data collection" about environmental conditions? Does it involve manipulation of some type of object (e.g., an ambulatory assistive device, a school backpack, shopping bags, suitcases)? Is it occurring in a familiar and predictable environment (e.g., at home) or in a more unpredictable and challenging "open" environment such as a busy school, supermarket, mall, or other public space? The task demands of locomotion in complex and challenging environments create more demand on the CNS structures involved in motor control (perceptual-motor function, motor planning, cerebellar "error control"), as well as on the musculoskeletal "effectors" (muscles and tendons, joints, ligaments, and bones) that enact the motor plan necessary for successful completion of the task that relies on body transport.[96]

The use of a limb segment can also be defined by the nature of the task and the circumstances in which the movement is performed.[97] Upper extremity functional tasks can involve one or more components: reaching, grasping, releasing, manipulation, or any combination of these four purposes. Upper extremity tasks can also be defined by considering the function to be accomplished by the movement: grooming, dressing, meal preparation, self-care, or writing. Many upper extremity mobility tasks are founded on effective postural control (e.g., making appropriate anticipatory postural adjustments as the COM shifts while throwing, lifting, lowering, or catching an object). Complex mobility tasks require simultaneous locomotion and segmented use of extremities (e.g., reaching for the doorknob while ascending the steps toward the front door, throwing or catching a ball while running during a football or baseball game).

Coordination can be thought of as the efficacy of execution of the movement necessary to complete a task.[66,76,96] A well-coordinated movement requires effective simultaneous control of many different dimensions of movement: the accuracy of a movement's direction and trajectory; the timing, sequencing, and precision of muscle activation; the rate and amplitude of force production; the interaction of agonistic and antagonistic muscle groups; the ability to select and manage the type of contraction (concentric, holding, or eccentric) necessary for the task; and the ability to anticipate and respond to environmental demands during movement. Coordination can be examined by considering the individual's ability to initiate movement, sustain movement during the task or activity, and terminate movement according to task demands.

For movement and coordination to be functional one must have adequate muscle performance that is flexible/adaptable to varying demands. Mobility or transport tasks cannot be performed independently (safely) unless the individual is (1) able to *transition* into and out of precursor positions (e.g., getting up from the floor into a standing position, rising from a chair); (2) *initiate* or begin the activity (e.g., take the first step); (3) *sustain* the activity (control forward progression with repeated steps); (4) *change direction* as environmental conditions demand (e.g., step over or avoid an obstacle); (5) *modulate speed* as environmental conditions demand (e.g., increase gait speed when crossing the street); and (6) safely and effectively stop or *terminate* the motion, returning to a precursor condition or position (quiet standing, return to sitting).

For individuals with neuromuscular disorders who have difficulty with muscle performance because of abnormal underlying tone or poor motor control, coordination of functional movement can be compromised in several ways. In order to approach and complete a movement task, the individual might rely on "abnormal" patterns of movement with additional effort and energy cost. Many individuals with hypertonicity initiate movement with strong bursts of muscle contractions but have difficulty sustaining muscle activity and force of contraction through the full ROM necessary to perform a functional movement.[66,98] Deficits in timing and sequencing of muscle contractions, as well as difficulty with dissociation of limb and body segments, also contribute to difficulty with performance of functional tasks. An adult with hemiplegia following a cerebrovascular accident (CVA) may be able to initiate a reach toward an object but not be able to bring the arm all the way to the target.[15] The same individual may have difficulty with timing and segmentation, leading to inability to open the hand before reaching the target in preparation for grasping the object. The muscle performance of many children with CP is compromised by inappropriate sequencing of muscle contractions when activation of synergists and antagonists happens simultaneously.[98] Conversely, an individual with hypotonus who has difficulty with stabilization often moves quickly with diminished accuracy and coordination.

MANAGEMENT OF NEUROMUSCULAR IMPAIRMENTS

Rehabilitation professionals use a variety of examination strategies to determine the nature and extent of impairment, across systems, associated with a particular pathological condition, to determine an appropriate movement-related physical therapy diagnosis, determine potential outcomes (prognosis), and structure an appropriate plan of care.[7,99-102] Strategies include response to deep tendon reflex testing; sensory and perceptual testing; response to passive movement of the limb at varying speeds; the ability to initiate, sustain, temper, and release muscular contraction; observation/classification of patterns of muscle activation during volitional movement; and functional performance on daily tasks. A comparison of definitions/descriptors used to quantify tone is presented in Table 12-6.[103-106] Importantly, ratings of reflex response and severity of abnormal tone (as measured by resistance to passive movement) do not accurately reflect the degree of functional ability or functional limitation.[107-110] Additional determinants of functional ability in individuals with abnormal tone include strength, sensation and perception, and the ability to isolate (dissociate) limb segments during voluntary movement.

Orthoses are one of many possible intervention strategies for persons with neuromotor/neurosensory system impairment.[111-113] Orthoses are used to align or position limb segments for more efficient function (e.g., an ankle-foot orthosis to provide prepositioning of the foot during swing limb advancement and stability during the stance phase of gait), influence abnormal tone (tone-inhibiting designs), provide external support and reduce the likelihood of secondary musculoskeletal impairments (especially in growing children), protect a limb following orthopedic surgery performed to correct deformity or instability, and as an adjunct following pharmacological intervention with botulinum toxin.[114-117]

Medical management of CNS dysfunction often includes prescription of *pharmacological agents*. Physicians can select from a range of centrally acting tone-inhibiting medications (e.g., baclofen [Lioresal]) or pharmacological interventions that target lower motor neurons, peripheral nerves, or muscle (e.g., botulinum toxin injection, intrathecal baclofen) for individuals with significant hypertonicity.[118-124] A summary of pharmacological agents used in the manage-

Table 12-6
Comparison of Commonly Used Rating Scales for Muscle Tone

DEEP TENDON REFLEX RESPONSE RATING[103]

Score	*Descriptor*
0	No reflex response, absent
+	Elicited only with reinforcement (Jendrassik maneuver)
1 +	Present but diminished reflex response
2 +	"Normal" reflex response
3 +	Brisk and exaggerated reflex response
4 +	Several beats of clonus observed
5 +	Sustained clonus

MODIFIED ASHWORTH SCALE[104] **(FOR INDIVIDUALS WITH HYPERTONICITY)**

Score	*Descriptor*
0	No increase in tone (normal)
1	Slight increase in tone: "catch and release" on passive elongation, or minimal resistance to passive elongation at end range
1+	Slight to moderate increase in tone: "catch and release" on passive movement, with some resistance to further elongation through less than half of range of motion
2	Moderate increase in tone: resistance to passive range of motion through most of range of motion, but limb can be easily moved
3	Considerable increase in tone: passive movement is difficult, requiring effort by examiner
4	Rigidity: limb held stiffly in either flexed or extended posture

CLINICAL ASSESSMENT OF TONE[105]

Score	*Descriptor*
0	Flaccidity (no tone)
1+	Hypotonia (decrease in tone)
2+	Normal
3+	Mild to moderate hypertonia (increase in tone)
4+	Severe hypertonia

UNIFIED PARKINSON'S DISEASE RATING SYSTEM[106]

Score	*Descriptor*
0	No apparent rigidity on passive movement
1	Minimal rigidity; activated by movement of other limb segments
2	Mild-to-moderate rigidity
3	Marked rigidity, but full range of motion possible
4	Severe rigidity, range of motion limited; passive range of motion requires effort by examiner

ment of muscle spasm after musculoskeletal injury, hypertonicity resulting from CNS disease, Parkinson's disease, MS, and seizure is presented in Table 12-7.

Alternatively, physicians may recommend various neurosurgical or orthopedic *surgical procedures* (e.g., neurotomy, tendon lengthening with or without derotation osteotomy, arthrodesis, dorsal rhizotomy, deep brain stimulation) to correct deformity, improve flexibility, or reduce level of abnormal tone[77,125-128] in an effort to enhance mobility and improve performance of functional tasks. Despite pharmacological and positioning interventions, musculoskeletal deformities can still develop, particularly in the growing child. Surgical interventions are used to correct musculoskeletal defaults of the spine and limbs, realign joints for better mechanical advantage, improve ease of caregiving and hygiene management, promote cosmesis, or reduce and prevent pain.[76]

Prevalent surgical interventions include muscle lengthening procedures; tendon lengthening, tendon transfers, and tenotomies; osteotomies and fusions; and neurectomies. Surgical interventions such as muscle and tendon procedures for the lower limbs are indicated in ambulatory

Text continued on page 315.

Table 12-7
Pharmacological Interventions for Individuals with Neurological and Neuromuscular System Impairments

Purpose	*Trade Names*	*Generic Name (Action)*	*Administration*	*Indications*	*Possible Adverse Effects*
Management of dystonia and CNS-related spasm	Neuroblock	Botulinum B toxin	Intramuscular	Facial spasm, spasmodic torticollis, blepharospasm	Ptosis, eye irritation, diplopia, bruising, weakness of neck muscles, dysphagia, dry mouth
Management of local muscle spasm	Paraflex Parafon Forte Remulon-S	Chlorzoxazone (centrally acting inhibitor of muscle spasm due to pain)	Oral	Muscle spasm (short-term use related to musculoskeletal injury)	Drowsiness, dizziness, headache, malaise, tremor, nausea, GI dysfunction
	Flexeril	Cyclobenzaprine hydrochloride (local action at muscle)	Oral	Muscle spasm (short-term use related to musculoskeletal injury)	Drowsiness, dry mouth, dizziness, fatigue, asthenia, nausea, headache, blurred vision, confusion
	Norflex/Norgesic Banflex, Flexoject, Flexon, Marflex, Myolin, Myophen, Neocyten, Orphenate, Qualaflex, Tega-flex	Orphenadrine citrate (analgesic, anticholinergic)	Oral or injection	Muscle spasm (short-term use related to musculoskeletal injury)	Disorientation, restlessness, irritability, weakness, drowsiness, headache, dizziness, hallucination, insomnia
	Skelaxin	Metaxalone (local action at muscle)	Oral	Muscle spasm (short-term use related to musculoskeletal injury	Drowsiness, dizziness, headache, nervousness, irritibility
	Soma, Chinchen, Flexatoll, Muslax, Neotica, Rela, Scutamil-C	Carisoprodol (centrally acting inhibitor of reticulospinal and spinal interneuron)	Oral	Muscle spasm and pain (short-term use related to musculoskeletal injury	Drowsiness, extreme weakness, transient quadriplegia, dizziness, ataxia, temporary visual loss, diplopia, dysarthria, agitation, confusion
	Robaxin, Carbocol, Forbaxin, Methocarb	Methocarbamol (CNS depression/ sedative)	Oral or injection	Muscle spasm and pain (short-term use related to musculoskeletal injury)	Anaphylaxis, fever, headache, bradycardia, hypotension, amnesia, confusion, diplopia, dizziness, drowsiness, incoordination, nystagmus, vertigo, seizure

Continued

Table 12-7
Pharmacological Interventions for Individuals with Neurological and Neuromuscular System Impairments—cont'd

Purpose	*Trade Names*	*Generic Name (Action)*	*Administration*	*Indications*	*Possible Adverse Effects*
Management of hypertonicity	Botox Dysport	Botulinum A toxin	Intramuscular or perineural injection Intrathecal	Chronic, severe spasticity Dystonia (e.g., spasmodic torticollis)	Muscle weakness
	Dantrium	Dantrolene sodium (direct-action muscle relaxant)	Oral Injection	Chronic, severe spasticity of UMN origin	Drowsiness, dizziness, weakness, malaise, fatigue, nervousness, nausea, headache
	Disipal Robaxin	Orphenadrine Methocarbamol	Oral Injection	Short-term relief of muscle spasm or spasticity	Sedation/drowsiness, light-headedness, fatigue, dizziness, nausea, restlessness
	Valium	Diazepam (acts at limbic system, thalamus, hypothalamus)	Oral Injection	Short-term relief of muscle spasm or spasticity	Drowsiness, fatigue, ataxia, confusion, depression, diplopia, dysarthria, tremor
	Ethyl alcohol	Ethyl alcohol	Intramuscular or perineural injection	Severe spasticity	
	Lioresal	Baclofen (possibly inhibition of spinal cord reflexes)	Oral Injection, Intrathecal	Chronic, severe spasticity from conditions including SCI, acquired brain injury, cerebral palsy, MS	Sedation, hypotension, dizziness, ataxia, headache, tremor, nystagmus, paresthesia, diaphoresis, muscular pain/weakness
	Phenol	Phenol	Intramuscular or perineural injection	Severe lower limb spasticity Pain control	Damage to other neural structures
	Zanaflex	Tizanidine sodium (centrally acting α-adreergic agonist)	Oral	Spasticity from MS or SCI	Sedation/drowsiness, fatigue, dizziness, mild weakness, nausea, hypotension, GI irritation

Table 12-7
Pharmacological Interventions for Individuals with Neurological and Neuromuscular System Impairments—cont'd

Purpose	*Trade Names*	*Generic Name (Action)*	*Administration*	*Indications*	*Possible Adverse Effects*
Management of MS	Medrol, Meprolone, Depo-Medrol, Depopred, Duralone	Methylprednisolone (corticosteroid)	Oral Injection Intravenous	During acute exacerbation	Cushing's syndrome, hypertension, confusion, muscle wasting, insomnia, psychosis, GI irritation, osteoporosis, delayed wound healing
	(Numerous brand names)	Hydrocortisone (corticosteroid)	Oral	During acute exacerbation	Electrolyte imbalance, CHF, weakness, atrophy, Achilles tendon rupture, osteoporosis, papilledema, vertigo, headache
	Decadron, Hexadrol, Maxidex, Mymethasone	Dexamethasone, (corticosteroid)	Oral Injection Intravenous	During acute exacerbation	Electrolyte disturbances, weakness, atrophy, osteoporosis, seizure, increased intracranial pressure, vertigo, headache, Cushing's syndrome
	Aristocort, Kenacort, Aristo-Pak	Triamcinolone Triamcinolone diacetate (corticosteroid)	Oral	During acute exacerbation Optic neuritis	Electrolyte disturbances, CHF, hypokalemia, weakness, myopathy, osteoporosis, convulsions, papilledema, vertigo, headache
	Avonex, Rebif, Betaseron, Actimmune	Beta-1a-interferon Beta-1b-interferon (antiviral, immunomodulator)	Injection	To reduce frequency/ severity of exacerbations for persons with relapsing/ remitting MS	Injection site reaction, anxiety, confusion, seizure
	Copaxone	Glatiramer acetate (immunosuppressant)	Injection	To reduce frequency/ severity of exacerbations for persons with relapsing/ remitting MS	On injection: flushing, chest pain, palpitation, tachycardia, dyspnea After injection: nausea, edema, syncope, asthenia, headache, tremor, diaphoresis, hypotonia, arthralgia, seizure

Continued

Table 12-7
Pharmacological Interventions for Individuals with Neurological and Neuromuscular System Impairments—cont'd

Purpose	*Trade Names*	*Generic Name (Action)*	*Administration*	*Indications*	*Possible Adverse Effects*
Management of MS (cont'd)	Symmetrel, Contenton, Topharmin, Symadine	Amantadine hydrochloride (antiviral, dopaminergic)	Oral	To manage fatigue associated with chronic MS, and drug-induced extrapyramidal symptoms	Nervousness, restlessness, tremor, dizziness, seizure, headache, blurred vision, GI disturbances, edema, dry mouth, diaphoresis, tics
	Novantrone	Mitoxantrone hydrochloride (antineoplastic)	Intravenous every 3 mo	To reduce frequency/ severity of exacerbation for persons with significant relapsing/remitting MS	Ventricular cardiac dysfunction, myelosuppression
Management of Parkinson's disease	Sinemet, Atamet, Cinetol, L-dopa-C	Carbidopa-levodopa (dopaminergic)	Oral	Idiopathic Parkinson's disease	Dyskinesia, ataxia, gait disturbances, agitation, postural hypotension, dizziness, drowsiness, headache, dysphagia, diplopia, fatigue, urinary incontinence
	Eldepryl, Carbex, Deprenyl, Alzene	Selegiline hydrochloride (dopaminergic, MAOI)	Oral	Used with or without Sinemet/L-dopa for idiopathic Parkinson's disease	Hypotension, nausea, headache, tremor, dizziness, muscle cramps, joint pain, agitation
	Comtan	Entacapone (COMT inhibitor)	Oral	As adjunct to levodopa in in idiopathic Parkinson's disease	Nausea, abdominal pain, dry mouth, dyskinesia, dystonia, hyperkinesia, dizziness
	Tasmar	Tolcapone (COMT inhibitor)	Oral	Adjunct to L-dopa-carbidopa	Hypotension/syncope, hallucinations, dyskinesia, diarrhea
	Permax	Pergolide mesylate (dopamine receptor agonist)	Oral	Idiopathic Parkinson's disease	Body pain, nausea, dyskinesia, somnolence, diplopia, dyspnea, drowsiness, hypotension
	Mirapex	Pramipexole dihydrochloride (dopamine receptor agonist)	Oral	Idiopathic Parkinson's disease	Nausea, drowsiness, dizziness, dyskinesia, edema

Table 12-7
Pharmacological Interventions for Individuals with Neurological and Neuromuscular System Impairments—cont'd

Purpose	*Trade Names*	*Generic Name (Action)*	*Administration*	*Indications*	*Possible Adverse Effects*
Management of Parkinson's disease (cont'd)	Requip	Ropinirole hydrochloride (dopamine receptor agonist)	Oral	Adjunct to levodopa in idiopathic Parkinson's disease	Nausea, abdominal pain, edema, drowsiness, dyskinesia, confusion, hypotension
	Parlodel	Bromocriptine mesylate (dopamine receptor agonist)	Oral	Adjunct to levodopa in idiopathic and postencephalitic Parkinson's disease	Hypotension, confusion, hallucination
	Contenton, Mantadan, Shikitan, Symmetrel, Topharmin	Amantadine hydrochloride (possibly anticholinergic: enhances dopamine sensitivity within CNS)	Oral	Symptoms of Parkinson's disease Drug-induced extrapyramidal symptoms	Depression, nervousness, dizziness, blurred vision, edema, hallucination, orthostatic hypotension, difficulty concentrating, anorexia, seizure
	Artane, Aparkane, Tremin, Trihexane, Trihexidyl, Trihexy, Tritane	Trihexyphenidyl hydrochloride (anticholinergic)	Oral	Idiopathic Parkinson's disease Drug-induced extrapyramidal symptoms May be used with levodopa	Dry mouth, GI disturbances, dizziness, blurred vision, urinary retention, nervousness, confusion, sedation
	Akineton	Biperiden hydrochloride (anticholinergic)	Oral	Adjunct to other anti-Parkinson's medications	Dry mouth, blurred vision, drowsiness, euphoria, postural hypotension, agitation
	Cogentin	Benztropine mesylate (anticholinergic)	Oral	Idiopathic Parkinson's disease Drug-induced extrapyramidal symptoms	Dry mouth, GI disturbances, dizziness, blurred vision, urinary retention, nervousness, confusion, sedation
	Benadryl	Diphenhydramine hydrochloride (anticholinergic)	Oral	Mild/early idiopathic Parkinson's, drug-induced Parkinson's, often in combination with other centrally acting anticholinergics	Sedation, sleepiness, dizziness, incoordination, fatigue, confusion, restlessness, tremor, irritability, insomnia, diplopia, vertigo, tinnitus

Continued

Table 12-7
Pharmacological Interventions for Individuals with Neurological and Neuromuscular System Impairments—cont'd

Purpose	*Trade Names*	*Generic Name (Action)*	*Administration*	*Indications*	*Possible Adverse Effects*
Management of myasthenia gravis	Mytelase	Ambenonium chloride (cholinesterase inhibitor)	Oral	Myasthenia gravis	Varies with individual's sensitivity to cholinergic medications
	Mestinon	Pyridostigmine bromide (cholinesterase inhibitor)	Oral Injection	Myasthenia gravis	Nausea, vomiting, increased peristalsis, increased salivation, diaphoresis, muscle cramps, fasciculation, weakness
Management of seizures	Luminal, Solfoton	Phenobarbital (anticonvulsant, barbiturate, sedative/hypnotic)	Oral Injection	Status epilepticus All seizure types, excluding absence seizures	Drowsiness, lethargy, agitation, confusion, ataxia, hallucination, bradycardia, hypotension, nausea
	Dilantin, Diphen, Diphentoin, Dyatoin, Phenytex	Phenytoin sodium (anticonvulsant, hydantoin)	Oral Injection	Status epilepticus Tonic-clonic seizures, simple complex seizures (excluding absence seizures)	Ataxia, slurred speech, confusion, insomnia, nervousness, hypotension, nystagmus, diplopia, nausea, vomiting
	Diamox	Acetazolamide (carbonic anhydrase inhibitor)	Oral	Absence seizure, myoclonic seizure	Drowsiness, dizziness
	Depakote	Divalproex sodium (anticonvulsant)	Oral	Complex partial seizures, absence seizures, as adjunct with other types of seizures	Headache, asthenia, nausea, somnolence, tremor, dizziness, diplopia, risk of hepatotoxicity,
	Depacon	Sodium valproate (anticonvulsant)	Oral Injection	All types of seizures	Ataxia, tremor, sedation, nausea, edema, hyperactivity, weakness, incoordination, risk of hepatotoxicity
	Depakene	Valproic acid (anticonvulsant)	Oral	Absence seizures, As adjunct for other seizure types	Nausea, sedation, ataxia, headache, nystagmus, diplopia, asterixis, dysarthria, dizziness, incoordination, depression, hyperactivity, weakness, risk of hepatic toxicity

Table 12-7
Pharmacological Interventions for Individuals with Neurological and Neuromuscular System Impairments—cont'd

Purpose	*Trade Names*	*Generic Name (Action)*	*Administration*	*Indications*	*Possible Adverse Effects*
	Gabitril	Tiagabine hydrochloride (anticonvulsant)	Oral	Partial seizures	Generalized weakness, dizziness, tiredness, nervousness, tremor, distractibility, emotional lability
	Lamictal	Lamotrigine (anticonvulsant)	Oral	Partial seizures Tonic-clonic seizures	Dizziness, headache, ataxia, drowsiness, incoordination, insomnia, tremors, depression, anxiety, diplopia, blurred vision, GI disturbances, agitation, confusion, rash
	Mysoline	Primidone (anticonvulsant)	Oral	All seizure types, except absence seizures Essential tremor	Ataxia, vertigo, drowsiness, depression, inattention, headache, nausea, visual disturbances
	Neurontin	Gabapentin (anticonvulsant)	Oral	Partial seizures Neuropathic pain	Drowsiness, dizziness, ataxia, fatigue, nystagmus, nervousness, tremor, diplopia, memory impairment
	Rivotril, Klonopin	Clonazepam (anticonvulsant)	Oral Injection	Myoclonic seizures Absence seizures, akinetic seizures	Drowsiness, dizziness, ataxia, dyskinesia, irritability, disturbances of coordination, slurred speech, diplopia, nystagmus, thirst
	Tegretol, Convuline, Atretol, Epitol, Macrepan	Carbamazepine (anticonvulsant)	Oral	Complex-partial seizures Tonic-clonic seizures Trigeminal neuralgia Bipolar disorder	Ataxia, diplopia, drowsiness, fatigue, dizziness, vertigo, tremor, headache, nausea, dry mouth, anorexia, agitation, rashes, photosensitivity, heart failure

Continued

Table 12-7
Pharmacological Interventions for Individuals with Neurological and Neuromuscular System Impairments—cont'd

Purpose	*Trade Names*	*Generic Name (Action)*	*Administration*	*Indications*	*Possible Adverse Effects*
	Topamax	Topiramate (anticonvulsant)	Oral	Partial seizures, adjunct to primary generalized tonic-clonic seizures	Ataxia, confusion, dizziness, fatigue, paresthesia, emotional lability, confusion, diplopia, nausea
	Trileptal	Oxcarbazepine (anticonvulsant)	Oral	Partial seizures Tonic-clonic seizures	Ataxia, drowsiness, nausea, dizziness, headache, agitation, memory impairment, asthenia, ataxia, confusion, tremor, nystagmus
	Zarontin, Thosutin	Ethosuximide (anticonvulsant, succinimide)	Oral	Absence seizures	Drowsiness, headache, fatigue, dizziness, ataxia, euphoria, depression, myopia, nausea, anorexia
	Valium, Dizac, Valrelease	Diazepam (anxiolytic, benzodiazepines)	Injection	Status epilepticus, severe/recurrent seizures	Drowsiness, fatigue, ataxia, confusion, depression, dysarthria, fatigue, syncope, tremor, vertigo

CHF, Congestive heart failure; *COMP,* inhibitor of catechol-O-methyltransferase; *GI,* gastrointestinal; *MAOI,* monoamine oxidase inhibitor; *MS,* multiple sclerosis; *SCI,* spinal cord injury; *UMN,* upper motor neuron.

children with spasticity (typically those with diplegia or hemiplegia) and are generally performed after walking is developed and a gait pattern has been established, usually between 5 and 7 years of age.[76] The surgical interventions that address structural alignment such as osteotomies and fusions are more typical in nonambulatory children (those with significant quadriplegia) and are generally deferred until after 10 years of age.[76] However, corrections for bony deformities of the foot or torsions of the tibia may be performed for ambulatory children after a consistent gait pattern has emerged with walking.

Individuals with significant spasticity are commonly managed with a combination of these strategies to most effectively diminish the impairment, improve functional ability, and help them participate in activities that are important to them.[129,130] Increasingly, instrumented gait analysis is being used to inform clinical decision making in selecting the most appropriate intervention or combination of interventions for ambulatory individuals with functional limitation secondary to neuromuscular pathologies and their associated secondary impairments.[131-138]

Management of Hypertonicity: Rehabilitation

Physical therapists use adaptive equipment and orthoses as integral components and strategies for managing hypertonicity. These tools are used to (1) promote joint alignment and minimize contracture development, (2) provide individuals with a variety of comfortable and safe positions in which they can sleep, eat, travel, work, or play, (3) provide positioning that assists the best voluntary limb movement, and (4) provide alternative methods for mobility.

A major concern among physical therapists is management of the risk for developing secondary musculoskeletal impairments in the presence of hypertonicity.[98,139,141] Passive stretching programs are generally ineffective by themselves as a management strategy for reducing risk of contracture development.[98,142] Prolonged positioning for several hours a day is a critical adjunct to stretching.[141,143] Adaptive equipment can be used to provide structural alignment for prolonged periods of time to maintain extensibility of muscles, decrease the effect of muscle imbalance across joints, and provide postural support. An example of this is an adaptive seating system that could provide upright postural support for sitting; maintain spinal alignment and pelvic positioning; maintain hip, knee, and ankle positions; and promote the best position for upper extremity function.[144-149] Positioning devices for supported standing are often used to maintain extensibility of muscles, promote bone mineral density through weight bearing, and promote musculoskeletal development such as acetabular depth in a developing child with hypertonicity.[150] Other examples of positioning devices include "side lyers," prone and supine systems, bathing and toileting seating systems, and a variety of mobility alternatives such as gait trainers.[151-153] Although there are many options for adaptive equipment designed to assist function and caregiving for persons with neuromuscular dysfunction, knowledge about options and limitations in funding limit access for many who might otherwise benefit from such devices.[154,155]

Serial corrective casts have long been used as a primary intervention for individuals with significant hypertonus to provide a prolonged elongation of soft tissue over a long time period. They increase the length of a contracted muscle and its supportive tissues and "reset" the threshold for response to stretch reflex.[156-161] Some splints or dynamic orthoses are used primarily at night to provide 8 or more hours of stretch on a regular basis; others can be worn during daily activities to provide a longer period of stretch (Figure 12-11). More recently, serial casting and dynamic splinting have been used in conjunction with pharmacological interventions for management of spasticity in both children and adults with severe hypertonicity (Figure 12-12).[141,161-165] Although the pharmacological agent may reduce the degree of spasticity in hypertonic muscles, concomitant shortening of the muscles and tendons must be addressed while the neurological influence is altered, as should concomitant deficits in other dimensions of muscle performance and motor control.[166-170] A young child with spastic diplegic CP, for example, may receive botulinum injections to the gastrocnemius and soleus muscles to reduce severity of spasticity, as an alternative to early orthopedic surgery.[171-173]

Selecting the Appropriate Orthosis

Rehabilitation professionals play an active role in deciding what type of orthosis would be most appropriate for an individual with neuromuscular impairment. A number of factors contribute to the decision-making process (Table 12-8); the collective wisdom of physical and occupational therapists, orthotists, physicians, family, and the patient who might benefit from orthotic intervention is necessary for appropriate and effective casting or orthotic intervention.[7,111,174-178]

The primary goal of orthotic *prescription* is to select the device and components that will best improve function, given the individual's pathology and prognosis, impairments, functional limitation, and the abilities or activities that he or she needs or wants to accomplish now and over time. To do this, the cast, splint, or orthosis might provide external support, control or limit ROM, optimally position a limb for function, reduce risk of secondary musculoskeletal complications, or provide a base for adaptive equipment that would make function more efficient. What evidence is available to support clinical decision making with respect to orthotic prescription? Although many professionals rely on expertise gained by working with persons with neuromotor impairment over years of clinical practice, a growing number of articles on orthotic design for particular patient

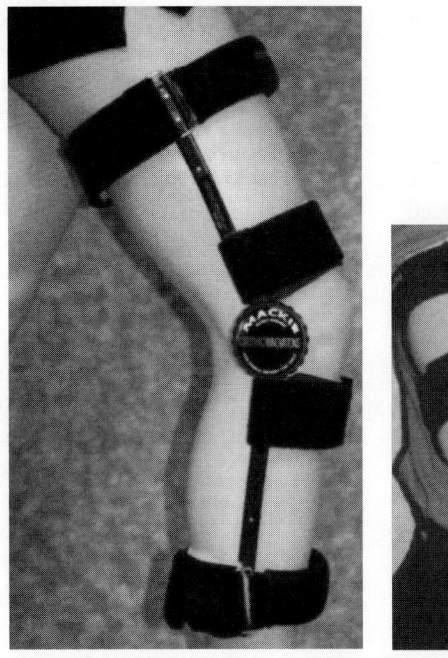
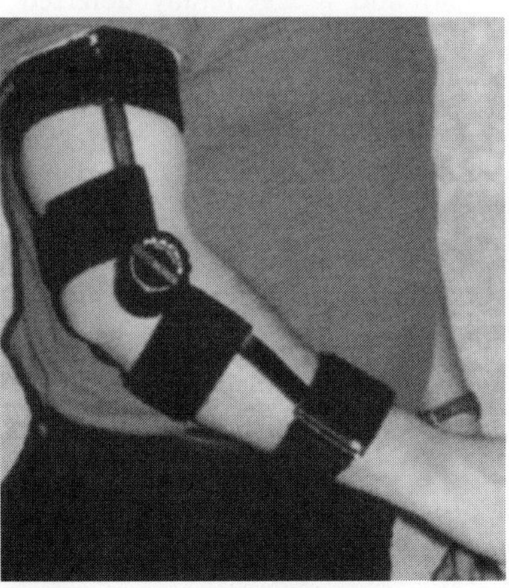

Figure 12-11
*Examples of dynamic orthoses used to provide prolonged "stretch" to tissues contributing to joint contracture at the knee (**A**) and elbow (**B**). These types of orthoses can be used for persons with both musculoskeletal and neuromuscular pathologies that have resulted in joint contracture and may be used as an adjunct to surgical and pharmacological interventions for persons with hypertonicity. (Courtesy Ortho Innovations, Rochester, Minn.)*

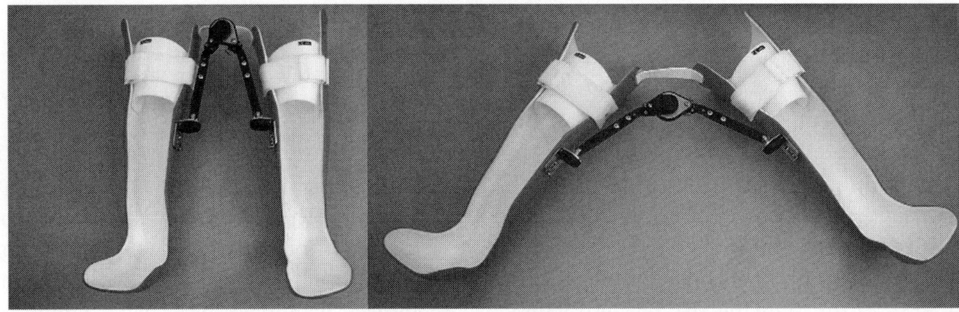

Figure 12-12
Example of a custom molded orthosis, worn in the immediate postoperative period and later during sleep, designed to enhance range of motion following botulinum toxin type A injection. The goal was to reduce hypertonicity and delay corrective orthopedic surgery, for a child with spastic cerebral palsy. (Courtesy Ultraflex systems Inc, Downingtown, Pa.)

populations in the rehabilitation and orthotic research literature are available to guide decision making, not only for individuals with hypertonicity[114,179-192] but also for those with spinal cord injury,[193,194] myelomeningocele,[195-198] and muscular dystrophy.[199-202]

If the primary goal of orthotic *intervention* is to improve safety and functionality during ambulation, it is imperative to identify where in the gait cycle abnormal tone or muscle performance is impaired (readers are referred to Chapter 3 for more information on critical events in each subphase of gait, as well as detailed information about strategies to examine gait). Systematic consideration of a series of questions can help identify where within the gait cycle (considering both stance and swing phases) problems occur.[203-205]

Preparing for initial contact requires asking the following:

- How well prepared is the limb (especially the ankle/forefoot) for initial contact?
- What factors (e.g., abnormal tone, limited ROM, joint instability, inadequate strength or power, abnormal pattern of movement) compromise prepositioning for this individual?
- What orthotic options might address difficulty with prepositioning of the limb for effective initial contact?

Table 12-8
Components of a Physical Therapy Examination and Evaluation in Preparation for Serial Casting, or Prescription/Fitting of Appropriate Splint or Orthoses

Component	*Dimension*	*Examination Strategy*
History and current condition	Duration of presenting problem	Review of medical record, interview with patient/caregivers
	Previous and concurrent pharmacological management	Review of medical record, interview with patient/caregivers, consultation with clinical colleagues
	Previous and concurrent orthopedic or neurosurgical management	Review of medical record, interview with patient/caregivers, consultation with clinical colleagues
	Previous orthotic management	Review of medical record, interview with patient/caregivers, consultation with clinical colleagues
	Current health status and comorbidities	Review of medical record, interview with patient/caregivers, consultation with clinical colleagues
	Goals and expected outcomes of proposed intervention	Interview with patient/caregivers, consultation with clinical colleagues
Biomechanical condition	Actual joint ROM	Goniometric measurement
Targeted joint Proximal joints Distal joints	Flexibility of multijoint muscles (muscle shortening)	Passive ROM, elongation of tissues
	End feel	Gentle overpressure at end of available ROM
	Integrity of ligaments and other supportive structures	Various orthopedic "special tests" appropriate to joint being examined
	Alignment of joint	Radiograph, goniometry
	Torsion/rotation of long bones of targeted limb	Various orthopedic special tests
	Other deformities at neighboring joints, spine	Radiograph, goniometry
	Overall postural alignment	Spatial relationships of head, upper trunk/limb girdle, mid trunk, lower trunk/pelvic girdle, extremity; symmetry
	Anthropomorphic characteristics	Height, limb length and girth, weight, body mass
Neuromotor status/ motor control	Resting tone	Reaction to passive movement, at various speeds, palpation, tone scales (e.g., Modified Ashworth)
	Response to deep tendon reflexes	Pattern of response (distal–proximal), symmetry of response (right–left) amplitude of response
	Response to change in position	Degree of influence of "abnormal" developmental reflexes
	Postural tone	Readiness to support trunk or body segment in various antigravity positions

Continued

Table 12-8
Components of a Physical Therapy Examination and Evaluation in Preparation for Serial Casting, or Prescription/Fitting of Appropriate Splint or Orthoses—cont'd

Component	*Dimension*	*Examination Strategy*
	Postural control	Stability in static positions; ability to implement anticipatory responses during functional activities and in transitions between positions; ability to implement appropriate equilibrium or protective responses in response to perturbation
	Recruitment/grading of contraction	Ability to control concentric, holding, or eccentric contraction Ability to initiate, sustain, and terminate contraction
	Relationships of agonist/antagonist	Ability to grade activity of agonist and antagonistic muscles (within limb, within limb-girdle musculature, within trunk during functional activities)
	Dexterity, coordination, agility	Observation of performance during functional activities, special tests, developmental scales and profiles
	Dissociation of segments	Ability to perform isolated movement of limb segment, ability to isolate limb movement from trunk movement Influence of abnormal synergistic movement patterns
Muscle performance	Strength	Ability to develop force Manual muscle test, hand-held goniometer
	Power	Rate of force development during functional activities; isokinetic testing
	Muscle endurance	Ability to sustain muscle activity over time Rate and degree of muscle fatigue development during functional activity
Integumentary integrity	Status of skin	Inspection; palpation; documentation of scarring, callus, previous vascular or neuropathic wounds; documentation of pressure-sensitive areas
	Sensory integrity	Ability to detect injury to skin (protective sensation) Paresthesia, possible peripherally based or CNS sensory impairment
Gait analysis	Uses of assistive devices or need for human assistance	Typical use on various surfaces and multiple environmental conditions
	Observational/descriptive (with and without orthoses)	Comparison to age-matched typically functioning peers, established norms Identification of primary and compensatory deviations
	Kinetics: time and distance measures	Velocity, cadence, stride and step length, step width, stride and step time, stance and swing time, single-limb and double-limb support time

Table 12-8
Components of a Physical Therapy Examination and Evaluation in Preparation for Serial Casting, or Prescription/Fitting of Appropriate Splint or Orthoses—cont'd

Component	*Dimension*	*Examination Strategy*
	Kinematic measures	Video analysis to determine joint angles, combined with force plate analysis to determine moments, torques, pattern of progression of center of mass
	Pattern of muscle activity during ambulation	Surface electromyography during instrumented gait analysis
	Aerobic capacity during ambulation	Cardiac and respiratory response to increasing or sustained activity, pulse oximetry, ratings of perceived exertion, other clinical measures (e.g., 6-minute walk)
Functional activities that would be affected by cast, splint, or orthosis	Mobility tasks	Strategies used during transitions to/from floor, sit to stand, car/bathroom transfers, other instrumental activities of daily living
	Activities of daily living/self-care	Donning/doffing device, transfers, bathing, feeding, etc.
	School or work-related activities	Typical demands and barriers encountered (self-report, interview with caregivers, observation)
	Leisure or play activities	Typical demands and barriers encountered (self-report, interview with caregivers, observation)

CNS, Central nervous system; *ROM*, range of motion.

Questions regarding the transition into loading response follow:

- Can the individual effectively load the limb (i.e., transfer weight onto the limb)?
- Can the individual effectively accomplish "shock absorption" (with eccentric activity of quadriceps)?
- How does the individual accomplish controlled lowering of the foot (first rocker of gait, with eccentric contraction of the anterior tibialis) during loading response?
- What factors (e.g., abnormal tone, limited ROM, joint instability, inadequate strength or power, abnormal pattern of movement) compromise loading of the limb for this individual?
- What orthotic options might address difficulty with loading of the limb?

Questions for going from loading response into midstance follow:

- Can the tibia move forward over the foot (with eccentric activity of the gastrocnemius and soleus complex) (second rocker of gait) from loading response into midstance (and continuing into terminal stance)?
- How well can the individual control the position of the knee in the sagittal plane (knee extension) as the COM moves from behind the knee joint axis in the transition from loading response into midstance?
- How well can the individual control the position of the hip and pelvis in the frontal plane (keeping the pelvis level) during single limb stance?
- What factors (e.g., abnormal tone, limited ROM, joint instability, inadequate strength or power, abnormal pattern of movement) compromise forward progression or single limb stability, or both, during early stance for this individual?
- What orthotic options might address difficulty with stability in the first part of the stance phase for this individual?

Questions for going from midstance into terminal stance follow:

- Can the individual convert the foot from "mobile adaptor" to "rigid lever" for an effective heel rise?
- Is there continued forward progression of the pelvis, with apparent hip extension, to prepare the limb for the start of the swing phase (i.e., trailing limb position) and to allow completion of an effective stride of the opposite limb?
- What factors (e.g., abnormal tone, limited ROM, joint instability, inadequate strength or power, abnormal pattern

of movement) compromise forward progression or single limb stability, or both, during late stance for this individual?
- What orthotic options might address difficulty with stability in the second part of the stance phase for this individual?

Questions for going from terminal stance into preswing follow:
- Can the individual "roll over" the first metatarsal head to accomplish the third rocker of gait?
- Can the individual transfer weight from what has been the stance limb onto the opposite limb that has just begun its loading response?
- Does sufficient knee flexion occur to preposition the limb for initiation of initial swing?
- What factors (e.g., abnormal tone, limited ROM, joint instability, inadequate strength or power, abnormal pattern of movement) compromise controlled unweighting of the limb coming out of stance and its preparation for initial swing for this individual?
- What orthotic options might address difficulty with preparation for the swing phase for this individual?

Questions for going from preswing into initial swing and midswing follow:
- How does the individual accomplish "swing limb shortening" for toe clearance in early swing phase? Is there sufficient dorsiflexion, knee flexion, and hip flexion?
- What factors (e.g., abnormal tone, limited ROM, inadequate strength or power, abnormal pattern of movement) compromise the individual's ability to relatively shorten the swing limb and continue forward progression of the COM?
- What orthotic options might address difficulty with relative limb shortening for toe clearance in the early part of swing?

Questions for going from midswing into terminal swing (toward initial contact) follow:
- How does the individual control momentum of the lower leg during forward progression of the limb in late swing? Can knee flexors eccentrically control advancement of the tibia in preparation for initial contact?
- Can the individual effectively "preposition" the foot in preparation for heelstrike at initial contact?
- Is there sufficient stance phase stability of the opposite limb for an effective stride length of the swinging limb?
- What factors (e.g., abnormal tone, limited ROM, inadequate strength or power, abnormal pattern of movement) compromise continued forward progression and preparation for initial contact during late swing phase for this individual?
- What orthotic options might address difficulty with continued forward progression and preparation for initial contact for this individual?

Rehabilitation professions must recognize that no orthosis will "normalize" gait for persons with neurologically based gait difficulties. Whenever an external device is placed on a limb, it is likely to "solve" one problem while at the same time creating other constraints on limb function. The therapist, orthotist, and patient collectively problem solve during the prosthetic prescription phase to prioritize the difficulties the individual is having during gait and then select the design and components that will allow the person to be most functional while walking, with the least additional constraint on other mobility and functional tasks.

The rehabilitation team at Rancho Los Amigos National Rehabilitation Center has developed an algorithm that is particularly useful in guiding clinical decision making and sorting through possible orthotic options for adults with neuromotor impairment (ROADMAP: Recommendations for Orthotic Assessment, Decision Making, and Prescription).[111] When considering orthotic interventions for persons having difficulty with ambulation, this team suggests asking the following questions:

1. Is there adequate ROM in the lower extremities to appropriately align or position limb segments in each subphase of gait?
2. Does the individual have the motivation and cognitive resources necessary to work toward meeting the goal of ambulation?
3. Does the individual have enough endurance (cardiovascular and cardiopulmonary resources) to be able to functionally ambulate? If endurance is not currently sufficient, might it be improved by a concurrent conditioning program?
4. Does the individual have adequate upper extremity, trunk, and lower extremity strength; power; motor control; and postural control for ambulation (with an appropriate assistive device, if necessary)? If these dimensions of movement are not currently sufficient, might they be improved with concurrent rehabilitation intervention?
5. Is there sufficient awareness of lower limb position (proprioception, kinesthesia) for controlled forward progression in gait? If not, might alternative sensory strategies be learned or used to substitute for limb position sense?

If the answers to *most* of these questions are "yes," the individual is considered to be a candidate for orthotic intervention. The next determinant is knee control and strength: If the individual has 3+ or better knee extension strength, even if there is impaired proprioception in the involved limb, then an ankle-foot orthosis may be appropriate. If there is impairment of strength or of proprioception (or both), then the team is more likely to recommend a knee-ankle-foot orthosis. The reader is referred to Box 12-1 for an example of a decision tree used to guide the selection of components.

Especially important is that the individual who will use the orthosis and caregivers, as appropriate, are actively involved in the decision-making process. To make an informed decision, the person needing an orthosis must understand both the benefits and constraints associated with

Box 12-1 *Decision Tree for Orthotic Options*

IS A KNEE-ANKLE-FOOT ORTHOSIS (KAFO) INDICATED?

Is there at least 3+/5 strength in quadriceps bilaterally?
Is proprioception intact bilaterally?
If yes: continue assessment for AFO
If no: KAFO may improve gait, continue assessment process

Which KAFO components are the most appropriate?

Is there at least 3+/5 strength in one lower extremity?
Is proprioception intact in at least one lower extremity?
If no: consider trial of bilateral KAFOs or a reciprocal gait orthosis
If yes: unilateral KAFO may be indicated—continue assessment to determine if knee locking mechanism necessary

Can the knee be fully extended, without pain, during stance?
If no: consider KAFO with knee lock
If yes: consider KAFO with variable knee mechanism and continue assessment

Is there at effective active control of knee extension during stance?
If no: consider stance control knee mechanism
If yes: consider free motion knee mechanism

Continue with ankle-foot orthosis (AFO) decision tree to determine appropriate ankle control strategy

IS AN AFO INDICATED?

Is there impairment of ankle strength?
Is there impairment of proprioception?
Is there hypertonicity of plantar flexors?
(or a combination of all of the above?)
If no: may not require lower extremity orthosis
If yes: lower extremity orthosis may improve gait—continue assessment process

Which AFO design and components are the best option?

Does impaired strength hamper foot position in stance or swing?
Does impaired proprioception hamper foot placement in stance or swing?
Does hypertonicity/spasticity hamper foot position in stance or swing?
If no: consider adjustable articulating ankle joint (allows full dorsiflexion [DF] and plantar flexion [PF])
If yes: consider limiting or blocking ankle motion, continue assessment process

Is there more than minimal impairment of static and dynamic postural control in standing?
Is there significant spasticity?
Is proprioception significantly impaired?
If no: consider adjustable articulating ankle joint that blocks PF beyond neutral ankle position and continue assessment
If yes: consider solid-ankle AFO or adjustable articulating ankle that is fully locked (consider rocker bottom shoe)

Is there also plantar flexion strength ≤ 4 in standing?
Is there also excessive knee flexion and dorsiflexion during stance?
Is there also excessive plantar flexion with knee hyperextension during stance?
If no: consider adjustable articulating ankle joint with PF stop, and continue assessment
If yes: consider adjustable articulating ankle joint with PF stop and limited DF excursion, and continue assessment

Is there also dorsiflexion strength ≤ 4 in standing?
If no: consider adjustable articulating ankle with PF stop, limited DF excursion in stance, no DF assist necessary
If yes: consider adjustable articulating ankle with PF stop, limited DF excursion, and DF assist for effective swing phase

the orthotic designs and components being considered. He or she must be able to consider the range of orthotic options, as well as concomitant medical/surgical intervention and additional rehabilitation interventions that might affect his or her ability to walk. The entire team must consider what the individual who will be wearing the orthosis wants to accomplish, as well as the preferences he or she might have in terms of ease of donning/doffing, wearing schedule, and cosmesis of the device being recommended. Beginning with a "trial" orthosis, perhaps a prefabricated or multi-adjustable version, is helpful before finalizing the orthotic prescription, especially if it is unclear whether ambulation will be possible in the long run. Certainly, most individuals with neuromuscular conditions that compromise their ability to walk benefit from a chance to experience what ambulation with an orthosis requires, given their individual constellation of impairments. Some may decide that using orthoses and an appropriate assistive device for functional ambulation throughout the day meets their mobility needs. Others may opt, because of the energy cost of walking with knee-ankle-foot orthoses or hip-knee-ankle-foot orthoses, to use a wheelchair for primary mobility and reserve the use of orthoses to exercise bouts aimed at building cardiovascular endurance. Finally, some may decide that orthotic intervention will not meet their needs and pursue other avenues to address mobility and endurance issues.

CASE EXAMPLE 1

T. H.: A Young Child with Spastic Diplegic Cerebral Palsy

T. H. is a 4-year-old child who was born prematurely at 32 weeks of gestation and diagnosed with spastic diplegic CP at 10 months of age. She is being evaluated for potential botulinum A injection as a strategy to manage significant extensor hypertonicity that is increasingly limiting her ability to ambulate as she grows. At present she uses bilateral articulating ankle-foot orthoses with a plantar flexion stop and a posterior rolling walker for locomotion at her early intervention program; she prefers bunny hopping in quadruped for mobility at home. Her articulating orthoses allow her to transition to and from the floor as she plays and is in school; however, they do not prevent her from assuming a "crouch" gait position, especially as she tires after a full day of activity. She has been monitored in a CP clinic at the regional children's hospital; the team is concerned that she is developing rotational deformity of the lower extremities, as well as plantar flexion contracture and forefoot deformity due to her long-standing hypertonicity.

Questions to Consider

- In which subphases of the gait cycle is function or safety compromised when T. H. ambulates without her orthoses?
- In what way does T. H.'s abnormal tone contribute to her difficulty with locomotion/ambulation? What strategies would be useful in documenting/assessing her abnormal tone?
- In what ways does T. H.'s impaired motor control contribute to her difficulty with locomotion/ambulation? What are the most likely dimensions of her impairment in motor control, given her diagnosis of spastic diplegia?
- In what ways does T. H.'s impaired muscle performance contribute to her difficulty with locomotion/ambulation? What are the most likely dimensions of her impairment in muscle performance, given her diagnosis of spastic diplegia?
- Are there primary or secondary musculoskeletal impairments that are influencing her function and safety during ambulation? How do her age and future growth influence her risk of developing secondary impairments?
- Given her constellation of impairments, what compensatory strategies is T. H. likely to use to accomplish the task of locomotion?
- Which of T. H.'s anticipated or observed impairments are remediable? Which will require accommodation?
- What orthotic options (design, components) are available to address T. H.'s impairment of locomotion and related functional limitations? What are the pros and cons of each?
- What alternative or concurrent medical (surgical/pharmacological) interventions might assist improvement in safety and function for T. H.?
- What additional rehabilitation interventions might assist improvement in function and safety for T. H.?
- How do you anticipate T. H.'s orthotic needs might change as she develops and grows?
- What outcome measures can be used to assess efficacy of orthotic, therapeutic, pharmacological, or surgical intervention for T. H.?

CASE EXAMPLE 2

J.T. : A Child with Spastic Quadriplegic Cerebral Palsy

J. T. is an 11-year-old boy with significant spastic quadriplegic CP who is in the midst of a preadolescent growth spurt. He currently uses a custom seating system in a power wheelchair for self-directed mobility at school and in the community. At home he divides his time between his chair and rolling/crawling on the floor. J. T.'s mom reports that it is becoming increasingly difficult to assist him in transfers into the family's sport utility vehicle and help him with self-care activities because of upper extremity flexor tightness, an increasing knee flexion contracture, and plantar flexion tightness.

In addition, when supine, J. T.'s resting position is becoming more obviously "windswept." He attends physical therapy at school several times each week to help him with functional abilities in the classroom and around campus, with additional outpatient visits focusing on improving motor control and muscle performance. Both of his therapists are becoming concerned about his increasing limitation in ROM, as well as the risk of increasing rotational deformity and hip dysfunction as he grows. His outpatient therapist accompanies J. T. and his mother to the CP orthotics clinic at the regional children's medical center to explore the possibility of functional bracing or dynamic orthoses, or both, to manage the musculoskeletal complications that are developing because of his spasticity. They also have questions about surgical or pharmacological intervention.

Questions to Consider

- In what way does J. T.'s abnormal tone contribute to his difficulty with mobility/locomotion and other functional activities?
- In what ways does J. T.'s impaired motor control contribute to his difficulty with functional activities?
- In what ways does J. T.'s impaired muscle performance contribute to his difficulty with functional activities?
- Are any primary or secondary musculoskeletal impairments influencing J. T.'s function and safety during mobility and transfer tasks?

- Given his constellation of impairments, what compensatory strategies is J. T. likely to use to accomplish his functional tasks at school and at home?
- Which of J. T.'s anticipated or observed impairments are remediable? Which will require accommodation?
- What orthotic options (design, components) are available to address J. T.'s impairments and functional limitations? What are the pros and cons of each?
- What alternative or concurrent medical (surgical/pharmacological) interventions might assist improvement in safety and function for J. T.?
- What additional rehabilitation interventions might assist improvement in function and safety for J. T.?
- How do you anticipate J. T.'s orthotic needs might change as he develops and grows?
- What outcome measures can be used to assess efficacy of orthotic, therapeutic, pharmacological, or surgical intervention for J. T.?

CASE EXAMPLE 3

P.G.: A Young Adult with Acquired Brain Injury and Decerebrate Pattern Hypertonicity

P. G. is a 17-year-old girl who sustained significant closed-head injury in a motor vehicle accident 3 weeks ago. She was admitted to the brain injury unit at the regional rehabilitation hospital earlier this week. Now functioning at a Rancho Los Amigos Cognitive Level 5 (confused and inappropriate), P. G. exhibits significant decorticate posturing whenever she attempts to move volitionally (R > L), with marked limitations in passive ROM at the elbow and wrist, as well as equinovarus at the ankle, both of which are limiting her ability to stand and effectively propel her wheelchair. She is most focused and responsive to intervention when involved in ambulation-oriented activities. Currently, her hypertonicity is being managed with oral baclofen (Lioresal). However, her therapists are concerned that contracture formation continues. During rehabilitation rounds the physiatrist, neurologists, and therapists agree that a trial of serial casting should be added to her regimen to "jumpstart" her rehabilitation.

Questions to Consider

- In which subphases of the gait cycle is function or safety compromised when G. P. attempts to ambulate?
- In what way does G. P.'s abnormal tone contribute to her difficulty with locomotion/ambulation? What strategies would be useful in documenting/assessing her abnormal tone?
- In what ways does G. P.'s impaired motor control contribute to her difficulty with locomotion/ambulation? What are the most likely dimensions of her impairment in motor control, given her diagnosis of acquired brain injury?
- In what ways does G. P.'s impaired muscle performance contribute to her difficulty with locomotion/ambulation? What are the most likely dimensions of her impairment in muscle performance, given her diagnosis of acquired brain injury?
- Are any primary or secondary musculoskeletal impairments influencing her function and safety during ambulation? What do you think is likely to develop as she recovers from her head injury?
- Given her constellation of impairments, what compensatory strategies is G. P. likely to use to accomplish the task of locomotion?
- Which of G. P.'s anticipated or observed impairments are remediable? Which will require accommodation?
- What orthotic options (design, components) are available to address G. P.'s impairment of locomotion and related functional limitations? What are the pros and cons of each?
- What alternative or concurrent medical (surgical/pharmacological) interventions might assist improvement in safety and function for G. P.?
- What additional rehabilitation interventions might assist improvement in function and safety for G. P.?
- How do you anticipate G. P.'s orthotic needs might change as she recovers over the next year?
- What outcome measures can be used to assess efficacy of orthotic, therapeutic, pharmacological, or surgical intervention for G. P.?

CASE EXAMPLE 4

Two Individuals with Recent Stroke

You work in the short-term rehabilitation unit associated with the regional tertiary care hospital in your area. This week two gentlemen recovering from stroke/brain attack sustained 3 days ago were admitted to the unit for a short stay in preparation for discharge home. Both indicate that their primary goals at this time are to be able to walk functional distances within their homes, manage stairs to enter/leave the house, and get to bedrooms on the second floor. You anticipate that they will receive intensive rehabilitation services for 5 to 8 days, with follow-up with home care after discharge.

M. O., who is 73 years old with a history of hypertension, mild chronic obstructive pulmonary disease, and an uncomplicated myocardial infarction 2 years ago, has been diagnosed with a lacunar infarct within the left posterior limb of internal capsule. On passive motion, he has been given modified Ashworth scores of "3" in his right upper extremity and "2" in his right lower extremity. When asked to bend his knee (when supine) he demonstrates difficulty initiating flexion, and when he finally begins to move, his ankle, knee, and hip move in a mass-flexion pattern; he is unable to isolate limb segments. When asked to slowly lower his leg to the bed, he "shoots" into a full lower extremity synergy pattern. He rises from sitting to standing with verbal and tactile cueing, somewhat asymmetrically relying on his left extremities. Once upright, he can shift his center of mass to the midline, holding an effective upright posture. With encouragement and facilitation, he can shift weight toward his right in preparation for swing-limb advancement of the left lower extremity, and he is pleased to have taken a few steps, however short, in the parallel bars. Before his infarct, he was an avid golfer and enjoyed bowling. He is fearful that he will never be able to resume these activities.

E. B., 64, is a recently retired car mechanic with an 8-year history of diabetes mellitus, previously controlled by diet and oral medications but requiring insulin since his stroke. MRI indicates probable occlusion in the right posterior-inferior branch of the middle cerebral artery, with ischemia and resultant inflammation in the parietal lobe. Because E. B. has been afraid of hospitals for most of his life, he resisted seeking medical care as his symptoms began, arriving at the emergency department 12 hours after onset of hemiplegia. He currently displays a heavy, hypotonic, somewhat edematous left upper extremity. He is unusually unconcerned about the fact that he has had a stroke and tells you that he should be able to function "well enough" when he returns home to his familiar environment. On examination he demonstrates homonymous hemianopsia, especially of the lower left visual field, and impaired kinesthetic awareness of his left extremities. You observe that he appears to be unaware when his lower upper extremity slips off the tray table of his wheelchair and his fingers become entangled in the spokes of the wheel as he propels forward using his right leg. When assisted to standing in the parallel bars, he does not seem to be accurately aware of his upright position, requiring moderate assistance to keep from falling to the left. When asked to try to walk forward a few paces, he repeatedly advances his right lower extremity, even when prompted to consider the position and activity of his lower left extremity.

Questions to Consider

- In what ways are the stroke-related impairments observed in these two gentlemen similar or different? How can you explain these differences?
- In what subphases of the gait cycle is function or safety compromised when each of these gentleman attempts to ambulate?
- In what way does each gentleman's abnormal tone contribute to his difficulty with locomotion/ambulation? What strategies would be useful in documenting/assessing the severity and type of their abnormal tone?
- In what ways does each gentleman's impaired motor control contribute to his difficulty with locomotion/ambulation? What are the most likely dimensions of each man's impairment in motor control, given his etiology and location of stroke?
- In what ways does each gentleman's impaired muscle performance contribute to his difficulty with locomotion/ambulation? What are the most likely dimensions of each man's impairment in muscle performance, given his etiology and location of stroke?
- Are any primary or secondary musculoskeletal impairments influencing each man's function and safety during ambulation? How does each man's age and concomitant medical conditions influence his risk of developing secondary impairments?
- Given each gentleman's constellation of impairments, what compensatory strategies is each likely to use to accomplish the task of locomotion?
- Which of each gentleman's anticipated or observed impairments are remediable? Which will require accommodation?
- What orthotic options (design, components) are available to address each gentleman's impairment of locomotion and related functional limitations? What are the pros and cons of each?
- What alternative or concurrent medical (surgical/pharmacological) interventions might assist improvement in safety and function for each individual?
- What additional rehabilitation interventions might assist improvement in function and safety for M. O. and E. B.?
- How do you anticipate each gentleman's orthotic needs might change as he recovers from CNS damage?
- What outcome measures can be used to assess the efficacy of orthotic, therapeutic, pharmacological, or surgical intervention for each gentleman?

CASE EXAMPLE 5

Z. C.: A Young Adult with Incomplete Spinal Cord Injury

Z. C. is a 23-year-old man who sustained an incomplete C7 spinal cord injury 3 weeks ago when he lost control and crash-landed during a failed acrobatic stunt during a "half-pipe" snowboard competition at a local ski resort. After being stabilized on site, he was quickly airlifted to a regional spinal cord injury/trauma center. Methylprednisolone was administered within 1.5 hours of injury, and his cervical fractures were repaired by fusion (C5 through T1) the day after injury; he now wears a Miami J cervical orthosis. He was admitted to your rehabilitation center 5 days ago. He demonstrates no activity of triceps brachii bilaterally but reports dysesthesia in the C7 and C8 dermatomes and can point his index finger on the left. He is aware of lower limb position in space and can activate toe flexors and extensors, plantar flexors, knee extensors, and hip flexors and abductors at 2+/5 levels of strength. Deep tendon reflex at the Achilles heel is brisk bilaterally, while more proximal lower extremity reflexes are diminished. He demonstrates positive Babinski reflex bilaterally. Biceps and wrist extensor deep tendon reflexes, initially diminished, are now more consistently rated 2+; the triceps reflex, initially diminished, is now quite brisk. He requires moderate assistance of 1 to come to sitting from supine but can hold a static posture in sitting, demonstrating a limited sway envelope when attempting to shift his weight anteriorly, posteriorly, and mediolaterally. He requires moderate assistance of 1 to rise from seated in his wheelchair to standing position in the parallel bars. He is determined to "walk" out of the facility on discharge, anticipated after 3 more weeks of rehabilitation.

Questions to Consider

- Given Z. C.'s history and present point in recovery from spinal cord injury, what is the anticipated prognosis concerning his functional performance and ability to ambulate?
- In what subphases of the gait cycle is function or safety likely to be compromised when Z. C. attempts to ambulate?
- In what way does Z. C.'s abnormal tone contribute to his difficulty with locomotion/ambulation? What strategies would be useful in documenting/assessing the severity and type of his abnormal tone?
- In what ways does Z. C.'s impaired motor control contribute to his difficulty with locomotion/ambulation? What are the most likely dimensions of Z. C.'s impairment in motor control, given his etiology and level of injury?
- In what ways does Z. C.'s impaired muscle performance contribute to his difficulty with locomotion/ambulation? What are the most likely dimensions of his impairment in muscle performance, given his etiology and level of injury?
- Are any primary or secondary musculoskeletal impairments likely to influence Z. C.'s function and safety during ambulation? How do Z. C.'s age and concomitant medical conditions influence his risk of developing secondary impairments?
- Given Z. C.'s constellation of impairments, what compensatory strategies is he likely to use to accomplish the task of locomotion?
- Which of Z. C.'s anticipated or observed impairments are remediable? Which will require accommodation?
- What orthotic options (design, components) are available to address Z. C.'s difficulty with locomotion and related functional limitations? What are the pros and cons of each?
- What alternative or concurrent medical (surgical/pharmacological) interventions might assist improvement in safety and function?
- What additional rehabilitation interventions might assist improvement in function and safety for Z. C.?
- How do you anticipate Z. C.'s orthotic needs might change as he recovers from his spinal cord injury?
- What outcome measures can be used to assess the efficacy of orthotic, therapeutic, pharmacological, or surgical intervention for Z. C.?

SUMMARY

This chapter has reviewed the functions and roles of structures and systems in both the central and peripheral nervous systems, the impairments that are likely to occur when particular structures or systems are damaged by injury or disease process, abnormalities of tone and motor control that influence an individual's ability to ambulate and affect the likelihood of developing secondary musculoskeletal impairments, and some of the pharmacological and surgical options that are available to manage hypertonicity and correct deformity that may develop over time. Strategies to determine where in the gait cycle an individual with various neuromotor impairments is likely to have difficulty have been explored, as well as which orthotic options might best address the limitations the individual faces. Although this has provided a strong foundation for physical therapy examination and evaluation, it has not taken the process into the "intervention" dimension of patient/client management. What the reader needs to do next is consider physical therapy interventions that will focus on wearing, using, and caring for the orthosis that is prescribed. These include, but are not limited to, (1) strategies to enhance motor learning when a new ambulatory aid (orthosis and/or assistive device) is introduced; (2) practice using the device under various environmental conditions (surfaces, obstacles, people moving within the environment); and (3) the ability to use the orthosis and ambulatory assistive device during functional activities beyond walking at comfortable gait speed.

REFERENCES

1. Who are physical therapists, and what do they do? Guide to physical therapist practice. *Phys Ther* 81(1):39-50, 2001.
2. Mueller MJ, Kaluf KS. Tissue adaptation to physical stress: a proposed "physical stress theory" to guide physical therapist practice, education and research. *Phys Ther* 82(4):383-403, 2002.
3. Bradley WG, Daroff RB, Fenichel G, et al. *Neurology in Clinical Practice,* 4th ed. Boston: Butterworth-Heinemann, 2003.

4. Weiner WJ, Lang KE. *Behavioral Neurology of Movement Disorders*. Philadelphia: Lippincott Williams & Wilkins, 2005.
5. Gilman S, Newman SW. Neurological diagnostic tests. In Gilman S, Newman SW (eds), *Manter & Gatz Essentials of Clinical Neuroanatomy and Neurophysiology,* 19th ed. Philadelphia: FA Davis, 2003. pp. 241-245.
6. Kiernan JA. Imaging techniques and neuroanatomical research methods. In Kiernan JA (ed), *Barr's The Human Nervous System: An Anatomical Viewpoint,* 8th ed. Philadelphia: Lippincott Williams & Wilkin, 2005. pp. 52-62.
7. What type of tests and measures do physical therapists use? Guide to physical therapist practice. *Phys Ther* 2001;81(1):51-103.
8. Lazarro RT, Roller M, Umphred DA. Differential diagnosis phase 2: examination and intervention of disabilities and impairments. In Umphred DA (ed), *Neurological Rehabilitation*, 4th ed. St. Louis: Mosby, 2001. pp. 43-55.
9. Nelson CA. Cerebral palsy. In Umphred DA (ed), *Neurological Rehabilitation*, 4th ed. St. Louis: Mosby, 2001. pp. 259-286.
10. Adams AC. *Neurology in Primary Care.* Philadelphia: F.A. Davis, 2001.
11. Shumway-Cook A, Woollacott MH. Physiology of motor control. In Shumway-Cook A, Woollacott MH (eds), *Motor Control: Theory and Practical Applications.* Philadelphia: Lippincott Williams & Wilkins, 2001. pp. 50-90.
12. Stein DG, Brailowsky S, Will B. *Brain Repair,* New York: Oxford, 1995.
13. Shumway-Cook A, Woollacott MH. Physiological basis of motor learning and motor recovery. In Shumway-Cook A, Woollacott MH (eds), *Motor Control: Theory and Practical Applications.* Philadelphia: Lippincott Williams & Wilkins, 2001. pp. 91-109.
14. Alarcon F, Zijlmans JC, Duenas G, et al. Post-stroke movement disorders: report of 56 patients, *J Neurol Neurosurg Psychiatr* 2004;75(11):1568-1574.
15. Ryerson SD. Hemiplegia. In Umphred DA (ed), *Neurological Rehabilitation,* 4th ed. St. Louis: Mosby, 2001. pp. 741-789.
16. Bear MF, Connors BW, Paradiso MA. Brain control of movement. In Bear MF, Connors BW, Paradiso MA (eds), *Neuroscience: Exploring the Brain,* 3rd ed. Philadelphia: Lippincott Williams & Wilkins, 2006. pp. 451-478.
17. Koski L, Iacoboni M, Mazziotta CJ. Deconstructing apraxia: understanding disorders of intentional movement after stroke. *Curr Op Euro* 2002;15(1):71-77.
18. Bhidayasiri R, Truong DD. Chorea and related disorders. *Postgrad Med J* 2005;80(947)L527-534.
19. Hallett M. *Movement Disorders: Handbook of Clinical Neurophysiology.* Philadelphia: Elsevier, 2003.
20. Weiner WJ, Lang KE. *Behavioral Neurology of Movement Disorders.* Philadelphia: Lippincott Williams & Wilkins, 2005.
21. Jankovic JJ, Euardo T. *Parkinson's Disease and Movement Disorders.* Philadelphia: Lippincott Williams & Wilkins, 2002.
22. Kiernan JA. Motor systems. In Kiernan JA (ed), *Barr's the Human Nervous System*, 8th ed. Philadelphia: Lippincott Williams & Wilkins, 2005. pp. 374-390.
23. Gilman S, Newman SW. Cerebellum. In Gilman S, Newman SW (eds), *Manter & Gatz Essentials of Clinical Neuroanatomy and Neurophysiology,* 10th ed. Philadelphia: F.A. Davis, 2003. pp. 135-146.
24. Melnick ME, Oremland B. Movement dysfunction associated with cerebellar problems. In Umphred DA (ed), *Neurological Rehabilitation*, 4th ed. St. Louis: Mosby, 2001. pp. 717-740.
25. Bear MR, Connors BW, Paradiso MA. The somatic sensory system. In Bear MF, Connors BW, et al (eds), *Neuroscience: Exploring the Brain,* 3rd ed. Philadelphia: Lippincott Williams & Wilkins, 2006. pp. 387-422.
26. Newton RA. Neural systems underlying motor control. In Montgomery PC, Connelly BH (eds), *Clinical Applications for Motor Control.* Thorofare, NJ: Slack; 2003. pp. 53-77.
27. Kiernan JA. Functional localization in the cerebral cortex. In Kiernan JA (ed), *Barr's The Human Nervous System, An Anatomical Viewpoint,* 8th ed. Philadelphia: Lippencott Williams & Wilkins, 2005. pp. 254-274.
28. Zucker-Levin A. Sensory and perceptual issues related to motor control. In Montgomery PC, Connolly BH (eds), *Clinical Applications for Motor Control.* Thorofare, NJ: Slack, 2003. pp. 207-243.
29. Zoltan, B. *Vision, Perceptions and Cognition: A Manual for the Evaluation and Treatment of the Neurologically Impaired Adult,* 3rd ed. Thorofare, NJ: Slack, 1996.
30. Kiernan JA. The visual system. In Kiernan JA (ed), *Barr's The Human Nervous System, an Anatomical Viewpoint,* 8th ed. Philadelphia: Lippincott Williams & Wilkins, 2005. pp. 337-352.
31. Kolbe H, Fernandez E, Nelson R. Webvision: the organization of the retina and visual system. Retrieved February 2003, at http://retina.umh.es/Webvision.
32. Chaikin LE. Disorders of vision and visual perception. In Umphred DA (ed), *Neurological Rehabilitation,* 4th ed. St. Louis: Mosby, 2001. pp. 821-853.
33. Goodale MA, Westwood DA. An evolving view of duplex vision: separate but interacting cortical pathways for perception and action. *Curr Opin Neurobiol* 2004;14(2):203-211.
34. Schmidt RA, Lee TD. Central contributions to motor control. In Schmidt RA, Lee TD (eds), *Motor Control and Learning: A Behavioral Emphasis,* 3rd ed. Champaign, IL: Human Kinetics, 2005. pp. 131-169.
35. Scheiman M. *Understanding and Managing Visual Deficits: A Guide for Occupational Therapists.* Thorofare, NJ: Slack, 1997.
36. Ross RT. Higher cortical functions: intelligence and memory. In Ross RT (ed), *How to Examine the Nervous System,* 3rd ed. Stamford, CT: Appleton & Lange, 1999. pp. 197-204.
37. Struss DT. Biological and psychological development of executive functions. *Brain Cog* 1992; 20(1):8-23.
38. Winkler PA. Traumatic brain injury. In Umphred DA (ed), *Neurological Rehabilitation,* 4th ed. St. Louis: Mosby, 2001. pp. 416-447.
39. Umphred DA. The limbic system: influence over motor control and learning. In Umphred DA (ed), *Neurological Rehabilitation,* 4th ed. St. Louis: Mosby, 2001. pp. 148-177.
40. Bear MF, Connors BW, Paradiso MA. Motivation. In Bear MF, Connors BW, Paradiso MA (eds), *Neuroscience: Exploring the Brain,* 3rd ed. Philadelphia: Lippincott Williams & Wilkins, 2006. pp. 509-531.
41. Bear MF, Connors BW, Paradiso MA. Brain mechanisms of emotion. In Bear MF, Connors BW, Paradiso MA. *Neuroscience: Exploring the Brain,* 3rd ed. Philadelphia: Lippincott Williams & Wilkins, 2006. pp. 563-583.

42. Bear MF, Connors BW, Paradiso MA. Memory systems. In Bear MF, Connors BW, Paradiso MA (eds), *Neuroscience: Exploring the Brain,* 3rd ed. Philadelphia: Lippincott Williams & Wilkins, 2006. pp. 725-759.
43. Light KE. Issues of cognition for motor control. In Montgomery PC, Connolly BH (eds), *Clinical Applications for Motor Control.* Thorofare, NJ: Slack, 2003. pp. 245-268.
44. Kiernan JA. Reticular formation. In Kiernan JA (ed), *Barr's The Human Nervous System: an Anatomical Viewpoint,* 8th ed. Philadelphia: Lippincott Williams & Wilkins; 2005. pp. 156-173.
45. Parvizi J. Consciousness and the brainstem. *Cognition* 2000;79(1-2):135-160.
46. Dandan IS. Altered consciousness. *Top Emerg Med* 2004;26(3):242-253.
47. Gilman S, Newman SW. Autonomic nervous system. In Gilman S, Newman SW (eds), *Manter & Gatz Essentials of Clinical Neuroanatomy and Neurophysiology,* 10th ed. Philadelphia: F.A. Davis; 2003. pp. 33-39.
48. Bear MF, Connors BW, Paradiso MA. Chemical control of the brain and behavior. In Bear MF, Connors BW, Paradiso MA (eds), *Neuroscience: Exploring the Brain,* 3rd ed. Philadelphia: Lippincott Williams & Wilkins, 2006. pp. 481-508.
49. Bear MF, Connors BW, Paradiso MA. Spinal control of movement. In Bear MF, Connors BW, Paradiso MA (eds), *Neuroscience: Exploring the Brain,* 3rd ed. Philadelphia: Lippincott Williams & Wilkins, 2006. pp. 423-478.
50. Joggi A, Birch R, Dean L, et al. Peripheral nerve injuries. In Stokes M (ed), *Physical Management in Neurological Rehabilitation,* 2nd ed. Edinburgh: Mosby; 2004. pp. 153-175.
51. Nolan MF. *Introduction to the Neurological Examination.* Philadelphia: F.A. Davis, 1996.
52. Shumway-Cook A, Woollacott MH. A conceptual framework for clinical practice. In Shumway-Cook A, Woollacott MH (eds), *Motor Control: Theory and Practical Applications,* 2nd ed. Philadelphia: Lippincott Williams & Wilkins, 2001. pp. 110-126.
53. Meythaler JM. Concept of spastic hypertonia. *Phys Med Rehabil Clin North Am* 2001;12(4):725-732.
54. Adams MM, Hicks AL. Spasticity after spinal cord injury. *Spinal Cord* 2005;43(10):577-586.
55. Barnes MP. Medical management of spasticity in stroke. *Age Ageing* 2001;30(2):13-16.
56. Haselkorn JK, Loomis S. Multiple sclerosis and spasticity. *Phys Med Rehabil Clin North Am* 2005;16(2):467-481.
57. Stuberg W, DeJong S, Ginsburg GM. Contracture management of children with neuromuscular disabilities. Educational session at the American Physical Therapy Association Combined Sections Meetings, San Diego, February 4, 2006.
58. Byl N, Gerber J, Mohamed O, et al. Effectiveness of sensory and motor rehabilitation of the upper limb following principles of neuroplasticity: patients stable post stroke. *Neural Rehabil Neural Repair* 2003;17(3):176-191.
59. Fahn S, Bressman SB, Marsden CD. Classification of dystonia. *Adv Neurol* 1998;78(1):1-10.
60. Guiliani CA. Spasticity and motor control. In Montgomery PC, Connolly BH (eds), *Clinical Applications for Motor Control.* Thorofare, NJ: Slack; 2003. pp. 309-332.
61. Guttman M. Current concepts in the diagnosis and management of Parkinson's disease. *CMAJ* 2003;168(3), 293-301.
62. Miller JL. Parkinson's disease primer. *Geriatr Nurs* 2002;23(2):69-75.
63. Westcott SL, Goulet C. Neuromuscular system: structures, functions, diagnoses, and evaluation. In Effgen SK (ed), *Meeting the Physical Therapy Needs of Children.* Philadelphia: F.A. Davis, 2005. pp. 185-244.
64. Dawson P. Hypotonia—sign or condition? What physiotherapists need to know. *S Afr J Physiother* 2004;60(3):15-21, 31-22.
65. Pilon JM, Sadler GR, Bartlett DJ. Relationship of hypotonia and joint laxity to motor development during infancy. *Pediatric Phys Ther* 2000;12(1):10-15.
66. Fitzgerald D, Stokes M. Muscle imbalance in neurological conditions. In Stokes M (ed), *Physical Management in Neurological Rehabilitation,* 2nd ed. Edinburgh: Mosby; 2004. pp. 501-516.
67. Sheerin F. Spinal cord injury: acute care management. *Emerg Nurse* 2005;12(10):26-34.
68. Dumont RJ. Acute spinal cord injury, part I: pathophysiologic mechanisms. *Clin Neuropharmacol* 2001;24(5):254-264.
69. Adams RD, Victor M, Ropper AH. Motor paralysis. In Adams RD, Victor M, Ropper AH (eds), *Principles of Neurology,* 6th ed. New York: McGraw-Hill, 1997. pp. 49-63.
70. Schneider JW, Krosschell KJ. Congenital spinal cord injury. In Umphred DA (ed), *Neurological Rehabilitation,* 4th ed. St. Louis: Mosby, 2001. pp. 449-476.
71. Atrice MB, Morrison SA, McDowell SL, et al. Traumatic spinal cord injury. In Umphred DA (ed), *Neurological Rehabilitation,* 4th ed. St. Louis: Mosby, 2001. pp. 477-530.
72. Adams RD, Victor M, Ropper AH. Viral infections of the nervous system. In Adams RD, Victor M, Ropper AH (eds), *Principles of Neurology,* 6th ed. New York: McGraw-Hill, 1997. pp. 742-776.
73. Adams RD, Victor M, Ropper AH. Diseases of the peripheral nerves. In Adams RD, Victor M, Ropper AH (eds), *Principles of Neurology,* 6th ed. New York: McGraw-Hill, 1997. pp. 1302-1369.
74. Kandel ER, Schwartz JH, Jessell TM. Transmitter release. In Kandell ER, Schwartz JH, Jessell TM (eds), *Principles of Neural Science,* 4th ed. New York: McGraw-Hill, 2000. pp. 253-279.
75. Adams RD, Victor M, Ropper AH. Abnormalities of movement and posture due to disease of the basal ganglia. In Adams RD, Victor M, Ropper AH (eds), *Principles of Neurology,* 6th ed. New York: McGraw-Hill, 1997. pp. 64-83.
76. Olney SJ, Wright MJ. Cerebral palsy. In SK Campbell, DW Vander Linden, Palisano RJ (eds.), *Physical Therapy for Children* 3rd ed., St. Louis: Saunders, 2006. pp. 625-664.
77. Staheli LT. *Pediatric Orthopaedic Secrets,* 2nd ed. Philadelphia: Hanley & Belfus, 2003.
78. Shumway-Cook A, Woollacott MH. Normal postural control. In Shumway-Cook A, Woollacott MH (eds), *Motor Control Theory and Practical Applications,* 2nd ed. Philadelphia: Lippincott Williams & Wilkins, 2001. pp. 163-191.

79. Allison L, Fuller K. Balance and vestibular disorders. In Umphred DA (ed), *Neurological Rehabilitation,* 4th ed. St. Louis: Mosby, 2001. pp. 616-660.
80. Seeger MA. Balance deficits: examination, evaluation and intervention. In Montgomery PC, Connelly BH (eds), *Clinical Applications for Motor Control,* Thorofare, NJ: Slack, 2003. pp. 271-306.
81. Newton R. Review of tests for standing balance abilities. *Brain Inj* 1989;3(4):335-343.
82. Panzer VP. Biomechanical assessment of quiet standing and changes associated with aging. *Arch Phys Med Rehabil* 1995;76(2):151-157.
83. Nashner L. Sensory, neuromuscular, and biomechanical contributions to human balance. In Duncan P (ed), *Balance: Proceedings of the APTA Forum.* Alexandria, VA: American Physical Therapy Association, 1990. pp. 5-12.
84. Horak FB. Clinical measurement of postural control in adults. *Phys Ther* 1987;67(12);1881-1885.
85. Shumway-Cook A, Horak FB. Assessing the influence of sensory interaction on balance: suggestion from the field. *Phys Ther* 1986;66(10):1548-1550.
86. Duncan PW, Studenski S, Chandler J et al. Functional reach: a new clinical measure of balance. *J Gerontol* 1990;45(6):M192-197.
87. Newton RA. Validity of the multi-directional reach test: a practical measure for limits of stability in older adults. *J Gerontol* 2001;56A(4):M248-252.
88. Bartlett D, Birmingham T. Validity and reliability of a pediatric reach test. *Pediatr Phys Ther* 2003;15(2):84-92.
89. Washington K, Shumway-Cook A, Price R, et al. Muscle responses to seated perturbations for typically developing infants and those at risk for motor delays. *Dev Med Child Neurol* 2004;46(10):681-688.
90. Sang IL, Woollacott M. Association between sensorimotor function and functional and reactive balance control in the elderly. *Age Ageing* 2005;34(4):358-363.
91. Mackey DC, Robinovitch SN. Postural steadiness during quiet stance does not associate with ability to recover balance in older women. *Clin Biomech* 2005;20(8):776-783.
92. Shumway-Cook A, Woollacott MH. Abnormal postural control. In Shumway-Cook A, Woollacott MH (eds), *Motor Control Theory and Practical Applications,* 2nd ed. Philadelphia: Lippincott Williams & Wilkins, 2001. pp. 248-270.
93. Shumway-Cook A, Woollacott MH. Abnormal mobility. In Shumway-Cook A, Woollacott MH (eds), *Motor Control Theory and Practical Applications,* 2nd ed. Philadelphia: Lippincott Williams & Wilkins, 2001. pp. 368-396.
94. Shumway-Cook A, Woollacott MN. Abnormal reach, grasp, and manipulation. In Shumway-Cook A, Woollacott MH (eds), *Motor Control Theory and Practical Applications,* 2nd ed. Philadelphia: Lippincott Williams & Wilkins, 2001. pp. 497-516.
95. Stout JL. Gait: development and analysis. In Campbell SK, Vander Linden DW, Palisano RJ (eds), *Physical Therapy for Children,* 3rd ed. St. Louis: Mosby, 2006. pp. 161-190.
96. Shumway-Cook A, Woollacott MH. Control of normal mobility. In Shumway-Cook A, Woollacott MH (eds), *Motor Control Theory and Practical Applications,* 2nd ed. Philadelphia: Lippincott Williams & Wilkins, 2001. pp. 305-337.
97. Shumway-Cook A, Woollacott MH. Normal reach, grasp and manipulation. In Shumway-Cook A, Woollacott MH (eds), *Motor Control Theory and Practical Applications,* 2nd ed. Philadelphia: Lippincott Williams & Wilkins, 2001. pp. 447-470.
98. Olney SJ, Wright MJ. Cerebral palsy. In Campbell SK, Vander Linden DW, Palisano RJ (eds), *Physical Therapy for Children,* 3rd ed. St. Louis: Mosby, 2006. pp. 625-679.
99. Kersten P. Principles of physiotherapy assessment and outcome measures. In Stokes M (ed), *Physical Management in Neurological Rehabilitation,* 2nd ed. Edinburgh: Mosby; 2004. pp. 29-46.
100. Orlin MN, Lowes LP. Musculoskeletal system: structure, function, and evaluation. In Effgen SK (ed), *Meeting the Physical Therapy Needs of Children,* Philadelphia: F.A. Davis, 2005. pp. 131-154.
101. Westcott SL, Goulet C. Neuromuscular system: structures, functions, diagnoses, and evaluation. In Effgen SK (ed), *Meeting the Physical Therapy Needs of Children,* Philadelphia: F.A. Davis, 2005. pp. 185-244.
102. Lazaro RT, Roller M, Umphred DA. Differential diagnosis phase 2: examination and evaluation of disabilities and impairments. In Umphred DA (ed), *Neurological Rehabilitation,* 4th ed. St. Louis: Mosby, 2001. pp. 43-55.
103. Fuller G. *Neurological Examination Made Easy.* Edinburgh: Churchill Livingstone, 1999.
104. Bohannon RW, Smith MB. Interrater reliability of a modified Ashworth scale of muscle spasticity. *Phys Ther* 1987;67(2):206-207.
105. O'Sullivan SB. Assessment of motor function. In O'Sullivan SB, Schmitz TJ (eds), *Physical Rehabilitation: Assessment and Treatment,* 4th ed. Philadelphia: F.A. Davis, 2001. pp. 177-212.
106. Fahn S, Elton RL. Unified Parkinson's disease rating scale. In Fahn S, Marsden CD, Goldstein M, et al (eds), *Recent Development in Parkinson's Disease,* New York: Macmillan, 1987. pp. 153-163.
107. Fellows SJ, Kaus C, Thilman AF. Voluntary movement of the elbow in spastic hemiparesis. *Ann Neurol* 1994;36(3):397-407.
108. Zackowski KM, Dromerick AW, Sahrman SA, et al. How do strength, sensation, spasticity, and joint individuation relate to the reaching deficits of people with chronic hemiparesis? *Brain* 2004;127(5):1035-1046.
109. Chambers HG. Treatment of functional limitations at the knee in ambulatory children with cerebral palsy. *Eur J Neurol* 2001;8(s5):59-74.
110. Richardson D. Physical therapy in spasticity. *Eur J Neurol* 2002;9(s1):17-22.
111. Eberly V, Kubota K, Weiss W. To brace or not to brace: making evidenced based decisions with our clients with neurological impairments. Session handouts, American Physical Therapy Association Combined Sections Meeting, San Diego, February 2, 2006.
112. Racette W. Orthotics: evaluation, prognosis, and intervention. In Umphred DA (ed), *Neurological Rehabilitation,* 4th ed. St. Louis: Mosby; 2001. pp. 937-950.
113. Edelstein JA, Bruckner J. *Orthotics: A Comprehensive Clinical Approach.* Thorofare, NJ: Slack, 2002.
114. deWitt DCM, Buurke JH, Nijlant JMM, et al. The effect of an ankle foot orthosis on walking ability in chronic stroke patients: a randomized controlled trial. *Clin Rehabil* 2004;18(5):550-557.

115. Katz K. Early mobilization after sliding Achilles tendon lengthening in children with spastic cerebral palsy. *Foot Ankle Int* 2000;21(12):1011-1014.
116. Park ES, Sussman M. Effects of dynamic ankle-foot orthoses on standing in children with severe spastic diplegia. *Int J Ther Rehabil* 2005;12(5):200-207.
117. Bottos M, Benedetti MG, Salucci P, et al. Botulinum toxin with and without casting in ambulant children with spastic diplegia: a clinical and functional assessment. *Dev Med Child Neurol* 2003;45(11):758-762.
118. O'Donnell M, Armstrong R. Pharmacologic interventions for management of spasticity in cerebral palsy. *Ment Retard Dev Disabil Res Rev* 1997;3(2):204-211.
119. Gladson B. Antispasticity medications and skeletal muscle relaxants. In Gladson B (ed), *Pharmacology for Physical Therapists.* St. Louis: Saunders Elsevier; 2006. pp. 327-344.
120. Khanderia M. Drug treatments in neurological rehabilitation. In Stokes M (ed), *Physical Management in Neurological Rehabilitation,* 2nd ed. Edinburgh: Mosby, 2004. pp. 469-485.
121. Smith TJ, Runion H. The impact of drug therapies on neurological rehabilitation. In Umphred DA (ed), *Neurological Rehabilitation,* 4th ed. St. Louis: Mosby; 2001. pp. 951-961.
122. Hagglund A. Prevention of severe contractures might replace multilevel surgery in cerebral palsy; results of a population-based health care programme and new techniques to reduce spasticity. *J Ped Orthop B* 2005;14(4):269-273.
123. Koman LA, Paterson-Smith B, Balkrishnan R. Spasticity associated with cerebral palsy in children; guidelines for the use of Botulinum A toxin. *Pediatr Drugs* 2003;5(1):1-23.
124. Skidmore-Roth L. *Mosby's 2006 Nursing Drug Reference.* St. Louis: Mosby, 2005.
125. Buffenoir K. Spastic equinus foot: multicenter study of the long term results of tibial neurotomy. *Neurosurgery* 2004;55(5):1130-1137.
126. Karol LA. Surgical management of the lower extremity in ambulatory children with cerebral palsy. *J Am Acad Orthop Surg* 2004;12(3):196-203.
127. Sayli U, Avci S. Multiple simultaneous approach in lower extremity spasticity surgery. *J Musculoskel Res* 2000;4(3): 221-229.
128. Noonan KJ, Jones J, Pierson J, et al. Hip function in adults with cerebral palsy. *J Bone Joint Surg Am* 2004;86(12): 2607-2613.
129. Gormley ME, Krach L, Paccini L. Spasticity management in the child with spastic quadriplegia. *Eur J Neurol* 2001;5(8):127-135.
130. Woo R. Spasticity: Orthopedic Perspective. *J Child Neurol* 2001;16(1):47-53.
131. Fuller DA. The impact of instrumented gait analysis on surgical planning: treatment of spastic equinovarus deformity of the foot and ankle. *Foot Ankle Int* 2002;23(8):738-743.
132. Kay RM. Outcome of gastrocnemius recession and tendo-achilles lengthening in ambulatory children with cerebral palsy. *J Pediatr Orthop B* 2004;13(2):92-98.
133. Smith PA. Gait analysis for children and adolescents with spinal cord injuries. *J Spinal Cord Med* 2004;27(Suppl): S44-49.
134. Pirpiris M. Femoral derotation osteotomy in spastic diplegia: proximal or distal? *J Bone Joint Surg Br* 2003;85B(2):265-272.
135. Kay RM. Outcome of medial vs. combined medial and lateral hamstring lengthening surgery in cerebral palsy. *J Pediatr Orthop* 2002;22(2):169-172.
136. Perry J. The use of gait analysis for surgical recommendations in traumatic brain injury. *J Head Trauma Rehabil* 1999;14(2):116-135.
137. Horn TS. Effect of intrathecal baclofen bolus injection on temporospatial gait characteristics in patients with acquired brain injury. *Arch Phys Med Rehabil* 2005;86(6):1127-1133.
138. Chantraine R. Effect of rectus femoris motor branch block on post-stroke stiff legged gait. *Acta Neurol Belg* 2005;105(3):171-177.
139. Gajdosik CG, Gajdoski RL. Musculoskeletal development and adaptation. In Campbell SK, Vander Linden DW, Palisano RJ (eds), *Physical Therapy for Children,* 3rd ed. St. Louis: Saunders, 2005. pp. 191-216.
140. What types of interventions do physical therapists provide? Guide to physical therapist practice. *Phys Ther* 2001;18(1):105-121.
141. Pflett PJ. Rehabilitation of spasticity and related problems in childhood cerebral palsy. *J Paediatr Child Health* 2003;39(1):6-14.
142. Cadenhead SL, McEwen IR, Thomson DM. Effect of passive range of motion exercises on lower extremity goniometric measurements of adults with cerebral palsy. *Phys Ther* 2002;82(7):658-699.
143. Tardieu C, Lespargot A, Tabary C, et al. For how long must the soleus muscle be stretched each day to prevent contracture? *Dev Med Child Neurol* 1998;30(1):3-10.
144. Deitz V. Gait disorder in spasticity and Parkinson's disease. *Adv Neurol* 2001;87(2):143-154.
145. Redstone F. The importance of postural control for feeding. *Pediatr Nurs* 2004;Mar-Apr;30(2):97-100.
146. McDonald R, Surtees R, Wirz S. The International Classification of Functioning, Disability and Health provides a model for adaptive seating interventions for children with cerebral palsy. *Br J Occup Ther* 2004;67(7):293-302.
147. Kanyer B. Meeting the seating and mobility needs of the client with traumatic brain injury. *J Head Trauma Rehabil* 1992;7(3):81-93.
148. Herman JH, Lange ML. Seating and positioning to manage spasticity after brain injury. *Neurorehabilitation* 1999;12(2):105-117.
149. Taylor SJ. Innovations in practice: an overview of evaluation for wheelchair seating for people who have had stroke. *Top Stroke Rehabil* 2003;10(1):95-99.
150. Gudjonsdottir B, Mercer VS. Effects of a dynamic versus static prone stander on bone mineral density and behavior in four children with severe cerebral palsy. *Pediatr Phys Ther* 2002;14(1):38-46.
151. Hong CW. Assessment for and provision of positioning equipment for children with motor impairments. *Int Ther Rehabil* 2005;12(3):126-131.
152. Jones MA, Gray S. Assistive technology: positioning and mobility. In Effgen SK (ed), *Meeting the Physical Therapy Needs of Children.* Philadelphia: F.A. Davis, 2005. pp. 455-474.
153. Thorton H, Kilbride C. Physical management of abnormal tone and movement. In Stokes M (ed), *Physical Management*

in Neurological Rehabilitation, 2nd ed. Edinburgh: Mosby, 2004. pp. 431-450.

154. Beatty PW, Hagglund KJ, Neri MT, et al. Access to health care services among people with chronic or disabling conditions: patterns and predictors. *Arch Phys Med Rehabil* 2003;84(10): 1417-1425.
155. Bingham SC, Beatty PW. Rates of access to assistive equipment and medical rehabilitation services among people with disabilities. *Disabil Rehabil* 2003;25(9):487-490.
156. Cottalorda J, Gautheron V, Metton G, et al. Toe walking in children younger than six years with cerebral palsy: the contribution of serial corrective casts. *J Bone Joint Surg* 2000;82B(4):541-544.
157. Brouwer B, Davidson LK, Olney SJ. Serial casting in idiopathic toe-walkers and children with spastic cerebral palsy. *J Pediatr Orthop* 2000;20(2):221-225.
158. Phillips WE, Audet M. Use of serial casting in the management of knee joint contractures in an adolescent with cerebral palsy. *Phys Ther* 1990;70(8):521-523.
159. Brouwer B, Wheeldon RK, Allum J. Reflex excitability and isometric force production in cerebral palsy: the effect of serial casting. *Dev Med Child Neurol* 1998;40(2): 168-175.
160. Conine TA, Sullivan T, Mackie T, et al. Effect of serial casting for the prevention of equinus deformity in patients with acute head injury. *Arch Phys Med Rehabil* 1990;71:310-312.
161. Wilton J. Casting, splinting, and physical and occupational therapy of hand deformity and dysfunction in cerebral palsy. *Hand Clin* 2003;19(4):573-584.
162. Kay RM, Rethlefsen SA, Fern Buneo A. Botulinum toxin as an adjunct to serial casting treatment in children with cerebral palsy. *J Bone Joint Surg* 2004;86(11):2377-2384.
163. Stoeckmann T. Casting for the person with spasticity. *Top Stroke Rehabil* 2001;8(1):27-35.
164. Boyd R, Havys RM. Current evidence for the use of botulinum toxin A in the management of children with cerebral palsy: a systematic review. *Eur J Neurol* 2001; 8(Suppl 5):S1-S20.
165. Gaebler-Spira D, Revivo G. The use of botulinum toxin in pediatric disorders. *Phys Med Rehabil Clin North Am* 2003;14(4):703-725.
166. Marushi M. Cerebral palsy in adults: independent effects of muscle strength and muscle tone. *Arch Phys Med Rehabil* 2001;82(5):637-641.
167. Dodd KJ, Taylor NF, Damiano DL. A systematic review of the effectiveness of strength-training programs for people with cerebral palsy. *Arch Phys Med Rehabil* 2002;83(8): 1157-1164.
168. Haslekorn JK, Loomis S. Multiple sclerosis and spasticity. *Phys Med Rehabil Clin North Am* 2005;16(2):467-481.
169. Morris SL, Dodd KJ, Morris ME. Outcomes of progressive resistance strength training following stroke; a systematic review. *Clin Rehabil* 2004;18(1):27-39.
170. Foran JR, Steinman S, Barash I, et al. Structural and mechanical alterations in spastic skeletal muscle. *Dev Med Child Neurol* 2005;47(10):713-717.
171. Corry IS, Cosgrove AP, Duffy CM, et al. Botulinum toxin A compared with stretching casts in the treatment of spastic equinus: a randomized prospective trial. *J Pediatr Orthop* 1998;18(30):304-311.
172. Hagglund G, Anderson S, Duppe H, et al. Prevention of severe contractures might replace multilevel surgery in cerebral palsy: results of a population-based health care programme and new techniques to reduce spasticity. *J Pediatr Orthop* 2005;14(4):269-273.
173. Molenaers G, Desloovere K, Fabry G, et al. The effects of quantitative gait assessment and botulinum toxin A on musculoskeletal surgery in children with cerebral palsy. *J Bone Joint Surg* 2006;88A(1):161-170.
174. Leahy P. Precasting worksheet: an assessment tool. *Phys Ther* 1988;68(1):72-74.
175. Nawoczenski DA. Introduction to orthotics: rationale for treatment. In Nawoczenski DA, Eppler ME (eds), *Orthotics in Functional Rehabilitation of the Lower Limb.* Philadelphia: Saunders, 1997. pp. 1-13.
176. Hanna D, Harvey RL. Review of preorthotic biomechanical considerations. *Top Stroke Rehabil* 2001;7(4):29-37.
177. Buckon CE, Thomas SS, Jakobson-Huston S, et al. Comparison of three ankle foot orthoses configurations for children with spastic diplegia. *Dev Med Child Neurol* 2004;46(9):590-598.
178. Teasell RW. Physical and functional correlations of ankle foot orthoses use in the rehabilitation of stroke patients. *Arch Phys Med Rehabil* 2001;82(8):1047-1049.
179. Smiley SJ, Jacobsen FS, Mielke C, et al. A comparison of the effects of solid ankle, articulated, and posterior leaf-spring ankle foot orthoses and shoes alone on gait and energy expenditures in children with spastic diplegic cerebral palsy. *Orthopedics* 2002;25(4):411-415.
180. Carlson WE, Vaughan CL, Damiano DL, et al. Orthotic management of gait in spastic diplegia. *Phys Med Rehabil* 1997;76(3):219-225.
181. Buckon CE. Comparison of three ankle foot orthosis configurations for children with spastic hemiplegia. *Dev Med Child Neurol* 2001;43(6):371-378.
182. Radtka SA. A comparison of gait with solid, dynamic, and no ankle foot orthoses in children with spastic diplegia. *Phys Ther* 1997;77(4):395-409.
182. Wang R, Yen L, Wang M, et al. Effects of ankle foot orthoses on balance performance in patients with hemiparesis of different durations. *Clin Rehabil* 2005;19(1):37-44.
183. Park ES, Park CI, Chang HJ, et al. The effect of hinged ankle-foot orthoses on sit-to-stand transfer in children with spastic cerebral palsy. *Arch Phys Med Rehabil* 2004;85(12): 2053-2057.
184. Zablotny CM. Use of orthoses for the adult with neurological involvement. In Nawoczenski DA, Eppler ME (eds), *Orthotics in Functional Rehabilitation of the Lower Limb.* Philadelphia: Saunders, 1997. pp. 205-243.
185. Stanger M. Use of orthoses in pediatrics. In Nawoczenski DA, Eppler ME. *Orthotics in Functional Rehabilitation of the Lower Limb.* Philadelphia: Saunders, 1997. pp. 245-372.
186. Oatis CA, Cipriany-Dacko BH. Perspectives on examination, evaluation, and intervention for disorders of gait. In Montgomery PC, Connolly BH (eds). *Clinical Applications for Motor Control.* Thorofare, NJ: Slack, 2003. pp. 335-363.
187. Beals RB. The possible effects of solid ankle foot orthoses on trunk posture in the non-ambulatory cerebral palsy population: a preliminary evaluation. *J Prosthet Orthot* 2001;13(2):34.

188. Crenshaw S, Herzog R, Castagno P, et al. The efficacy of tone reducing features in orthotics on the gait of children with spastic diplegic cerebral palsy. *J Pediatr Orthop* 2000;20(2): 210-216.
189. Lohman M, Goldstein H. Alternative strategies in tone-reducing AFO design. *J Prosthet Orthot* 1993;5(1):1.
190. Thompson NS, Taylor TC, McCarthy KR, et al. Effect of a rigid ankle foot orthosis on hamstring length on children with hemiplegia. *Dev Med Child Neurol* 2002;44(1):51-57.
191. Yamanaka T, Ishii M; Suzuki H. Short leg brace and stroke rehabilitation. *Top Stroke Rehabil* 2004;11(3):3-5.
192. Cattaneio D, Marazzini F, Crippa A, et al. Do static or dynamic AFOs improve balance? *Clin Rehabil* 2002;16(8):894-899.
193. Edelstein JE. Orthotic options for standing and walking. *Top Spinal Cord Inj Rehabil* 2000;5(4):11-23.
194. Atrice MB. Lower extremity orthotic management for the spinal cord injured client. *Top Spinal Cord Inj Rehabil* 2000;5(4):1-10.
195. Thomas SS, Buckon CE, Melchionni J, et al. Longitudinal assessment of oxygen cost and velocity in children with myelomeningocele: comparison of the hip knee ankle foot orthosis and the reciprocating gait orthosis. *J Pediatr Orthop* 2001;21(6):798-803.
196. Stallard J, Lomas B, Woollam P, et al. New technical advances in swivel walkers. *Prosthet Orthot Int* 2003;27(2):132-128.
197. Katz-Leurer M, Weber C, Smerling-Kerem J, et al. Prescribing the reciprocal gait orthosis for myelomeningocele children: a different approach and clinical outcome. *Pediatr Rehabil* 2004;7(2):105-109.
198. Polliack AA, Elliot S, Landsberger SE, et al. Lower extremity orthoses for children with myelomeningocele: user and orthotist perspectives. *J Prosthet Orthot* 2001;13(4):123-129.
199. Bakker JP, deGroot IJ, Beckerman H, et al. The effects of knee ankle foot orthoses in the treatment of Duchenne muscular dystrophy: review of the literature. *Clin Rehabil* 2000;14(4):343-359.
200. Siegel IM, Bernardoni G. Orthotic management of equinus in early Duchenne muscular dystrophy. *J Neuro Rehab* 1997;11(1):1-5.
201. Taktak DM, Bowker P. Lightweight modular knee ankle foot orthoses for Duchenne muscular dystrophy: design, development, and evaluation. *Arch Phys Med Rehabil* 1995;76:1156-1162.
202. Siegel IM. Kinematics of gait in Duchenne muscular dystrophy: implications of orthotic management. *J Neuro Rehab* 1997;11(3):169-173.
203. *Observational Gait Analysis,* Downey, CA: Pathokinesiology Service & Physical Therapy Department, Rancho Los Amigos Medical Center, 1993.
204. Inman VT, Ralston HJ, Todd F. *Human Walking.* Baltimore: Williams & Wilkins, 1981.
205. Craik RL, Oatis CA. *Gait Analysis: Theory and Application.* St. Louis: Mosby, 1995.

al plateau (Figure 13-1). These menisci increase ·ity of the tibial articular surface, enhancing con- f articulation with the femoral condyles to facili- al gliding and distribute weight-bearing forces knee during gait and other loading activities.[4] The

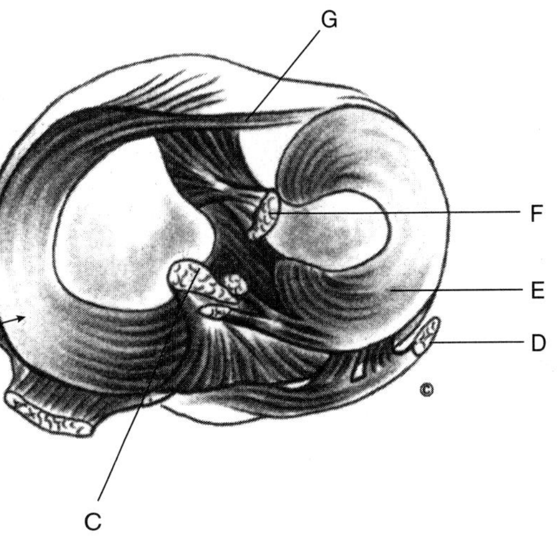

Figure 13-1
*v of the surface of the tibia, we can identify the 'ateral ligament (**A**), the C-shaped medial meniscus e medial tibial plateau (**B**), the posterior cruciate /ith the accessory anterior and posterior noral ligaments (**C**), the tendon of the popliteus), the circular lateral meniscus on the smaller al plateau (**E**), the anterior cruciate ligament as it ird the inside of the lateral femoral condyle (**F**), insverse ligament (**G**). (From Greenfield BH.* tion of the Knee: A Problem Solving Approach. *ia: F.A. Davis, 1993.)*

menisci also play an important role in nutrition and lubrication of the articular surfaces of the knee joint.

Although contraction of the quadriceps and knee flexor muscle groups produces compressive forces that help to stabilize the knee, most of the knee's stability is provided by two sets of ligaments. The collateral ligaments counter valgus and varus forces that act on the knee. The cruciate ligaments check translatory forces that displace the tibia on the femur. The location of attachments makes each of these ligaments most effective at particular places in the knee's normal arch of motion.[4]

Medial Collateral Ligament

The medial (tibial) collateral ligament (MCL) is a strong, flat, membranous band that overlays the middle portion of the medial joint capsule (Figure 13-2, *A*). It is most effective in counteracting valgus stressors when the knee is slightly flexed to fully extended. Approximately 8 to 10 cm in length, it originates at the medial epicondyle of the femur and attaches to the medial surface of the tibial plateau. The MCL can be subdivided into a set of oblique posterior fibers and anterior parallel fibers.

A bundle of meniscotibial fibers, also known as the *posterior oblique ligament*, runs deep to the MCL, from the femur to the midperipheral margin of the medial meniscus and toward the tibia. These fibers connect the medial meniscus to the tibia and help to form the semimembranosus corner of the medial knee.

Lateral Collateral Ligament and Iliotibial Band

The lateral (fibular) collateral ligament (LCL) resists varus stressors and lateral rotation of the tibia and is most effective when the knee is slightly flexed. The LCL runs from the lateral femoral condyle (the back part of the outer tuberosity

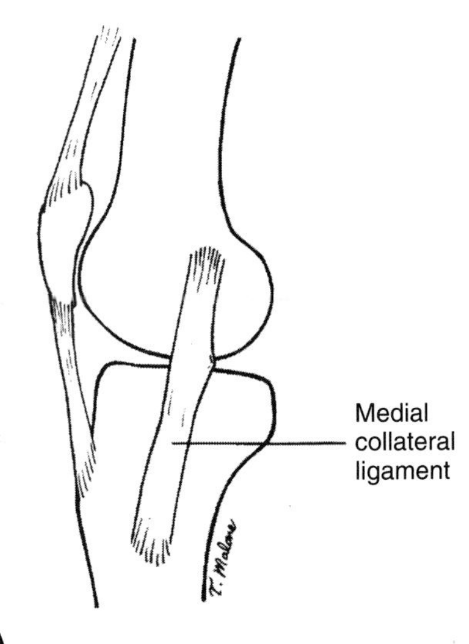

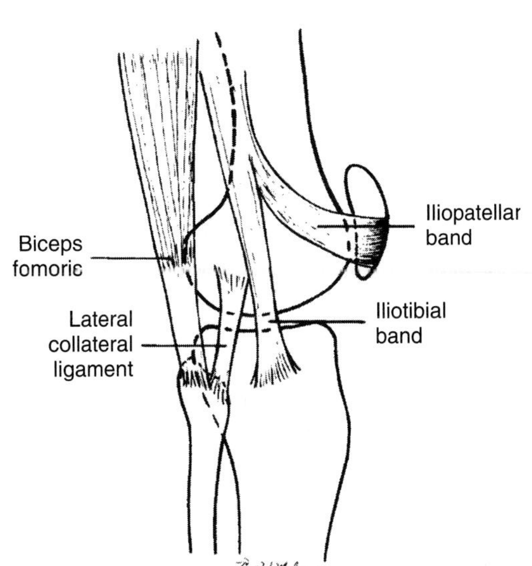

Figure 13-2
*f the medial collateral ligament (**A**) and lateral collateral ligament and iliotibial band (**B**). (From Norkin CC, Levangie* Structure and Function: A Comprehensive Analysis, *ed 2. Philadelphia: F.A. Davis, 1992.)*

13

Orthotic Options for Knee Instabil
and Pain

JOHN F. KNECHT AND ELLEN WETHERBEE

LEARNING OBJECTIVES

On completion of this chapter, the reader will be able to do the following:

1. Describe the normal anatomical structure and biomechanical function (kinematic and kinetic) of the human tibiofemoral and patellofemoral joints.
2. Explain the most common mechanisms of injury to the knee.
3. Compare and contrast the purposes, indications, and limitations of rehabilitative, functional, and prophylactic knee orthoses.
4. Identify the force vectors used to control knee motion used in various designs of knee orthoses.
5. Use evidence of efficacy of various knee orthoses to select the most appropriate device for a given injury to the knee.

Although knee orthoses have long been used as a means of protection and stabilization of the knee joint, their effectiveness in preventing ligamentous injury or in stabilizing a knee with ligamentous insufficiency has not been well supported by research findings.[1,2] In 1984 the American Academy of Orthopaedic Surgeons developed a classification system that groups knee orthoses by their intended function.[3] Prophylactic knee orthoses are designed to reduce the risk of knee injury for individuals engaged in "high-risk" activities, especially those who have a history of previous knee dysfunction. Rehabilitative knee orthoses are used to protect a knee that has been injured or surgically repaired until adequate tissue healing has occurred. Functional knee orthoses (FKOs) are intented to provide biomechanical stability when ligaments are unable to do so during daily activities. This functional classification system continues to be helpful for physical therapists (PTs), orthotists, and athletic trainers who work with patients who have knee dysfunction.

ANATOMY

To select the most appropri knee dysfunction, a clinician of normal knee structure an chapter begins with a revi mechanical stability of the and the physiological an tibiofemoral and patellofem tional goals of prefabrica orthoses and indications for ment of common knee i examined next. Finally the clinical decision making in tional orthosis for active p mentous instability of the kn

Tibiofen

The knee joint is a hinge medial and lateral condyles o lateral tibial plateau. Becaus of the condyles, the instanta extension motion changes t open chain movements (foo tibia rotates around the fen movements (foot-on-the-gr "locking" mechanism is pres sion, as the longer medial fe on the articular surfaces of t an adducted femur and re vulnerability to valgus stress ties. The capsule that encas by the collagen-rich medial medial and lateral menisci ring-shaped disks that are att

of the til the conc gruency tate nor within th

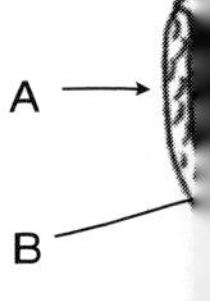

In this vi medial c on the la ligament meniscof muscle (I lateral tib twists tov and the t Rehabilit *Philadelp*

Positions PK. Joint

of the femur) to the proximal lateral aspect of the fibular head (see Figure 13-2, *B*). The tendon of the popliteus muscle and the external articular vessels and nerves pass beneath this ligament.

The iliotibial band (ITB) is positioned slightly anterior to the LCL and is taut in all ranges of knee motion. Although the ITB's position allows it to stabilize against varus forces, as does the LCL, the ITB also appears to assist the anterior cruciate ligament (ACL), preventing posterior displacement of the tibia when the knee is extended.[5]

Anterior Cruciate Ligament

The ACL runs at an oblique angle between the articular surfaces of the knee joint and acts to prevent forward shift and excessive medial rotation of the tibia as the knee moves toward extension (Figure 13-3; see also Figure 13-1). The ACL attaches to the tibia in a fossa just anterior and lateral to the anterior tibial spine and to the femur in a fossa on the posteromedial surface of the lateral femoral condyle. The ACL's tibial attachment is somewhat wider and stronger than its femoral attachment. Some authors divide the fasciculi that make up the broad, slightly flat ACL into two or three distinct bundles. The ligament's anteromedial band, with fibers running from the anteromedial tibia to the proximal femoral attachment, is most taut in flexion and relatively lax in extension. The posterolateral bulk (PLB), which begins at the posterolateral tibial attachment, is most taut in extension and relatively lax in flexion. An intermediate bundle of transitional fibers between the anteromedial band and PLB tends to tighten when the knee moves through the midranges of motion. This arrangement of fibers ensures tension in the ACL throughout the entire range of knee motion. The ACL is most vulnerable to injury when the femur rotates internally on the tibia when the knee is flexed and the foot is fixed on the ground during weight-bearing activities.[6]

Posterior Cruciate Ligament

The posterior cruciate ligament (PCL) restrains posterior displacement of the tibia in its articulation with the femur, especially as the knee moves toward full extension.[4] The PCL is shorter and less oblique in orientation than the ACL; it is the strongest and most resistant ligament of the knee. PCL fibers run from a slight depression between articular surfaces on the posterior tibia to the posterolateral surface of the medial femoral condyle (see Figures 13-1 and 13-3). Like the ACL, the PCL can be divided into anterior and posterior segments. The larger anterior medial band is most taut between 80 and 90 degrees of flexion and is relatively lax in extension. The smaller PLB travels somewhat obliquely across the joint, becoming taut as the knee moves into extension. The PCL plays a role in the locking mechanism of the knee, as tension in the ligament produces lateral (external) rotation of the tibia on the femur in the final degrees of knee extension. The PCL may also assist the collateral ligaments when varus or valgus stressors are applied to the knee.[4]

The meniscofemoral ligament, stretching between the posterior horn of the lateral meniscus and the lateral surface of the medial femoral condyle, along with fibers of the PCL, has sometimes been described as a *third cruciate ligament.*[7] The anterior meniscofemoral band (Humphry's ligament) runs along the medial anterior surface of the PCL and may be up to one-third its diameter. The posterior meniscofemoral band (Wrisberg's ligament) lies posterior to the PCL and may be as much as one-half its diameter. The meniscofemoral ligaments act to pull the lateral meniscus forward during flexion of the weight-bearing knee, to maintain as much articular congruency as possible with the lateral femoral condyle.

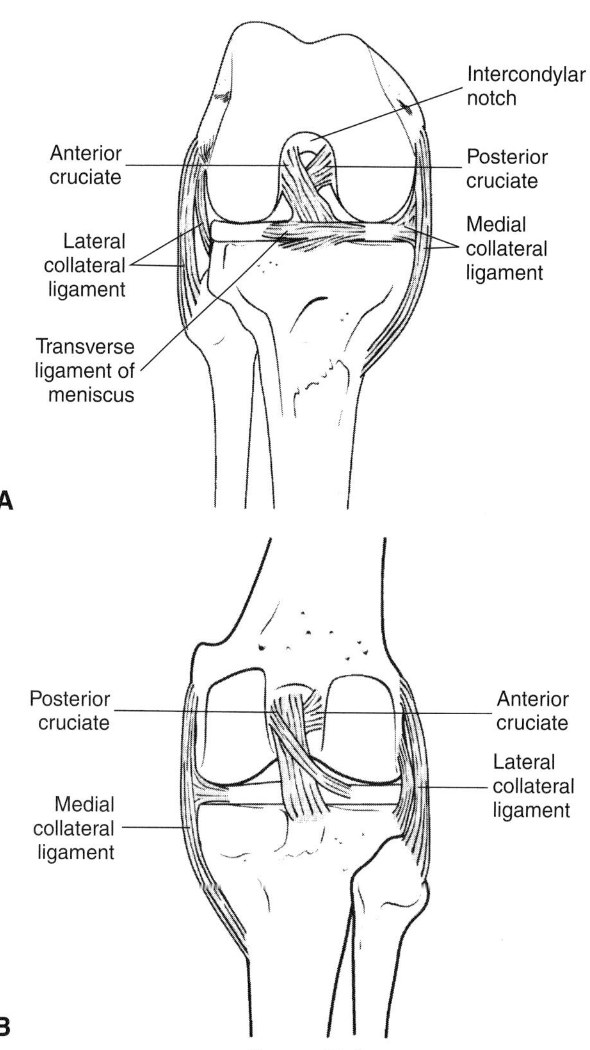

Figure 13-3

A, *Anterior view of the tibiofemoral joint in 90 degrees of knee flexion showing the menisci and the ligamentous structures that stabilize the knee.* ***B,*** *Posterior view of the knee in extension. (From Antich TJ. Orthoses for the knee; the tibiofemoral joint. In Nawoczenski DA, Epler ME [eds],* Orthotics in Functional Rehabilitation of the Lower Limb. *Philadelphia: Saunders, 1997.)*

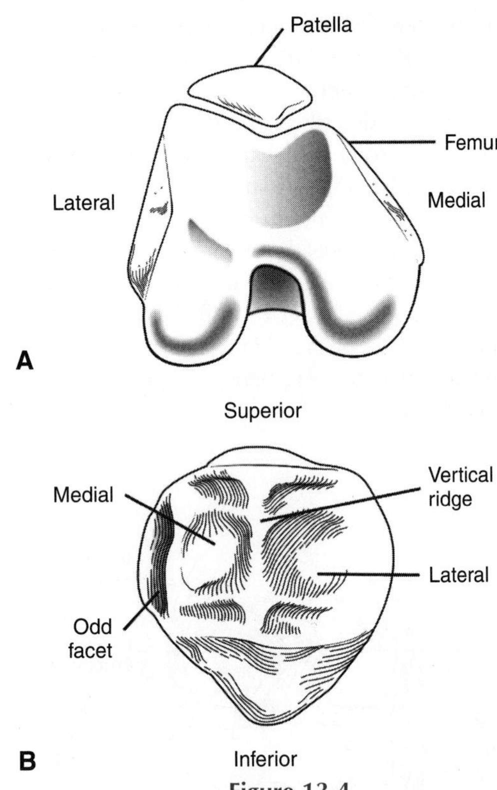

Figure 13-4

A, *The normal position of the patella in the intercondylar groove of the distal femur.* **B,** *Underside of the patella with its three facets and vertical ridge. (From Belyea BC. Orthoses for the knee: The patellofemoral joint. In Nawoczenski DA, Epler ME [eds],* Orthotics in Functional Rehabilitation of the Lower Limb. *Philadelphia: Saunders, 1997. pp.32-33.)*

Posterolateral Corner of the Knee

The lateral meniscus is somewhat more mobile than the medial meniscus because of the anatomy of the posterolateral corner of the knee. The arcuate complex and posterolateral corner run from the styloid process of the fibula, joining the posterior oblique ligament on the posterior aspect of the femur and tibia. The arcuate ligament is firmly attached to the underlying popliteus muscle and tendon. The tendon of the popliteus muscle separates the deep joint capsule from the rim of the lateral meniscus.

Patellofemoral Joint

The *patella*, a sesamoid bone embedded in the tendon of the quadriceps femoris, is an integral part of the extensor mechanism of the knee. The patella functions as an anatomical pulley, increasing the knee extension moment created by contraction of the quadriceps femoris by as much as 50%. It also guides the forces generated by the quadriceps femoris to the patellar ligament, protects deeper knee joint anatomy, protects the quadriceps tendon from frictional forces, and increases the compressive forces to which the extensor mechanisms can be subjected.[8-11]

Table 13-1

Classification of Patellar Types, Listed from Most to Least Stable

Patellar Type	*Description*
I	Equal medial and lateral facets, both slightly concave
II	Small medial facet, both facets slightly concave
II/III	Small, flat medial facet
III	Small, slightly convex medial facet
IV	Very small, steeply sloped medial facet, with medial ridge
V (Jagerhut)	No medial facet, no central ridge

Although the anterior surface of the patella is convex, the posterior surface has three distinct anatomical areas: lateral, medial, and "odd" facets. The lateral and medial facets are separated by a vertical ridge. The odd facet articulates with the medial condyle at the end range of knee extension (Figure 13-4). The posterior patellar surface is covered with hyaline articular cartilage, except for the distal apex, which is roughened for the attachment of the patellar tendon. Pressure between the patella and trochlear groove of the femur increases substantially as the knee flexes. During knee flexion, the patella moves in a complex but consistent three-dimensional pattern of flexion/extension rotation, medial/lateral rotation, medial/lateral tilt (also described as wavering), and a medial/lateral shift relative to the femur.[9,11] These motions occur biomechanically in the X, Y, and Z planes.

The stability of the patella is derived from the patellofemoral joint's static structural characteristics and dynamic (muscular) control. Static stability is a product of the anatomy of the patella, the depth of the intercondylar groove, and the prominent and longer lateral condyle of the femur. The sulcus angle, formed by the sloping edges of the condyles, is normally between 114 and 120 degrees; however, it can vary significantly from person to person.[12] Wiberg[13] divides the patellofemoral joint into six types based on the size and shape of facets (Table 13-1). The depth of the patellar trochlea and the facet pattern are important in patellar stability.

Dynamic stability of the patellofemoral joint is derived primarily from activity of the quadriceps femoris, as well as from the tensile properties of the patellar ligament (Figure 13-5). The four components of the quadriceps muscle act together to pull the patella obliquely upward along the shaft of the femur, whereas the patellar ligament anchors it almost straight downward along the anatomical axis of the lower leg. The tibial tubercle is typically located at least 6 degrees lateral to the mechanical axis of the femur.

Because the structure of the patellofemoral articulation and the muscular and ligamentous forces that act on the

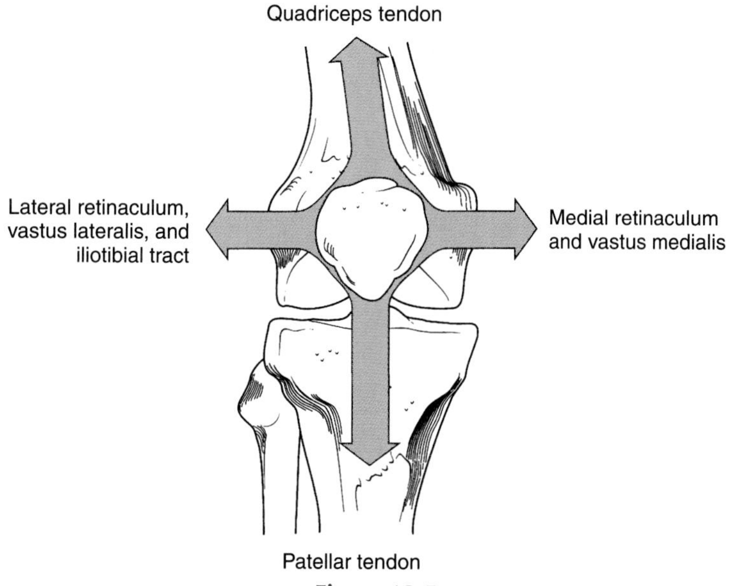

Figure 13-5

Structures that provide dynamic stability for the patella. (From Belyea BC. Orthoses for the knee: the patellofemoral joint. In Nawoczenski DA, Epler ME [eds], Orthotics in Functional Rehabilitation of the Lower Limb. *Philadelphia: Saunders, 1997.)*

patella are complex, patellar dynamics involve much more than simple cephalocaudal repositioning as the knee is flexed or extended. Van Kampen and Huiskes[11] describe the three-dimensional motions of the patella as flexion rotation, medial rotation, wavering tilt, and lateral shift. All of these patellar movements (except flexion) are influenced by the rotation of the tibia and the dynamic stabilization of the muscles that act on the patella.

BIOMECHANICS OF KNEE MOTION

Evaluating and managing knee injuries requires an in-depth understanding of the biomechanical characteristics of the knee joint. The *kinematics of the knee* describe its motion in terms of the type and location and the magnitude and direction of the motion.[14] The *kinetics of the knee* describe the forces that act on the knee, causing movement.[14] Kinetic forces are classified as either external forces that work on the body (e.g., gravity) or as internal, body-generated forces (e.g., friction, tensile strength of soft tissue structures, muscle contraction).

Motion in the tibiofemoral joint can be best understood by separating the motion into its physiological and accessory components. Physiological motion can be controlled consciously, most often through voluntary contraction of muscle. Osteokinematic (bone movement) and arthrokinematic (joint surface motion) are examples of physiological motion. Accessory motion occurs without conscious control and cannot be reproduced voluntarily. Joint play, which is elicited by passive movement during examination of a joint, is an example of an accessory motion. The magnitude and type of accessory motion possible are determined by the characteristics of a particular articulation and the tissue properties that surround it.

An important accessory component motion of the tibiofemoral joint is its *screw home*, or locking mechanism. In the final degrees of knee extension, the tibia continues to rotate around the large articular surface of the medial femoral condyle. This motion cannot be prevented or changed by volitional effort; it is entirely the result of the configuration of the articular surfaces. When the knee is flexed to or beyond 90 degrees, however, conscious activation of muscles can produce physiological (osteokinematic) external (lateral) or internal (medial) rotation of the tibia on the femur.

Three osteokinematic motions are possible at the tibiofemoral joint. Knee flexion and extension occurs in the sagittal plane around an axis in the frontal plane (X axis). Internal and external rotation of the tibia on the femur (or vice versa) occurs in the transverse plane around a longitudinal axis (Y axis). Abduction and adduction occur in the frontal plane around a horizontal axis (Z axis). The arthrokinematic movements of the tibiofemoral joint are rolling, gliding, and sliding (Figure 13-6). It is noteworthy that the roll-glide ratio is not constant during tibiofemoral joint motion: Approximately 1:2 in early flexion, the roll-glide ratio becomes almost 1:4 in late flexion.[15] Rolling and gliding occur primarily on the posterior portion of the femoral condyles. In the first 15 to 20 degrees of flexion, a true rolling motion of the femoral condyles occurs in concert with the tibial plateau. As the magnitude of flexion increases, the femur begins to glide posteriorly on the tibia. Gliding becomes more significant as flexion increases.[7]

From a kinematic standpoint, the ACLs and PCLs operate as a true "gear" mechanism controlling the roll-glide motion of the tibiofemoral joint. With rupture of either or both of the cruciate ligaments, the gear mechanism becomes ineffective and the arthrokinematic motion is altered. In an ACL-deficient knee, the femur is able to roll beyond the posterior half of the tibial plateau, increasing the likelihood of damage or tear of the posterior horn of the medial or lateral meniscus.

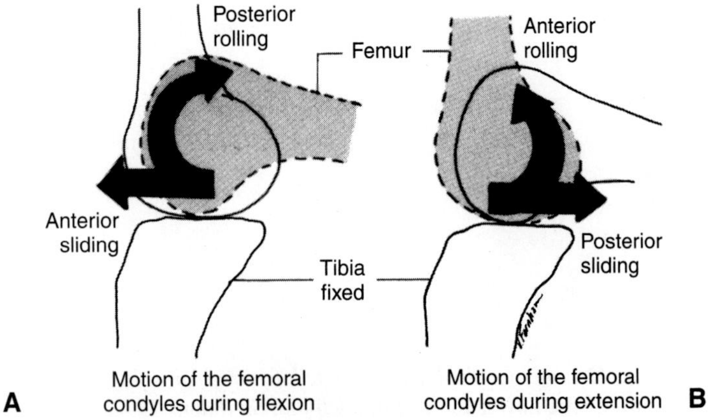

Because the knee has characteristics of a hinge joint and an arthrodial joint, two types of motion (translatory and rotatory) can occur in each plane of motion (sagittal, frontal/coronal, transverse). For this reason, knee motion is described as having 6 degrees of freedom. The three translatory motions of the knee include anteroposterior translation of 5 to 10 mm, mediolateral translation of 1 to 2 mm, and compression-distraction motion of 2 to 5 mm. The three rotatory motions occur in flexion/extension, varus/valgus, and internal (medial)/external (lateral) rotation.[4,15] Hinge design of an orthosis is discussed further in this chapter to help control these motions. Single, dual, or multiple hinged orthoses that do not conform with the anteroposterior translations or roll back and the rotation of the joint exert adverse mechanical effects.[16]

Figure 13-6

Diagram of femoral motion on a fixed tibia. ***A,*** *As the knee flexes, the femoral condyles roll posteriorly* (curved arrow) *while gliding/sliding forward* (straight arrow). ***B,*** *As the knee extends, the condyles roll forward* (curved arrow) *while gliding posteriorly* (straight arrow). *(From Norkin CC, Levangie PK.* Joint Structure and Function: A Comprehensive Analysis, *ed 2. Philadelphia: F.A. Davis, 1992.)*

ORTHOSES FOR THE KNEE

Table 13-2 lists some of the many knee orthoses that are commercially available for health professionals in sports medicine. Some are designed to immobilize the knee after surgical repair of damaged or ruptured ligaments or menisci during the acute phases of healing. *Rehabilitative orthoses* are designed to protect the knee and allow progressive increase in active range of motion (ROM) during rehabilitation.

Table 13-2
Examples of Knee Orthoses by Category and Manufacturer

Manufacturer	*Rehabilitative Knee Orthoses*	*Functional ACL/PCL*	*Functional Osteoarthritis*	*Prophylactic*	*Patellofemoral*
Bauerfeind USA Kennesaw, Ga. (800) 423 3405 www.bauerfeindusa.com		Softech Genu	Softtech OA		Genutrain P3 Comprifix
Bledsoe by Medical Technology Grand Prairie, Tex. (888) 253-3763 www.bledsoebrace.com	Extender Leverlock OR Knee Revolution	Ultimate Dynamic U^2CI Kneecage Forcelite	Thruster Aligner		Bledsoe Sport Max
Brace International Atlanta, Ga. (800) 545-1161 ww.braceint.com					FLUK Infrapatellar Strap
Cropper Medical, Inc./ Bio Skin Ashland, Ore. (541) 488-0600 ww.bioskin.com					Bioskin "Q"

Continued

Table 13-2
Examples of Knee Orthoses by Category and Manufacturer—cont'd

Manufacturer	*Rehabilitative Knee Orthoses*	*Functional ACL/PCL*	*Functional Osteoarthritis*	*Prophylactic*	*Patellofemoral*
dj Orthopedics, Inc. Vista, Calif. (800) 336-6569 www.djortho.com	Total RO ELS IROM	Defiance Forcepoint Armor Legend 4titude Playmaker	Defiance Montana Adjustor Opal	Protective-Knee Guard Playmaker	TruPull Advantage H-Buttress Air Donjoy Ontrack
Generation II USA, Inc./Ossur Bothell, Wash. (800) 462-7252 www.gen2.com		Generation II 3DX Matrix Extreme Select GII Trainers	Unloader Select Unloader Adj Unloader Spirit Unloader Bi-Com^{pf}		Patellar Stabilizer
Innovation Sports, Inc. Irvine, Calif. (800) 222-4284 www.isports.com	Sentry Knee MD Quicklock Option	CTi Edge C180 XCI Aspire CTI^2	CTI^{2}OA		Powerflex Donut Stabilizer Lateral J Stabilizer
McDavid Sports/ Medical Products Woodridge, Ill. (800) 237-8254 www. mcdavidinc.com				428 Pro Stabilizer	
Omni LifeScience/ Bodyworks North Springville, Utah (800) 448-6664 www.bw-omni.com		Icon RT and XC Rage RT and XC	V-Force		
Pro Orthopedic Devices, Inc Tuscon, Ariz. (800) 523-5611 www.proorthopedic.com					Dr. "U" Universal Patellar Brace Stabilizing Sleeve Patellar Strap
Seattle Orthopedic Group Poulsbo, Wash. (800) 248-6463 www.soginc.com		Lenox Hill Precision Lenox Hill Spectra			
Townsend Design Bakersfield, Calif. (800) 700-2722 www.townsenddesign.com	ROM EZROM	Airtownsend Ultraair Premier Series Rebel Series TS Series	Reliever Series		Neoprine Sports Brace

ACL, Anterior cruciate ligament; *PCL,* posterior cruciate ligament.

FKOs provide additional protection as rehabilitation is completed and a patient returns to normal activities. A final group, *prophylactic knee orthoses,* are intended to prevent injury (or at least lessen the extent of injury) in athletes who are at risk of injury during competition. Given the complexity of the knee joint (with its polycentric axis of rotation for flexion/extension, asymmetry of the lateral and medial compartments, and the arrangement of its muscular and ligamentous attachments), most orthotic designs cannot support, protect, or stabilize the knee with the same efficiency as its own physiological motion.

Rehabilitation Knee Orthoses

Orthoses used in the postoperative and early rehabilitation of patients who have had surgical repair of damaged ligaments are designed to control knee motion carefully to minimize excessive loading on healing tissues (Figure 13-7).[3] Although many rehabilitation knee orthoses are on the market, an effective orthosis has several important characteristics. The orthosis must be adjustable to accommodate for changes in limb girth due to edema or to atrophy. It must remain in the desired position on the limb during upright and sitting activities. It must be comfortable to wear, easy to don and doff, durable, and economical. Most physicians require an adjustable knee unit so that "free" active ROM can be increased incrementally as the patient's condition improves. The ability to move in carefully controlled ranges of motion is thought to improve ligamentous strength and to minimize the risk of scar formation in the intracondylar notch that is associated with flexion contractor.[15]

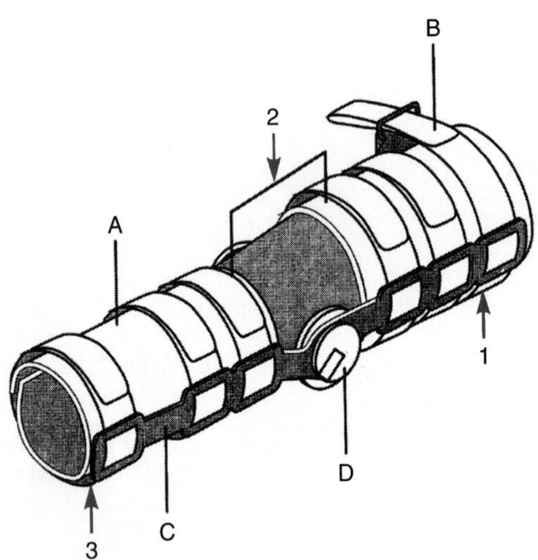

Figure 13-7
The components of most commercially available rehabilitation knee orthoses include open cell foam interface that encase the calf and thigh (A) *and nonelastic, adjustable Velcro strap for closures* (B)*; lightweight metal, composite, or plastic sidebars* (C)*; and single-axis or polycentric hinge that can be locked or adjusted to allow or restrict motion within the therapeutically desired range of motion* (D)**.** *The force systems of these orthoses apply a pair of anteriorly directed forces at the proximal posterior thigh* (1) *and distal posterior calf* (3)*, against a posteriorly directed force* (2) *applied over or on either side of the patella. Varus and valgus stressors are resisted by the sidebars. (From Trautman P. Lower limb orthoses. In Redford JB, Basmajian JV, Trautman P [eds],* Orthotics: Clinical Practice and Rehabilitation Technology. *New York: Churchill Livingstone, 1995.)*

Functional Knee Orthoses

Use of knee orthoses as functional braces parallels the development of the discipline of sports medicine since the early 1970s.[17] Before 1970, orthoses designed for patients with neuromuscular dysfunction were adapted in an attempt to meet the needs of injured athletes with a functionally unstable knee. Typically, the adapted orthosis was cumbersome and significantly impaired the quality of the athlete's performance. To assist professional athletes in quickly and safely returning to competition, the sports medicine community explored alternative orthotic interventions to manage an unstable knee. The development of FKOs as alternatives to surgery (which often sidelined athletes for considerable periods of time) was especially welcomed.[18]

One of the first FKOs, The Lenox Hill Derotation Knee Brace, was developed by Nicholas and Castiglia of Lenox Hill Hospital in the early 1970s to protect the chronically unstable knees of football quarterback Joe Namath.[19] The Lenox Hill orthosis was the primary design that was commercially available until the late 1970s. The original orthosis had medial and lateral uprights, a single-axis knee joint with a medial fulcrum pad, a broad elastic thigh and calf cuff and strap to hold the orthosis in place, and a set of derotation straps to control movement of the tibia on the femur. This orthosis was designed to control mediolateral instability, rotational instability, and multiple ligament impairment.[20] Subsequent versions of the Lenox Hill orthosis are available in standard, lightweight, and ultra-lightweight versions, with a dial-lock option to adjust available ROM and with protective undersleeves and oversleeves (Figure 13-8).

The original design has evolved considerably. More than three dozen functional braces are being manufactured in today's sports medicine market (see examples in Table 13-2), most of which are based on a lightweight rigid suprastructure made from carbon composite or titanium alloy. Many use adjustable elasticized or Velcro strapping to apply a four-point stabilizing force and to hold the orthosis in position on the limb. Some have polycentric knee units; others allow variable flexion control or assisted extension. The basic design and components of most commercially available FKOs are shown in Figure 13-9.

Unfortunately, systematic critical evaluation of the efficacy of FKOs has not kept pace with the development of

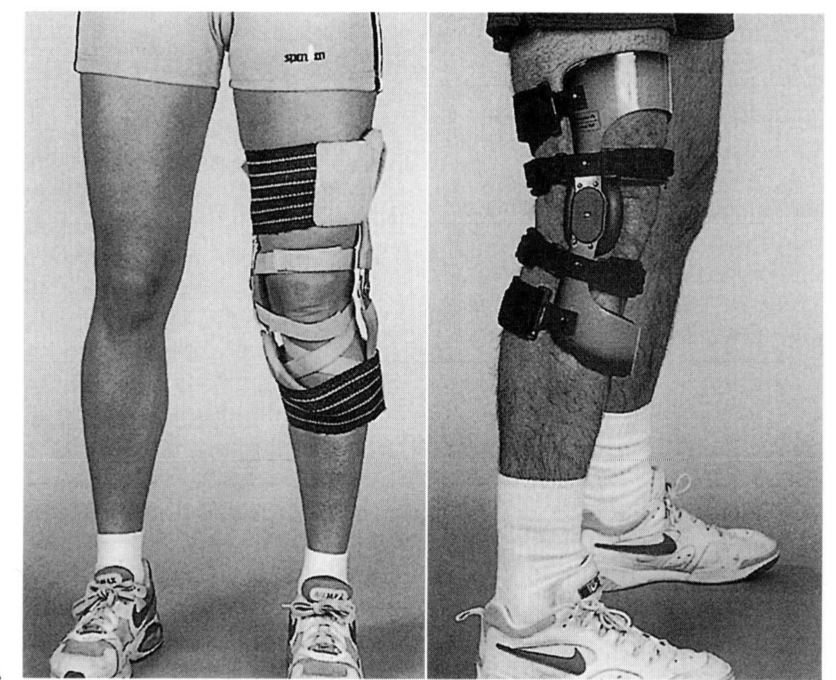

Figure 13-8

*Comparison of the original **(A)** and current **(B)** Lenox Hill Derotation Orthosis. (From Nawoczenski DA, Epler ME [eds],* Orthotics in Functional Rehabilitation of the Lower Limb, *Philadelphia: Saunders, 1997.)*

new designs; there is a paucity of clinical and laboratory research defining the indications for, roles of, or outcomes of use for these functional braces.[18]

Functional Knee Orthoses and Performance

Current available literature can be characterized by two major approaches to comparing braced and unbraced performances: (1) maximal effort tests, in which subjects performed at maximal intensity and the criterion measure was an overall performance measure such as distance hopped or the time to run a specified distance and (2) matched effort tests, in which subjects perform at submaximal intensity and the criterion measures tend to be specific variables such as muscle activation patterns determined via electromyography (EMG) or ground reaction forces determined via force plate.[21] Nemeth and colleagues[22] studied six expert downhill skiers who had sustained ACL injuries. Surface electrodes were used with an eight-channel telemetric EMG system to collect recordings from the vastus medialis, bicep femoris, semimembranosus, semitendinosus, and gastrocnemius medialis muscles from both legs. Without a brace, the EMG activity level of all muscles increased during knee flexion. With a brace, the EMG activity increased in midphase during the upward push for the weight transfer and the peak activity occurred closer to knee flexion in midphase. Nemeth and colleagues[22] suggest the brace caused an increase in afferent input from proprioceptors, resulting in

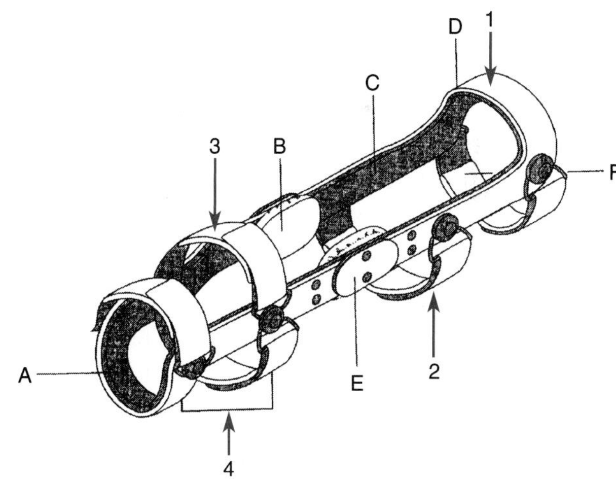

Figure 13-9

Components of most contemporary functional knee orthoses include the calf section/cuff with its closure (A)*; medial or lateral condylar pads, or both* (B)*; medial and lateral uprights* (C)*; the thigh section/cuff with its closure* (D)*; an adjustable knee hinge* (E)*; and the thigh strap* (F)*. The stabilizing forces that are typically applied by the orthosis include a posterior force over the anterior proximal thigh* (1)*, an anterior force on the distal posterior femur* (2)*, a posterior force at the proximal anterior tibia* (3)*, and an anterior force at the midshaft of the posterior tibia* (4)*. (From Trautman P. Lower limb orthoses. In Redford JB, Basmajian JV, Trautman P [eds],* Orthotics: Clinical Practice and Rehabilitation Technology. *New York: Churchill Livingstone, 1995. p. 31.)*

an adaptation of motor control patterns secondarily modifying EMG activity and timing.

A number of researchers have investigated the impact of functional braces on performance and endurance in uninjured and previously injured athletes. Stephens[23] found little impact on speed of running in uninjured collegiate basketball players during straight line running tasks (end line to foul line, full court) when comparing performance in two functional braces to nonbraced speed. Although these results are positive, the in-brace time and types of activity used for the study were significantly different from those of an active, full-length basketball game.

Highgenboten and colleagues[24] found a 3% to 6% increase in metabolic cost during steady-state treadmill running when functional braces were worn. Subjects also had higher ratings of perceived exertion when exercising with the brace. These effects were attributed to the weight of the brace. In addition, research by Wojtys and colleagues[25] showed that most braces appear to slow hamstring muscle reaction times at voluntary levels. Evidence from these maximal-effort and matched-effort performance tests suggests no advantage to use of FKOs.

Most functional knee braces weigh close to 1 lb. Despite the use of lightweight materials that are resilient to various forces, it is possible that long in-brace times can lead to fatigue or injuries to other areas that compensate for the added weight of the orthosis. This may explain the increase in injuries of the foot and ankle reported by Grace and associates[26] in athletes who wore braces. Styf and colleagues[27] studied changes in intramuscular pressures within the anterior compartment of the leg at rest, during exercise, and after exercise, comparing three orthoses. Intramuscular pressures at rest and muscle relaxation pressure during exercise were higher when subjects wore each of the orthoses. To evaluate whether distal strapping was responsible for this increase in pressure, distal straps were removed and subjects retested. Intramuscular pressure and muscle relaxation pressure returned to levels that were similar to nonbraced levels. This study demonstrates the subtle yet potentially important impact of orthoses on muscle function that may contribute to injury; external compression elevates the intramuscular pressure beneath the thigh and leg straps. Local muscle blood flow is impaired by the increased intramuscular pressure, which leads to decreased oxygen tension and impaired muscle function.[28] This could possibly be the reason for premature leg muscle fatigue that has been reported in other experimental studies on individuals using knee braces.[27,29,30]

Prophylactic Knee Orthoses

In the 1990s debate was considerable concerning the potential benefits or effectiveness of orthoses designed to prevent knee injuries or minimize the severity of injury for athletes involved in high-risk injury activities.[26,31-33] The objective of wearing a prophylactic knee orthosis (PKO) is to provide protection to the soft tissue restraints of the knee. Most commonly, these braces have been worn by athletes who are exposed to lateral impacts.

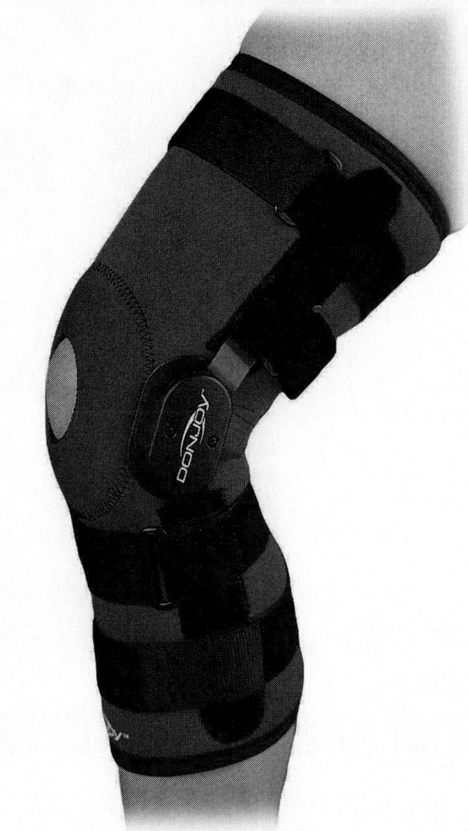

Figure 13-10
An example of a prophylactic knee orthosis, designed to reduce risk of knee injury for athletes during practice and competition situations. (Courtesy dj Orthopedics, Inc., Vista, Calif.)

Lateral impacts can result in MCL and cruciate ligament injuries.[34] Prophylactic orthoses are designed to protect the integrity of medial knee structures. Most prophylactic designs have a hinged lateral frame, held in place by a set of thigh and calf cuffs or straps. The hinge may be single axis, dual axis, or polycentric; many designs have also incorporated a hyperextension stop for further protection of the athlete's knee against forceful hyperextension injury (Figure 13-10). Some designs use a plastic shell with medial and lateral uprights and polycentric hinges.[35]

CASE EXAMPLE 1

A High School Football Player

J. P., 17, and his father come into a sports medicine and rehabilitation practice for a professional opinion regarding the potential benefits of wearing a knee brace during football games and practices. J. P. is an outstanding tight end on his high school football team and is being considered for a football scholarship by college recruiting personnel. He has no history of injury preventing him from playing or practicing football. However, father and son know that football players are susceptible to experiencing lateral blows at the knee, making them vulnerable to knee ligament injuries. J. P.'s father is concerned that his son's ability to play college football might be compromised if he were to injure his knee. He wants to know whether wearing a prophylactic knee orthosis (PKO) could reduce the likelihood that J. P. will sustain a severe knee injury.

Questions to Consider

- Given J. P.'s history and current presentation, what additional tests and measures would provide helpful information to use in your evaluation process?
- What is your movement dysfunction–related diagnosis for J. P.?
- What is the rehabilitation prognosis for J. P.? What are his goals for intervention? What are your rehabilitation goals? How long to do you think it will take to achieve any goals that you and J. P. agree upon?
- What is the current evidence in clinical research literature about the efficacy of PKOs in reducing the incidence and severity of knee injuries in college football players?
- How does wearing a PKO affect performance during athletic competition? What are the risks associated with wearing a PKO during athletic competition?
- Based on J. P.'s goals and expectations, your understanding of the risk of injury for football players, and evidence available in the clinical research literature, what recommendations would you make for intervention at this point? Is the evidence convincing enough that you would recommend this athlete to wear a PKO?
- Of the various PKO designs available, which might be most appropriate for this college-bound football player?
- How will you assess whether J. P.'s goals have been met?
- What type of follow-up would you recommend for J. P.?

Prophylactic knee orthoses are available "off the shelf" or can be custom molded for the individual athlete. Clinical practice and research have not yet resolved the debate about the efficacy of prophylactic orthoses. Questions remain about the relationship between the biomechanical characteristics of the orthoses and the anatomical knee, the response of the orthosis to valgus loading, the impact of the orthosis on the continuum of locomotion (walking to running), and the ability of the orthosis to prevent injuries during activity as intended by its design.

Biomechanical Performance of Prophylactic Knee Orthosis

Many studies that have investigated the biomechanical performance of prophylactic braces have used either cadaver knees or mechanical surrogate models of the knee. Most studies have concluded that protection of the MCL has been inconsistent and only borderline at best.[32,36-40] Many health care providers are concerned about how the orthosis might preload the MCL before normal physiological loading.[36,38,39] Our understanding of the interaction between the orthosis and knee tissues is based on the properties of human tissue and of brace materials under static and dynamic loading conditions.

Manufacturers report high resistance of the braces to laterally directed impact loading; however, the research design and methodology on which these claims are based are often poor or flawed. In some cases the braces are actually less rigid and resistant to derangement during loading than the anatomical knee itself. The ability of a knee orthosis prepositioned in flexion to protect against major ligament damage is uncertain.[41] Joint line clearance during brace deformation is an additional concern. Theoretically, the prophylactic brace is designed to transmit valgus loads on the knee over the greatest possible area to dissipate the forces away from susceptible ligaments effectively.[33,38,39] The orthotic hinge forms a bridge over the joint line; its sites of attachment are best placed as far as possible on the proximal femur and distal tibia. Clearance between the hinge and the joint must be adequate. Contact between the hinge and the joint creates a three-point bending system centered at the joint, inadvertently preloading the MCL.[38,39]

Evidence of Efficacy of Prophylactic Knee Orthoses

Many studies have tried to determine the effectiveness of PKOs in preventing knee ligament injuries in football players.[26,42-45] In 1987 Teitz and colleagues[45] reported on data collected in 1984 and 1985 regarding football players from National Collegiate Athletic Association (NCAA) Division I schools. Players who wore PKOs had more knee injuries than players who did not wear these braces. This study, however, did not control for players' history of prior knee injury.[45] In 1986, Hewson and associates[42] reported findings on University of Arizona football players from a study that spanned 8 years. The injury records of 4 academic years in which players wore PKOs were compared with the preceding

4 years in which players did not use PKOs. It was mandatory for the players who were at the greatest risk of injury (linebackers, defensive linemen, tight ends) to wear PKOs in the years when brace wear was being monitored in this study. The results indicated that, when comparing groups of braced players to unbraced players, there were no reductions in the number, rate, or type of knee injuries that players sustained.[42]

The results of a 3-year study of NCAA Division I college football players in the Big Ten Conference by Albright and colleagues[46] were slightly different. This research indicated that players who wore PKOs experienced lower rates of MCL injuries than their unbraced peers. These trends were evident only when influential factors such as playing position, skill level of the player, and session (game or practice) in which the injury was sustained were considered in the analysis. Starting players and those who were substitutes in line positions, linebackers, and tight end positions had lower injury rates in practices and games. However, backs, receivers, and kickers had higher injury rates in games when using a PKO.[46]

The implication that the benefits of PKO use may be related to player position is also suggested in a study by Sitler and associates.[44] Participants in this study included young men in an eight-man intramural tackle football program at the United States Military Academy at West Point, N.Y., between 1986 and 1987. Variables such as the athletic shoe, playing surface, knee injury history, type of brace, and injury assessment and documentation were all controlled. Subjects wearing PKOs while on defense had significantly fewer knee injuries than their nonbraced counterparts. No significant differences for these parameters were noted when players were on offense.[44]

Researchers and athletic trainers have concerns about the risk of injury to other areas of the limb when these orthoses are worn during competition. In a two-season prospective study of potentially protective benefits of prophylactic bracing in a sample of 580 high school football players, Grace and colleagues[26] found a dramatic increase in the number of injuries of the ankle and foot among athletes who wore the braces. In contrast, Sitler and associates[44] found no significant difference in the frequency of ankle injuries between a knee brace group and a control group of military cadets. Additionally, the severity of MCL and ACL knee injury was not reduced with the use of unilateral-biaxial prophylactic knee braces.[44]

The variability of these findings makes an unequivocal statement regarding the need for high school and college athletes to wear a PKO difficult. The research is confusing because data collection cannot take into account annual variations in coaching techniques or completely control the data collection methods employed by all of the schools participating in the studies. Furthermore, injury diagnosis among these studies is not standardized, making a comparison of study results problematic.[34] Many studies have methodological problems and limited sample size that hinder interpretation of their findings.[47-51] Despite the inconsistency of research methods and findings, however, France and Paulos[34] concluded that there is sufficient evidence that bracing can be beneficial in reducing the number of MCL injuries sustained from direct lateral blows to the knee, especially when the knee is near full extension. They recommend that a PKO be carefully fit so that the hinge maintains its position at the lateral joint line during activity, that the brace provides enough clearance from the joint line during impact, and that the materials used in the brace construction are sufficient to control the amount of impact delivered to the knee.[34] The literature does not provide enough information about the protection that these braces offer to the other soft tissue structures of the knee.

If prophylactic braces are intended to prevent or reduce the severity of injury, clinicians and brace manufacturers must work to be responsible for critical evaluation of these devices to define better their appropriate use and outcomes. At present clinicians must hold vendors accountable for their products, requesting well designed and clearly reported quantitative studies to support the narrative accounts in marketing brochures about design criteria.

INFORMED CLINICAL DECISION MAKING

Because so many FKOs are currently marketed, evaluation of the information published in marketing literature is challenging and often frustrating for clinicians and surgeons when research support is not always available. Remaining well informed is also challenging, because orthotic designs are constantly being modified and "improved." Making a sound decision about which design can best meet the stability and activity needs of a given individual can be a daunting task and must not be based on which sales representative most recently shared information or which orthosis is currently the most popular choice. Although patients may seek a functional orthoses to protect their knees or to improve their performance, many do not have the knowledge or resources to understand the specifics and idiosyncrasies of each brace. To make an informed decision, the clinician must consider a patient's specific injuries and patterns of instability, the present and anticipated strength and bulk of the muscles around the injured knee, and the activities and likely mechanism of being reinjured in the patient's preferred sports activities.

Decisions about orthotic options must be made deliberately, with discussion involving the patient, PT, or athletic trainer, orthotist, brace manufacturer, and physician. Quick decisions about an FKO, made without careful evaluation of the match between the patient's needs and the orthotic design, lead to frustration and dissatisfaction for all involved.

In evaluating information about knee orthoses published in the literature, health professionals must look closely at research design and methodology and evaluate the clinical relevance of the conclusions drawn from study results. They should consider three important questions:

1. Did the study evaluate the orthosis under static conditions or during dynamic use?
2. Did the study use cadaver models or physiologically active joints in the evaluation of orthotic performance?
3. Did the study test reconstructed ACL knees in the use of knee orthosis?

Many of the most frequently cited studies evaluate brace performance under static conditions, specifically the ability of particular orthoses to prevent anterior excursion of the tibia on the femur as measured by standard clinical tests for ligamentous instability (e.g., Lachman's, pivot shift, Losee's tests). Some studies have used electronic and mechanical instrumentation to evaluate orthotic performance more precisely under static and controlled dynamic conditions. Although many studies demonstrate the efficacy of knee orthoses in prevention of excessive anterior excursion under static conditions, to generalize these static results to dynamic activity for patients with ACL-deficient knees is foolhardy. An orthosis' ability to provide a degree of stability for the knee under static conditions does not guarantee that it can also stabilize the knee during high demand activity. The low load levels applied to knee ligaments during static or cadaver model testing do not accurately reflect load levels during functional and athletic activities. Decisions to choose a particular orthosis on the basis of this type of research alone are not well informed.

Today the selection of a functional brace is even more challenging because insurance companies dictate where and from which vendor consumers can get their braces made, either for custom or off-the-shelf models. This limits the choice and type of brace used and puts the patient in a one-brace-for-all scenario.

Another dilemma facing clinicians is that the aggressive rehabilitation protocols for ACL reconstruction currently being used show close to normal range and strength by the third to sixth month. Currently, whether to have the patient jump, hop, turn, or twist is a complex decision based on many factors, including the strength of the ACL graft, graft fixation, and known biological factors that affect healing. A knee joint that is stabilized by a strong isometric graft and that goes through a controlled rehabilitation program should not need a functional brace. The most important part of the patient's return to activity and work is the physical rehabilitation or surgery, or both.

HINGE DESIGN

Hinge options for knee orthoses range from simple single-axis (unicentric) designs to complex four-bar polycentric designs. Most commercially available off-the-shelf FKOs have hinges in one of three categories: (1) the single-axis hinge, (2) the posterior offset hinge, or (3) the polycentric or genucentric hinge.

All single-axis/unicentric hinges act as a simple hinge; a unicentric hinge becomes incongruent with the anatomical joint axis as the instantaneous axis of rotation of the knee changes with movement through the ROM. Posterior offset designs attempt to improve the match between orthotic and anatomical axis of motion by approximating the location of the sagittal radius of curvature of the posterior femoral condyles as it articulates with the tibia in flexion.[52] Polycentric designs attempt to replicate the instantaneous axis of rotation of the anatomical knee joint, using two geared surfaces that mechanically constrain motion into a defined path.[53] Theoretically, polycentric or genucentric hinges are better able than unicentric hinge designs to match the rolling and gliding of the tibiofemoral joint as the knee flexes and extends. This closer match to physiological motion is meant to reduce pistoning, discomfort, and slippage of the orthosis on the limb during activity.

When considering which hinge design to select, remember that the soft tissue of the knee between the orthosis and the bone compromises the impact of any hinge on the kinematics of the knee. The most important characteristic of the hinge is its ability to transfer load during activity. Poorly designed or constructed hinges, or those made of weak or pliable materials, cannot effectively accomplish this task, and abnormal translations and rotations will not be well controlled. The work of Lew and colleagues[53] demonstrated greater variation in the pistoning constraint forces in a particular joint design than across designs when three orthoses were compared during specific activities.

Regalbuto and associates[54] evaluated the performance of four hinge designs fit into a custom-fit knee orthoses in three healthy subjects. Each subject wore the orthosis while performing a squat, an 8-inch step-up, a stand-to-sit activity, and an open-chain knee extension exercise. The researchers found that accurate hinge placement was a more important influence on function and comfort than hinge kinematics. Differences in kinematics among the four designs were masked by the compliance of the soft tissues between the brace cuffs and the bones of the knee.

FUNCTIONAL ORTHOSES FOR ACL INSUFFICIENCY

PTs are often involved in conservative and postsurgical rehabilitation for patients with ACL insufficiency. For more than 20 years, FKOs have been used to prevent forward subluxation of the tibia on the femur for patients with ACL insufficiency. Various designs have evolved to be used for partial ACL tears or for complete ACL rupture (Figure 13-11).

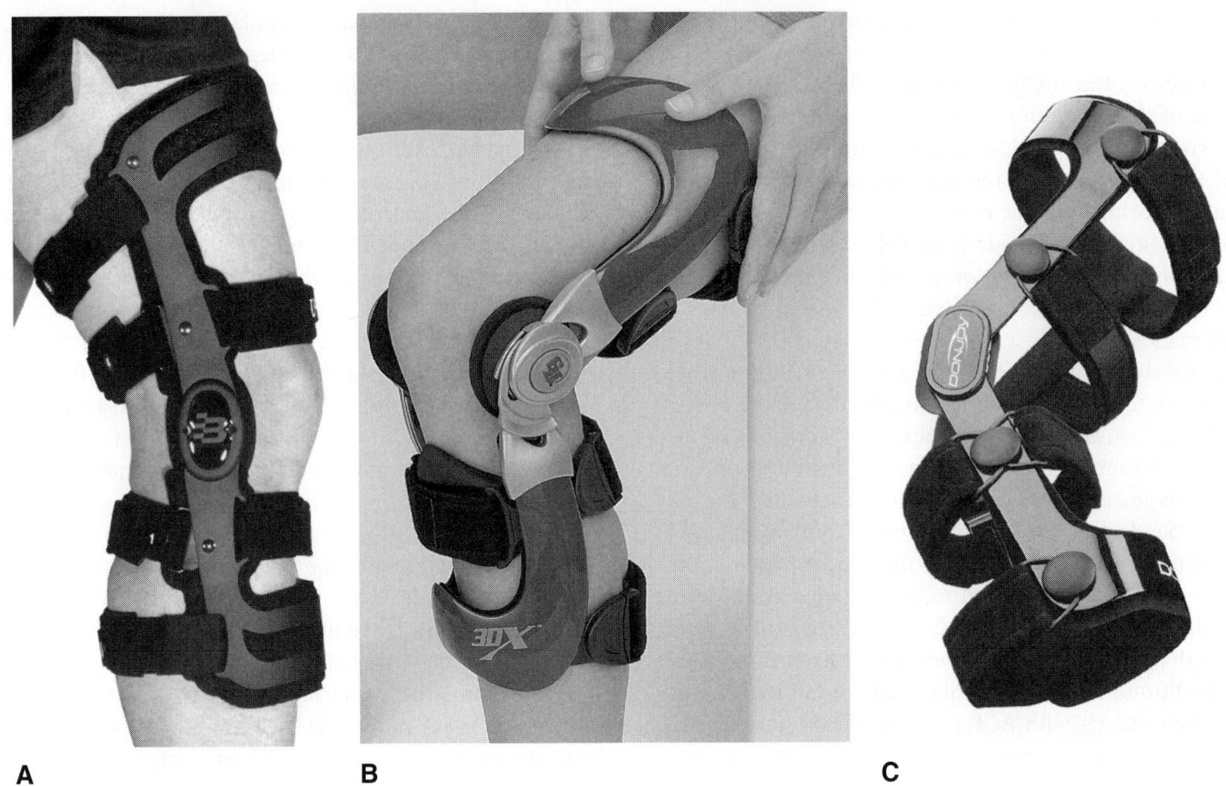

Figure 13-11
Examples of commercially available, custom-fit functional knee orthoses. ***A,*** *The Bledsoe Ultimate CI.* ***B,*** *The Generation II 3DX.* ***C,*** *The Donjoy 4titude. (****A,*** *Courtesy Bledsoe Brace Systems, Grand Prairie, Tex.;* ***B,*** *courtesy Ossur/Generation II, Viejo, Calif.;* ***C,*** *courtesy dj Orthopedics, Vista, Calif.)*

Biomechanical Performance of Functional Knee Orthoses for Anterior Cruciate Ligament Insufficiency

For patients with an ACL tear or deficiencies, or both, a primary goal of bracing is to control the excessive anterior drawer movement of the tibia. Numerous research studies have attempted to evaluate whether these orthoses are effective in controlling tibial movement. One strategy is to use cadaver models to evaluate the efficacy of FKOs for support of the ACL.[55,56] The major drawback of this type of study, however, is the difference between living and preserved tissue. Because active muscle contraction and normal soft tissue compliance contribute to strain on the ACL, the lack of active musculature and compliance changes in soft tissue around the knee limit the application of cadaver study findings. Similarly, the magnitude and sequence of muscle contraction alter the stiffness between the brace and the soft tissue of the leg. It is impossible to reproduce this interface in cadaver studies.

Another strategy is to compare forward excursion of the tibia on the femur by using clinical tests of knee instability performed on a subject with and without bracing.[17,41,57] Wojtys and colleagues[58,59] conducted two studies in which anterior tibial translation was measured while subjects were seated on an ischial support, in both braced and unbraced conditions. Patients were instructed to stay relaxed throughout a test in which the tibia was forced anteriorly. Reflexive contraction of the hamstrings, quadriceps, and gastrocnemius muscles to this initial perceived force occurred more quickly in the braced than the unbraced condition. However, these muscles reacted more slowly in the braced condition when patients were told to actively resist this movement as soon as they perceived it. Beynnon and colleagues[60] found no significant improvement in subjects' ability to detect passive anterior tibial translation in braced conditions when subjects were tested in a seated position.

Given the conflicting results of these studies, drawing a clinical conclusion regarding the effects of bracing on anterior tibial translation in patients with ACL deficient knees is difficult. Although the studies seem to indicate that subjects' ability to perceive passive anterior tibial motion did not improve, one must also consider that subjects were tested in nonfunctional, non–weight-bearing conditions versus dynamic situations. Additionally, the relationship between static testing and actual physiological loading during sport activity has not been well established. Noyes and associates[55] have demonstrated that manual examination cannot duplicate the magnitude of force that is present during activity.

Although static and cadaver studies have been the first step in critically evaluating the efficacy of FKOs for patients with ACL insufficiency, the most informative research would be done in vivo. This is especially important because static and cadaver studies cannot replicate the real-life physiological loading that occurs in the knee during activities.[55,56,61-64] The next challenge for clinical researchers is to develop methodology to evaluate FKOs worn during functional activities.

Evidence of Efficacy of Functional Knee Orthoses for Anterior Cruciate Ligament Insufficiency

In 1997 Kramer and colleagues[21] published a review of research conducted between 1982 and 1992 that summarized the evidence regarding use of FKOs on dynamic performance. Collectively, these studies did not provide overwhelming evidence to support or refute the use of FKOs by individuals with ACL-deficient knees. This review cited 16 maximal-effort, experimental situations in which subjects' performance in braced and unbraced conditions for a one-leg hop test, figure-of-eight runs, stair climbing, sprinting, and agility was recorded. Results across the studies were mixed: FKOs either improved, hindered, or had no effect on performance.

The review also summarized the results of several matched effort tests that measured biomechanical variables. The variables assessed in these studies included ground reaction forces, ROM, EMG, joint moment, and power. Interpreting whether FKO use was advantageous or disadvantageous for wearers was difficult because the studies did not assess how changes in measured variable affected overall performance. Three of the matched effort studies demonstrated that bracing subjects during testing resulted in detrimental effects on energy costs. Overall, this literature review noted that five of the included studies indicated that many of the subjects reported feeling more stable when wearing the FKO. Given the mixed results of these studies, a conclusive statement about whether or not patients with ACL deficiency should expect enhanced performance when wearing FKOs cannot easily be made.

The ability for subjects to control anterior tibial translation during functional testing was examined by Ramsey and associates.[65] This study demonstrated negligible reduction in the anterior drawer movement of the tibia between braced and unbraced conditions when patients performed horizontal, one-legged jumps.

Another strategy is to evaluate muscle function when subjects with ACL deficiency use an FKO. Branch and colleagues[66] found little difference in electromyographic firing patterns between testing in subjects who were braced and unbraced. Because muscle activity was similarly reduced under both conditions (as referenced to an ACL intact limb), the researchers suggest that functional knee orthoses do not have a significant proprioceptive influence on muscle function. A study by Wu et al[67] looked at 31 subjects who had undergone a unilateral ACL reconstruction with three bracing conditions: (1) a manufactured brace, (2) a mechanical placebo brace, and (3) no brace. Using an isokinetic machine to measure specific knee joint angles and peak torques, they found that knee bracing can improve static proprioception but not muscle function. The manufactured and mechanical placebo brace groups performed better than the no-brace group. The apparent improvement in proprioception with knee bracing was not due to the mechanical restraining action of the brace.[67] Other studies show similar results when measuring proprioceptive improvement on ACL-reconstructed knees when doing functionally relevant tasks.[68,69]

Nemeth and associates[22] studied the effects of bracing and not bracing during a series of downhill ski runs by six downhill skiers who had ACL-deficient knees. Surface electrodes were placed over the muscle bellies of vastus medialis, gastrocnemius medialis, biceps femoris, and semimembranosus and semitendinosus muscles to record activity during skiing and determine any differences in the patterns of muscle firing between braced and unbraced conditions. Statistical analysis did not reveal significant differences among subjects' muscle response in either condition. However, subjects with greater knee instability, compared with subjects with less knee instability, had increased levels of lateral hamstring muscle activity during knee flexion when wearing braces. In theory, this muscle activation may help control excessive anterolateral shifting of the tibial plateau, thus helping the patient feel greater lower-extremity stability. Despite the lack of definitive results in this study, all subjects who wore the FKO reported feeling safer and more stable while skiing.

Another study by Ramsey and associates[70] examined the muscle firing patterns of rectus femoris, semitendinosus, biceps femoris, and the lateral head of the gastrocnemius of four subjects with ACL-deficient knees who did or did not wear braces during one-legged jumps. They also measured anterior tibial displacement during the testing activity. Interestingly, their findings indicated that the subjects who wore braces demonstrated decreased levels of hamstring activity and increased levels of quadriceps activity. The braced condition resulted in small reductions of anterior displacement in two subjects, no change in one subject, and small increases in this translation for one subject.

Cook and colleagues[71] compared the ability of subjects with absent ACLs ($n = 14$) to perform running and cutting maneuvers with and without a commercially available orthosis. Subjects' performance with the orthosis was objectively and subjectively better. In a similar study that compared the performance of subjects with ACL deficiency in several orthoses, Marans and colleagues[72] reported improved performance in two of the six orthoses evaluated.

Numerous studies have examined the metabolic cost, using dynamic analysis of orthotic use to test the validity and reliability of functional knee braces on ACL-insufficient knees.[24,73] Whether the slight increase in energy requirements noted is offset by protection and improved function while wearing the orthosis is not yet understood.

The authors of these studies who examined the effects of bracing subjects with ACL-deficient knees during dynamic test conditions suggest that there may be afferent inputs to the central nervous system from knee proprioceptors and the brace-skin-bone interface. This neural input may evoke adaptive motor responses when patients wear the knee brace during functional activities. The number of subjects used in each study was fewer than 10, making it difficult to draw conclusions if each study is considered independently. Collectively, however, the results of each study are similar, which may help the PT formulate an opinion about the merits of using a brace on an ACL-deficient knee.

CASE EXAMPLE 2

An Individual with a Recent Anterior Cruciate Ligament Tear

R. S., 43, comes to physical therapy 4 weeks after injuring his right knee while skiing. Three days after his injury, he was evaluated by an orthopedic surgeon and referred for magnetic resonance imaging (MRI). The MRI confirmed a tear to his anterior cruciate ligament (ACL). At the initial physical therapy visit R. S. complains that his leg has "given out" several times while he was descending stairs or pivoting from his right leg.

R. S. says his goal is to regain enough confidence in his knee so that he can ski three to four times a season with his family and play modest recreational sports with his two young sons. Although he had discussed the option of surgery with the surgeon, he wants to see if he can rehabilitate his knee enough to avoid the recovery associated with the surgery. R. S. wonders if a specialized knee brace could help him maintain the stability of his knee during recreational activities. He says he has heard conflicting information about whether knee braces are beneficial, and he wants advice from a physical therapist about the merits of obtaining such a brace.

The physical therapist wants to find evidence to support whether R. S. should invest in a functional knee orthosis brace (FKO) to enhance his knee stability. The clinical question that directs review of the evidence is this: "Will a brace designed for patients with ACL-deficient knees enhance the control and stability of the knee during recreational activities?"

Questions to Consider

- Given this patient's history and current presentation, what additional tests and measures would provide helpful information to use in your evaluation process?
- What is your movement dysfunction–related diagnosis for this patient?
- What might the prognosis be for R. S.? What are his goals for intervention? What are your rehabilitation goals? How long do you think it will take to achieve the goals that you and R. S. agree upon?
- What is the role of exercise or FKO, or both, in the conservative management of a patient like R. S. with a recent ACL tear?
- What evidence is available in the clinical research literature about the efficacy of FKO to protect the integrity of an ACL-deficient knee? What evidence is available about the impact of an FKO on function for individuals with ACL-deficient knees?
- On the basis of this patient's goals and expectations, your understanding of the underlying disease process, and evidence from the clinical research literature, what recommendations would you make for intervention at this point?
- Is the evidence convincing enough, given the level of impairment that R. S. demonstrates and his prognosis, to warrant recommending the purchase an FKO to wear during recreational activities?
- Of the various FKO designs available, which might be most appropriate for this individual seeking conservative management of his ACL injury and rehabilitation?
- How will you assess whether this patient's rehabilitation goals have been met?
- What type of follow-up would you recommend for this patient?

Recommendations for the Patient with Anterior Cruciate Ligament Insufficiency

After reviewing the evidence, the PT tells R. S. that the research to support or refute the use of an FKO is equivocal. Evidence suggests that some patients feel more stable when they wear a brace, yet it is unknown whether their feelings of enhanced stability are due to biomechanical or neuromuscular changes that are the result of FKO wear. The PT recommends that R. S. rehabilitate his knee through participation in an exercise program before returning to any recreational activity.

Role of Exercise in Anterior Cruciate Ligament Rehabilitation

Some literature supports the premise that hamstrings and gastrocnemius muscles assist in stabilizing ACL-deficient knees,[74-76] and also that patients with ACL-deficient knees benefit from closed kinetic chain exercise programs and perturbation training.[77,78] If the patient perceives the need for an FKO after participating in a rehabilitation program, the PT can recommend braces that are available while cautioning the patient to continue with a home strengthening program.

ORTHOSES FOR OSTEOARTHRITIS

Narrowing of the medial or lateral compartment of the knee is a common source of discomfort and pain for many adults. Osteoarthritis is a condition where the collagen fibers of the articular cartilage are compromised. The breakdown of the articular cartilage in the medial or lateral compartment results in the uneven distribution of the load forces.[79] Currently there are five general methods of management for osteoarthritis:

1. Pharmaceuticals
2. Surgery: unicompartmental or total knee arthroplasty
3. Orthoses
4. Injections
5. Use of valgus or varus knee orthoses

Valgus and varus knee bracing evolved in the early 1990s with the theory that, by unloading the medial or lateral compartment, pain could be altered enough to ward off surgery and prolong the function of an osteoarthritic knee.

Most individuals with osteoarthritis of the knee demonstrate functional losses and report pain when the knee is loaded during the stance phase of gait, beginning at heel strike and ending with toe off. Biomechanical analysis on healthy subjects reveals that loading in the knee is 62% on the medial side and 38% on the lateral side during stance; in those with a varus deformity associated with medial joint osteoarthritis, the medial compartment loading can increase to 100% of the total compressive load on the knee joint during this phase of gait.[80] On the basis of this premise, the conservative and surgical strategy in treating these individuals is to reduce the load on the medial side of the joint in an effort to reduce the patient's painful symptoms.[80]

Valgus (unloading) orthoses (Figure 13-12) are designed to unload the medial knee compartment noted to have degenerative changes and provide a similar type of advantage as realignment osteotomy.[80] These orthoses unload the medial compartment of the knee through use of adjustable tension straps crossing the lateral aspect of the knee joint; lateral condylar pads; or lateral hinge systems, which are fixed to a brace shell at the calf and thigh.[80-82]

Evidence of Efficacy of Valgus Orthoses

Research over the past 10 years has attempted to validate manufacturers' claims that valgus and varus bracing will

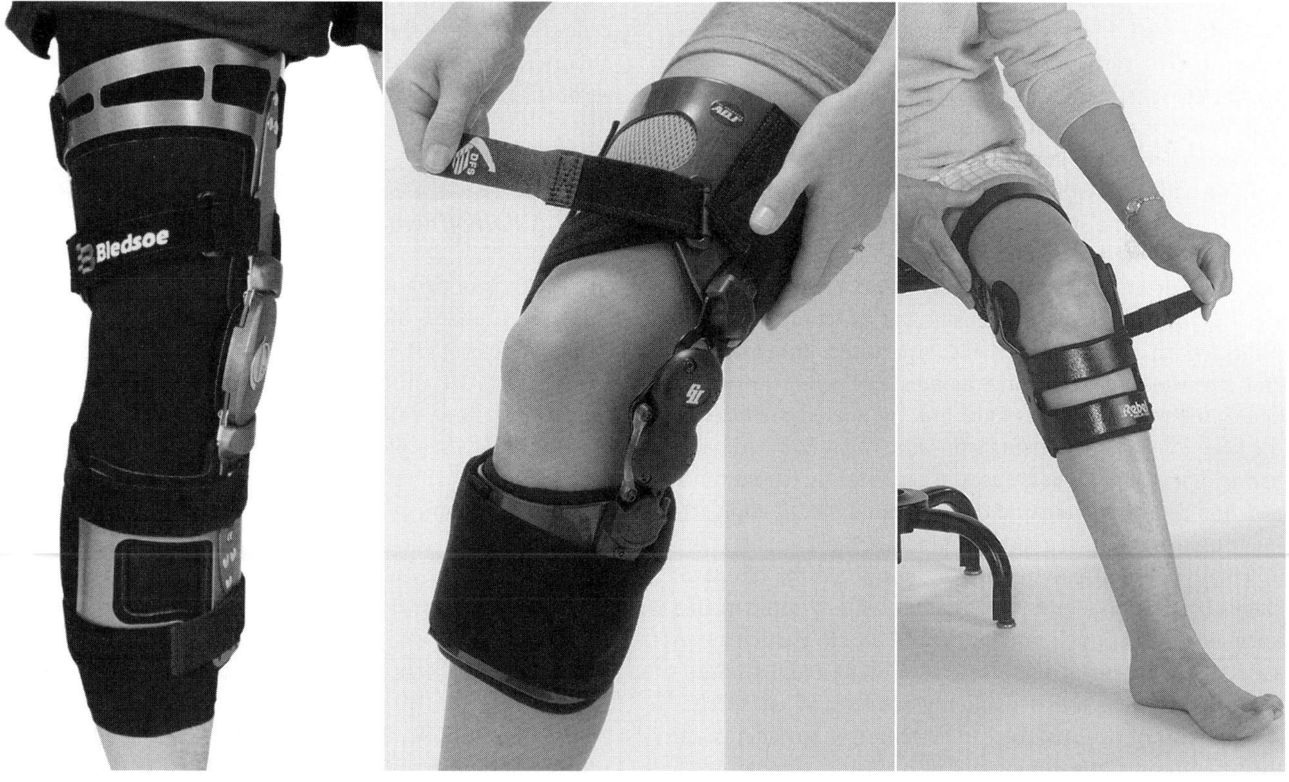

A B C

Figure 13-12

Examples of functional knee orthoses designed to unload medial compartment of the knee for individuals with painful osteoarthritis. ***A,*** *The Thruster 2.* ***B,*** *The Generation II Unloader.* ***C,*** *The Reliever OTS. (****A,*** *Courtesy Bledsoe Brace Systems, Grand Prairie, Tex.;* ***B,*** *courtesy Ossur/Generation II, Viejo, Calif.;* ***C,*** *courtesy Townsend Design, Bakersfield, Calif.)*

achieve significant reductions in the amount of pain and swelling in the involved joint region. Pollo[83] looked at nine subjects (mean age 46 ± 11 years) with a varus mechanical alignment of 0 to 10 degrees. Each subject was tested during walking with and without a commercially available brace. Kinematic and kinetic data were recorded with a video-based, six-camera Motion Analysis System in conjunction with two Bertec force platforms. Comparisons were made at the initial test and at the 3-month follow-up. Wearing the commercially available brace resulted in a statistically significant improvement in pain and function along with a reduction in the external varus moment about the knee. Other authors[85] have found similar results with unicompartmental osteoarthritis and the improved function that the valgus brace affords to the patients.

A study by Katsuragawa and colleagues[85] demonstrated an increase in bone mineral density more in the lateral tibial condyle than the medial due to the transfer of forces across the knee joint from the medial to the lateral side after use of a valgus orthosis. Research by Horlick and associates[86] demonstrated a significant reduction of pain when patients wore a valgus brace but did not find a change in functional status or in the femoral-tibial angle and joint space as viewed via radiographs.

Self and colleagues[80] examined the effects of valgus knee bracing on the varus moment at the knee during level gait on five patients who had confirmed medial compartment knee arthrosis. The varus moment causes greater loading on the medial compartment and may be responsible for the pain that patients with medial knee arthrosis experience. The researchers collected kinematic data on subjects' patterns of walking with and without their orthoses. The use of a valgus brace reduced the net varus moment on the medial compartment of the knee during the time when this moment was typically at its maximum load.[80] Lindenfeld and associates[81] examined the pain intensity and function scores for subjects with confirmed medial compartment knee arthrosis and persistent pain during ambulation. They hoped to determine whether valgus knee bracing altered the loads at the knee joint. Most patients who wore the prescribed brace had excellent clinical responses in terms of increased function and decreased pain and demonstrated medial compartment unloading during radiographic testing.[81]

Finally Hewett and colleagues[82] examined the effects of valgus bracing on a group of 19 adults with chronic medial knee joint pain, which limited their ability to participate in sports or perform activities of daily living (ADLs). Study participants were assessed after 9 weeks and again after about 1 year of orthotic wear to determine if any changes in their symptoms and function had occurred. Fifteen of 18 subjects reevaluated after 9 weeks reported reduction in their pain symptoms or an increase in walking tolerance, or both. Thirteen patients continued to wear their braces for an average of 1 year. Ten of these patients felt an improvement in pain or function after using the brace, the most dramatic of which related to the amount of time participants could walk before the onset of pain. Wearing the orthosis, however, did not have much impact on returning participants to sports activities. Moreover, despite the improvements in symptoms and function for many patients, gait analysis did not reveal any changes in loading at the varus moment or any gait adaptations during brace wear.[82]

These studies, reviewed independently, include relatively small numbers of subjects, but the conclusions in all studies regarding patients who wore valgus braces to control the detrimental effects of medial tibiofemoral arthrosis were similar. If pain associated with medial joint compartment arthritis is related to varus loading of the knee joint, it appears that valgus bracing can be effective in controlling some of the painful symptoms associated with this pathosis.

The impact of valgus bracing on function and gait kinematics is not as clear. Despite the conflicting evidence regarding the influence that these braces have on gait kinematics and joint loading, evidence seems to support the notion that patients may benefit from valgus brace wear to diminish pain and increase function if these individuals do not want surgery as an immediate option.

Evidence clearly indicates that weakness of the quadriceps muscle is related to osteoarthritic conditions at the knee joint.[87,88] In a review of research related to guidelines for management of osteoarthritis in the knee, Hochberg and colleagues[89] cited the need for patients to participate in quadriceps strengthening and ROM exercises, as well as aerobic conditioning exercises.

CASE EXAMPLE 3

A Patient with Osteoarthritis of the Knee

R. P., 55, is undergoing 6 weeks of physical therapy with the goal of managing his right knee pain. An orthopedic surgeon referred R. P. to physical therapy with a diagnosis of degenerative joint disease. R. P. has a 1-year history of increasing knee pain, concentrated around the medial joint line. His symptoms have worsened to the point that he feels compromised in his activities of daily living (ADLs). R. P. underwent a partial medial meniscectomy 4 years before the onset of his knee pain. Before his referral to physical therapy, x-rays revealed medial tibiofemoral knee arthrosis.

R. P. reports that he cannot stand for more than 10 minutes or walk more than 30 minutes. His goals are to walk 60 minutes on a level surface for exercise and stand for 45 minutes. R. P. attends the physical therapy clinic three times per week; his program emphasizes quadriceps strengthening and exercises to maintain his knee range of motion. After 4 weeks of therapy, R. P. feels that there has been little change in his function. The referring physician recommends surgery because R. P.'s symptoms have not changed. R. P., however, does not want to consider surgery because of the length and intensity of postoperative rehabilitation. He asks if any other interventions might be considered to manage his knee pain.

Questions to Consider

- Given this patient's history and current presentation, what additional tests and measures would provide useful information in your evaluation process?
- What is your movement dysfunction–related diagnosis for this patient?
- What might the prognosis be for this patient? What are the patient's goals for intervention? What are your rehabilitation goals? How long do you think it will take to achieve the goals that you and the patient agree upon?
- On the basis of the patient's goals and expectations, as well as your understanding of the underlying disease process, what recommendations would you make for intervention at this point? What "evidence" from the clinical research literature supports your recommendations? Why have you chosen and prioritized these possible interventions?
- How will you assess whether patient and rehabilitation goals have been met?
- What type of follow-up would you recommend for this patient?

Recommendations for a Patient with Osteoarthritis of the Knee

After reviewing the evidence, and in light of R. P.'s goals for intervention, the physical (PT) therapist recommends that wearing a valgus brace may diminish R. P.'s knee pain and improve his function in standing and walking. R. P. and the PT consult with an orthotist to select the most appropriate orthosis. The PT and orthotist caution the R. P., however, that there is little evidence to suggest how long the potentially positive effects of this brace wear will last. The PT encourages R. P. to continue exercising on a regular basis because there is clear evidence that weakness of the quadriceps muscle is related to osteoarthritic conditions at the knee joint. The PT and R. P. agree on a home exercise program that includes range of motion, aerobic, and quadriceps resistive exercise and discuss appropriate intensity. The PT helps R. P. understand that brace wear and exercise should not induce increased pain or swelling or loss of function and instructs him to return to his physician, PT, or orthotist for follow-up.

ORTHOSES FOR PATELLOFEMORAL DYSFUNCTION

Just as evidence to support prophylactic and functional orthoses for tibiofemoral joint instability is inadequate, research support for the efficacy of patellofemoral taping and bracing is lacking. Nevertheless, orthotic management of patellofemoral dysfunction has become widespread in athletic and nonathletic practice environments. The need for well-designed clinical research studies is pressing.

Physical therapy interventions for patients with patellofemoral stress syndrome (PFSS) are most often directed at reducing systems. Intervention may include modalities such as phonophoresis directed at the posteromedial aspect of the patella, as well as soft tissue stretching to enhance medial patella gliding and extensibility of the soft tissue along the lateral aspect of the patella. An exercise program, guided by the patient's tolerance, typically focuses on rectus femoris flexibility, as well as strengthening exercises (especially eccentric) for the quadriceps muscle group.

Patellofemoral orthoses are often used as adjuncts to exercise to do the following:

1. Provide pain relief and improve function for patients with PFSS.
2. Prevent or control patellar subluxation or dislocation in patients with patellar tracking problems.
3. Provide pain relief and support healing for patients with patellar tendonitis of the quadriceps or patellar tendon and for patients with Osgood-Schlatter disease.
4. Manage patients with chondromalacia and other symptomatic degenerative articular changes of the patellofemoral joint.[92]

Various knee orthoses are designed to control the pain associated with PFSS. Typically, these braces consist of an elasticized or neoprene sleeve worn over the knee (Figure 13-13). Most have a circular opening to accommodate the patella and a semicircular, crescent-shaped buttress that is sewn in place or held by Velcro closures and reinforcing straps. The purpose of the buttress and straps is to stabilize the position of the patella as it slides in the intracondylar groove during knee motion.[10] The goal of the PFSS orthoses is to control the undesirable, excessive lateral movement of the patella that is thought to be the underlying cause of PFSS. Some of these braces have a hinge system that, theoretically, resists knee extension, thus reducing the potential for the unfavorable coupling effect of knee extension and excessive lateral patella excursion.[34] Other braces allow the buttress to be positioned in a number of positions around the patella, depending on the type of patella malalignment the patient demonstrates.[93] Another design uses a curved, vinyl-covered strap worn snugly at the patellar tendon to support and elevate the patella during activity for more efficient tracking.[94] Normalization of tracking can, theoretically, minimize abnormal compressive forces on the articular surfaces, reduce the likelihood of further degenerative changes, and provide relief of symptoms.[95]

Biomechanics of Patellofemoral Orthoses

The mechanism for pain in those who suffer PFSS is unclear. Various theories propose that pain can be caused from

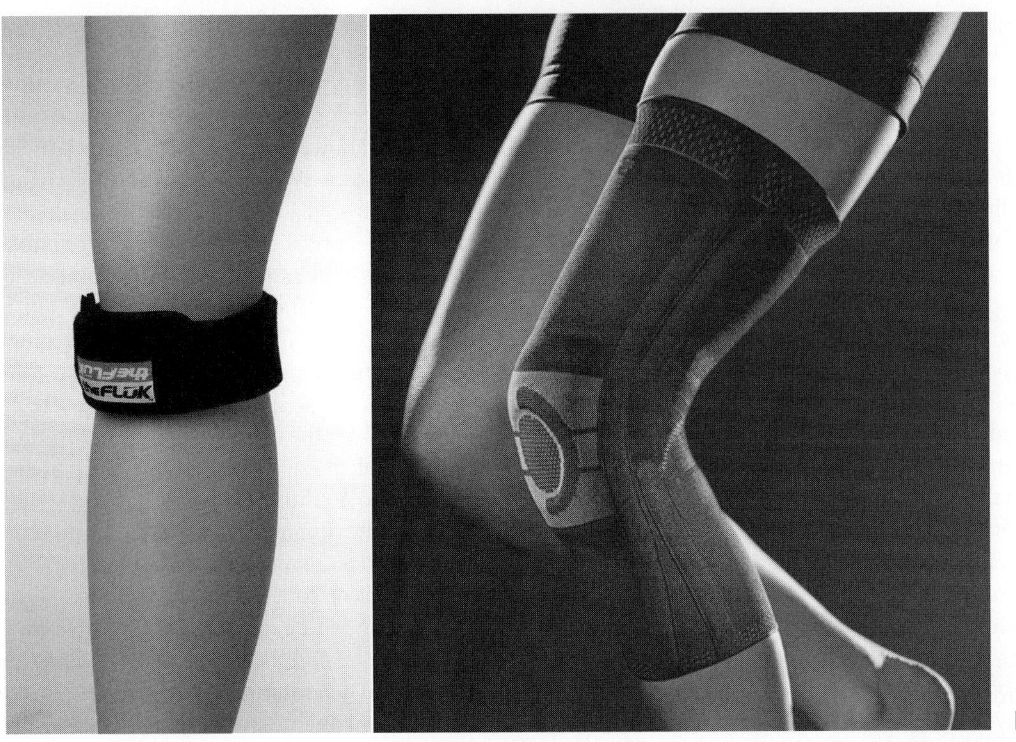

Figure 13-13
Examples of orthoses used for patellofemoral stress syndrome or patellar tracking problems, or both. ***A,*** *The FLUK infrapatellar strap.* ***B,*** *The Genutrain orthosis. (****A,*** *Courtesy Brace International, Atlanta, Ga.;* ***B,*** *courtesy Bauerfeind USA, Kennesaw, Ga.)*

patellar maltracking, tightness of the surrounding soft tissues, or less than optimal firing of various aspects of the quadriceps.[96] On the basis of these assumptions, several studies have examined the effect of patellofemoral orthoses on the biomechanical function of the patellofemoral joint. Powers and colleagues[96] studied 10 female subjects with 12 symptomatic patellae, all of whom had a kinematic MRI procedure that documented lateral subluxation in their knees. The subjects performed resisted knee extension during MRI, which recorded patella movement in braced and unbraced conditions. The patellofemoral orthosis used in this study had no significant effect on patella tracking (i.e., patellar tilt or medial/lateral displacement) from 45 to 0 degrees of knee flexion. The research did show a subtle patellar position change in the sulcus angle of the patella such that the patella moved to a shallower portion of the trochlear groove when the knees were braced.[96]

Tim[97] used a Protonics orthosis, a brace that can be set to offer resistance to the knee flexor and extensor muscle groups while subjects perform functional activities such as walking. Patients who wore the brace as much as possible for 4 weeks experienced a reduction in patellofemoral pain and improvement in patellofemoral congruence.[97] A systematic review by D'hondt and associates[98] concluded that the strength of the scientific evidence to support the use of patellofemoral orthoses is limited. The authors stated that one must take clinicians' clinical expertise and patient preferences into account when prescribing a knee orthosis.

Evidence of Efficacy of Patellofemoral Orthoses

Numerous studies have examined the effectiveness of these braces. It has been difficult to make comparisons of the research because different braces have been used and the measured outcomes also vary within these studies.

In a longitudinal study of 25 patients with unilateral retropatellar pain syndrome, Reikeras[99] found patellofemoral bracing to be minimally effective for symptom relief and return to functional activities. In contrast, comprehensive conservative management of chondromalacia[100] and patellofemoral pain[101]—staged for acute symptom management, exercises to build flexibility and strength, maintenance exercise for eccentric control and muscular endurance, and return to activity using patellofemoral bracing—were effective for 77% to 82% of patients. A preliminary report by Crocker and Stauber[102] demonstrated that use of a patellar stabilizing brace enabled four of five subjects to generate normal strength curves and increased power during isokinetic testing. Subjects in this study also experienced improved performance in functional and sport activities when wearing the patellofemoral brace. In a larger study, 59 of 62 patients with diagnoses of patellar subluxation, patellofemoral arthritis, or Osgood-Schlatter disease were able to perform activities that typically provoked symptoms (pivoting, running, stair climbing, and long-distance walking) when wearing patellofemoral braces.[10]

Although some of these results are encouraging, the use of a patellofemoral brace as the primary intervention for patients with patellofemoral pain is not well supported. Conservative management strategies with established efficacy include activity modification, limited use of nonsteroidal antiinflammatory medications, and strengthening and flexibility exercises. Further clinical research to evaluate carefully the added benefit of patellofemoral bracing in the conservative management of patellofemoral dysfunction is necessary.

The literature regarding the appropriate rehabilitation protocol for management of PFSS is inconsistent. A systematic review by Crossley and associates,[103] which examined the efficacy of numerous nonpharmacological and nonsurgical physical interventions for PFSS, illustrates this notion. The authors' recommendation, based on evidence from studies included in this review, is that stretching exercises, patient education, and quadriceps strengthening including eccentric exercises should be included in a physical therapy program. However, the evidence to support these protocols is inconclusive.[103]

A study by Finestone and colleagues[104] demonstrated that a group of army recruits having patellofemoral pain had diminished symptoms with use of a simple elastic sleeve or an elastic sleeve with a silicone patella ring, compared with a control group without braces. However, 80% of the recruits who did not receive braces were found to be asymptomatic at a 2-month follow-up visit.[104] In a study by Greenwald and colleagues,[105] subjects who wore a brace with a neoprene undersleeve and plastic exoskeleton with an extension stop reported that use of this brace significantly reduced the frequency and severity of their pain. BenGal and associates[106] demonstrated that there might be some evidence to support the use of a knee brace to prevent anterior knee pain.

CASE EXAMPLE 4

A Patient with Patellofemoral Stress Syndrome

T. L., 35, has been referred to physical therapy with a diagnosis of right patellofemoral stress syndrome (PFSS). She has had a diffuse ache around her anterior right patella for the past 2 months. About 1 month before the onset of pain, T. L. started a walking exercise program. She had increased her mileage gradually to the point that she was walking 2 miles, four times per week. After 1 month in the program, T. L. began experiencing right knee pain after completing her walk. This pain resolved approximately 1 hour after stopping the activity. She continued to walk but noticed that her pain got progressively worse over the next 2 months. Currently, T. L. reports that she experiences pain in her right knee if she sits with her knee flexed more than 45 minutes, when ascending and descending stairs, and when she walks more than half a mile.

Examination reveals that T. L. has pain on palpation of the posteromedial aspect of the patella. She also has a positive Ely's test, a measurement of rectus femoris tightness.[90] On visual inspection, the patella orientation is consistent in demonstrating some malalignments. At 20 degrees' knee flexion, T. L.'s patella sits 10 mm closer to the lateral femoral epicondyle than the medial femoral epicondyle. When T. L. is positioned supine with her knee extended, the medial border of the patella is higher than the lateral border. These patterns of patella alignment may contribute to the symptoms of PFSS.[91]

Questions to Consider

- Given this patient's history and current presentation, what additional tests and measures would provide helpful information to use in your evaluation process?
- What is your movement dysfunction–related diagnosis for this patient?
- What might the prognosis be for this patient? What are the patient's goals for intervention? What are your rehabilitation goals? How long do you think it will take to achieve the goals that you and the patient agree upon?
- On the basis of the patient's goals and expectations, as well as your understanding of the underlying disease process, what recommendations would you make for intervention at this point? What "evidence" from the clinical research literature supports your recommendations? Why have you chosen and prioritized these possible interventions?
- How will you assess whether patient and rehabilitation goals have been met?
- What type of follow-up would you recommend for this patient?

Recommendations for a Patient with Patellofemoral Stress Syndrome

T. L. states that her pain has decreased after her course of therapy. She has greater sitting tolerance; can ascend and descend stairs with no pain; and has increased her walking distance to 1 mile, four times a week. She experiences mild discomfort at the end of her walk, but this resolves within a half hour. T. L.'s goal is to increase her walking distance to that of her original exercise program, yet she is concerned that her symptoms will reoccur. She asks the therapist whether wearing a knee orthosis during exercise would be beneficial. The therapist recommends a patellofemoral brace with a lateral buttress. This orthosis would minimize T. L.'s excessive lateral patella tracking and, hopefully, reduce her pain. The therapist also strongly recommends that T. L. continue with her exercise program for stretching and strengthening her quadriceps muscle, even as her walking time and distance increases.

SUMMARY

This chapter reviewed the normal structure and function of the tibiofemoral and patellofemoral joints, with special attention to the role of the collateral and cruciate ligaments in the arthrokinematics and osteokinematics of the knee joint. The three types of knee orthoses for the tibiofemoral joint are rehabilitation orthoses, functional orthoses, and prophylactic orthoses. A review of the literature reveals a gap between what many of these orthoses are designed to do and evidence of their efficacy. This chapter identified research strategies that are most frequently used in the study of knee orthoses and discussed problems with research design, methods, and generalizability to patients and athletes involved in dynamic activities. Similar problems exist when the role of patellofemoral orthoses in sports medicine and rehabilitation are considered.

After reading this chapter, health care professionals should be better able to evaluate the intent and design of knee orthoses and to ask for clinically applicable evidence of efficacy from brace designers and manufacturers. Clinicians also have an opportunity to contribute to the understanding of the impact of knee orthoses in rehabilitation and long-term management of patients with ligamentous instability by participating in clinical research.

REFERENCES

1. Cawley PW. *Is Knee Bracing Really Necessary? A Review of Current Research on Brace Function, the Natural History of Graft Remodeling, and Physiologic Implications.* Carlsbad, CA: Smith & Nephew Donjoy Biomechanics Research Laboratory, 1989.
2. Trautman P. Lower limb orthoses. In Redford JB, Basmajian JV, Trautman P (eds), *Orthotics: Clinical Practice and Rehabilitation Technology.* New York: Churchill Livingstone, 1995. pp. 13-54.
3. Drez D, DeHaven K, D'Ambrosia R. *Knee Braces Seminar Report.* Chicago, American Academy of Orthopaedic Surgeons, 1984.
4. Levangie PK, Norkin CC. The knee complex. In *Joint Structure and Function: A Comprehensive Analysis,* ed 3. Philadelphia: F.A. Davis, 2001.
5. Antich TJ. Orthoses for the knee: the tibiofemoral joint. In Nawoczenski DA, Epler ME (eds), *Orthotics in Functional Rehabilitation of the Lower Limb.* Philadelphia: Saunders, 1997. pp. 57-76.
6. Terry GC, Hughston JC, Norwood LA. Anatomy of the iliopatellar band and iliotibial tract. *Am J Sports Med* 1986;14(1):39-45.
7. Greenfield BH. Functional anatomy of the knee. In Greenfield BH (ed), *Rehabilitation of the Knee: A Problem Solving Approach.* Philadelphia: Davis, 1993. pp. 1-42.
8. Cox AJ. Biomechanics of the patellofemoral joint. *Clin Biomech (Bristol, Avon)* 1990;5:123-130.
9. Grabiner MD, Koh TJ, Draganich LF. Neuromechanics of the patellofemoral joint. *Med Sci Sports Exerc* 1994;26(1):10-21.
10. Palumbo PM. Dynamic patellar brace: a new orthosis in the management of patellofemoral disorders. *Am J Sports Med* 1981;9(1):45-49.
11. Van Kampen A, Huiskes R. The three-dimensional tracking pattern of the human patella. *J Orthop Res* 1990;8(3): 372-382.
12. Larson RL, Cabaud HE, Slocum DB, et al. The patellar compression syndrome: surgical treatment by lateral retinacular release. *Clin Orthop* 1978; July/Aug (134):158-167.
13. Wiberg G. Roentgenographic and anatomic studies on the femoropatellar joint: with special references to chondromalacia patellae. *Acta Orthop Scand* 1941; 12:319-409.
14. Levangie PK, Norkin CC. Basic concepts in biomechanics. In *Joint Structure and Function: A Comprehensive Analysis,* ed 3. Philadelphia: F.A. Davis, 2001.
15. Muller W. *The Knee: Form, Function, and Ligament Reconstruction.* Berlin: Springer-Verlag, 1985.
16. Regalbuto MA, Rovic JS, Walker PS. The forces in a knee brace as a function of hinge design and placement. *Am J Sports Med* 1989;17(4):535-543.
17. Bassett GS, Fleming BW. The Lenox Hill brace in anterolateral rotatory instability. *Am J Sports Med* 1983;11(5):345-348.
18. Branch TP, Hunter RE. Functional analysis of anterior cruciate ligament braces. *Clin Sports Med* 1990;9(4):771-797.
19. Nicholas JA. Bracing the anterior cruciate ligament deficient knee using the Lenox Hill derotation brace. *Clin Orthop* 1983; Jan/Feb (172):137-142.
20. Beets CL, Clippinger FW, Hazard PR, Vaugh DW. Orthoses and the dynamic knee: a basic overview. *Orthot Prosthet* 1985;39(2):33-39.
21. Kramer JF, Dubowitz T, Fowler P, et al. Functional knee braces and dynamic performance: a review. *Clin J Sport Med* 1997;7(1):32-39.
22. Nemeth G, Lamontagne M, Tho KS, Eriksson E. Electromyographic activity in expert downhill skiers using functional knee braces after anterior cruciate ligament injuries. *Am J Sports Med* 1997;25(5):635-641.
23. Stephens DL. The effects of functional knee braces on speed in collegiate basketball players. *J Orthop Sports Phys Ther* 1995;22(6):259-262.
24. Highgenboten CL, Jackson A, Meske N. The effects of knee brace wear on perceptual and metabolic variables during horizontal treadmill running. *Am J Sports Med* 1991;19(6):639-643.
25. Wojtys EM, Kothari SU, Huston LJ. Anterior cruciate ligament functional brace use in sports. *Am J Sports Med* 1996;24(4):539-546.
26. Grace TG, Skipper BJ, Newberry JC, et al. Prophylactic knee braces and injury to the lower extremity. *J Bone Joint Surg* 1988;70A(3):422-427.
27. Styf JR, Nakhostine M, Gershuni DH. Functional knee braces increase intramuscular pressures in the anterior compartment of the leg. *Am J Sports Med* 1992;20(1):46-49.
28. Styf J. The effects of functional knee bracing on muscle function and performance. *Sports Med* 1999;28(2):77-81.
29. Sforzo GA, Chen NM, Gold CA, et al. The effect of prophylactic knee bracing on performance. *Med Sci Sports Exerc* 1989;21(3):254-257.

30. Styf JR, Lundin O, Gershuni DH. Effects of a functional knee brace on leg muscle function. *Am J Sports Med* 1994;22(6):830-834.
31. Black KP, Raasch WG: Knee braces in sports. In Nicholas JA, Hershman EB (eds), *The Lower Extremity and Spine in Sports Medicine,* ed 2. St. Louis: Mosby, 1995. pp. 987-998.
32. Erickson AN, Yasuda K, Beynnon B. An in vitro dynamic evaluation of prophylactic knee braces during lateral impact loading. *Am J Sports Med* 1993;21(1):26-35.
33. Garrick JG, Requa RK. Prophylactic knee bracing. *Am J Sports Med* 1987;15(5):471-476.
34. France PE, Paulos LE. Knee bracing. *J Am Acad Orthop Surg* 1994;2(5):281-287.
35. Edelstein JE, Bruckner J. *Orthotics: A Comprehensive Clinical Approach.* Thorofare, NJ: Slack, Inc; 2002. pp. 59-71.
36. Baker BE, VanHanswyk E, Bogosian SP, et al. The effect of knee braces on lateral impact loading of the knee. *Am J Sports Med* 1989;17(2):182-186.
37. Baker BE, VanHanswyk E, Bogosian SP. A biomechanical study of the static stabilizing effect of knee braces on medial stability. *Am J Sports Med* 1987;15(6):566-570.
38. France EP, Paulos LE, Jayaraman G, Rosenberg TD. The biomechanics of lateral knee bracing. Part II: Impact response of the braced knee. *Am J Sports Med* 1987;15(5):430-438.
39. Paulos LE, France EP, Rosenberg TD, et al. The biomechanics of lateral knee bracing. Part I: response of the valgus restraints to loading. *Am J Sports Med* 1987;15(5):419-429.
40. Paulos LE, Cawley PW, France EP. Impact biomechanics of lateral knee bracing. The anterior cruciate ligament. *Am J Sports Med* 1991;19(4):337-342.
41. Cawley PW, France EP, Paulos LE. Comparison of rehabilitative knee braces. A biomechanical investigation. *Am J Sports Med* 1989;17(2):141-146.
42. Hewson GF, Mendini RA, Wang JB. Prophylactic knee bracing in college football. *Am J Sports Med* 1986;14(4):262-266.
43. Rovere GD, Haupt HA, Yates CS. Prophylactic knee bracing in college football. *Am J Sports Med* 1987;15(2):111-116.
44. Sitler M, Ryan J, Hopkinson W, et al. The efficacy of a prophylactic knee brace to reduce injuries in football. A prospective, randomized study at West Point. *Am J Sports Med* 1990;18(3):310-315.
45. Teitz CC, Hermanson BK, Kronmal RA, Diehr PH. Evaluation of the use of braces to prevent injury to the knee in collegiate football players. *J Bone Joint Surg Am* 1987;69A(1):2-9.
46. Albright JP, Powell JW, Smith W, et al. Medial collateral ligament knee sprains in college football. *Am J Sports Med.* 1994;22(1):12-18.
47. Borsa PA, Lephart SM, Fu FH. Muscular and functional performance characteristics of individuals wearing prophylactic knee braces. *J Athl Train* 1993;28(4):336-342.
48. Liggett CL, Tandy RD, Young JC. The effects of prophylactic knee bracing on running gait. *J Athl Train* 1995;30(2):159-161.
49. Osternig LR, Robertson RN. Effects of prophylactic bracing on lower extremity joint position and muscle activation during running. *Am J Sports Med* 1993;21(5):733-737.
50. Van Horn DA, Makinnion JL, Witt PL. Comparison of the effects of the Anderson knee stabler and McDavid knee guard on the kinematics of the lower extremity during gait. *J Orthop Sports Phys Ther* 1988;9(7):254-260.
51. Veldhuizen JW, Koene FM, Oostvogel HJ. The effects of a supportive knee brace on leg performance in healthy subjects. *Int J Sports Med* 1991;12(6):577-580.
52. Gardner HF, Clippinger FW. A method for location of prosthetic and orthotic knee joints. *Artif Limbs* 1979;13(2):31-35.
53. Lew WD, Patrnchak CM, Lewis JL, et al. A comparison of pistoning forces in orthotic knee joints. *Orthot Prosthet* 1984;36(2):85-95.
54. Regalbuto MA, Rovick JS, Walker PS. The forces in a knee brace as a function of hinge design and placement. *Am J Sports Med* 1989;17(4):535-542.
55. Noyes FR, Grood ES, Butler DL, Malek M. Clinical laxity tests and functional stability of the knee: biomechanical concepts. *Clin Orthop* 1980;146:84-89.
56. Wojtys EM, Loubert PV, Samson SY, Viviano DM. Use of a knee-brace for control of tibial translation and rotation. *J Bone Joint Surg Am* 1990;72A(9):1323-1329.
57. Colville MR, Lee CL, Ciullo JV. The Lenox Hill brace. An evaluation of effectiveness in treating knee instability. *Am J Sports Med* 1986;14(4):257-261.
58. Wojtys E, Kothari W, Huston L. Anterior cruciate ligament functional brace use in sports. *Am J Sports Med* 1996;24(2):539-546.
59. Wojtys E, Huston L. "Custom-fit" versus "off-the-shelf" ACL functional braces. *Am J Knee Surg* 2001;14(3):157-162.
60. Beynnon B, Ryder S, Konradsen L, et al. The effect of anterior cruciate ligament trauma and bracing on knee proprioception. *Am J Sports Med* 1999;27(2):150-155.
61. Beck C, Drez D, Young J, et al. Instrumented testing of functional knee braces. *Am J Sports Med* 1986;14(4):253-256.
62. Beynnon BD, Pope MH, Wertheimer CM, et al. The effect of functional knee-braces on strain on the anterior cruciate ligament in vivo. *J Bone Joint Surg Am* 1992;74A(9):1298-1312.
63. Jonsson H, KarrhoRS J. Brace effects on the unstable knee in 21 cases. A roentgen stereophotogrammetric comparison of three designs. *Acta Orthop Scand* 1990;61(4):313-318.
64. Mishra DK, Daniel DM, Stone ML. The use of functional knee braces in the control of pathologic anterior knee laxity. *Clin Orthop* 1989;April(241):213-220.
65. Ramsey D, Lamontagne M, Wretenberg P, et al. Assessment of functional knee bracing: an in vivo three-dimensional kinematic analysis of the anterior cruciate deficient knee. *Clin Biomech (Bristol, Avon)* 2001;16(1):61-70.
66. Branch TP, Hunter RE, Donath M. Dynamic EMG analysis of anterior cruciate deficient legs with and without bracing during cutting. *Am J Sports Med* 1989;17(1):35-41.
67. Wu GK, Ng GY, Mak AF. Effects of knee bracing on the sensorimotor function of subjects with anterior cruciate ligament reconstruction. *Am J Sports Med* 2001;29(5):641-645.
68. Moller E, Forssblad M, Hanson L, et al. Bracing versus nonbracing in rehabilitation after anterior cruciate ligament reconstruction: a randomized prospective study with 2-year follow-up. *Knee Surg Sports Traumatol Arthrosc* 2001;9(2):102-108.
69. Wu GK, Ng GY, Mak AF. Effects of knee bracing on the

functional performance of patients with anterior cruciate ligament reconstruction. *Arch Phys Med Rehab* 2001;82(2):282-285.

70. Ramsey D, Wretenberg P, Lamontagne M, Nemeth G. Electromyographic and biomechanic analysis of anterior cruciate ligament deficiency and functional knee bracing. *Clin Biomech (Bristol, Avon).* 2003;18(1):28-34.
71. Cook FF, Tibone JE, Redfern FC. A dynamic analysis of a functional brace for anterior cruciate ligament insufficiency. *Am J Sports Med* 1989;17(4):519-524.
72. Marans HJ, Jackson RW, Piccinin J, et al. Functional testing of braces for anterior cruciate ligament-deficient knees. *Can J Surg* 1991;34(2):167-172.
73. Zetterlund AE, Serfass RC, Hunter RE. The effect of wearing the complete Lenox Hill derotation brace on energy expenditure during horizontal treadmill running at 161 meters per minute. *Am J Sports Med* 1986;14(1):73-76.
74. Yanagawa T, Shelburne K, Serpas F, Pandy M. Effect of hamstrings muscle action on stability of anterior cruciate ligament-deficient knee in isokinetic extension exercise. *Clin Biomech (Bristol, Avon).* 2002;17(9-10):705-712.
75. Giove TP, Miller SJ III, Kent BE, et al. Higher levels of sports participation in patients whose hamstring strength was equal to or greater than quadriceps. *J Bone Joint Surg Am* 1983;65(2):184-192.
76. Lass P, Kaalund S, leFevre S, et al. Muscle coordination following rupture of anterior cruciate ligament. Electromyographic studies of 14 patients. *Acta Orthop Scand* 1991;62(1):9-14.
77. Kirst J, Gillquist J. Sagital plane knee translation and electromyographic activity during closed and open kinetic chain exercise in anterior cruciate ligament-deficient patients and control subjects. *Am J Sports Med* 2001;29(1):72-82.
78. Chmieleski TL, Rudolph KS, Snyder-Mackler L. Development of dynamic knee stability after acute anterior cruciate ligament injury. *J Electromyogr Kinesiol* 2002;12(4):267-274.
79. Loomer R, Horlick S. Valgus knee bracing for medial gonarthrosis. *Clin J Sport Med* 1993;3:251-255.
80. Self B, Greenwald RM, Pflaster D. A biomechanical analysis of a medial unloading brace for osteoarthritis in the knee. *Arthritis Care Res* 2000;14(4):191-197.
81. Lindenfeld T, Hewett T, Andriacchi TP. Joint loading with valgus bracing in patients with varus gonarthrosis. *Clin Orthop Rel Res* 1997; Nov(344):290-297.
82. Hewett TE, Noyes FR, Barber-Westin SD, Heckmann TP. Decrease in knee joint pain and increase in function in patients with medial compartment arthrosis: a prospective analysis of valgus bracing. *Orthopedics* 1998;21(2):131-138.
83. Pollo FE, Otis JC, Wickiewicz TL, Warren RF. Biomechanical analysis of valgus bracing for the osteoarthritic knee. Presented at the first conference of the North American Clinical Gait Laboratory, Portland, 1994.
84. Kirkley A, Webster-Bogaert S, Litchfield R, et al. The effects of bracing on varus gonarthrosis. *J Bone Joint Surg Am* 1999;81(4):539-548.
85. Katsuragawa Y, Fukui N, Nakamura K. Change of bone density with valgus knee bracing. *Int Orthop* 1999;23(3): 164-167.
86. Horlick SG, Loomer RL. Valgus knee bracing for medial gonarthrosis. *Clin J Sports Med* 1993;3(4)251-255.
87. Slemenda C, Brandt KD, Heilman DK, et al. Quadriceps weakness a primary risk factor for knee pain. *Ann Intern Med* 1997;127(2):97-104.
88. Hurley MV. The role of muscle weakness in pathogenesis of osteoarthritis. *Rheum Dis Clin North Am* 1999;25(2):283-98.
89. Hochberg MC, Altman RD, Brandt KD, et al. Guidelines for the medical management of osteoarthritis. *Arthritis Rheum* 1995;38(11):1541-1546.
90. Magee DJ. *Hip in Orthopedic Physical Assessment.* Philadelphia: Saunders, 2002. p. 632.
91. McConnell J. Management of patellofemoral problems. *Man Ther* 2000;1(2):60-66.
92. Belyea BC. Orthoses for the knee: the patellofemoral joint. In DA Nawoczenski, ME Eppler (eds), *Orthotics in Functional Rehabilitation of the Lower Limb.* Philadelphia: Saunders, 1997. pp. 31-56.
93. Paluska SA, McKeag DB. Knee braces: current evidence and medical recommendations for their use. *Am Fam Physician* 2000;61(2): 411-417.
94. Levine J, Splain S. Use of the infrapatellar strap in the treatment of patellofemoral pain. *Clin Orthop* 1979;March/April(139):179-181.
95. Levine J. A new brace for chondromalacia patella and kindred conditions. *Am J Sports Med* 1978;6(3):137-140.
96. Powers CM, Shellock FG, Beering TV, et al. Effect of bracing on patellar kinematics in patients with patellofemoral joint pain. *Med Sci Sports Exerc* 1999;31(12):1714-1720.
97. Timm K. Randomized controlled trial of Protonics on patellar pain, position, and function. *Med Sci Sports Exerc* 1998;30(5): 665-670.
98. D'hondt NE, Struijs PA, Kerkhoffs GMJ, et al. Orthotic devices for treating patellofemoral pain syndrome. *Cochrane Database Sys Rev* 2003;(2).
99. Reikeras O. Brace with a lateral pad for patellar pain: 2 year follow-up of 25 patients. *Acta Orthop Scand* 1990;61(4):319-320.
100. DeHaven KE, Lolan WA, Mayer PJ. Chondromalacia patellae in athletes: clinical presentation and conservative management. *Am J Sports Med* 1979;7(1):5-11.
101. Malek M, Mangine R. Patellofemoral pain syndromes: a comprehensive and conservative approach. *J Orthop Sports Phys Ther* 1981;2(3):108-116.
102. Crocker B, Stauber WT. Objective analysis of quadriceps force during bracing of the patella: a preliminary study. *Aust J Sci Med Sport* 1989;21:25-28.
103. Crossley K, Bennell K, Green S, McConnell J. A systematic review of physical interventions for patellofemoral pain syndrome. *Clin J Sports Med* 2001;11(2):103-110.
104. Finestone A, Radin EL, Lev B, et al. Treatment of overuse patellofemoral pain. Prospective randomized controlled clinical trial in a military setting. *Clin Orthop Rel Res* 1993;Aug(293):208-210.
105. Greenwald, AE, Bagley AM, France P, et al. A biomechanical and clinical evaluation of a patellofemoral knee brace. *Clin Orthop Rel Res* 1996;March(324):187-195.
106. BenGal S, Lowe J, Mann G, et al. The role of the knee brace in the prevention of anterior knee pain syndrome. *Am J Sports Med* 1997;25(1):118-122.

14

Orthotics in the Rehabilitation of Congenital, Developmental, and Trauma-Related Musculoskeletal Impairment of the Lower Extremities

MICHELLE M. LUSARDI, WILLIAM J. BARRINGER, AND MELVIN L. STILLS

LEARNING OBJECTIVES

On completion of this chapter, the reader will be able to do the following:

1. Describe the most common musculoskeletal injuries that occur at various points in the lifespan.
2. Describe orthotic intervention for congenital and growth-related musculoskeletal impairments.
3. Classify fracture of bone by type and severity, and describe the interventions most often used by orthopedists and orthopedic surgeons on the basis of fracture type.
4. Delineate the roles of health care team members in the rehabilitation and orthotic management of individuals with congenital and acquired musculoskeletal impairment.

Orthoses play a significant role in orthopedic and rehabilitative care of individuals with many different types of musculoskeletal pathologies and impairments. Dysfunction of the musculoskeletal system can be the result of congenital or developmental disorders or can be acquired as a result of overuse injury, systemic disease, infection, neoplasm, or trauma at any point in the lifespan. This chapter focuses on the use of orthoses to manage congenital and developmental musculoskeletal problems in children and fractures of long bones of the lower extremity. Readers are referred to Chapter 13 for more information about orthoses in the management of knee pain and arthritis, Chapter 15 for more information about orthoses in the management of osteoporosis, Chapter 17 for information about orthoses for the upper extremity and hand, and Chapter 31 for an overview of the management of congenital limb deficiencies.

The understanding of how orthoses are helpful in the care of those with musculoskeletal impairments is founded on knowledge of the development and physiology of musculoskeletal tissues (bone, cartilage, ligaments, menisci, muscles, and their tendons or aponeuroses); the kinesiological relationships among these tissues; and an understanding of how these tissues remodel in response to physical stressors (forces).[1,2] The study begins with an overview of the anatomy of bone, its growth and remodeling, and a description of principles underlying the rehabilitation (examination and intervention) of persons with disorders of bone. Then the authors look specifically at disorders of the hip joint and orthotic/orthopedic strategies for limb fractures.

BONE STRUCTURE AND FUNCTION

In anatomy classes and texts, students learn that the mature adult human skeleton is composed of 206 bones (Figure 14-1), ranging from the long bones of the extremities, the blocklike vertebrae of the spine, the encasing protective ribs and skull, and the multiarticulating carpals and tarsals of the wrist and ankles that enable positioning of the hands and feet for functional activities.[3,4] Bony prominences developed from the force of muscle contraction at the point of attachment are identified.[1] Students scrutinize articular surfaces to understand how joints move, consider the hyaline cartilage that protects the joint from repeated loading during activity, and learn to examine the ligaments that maintain alignment for normal joint function. From a skeletal model or examination of bone specimens in anatomy laboratory, it is not intuitively apparent that living bone is a dynamic and

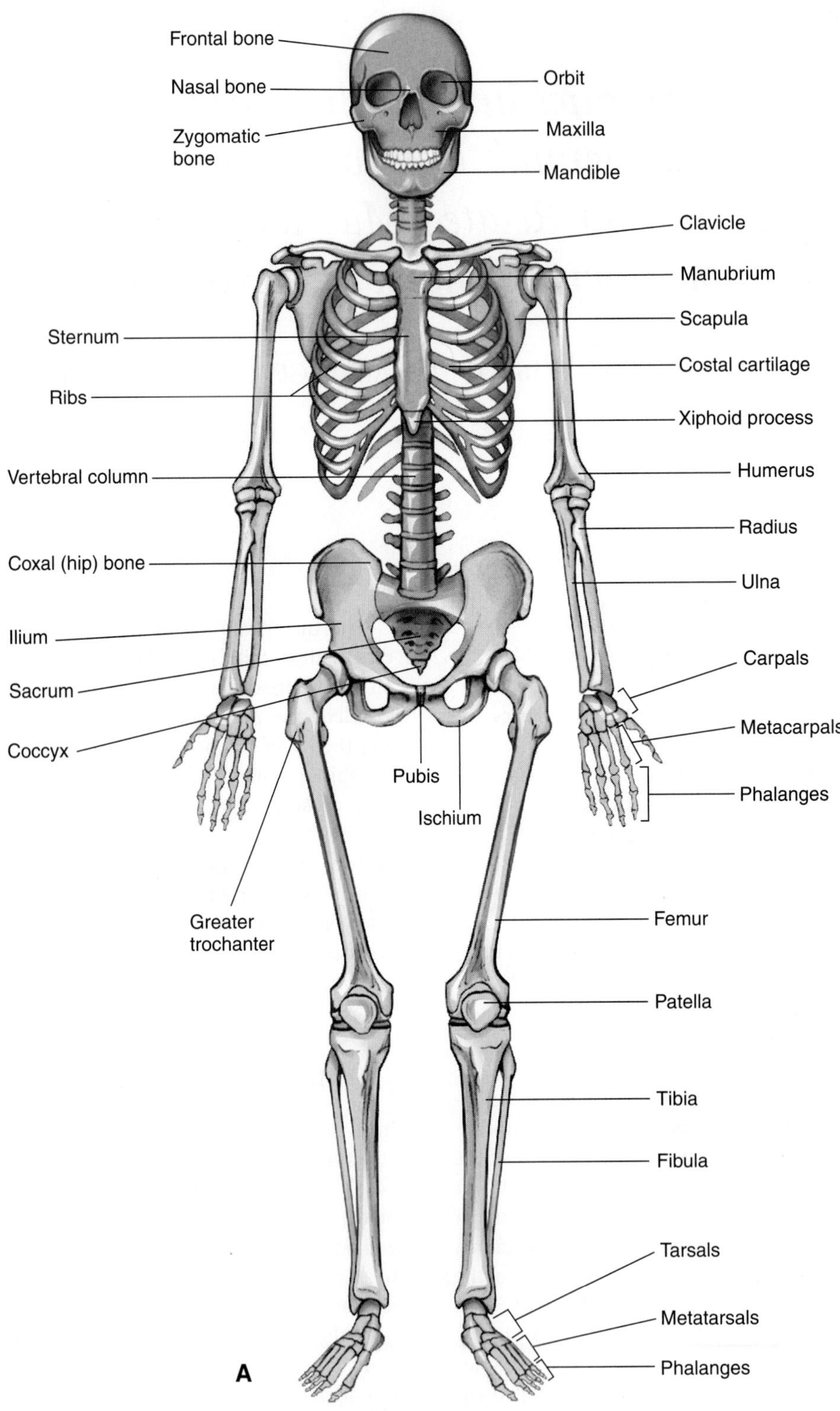

Figure 14-1

The bones of the human skeleton. ***A,*** *Anterior view. (From Thibodeau GA, Patton KT.* Anatomy and Physiology, *5th ed. St. Louis: Mosby, 2003.)*

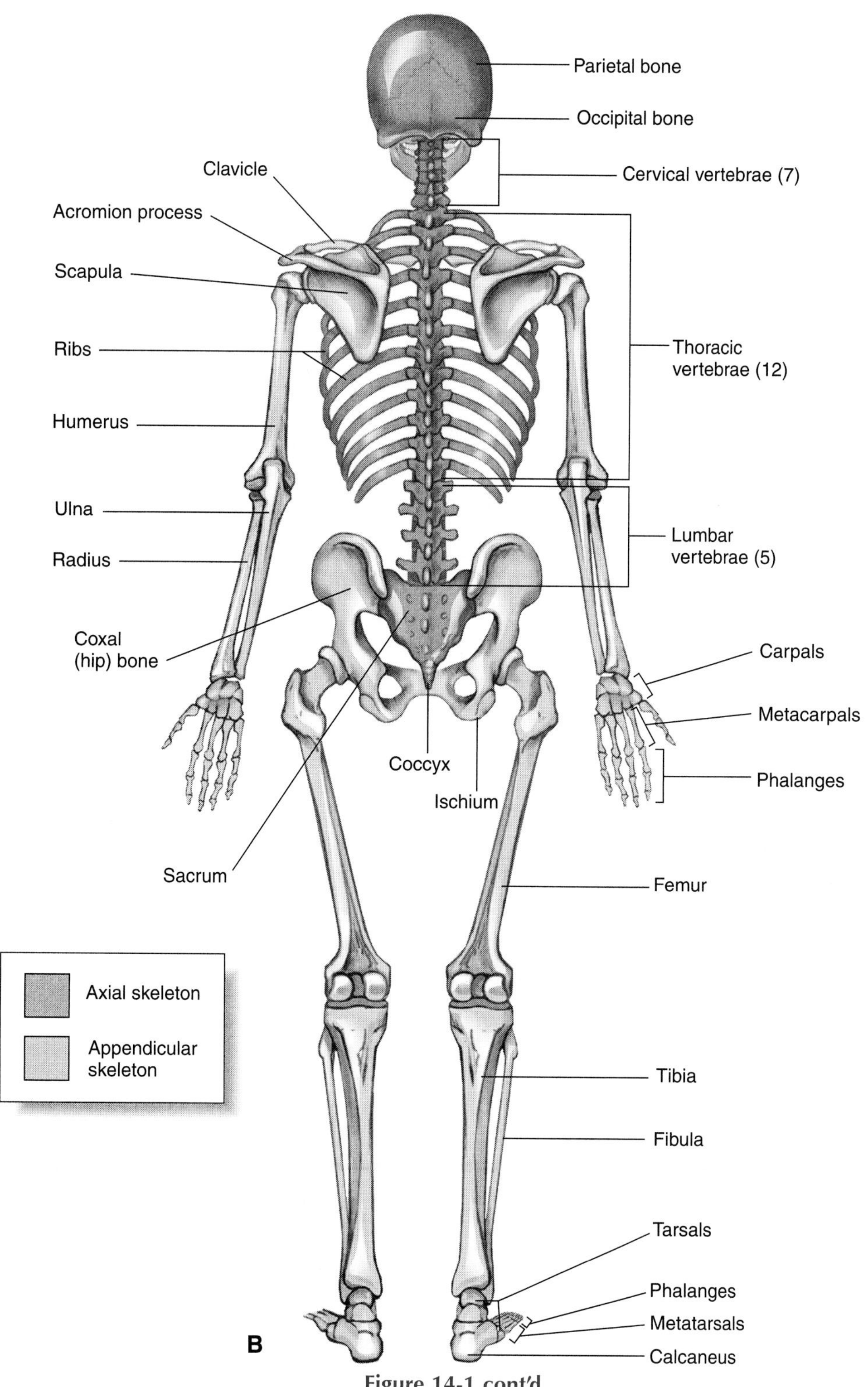

Figure 14-1 cont'd

B, Posterior view. (From Thibodeau GA, Patton KT. Anatomy and Physiology, *5th ed. St. Louis: Mosby, 2003.)*

metabolically active tissue serving multiple purposes and physiological roles.[5] These include storage and homeostasis of calcium, phosphate, magnesium, sodium, and carbonate (via ongoing osteoblastic and osteoclastic activity in conjunction with kidney function); production of erythrocytes, granular leukocytes, and platelets in the marrow; physical growth and development (by responsiveness to the pituitary's hormones at the epiphyseal plate); providing a protective and functional frame for the organs of the thorax and abdomen (how would people breathe without ribs?); and supporting body weight when the body is still and when it is moving during functional activities.[6]

Bone is a dense, regular, connective tissue derived from embryonic mesoderm. It contains a combination of specialized cells (osteoblasts, osteocytes, osteoclasts) embedded in a matrix of minerals (70%), protein (22%), and water (8%). The many bones of the human body can be described as long or short tubular bone (e.g., the femur, tibia, metarsals, phalanges), flat bone (e.g., the pelvis or skull), irregular bone (e.g., the tarsals and carpals), sesamoid bone embedded within tendons (e.g., patella), or accessory bones (e.g., ossicles of the middle ear). Alternatively, they can be classified as primarily cortical (dense) or cancellous (trabecular) bone on the basis of the density and arrangement of their components. Long bones are subdivided into regions, each of which has its own blood supply (Figure 14-2). The *diaphysis* (shaft) is supplied by one or more nutrient arteries that penetrate the layers of the bony cortex, dividing into central longitudinal arteries within the marrow cavity. The flared *metaphyses* serve as an area of transition from cortical to cancellous bone and are supplied by separate metaphysical arterioles. The *epiphyses* are metabolically active areas of cancellous bone with supportive trabeculae, with an extensive capillary network derived from epiphyseal arteries. The epiphysis is actively remodeled over the lifespan in response to weight bearing and muscle contraction during activity.[7] In childhood and adolescence, before skeletal maturation, the bony metaphyses and epiphyses are connected by cartilaginous *epiphyseal (growth) plate*, which calcifies and fuses after puberty in early adulthood. The *periosteum* is a layer of less dense, vascularized connective tissue that overlies and protects the external surface of all bone and houses osteoblastic cells necessary for bone deposition and growth. The periosteum is replaced by articular (hyaline) cartilage within the joint capsule. The *endosteum*, a thin connective tissue lining of the marrow cavity of long bones and the internal spaces of cancellous bone of the marrow space, also houses osteoblasts. Both linings are active as part of osteogenesis during growth and fracture healing.

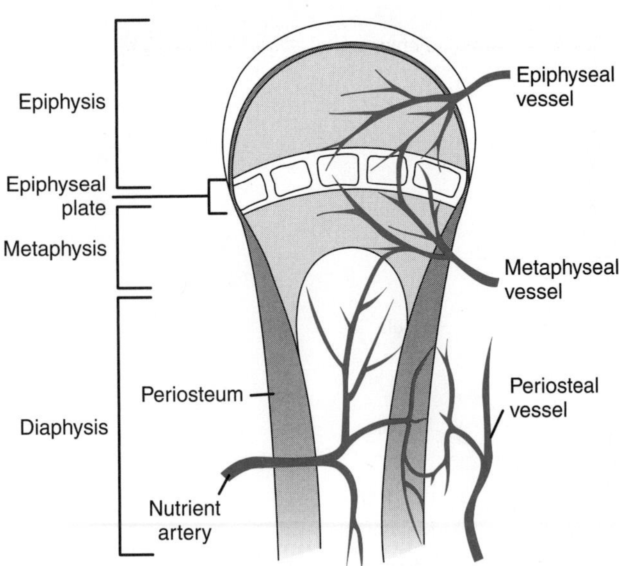

Figure 14-2

Diagram of the regions (epiphysis, epiphyseal plate, metaphysis, and diaphysis) of a long bone and their arterial vascular supply. (Modified from Lundon K. Orthopedic Rehabilitation Science, Principles for Clinical Management of Bone. *Boston: Butterworth Heinemann, 2000.)*

Cortical bone is the most highly mineralized type of bone found in the shafts (diaphysis) of the long bones of the body and serves as the outer protective layer of the metaphysis and epiphysis of tubular bone, as well as the external layers of flat, irregular, and sesamoid bones. Most of the bones in the human skeleton (80% to 85%) are primarily cortical with cancellous/trabecular bone in the metaphyseal and epiphyseal region. Cross section of a long tubular bone reveals three layers of cortical bone: the inner or endosteal region next to the marrow cavity, the metabolic intracortical or haversian region with its haversian canals surrounded by concentric layered rings (osteons) and Volkmann's canals containing a perpendicularly arranged anastomosing capillary network, and the dense outer periosteal region (Figure 14-3, *A* and *B*).

Cancellous (trabecular) bone with its "honeycomb" or "spongy" appearance is much more metabolically active and much less mineralized than cortical bone. Cancellous bone is composed of branching bony spicules (trabeculae) arranged in interconnecting lamellae to form a framework for weight-bearing (Figure 14-4, *A*). In the vertebral bodies, for example, trabeculae are arranged in an interconnecting horizontal and vertical network oriented perpendicular to the lines of weight-bearing stress into a boxlike shape (see Figure 14-4, *B*). In contrast, trabeculae in the proximal femur form an arch-like structure to support weight-bearing forces between the hip joint and femoral shaft (Figure 14-4, *C*). In living bone, cavities between trabeculae are filled with bone marrow.

Three types of cells are found embedded within the various compartments of bone. *Osteoblasts*, bone building cells, synthesize and secrete the organic matrix of bone (osteoid) that mineralizes as bone matures. They are located under periosteum and endosteum and are active in times of bone growth and repair. *Osteocytes* are matured and inactive osteoblasts that have become embedded within bone matrix. Osteocytes remain connected to active osteoblasts via long

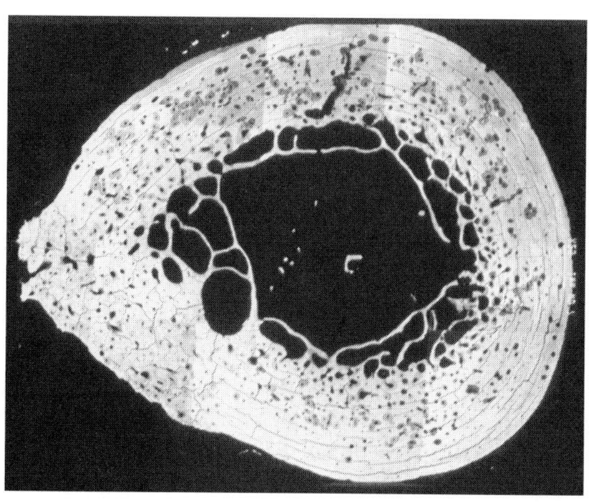

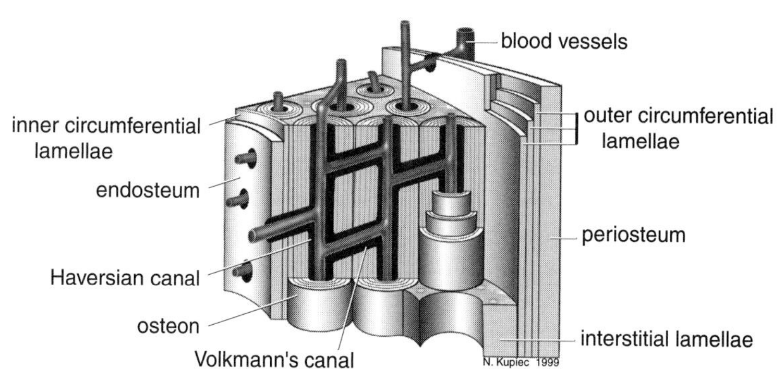

Figure 14-3

A, *A cross section through the diaphysis of a long bone, with the external periosteal layer, the middle haversian/intracortical layer, the inner endosteal layer, and the marrow cavity.* ***B,*** *Diagram of a cross section through the diaphysis of a long bone. (From Lundon K.* Orthopedic Rehabilitation Science: Principles for Clinical Management of Bone. *Boston: Butterworth-Heinemann, 2000.)*

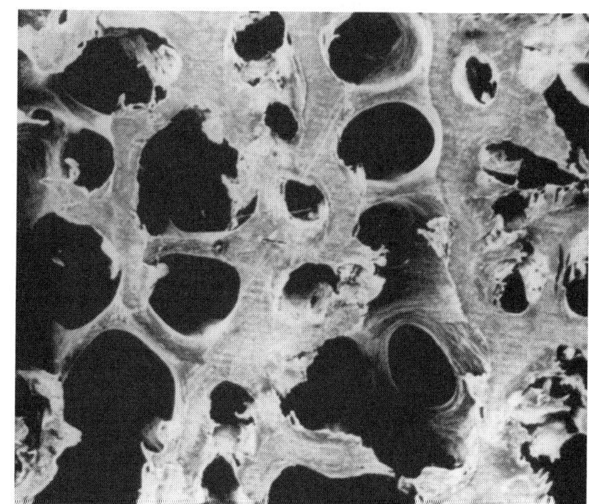

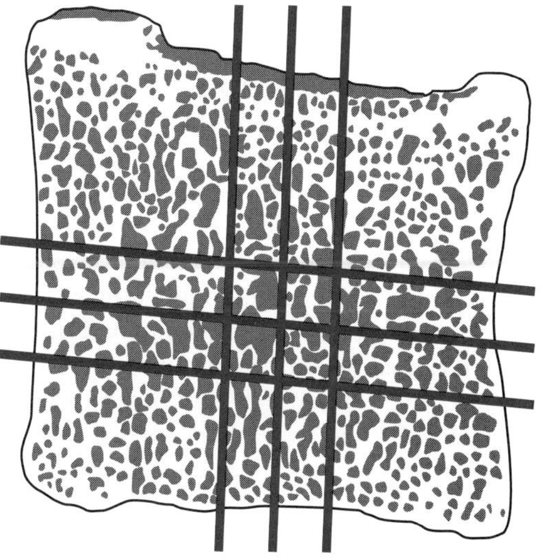

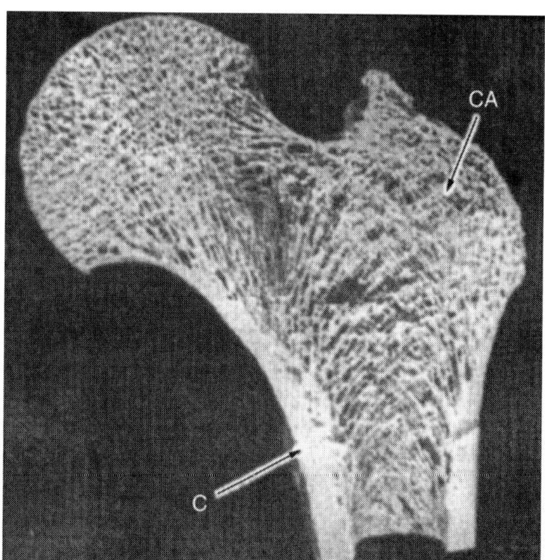

Figure 14-4

A, *Scanning electron microscope view of cancellous/trabecular bone. (From Lundon K.* Orthopedic Rehabilitation Science: Principles for Clinical Management of Bone. *Boston, Butterworth-Heinemann, 2000.)* ***B,*** *The trabecular pattern in a healthy lumbar vertebra demonstrates bone tissue's response to vertical and horizontal forces during upright activity.* ***C,*** *The relationship of form and function is demonstrated by the arched "bridgelike" trabecular pattern in this cross section of the proximal femur. (From Lundon K.* Orthopedic Rehabilitation Science: Principles for Clinical Management of Bone. *Boston: Butterworth Heinemann, 2000.)*

dendritic processes running through the canaliculi (small channels) within the bone matrix. Both osteoblasts and osteocytes are responsive to circulating growth hormones, growth factors, and cytokines, as well as mechanical stressors and fluid flow within the bone itself.[8,9] Osteocytes are thought to be involved in mineral exchange, detection of strain and fatigue, and control of mechanically induced remodeling.[10] Osteoclasts, derived from precursor cells in bone marrow, are macrophage-like cells that can move throughout bone to resorb bone by releasing minerals from the matrix and removing damaged organic components of bone.[11,12]

The epiphyses of long bones, the vertebrae, and large flat bones house nociceptors and mechanoreceptors and a network of afferent sensory neurons that contribute to exteroceptive (primarily pain) pathways.[13] The periosteum has a particularly rich neural network with branches that continue along with penetrating nutrient arteries into the haversian canals into the diaphysis.

BONE GROWTH AND REMODELING OVER THE LIFESPAN

During childhood and adolescence, growth occurs through the process of *modeling*, in which bones increase in length and diameter and are reshaped until the epiphyseal plates calcify and skeletal maturity is achieved (typically in midadolescence for females and early adulthood for males).[14] In adulthood, bone health is maintained by the ongoing process of *remodeling*, in which there is a balance and coupling between osteoblastic deposition of new bone substance and osteoclastic resorption of existing bone.[15] This ongoing process of "turnover" means that the internal architecture of living bone is actively restructured and replaced at a rate of approximately 5% per year in cortical bone and up to 20% per year in cancellous bone.[5] The rate of bone formation, resorption, and turnover is influenced by both systemic hormones and other substances (e.g., parathyroid hormone, calcitonin, vitamin D from the kidney, growth hormone, adrenocorticosteroids, estrogen, progesterone, androgens); local cell-derived growth factors; and availability of essential nutrients (calcium, fluoride, vitamin A, vitamin D, and vitamin E).[16-18] These substances, along with blood or urinary levels of certain enzymes active during turnover and metabolites of bone resorption, are monitored as "biomarkers" to track progression of bone diseases associated with high rates of bone resorption (e.g., Paget's disease, osteoporosis, hyperparathyroidism) and to determine efficacy of medical-pharmaceutical interventions for these diseases.[19-21]

In the prenatal period and in infancy, the flat bones of the skull develop as the fetal mesenchyme that forms as the periosteum begins to ossify (intramembranous ossification). Most long bones, as well as the vertebrae and pelvis, develop from a cartilaginous framework or template: in this process of endochondral bone formation, cartilage cells mature and eventually ossify.[7] During childhood and adolescence, bones grow in both length and diameter and are dynamically modeled toward their mature configurations.[22] During puberty, accumulation of bone mass accelerates; by the end of puberty as much as 90% of mature bone mass is established.[23] For young children with abnormal skeletal development, orthoses attempt to capitalize on the dynamic modeling process, applying external forces to influence bone shape and length.[24] For approximately 15 years following puberty, after closure of the epiphyseal plates of the long bones, bone mass continues to increase—a process described as *consolidation*.[22] Gender differences in peak bone mass have been well documented: average peak bone mass in women is approximately 20% less than that of men. Early in the midlife period, both men and women enter a period of gradual endochondral bone loss that appears to be genetically determined; the rate of bone loss is also influenced by hormonal status, nutrition, smoking and alcohol use, and activity level.[25-28] It is estimated that males will lose between 15% and 40% of cancellous bone mass and 5% to 15% of cortical bone mass over their lifetime. In women, menopause accelerates the rate of bone loss; there may be up to a 50% decrease from peak cancellous bone mass and 30% decrease in cortical bone mass over their lifetimes.[29] Significant loss of bone mass is associated with increasing vulnerability to fracture, especially among postmenopausal women.

ORTHOSES IN THE MANAGEMENT OF HIP DYSFUNCTION

Hip orthoses are important in the management of hip disorders in infants and children, as well as in the postsurgical care of children and adults. An understanding of the designs of and indications for various hip orthoses is essential for physicians and rehabilitation professionals working with individuals who have orthopedic problems of the pelvis, hip joint, or proximal femur. For children with developmental dysplasia of the hip (DDH) or Legg-Calvé-Perthes disease (LCPD), hip orthoses are the primary intervention for prevention of future deformity and disability. Hip orthoses are essential elements of postoperative care and rehabilitation programs for children with musculoskeletal and neuromuscular conditions who have had surgical intervention for bony deformity or soft tissue contracture. Hip orthoses can also be major postoperative interventions for adults who have had repair of a traumatic injury or a complex total hip arthroplasty. The efficacy of orthotic intervention is influenced by patient and caregiver adherence: The key to successful use of these orthoses is clear, and open communication exists among the physician, therapist, orthotist, and family concerning the primary goals of the orthosis, its proper application and wearing schedule, and the possible difficulties that may be encountered. Positive health care outcomes and happy patients and families are contingent on the ability of the health care team to communicate.

When Are Hip Orthosis Indicated?

Most nontraumatic hip joint dysfunction or pathology occurs either in childhood or in late adult life and is frequently related to one or more of the four following factors:

1. Inadequate or ineffective development of the acetabulum and head of the femur in infancy
2. Avascular necrosis of the femoral head associated with inadequate blood supply during childhood
3. Loss of cartilage and abnormal bone deposition associated with osteoarthritis
4. Loss of bone strength and density in osteoporosis

Orthotic intervention is an important component in the orthopedic management of many of these conditions. Most often, hip orthoses are used to protect or position the hip joint by limiting motion within a desirable range of flexion/extension and abduction/adduction. It is important to note that hip orthoses alone are not effective in controlling internal/external rotation of the hip joint. If precise rotational control is desired, a hip-knee-ankle-foot orthosis (HKAFO) must be used.

Hip Structure and Function

The hip (coxofemoral) joint is a synovial joint formed by the concave socketlike acetabulum of the pelvis and the rounded ball-like head of the femur (Figure 14-5). Because of the unique bony structure of the hip joint, movement is possible in all three planes of motion: flexion/extension in the sagittal plane, abduction/adduction in the frontal plane, and internal/external rotation in the transverse plane. Most functional activities blend movement of the femur on the pelvis (or of the pelvis on the femur) across all three planes of motion.

The hip joint has two important functions. First, it must support the weight of the head, arms, and trunk during functional activities (e.g., erect sitting and standing, walking, running, stair climbing, transitional movements in activities of daily living). Second, it must effectively transmit forces from the pelvis to the lower extremities during quiet standing, gait, and other closed chain activities.[30]

The acetabulum is formed at the convergence of the pubis, ischium, and ilium. Its primary orientation is in the

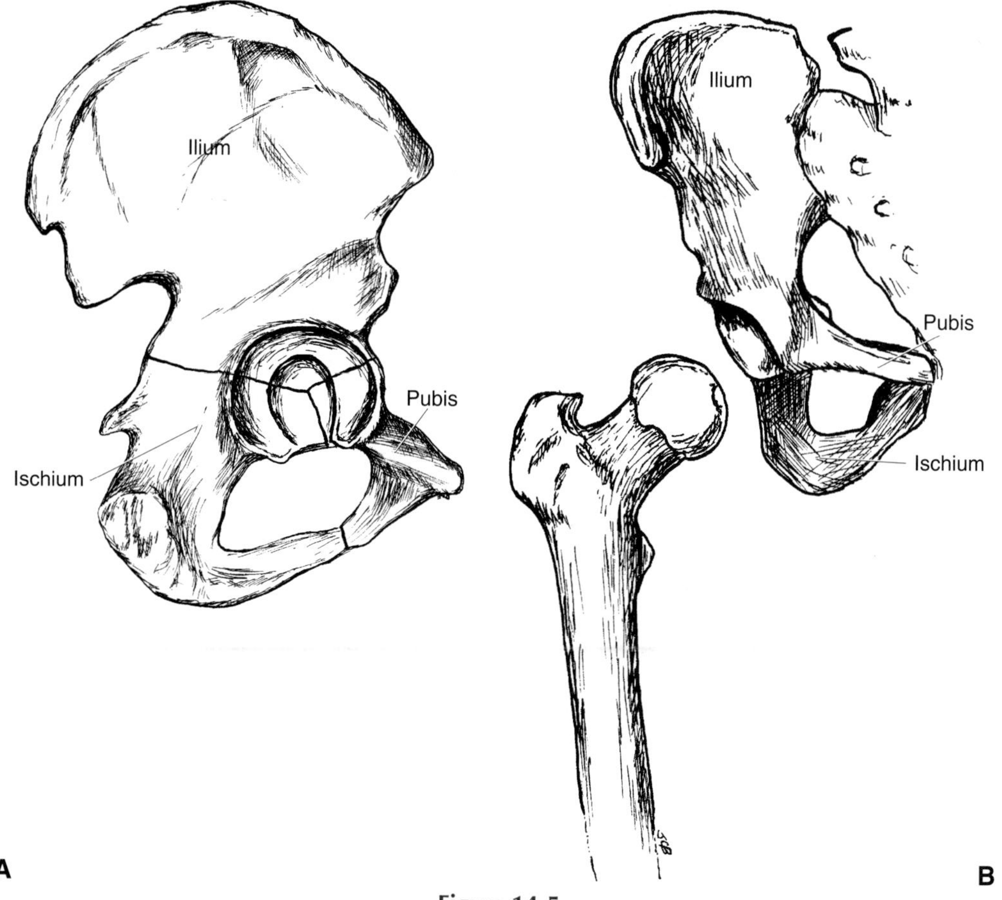

Figure 14-5

*Anatomy of the hip joint. **A,** The articular surface of the socketlike acetabulum, a horseshoe-shaped area covered by hyaline cartilage, is extended by the acetabular labrum. **B,** The proximal femur is angled to seat the femoral head optimally within the acetabulum, to support the upper body and to transmit loading forces to or from the lower extremity.*

vertical, facing laterally, but it also has a slight inferior and anterior tilt. Developmentally, the depth of the acetabulum is dynamically shaped by motion of the head of the femur during leg movement and weight bearing. The acetabulum is not fully ossified until late adolescence or early young adulthood. The *articular surface of the acetabulum* is a horseshoe-shaped, hyaline cartilage–covered area around its anterior, superior, and posterior edges. A space along the inferior edge, called the *acetabular notch*, is nonarticular and has no cartilage covering. The *acetabular labrum* is a fibrocartilaginous ring that encircles the exterior perimeter of the acetabulum, increasing joint depth and concavity. The center of the acetabulum, the *acetabular fossa*, contains fibroelastic fat and the ligamentum teres, and is covered by synovial membrane.

The femoral components of the hip joint include the femoral head, the femoral neck, and the greater and lesser trochanters. The spherical articular surface of the femoral head is covered with hyaline cartilage. Because the femoral head is larger and somewhat differently shaped than the acetabulum, some portion of its articular surface is exposed in any position of the hip joint. The femur and acetabulum are most congruent when positioned in a combination of flexion, abduction, and external rotation. The proximal femur, composed of trabecular bone, is designed to withstand significant loading while also permitting movement through large excursions of range of motion. The orientation of the femoral head and neck in the frontal plane, with respect to the shaft of the femur, is described as its *angle of inclination* (Figure 14-6).

In infancy the angle of inclination may be as much as 150 degrees but decreases during normal development to approximately 125 degrees in midadulthood and to 120 degrees in later life.[31] The orientation of the proximal femur to the shaft and condyles in the transverse plane, called the *angle of anteversion*, is also a key determinant of hip joint function (Figure 14-7). Anteversion may be as much as 40 degrees at birth, decreasing during normal development to approximately 15 degrees in adulthood.[31] These two angulations determine how well the femoral head is seated within the acetabulum and, in effect, the biomechanical stability of the hip joint. The functional stability of the hip joint is supported by a strong fibrous joint capsule and by the iliofemoral and pubofemoral ligaments. Fibers of the capsule and ligaments are somewhat obliquely oriented, becoming most taut when the hip is in an extended position.

Infants and Children with Developmental Dysplasia of the Hip

DDH is the current terminology for a condition previously called *congenital dislocation of the hip.* This new term includes a variety of congenital hip pathologies including dysplasia, subluxation, and dislocation. This terminology is preferred, as it includes those infants with normal physical examination at birth who are later found to have a subluxed or dislocated hip, in addition to those who are immediately identified as having hip pathologies.[32-34]

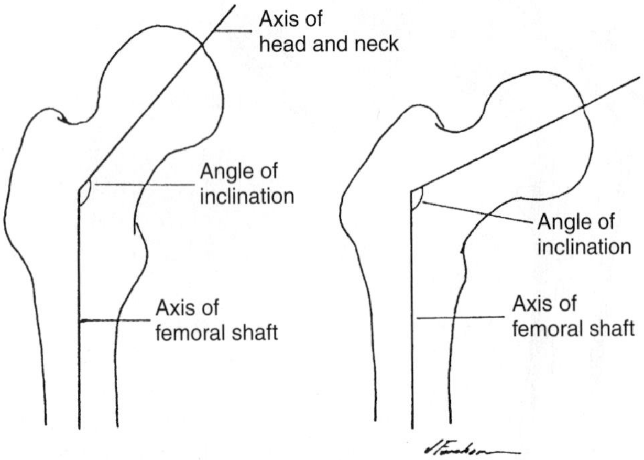

Axis of head and neck
Angle of inclination
Axis of femoral shaft
Angle of inclination
Axis of femoral shaft

Figure 14-6

***A,** Normal angle of inclination between the neck and shaft of the femur is 125 degrees in adults. A pathological increase in the angle of inclination is called coxa valga, and a pathological decrease in the angle of inclination **(B)** is called coxa vara. (From Norkin CC, Levangie PK (eds). The hip complex. In* Joint Structure and Function: A Comprehensive Analysis, *2nd ed. Philadelphia: F.A. Davis, 1992. p. 305.)*

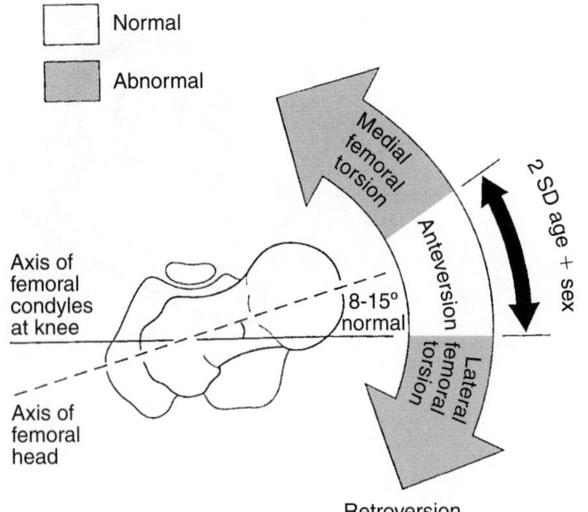

Figure 14-7

Normal relationship between the axis of the femoral neck and the axis of the femoral condyles (viewed as if looking down the center of the femoral shaft) is between 8 and 15 degrees. Excessive anteversion leads to medial (internal) femoral torsion. Insufficient angulation, retroversion, is associated with lateral (external) femoral torsion. (From Staheli LT. Orthop Clin North Am *1980;11:40.)*

Incidence and Etiology of Developmental Dysplasia of the Hip

Instability of the hip due to DDH occurs in 11.7 of every 1000 live births, with most of these classified as hip subluxation (9.2/1000), followed by true dislocation (1.3/1000) and dislocatable hips (1.2/1000).[33,35] Hip dislocation is more common in girls (70%) than in boys and among white than among black newborns. Approximately 20% of all hip dislocations are associated with breech presentation, although the incidence of breech presentation in the normal population is approximately 4%.[36] A familial tendency is also found: DDH is much more likely to occur when an older sibling has had congenital subluxation or dislocation. The risk of dysplasia increases with any type of intrauterine malpositioning leading to extreme flexion and adduction at the hip. This occurs more commonly during first pregnancies, if and when tightness of maternal abdominal or uterine musculature is present, when the infant is quite large, or when insufficient amniotic fluid restricts intrauterine motion.[32,37] A higher incidence of DDH is also found among newborns with other musculoskeletal abnormalities including torticollis, metatarsus varus, clubfoot, or other unusual syndromes.

At birth the acetabulum is quite shallow, covering less than half of the femoral head. In addition, the joint capsule is loose and elastic. These two factors make the neonate hip relatively unstable and susceptible to subluxation and dislocation. Normal development of the hip joint in the first year of life is a function of the stresses and strains placed on the femoral head and acetabulum during movement. In the presence of subluxation or dislocation, modeling of the acetabulum and femoral head is compromised. The most common clinical sign of DDH is limitation in hip abduction.[38] On clinical examination, a "click" (Ortolani sign) felt when upward pressure is applied at the level of the greater trochanter on the newborn or infant's flexed and abducted hip (Figure 14-8) indicates that a dislocated hip has been manually reduced.[39] The goal of orthotic management in developmental dysplasia is to achieve optimal seating of the femoral head within the acetabulum while permitting the kicking movements that assist shaping of the acetabulum and femoral head for stability of the hip joint.[40-41] This is best achieved if the child is routinely positioned in flexion and abduction at the hip. If DDH is recognized early, and appropriate intervention initiated, the hip joint is likely to develop normally. If unrecognized and untreated, DDH often leads to significant deformity of the hip as the child grows, resulting in compromised mobility and other functional limitations.

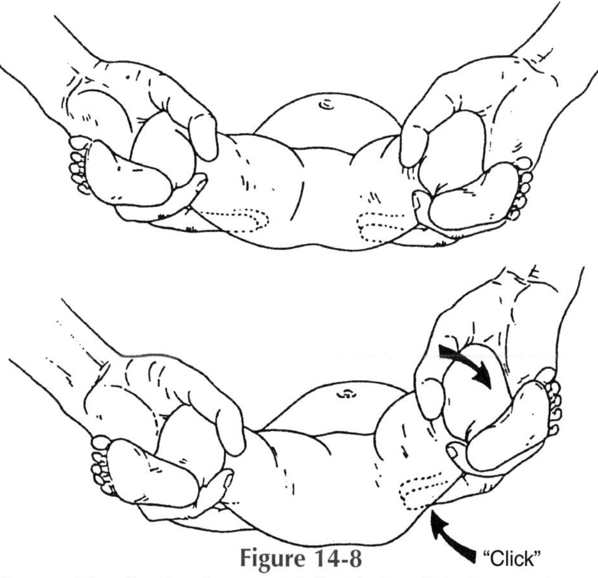

Figure 14-8

Test position for developmental dysplasia of the hip in the newborn. ***A,*** *The hip is moved into flexion, adduction, and internal rotation.* ***B,*** *A "click" when upward pressure is applied at the greater trochanter suggests that the dislocation has been reduced. (From Magee DJ.* Orthopedic Physical Assessment, *3rd ed. Philadelphia: Saunders, 1997. p. 477.)*

Early Orthotic Management of Developmental Dysplasia of the Hip: Birth to 6 Months

In 1958 Professor Arnold Pavlik of Czechoslovakia described an orthosis for the treatment of dysplasia, subluxation, and dislocation of the hip.[42,43] The orthosis he developed, the Pavlik harness, relies on hip flexion and abduction to stabilize the hip at risk. In the United States it has become widely accepted as an effective treatment for the unstable hip in neonates from birth to 6 months of age.

At first glance the Pavlik harness seems a confusing collection of webbing, hook-and-loop material, padding, and straps. In reality, this dynamic orthosis (Figure 14-9) has three major components:

1. A shoulder and chest harness that provides a proximal anchor for the device
2. A pair of booties and stirrups used as the distal attachment
3. Anterior and posterior leg straps between chest harness and booties used to position the hip joint optimally

The anterior strap allows flexion but limits extension, whereas the posterior strap allows abduction but limits adduction. The child is free to move into flexion and abduction, the motions that are most likely to assist functional shaping of the acetabulum in the months after birth.[42-44] To be effective, however, the fit of the harness must be accurately adjusted for the growing infant and the orthosis must be properly applied. Because of this, the family caregiver must be involved in an intensive education program when the newborn is being fit with the Pavlik harness. Nurses, physical and occupational therapists, pediatricians, and orthopedic residents who work with newborns also need to understand the function and fit of this important orthosis. The guidelines for properly fitting a Pavlik harness include the following key points[40,45]:

1. The shoulder straps cross in the back to prevent the orthosis from sliding off the infant's shoulders.

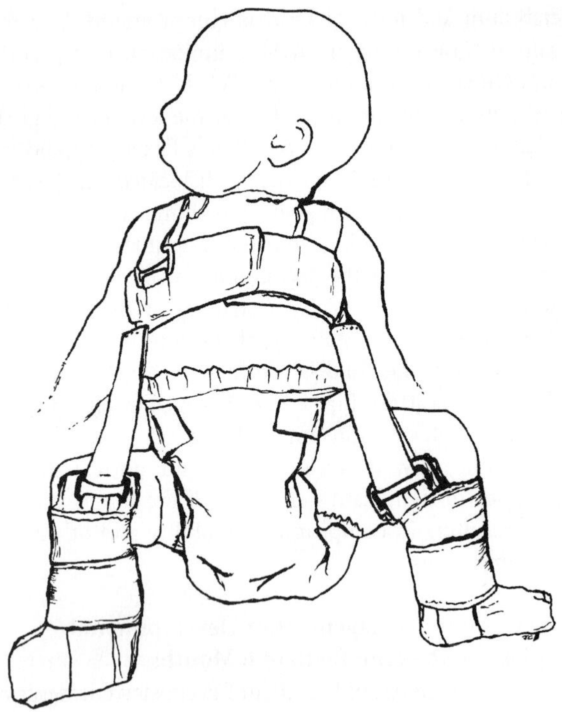

Figure 14-9

A Pavlik harness positions the infant's lower extremities in hip flexion and abduction, in an effort to position the femoral head optimally within the acetabulum, assisting normal bony development of the hip joint. The anterior leg straps allow hip flexion but limit hip extension; the posterior flaps allow abduction but limit adduction.

2. The chest strap is fit around the thorax at the infant's nipple line.
3. The proximal calf strap on the bootie is fit just distal to the knee joint.
4. The anterior leg straps are attached to the chest strap at the anterior axillary line.
5. The posterior leg straps are attached to the chest strap just over the infant's scapulae.

In a correctly fit orthosis, the lower extremity is positioned in 100 to 120 degrees of hip flexion, as indicated by the physician's evaluation and recommendation. The limbs are also positioned in 30 to 40 degrees of hip abduction. The distance between the infant's thighs (when the hips are moved passively into adduction) should be no more than 8 cm to 10 cm. In a well-fit orthosis, extension and adduction are limited, whereas flexion and abduction are freely permitted: The infant is able to "kick" actively within this restricted range while wearing the orthosis. This position and movement encourage elongation of adductor contractures, which in turn assists in the reduction of the hip and enhances acetabular development. Three common problems indicate that the fit of the harness requires adjustment[40,46]:

1. If the leg straps are adjusted too tightly, the infant cannot kick actively.
2. If the anterior straps are positioned too far medially on the chest strap, the limb is positioned in excessive adduction rather than the desired abduction.
3. If the calf strap is positioned too far distally on the lower leg, it does not position the limb in the desired amount of hip flexion.

Optimal outcomes in infants with DDH are associated with early aggressive intervention of the unstable hip using the Pavlik harness.[47,48] Families and health care professionals must seek proper orthopedic care to avoid misdiagnosis and mistreatment. One of the most common misdiagnoses is mistaking dislocation for subluxation and implementing a triple- or double-diapering strategy for intervention. Although this strategy does position the infant's hip in some degree of flexion and abduction, bulky diapers alone are insufficient for reducing dislocation.

Initially, most infants wear the Pavlik harness 24 hours a day. The parents can be permitted to remove the harness for bathing, at the discretion of the orthopedist. Importantly, especially early in treatment, the fit and function of the orthosis must be reevaluated frequently to ensure proper position in the orthosis. The many straps of the Pavlik harness can be confusing to the most caring of families. The proper donning and doffing sequence should be thoroughly explained and demonstrated to the family. Additional strategies to enhance optimal reduction of the hip such as prone sleeping should be encouraged.

Families must be instructed in proper skin care and in bathing the newborn or infant wearing the orthosis. Initially, they may be advised to use diapers, but not any type of shirt, under the orthosis. The importance of keeping regularly scheduled recheck appointments for effective monitoring of hip position and refitting of the orthosis as the infant grows cannot be overstressed to the parents or caregivers.[48-50] Missed appointments often result in less than optimal positioning of the femoral head with respect to the acetabulum, a less than satisfactory outcome of early intervention, and the necessity of more involved treatment procedures as the child grows.

Over time, when hip development is progressing as desired, the wearing schedule can be decreased to night and naptime wear. This often welcomed change in wearing time can begin as early as 3 months of age if x-ray, ultrasound, and physical examination demonstrate the desired bone development. When the orthopedist determines that the hip is normal according to radiographs and ultrasound and is satisfied with the clinical examination, the orthosis can be discontinued. If development of the hip is slow or the infant undergoes rapid growth, it may be advisable to continue the treatment with another type of hip abduction orthosis designed for older and larger babies, to maintain the position of flexion and abduction for a longer period of time.

Management of Developmental Dysplasia of the Hip: 6 Months and Beyond

For older infants and toddlers (6 to 18 months) whose DDH was unrecognized or inadequately managed early in infancy, intervention is often much more aggressive and may include an abduction brace, traction, open or closed reduction, and hip spica casting.[33,51] For infants who are growing quickly or whose bone development has been slow, an alternative to the Pavlik harness is necessary. After the age of 6 months, especially as the infant begins to pull into standing in preparation for walking, the Pavlik harness can no longer provide the desired positioning for reduction. Often, the infant is simply too large to fit into the harness. By this time, families who have been compliant with harness application and wearing have grown to dislike it and are ready for other forms of intervention.

A custom-fit prefabricated thermoplastic *hip abduction orthosis* is often the next step in orthotic management of DDH. This orthosis consists of a plastic frame with waist section and thigh cuffs, waterproof foam liner, and hook-and-loop material closures. The static version is fixed at 90 degrees of hip flexion and 120 degrees of hip abduction (Figure 14-10). An adjustable joint can be incorporated into the abduction bar; however, hip flexion is maintained at 90 degrees. This orthosis appears to be static, but the child is able to move within the thigh sections while the "safe zone" for continued management of hip position is maintained.

Many families view the hip abduction orthosis as an improvement over the Pavlik harness: The caregivers and the infant are free from cumbersome straps, the orthosis is easily removed and reapplied for diaper changing and hygiene, and the orthosis itself is waterproof and easier to keep clean. Parents and caregivers can hold the infant without struggling with straps, and the baby is able to sit comfortably for feeding and play.

Because most hip abduction orthoses are prefabricated, the knowledge and skills of an orthotist are necessary to ensure a proper custom fit for each child. To determine what the necessary modifications are, the orthotist evaluates three areas:

1. *The length of the thigh cuffs.* Thigh cuffs are trimmed proximal to the popliteal fossae. Cuffs that are too long can lead to neurovascular compromise if the child prefers to sleep in a supine position, as the risk of compression of the legs against the distal edge of the cuffs is present.
2. *The width of the anterior opening of the waist component.* Although the plastic is flexible, the opening may need to be enlarged for heavy or large-framed infants.
3. *The foam padding of the thigh and waist components.* All edges must be smooth to avoid skin irritation or breakdown, and the circumference of the padding should fit without undue tightness.

Modifications may require reheating or trimming of the plastic or foam padding. Usually this fitting takes place in the orthotist's office or the clinic setting, where the necessary tools are readily available. Once the fit is evaluated and modified as appropriate for the individual child, the parents or caregivers are instructed in proper donning/doffing and orthotic care.

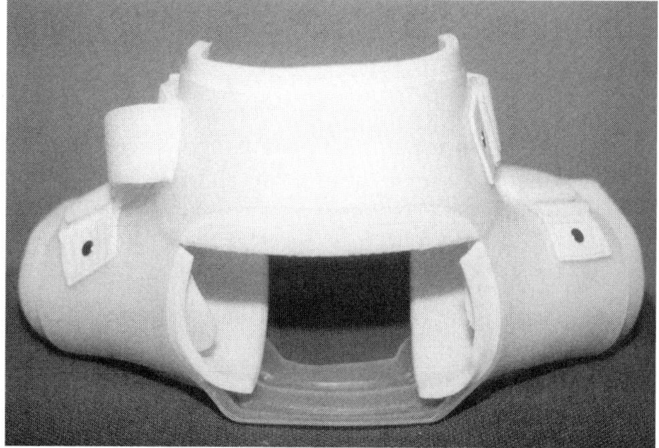

Figure 14-10
A posterior view of a static hip abduction orthosis, which positions the infant in 90 degrees of hip flexion and 120 degrees of abduction.

The static hip abduction orthosis is used in either of two ways. First, the orthosis may be a continuation of the course of treatment established by the Pavlik harness, as determined by the orthopedist's evaluation of the child's hip. As a continuation of treatment, the orthosis can be worn day and night; most often, however, it is reserved for nighttime use while the child is sleeping.[38,40,51] The use of the orthosis at night is believed to assist development of acetabular growth cartilage. If the orthosis is worn consistently for several months and evidence of effective reduction and reshaping of the joint is present, it is less likely that more aggressive forms of treatment will be necessary as the child grows.

The second application for the hip abduction orthosis is for follow-up management for children with DDH who require an orthopedic intervention such as traction, surgical reduction, or casting. In this case the orthosis provides external stability to the hip during the postoperative weeks and months, while the baby regains range of motion and continues to grow and progress through the stages of motor development. This extra stability reduces parental and physician concern about dislocation and other undesired outcomes of the orthopedic procedure.

The static hip abduction orthosis has obvious advantages over plaster or synthetic hip spica casts including greater ease in diaper hygiene and bathing and is often welcomed by families as a positive next step in treatment. Fitting requires the knowledge and skills of an orthotist familiar with proper fitting techniques and who can manage potentially irritable babies just freed from a confining hip spica cast.

Goals of Orthotic Intervention for Children with Developmental Dysplasia of the Hip

To be effective, orthotic intervention for DDH must have a set of clearly described treatment objectives against which success can be measured. The components necessary for effective orthotic interventions for children with DDH include the following:

1. Clearly presented verbal, psychomotor, and written instructions for the child's family or caregivers, with an additional goal of minimizing stress in an already stressful situation.
2. Effective communication among members of the health care team about the appropriate use and potential pitfalls of the orthosis. This often includes education about the orthosis provided by the orthotist and careful monitoring of family compliance and coping by all members of the team (orthotists, orthopedists, pediatricians, therapists, nurses, and other health professionals who may be involved in the case).
3. Safe and effective hip reduction to minimize the necessity of more aggressive casting or surgery. This requires proper orthotic fit and adjustment, as well as consistency in wearing schedules.

The ultimate goal is to facilitate normal development of the hip joint, providing the child with a pain-free, stable, functional hip that will last throughout his or her lifetime.

Complications of Orthotic Management of Developmental Dysplasia of the Hip

In most cases the Pavlik harness, perhaps followed by abduction splint use as the child grows, is a successful intervention for DDH. A small percentage of infants with DDH managed by the Pavlik harness (<8%) develop complications, the most serious of which is avascular necrosis.[33,49-54] Children who have complications differ from those without complications in a number of ways. They tend to have larger acetabular angles (>35 degrees) and less total coverage of the femoral head within the acetabulum (<20%) on radiography or ultrasound,[49,50] have an irreducible dislocation at initiation of orthotic intervention,[50] have delayed diagnosis and intervention (older than 3 months of age),[49] and have not demonstrated a prior ossific nucleus on radiograph or ultrasound.[52,55]

Orthotic Management of Legg-Calvé-Perthes Disease

LCPD is a hip pathology that affects otherwise healthy school-aged children. Although the clinical signs and symptoms of LCPD, as they differ from tuberculosis involving the hip, were first described by Arthur T. Legg in 1910,[56] the etiology of this condition is not clearly understood and its treatment and orthopedic management continue to be controversial. The hallmark of LCPD is a flattening of the femoral head, often accompanied by avascular necrosis. Left untreated, LCPD leads to permanent deformity and osteoarthritis in the adult hip. The disease is four times as common in boys between the ages of 4 and 8 years old as in girls, although outcomes in girls tend to be less satisfactory.[57-59] LCPD generally involves only one hip; only approximately 12% of cases are bilateral. It is rare within the black population. Several options for orthotic management of LCPD have evolved. All are designed to help maintain a spherical femoral head and normal acetabulum.

Etiology of Legg-Calvé-Perthes Disease

The etiology of LCPD remains controversial more than 90 years after it was first described. Most researchers believe that LCPD is a result of some event or condition that compromises blood flow to the femoral head and leads to avascular necrosis. The exact mechanism that triggers this compromise is unknown. Some theories focus on an acute trauma that damages the vascular system of the femoral head, whereas others suggest that repeated episodes of a transient synovitis may compromise blood flow.[58,60,61] Another theory suggests an abnormality of thrombolysis in children who develop LCPD.[62] A genetic predisposition to delayed bone age that exposes vessels to high rates of compression as they pass through cartilage to the bony head has also been suggested.[60] Although the exact etiology of LCPD remains a mystery, it is certainly linked to episodes of avascular necrosis in the femoral head. The goal of intervention in children with LCPD is to assist revascularization of the femoral head and to restore normal anatomical shape and alignment of the hip joint.

Evaluation and Intervention for Legg-Calvé-Perthes Disease

LCPD should be suspected in children with one or more of the following signs or symptoms[63,64]:

1. A noticeable limp, often with a positive Trendelenburg's sign
2. Pain in the hip, groin, knee, or a combination of these locations
3. Loss of range of motion of the hip joint

When these symptoms are present, radiographic, ultrasound, or magnetic resonance imaging studies of the hip are used to discriminate between LCPD (Figure 14-11) and other hip disorders (e.g., slipped capital femoral epiphysis, fracture, rheumatic disease, infection).[65] These studies are used by the orthopedist to determine severity and progression of the disease, considering stage of disease, shape of femoral head, degree of congruence with the acetabulum, and length and angle of the femoral neck.[66,67] A variety of classification systems have been developed to rate severity of involvements. The Catterall system describes four groups on the basis of the location of involvement and identifies four "head at risk" signs for the orthopedist or radiologist to focus on in interpreting radiographs.[68] Studies of the inter-rater and concurrent reliability of the Catterall systems have not all been positive.[69-71] The Salter-Thompson system rates severity of involvement on the basis of the location and extent of subchondral fracture that may be observed early in the disease process.[72,73] The Herring system examines the condition of the lateral pillar of the femoral head on radiographs.[65,71,74] The reader is referred to texts on orthopedic conditions in pediatrics for further information about classification.[60,61]

LCPD is a self-limiting process that often resolves in 1 to 3 years. The disease progresses through three stages:

1. Necrotic stage: avascular necrosis
2. Fragmentation stage: resorption of damaged bone
3. Healing/reparative stage: revascularization, reossification, and bony remodeling

Factors that influence the eventual outcome of the disease include age at onset, severity of damage to the femoral head and epiphysis, and quality of congruency of the acetabulum and femoral head.[58-61]

Because the disease process is self-limiting, the optimal intervention strategy is controversial. The three most commonly used avenues of treatment for LCPD are observation, surgical intervention, and conservative orthotic management. Decisions about treatment are often guided by age of the child, extent of femoral head deformity, and severity of incongruency between the femoral head and acetabulum.[60,61,75]

For children with minimal bony deformity, observation and exercise may be the most appropriate intervention.[76] Because the child is likely to continue to limp until sufficient revascularization and remodeling have occurred (which may require several years), parents may be uneasy, preferring instead a more aggressive intervention. Parents are reassured when close clinical follow-up is performed, with periodic reexamination by x-ray evaluation to monitor progression of the disease process.

Surgical intervention is based on the principle of containment, optimally positioning the femoral head within the acetabulum. Proximal femoral derotation osteotomy is used to decompress and center the femoral head within the acetabulum for more functional weight bearing in an extended position.[77-78] A pelvic osteotomy, which repositions the acetabulum over the femoral head, is sometimes necessary when a significantly enlarged or subluxed femoral head cannot be effectively repositioned by femoral derotation osteotomy.[79,80] Shelf arthroplasty to reshape the acetabulum to better accept the femoral head has also been used as an intervention.[81,82] The outcome of surgery is likely to be most positive for children who have full hip range of motion preoperatively. Parents must understand the goals and risks of the surgical procedure and must be actively involved in postoperative rehabilitation efforts.

The goal of conservative orthotic management of LCPD is similar to that of surgical intervention: to contain the femoral head within the acetabulum during the active stages of the disease process so that optimal remodeling can occur.[41,83] Much debate has taken place concerning whether surgery or orthotic intervention is most efficacious. If both are viable methods of treatment, the end result should be the same: a well-shaped femoral head and pain-free hip. Comparing the efficacy of surgical versus orthotic management of LCPD is challenging because of differences in study design and definition of control for variables such as age of onset, duration of the disease, gender, and inadequate interobserver reliability of classification systems.[83,84] Although two reports published in 1992 question the efficacy of orthotic treatment,[85,86] other studies advocate orthotic treatment even in severe cases of the disease. Because studies have reported success, as well as lack of success for all three types of intervention (noncontainment/observation, surgery, and the use of orthoses), the most appropriate management of LCPD has not been clearly determined.

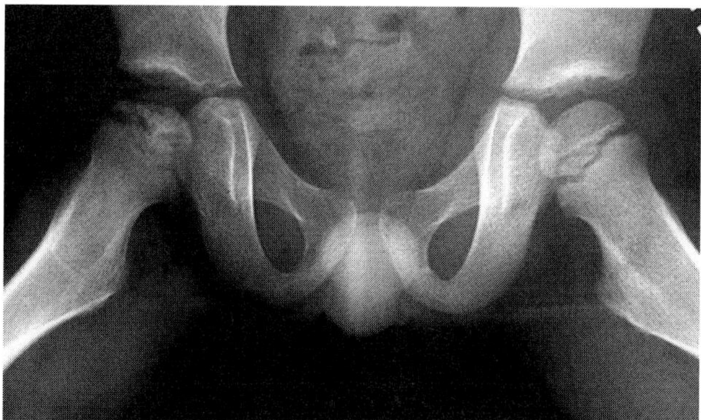

Figure 14-11
A radiograph of a child with Legg-Calvé-Perthes disease, comparing the shape and density of the head of the femur and of the capital epiphysis on the "normal" (right side of image) and affected (left side of image) right hip.

Orthotic Management in Legg-Calvé-Perthes Disease

Currently the most commonly used orthosis in the inoperative management of LCPD is the *Atlanta/Scottish-Rite* hip abduction orthosis (Figure 14-12). The design of this orthosis allows the child to walk and be involved in other functional activities while containing the femoral head in the acetabulum with abduction of the hips.[87-89] The Atlanta/Scottish-Rite orthosis has three components: a pelvic band, a pair of single-axis hip joints, and a pair of thigh cuffs. An abduction bar may also be included, interconnecting the thigh cuffs with a ball-and-socket joint as an interface. This orthosis holds each hip in approximately 45 degrees of hip abduction, permits flexion and extension of the hip, and can be worn over clothing. While in the orthosis the hips are abducted and flexed, but the patient has no limitation in knee range of motion and therefore can sit or walk without difficulty. The orthosis is not designed to control internal rotation of the hip. This type of orthosis is most effective if the child who is wearing it has close to normal range of motion at the hip joint. Limitations in

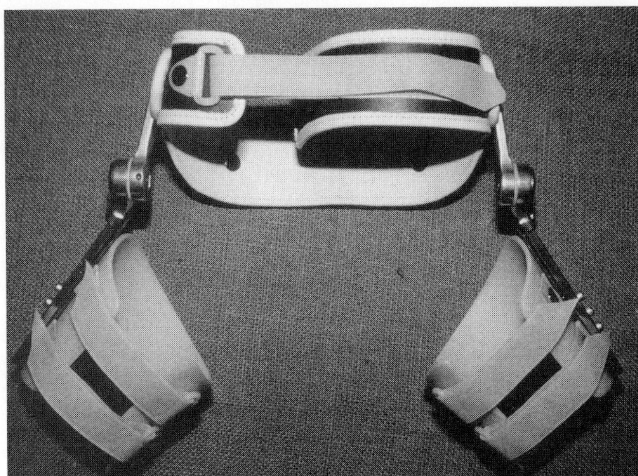

Figure 14-12
The Atlanta/Scottish-Rite hip abduction orthosis (anterior view), used in the conservative management of Legg-Calvé-Perthes disease. This orthosis has three components: the pelvic band, the free-motion hip joints, and the thigh cuffs. An abduction bar can be placed between the thigh cuffs to provide extra stability in the desired position of 45 degrees of hip abduction.

range of motion cause the child to stand asymmetrically in the orthosis, which effectively reduces the amount of abduction and containment of the femoral head.

Historically (in the 1960s and 1970s), a number of other orthoses were developed on the basis of the principles of containment of the femoral head. The Toronto orthosis (Figure 14-13, *A*) and the Newington orthosis (Figure 14-13, *B*) hold both limbs in 45 degrees of abduction with internal rotation, but unlike the Atlanta/Scottish Rite orthosis, require the use of crutches for safe mobility.[90,91] Both of these orthoses are cumbersome to wear and significantly affect the ease of daily function. Because the efficacy of the Atlanta Scottish-Rite orthosis is as high as or higher than the efficacy of the Toronto and Newington orthoses, the latter two orthoses are not commonly used in current management of children with LCPD.[41,92]

If the disease process progresses and the hip begins to lose additional range of motion, the orthotist may be the first to recognize this problem. The parents may bring the child to the clinic for an orthotic adjustment because the thigh cuffs have become uncomfortable. If loss of additional range of motion is noticed by parents or by therapists who are working with the child, an immediate referral to the orthotic clinic or physician is necessary. The Atlanta/Scottish-Rite orthosis is not designed to increase range of motion; its primary function is to hold the hips in abduction comfortably. Using the orthosis to restore range of motion defeats the purpose of the orthotic design and compromises treatment principles.

Communication among the orthopedist, orthotist, therapist, and family is essential. Parents must understand that this is a demanding form of treatment. Typically, the orthosis is worn continually for 12 to 18 months. Once radiographic evidence of femoral head reossification is seen, time in the orthosis is gradually reduced.

Absolute compliance with the wearing schedule is necessary for maximum effectiveness: A well-designed and well-fit orthosis can only work if it is being used. The first few days and weeks in the orthosis are often stressful for the parent and the child. With the hips held in an abducted position, routine tasks including walking may require assistance until the child learns effective adaptive strategies. Physical therapists may work with the child on crutch-walking techniques on level surfaces, stairs, inclines, and uneven surfaces. They may make suggestions for adaptation of the home and school environments so that sitting and transitions from flooring, chairs, and standing quickly become manageable. If family education and support efforts are effective and enable parents and children to weather this difficult initial stage in orthotic management well, the likelihood of compliance in the remaining months of intervention is significantly enhanced.

Pediatric Postoperative Care

Numerous musculoskeletal and neuromuscular conditions, in addition to LCPD and developmental dysplasia, may necessitate surgical intervention for children with hip and lower extremity dysfunction or deformity. Orthoses that control hip and leg position are often used in the weeks and months after surgery as an alternative to traditional plaster casts or as a follow-up strategy once casts are removed. Although a cast may be applied in the operating room for immediate postoperative care, orthoses are often fit soon afterward and effectively shorten the time that a child spends in a cast. Hip orthoses are used when immobilization and support will be required for a long period of time, when complications arise, or when a child's special needs demand their use.

One of the major benefits of an orthosis (as compared with a plaster cast) is in regard to hygiene, especially for children who have not yet developed consistent bladder and bowel control. Additional benefits of postoperative hip orthoses include the following:

1. Being much lighter than traditional casts, hip orthoses reduce the burden of care for parents and caregivers who must lift or carry the child.
2. Hip orthoses can be removed for inspection of surgical wounds and for bathing and skin care.
3. Hip orthoses can be removed for physical therapy, range of motion, mobilization, strengthening, or other appropriate interventions.
4. Thermoplastic orthoses are waterproof; therefore residues of perspiration or urine can be easily cleaned and sanitized with warm soap and water.

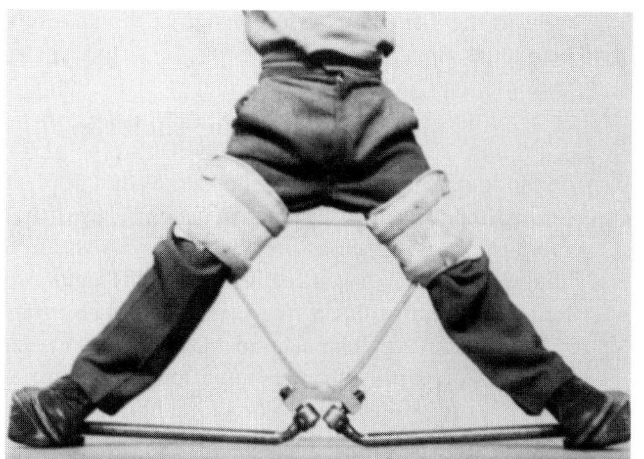

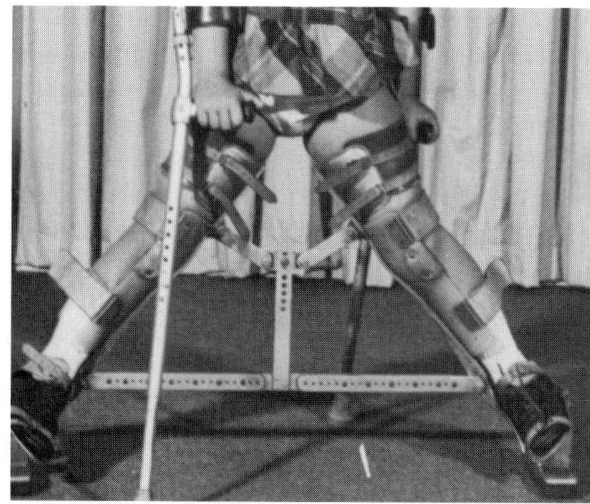

Figure 14-13

*Earlier designs for hip abduction knee-ankle-foot orthoses used to manage Legg-Calvé-Perthes disease. The Toronto hip-knee-ankle foot orthosis (**A**) and Newington orthoses (**B**) were more cumbersome to don and to function with than the Atlanta/Scottish-Rite hip abduction orthoses. (From Goldberg B, Hsu JH (eds).* Atlas of Orthotics and Assistive Devices, *3rd ed. St. Louis: Mosby, 1997.)*

5. A well-fit orthosis is less likely to cause skin irritation or breakdown and, unlike a cast, can often be adjusted if areas of impingement develop.
6. The position and amount of abduction can be easily adjusted.
7. A hip orthosis can be custom designed for a patient with complicated needs, especially those who have had multiple surgical procedures.

Postoperative Hip Orthoses

Two basic designs are available for children's postoperative orthoses. The first is composed of thigh cuffs that fit between the knee and hip joint, an abduction bar, and hook-and-loop material closures (Figure 14-14). This orthosis can be fabricated from measurements taken before surgery and fit with no delay as soon as the cast is removed. It can also be fit in lieu of a cast if the surgical procedure was minor or when static positioning of the hip is required. This type of orthosis is commonly used after adductor release or varus osteotomy with adductor release or for the management of a septic hip. A postoperative hip orthosis is most often used for extended periods of nighttime-only wear but in some circumstances can also be worn during the day.[93] In many clinics this orthosis is used after hip procedures in children with cerebral palsy.

Parents and caregivers find the postoperative hip orthosis a welcome relief from a cast. Despite its simple appearance, families should be given special instructions about how the orthosis is worn and cared for. It can be worn over clothing or pajamas or next to the skin if necessary. It should not cause skin irritation or discomfort on either side of the hip joint. If the patient experiences any hip joint pain, the orthotist should consult with the orthopedist to determine if the angle of abduction can be safely adjusted. Overzealous attempts to abduct the hip can cause pain and reduce compliance. Occasionally, this orthosis may be difficult to keep in place even though it has been properly fit. A simple suspension belt can be added to ensure optimal positioning.

The second option for postoperative care is a modification of a knee-ankle-foot orthosis. This orthosis is composed of two thermoplastic knee-ankle-foot orthoses without knee joints but with an abduction bar and hook-and-loop material closures (Figure 14-15). Fabrication of this type of orthosis requires that plaster impressions be taken: Simple length and circumferential measurements are not adequate to ensure proper fit. Ideally, these impressions are taken at the first postoperative cast change. The orthosis is then fabricated, and fitting occurs during the next clinic appointment. Taking the impressions before surgery is not advisable. Postoperatively, each joint will be at a new angle, compromising the fit of the orthosis based on preoperative impressions. This type of orthosis is recommended for patients who have had bony procedures around the hip, as well as extensive soft tissue procedures such as hamstring or heel cord release, which require protection in the early stages of healing. In our clinic, this orthosis is most often used for children with cerebral palsy or myelomeningocele. In some circumstances, when more precise control of the hip joint is desirable, the orthosis can be extended upward to include the pelvis.

Because of the intimate fit of this orthosis, parents and caregivers must be given careful education concerning proper fit and cleaning. Especially important is a careful inspection of the posterior aspect of the calcaneus: This area is vulnerable to skin breakdown from prolonged pressure and may be overlooked during skin checks that focus on the healing surgical wounds. Because the foam lining and thermoplastic material do not "breathe," perspiration cannot effectively evaporate. The orthosis should be removed periodically for cleaning to minimize the risk of skin maceration or infection from microorganisms that thrive in warm moist environments.

The postoperative orthosis has proven useful in the overall orthopedic management of children with musculoskeletal or neuromuscular diseases. The orthosis is an effective substitute for heavy casts, especially when skin irritation and incontinence are concerns. The postoperative hip orthosis helps to ensure healing in the optimal joint position and reduces the likelihood of recurrence of the deformity that prompted surgical intervention.

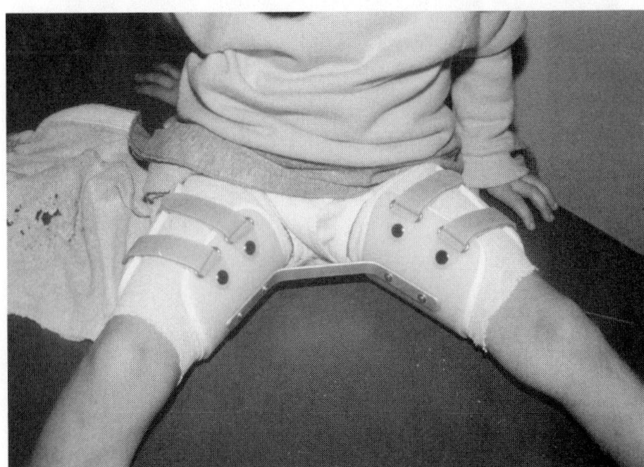

Figure 14-14
A postoperative hip abduction orthosis has two components: a pair of thigh cuffs held in position by an abduction bar.

Management of the Adult Hip

Orthotic intervention for the hip in the adult population is limited, focusing on two groups of patients. Hip orthoses are most commonly used as postsurgical and postcast care of adult patients who have sustained a complex hip or proximal femoral fracture from a traumatic event such as a motor vehicle accident, industrial accident, or fall. In some circumstances a hip orthosis can be used for older adults after a total hip procedure, revision of a total hip, or fracture associated with total hip arthroplasty.[94,95] Although injury that affects the hip can occur at any point in the lifespan, most adults with trauma-related fractures who are managed with hip orthoses are young and middle aged, and many of those who are undergoing a new or revised total joint arthroplasty are 65 years or older. As the number of older adults increases in the U.S. population, so will the number of hip fractures. One estimate suggests that as many as 512,000 hip fractures will occur in the United States by the year 2040.[96]

In both of these circumstances, stabilization of the orthopedic injury and rehabilitation planning are important issues. Patients with this type of injury of the hip often require extensive physical therapy programs. Clinicians must understand age-related pathophysiological changes that affect the healing musculoskeletal system, the impact and detrimental effects of prolonged bed rest, and the optimal

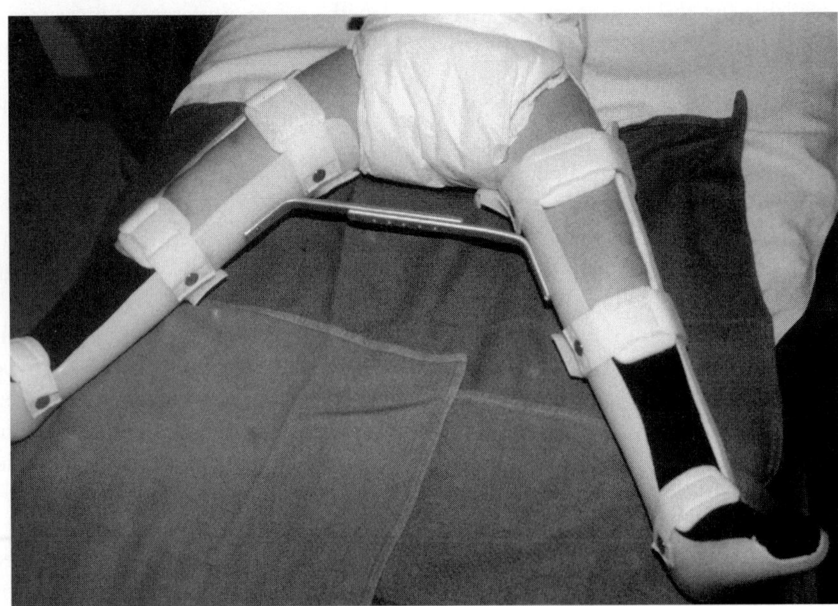

Figure 14-15
For postoperative management of children after extensive bony and soft tissue surgery, knee-ankle-foot orthoses with the addition of an abduction bar are often used subsequent to cast removal. Rotation of the hip is well controlled by the intimate fit of the orthosis including the ankle-foot complex. When precise control of the hip is necessary, the postoperative hip abduction orthosis encompasses the pelvis as well.

point at which an orthosis should be integrated into the overall treatment plan.

Total Hip Arthroplasty

Although a hip orthosis is usually not indicated in most simple, elective total hip arthroplasties, in some circumstances this orthosis can assist healing and rehabilitation. Hip orthoses can be used for patients with significant osteoporosis in whom femoral fracture occurs during total joint surgery or for those who require emergency total joint replacement as a result of trauma. Hip orthoses are also used for patients who are undergoing revision of a total hip replacement as a consequence of recurrent dislocation or of aseptic loosening of the femoral component. If control of rotation is desired, an HKAFO can be prescribed to provide additional support and protection to healing structures.

Most HKAFOs have a pelvic band and belt and an adjustable hip joint that can be locked or can allow free motion or limit motion within a specific range (Figure 14-16). An adjustable anterior panel can be added to the thigh section if a fracture has occurred during the surgical procedure and requires additional protection. The knee joint can also be locked, free motion, or adjustable for specific ranges of motion, depending on the patient's need. The ankle-foot orthosis component is necessary to provide maximum control of unwanted rotation of the hip.

Typically, HKAFOs are custom fabricated on the basis of an impression of the patient's limb. This increases the likelihood of an optimal fit and allows customization of the orthosis to meet the specific needs of the patient. If this approach is not amenable to certain health care environments, prefabricated custom-fit HKAFOs and hip orthoses are available as alternatives to custom-molded orthoses.[95] These orthoses are fabricated from components that are then custom fit on the basis of the patient's limb measurements. Most postoperative hip orthoses are designed to limit flexion and adduction of the hip joint (Figure 14-17). They try to prevent dislocation by supporting the optimal position of the hip joint within a safe range of motion and by providing a kinesthetic reminder when patients attempt to move beyond these ranges.[95] Many of the prefabricated hip orthoses that are commercially available are unable to provide maximum control of rotation because they do not encompass the foot. Careful evaluation of the patient is required to determine which alternative is most appropriate. In both cases the orthosis is worn whenever the patient is out of bed and, in some instances, while the patient is in bed as well. The orthosis is usually worn for at least 8 weeks after total hip revision.

Because lower extremity orthoses add weight to a lower extremity that is already compromised, orthotists must be sensitive to the selection of lightweight materials and components. This is especially true for older patients, who may have limited endurance because of cardiac or respiratory disease. Although the initial orthosis may restrict joint motion to provide external stability to a vulnerable hip joint, the orthotic hip, knee, and ankle joints can be adjusted to meet the patient's needs as the rehabilitation program progresses. Hip orthoses and HKAFOs may be important adjuncts for rehabilitation in the following ways:

1. A well-fit hip orthosis provides protection against dislocation in patients who are predisposed to this problem.
2. Hip orthoses protect and support healing fracture sites, often allowing earlier mobility and gait training than would otherwise be possible.
3. Early and safe weight bearing for older patients with dislocation or fracture reduces the risk of secondary complications associated with prolonged bed rest or immobility.
4. The orthotic hip, knee, and ankle joints can be adjusted to restrict or permit motion to match the patient's specific needs at initial fitting and as the treatment program progresses.

Following surgical intervention after fracture or total joint arthroplasty, the focus of the rehabilitation program shifts to

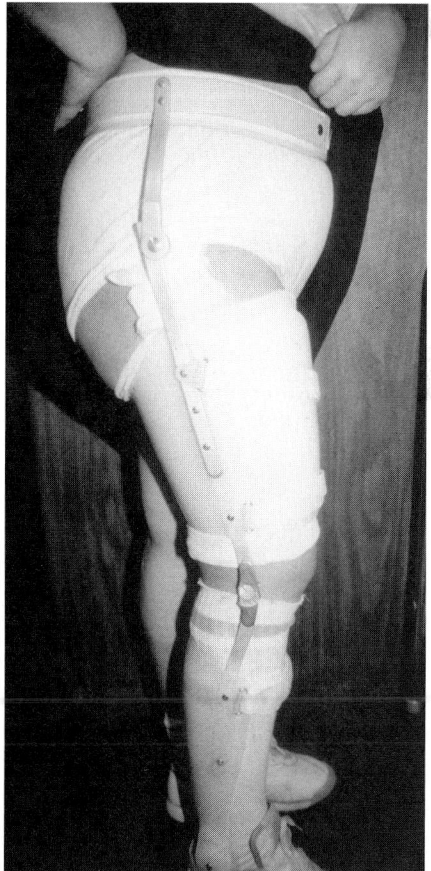

Figure 14-16

Lateral view of a hip-knee-ankle-foot orthosis, prescribed for postoperative management after a complex total hip arthroplasty. Note the pelvic band, free hip joint, supportive thigh cuff, and free knee joint. The ankle-foot orthosis component is necessary for effective control of rotary forces through the femur and hip joint.

mobility training, strengthening, flexibility, and endurance. The decision to recommend a hip orthosis is individual, influenced by the severity of the musculoskeletal problem, the patient's particular circumstances, and the experience and preferences of the health professionals involved in postoperative care. Few definitive guidelines or documentation are available concerning the efficacy of hip orthoses in the postoperative management of hip fracture or arthroplasty. An orthosis is best used to augment the goals of rehabilitation including the return to preoperative ambulatory status, safe and protected weight bearing during activities of daily living, facilitation of union of the fracture site, and ultimately return to presurgical social and self-care independence.

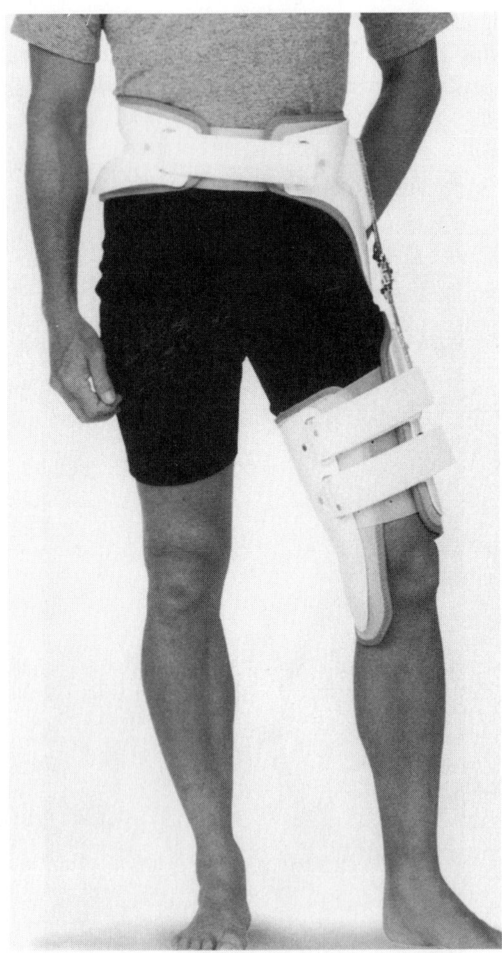

Figure 14-17
A postoperative hip abduction orthosis has three components. The proximal component is a padded pelvic band with a lateral extension and anterior closure that fits snugly around the upper pelvis. The distal component is a thigh cuff with a medial extension across the medial knee joint. These two pieces are connected by uprights and an adjustable hip joint, angled toward hip abduction and adjusted to limit hip flexion or extension. (From Orthomerica Newport. JPO 1995;7[1]:advertisement on front cover.)

Posttrauma Care

The other group of individuals who may benefit from hip orthoses are those who have experienced traumatic fractures of the femur, hip, or pelvis as a result of motor vehicle accidents, industrial accidents, or falls from great heights. Most of these patients are fit with their orthosis after stabilization of the fracture with internal fixation. The HKAFO is similar in design to the orthosis described for older patients after hip fracture or arthroplasty. Depending on the need for external support and stability, the hip joint can be locked to prevent flexion and extension or may allow motion within a limited range. For some patients, it may be necessary to incorporate a lumbosacral spinal orthosis to achieve the desired control of pelvic and hip motion. The ankle-foot orthosis component provides control of hip rotation in the transverse plane.

When complete immobilization is warranted after orthopedic trauma of the lower spine, pelvis, and hip, a custom-molded thermoplastic version of a hip spica cast can be fabricated (Figure 14-18). This hip orthosis has anterior and posterior components, extending from the mid- to lower thoracic trunk to just above the femoral condyles of the fractured extremity and to the groin of the intact extremity. This design provides maximum stability and can be used in lieu of or after casting. The position of the lower extremity within the orthosis is determined by the type and extent of the surgical repair. When the patient is lying in the supine position, the anterior component can be removed for skin inspection and personal care. Similarly, the posterior component can be removed when the patient is prone. This is an advantage for patients with open wounds or difficulty with continence and is especially appreciated if immobilization will be required for an extended period.

Many patients who are recovering from musculoskeletal trauma involving the pelvis and hip joint require physical therapy for gait and mobility training after surgery and an intensive rehabilitation program to regain preinjury muscle strength, range of motion, and functional status. The orthopedic surgeon and therapists, as well as the patient and family, must clearly understand the advantages provided and the mobility limitations imposed by postsurgical hip orthoses. An optimal orthosis can assist rehabilitation if fabricated with lightweight but durable components that can be adjusted as the patient progresses, while meeting the individual patient's need for stability or supported mobility of the hip. An appropriate hip orthosis also enhances early mobility and protected weight bearing, reducing the risk of loss of function related to bed rest and deconditioning.

FRACTURE MANAGEMENT

A fracture occurs when there is disruption in the continuity of bone and its associated cartilage.[97] Fractures are common consequences of trauma from falls, sports, work-related injuries, motor vehicle accidents, or violence.[98-100] Many disorders and diseases (e.g., osteopenia, malnutrition, paralysis, osteoporosis), as well as primary or metastatic malignancies of bone, increase vulnerability to fracture.[101,102] Habitual activity level over the lifespan, health habits (e.g., smoking), and gender and age (e.g., bone density and menopausal status) influence bone density and, subsequently, the risk of fracture during daily activity.[103-106] Orthopedic intervention for fractures is dictated by the severity of the fracture, as well as etiology. Simple fractures, those with minimal fragmentation or displacement, are often managed with closed reduction followed by a period of immobilization in a plaster or fiberglass cast or a custom-fit, prefabricated fracture orthosis until bony union is achieved.[107] More complex fractures, those with multiple fragments or significant displacement, often require open (surgical) reduction with internal fixation (with screws, plates, or prosthetic replacement) (ORIF) or stabilization in an external rigging or frame until there has been sufficient bony repair.[108]

The care provided to individuals recovering from a fracture is founded on understanding the mechanism of injury, fracture classification, and process of bone repair and healing.[109,110] The orthopedic surgeon and orthotist choose from a variety of casts, cast braces, splints, and fracture orthoses to provide the most effective fracture management strategy for each patient on the basis of the fracture type and location, degree of reduction, skin condition, mobility needs, and likelihood of compliance. Geographical and personal preferences regarding design, device selection, and treatment influence the choice of fracture management strategy, as do the training and experience of the health professionals involved. Few strategies for immobilization can provide 100% rigid fixation. Absolute immobilization is only possible with direct skeletal attachment. A variety of factors influence the quality of fit and function of any cast, cast brace, splint, or fracture orthosis. Each device has the potential to contribute to a successful result, but only if used appropriately, with absolute attention to detail by each of the treatment team members.

Mechanisms of Fracture Healing

Three distinct stages of physiological fracture repair occur: inflammation, repair, and remodeling.[110] Fracture damages bone; its periosteum; nutrient vessels; marrow; and, often, surrounding soft tissue and muscle. Disruption of vascular supply leads to ischemia and necrosis of bone cells and other injured tissues. These damaged tissues release inflammatory mediators into intracellular space, triggering an *inflammatory response*: a shift in plasma from capillary to intracellular space leads to significant edema. Migration of polymorphonuclear leukocytes, macrophages, and lymphocytes to the injured area is the first step in clearing necrosis. A hematoma forms; in a simple nondisplaced fracture on the shaft of a long bone, this hematoma provides the initial "reconnection of" edges of the fracture (Figure 14-19, *A*). In more complex fractures, the process of reducing the fracture to align bony fragments further irritates tissues, augmenting the inflammatory response that is the first necessary step in fracture healing. This initial inflammatory response to fracture can last 5 or more days, depending on the severity of injury and extent of tissue disruption.

The next stage of healing is the *repair stage*, a period of cell migration, proliferation, and granulation. The combination of chemotactic factors and bone matrix proteins released by damaged bone and during inflammation triggers the initiation of bony repair. The hematoma organizes into a fibrin "scaffold," and cells within the hematoma begin to release growth factors and other proteins that trigger cell migration and proliferation of osteoblasts from the periosteum and endosteum, as well as synthesis of a fracture callus matrix for bony repair (Figure 14-19, *B* and *C*).[111] Initially the pH of the area around the fracture is acidic, and the fracture callus is primarily cartilaginous. As the repair stage progresses, the pH becomes more alkaline, creating an environment that enhances activity of the alkaline phosphatase enzyme, and subsequently mineralization of the cartilage of the fracture callus into woven bone tissue (Figure 14-19, *D*). The deposition of new cartilage within the callus is accompanied by both endochondral and intramembranous ossification. Clinical union of the fracture during the repair stage can last up to 3 months postinjury (hence the need for long periods of immobilization).

The final stage of healing is the *remodeling stage*, during which the new bone woven within the callus is reshaped into the more mature lamellae of long bone and excess callus resorbed. During this phase osteoclasts are active to reshape trabeculae and lamellae along the lines of weight-bearing

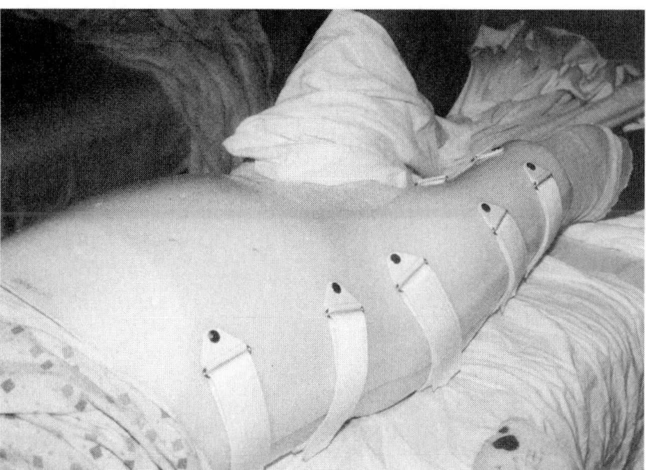

Figure 14-18
A postoperative custom-molded hip orthosis is sometimes used instead of a plaster hip spica cast when complete immobilization of the hip joint is required.

forces. The process of maturation of the callus into a fully repaired bone can last a year or more, especially in complex fractures, whether managed by casting or ORIF. Factors that influence the duration of the remodeling stage include age, severity of injury, nutritional status, concurrent chronic illness, and medication use (especially corticosteroids).[112]

Fracture Classifications

Fractures are classified as either open or closed injuries on the basis of the disruption of the skin and soft tissue surrounding the injured bone.[113] In a *closed fracture*, the soft tissue envelope of muscles and skin around the bone fracture site is completely intact. Although muscle around the fracture site may be significantly damaged, the intact skin provides a barrier that prevents bacterial invasion of the injured muscle or bone. When an *open* or *compound* fracture occurs, the soft tissue envelope has been violated: The wound leaves muscle and fractured bone open to the environment and susceptible to infection. In many cases bone may actually protrude through the skin. Open injuries are orthopedic emergencies; patients are quickly taken to the operating room for débridement of the wound and fracture. Severely damaged or contaminated tissue is removed, and the wound is carefully cleaned in an effort to avoid infection and provide optimal circumstances for healing.[108] The fracture is then stabilized with a cast or surgical implant.

Gustilo and Anderson have developed a classification system that rates the severity of open or compound fractures.[113] The least severe is a type I injury, in which a small wound (1 cm) communicates with the fracture. The wound in a type II fracture is between 1 cm and 12 cm, and significant soft tissue injury may be present underneath the laceration or wound. In a more severe, type III injury, the wound diameter is greater than 12 cm and barely enough muscle or skin is present to cover the injured or fractured bone adequately. Type III open fractures are subdivided into another three categories—A, B, and C—on the basis of whether the soft tissue can cover the bone and whether neurological or vascular involvement is present in association with the open fracture.

The particular location and pattern of fracture determine whether the fracture is stable and can be effectively managed with an external cast, or unstable, requiring surgical intervention. A fracture with concurrent joint dislocation creates an extremely unstable condition, most often requiring anesthesia or surgery for reduction and management of the fracture/dislocation and a long period of rehabilitation.

Fractures (whether closed and open) are described as *displaced* or *nondisplaced* on the basis of the degree of malalignment or overlap that is observed on a radiograph (Figure 14-20). They are described as *complete* or *incomplete*, depending on whether the bone has fully transected. In children a "greenstick" fracture is an incomplete oblique or spinal fracture that extends only partially through bone. Exact location of the fracture is also important: fractures of the diaphysis or metaphysis of a long cortical bone are *extraarticular* (Figure 14-21), while those involving the epiphysis within the joint capsule are *intraarticular.*

Extraarticular fractures can be *transverse* (mostly perpendicular to the axis of the bone), *oblique* (diagonal to the axis of the bone), or *spiral* (typically a result of torsional forces), depending on the direction of force contributing to the injury and the resulting alteration in bone configuration.

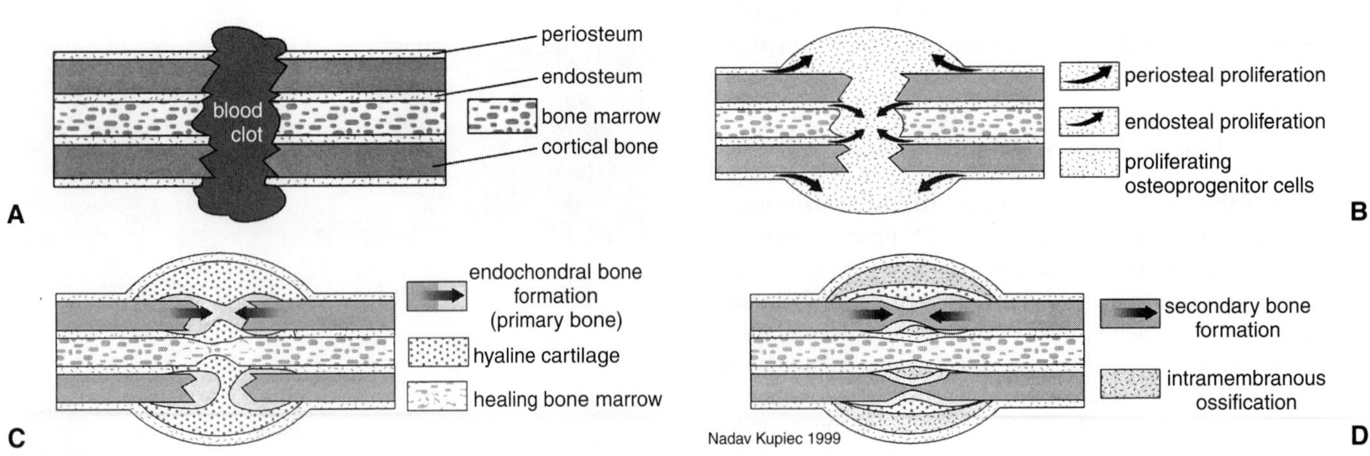

Figure 14-19

Healing and repair of a long bone fracture. ***A,*** *Disruption of blood vessels in the bone, marrow, periosteum, and surrounding tissue at the time of injury results in extravasation of blood at the fracture site and the formation of hematoma.* ***B,*** *Initiation and development of the fracture callus.* ***C,*** *Note the simultaneous occurrence of chondrogenesis, endochondral ossification, and intramembranous bone formation in different regions of the fracture site.* ***D,*** *Union of a long bone fracture. (From Lundon K.* Orthopedic Rehabilitation Science: Principles for Clinical Management of Bone. *Boston: Butterworth-Heinemann, 2000.)*

When one or more substantive fragments are seen on the radiograph, the fracture is *segmental;* if there are multiple small fragments, the fracture is *comminuted*. In high-impact, complex fractures there is often enough destruction of bone that there will be loss of bone length or substance. Fractures of the metaphysis are determined to be nondisplaced or displaced, simple, compressed, or comminuted (Figure 14-22). Before and during puberty (during times of rapid bone growth), there can be displacement of the proximal or distal epiphysis from the metaphysis through the cartilaginous epiphyseal plate (Figure 14-23); the proximal (subcapital) epiphysis of the femur is particularly vulnerable.

In the femur, fractures of the metaphysis are described as *intertrochanteric* extraarticular (linear or oblique, through or between the trochanters), *subcapital* intraarticular (across the neck of the femur), or *comminuted* (with multiple fragments of neck and or trochanters) (Figure 14-24); these fractures typically require ORIF or, if severe, replacement with a femoral prosthesis or even a total hip arthroplasty (Figure 14-25). Fractures of the acetabulum are the result of either a longitudinal force through the femur into the pelvis or an upward oblique lateral force through the greater trochanter; if the hip happens to be adducted at the time of injury, this may lead to posterior dislocation (Figure 14-26).

Intraarticular fractures are classified as linear, comminuted, impacted, or having a percent of bone loss (Figure 14-27); complex intraarticular fractures involve both proximal and distal components of the joint (Figure 14-28) and typically require ORIF.

Fractures of the pelvis are classified as *stable* or *unstable* on the basis of the extent of damage that disrupts the circumferential integrity of the pelvis (Figure 14-29). Persons with unstable fractures of the pelvis are at risk for life-threatening hemorrhage, as well as residual genitourinary or neurological complications, given the vessels, nerves, muscles, and organs that are housed within the pelvis.[114]

Fractures of irregularly shaped bones such as the tarsals and vertebrae tend to fall into three categories. *Stress fractures* result from repetitive loading of the bone, are often nondisplaced, and can disrupt either the inner scaffolding of the cancellous bone or the outer shell of cortical bone. Simple stress fractures typically heal well with immobilization; more complex stress fractures may require surgical stabilization. *Pathological fractures* occur when there is underlying disease (e.g., osteoporosis, Charcot's osteopathy, neoplasm) that compromises bone density or metabolism.

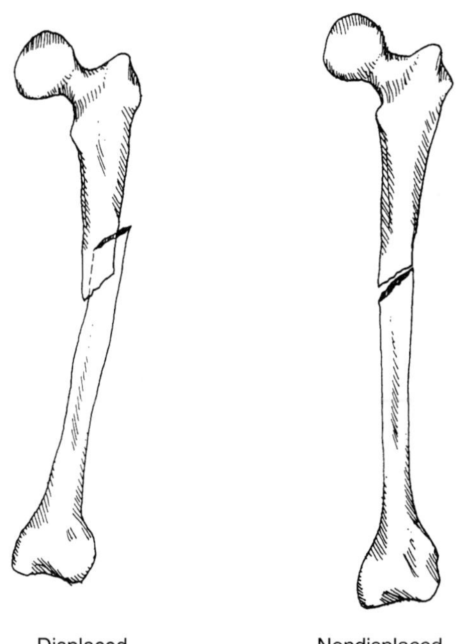

Figure 14-20
Diagram of a displaced and nondisplaced fracture of the diaphysis of the femur. (From Gustilo RB. The Fracture Classification Manual. *St. Louis: Mosby, 1991.)*

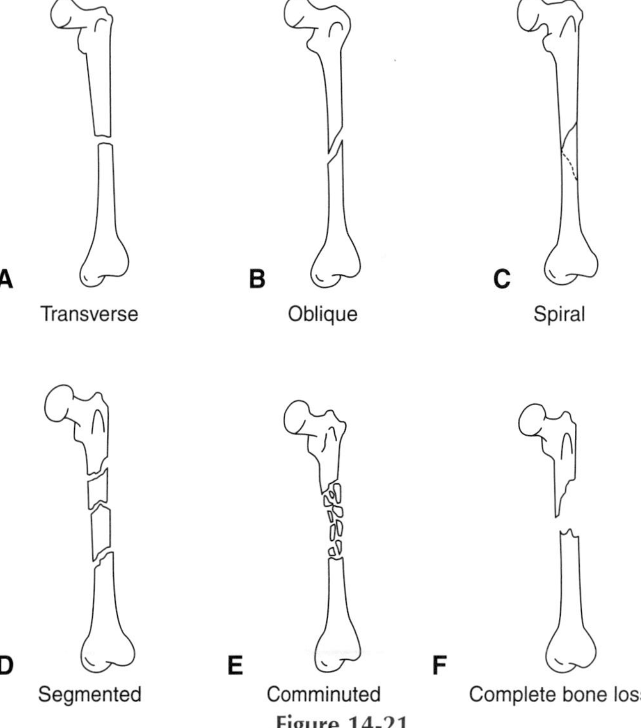

Figure 14-21
*Examples of types of long bone fractures, illustrated in the diaphysis of the femur: A transverse fracture (**A**) is primarily perpendicular to the long axis of the bone, while an oblique fracture (**B**) diagonally transects the bone. A spiral fracture (**C**) is the result of a rotary force during injury. Segmental fractures (**D**) have one or more noncontinuous segments, while a comminuted fracture (**E**) has multiple small fragments. In cases of significant trauma, there may actually be loss of bone substance (**F**). (Modified from Gustilo RB.* The Fracture Classification Manual. *St. Louis: Mosby, 1991.)*

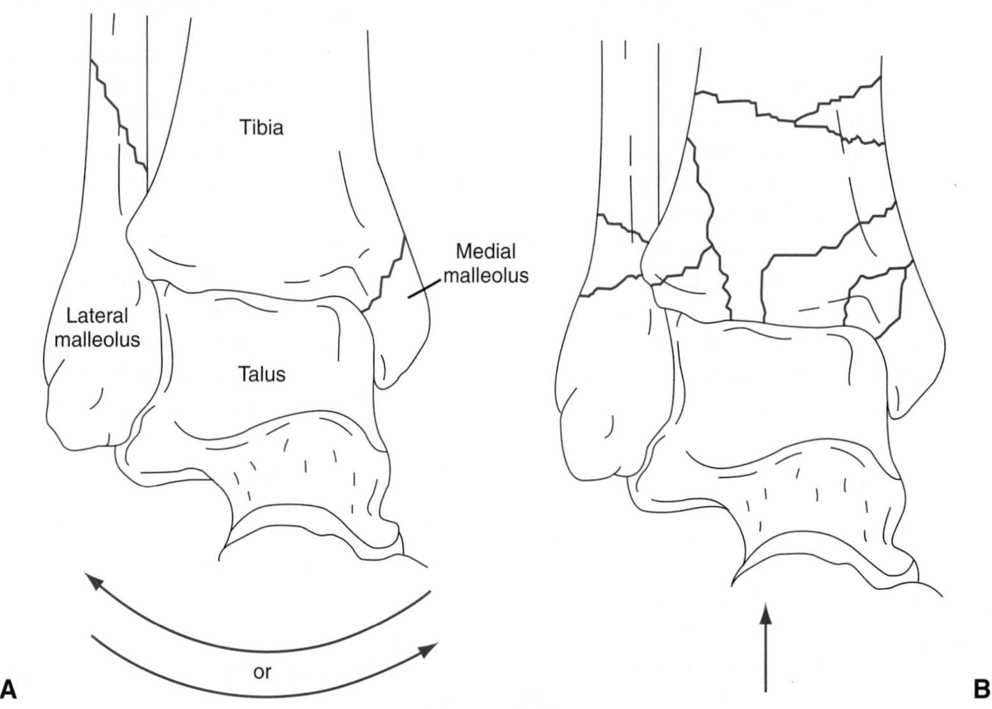

Figure 14-22

A, *Extraarticular metaphyseal fracture of the malleoli of the tibia and fibula is often the result of rotational injuries.*
B, *Intraarticular fractures of the ankle mortis (also called plafond or pylon fractures) result from high-energy compressive injury. (Modified from Clark CR, Bonfiglio M (eds).* Orthopaedics: Essentials of Diagnosis and Treatment. *Philadelphia: Churchill Livingstone, 1994.)*

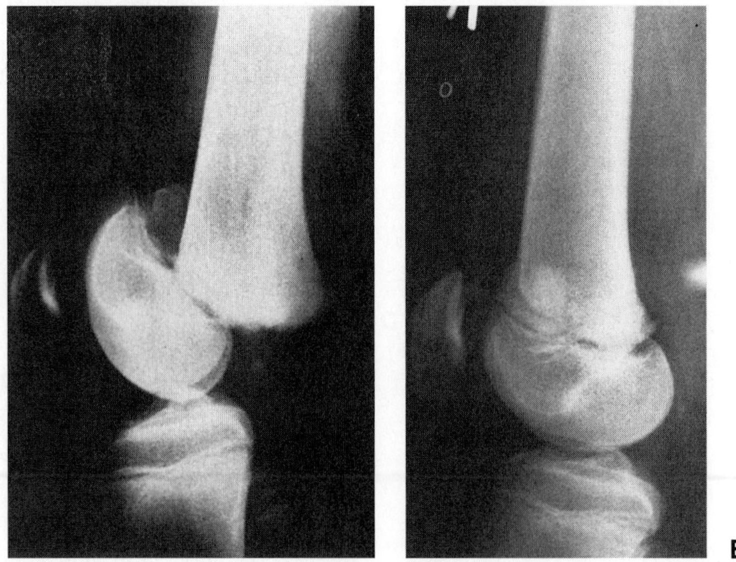

Figure 14-23

*Lateral view of an avulsed distal femoral condyle (**A**) before and (**B**) following closed reduction. (From CR Clark, M Bonfiglio (eds).* Orthopaedics: Essentials of Diagnosis and Treatment. *Philadelphia: Churchill Livingstone, 1994.)*

In pathological fractures the trabeculae are overwhelmed by the magnitude of force exerted through the bone, and the bone is compressed or fractured into fragments. Management of pathological fractures can be challenging, as bone healing is often compromised by the underlying disease process. *Traumatic fractures* are often comminuted; depending on severity, they may be managed by immobilization in a cast or orthosis, ORIF, or placement of an external fixation apparatus (Figure 14-30).

Casts and Splints

The primary goal of fracture management is to restore musculoskeletal limb function of the injured extremity with optimal anatomical alignment, functional muscle strength, sensory function, and pain-free joint range of motion. The most common methods used for immobilization of closed fractures include casts, splints, fracture orthoses, or a hybrid cast-orthosis.[107,115] Immobilization may also be used after ORIF of open fractures.

In choosing the appropriate immobilization strategy for an individual's fracture, the orthopedist considers several issues. The first is the stability of the fracture site and how well a device will be able to maintain fracture reduction and achieve the desired anatomical result. The condition of the skin and soft tissue is also an important consideration, especially if wounds are present that must be accessed for proper care. Limb volume must be evaluated, especially if edema is present or anticipated: How will limb size change over time in the device? Length of immobilization time varies as well: Is the device designed for a short-term problem, or will protection of the limb be necessary for an extended period? Will the device need to be removed for hygiene or wound care? Can the limb be unprotected while sleeping or when not ambulating? Availability (time to application) may also influence decision making. Casts and cast braces can be applied quickly. Custom orthoses need additional fabrication and fitting time; an alternative means of protection is often required while the device is being fabricated.

The individual's ability to comply consistently and reliably with weight-bearing restrictions and other aspects of fracture management must also be considered. Factors such as cognitive ability, emotional status, motivation, and physical ability, as well as the availability of assistance and environmental demands, influence the decision to provide additional external support. An unstable fracture managed by ORIF may not require additional support for those with

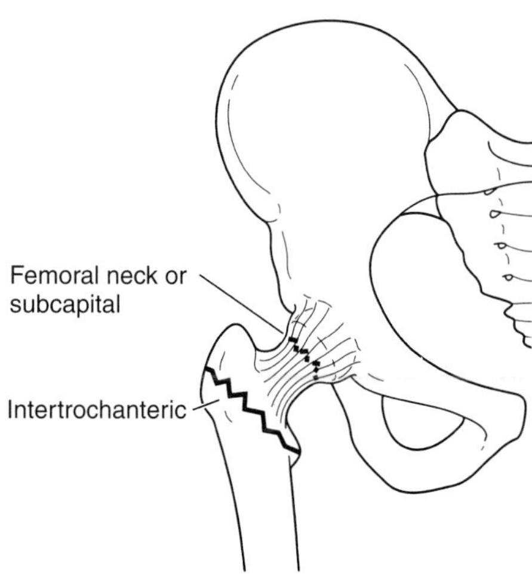

Figure 14-24
Femoral neck fractures are intracapsular and traverse the blood supply to the femoral head. Intertrochanteric fractures spare the blood supply but are a greater risk for failure of fixation. (From Clark CR, Bonfiglio M (eds). Orthopaedics: Essentials of Diagnosis and Treatment. *Philadelphia: Churchill Livingstone, 1994.)*

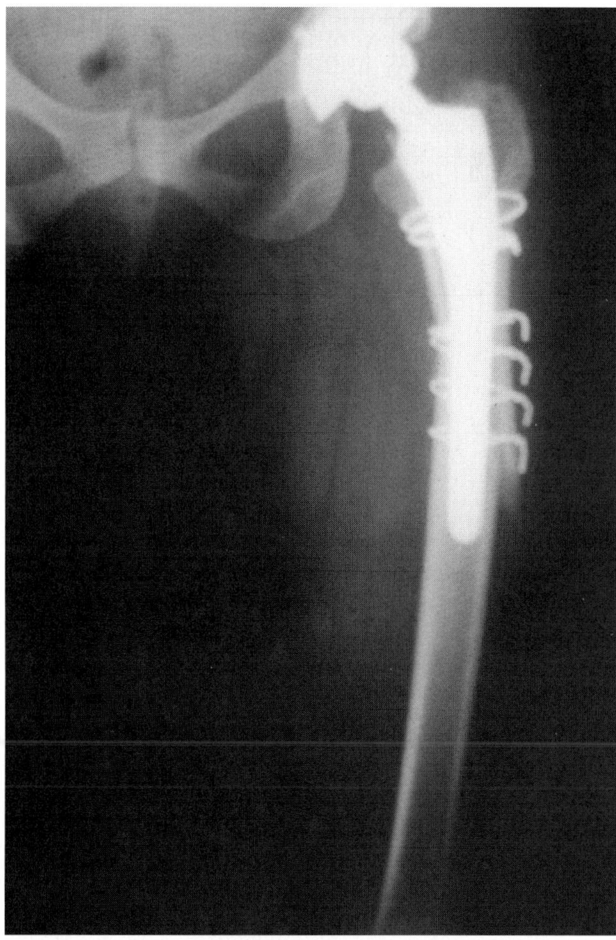

Figure 14-25
A radiograph of a repaired complex fracture of the proximal femur, with prosthetic total hip replacement and open reduction internal fixation with circumferentially wrapped wires to stabilize a spiral fracture of the proximal femoral diaphysis.

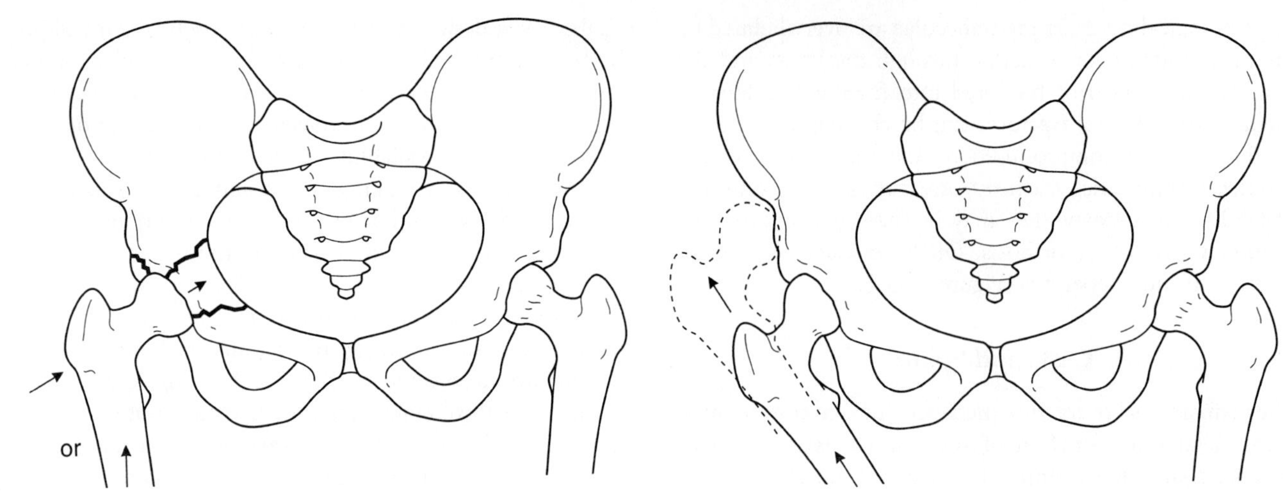

Figure 14-26

*A, Acetabular fractures occur from a lateral blow over the greater trochanter or a proximally directed force transmitted up the length of the femur. **B,** If the limb is injured with the hip in adduction and flexion, a posterior hip dislocation is likely. (From Clark CR, Bonfiglio M (eds).* Orthopaedics: Essentials of Diagnosis and Treatment. *Philadelphia: Churchill Livingstone, 1994.)*

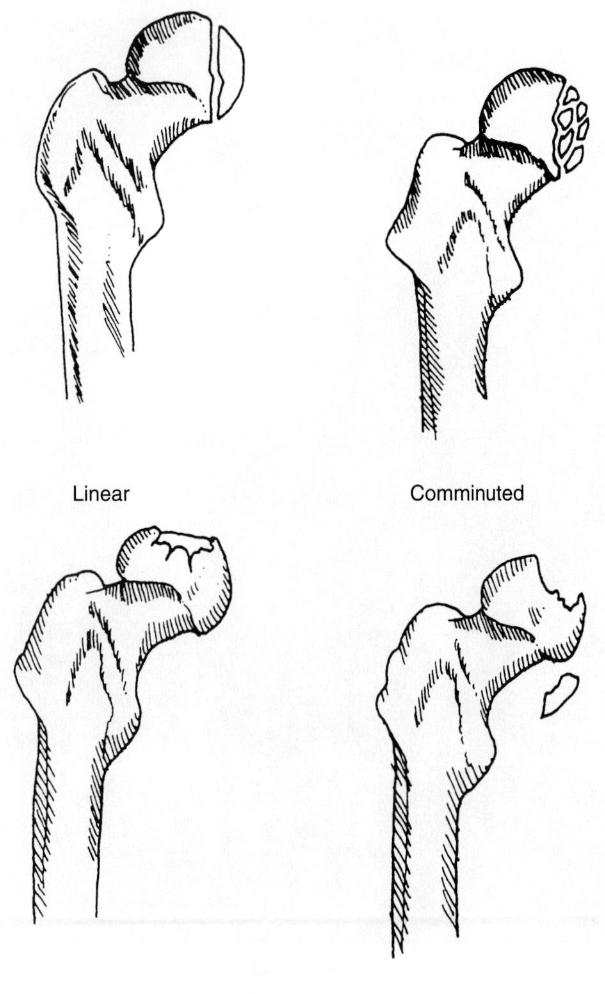

Figure 14-27

Examples of types of intraarticular fractures, using the head of the femur as an example. (From Gustilo RB. The Fracture Classification Manual. *St. Louis: Mosby, 1991.)*

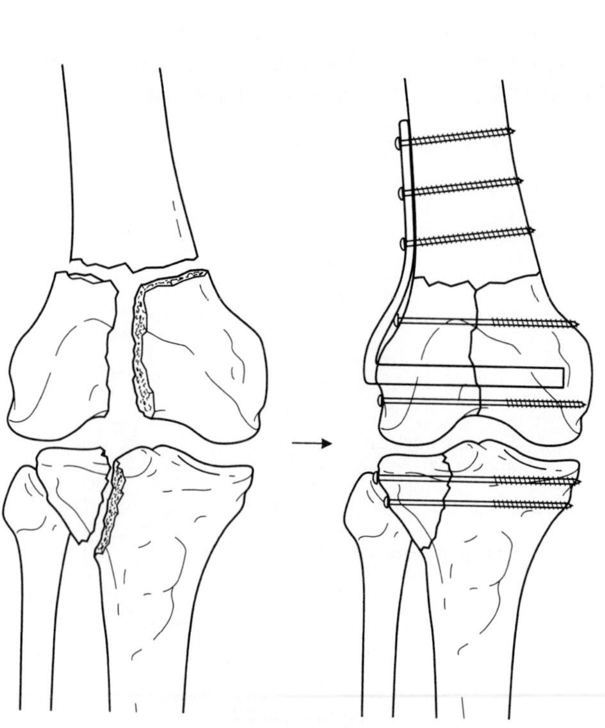

Figure 14-28

Major intraarticular fractures of the distal femur and proximal tibia are typically managed by surgical open reduction internal fixation using a combination of bone screws or nail and an external plate. (From Clark CR, Bonfiglio M (eds). Orthopaedics: Essentials of Diagnosis and Treatment. *Philadelphia: Churchill Livingstone, 1994.)*

sufficient strength and balance who have a clear understanding of the healing process. If the individual with a fracture cannot understand the need to protect the involved limb from excessive loading or is physically unable to do so, additional external support is essential. If compliance is questionable, the device of choice is usually a nonremovable cast or cast brace.

To effectively stabilize a fracture, the joints above and below the fracture site must be immobilized. The period of immobilization varies with fracture severity and location; in most cases the cast remains in place from 6 to 8 weeks or until a radiograph indicates that bone healing has progressed sufficiently for safe weight bearing and function. Although immobilization is essential for effective bone healing, it also has significant consequences on other tissues: while in a cast, patients are likely to develop significant joint stiffness (contracture), as well as disuse atrophy and weakness of the muscles of the immobilized limb. Once the cast is removed, rehabilitation professionals are called on to help the patient regain preinjury muscle performance, flexibility, and range of motion.

A *cast* is a rigid, externally applied device that provides circumferential support to an injured body part.[107] Casts immobilize a body segment to maintain optimal skeletal alignment (Figures 14-31 and 14-32). Once a cast has been applied, a radiograph can be used to assess the effectiveness of skeletal alignment. The cast may need to be modified, wedged, or replaced to improve alignment.[116]

A *splint* is a temporary supportive device, usually fabricated from rigid materials, held in position on the fractured extremity with bandages or straps. Splints can be used for temporary immobilization before casting or surgical stabilization. They can be used to maintain fracture reduction while waiting for swelling to diminish or fracture blisters to clear or to provide comfort. The most commonly used temporary fracture splint is called a *sugar tong splint*, a long, U-shaped, padded plaster splint named for its similarity to the tool used to pick up sugar cubes.[116]

Casting and Splinting Materials

Before the 1800s, fracture casts were made from linen bandages soaked in beaten egg whites and lime. The modern era in fracture care began with the discovery of plaster of Paris (calcium sulfate), first used in the Turkish Empire as reported by Eaton in 1798.[117] Plaster of Paris was used in Europe in the early nineteenth century, and a Flemish surgeon (Mathijsen) is credited with combining the use of plaster of Paris and cloth bandages to form casts for the treatment of fractures in 1852.[116-118]

Plaster of Paris is created when heat is used to dehydrate gypsum. When water is added to plaster of Paris powder, the dehydration process is reversed, and crystals of gypsum are formed again. The new crystals interlock in a chemical exothermic (heat-producing) process.[119] The setting process is complete when heat is no longer being produced, although the cast remains wet to the touch until the excess water used in the process evaporates. Maximum cast strength is not

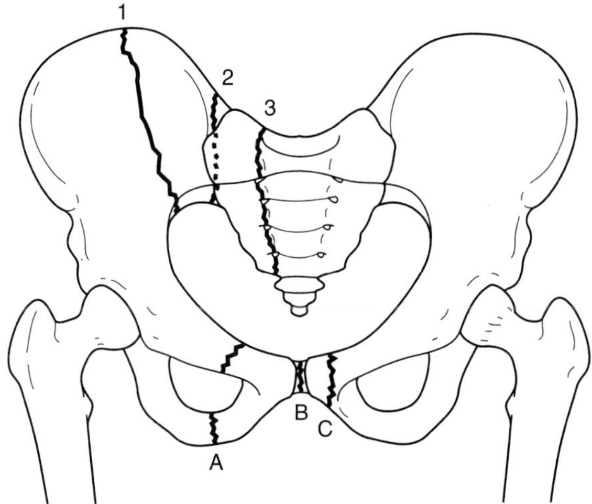

Figure 14-29
Unstable pelvic fractures occur when pubic rami fractures (A), *symphysis disruption* (B), *or pubic body fractures* (C) *are accompanied by fractures through the iliac wing* (1), *sacroiliac joint* (2), *or sacrum* (3). *(From Clark CR, Bonfiglio M (eds).* Orthopaedics: Essentials of Diagnosis and Treatment. *Philadelphia: Churchill Livingstone, 1994.)*

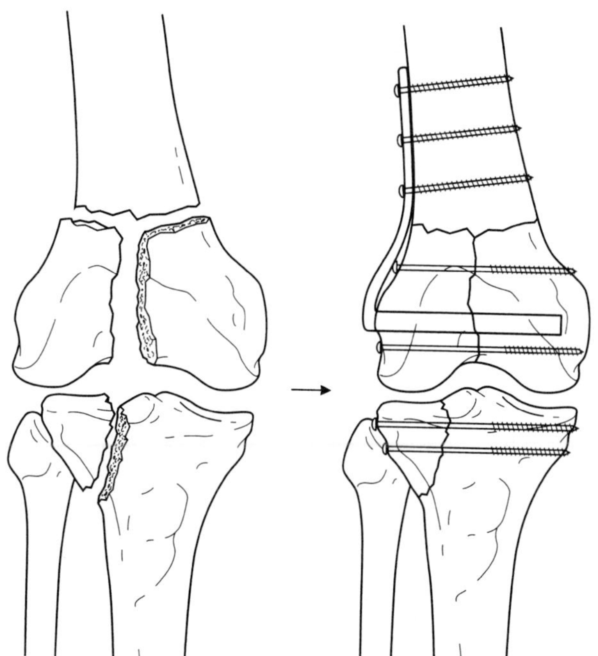

Figure 14-30
Open fractures of the tibial shaft often require skeletal stabilization with external fixation, as well as soft tissue repair. (From Clark CR, Bonfiglio M (eds). Orthopaedics: Essentials of Diagnosis and Treatment. *Philadelphia: Churchill Livingstone, 1994.)*

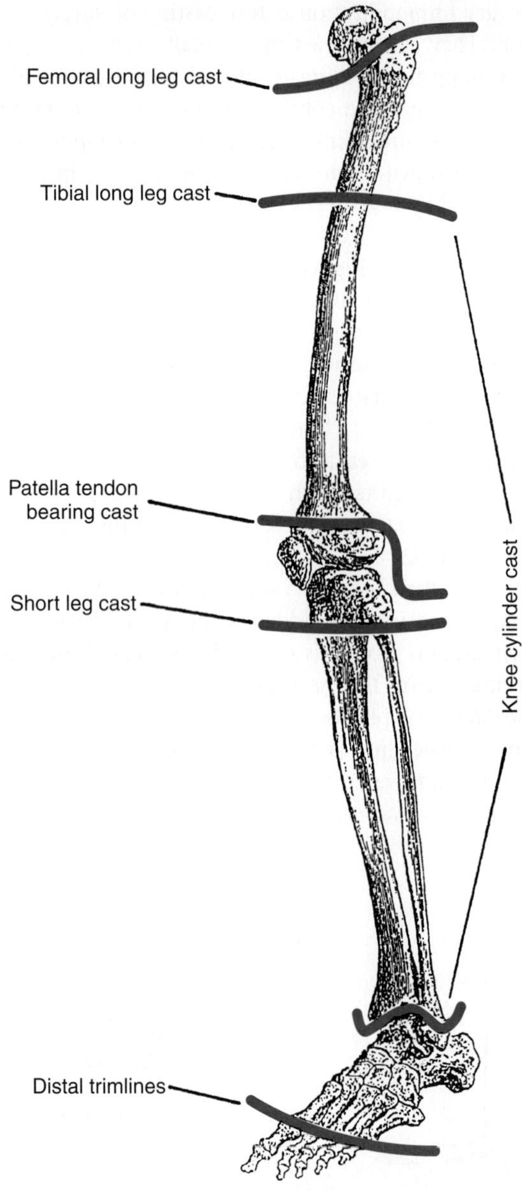

Figure 14-31
Proximal and distal trimlines used in standard lower extremity casts. Typically, the joints above and below the fracture site are immobilized. Trimlines can be extended to provide better control and stabilization.

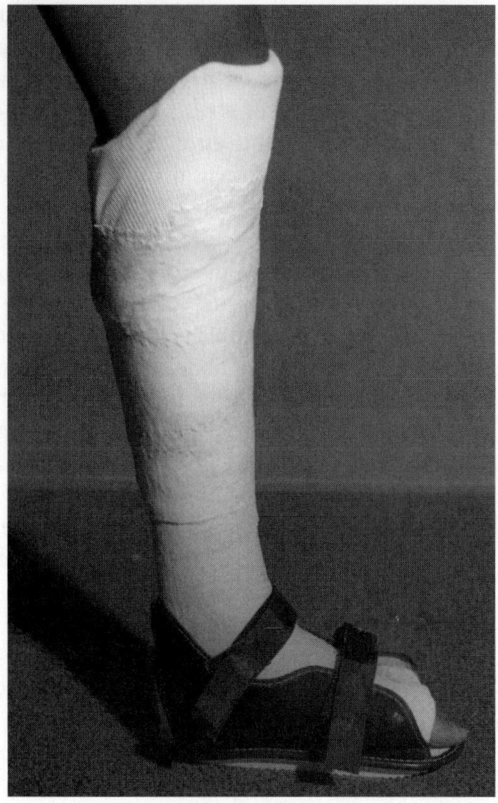

Figure 14-32
A medial view of a patellar tendon–bearing short leg cast. The proximal anterior area of the cast has been molded by pressing inward at the level of the patellar tendon, while the proximal posterior of the cast has been molded over the calf and then trimmed to allow knee flexion. (From Moore TJ: Functional bracing of lower extremity fractures. In Goldberg B, Hsu JD (eds). Atlas of Orthoses and Assistive Devices. St. Louis: Mosby; 1997.)

reached until the plaster is completely dry. Drying time varies with the thickness of the cast, ambient humidity, and the type of plaster used. In most instances maximum cast strength is reached in approximately 24 hours.

Various types of plaster of Paris with different working characteristics are available. Manufacturers may add accelerators to the material that shorten the setting time: The limb has to be held still for less time while the plaster sets. Although this may be advantageous when a cast is applied to the limb of an anxious child or when an unstable fracture is cast, it also means that less working time is available to manipulate the extremity and optimally shape the cast. Setting time can be prolonged slightly if cold water is used. If warm or hot water is used to reduce setting time, care must be taken to protect the limb from injury from the higher heat that can be generated during the setting process.[116] Cast temperatures as high as 68.5° C have been reached with water temperatures of 40° C; burns can occur if cast temperature is maintained at 44° C for 6 hours or more.[120,121] To minimize any potential for burns in cast or splint application, room temperature tepid water (24° C) is recommended. If higher water temperatures have been used, the newly casted limb must not be placed on a pillow or other type of support that is likely to retain or reflect heat. Cast burns can also occur when insufficient padding has been placed between the plaster of Paris and the surface of the skin. Cast burns are avoidable if simple procedures are followed.

Cast strength is determined by three factors: the type of casting material used, the thickness of the cast, and the effectiveness of lamination among the layers of the cast material. The cloth mesh material that serves as the "carrier" for the plaster of Paris provides little strength for the cast. A plaster cast must be kept absolutely dry to prevent it from becoming soft and ineffective in immobilization.

The difficulties associated with the use of plaster of Paris have led to the development of newer and improved casting materials. *Polyurethane-impregnated casting tapes* have gained widespread popularity because of their superior strength, light weight, shorter setting time, cleaner application, and low exothermic reaction. Polyurethane casts are also radiolucent, permitting x-ray evaluation of fracture site healing while the limb remains encased in the cast.

Polyurethane is a plastic material that can be impregnated into a fabric substrate. Although the polyurethane bonds the layers of substrate together, it is actually the substrate that determines the strength of the cast. A variety of substrate materials are available. The weave determines how elastic the material will be during cast application and how strong the cast will be when set. Cotton, polyester, fiberglass, polypropylene, and blends of these materials and others are used in synthetic casting tapes.[119,122,123]

Immersing the synthetic casting tape in room temperature water for 10 seconds begins a heat-producing exothermic reaction and causes the material to harden (polymerize). Setting is complete for most synthetic casting materials in 5 to 10 minutes. Because of this short setting time, the rolls of bandage material cannot be opened until they are ready to be applied as a cast. The application process requires skill and must move quickly to ensure adequate molding time. Unlike plaster of Paris, the plastic bandage does not need to be massaged to ensure proper lamination between the layers of material. Also unlike plaster of Paris, which can easily be washed from the hands or clothing, polyurethane is not easily removed: Adequate protective padding must be placed around the patient's limb, and protective gloves worn to safeguard the applicator's hands. Polyurethane resin in its natural state is tacky. An additive may be incorporated into the casting tape to reduce its tackiness. In some cases the manufacturer provides special gloves with an antitacky additive to further minimize the tack.[119] The exothermic polymerization of polyurethane resin produces much less heat (44.9° C in 40° C water) than that of setting plaster of Paris. In addition, heat is quickly dissipated so that burns are much less likely to occur when synthetic materials are used. To further minimize the risk of burns, immersion of cast tape in room temperature water (24° C) is recommended.[116,121,124]

Cast Application

Stockinet is the first layer of a cast, applied over the skin, before any padding is added. The most common stockinet material is cotton. Synthetic materials such as polyester or polypropylene can be chosen in place of cotton because they do not retain water like cotton materials do. Stockinet also helps to position dressings over wounds and provides extra circumferential control of soft tissue within the cast. Stockinet is folded over the proximal and distal edges to finish the cast (and prevent inadvertent removal of cast padding by a nonresponsible individual or a child).

Next, a layer of cast padding is added over the stockinet. A variety of materials are available to pad casts. Sheet cotton comes in various forms and is used to provide a barrier between the rigid walls of the cast and surface of the skin. Some cast materials have been elasticized for easier application and conformation, and others require more technique to ensure that they uniformly conform to the body part being casted.

Although synthetic cast tapes are not affected by water, cast padding or stockinet does retain water. The risk of skin maceration and breakdown is present if the inside of a cast remains damp for long periods of time. Some manufacturers market cast padding that reportedly permits exposure to water; however, manufacturer recommendations must be followed carefully.

The thickness of cast padding varies; $\frac{1}{8}$ to $\frac{1}{4}$ inch is sufficient for most individuals. The goal is to protect bony prominences and soft tissue from the rigid walls of the cast while effectively immobilizing the fracture site. Soft tissue usually does well with a fairly thin, uniform two- or three-layer wrap. Extra padding is added to smooth and protect the irregular surfaces around bony prominences. Excessive padding reduces the ability of the cast to provide adequate immobilization. A well-molded cast that accurately follows the anatomical contours of the extremity requires less padding. Cast padding also provides a barrier so that the cast can be removed more easily when it needs to be changed or is no longer necessary.

Lower Extremity Casts

The *short leg cast* is used in the management of fractures involving the distal tibia or fibula, or both; the ankle joint; or the rear foot or midfoot. The foot is positioned in a functional neutral ankle position (90 degrees) or in slight dorsiflexion. The foot can be casted in a plantarflexed position to accommodate repair of an Achilles tendon rupture. The proximal trimline falls at the level of the tibial tubercle; the distal trimline usually encloses the metatarsal heads. The area around the fibular head is protected by adding extra cast padding to minimize the risk of entrapment of the peroneal nerve. A cast shoe should be used to protect the bottom of the cast if weight bearing is to be permitted.

For persons with midshaft fractures of the tibia, a *patellar tendon–bearing cast* (PTB) may be applied. This design incorporates a patellar tendon bar, which directs some of the limb loading force to the external shell of the cast, thus protecting the full length of the tibia against bending moments (see Figure 14-32). This type of cast is not effective, however, in reducing axial loading of the tibia or hind foot. The PTB is most often used when extra stability is desired for individuals who will be allowed some degree of weight-bearing activity. The cast is applied with the ankle maintained in neutral or slightly dorsiflexed position, to minimize potential hyperextension moment at the knee in stance. Trimlines are similar to those used for a PTB transtibial prosthetic socket: at the midpatella (or sometimes suprapatella) anteriorly but trimmed and slightly flared posteriorly to permit knee flexion of at least 90 degrees. Proximally, the cast is well molded to the tibia in the area of the medial flare and around the patella.[125,126] Care must be taken to ensure that no pressure is placed on the peroneal nerve.

A *knee cylinder cast* is often applied when there have been fractures of the patella or surgical repair of the knee joint when the knee must be immobilized in full extension. To ensure the necessary stability for the knee joint, the proximal trimline encompasses the lower two thirds of the thigh and the distal trimline the entire tibial segment to just above the malleoli. The cast can be applied using either plaster of Paris or synthetic casting tape. To limit the risk of pistoning when the person wearing the cast is standing or walking, the cast is carefully molded to fit the contours of the medial femoral condyle.

For closed fractures of the upper tibia, knee joint, or lower femur, a *long leg cast* provides the necessary stability for healing. Depending on the site of fracture and its relative stability, the limb is immobilized in nearly full extension or in a bent knee position.[127] A straight knee cast is usually applied with a slight (5-degree) knee flexion angle to enhance patient comfort. Bent knee casts are usually chosen when non–weight bearing must be ensured during ambulation or to aid in controlling rotation of the tibia. With the relatively mobile arrangement of soft tissue that surrounds the femur, it is challenging to provide adequate immobilization, especially for persons who are particularly muscular or overweight. For this reason, control of rotational forces through the femur within a long leg cast is questionable. If the cast is being used to stabilize the tibia, the proximal trimline is at the junction of the middle and proximal third of the femur. If the cast is being used to stabilize the distal femur, the proximal trimline is at the level of the greater trochanter. Distally, the cast immobilizes the ankle and extends to a point just beyond the metatarsal heads. The fibular head should be well padded within the cast to minimize the risk of entrapment of the peroneal nerve.

A *hip spica cast,* which encases the hip and pelvis in addition to the lower extremity, is necessary for effective control of fractures of the proximal femur and of the hip joint[128] (Figure 14-33). The hip spica is the primary method of treatment of femoral fractures in children and is used in adults when a prefabricated hip orthosis is not appropriate. Several variations of the hip spica are available. In a single hip spica, the plaster or synthetic cast material is anchored around the entire pelvis and lower trunk but immobilizes only the hip and proximal femur of the involved side, allowing fairly

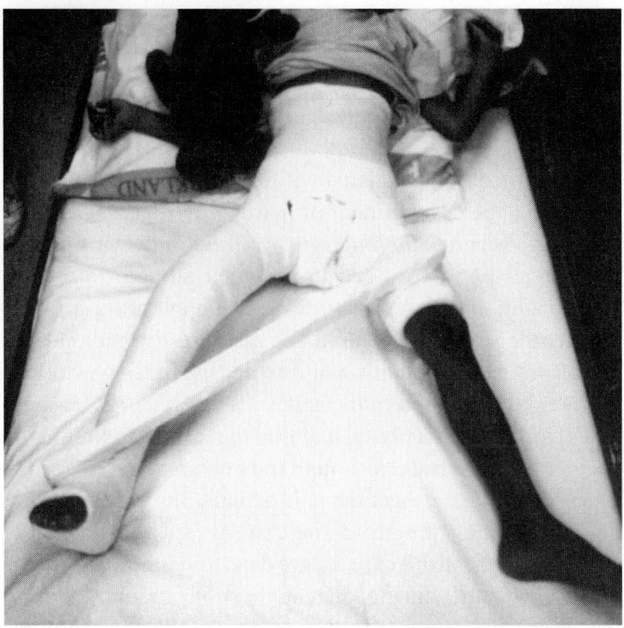

Figure 14-33
This child has been placed in a $1\frac{1}{2}$ hip spica cast to stabilize a fracture of the proximal femur. Note the opening for personal hygiene and the additional diagonal support bar incorporated between the short and long sections of the cast.

unrestricted hip motion of the opposite limb. In a $1\frac{1}{2}$ hip spica, the cast encases the entire lower extremity on the affected side, as well as the lower trunk, pelvis, and thigh on the uninvolved side. Usually the knee on the affected side is completely immobilized; however, an articulated knee joint can be incorporated if specific circumstances so dictate. In most instances the hip joint of the affected limb is immobilized in 30 degrees of flexion and 30 degrees of abduction, and the perineal edges are trimmed back to allow for personal care and hygiene. The knee is usually positioned in 30 degrees of flexion. The proximal cast encases the lower to middle trunk (to the level of the costal margin or nipple line), depending on the amount of spinal immobilization required. The $1\frac{1}{2}$ hip spica cast is often reinforced by the incorporation of a lightweight diagonal bar between the short and long extremity segments. Ambulation is possible but often quite challenging, requiring significant upper body strength to manage the adapted crutch-walking gait that the cast position makes necessary.

Cast Removal

A cast cutter with a vibrating disk is used to cut the cast during cast removal. Modern cast cutter blades reciprocate back and forth approximately $\frac{1}{8}$ inch in either direction. The vibrating blade easily cuts rigid materials such as metal, wood, plaster, or synthetic cast materials but does not cut through materials that are elastic or mobile. If used properly, a cast cutter does not cut skin. Incorrect or inappropriate use of a cast cutter can seriously cut or burn a patient. To reduce

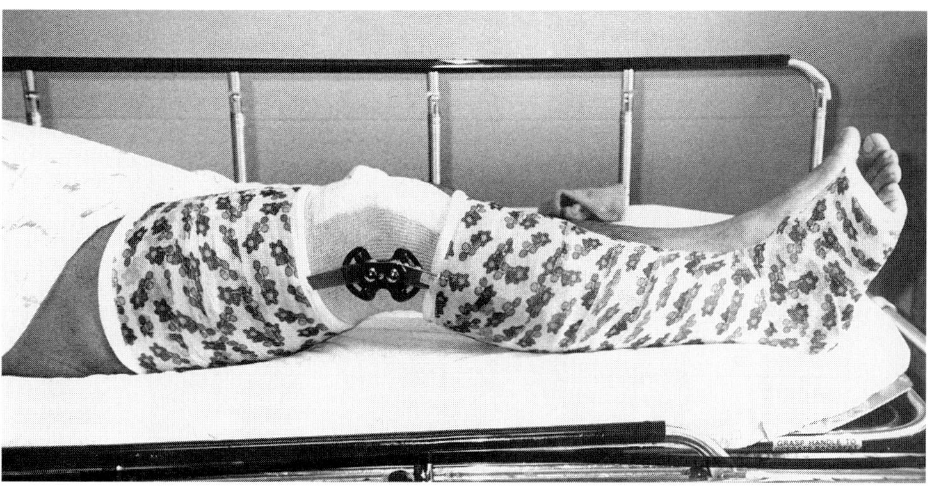

Figure 14-34
A tibial cast brace with polycentric adjustable range of motion hinges. The patient has undergone an open reduction internal fixation surgery after fracture of the tibial plateau. Note that synthetic cast tape is available in a wide variety of colors and patterns.

the risk of injury, the blade should not directly contact the patient's skin. Friction between the blade and cast significantly heats the blade, creating a potential for burns. A sharp new blade has less potential for burning the patient than does a blade that has become dull or worn out. The noise of the cast cutter can be quite frightening to children or other particularly anxious patients. A careful explanation and a demonstration of the cast cutter's action are the first steps in the process of cast removal.

To remove a cast safely, the cutter is used in a repetitive in-out motion, progressively opening the cast. This strategy reduces the risk of a cut or burn on the patient's skin.[129] The operator's thumb is used as a fulcrum as downward pressure is applied through the wrist. The thumb also controls the depth of the blade. Care is taken to avoid positioning the cast cutter in areas where skin is vulnerable: over a bony prominence or where significant edema or fragile healing skin is present. As the blade breaks through the inner wall of the cast, the sensation of reduced resistance to downward pressure, as well as a change in sound, occurs. Once an area of cast has been cut, the blade is repositioned farther along the cast and the process is repeated until the cast can be pried open completely. Bandage scissors are used to cut through padding and stockinet, and the limb is then extracted from the open cast. For infants and young children with small limbs, an alternative strategy can be used: A plaster of Paris cast can be removed by soaking in water. This method works particularly well when a corrective clubfoot cast is removed from an infant's limb.

Hybrid Cast Braces

Hybrid cast braces were first developed as a method of management of proximal tibial and distal femoral fractures near the knee just after World War I but then fell out of use until the mid-1960s[130-132] (Figure 14-34). In some centers the cast brace is the method of choice for the management of nondisplaced tibial plateau fractures. The cast brace is often used for additional support of fractures near the knee or of the femur that have been stabilized via ORIF surgery for external fixation (Figure 14-35). This method is also used to control motion after knee ligament injury or reconstruction.

Cast braces incorporate orthotic components (e.g., hinge joints, range of motion locks) into a plaster or synthetic cast in an effort to provide additional stability to a healing limb.[133-141] The cast brace can be applied using either plaster of Paris or synthetic cast materials. Depending on the nature of the fracture and its stability, the orthotic knee joints incorporated into the cast brace may be chosen to provide limited, controlled, or free-knee range of motion. Because the anatomical center rotation of the knee moves in an arc centered over the femoral condyles, it is essential that the mechanical joints be carefully aligned with the anatomical knee joint to reduce the abnormal stress that occurs across the joint and fracture site.[142,143]

Many orthotists and orthopedic surgeons choose a polycentric orthotic knee joint because its motion more closely follows anatomical motion and reduces the torque-related stress that results from a single-axis mechanical joint. Palpating the condyles on a patient who has had recent trauma about the knee is difficult; the midpatella is a somewhat less precise alternative landmark for alignment. A properly placed polycentric metal joint will be proximal to the joint line and slightly posterior to the midline. Orthotic knee joints are positioned close to but not quite contacting skin. This is especially important medially, where contact between the knees during functional activity is likely.

Medial and lateral uprights are incorporated into the cast above and below the orthotic knee joint to provide protection against unwanted varus and valgus stress and help

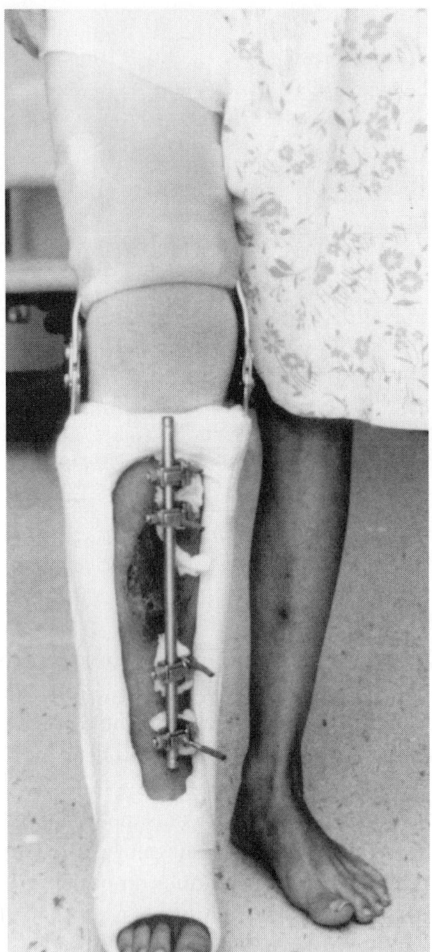

Figure 14-35
This cast brace provides medial/lateral stability for a comminuted grade 3 open tibial fracture. The length of the tibia is being maintained by an external fixation device. The patient also sustained a closed femoral fracture, which has been supported by an intramedullary rod fixation. Because the proximal portion of the cast must not terminate near a fracture line, the femoral portion of the cast has been extended up to the level of the trochanter to avoid stress on the femoral fixation.

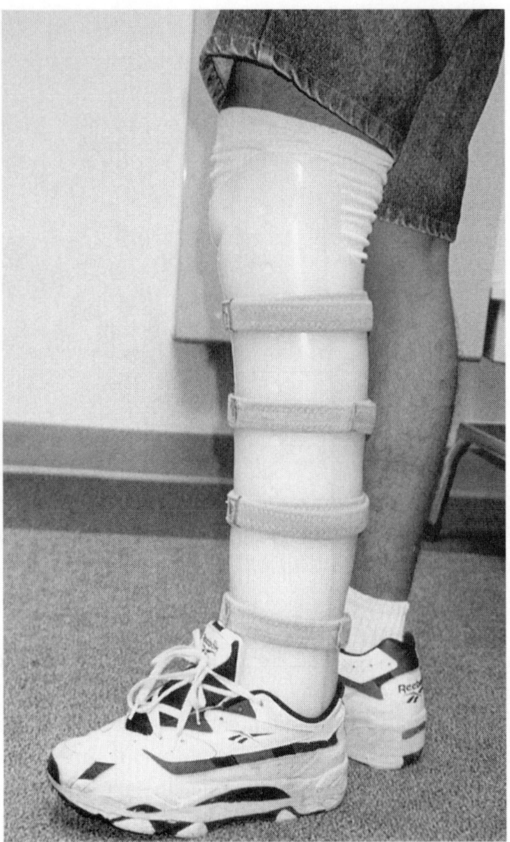

Figure 14-36
Ankle-foot fracture orthosis with a patellar tendon–bearing design incorporated to protect the tibia for bending moments during weight bearing. This patient was originally managed with an external fixation device, which had to be removed secondary to pin loosening before union of the fracture was solid. Note that the shoe has been modified with a cushion heel and rocker sole to compensate for a fixed ankle position and to improve forward progression during the stance phase of gait.

control anteroposterior displacement of the tibia or femur.

The distal tibial cast holds the ankle in a neutral position and extends distally to encompass the metatarsal heads. The proximal trimline of the tibial cast is typically at the tibial tubercle, and the distal trimline of the femoral cast is an equal distance from the midpatella. Posteriorly, both tibial and femoral casts are trimmed to permit at least 90 degrees of knee flexion. If warranted, a slight varus or valgus stress can be applied at the time of cast brace application, or a varus/valgus strap can be added to aid in unloading a knee compartment. For persons with fractures of the upper tibia and knee, the proximal component encases the lower two thirds of the femur. If fracture of the femur has occurred, the proximal component extends upward to the level of the greater trochanter. To be effective, careful molding of the proximal portion of the cast around the trochanter and medial wall is required. For fractures of the mid to upper femur, an orthotic hip joint and pelvic band must be added to ensure alignment and stability.

Fracture Orthoses

A custom-fabricated or custom-fit *fracture orthosis* is designed to maintain a body part in an optimal anatomical position, limit joint motion, and unload weight-bearing forces.[144-147] The major advantage of a fracture orthosis, as compared with a cast brace, is that the orthosis can be removed for wound or skin care. Fracture orthoses are fabricated from high-temperature thermoplastic materials. They are designed to provide total contact, circumferential control of a fracture while allowing the individual with

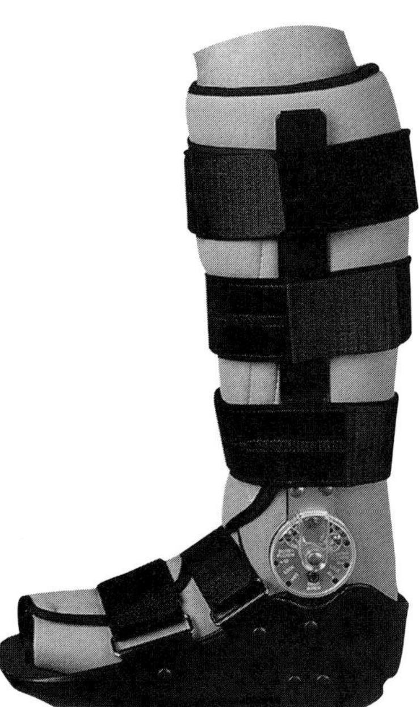

Figure 14-37
An example of a commercially available short leg walker with a rocker bottom sole that can be used for individuals with Achilles tendon repair, stable healing fractures of the distal tibia/fibula, ankle, or foot, or with severe ankle sprain. This particular walker has an orthotic ankle joint that can be preset to limit or allow motion at the ankle joint. (Courtesy DJ Orthopedics, Vista, CA.)

a healing fracture to have functional mobility. Fracture stability is enhanced in two ways: by hydrostatic pressure forces created as the rigid walls of the orthosis compress soft tissue and muscles in the extremity and by the lever arm created by extension of the orthosis above and below the fracture site. Fracture orthoses do not entirely unload the lower extremity during weight bearing. If complete unloading or reduced loading is required to protect the fracture site, an appropriate assistive device (crutches or a walker) and a single limb gait pattern must be used.[139]

Two types of fracture orthoses are available: (1) those that are custom fabricated from a mold of the patient's limb and (2) prefabricated orthoses that are custom fit to match the patient's needs. Because of the wide variation in anatomical characteristics among individuals, it is not always possible to use a prefabricated orthosis. Likewise, because of anatomical similarities in the human skeleton, it is not always necessary to create a custom-fabricated device. In certain instances an orthosis must be precisely fit to provide the desired stabilization of the fracture; in other cases the orthosis must be heavily padded so that a precise fit is less important. The orthotic prescription must clearly designate the motions to be permitted and controlled, the corrective forces to be applied, and a precise diagnosis and description of the fracture.

Types of Fracture Orthoses

Fracture orthoses are named by the joints they encompass and the motion that they are designed to control. An *ankle-foot orthosis (AFO) with an anterior shell* is used to control ankle and distal tibia motion (Figure 14-36). It encases the injured limb completely, limiting motion of the foot or ankle for patients with distal tibial or fibular fractures. The AFO fracture orthosis has two advantages: It can be removed for wound care and hygiene, and it can be worn with standard lace-up shoes if weight bearing is permitted. The application of a cushion heel and rocker sole may be necessary on the shoe to compensate for limited heel, ankle, and toe rocker motion during gait. Because total contact is essential, this thermoplastic orthosis is vacuum molded over a positive impression of the patient's limb. The anterior shell may be lined with soft-density foam to accommodate bony deformity or insufficient soft tissue. Perforated thermoplastic material is often used for the anterior section as a means of ventilation for patient comfort. The proximal anterior trimline is at the tibial tubercle. Adequate clearance must be provided for the head of the fibula and the peroneal nerve. The distal posterior section usually extends to just beyond the metatarsal heads on the plantar surface, whereas the anterior section is trimmed just proximally. A stocking or thin sock is worn to protect the skin and for comfort. The anterior section is held in place with a series of hook-and-loop material straps. Shoes must be worn if weight bearing is permitted.

A number of prefabricated *short leg walkers* are also commercially available; these devices are designed to substitute for a short leg cast and are intended to be removable by the patient. They are heavily padded and, if properly fit, provide excellent immobilization of the distal tibia, ankle, rear foot, and forefoot (Figure 14-37). The various designs are similar, but manufacturers' instructions should be followed to maximize their effectiveness. The short leg walker's advantage is that it can be removed for wound and skin care. Its disadvantage may be slightly less effective immobilization. The ankle is positioned at a neutral (90-degree) angle. Some designs have an adjustable orthotic ankle joint that permits a controlled, limited range of motion, to assist forward progression during walking. The components of a short leg walker include a rigid foot piece that is attached to a pair of metal or thermoplastic uprights and a proximal cuff that helps to suspend a foam liner. Short leg walkers are manufactured in various styles and sizes. To ensure proper fit, the manufacturer's recommendations must be followed carefully.

The *PTB fracture orthosis* is the removable version of the PTB cast, providing significant protection from bending and rotatory torque for the tibia during weight-bearing activities. This thermoplastic orthosis is most often vacuum molded over a positive mold of the patient's limb for optimal total contact fit. Ankle position within the orthosis is often in slight dorsiflexion, once again to minimize hyperextension moment at the knee during the stance phase of gait. Trimlines are similar to those of an AFO with anterior shell, with the proximal trimline extending somewhat more proximally to the proximal pole of the patella anteriorly, medially, and laterally. The posterior trimline should permit free knee flexion beyond 90 degrees. Hook-and-loop material straps are used to secure the anterior and posterior sections together. The anterior and the posterior sections can be hinged at the proximal edge for improved anteroposterior control.

The purpose of the *knee-ankle-foot fracture orthosis* is to provide long-term protection for fractures of the distal to middle femur or for fractures about the knee (Figure 14-38). This orthosis is often used as an alternative to a hybrid cast brace for persons who have had ORIF for fractures of the proximal tibia, knee, or distal femur. The orthosis is removable for wound care and personal hygiene and when protection is not required. Depending on the location of the fracture, the orthosis can be designed to limit range of motion or to permit full motion of the knee. Drop locks can be used to stabilize the knee in full extension during ambulation. The design of the orthosis also protects the knee from excessive mediolateral and anteroposterior shear stress during ambulation. If maximum stability is necessary, a solid-ankle design can be incorporated; if mobility of the ankle is desired, an articulated ankle joint with an appropriate motion stop mechanism can be used. The orthosis requires total contact within the femoral and tibial components. Proximal trimlines follow the anatomical contours of the proximal femur to the greater trochanter to provide femoral protection. To stabilize the knee or proximal tibia, encasement of the lower two thirds of the femur is sufficient. The orthosis alone cannot effectively unload the femur, tibia, or foot: If axial unloading is desired, appropriate assistive devices (crutches or walker) must be used.

For individuals with proximal femoral fractures, a hip joint and pelvic band are often incorporated into a total contact knee-ankle-foot orthosis in an effort to control motion and rotational forces through the femur (Figure 14-39). Depending on the patient's specific needs, hip flexion/extension motion can be restricted or free; abduction/adduction is usually restricted. The placement of the orthotic hip joint is approximately 1 cm anterior and 1 cm proximal to the tip of the greater trochanter in most adults. Knee and ankle motion can be free or limited, given the location and stability of the fracture. A variety of single-axis or polycentric orthotic hip joints can be incorporated. A pelvic belt is used to maintain the orthotic hip joint in proper functional position. The belt should fit midway between the crest of the ilium and the greater trochanter.

External Fixation Devices

External fixation devices have evolved primarily to care for complex open fractures that are most often the result of high-velocity injury or multiple trauma (see Figures 14-30 and 14-35).[149-152] In particular, external fixation is used for severe metaphyseal fractures, severe intraarticular fractures, when there has been nonunion, in cases of substantial bone loss with allograft, and for fractures in osteoporotic bone.[150,153] They are particularly useful when fracture disrupts pelvic stability.[154-156]

Pins are placed into bone on either side of the fracture and then clamped onto lightweight rods in an external frame. The external frame can be a single rod, a set of articulated rods that cross the joint axis, circumferential, or a combination of these options.[157-161] The goal is to provide optimal skeletal alignment while providing visual access to healing skin and muscle. The external fixator permits active range of motion of the joint above and below the fracture. It is removed when soft tissues have adequately healed and radiographs demonstrate healing of the fracture. Casts or orthoses can be used to provide immobilization after fixator removal to support and protect the fracture until healing is complete.

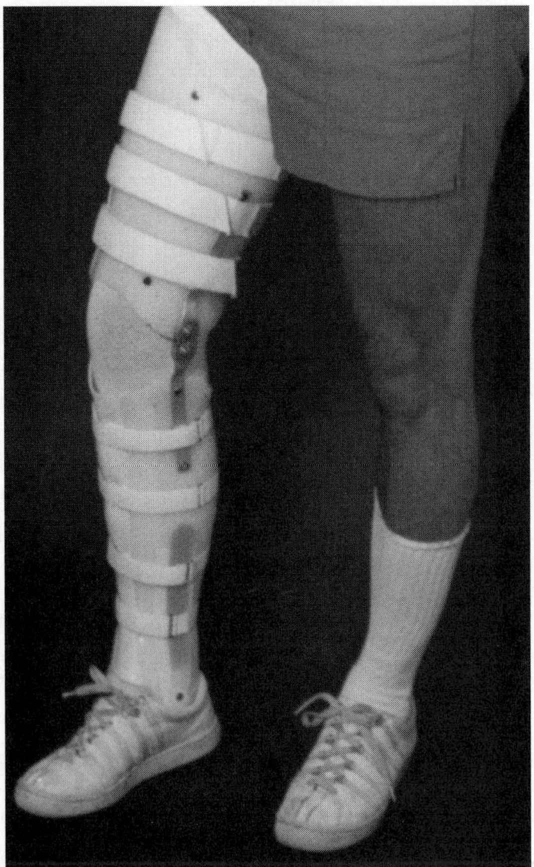

Figure 14-38
A prefabricated functional fracture orthosis must be adjusted regularly to ensure snug compression of soft tissues so that stability and alignment across the fracture will be maintained. (From Moore TJ: Functional bracing of lower extremity fractures. In Goldberg B, Hsu JD (eds). Atlas of Orthoses and Assistive Devices. *St. Louis: Mosby; 1997.)*

Postfracture Management and Potential Complications

The postfracture issues and complications that are of concern to the managing physician and rehabilitation team include vascular injury, compartment syndrome, appropriate weight-bearing status, loss of reduction, delayed or nonunion, infection, implant failure (for ORIF), compression neuropathy, and skin breakdown. Each patient who presents to the emergency department with a fracture must be assessed for potential vascular injury and risk of developing compartment syndrome by careful physical examination. Whether a splint, cast, surgical ORIF, or placement of external fixators has been used to stabilize the fracture, the condition of the extremity must be monitored carefully by the physician, rehabilitation professional, patient, and family caregivers.

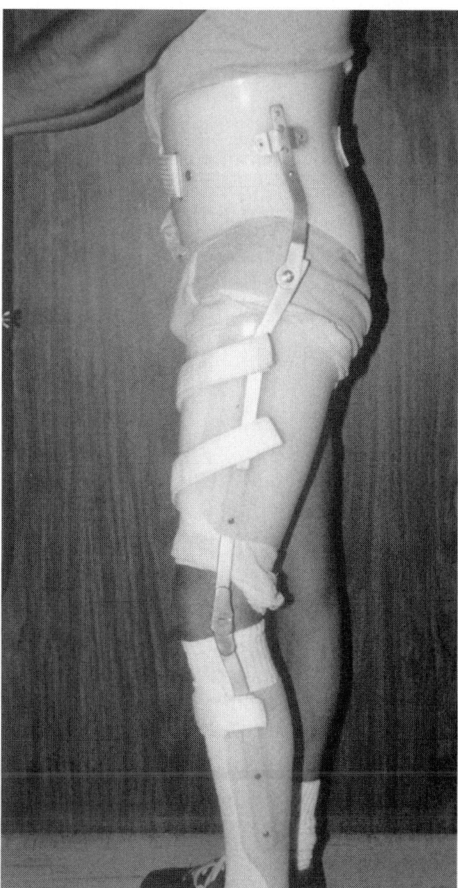

Figure 14-39
A lumbar sacral orthosis with an orthotic hip joint has been added to this knee-ankle-foot orthosis to provide better control of hip abduction/adduction and rotation while a proximal femoral fracture heals. The lateral uprights limit angulation through the healing femur during ambulation. Weight-bearing status is determined by the physician on the basis of the severity of the fracture and stability of the reduction.

Fractures or dislocations around joints may have a *concomitant arterial injury* that can bruise or completely disrupt an artery, compromising or completely interrupting blood flow beyond the site of fracture.[162-164] This creates a grave situation: The physician has a window of less than 6 to 8 hours in which to restore blood supply and nutrition to the distal muscle and bone before significant tissue death occurs. The longer the period of ischemia, the greater the likelihood of delayed healing, infection, and necrosis.

Compartment syndrome evolves when bleeding or inflammation exceeds the expansive capacity of semirigid muscle or soft tissue anatomical spaces (compartments) of the fractured limb.[165-167] Once interstitial pressure exceeds a critical level, blood vessels and muscle are compressed and oxygen supply to the muscles is significantly compromised. Irreversible muscle or nerve damage occurs if compartment syndrome continues for longer than 6 to 8 hours. Presenting signs and symptoms include extreme pain and significant swelling of the extremity with taut skin. Passive motion of the fingers or toes causes excruciating pain. Compartment syndrome is considered a medical emergency: The treating physician must be notified immediately so that a fasciotomy can be performed to relieve excessive compartment pressures. All health professionals who are involved in the treatment of extremity trauma should be aware of the signs and symptoms of compartment syndrome. If unrecognized and untreated, compartment syndrome has devastating results.

One of the most important considerations for lower extremity fractures is *weight-bearing status*. A patient's weight-bearing status (full weight bearing, weight bearing as tolerated, partial weight bearing, toe-touch weight bearing, or non–weight bearing) is determined by the physician on the basis of the stability of the fracture and the immobilization method used. Once a patient is stable after an operation or a cast has been applied and is properly set, rehabilitation professionals work with the patient and family on mobility and gait training. The rehabilitation professional selects the appropriate assistive device for a patient's weight-bearing status, given the patient's physical and cognitive status and the characteristics of his or her usual living environment. Communicating quickly to the referring physician any signs of developing complications or difficulty with compliance that might put the fracture site at risk is important.

Loss of reduction of the fracture is a serious complication and can occur whether a splint, cast, ORIF, or external fixator has been used to realign and stabilize the limb.[159,168-170] A progressive angular deformity or abnormal position of the limb suggests loss of reduction and must be quickly reported to the managing physician. Even if reduction appears to be appropriate, inadequate immobilization within a splint or cast can lead to delayed union, nonunion (nonhealing), or malunion (healing in an abnormal position).

Any patient who has sustained an open fracture is at risk of developing *infection* of skin, deep tissue and muscle, or even bone. Both intravenous and local antibiotics are administered in the emergency department and operating room to minimize likelihood of infection from contamination sustained at the time of injury.[171,172] Infections may also be iatrogenic.[172,173] An infection is a serious complication that requires aggressive antibiotic treatment or débridement, or both. If an infection occurs after ORIF, the implanted hardware may have to be removed and an external fixation device applied. For individuals with external fixation, the pins provide a tract for infectious organisms directly into bone.[174] Appropriate wound and pin care is essential to minimize the risk of infection.[175] Osteomyelitis, or infection of bone, is a serious situation that can result in deformity; joint destruction; and, in some circumstances, amputation.[176,177]

Patients who have undergone ORIF are at risk of *implant failure* if repeated loading exceeds the strength of the implant material and design.[178-180] Loosening or breakage of implanted screws, plates, or other devices also indicates excessive motion of the fracture site and increases the risk of delayed healing or nonunion. The patient's ability to function within weight-bearing limits established by the physician must be carefully assessed and monitored to reduce the risk of implant failure.

Complications also occur in patients whose fractures are managed by casting. The patient's neurovascular function is documented before cast application and carefully monitored while the cast is in place. In the distal lower extremity, the peroneal nerve is susceptible to prolonged pressure (compression-induced peroneal palsy) as it wraps around the head of the fibula.[107,127,181]

Complaints of edge pressure or toes being squeezed can be solved with cast modifications; however, excessive pressure and discomfort inside the cast often require removal and reapplication of a new cast.[182] On initial application, a cast is designed to have a snug but not tight fit. Signs of distal vascular compromise such as delayed capillary refill on compression of the nail bed suggest that the cast may be excessively tight.[107,182] It is not uncommon for cast fit to loosen over time as a result of several factors: Initial edema resolves, compressive forces modify soft tissue composition, disuse atrophy occurs, and cast padding compresses over time. Fit must be carefully monitored over time: A loose cast provides less control of the skeleton, and fracture reduction may be lost. Pistoning of a loose cast on the extremity is likely to lead to skin breakdown and shear over bony prominences.

Casts applied postoperatively while the patient is anesthetized are usually univalved (split down the front) to accommodate postoperative swelling.[108] Excessive swelling is accompanied by significant pain. Limb elevation is the first defense against excessive swelling and pain; however, the cast can be opened further or bivalved to relieve extreme pressure.[3] The risk of compartment syndrome must always be considered: If the patient experiences significant pain on passive motion of the fingers or toes, the physician must be contacted immediately. Failure to recognize and appropriately treat a compartment syndrome results in muscle necrosis and possible loss of the limb.[166]

Occasionally, a window can be cut into a cast to inspect a wound or relieve a pressure area. If the limb is edematous, it is likely that soft tissue will begin to protrude through the window, resulting in additional skin irritation and breakdown. For this reason, any piece of cast that is removed to make a window must be reapplied and secured to the cast after modifications have been made.[182]

Patients with foot pain try to reposition the foot within the cast to make it more comfortable. Inappropriate plantar flexion of the foot within the cast creates excessive pressure on the posterior heel and dorsum of the foot. Discomfort can be reduced if the patient is able to push the relaxed foot gently downward while pulling the cast upward, as if pulling on a boot. If this fails to relieve pressure, the cast must be removed and reapplied.[182]

Foreign objects introduced into a cast are the most common cause of discomfort and pressure. In an attempt to relieve itching of dry skin, patients are sometimes tempted to insert coat hangers, rulers, sticks, pens, and similar objects into the cast to scratch the itchy areas. This strategy often leads to displacement of cast padding, creating lumps and bumps where smooth surface contact is essential. Objects can break off or become trapped within the cast as well. The best way to relieve itching is by tapping on the cast or blowing cool air into it.

Another common complication is *skin maceration*, which is the result of prolonged exposure to water or a moist environment within the cast. Although, ideally, a cast is kept completely dry, many become wet at some point after application. Plaster casts that become wet lose significant stability and must be replaced. Synthetic casts can be towel dried as much as possible and then further dried using a cool setting on a blower or hairdryer.

SUMMARY

In this chapter the reader has discovered that orthoses play an important role in the management of traumatic (e.g., fracture) and developmental (e.g., DDH, LCPD) musculoskeletal conditions. Each member of the interdisciplinary rehabilitation team has a contribution to make to the care of individuals with pathologies of the musculoskeletal system, as well as shared responsibility to monitor for changes in function and potential complications. Although many prefabricated orthoses are available, knowledge of appropriate fit, design, and dynamics of the orthoses is essential so that the device will most closely match the intention of intervention. Precise communication about the goals of the orthosis (e.g., to fully immobilize the limb or to allow joint motion within a restricted range), wearing schedule (e.g., all the time or during particular activities), and weight-bearing status while using the orthosis has a major impact on efficacy of the orthotic intervention. All team members participate in patient and family education about the orthosis and its purpose, maintenance and cleaning, signs that indicate problems, and strategies to put in place should problems arise.

REFERENCES

1. Levangie PK. Biomechanical applications to joint structure and function. In Levangie PK, Norkin CC (eds), *Joint Structure and Function: A Comprehensive Analysis,* 4th ed. Philadelphia: F.A. Davis, 2005. pp. 3-68.
2. Mueller MJ, Maluf KS. Tissue adaptation to physical stress: a proposed "physical stress theory" to guide physical therapist practice, education, and research. *Phys Ther* 2002;82(4):383-403.
3. Williams PL (ed). *Gray's Anatomy,* 38th ed. New York: Churchill Livingstone, 1995.
4. Netter FH, Hansen JT. *Atlas of Human Anatomy,* 3rd ed. Teterboro, NJ: ICON Learning Systems, 2002.
5. Lundon K. Anatomy and biology of bone tissue. In *Orthopedic Rehabilitation Science: Principles for Clinical Management of Bone.* Boston: Butterworth-Heinemann, 2000. pp. 5-23.
6. Curwin S. Joint structure and function. In Levangie PK, Norkin CC (eds), *Joint Structure and Function: A Comprehensive Analysis,* 4th ed. Philadelphia: F.A. Davis, 2005. pp. 69-111.
7. Lundon K. Changes in bone across the lifespan. In *Orthopedic Rehabilitation Science: Principles for Clinical Management of Bone.* Boston: Butterworth-Heinemann, 2000. pp. 33-47.
8. Bidwell JP, Alvarez M, Feister H, et al. Nuclear matrix proteins and osteoblast gene expression. *J Bone Mineral Res* 1998;13(2):155-167.
9. Rodan GA. Control of bone formation and resorption: biological and clinical perspective. *J Cell Biochem* 1998; 30-31(Suppl):55-61.
10. Lanyon LE. Osteocytes, strain detection, bone modeling and remodeling. *Calcif Tissue Int* 1993;53(Suppl 1):S102-107.
11. Suda T, Nakamura I, Eijirio J, et al. Regulation of osteoclastic function. *J Bone Miner Res* 1997;12(6):869-879.
12. Blair HC. How the osteoclast degrades bone. *Bioessays* 1998; 20(10):837-846.
13. Payne R. Mechanisms and management of bone pain. *Cancer* 1997;80(Suppl 8):1608-1613.
14. Stevens DA, Williams GR. Hormone regulation of chondrocyte differentiation and endochondral bone formation. *Mol Cell Endocrinol* 1999;151(1-2):195-204.
15. Mundy GR. Bone resorption and turnover in health and disease. *Bone* 1987;8(Suppl 1):S9-S16.
16. Watkins BA. Regulatory effects of polyunsaturates on bone modeling and cartilage function. *World Rev Nutr Diet* 1998;83:38-51.
17. Rosen GJ. Insulin-like growth factors I and calcium balance: evolving concepts of an evolutionary process. *Endocrinology* 2003;144(11):4679-4681.
18. Lundon K. Physiology and biochemistry of bone tissue. In *Orthopedic Rehabilitation Science: Principles for Clinical Management of Bone.* Boston: Butterworth-Heinemann; 2000. pp. 25-32.
19. Jilka RL. Cytokines, bone remodeling, and estrogen deficiency; a 1998 update. *Bone* 1998;23(2):75-81.
20. Christenson RH. Biochemical markers of bone metabolism; an overview. *Clin Biochem* 1997;30(8):573-593.
21. Seibel MJ, Baylink DJ, Farley JR, et al. Basic science and clinical utility of biochemical markers of bone turnover—a Congress report. *Endocrinol Diabetes* 1997;105(3):125-133.
22. Riggs B, Melton L. Involutional osteoporosis. *N Engl J Med* 1986;314(26):1676-1686.
23. Sabateir JP, Guaydiersouquieres G, Laroche D, et al. Bone mineral acquisition during adolescence and early adulthood: a study of 574 healthy females 10-24 years of age. *Osteoporosis Int* 1996;6(2):141-148.
24. Crawford AH, Ayyangar R, Durrett GL. Congenital and acquired disorders. In Goldberg B, Hsu JH (eds), *Atlas of Orthoses and Assistive Devices,* 3rd ed. St. Louis: Mosby; 1997. pp. 479-500.
25. Shipman AJ, Guy GW, Smith I, et al. Vertebral bone mineral density, content and area in 8789 normal women aged 33-73 who have never had hormone replacement therapy. *Osteoporosis Int* 1999;9(5):420-426.
26. Stevens DA, Williams GR. Hormonal regulation of chondrocyte differentiation and endochondral bone formation. *Mol Cell Endocrinol* 1999;151(1-2):195-204.
27. Torgerson DJ, Campbell MK, Reid DM. Lifestyle, environmental, and medical factors influencing peak bone mass in women. *Br J Rheumatol* 1995;34(7):620-624.
28. Mazess RB, Barden HS. Bone density in pre-menopausal women: effects of age, dietary intake, physical activity, smoking, and birth control pills. *Am J Clin Nutr* 1991;53(1): 132-142.
29. WHO Scientific Group on Prevention and Management of Osteoporosis. Prevention and management of osteoporosis. *World Health Organ Tech Rep Ser* 2003;921:1-164.
30. Levangie PK. The hip complex. In Levangie PK, Norkin CC (eds), *Joint Structure and Function: A Comprehensive Analysis,* 4th ed. Philadelphia: F.A. Davis, 2005. pp. 355-392.
31. Steinberg ME (ed). *The Hip and Its Disorders.* Philadelphia: Saunders, 1991.
32. Guille JT, Pizzutillo PD, MacEvew GD. Development dysplasia of the hip from birth to six months. *J Am Acad Orthop Surg* 2000;8(4):232-242.
33. Vitale MG, Skaggs DL. Developmental dysplasia of the hip from six months to four years of age. *J Am Acad Orthop Surg* 2001;9(6):401-411.
34. Ilfeld FW, Westin GW, Makin M. Missed or developmental dislocation of the hip. *Clin Orthop* 1986;Feb(203):276-281.
35. Mubarik SJ, Leach JL, Wenger DR. Management of congenital dislocation of the hip in the infant. *Contemp Orthop* 1987;15:29-44.
36. Shapiro F. Developmental dysplasia of the hip. In Shapiro F (ed), *Pediatric Orthopedic Deformities: Basic Science, Diagnosis and Treatment.* San Diego: Academic Press, 2002. pp. 153-271.
37. Hesinger RN. Congenital dislocation of the hip; treatment in infancy to walking age. *Orthop Clin North Am* 1987;18(4):597-616.
38. Leach J. Orthopedic conditions. In Campbell SK, Vander Linden DW, Palisano RT (eds), *Physical Therapy for Children,* 2nd ed. Philadelphia: Saunders, 2000. pp. 398-428.

39. Lotito FM, Rabbaglietti G, Notarantonio M. The ultrasonographic image of the infant hip affected by developmental dysplasia with a positive Ortolani's sign. *Pediatr Radiol* 2002;32(6):418-22.
40. Walker JM. Musculoskeletal development: a review. *Phys Ther* 1991;71(12):878-889.
41. Riester JA, Eilert RE. Hip disorders. In Goldberg B, Hsu JD (eds), *Atlas of Orthotic and Assistive Devices,* St. Louis: Mosby, 1997. pp. 509-526.
42. Pavlik A. The functional method of treatment using a harness with stirrups as the primary method of conservative therapy for infants with congenital dislocation of the hip. *Clin Orthop* 1992;Aug(281):4-10.
43. Mubarak SJ. Pavlik: the man and his method. *J Pediatr Orthop* 2003;23(3):342-346.
44. Song KM, Lapinsky A. Determination of hip position in the Pavlik harness. *J Pediatr Orthop* 2000;20(3):317-319.
45. Wenger DR, Rang M. Developmental dysplasia of the hip. In Wenger DR, Rang M (eds), *The Art and Practice of Children's Orthopaedics*, 1st ed. New York: Raven, 1993. pp. 272-280.
46. Mubarak S, Garfin S, Vance R, et al. Pitfalls in the use of the Pavlik harness for treatment of congenital dysplasia, subluxation, and dislocation of the hip. *J Bone Joint Surg* 1981;63A(8):1239-1247.
47. Kim HW, Weinstein SL. Intervening early in developmental hip dysplasia: early recognition avoids serious consequences later. *J Musculoskel Med* 1998;15(2):70-72 and 77-81.
48. Harding MG, Harke HT, Bowen JR, et al. Management of dislocated hips with Pavlik harness treatment and ultrasound monitoring. *J Pediatr Orthop* 1997;17(2):189-198.
49. Inoue T, Naito M, Nomiyama H. Treatment of developmental dysplasia of the hip with the Pavlik harness: factors for predicting unsuccessful reduction. *J Pediatr Orthop B* 2001;10(3):186-191.
50. Leman JA, Emans JB, Millis MB, et al. Early failure of Pavlik harness treatment for developmental hip dysplasia: clinical and ultrasound predictors. *J Pediatr Orthop* 2001;21(3): 348-353.
51. Hedequist D, Kasser J, Emans J. Use of an abduction brace for developmental dysplasia of the hip after failure of the Pavlik harness. *J Pediatr Orthop* 2003;23(2):175-177.
52. Segal LS, Boal DK, Borthwick L, et al. Avasucular necrosis after treatment of DDH: the protective influence of the ossific nucleus. *J Pediatr Orthop* 1999;19(2):177-184.
53. Suzuki S, Kashiwagi N, Kasahara Y, et al. Avascular necrosis and the Pavlik harness: the incidence of avascular necrosis in three types of congenital dislocation of the hip as classified by ultrasound. *J Bone Joint Surg Br* 1996;78(4):631-635.
54. Carey TP, Guidera KG, Ogden JA. Manifestations of ischemic necrosis complicating developmental dysplasia. *Clin Orthop* 1992;Aug(281):11-17.
55. Luhman SJ, Schoenecker PL, Anderson AM, et al. The prognostic importance of the ossific nucleus in the treatment of congenital dysplasia of the hip. *J Bone Joint Surg Am* 1998;80(12):1719-1727.
56. Legg AT. An obscure affection of the hip joint. *Boston Med Surg J* 1910;162-202.
57. Canale ST. Osteochondroses. In Canale ST, Beatty JH (eds), *Operative Pediatric Orthopedics*. St. Louis: Mosby-Year Book, 1991. pp. 743-776.
58. Stulberg SD, Cooperman DR, Wallensten R. The natural history of Legg-Calvé-Perthes disease. *J Bone Joint Surg Am* 63(7):1095-1108.
59. Guille JT, Lipton GE, Szöke G, et al. Legg-Calvé-Perthes disease in girls: a comparison of results with those seen in boys. *J Bone Joint Surg* 1998;80A(9):1256-1263.
60. Herring JA, Tachdjian MO. *Tachdjian's Pediatric Orthopaedics,* 3rd ed. Philadelphia: Saunders, 2002.
61. Guile JT Bowen JR: Legg-Calvé-Perthes disease. In Dee R (ed), *Principles of Orthopaedic Practice*, 2nd ed. New York: McGraw-Hill, 1997. pp. 723-734.
62. Balasa VV, Gruppo RA, Glueck CJ, et al. Legg-Calvé-Perthes disease and thrombophilia. *J Bone Joint Surg Am* 2004;86(12):2642-2647.
63. Hamer AJ. Pain in the hip and knee. *BMJ* 2004;328(7447): 1067-1069.
64. Gerberg LF, Micheli LJ. Nontraumatic hip pain in active children. *Phys Sports Med* 1996;24(1):69-74.
65. Eich GF, Supertis-Furga A, Umbricht FS, et al. The painful hip: evaluation of criteria for clinical decision making. *Eur J Pediatr* 1999;158(11):923-928.
66. Herring JA, Kim HT, Browne R. Legg-Calvé-Perthes disease part 1: classification of radiographs with use of the modified lateral pillar and Stulberg classifications. *J Bone Joint Surg Am* 2004;86(10):2103-2121.
67. Yazici M, Aydingoz U, Aksoy MC, et al. Bipositional MR imaging for the evaluation of femoral head sphericity and containment in Legg-Calvé-Perthes disease. *Clin Imaging* 2002;26(5):342-346.
68. Catterall A. Natural history, classification, and x-ray signs in Legg-Calvé-Perthes disease. *Acta Orthop Belg* 1980;46(4):346-351.
69. Christensen F, Soballe K, Ejsted R, et al. The Catterall classification of Perthes disease: an assessment of reliability. *J Bone Joint Surg Br* 1986;68(4):614-615.
70. Hardcastle PH, Ross R, Hamalalnen M, et al. Catterall grouping of Perthes disease: an assessment of observer error and prognosis using the Catterall classification. *J Bone Joint Surg Br* 1980;62(4):428-431.
71. Ritterbusch JF, Shantharam SS, Gellnas C. Comparison of lateral pillar classification and Catterall classification of Legg-Calvé-Perthes disease. *J Pediatr Orthop* 1990;13(2): 200-202.
72. Salter RB, Thompson GH. Legg-Calvé-Perthes disease: the prognostic significance of the subchondral fracture and a two group classification of the femoral head involvement. *J Bone Joint Surg Am* 1984;66(4):479-489.
73. Sponseller PD, Desai SS, Mills MB. Abnormalities of proximal femoral growth after severe Perthes disease. *J Bone Joint Surg Br* 1989;71(4):479-489.
74. Podeszwa DA, Stanitski CL, Stanitski DF, et al. The effect of pediatric orthopedic experience on interobserver and intraobserver reliability of the Herring lateral pillar classification of Perthes disease. *J Pediatric Orthop* 2000;20(5):562-565.
75. Herring JA, Kim HT, Browne R. Legg-Calvé-Perthes disease part II: Prospective multi-center study on the effect of treatment outcome. *J Bone Joint Surg* 2004;86(10):2121-2134.
76. MacEwen GD. Conservative treatment of Legg-Calvé-Perthes disease conditions. In Fitzgerald FH (eds), *The Hip:*

Proceedings of the 13th Open Scientific Meeting of the Hip Society. St. Louis: Mosby, 1985. pp. 17-23.

77. Wenger DR, Ward WT, Herring JA. Current concepts review: Legg-Calvé-Perthes disease. *J Bone Joint Surg* 1991;73(5): 778-788.
78. Poussa M, Yrjonen T, Holkka V, et al. Prognosis after conservative and operative management of Perthes disease. *Clin Orthop* 1993;Dec(297):549-553.
79. Noonan KJ, Price CT, Kupiszewski SJ, et al. Results of femoral varus osteotomy in children older than 9 years of age with Perthes disease. *J Pediatr Orthop* 2001;21(2):198-204.
80. Paterson DC, Leitch JM, Foster BK. Results of innominate osteotomy in the treatment of Legg-Calvé-Perthes disease. *Clin Orthop* 1991;May (266):93-103.
81. Kruse RW, Gulle JT, Bowen JR. Shelf arthroplasty in patients who have Legg-Calvé-Perthes disease: a long term study of results. *J Bone Joint Surg Am* 1991;73(9):1338-1347.
82. Willett K, Hudson I, Catterall A. Lateral shelf acetabuloplasty: an operation for older children with Perthes disease. *J Pediatr Orthop* 1992;12(5):563-568.
83. Grzegorzeski A, Bowen JR, Guille JT, et al. Treatment of the collapsed femoral head by containment in Legg-Calvé-Perthes disease. *J Pediatr Orthop* 2003;23(1):15-19.
84. Herring JA. Current concepts review. The treatment of Legg-Calvé-Perthes disease; a critical review of the literature. *J Bone Joint Surg* 1994;76A(3):448-458.
85. Martinez AG, Weinstein SL, Deat FR. The weight bearing abduction brace for the treatment of Legg-Perthes disease. *J Bone Joint Surg* 1992;74A(1):12-21.
86. Meehan TL, Angel D, Nelson JM. The Scottish-Rite abduction orthosis for the treatment of Legg-Perthes disease. A radiographic analysis. *J Bone Joint Surg* 1992;74A(1): 2-12.
87. Purvis JM, Dimon JH, Meehan PL, et al. Preliminary experience with the Scottish Rite hospital abduction orthosis for Legg-Perthes disease. *Clin Orthop* 1980;July-Aug(150): 49-53.
88. Meehan PL, Angel D, Nelson JM. The Scottish Rite abduction orthosis for the treatment of Legg-Perthes disease: a radiographic analysis. *J Bone Joint Surg Am* 1992;74(1):2-12.
89. Martinez AG, Weinstein SL, Dietz FR. The weight bearing abduction brace for the treatment of Legg-Perthes disease. *J Bone Joint Surg Am* 1992;74(1):12-21.
90. Bobechko WP, McLaurin EA, Motloch WM. Toronto orthosis for Legg-Perthes disease. *Artif Limbs* 1968;12(2): 36-41.
91. Curtis HD Gunther SF, Gossling HR, et al. Treatment for Legg-Perthes disease with the Newington ambulation abduction brace. *J Bone Joint Surg* 1974;56(6):1135-1146.
92. Edelstein JE, Brukner J. *Orthotics: a Comprehensive Clinical Approach.* Thorofare, NJ: Slack, 2002.
93. Drennan JC. *Orthopaedic Management of Neuromuscular Disorders,* 1st ed. Philadelphia: Lippincott, 1983. p. 278.
94. Walker WC, Keyser-Marcus LA, Cifu DX, et al. Inpatient interdisciplinary rehabilitation after total hip arthroplasty surgery: a comparison of revision and primary total hip arthroplasty. *Arch Phys Med Rehabil* 2001;82(1):123-133.
95. Lima D, Magnus R, Paproshy WG. Team management of hip revision patients using a post-op hip orthosis. *J Prosthet Orthot* 1994;6(1):20-24.
96. Cummings SR, Rubin SM, Black D. The future of hip fractures in the United States: numbers, costs, and potential effects of postmenopausal estrogen. *Clin Orthop* 1991;March(252):163-166.
97. Schultz RJ. *The Language of Fractures,* 2nd ed. Baltimore: Williams & Wilkins, 1990.
98. Islam SS, Biswas RS, Nambiar AM, et al. Incidence and risk of work-related fracture injuries; experience of a state-managed worker's compensation system. *J Occup Environ Med* 2001;43(2):140-146.
99. Tiderius CJ, Landin L, Duppe H. Decreasing incidence of fractures in children. *Acta Orthop Scand* 1999;70(6): 622-626.
100. Estrada LS, Alonso JE, McGwin G, et al. Restraint use and lower extremity fracture in frontal motor vehicle collisions. *J Trauma* 2004;57(2):323-328.
101. Edwards BJ, Bunta AD, Madision LD, et al. An osteoporosis and fracture intervention program increases the diagnosis and treatment for osteoporosis for patients with minimal trauma fractures. *Jt Comm J Qual Patient Saf* 2005; 31(5)267-274.
102. Jacofsky DF, Haidukewych GJ. Management of pathological fractures of the proximal femur: state of the art. *J Orthop Trauma* 2004;18(7):459-460.
103. Ringsberg KA, Gardsell P, Johnell O, et al. The impact of long-term moderate physical activity on functional performance, bone mineral density, and fracture incidence in elderly women. *Gerontology* 2001;47(1):15-20.
104. Boden BP, Osbahr DC, Jimenez C. Low risk stress fractures. *Am J Sports Med* 2001;29(1):100-111.
105. Vanderschueren D, Boonen S, Bouillon R. Action of androgens versus estrogens in male skeletal homeostasis. *Bone* 1998;23(5):391-394.
106. Seeman E. Advances in the study of osteoporosis in men. In Meunier PH (ed), *Osteoporosis: Diagnosis and Management.* London: Dunitz; 1998. pp. 211-232.
107. Charnley J. *The Closed Treatment of Common Fractures,* 4th ed. London: Cambridge University Press, 2002.
108. Cole AS, McNally MA. The management of open fractures. In Bulstrode CJ, Buchwalker J, Carr A, et al (eds), *Oxford Textbook of Orthopedics and Trauma.* New York: Oxford University Press, 2002. pp. 1636-1651.
109. DeCoster TA. Fracture classification. In Bulstrode CJ, Buchwalker J, Carr A, et al (eds), *Oxford Textbook of Orthopedics and Trauma.* New York: Oxford University Press, 2002. pp. 1575-1580.
110. Lundon K. Injury, regeneration, and repair in bone. In *Orthopedic Rehabilitation Science: Principles for Clinical Management of Bone.* Boston: Butterworth-Heinemann, 2000. pp. 93-113.
111. Reddi AH. Initiation of fracture repair by bone morphogenetic proteins. *Clin Orthop* 1998;Oct(355 Suppl):S66-72.
112. Hayda RA, Brighton CT, Esterhai JL. Pathophysiology of delayed healing. *Clin Orthop* 1998;Oct(355 Suppl):S31-40.
113. Gustilo RB, Anderson JT. Prevention of infection in the treatment of one thousand and twenty-five open fractures of long bones. *J Bone Joint Surg* 1976;58(4):453-458.
114. Rose DD, Rowven DW. Perioperative considerations in major orthopedic trauma: pelvic and long bone fractures. *Am Assoc Nurse Anesth J* 2002;70(2):131-137.

115. Gugenheim JJ. External fixation in orthopedics. *JAMA* 2004;291(17):2122-2134.
116. Harkess JW, Ramsey WC, Harkess JW. Principles of fracture and dislocations. In Rockwood CA, Green DP, Bucholz RW (eds), *Rockwood and Green's Fractures in Adults,* vol 1, 3rd ed. Philadelphia: Lippincott Williams & Wilkins, 1991. pp. 1-180.
117. Bick EM. *Source Book of Orthopaedics.* New York: Hafner, 1968. pp. 286-287.
118. Wytch R, Mitchell C, Ratchie IK, et al. New splinting material. *Prosthet Orthot Int* 1987;11(1):42-45.
119. Richard RE. Polymers in fracture immobilization. In Salamore JC (ed), *The Polymeric Materials Encyclopedia.* Boca Raton, FL: CRC Press, 1996.
120. Wytch R, Ashcroft GP, Ledingham WM, et al. Modern splinting bandages. *J Bone Joint Surg* 1991;73(1):88-91.
121. Lavalette RN, Pope M, Dickstein H. Setting temperatures of plaster casts. *J Bone Joint Surg* 1982;64(6):907-911.
122. Wytch R, Mitchell CB, Wardlaw D, et al. Mechanical assessment of polyurethane impregnated fiberglass bandage for splinting. *Prosthet Orthot Int* 1987;11(3):128-134.
123. Wytch R, Ross N, Wardlaw D. Glass fiber versus non-glass fiber splinting bandages. *Injury* 1992;23(2):101-106.
124. Pope M, Callahan G, Leveled R. Setting temperature of synthetic casts. *J Bone Joint Surg* 1985;67A(2):262-264.
125. Mooney V. Cast bracing. *Clin Orthop* July/Aug 1974;(102):159-166.
126. Brown PW. The early weight-bearing treatment of tibial shaft fractures. *Clin Orthop* Nov/Dec 1974;(105):167-178.
127. Russell TA, Taylor JC, LaVelle DG. Fractures of the tibia. In Rockwood CA, Green DP, Bucholz RW (eds), *Rockwood and Green's Fractures in Adults.* 3rd ed, vol 2. Philadelphia: Lippincott Williams & Wilkins, 1991. pp. 1915-1982.
128. Beatty JH. Congenital anomalies of the hip and pelvis. In Crenshaw AH (ed), *Campbell's Operative Orthopaedics.* St. Louis: Mosby, 1987. pp. 2721-2722.
129. Hilt NE, Cogburn SB. Cast and splint therapy. In Hilt NE, Cogburn SB (eds), *Manual of Orthopaedics.* St. Louis: Mosby, 1980. pp. 459-516.
130. Pellegrini VD, Evarts CM. Complications. In Rockwood CA, Green DP, Bucholz RW (eds), *Rockwood and Green's Fractures in Adults,* 3rd ed, vol 1. Philadelphia: Lippincott Williams & Wilkins, 1991. pp. 390-393.
131. Connolly JF, Dahne E, Lafollette B. Closed reduction and early cast-brace ambulation in the treatment of femoral fractures. Part 2. *J Bone Joint Surg* 1973;55A(8):1581-1599.
132. Moll JH. The cast brace walking treatment of open and closed femoral fractures. *South Med J* 1973;66(3):345-352.
133. Lenin BE, Mooney V, Ashy ME. Cast-bracing for fractures of the femur. *J Bone Joint Surg* 1977;59S(7):917-923.
134. Maggot B, Gad DA. Cast bracing for fractures of the femoral shaft. *J Bone Joint Surg* 1981;63B(1):12-23.
135. Stills M, Christiansen K, Bucholz RW, et al. Cast bracing bicondylar tibial plateau fractures after combined internal and external fixation. *J Prosthet Orthot* 1991;3(3):106-113.
136. DeCoster TA, Nepola JU, El-khoura GY. Cast brace treatment of proximal tibia fractures. *Clin Orthop* 1988;231:196-204.
137. Sutcliffe JR, Wilson-Storey D, Mackinlay GA. Children's femoral fractures: the Edinburgh experience. *J R Coll Surg Edinb* 1995;40(6):411-415.
138. Segal D, Mallik AR, Wetzler MJ, et al. Early weight bearing of lateral tibial plateau fractures. *Clin Orthop Relat Res* 1993;Sept(294):232-237.
139. Tang SF, Au TL, Wong AM, et al. Modified fracture brace for tibial fracture with varus angulation: a case report. *Prosthet Orthot Int* 1995;Aug(2):115-119.
140. Hardy AE. The treatment of femoral fractures by cast-brace application and early ambulation. *J Bone Joint Surg* 1983;65(1): 56-65.
141. Hohl M, Johnson EE, Wiss DA. Fractures of the knee. In Rockwood CA, Green DP, Bucholz RW (eds), *Rockwood and Green's Fractures in Adults,* vol 2. Philadelphia: Lippincott Williams & Wilkins, 1991. pp. 1725-1761.
142. Kapandji IA. The knee. The physiology of the joints, 25th ed. New York: Churchill Livingstone, 1991. pp. 64-147.
143. Snyder-Macker L, Lewek M. The knee. In Levangie PK, Norkin CC (eds). *Joint Structure and Function—A Comprehensive Analysis,* 4th ed. Philadelphia: F.A. Davis, 2005. pp. 393-436.
144. Moore TJ. Functional bracing of lower extremity fractures. In Goldberg B, Hsu JD (eds), *Atlas of Orthoses and Assistive Devices,* 3rd ed. St. Louis: Mosby; 1997. pp. 401-408.
145. Goss J. Developments in orthotic deweighting technology. *Phys Med Rehabil Clin North Am* 2000;11(3):497-508.
146. Pritham Beatty JH. Congenital anomalies of the hip and pelvis. In Crenshaw AH (ed), *Campbell's Operative Orthopaedics.* St. Louis: Mosby, 1987. pp. 2721-2722.
147. Stills ML. Vacuum-formed orthosis for fractures of the tibia. *Orthot Prosthet* 1976;30(2):43-55
148. Sarmiento A. On the behavior of closed tibial fractures. *J Orthop Trauma* 2000;14(3):199-205.
149. Chapman MW. Open fractures. In Rockwood CA, Green DP, Bucholz RW (eds), *Rockwood and Green's Fractures in Adults,* 3rd ed, vol 1. Philadelphia: Lippincott Williams & Wilkins, 1991. pp. 223-264.
150. Pacheo RJ, Saleh M. The role of external fixators in trauma. *Trauma* 2004;6:143-160.
151. Weigel DP, Marsh JL. High energy fractures of the tibial plateau: knee function after longer follow-up. *J Bone Joint Surg Am* 2002;84(9):1541-1551.
152. Babar IU. External fixation in close comminuted femoral shaft fractures in adults. *J Coll Physicians Surg Pak* 2004;14(9):553-555.
153. Haidukewych GJ. Temporary external fixation for the management of complex intra- and periarticular fractures of the lower extremity. *J Orthop Trauma* 2002;16(9): 678-685.
154. Chui FY, Chuang TY, Lo WH. Treatment of unstable pelvic fractures: use of a transiliac sacral rod for posterior lesions and anterior lesions. *J Trauma* 2004;57(1):141-145.
155. Ponsen KJ, van Dijke, GA, Joosse P, et al. External fixators for pelvic fractures. *Acta Orthopaedica Scandinavica* 2003;74(2):165-171.
156. Yang AP, Iannacone WM. External fixation for pelvic ring disruptions. *Orthop Clin North Am* 1997;28(3): 331-344.
157. Hayek TE. External fixators in the treatment of fractures in children. *J Ped Orthopaed B* 2004;13(2):103-109.
158. Garcia-Cimbrelo E. Circular external fixators in tibial nonunions. *Clin Orthopaed Relat Res* 2004;1(419):65-70.

159. Gordon JE. A comparison of monolateral and circular external fixation of diaphysial tibial fractures in children. *J Pediatr Orthopaed* 2003;12(5):338-345.
160. Krieg JC. Proximal tibial fractures: current treatment, results, and problems. *Injury* 2003;34(Suppl 1):A2-10.
161. Robberts CS, Dodds JC, Perry K, et al. Hybrid external fixation of the proximal tibia: strategies to improve frame stability. *J Orthop Trauma* 2003;17(6):415-420.
162. Stannard JP, Sheils TM, Lopez-Ben RR, et al. Vascular injuries in knee dislocations: the role of physical examination in determining the need for arteriography. *J Bone Joint Surg Am* 2004;86(5):910-915.
163. Rozycki GS, Tremblay LN, Feliciano DV, et al. Blunt vascular trauma in the extremity: diagnosis, management, and outcome. *J Trauma Inj Infect Crit Care* 2003;55(5): 814-824.
164. Lin C, Wei F, Levin LS, et al. The functional outcome of lower-extremity fractures with vascular injury. *J Trauma Inj Infec Crit Care* 1997;43(3):480-485.
165. Olson SA, Rhorer AS. Orthopaedic trauma for the general orthopaedist: avoiding problems and pitfalls in treatment. *Clin Orthop Relat Res* 2005;April (433):30-37.
166. Altizer L. Compartment syndrome. *Orthop Nurs* 2004;23(6):391-396.
167. Leyes M, Torres R, Guillén P. Complications of open reduction and internal fixation of ankle fractures. *Foot Ankle Clin* 2003;8(1):131-147
168. Im GI, Shin YW, Song YJ. Potentially unstable intertrochanteric fractures. *J Orthop Trauma* 2005;19(1):5-9.
169. Narayanan UG, Hyman JE, Wainwright AM, et al. Complications of elastic stable intramedullary nail fixation of pediatric femoral fractures, and how to avoid them. *J Pediatr Orthop* 2004;24(4):363-369.
170. Borg T, Melander T, Larsson S. Poor retention after closed reduction and cast immobilization of low-energy tibial shaft spiral fractures. *Scand J Surg* 2002;91(2):191-194.
171. Zalavras CG, Patzakis MJ. Open fractures: evaluation and management. *J Am Acad Orthop Surg* 2003;11(3):212-219.
172. Benirschke SK, Kramer KA. Wound healing complications in closed and open calcaneal fractures. *J Orthop Trauma* 2004;18(1):1-6.
172. Khatod M, Botte MJ, Hoyt DB, et al. Outcomes in open tibia fractures: relationship between delay in treatment and infection. *J Trauma Inj Infect Crit Care* 2003;55(5): 949-954.
173. Weitz-Marshall AD, Bosse MJ. Timing of closure of open fractures. *J Am Acad Orthop Surg* 2002;10(6):379-384.
174. Parameswaran AD, Roberts CS, Seligson D, et al. Pin tract infection with contemporary external fixation: how much of a problem? *J Orthop Trauma* 2003;17(7):503-509.
175. Temple J, Santy J. Pin site care for preventing infections associated with external bone fixators and pins. *Cochrane Database Syst Rev* 2004;CD004551.
176. Thordarson DB, Ahlmann E, Shepherd LE, et al. Sepsis and osteomyelitis about the ankle joint. *Foot Ankle Clin* 2000;5(4):913-928.
177. Holtom PD, Smith AM. Introduction to adult posttraumatic osteomyelitis of the tibia. *Clin Orthop Relat Res* 1999;Mar(360):6-13.
178. Bedi A, Toan Le T. Subtrochanteric femur fractures. *Orthop Clin North Am* 2004;35(4):473-483.
179. Bhandari M, Audige L, Ellis T, et al. Operative treatment of extra-articular proximal tibial fractures. *J Orthop Trauma* 2003;17(8):591-595.
180. Sadowski C, Lübbeke A, Saudan M, et al. Treatment of reverse oblique and transverse intertrochanteric fractures with use of an intramedullary nail or a 95 degrees screw-plate: a prospective, randomized study. *J Bone Joint Surg Am* 2002;84(3):372-381.
181. Weiss AP, Schenck RC, Sponseller PD, et al. Peroneal nerve palsy after early cast application for femoral fractures in children. *J Pediatr Orthop* 1992;12(1):25-28.
182. Morgan S, Upton J. Plaster casting: patient problems and nursing care. Boston: Butterworth-Heinemann, 1990.

15

Orthotics in the Management of Spinal Dysfunction and Instability

THOMAS M. GAVIN, AVINASH G. PATWARDHAN, ALEXANDER J. GHANAYEM, AND ANTHONY RINELLA

LEARNING OBJECTIVES

On completion of this chapter the reader will be able to do the following:

1. Identify the three primary the goals of orthotic intervention for patients with spinal dysfunction.
2. Use correct nomenclature to describe commonly prescribed spinal orthoses for the neck, thorax, and pelvis.
3. Compare and contrast the mechanisms of action (degree of support or immobilization), in each plane of motion, provided by the various spinal orthoses described in the chapter.
4. Describe the roles of, options for, and limitations of orthotic and surgical intervention in the management of traumatic compression fractures, burst fractures, chance/slice "seat belt" fractures, and fracture dislocations of the spinal column.
5. Describe the roles of, options for, and limitations of orthotic, rehabilitation, and surgical intervention in the management of acute and chronic mechanical-discogenic and neurocompressive low back pain.
6. Describe the roles of, options for, and limitations of orthotics and rehabilitative intervention in the management of pathological vertebral fractures resulting from osteoporosis.
7. Apply knowledge of the kinesiology and biomechanics of the cervical spine in determining the appropriate cervical or cervicothoracic orthosis to manage instability of the upper, middle, and lower cervical spine.
8. Appreciate the importance of an appropriate immobilization and orthotic control system in the postoperative period following spinal fusion or repair, as well as the impact this may have on early rehabilitation activities.

Management of spinal dysfunction with an external device is not new or unique to the twentieth-century medical profession. The use of mechanical devices to treat pathological conditions of the spine has a long and rich history. The evidence from prehistoric bone findings is that humans began to use splints for weak limbs and broken bones as early as 9000 BC in the Paleolithic age. Crude lumbar supports constructed from tree bark have been recovered from the cliff dwellings of the pre-Columbian Indians.[1] The terms *scoliosis*, *lordosis*, and *kyphosis* were first used by Galen (131-201 AD), who used dynamic bracing and an exercise program to treat spinal deformity.[1]

In 1743 Nicholas Andry, a professor of medicine in Paris, suggested in his book *Orthopaedia*[2] the following strategy to straighten the spine in children:

"If the spine be crooked in the shape of an S, the best method you can take to mend it is to have recourse to the whale bone bodice, stuffed parts shall exactly answer to those protuberances which ought to be repressed, and these bodices must be renewed every 3 months at least." The term *orthopaedic* was taken from the title of Andry's book.

THE FUNCTION OF ORTHOSES

Since the appearance of the Milwaukee brace in the late 1940s, many different types of spinal orthoses have been developed, each to manage a particular spinal pathology. Most were named for the orthotist or clinician who first designed the orthosis or the city where it was developed. Currently spinal orthoses are named after the initials of the regions of the spine that are encompassed by the orthosis (Table 15-1). Orthoses may be made from thermoplastic materials and various metals and strapping materials or can be fabricated as soft garments from canvas. For soft garments the nomenclature usually includes a descriptor of the garment.

Despite differences in design, all spinal orthoses provide some common mechanisms of action. First, all spinal

Table 15-1
Nomenclature for Spinal Orthoses

Acronym	Name
Rigid Thermoplastic or Metal Orthoses, or Both	
SIO	Sacroiliac orthosis
LSO	Lumbosacral orthosis
TLSO	Thoracolumbosacral orthosis
CTLSO	Cervico-thoracolumbosacral orthosis
CTO	Cervicothoracic orthosis
CO	Cervical orthosis
Soft Garments and Supports	
SI belt	Sacroiliac belt
LS corset	Lumbosacral corset
DL corset	Dorsolumbar corset
Soft collar	Nonreinforced cervical collars made from foam or any low modulus material

orthoses reduce gross spinal motion (limiting bending and twisting of the torso) to some degree. Second, they stabilize individual motion segments, reducing the planar range of motion of one vertebra relative to those above and below. Third, they all apply closed chain force systems specifically designed to correct or prevent progression of vertebral column deformities and to stabilize instabilities. In addition, spinal orthoses are used to protect surgical constructs (e.g., fusions, implanted implementation, grafts) by preventing bending and twisting, thus reducing stresses at the bone-implant interface and in adjacent segments.

To optimize orthotic management, an orthotist must specifically diagnose the mechanical deficit, vertebral level, and magnitude (or severity) of the deformity and instability. Although spinal orthoses have proven to be safe and cost-effective treatments for spinal disorders, they require careful attention to detail and frequent follow-up adjustment and may lead to poor results if not fitted and worn properly.

Although many orthoses designed for lower and upper limbs are considered to be assistive devices, the majority of spinal orthoses are used for treatment of an instability or deformity. Success of spinal orthotic treatment (intervention) depends on a person's ability to properly wear the orthosis enough hours daily to facilitate optimal outcome. The mechanical stiffness and applied force systems of the orthosis may be considered *magnitude* of treatment, while wearing time might be considered *dosage* of treatment.[3]

The efficacy of spinal orthoses in the management of spinal dysfunction has been the focus of many recent research efforts. Over time the treatment effectiveness of orthoses for the prevention, correction, and stabilization of deforming curves that are secondary to idiopathic, neuromuscular, and congenital scoliosis; traumatic and pathological fractures; and postinfectious instabilities and tumors has been demonstrated both clinically and in the literature. Although the effectiveness of orthotic intervention for spinal deformity or fracture has been well documented,[4-9] the evidence for the role of orthotic intervention in the management of low back pain or postoperative protection of spinal implants is less clear.[10,11]

Current Concepts

The development of surgical procedures and hardware has yielded techniques to better instrument the spine to obtain optimal deformity correction or yield early stable fusion of one or multiple vertebral motion segments or functional spinal units (FSUs). However, some recent surgical methods that were once considered of sufficient mechanical integrity to completely eliminate the use of postoperative orthoses have not succeeded in many cases. Some surgical constructs are vulnerable to failure, and iatrogenic deformity still remains a risk that may be minimized with a well-fitted postoperative orthosis. Proper orthotic management results in treatment that (1) has minimal complications, (2) is cost efficient, and (3) is highly effective.

New materials and manufacturing techniques guided by engineering, biomechanics, physics, and mathematical principles have led to scientifically improved orthotic treatment with lighter and more cosmetic orthoses and will eventually lead to greater precision in the prediction of outcomes of orthotic management and a better understanding of the associated psychological and social issues associated with this treatment modality.

Team Approach

The goal of working in the team setting as opposed to the individual setting is ideal clinical management. It enables individual treatment of the person, not the treatment of a pathosis or instability. Increasingly in our current health care model, however, the team model is diminishing. Lack of a cohesive team approach usually results in a major lack of communication and nonuniform goals and may cause confusion and anxiety for the person with spinal instability, as well as the family.

Orthotic management of the spine is an effective, safe, and low-cost method to treat many persons with musculoskeletal disorders. However, it will be most successful when implemented by a cohesive clinical team.

Making Treatment Decisions

It is important to understand that the natural histories of the various disorders of the spine are different and that each case is individual, although many persons may present with similar diagnoses. Orthotic management is at the center of a pendulum between invasive and conservative treatment.

Table 15-2
A Model for Clinical Decision Making for the Management of Spinal Problems

	Healthy Spine	*Unhealthy Spine*
Stable spine	No intervention	Medical intervention Physical therapy Prophylactic orthosis Surgical intervention
Unstable spine	Surgical intervention Orthotic intervention Physical therapy	Medical intervention Physical therapy Orthotic intervention Surgical intervention

Clinicians should strive to keep the enthusiasm of executing and maintaining the conservative treatment even when the most optimal result is not achieved.

New interventions or treatments should be based on an understanding of the difference between the "healthy spine" and the "stable spine." A healthy spine is a purely biological concept, meaning that all the individual structures are normal and free of disease, but the spine still may present itself with deformity or instability such as idiopathic scoliosis. Therefore a biologically healthy spine may still have deformity, either stable or unstable. A stable spine refers to physics and biomechanical concepts. An unhealthy spine can be stable or unstable, in the presence or absence of deformity.

A healthy and stable spine that is deformed yet stable is preferable to an unhealthy spine that is stable, even with no deformity. When making treatment decisions, these two concepts should always be considered in a unified manner to arrive at an adequate diagnosis and subsequently plan an ideal treatment (Table 15-2). Frequently, many unsatisfactory treatments are chosen because clinicians concern themselves with one specific concern such as stability or deformity while overlooking pathology, or vice versa.

For instance, traumatic compression fractures may be present in a spine that is both healthy and stable whereas a burst fracture may cause instability in a spine that is still healthy. In contrast, a person with pathological fractures from osteoporosis or spinal neoplasms has an unhealthy spine that may or may not be stable.

THORACOLUMBOSACRAL ORTHOSES

Orthoses designed to control or support the lower spine and pelvis can be grouped into three categories: corsets, traditional metal and leather orthoses, or custom-fit or custom-molded thermoplastic orthoses.

Corsets and Supports

Fabric lumbosacral (LS) corsets, sacroiliac corsets, and thoracolumbar (dorsolumbar) corsets primarily function to reduce overall gross trunk motion. A snugly fit nonelastic LS or thoracolumbar corset compresses fluid and tissues of the abdomen and abdominal cavity, theoretically reducing axial loading of vertebral bodies. Pain that results from muscle strain is effectively managed with a corset, because the activity of spinal and abdominal muscles is reduced while the corset is being worn. However, long-term corset use can lead to muscle atrophy, ultimately increasing the chance of reinjury. For this reason, corsets are best used only during the acute phase of back pain.

Sacroiliac Corsets

Sacroiliac corsets are meant to support only the sacroiliac joint (Figure 15-1). With end points inferior to the waist and superior to the pubis, these garments encompass the pelvis but not the lower trunk. Sacroiliac corsets increase in abdominal circumferential pressure only slightly and are best used for persons with mild sacroiliac dysfunction.

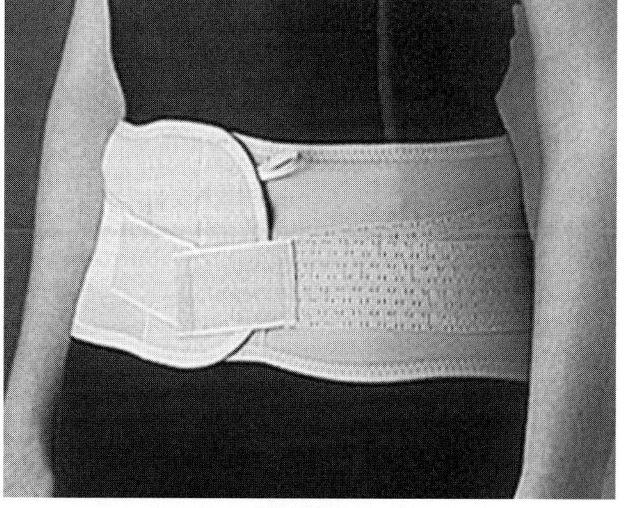

Figure 15-1
Because the sacroiliac belt is narrow, encompassing only the pelvis, it provides some support to the sacroiliac joint but not to the rest of the spine.

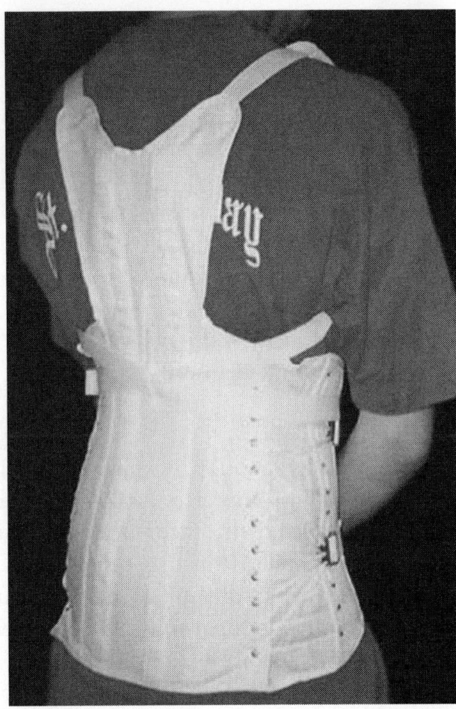

Figure 15-2
The dorsolumbar corset provides some control of gross trunk motion but does not prevent intervertebral motion of the thoracic or lumbar spine.

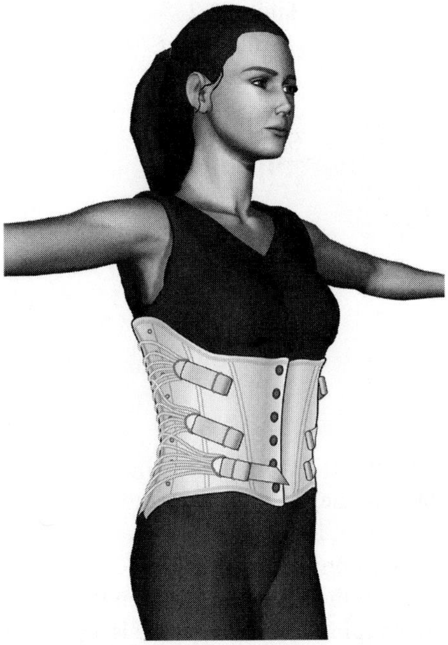

Figure 15-3
The lumbosacral corset is the most widely prescribed spinal orthosis, typically used in the management of acute low back pain. Stays are sewn into the corset to support the trunk. When adjusted appropriately to fit snugly, the lumbosacral corset limits motion of the lumbar spine and supports the abdomen. (Courtesy BioConcepts Orthotic Prosthetic Center, Burr Ridge, Ill.)

Because they are so narrow, sacroiliac corsets do not provide significant support to the spine.

Thoracolumbar Corsets

Because the thoracolumbar (dorsolumbar) corset encompasses much of the thoracic spine, leverage of the corset system is increased to control gross motion and to provide some resistance to flexion (Figure 15-2). The inferior borders of a thoracolumbar corset are the same as those of an LS corset. The superior posterior border terminates just inferior to the scapular spine. Shoulder straps create a posteriorly directed force aimed at resisting thoracic spine flexion. Although the thoracolumbar corset encloses much of the thoracic spine, its leverage is insufficient to prevent intervertebral thoracic or lumbar spinal motion. The corset serves primarily as a kinesthetic reminder to control such motion.

Lumbosacral Corsets

The LS corset is the most frequently prescribed supporting orthosis for patients with low back pain (Figure 15-3). Corsets are made from soft canvas or Dacron materials, fortified with rigid and flexible stays. These stays can be contoured to accommodate a deformity or can be straight to encourage postural correction. When donned properly, the LS corset can effectively limit much, but not all, motion of the lumbar spine; it cannot, however, achieve the same degree of gross and segmental immobilization of the spine as a rigid thoracolumbosacral orthosis (TLSO).[12]

LS corsets encompass the abdomen and the pelvis. In exerting circumferential pressure, they increase intracavitary pressure in the abdomen and transmit a three-point pressure system to the lumbar spine. Typically, the anterior borders of the LS corset are superior to the symphysis pubis and inferior to the xiphoid process. The posterior borders extend between the sacrococcygeal junction of the pelvis and the inferior angle of the scapulae.

LS corsets are most often used to manage acute low back pain; their efficacy in chronic low back pain is questionable. Corsets are designed to support the trunk in a neutral sagittal alignment, providing some gross motion reduction, bending prevention, and a minimal amount of midlumbar segmental immobilization. For disk-related pain at the level of L5-S1, other interventions are more effective. An orthosis with a thigh extension was shown to provide nearly complete symptomatic relief of discogenic pain at the L5-S1 junction (Figure 15-4) whereas patients with low back or leg pain secondary to spondylolysis or spondylolisthesis often have better pain relief with a TLSO fitted in lumbar flexion (Figure 15-5).[13]

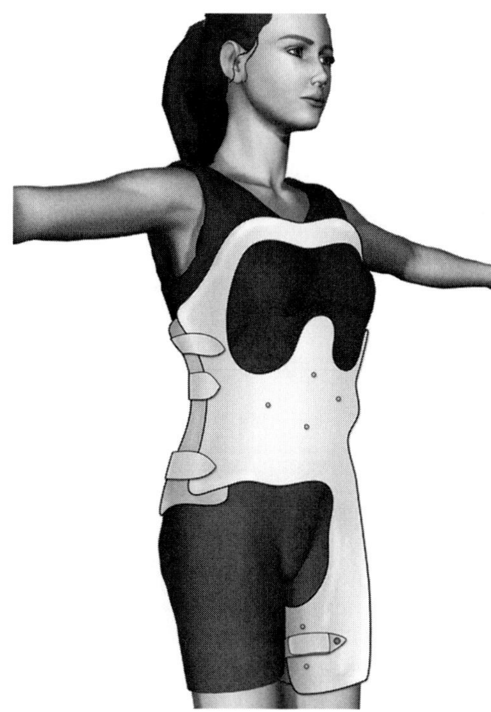

Figure 15-4

The thoracolumbosacral orthosis with a thigh spica may relieve pain caused by herniation at L5-S1 levels more effectively than a lumbosacral corset or orthosis. (Courtesy BioConcepts Orthotic Prosthetic Center, Burr Ridge, Ill.)

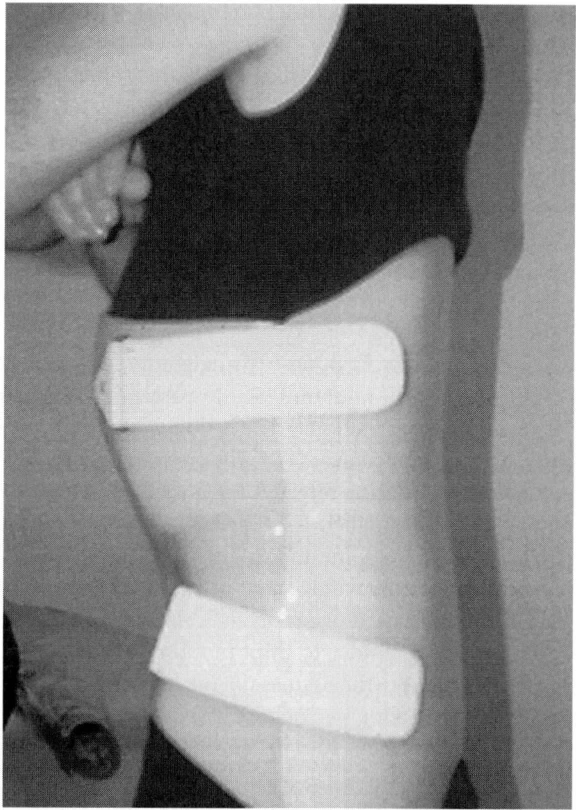

Figure 15-5

Individuals with back pain related to spondylolysis or spondylolisthesis may benefit from an LSO such as the Raney Flexion Lumbosacral Orthosis, because it can maintain the lumbar spine in flexion (posterior tilt).

Traditional Metal and Leather Spinal Orthoses

Traditional metal and leather spinal orthoses are designed to provide motion control and trunk support. They are custom fabricated to fit specific anatomical landmarks so that the orthoses have the best possible leverage against the trunk. Most designs for traditional spinal orthoses have a pelvic band; a thoracic band; and a set of lateral or paraspinal bars, or both.[14] These bands and bars are made from radiolucent aluminum alloys that are malleable yet stiff enough to hold their shape.

The *pelvic band* is fit closely at the posterior midline, with its inferior edge against the sacrococcygeal junction. The band is contoured or curved downward to contain the gluteal muscles on either side of the midline and to create the maximum possible leverage for control of the pelvis. The pelvic band wraps around the pelvis laterally, terminating just anterior to the midaxillary trochanteric line (MATL). A design variation proposed by Norton and Brown[15] has inferior projections from the lateral bars, terminating in disks over the trochanters, in an effort to improve motion control at the LS junction. A strap that fastens in the front connects to these disks to achieve additional leverage in the sagittal plane. The position of the disks also improves leverage for control of motion in the coronal plane.

The upper edge of the *thoracic band* is usually placed 24 mm below the inferior angle of the scapulae. The thoracic band is high and horizontal at the posterior midline and curves inferolaterally to provide relief for the scapulae. The thoracic band also wraps around the trunk laterally, ending just in front of the MATL at the lateral midline of the body.

When an orthotic design includes *paraspinal bars,* they are placed on either side of the posterior midline over the paraspinal muscle mass. Paraspinal bars on LS orthoses (LSOs) are vertical, spanning from the pelvic band to the thoracic band. For traditional TLSOs, the paraspinal bars end just inferior to the spine of the scapulae. If the orthosis has *lateral bars,* they are placed at the lateral midline of the trunk, following the MATL from the inferior edge of the pelvic band to the superior edge of the thoracic band. If the orthosis has an *interscapular band,* it is positioned within the lateral borders of the scapulae, with a bottom edge placed just above the inferior border of the scapulae.[16]

Most traditional metal and leather spinal orthoses have a corset front or anterior panel that is closed by laces, buckles, or Velcro straps. The anterior panel, if fastened correctly, increases abdominal intracavitary pressure similarly to how LS corsets do.

Sagittal Control Lumbosacral Orthoses: The Chairback Orthosis

The chairback lumbosacral orthosis (LSO), a spinal orthosis designed to control motion in the sagittal plane, has a thoracic and pelvic band connected by two paraspinal bars. A full-trunk corset is attached to the paraspinal bars. This orthosis is prescribed when the patient's condition requires reduction of gross and intersegmental flexion and extension motion of the trunk. Motion into forward trunk flexion is limited by a pair of posteriorly directed forces applied by the anterior corset, one at the xyphoid level and the other at the pubis. These forces oppose a single anteriorly directed force applied at the midpoint of the paraspinal bars. The force system for restriction of extension has two anterior-directed forces applied across the thoracic and pelvic bands that oppose a posterior-directed force applied at the midpoint of the corset panel. Increased intracavitary pressure can act to unload the spine and its disks by transmitting load onto soft tissue of the trunk.

This orthosis is used primarily for pain management and as a kinesthetic reminder to limit motion for persons with low back pain. The orthosis does not limit motion enough to stabilize the trunk for persons with spinal fractures.[17] The chairback LSO design can be converted to a TLSO by increasing the proximal length of the paraspinal bars and adding shoulder straps.

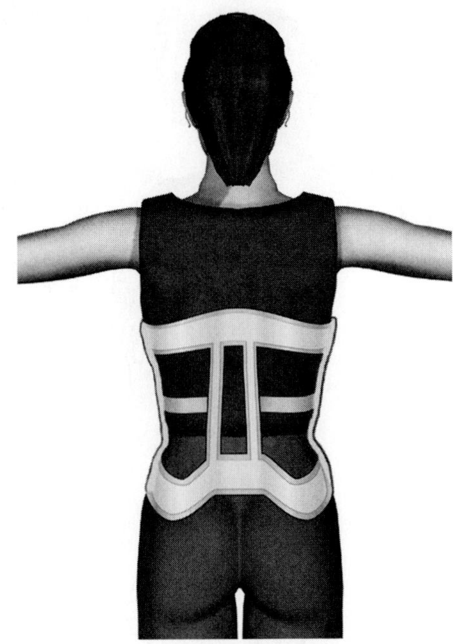

Figure 15-6
The traditional Knight lumbosacral orthosis (LSO) has both paraspinal and lateral bars to limit extension lateral flexion motion. Because a chairback LSO omits the lateral bars, it can control only sagittal plane extension. (Courtesy BioConcepts Orthotic Prosthetic Center, Burr Ridge, Ill.)

Sagittal-Coronal Control Lumbosacral Orthoses: The Knight Orthosis

When a pair of lateral bars is added to the orthosis, control of spinal motion is possible in the coronal (frontal), as well as the sagittal, planes (Figure 15-6).[14] This orthosis, also known as a Knight spinal orthosis, has thoracic and pelvic bands connected by a set of paraspinal bars and a set of lateral bars, with an anterior half-corset closure. Control of spinal flexion and extension is achieved by the same three-point force systems described for the chairback LSO. Lateral flexion of the trunk is controlled by medially directed forces at the edges of thoracic and pelvic bands, opposing a force at the midpoint of the opposite lateral bar.

This orthosis was originally designed for patients with tuberculosis of the spine but is now used primarily in the management of low back pain. It is sometimes prescribed for persons with stable noncompression fractures of the lumbar spine; however, this orthosis does not sufficiently control the pelvis or thorax when compression fractures or complex spinal injuries require more complete limitation of motion or total immobilization. The Knight LSO orthosis can also be fabricated as a TLSO Taylor orthosis if more support of the thoracic spine is necessary.

Extension Resist Orthoses: The Williams Orthosis

The Williams LSO is a dynamic orthosis that has a thoracic and a pelvic band, a pair of lateral bars, and a set of oblique bars positioned between the lateral bars and pelvic band (Figure 15-7). The attachments between the thoracic band and lateral bars are mobile; structural integrity is achieved by the firmly attached oblique bars. The articulation between the thoracic band and lateral bars allows the person to move into some trunk flexion in the sagittal plane. The nonarticulating connections between lateral bars and the pelvic band, reinforced by oblique bars and a snugly fit, inelastic pelvic strap, limits trunk extension.

The Williams LSO was originally designed as a treatment for spondylolisthesis and continues to be used in its management today.[18] Although flexion orthoses were once used for patients with lumbar disk herniation, recent work suggests that lordosis (lumbar extension) is more comfortable for patients and physiologically appropriate for reduction of herniation, so flexion orthoses are not suitable for this population.

Hyperextension Orthoses: The Jewett and CASH Orthoses

When compression fracture of the lumbar or low thoracic spine has occurred, it is important to limit trunk flexion during the healing process. Two orthoses that are designed specifically to limit flexion while encouraging trunk hyperextension are the Jewett TLSO flexion control orthosis and the CASH hyperextension orthosis (Figure 15-8).[19] Both orthoses are available in various styles and sizes from numerous manufacturers. The Jewett orthosis has an antero-

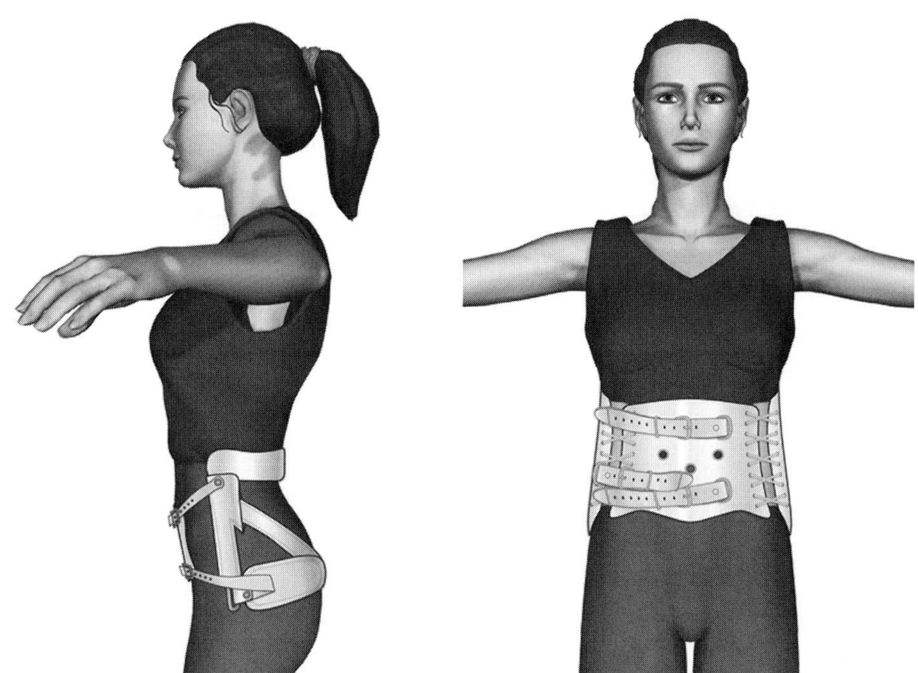

Figure 15-7

The dynamic Williams lumbosacral orthosis is designed to limit trunk extension while permitting some trunk flexion. It is most often used for individuals with spondylolisthesis.

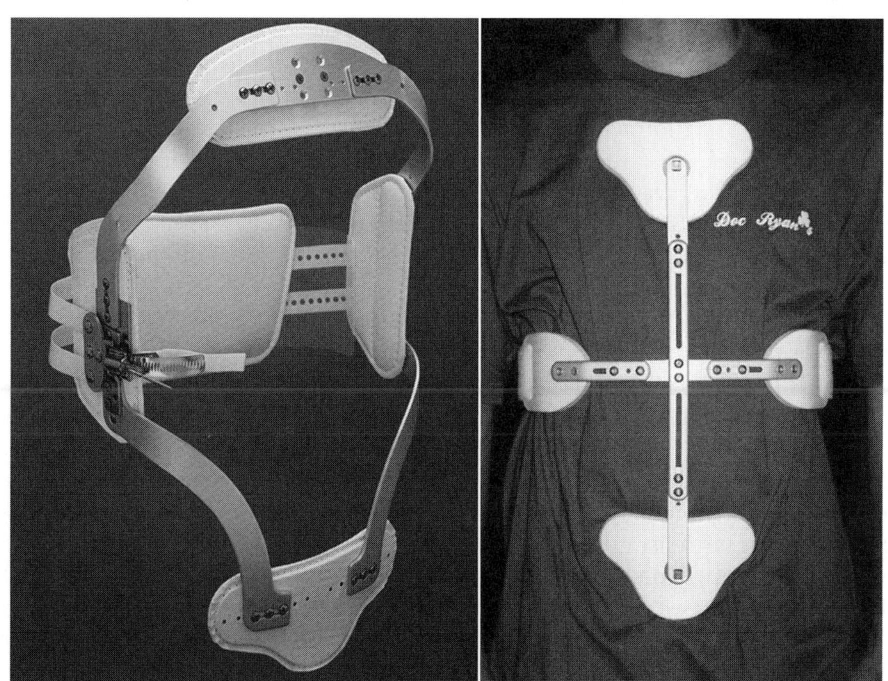

Figure 15-8

*The Jewett (**A**) and CASH (**B**) hyperextension orthoses are designed to limit trunk flexion but encourage hyperextension of low thoracic and upper lumbar vertebrae. Both are used for individuals with compression fractures of the low thoracic and lumbar spine.*

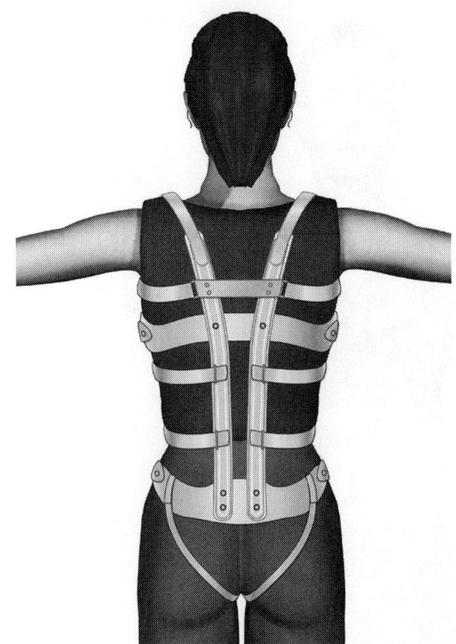

Figure 15-9
The Knight-Taylor thoracolumbosacral orthosis is designed to limit flexion, extension, and lateral flexion of the thoracis and lumbar spine. (Courtesy BioConcepts Orthotic Prosthetic Center, Burr Ridge, Ill.)

lateral aluminum frame with pads at the pubis, sternum, and lateral midline of the trunk and a posterior lumbar pad. Trunk flexion is limited by a single three-point pressure system, with posteriorly directed forces applied at the sternum and the pubis, which oppose an anteriorly directed force applied by the posterior lumbar pad. When the orthosis is well fitting, this force system prevents flexion of the spine but allows active hyperextension.

The CASH orthosis (cruciform anterior hyperextension orthosis) has an adjustable-length anterior cross with sternal and pelvic pads at the ends of the vertical bar as well as lateral pads and a posterior belt. The CASH orthosis uses the same three-point pressure system to control trunk flexion as the Jewett design.

Sagittal Control Thoracolumbosacral Orthoses: The Taylor Orthosis

The Taylor orthosis has a pelvic band, two paraspinal bars, an interscapular band, and a pair of axillary straps. The orthosis is designed to limit flexion and extension of the thoracic and lumbar spine. An anteriorly directed force is applied at the interscapular band to resist extension. The axillary straps apply posteriorly directed forces, which function to limit trunk flexion.[16]

Sagittal-Coronal Control Thoracolumbosacral Orthoses: The Knight-Taylor Orthosis

The sagittal-coronal control TLSO, a hybrid of the Knight LSO and the Taylor TLSO, has pelvic and thoracic bands, lateral bars, paraspinal bars that reach the spine of the scapula, an interscapular band, and a pair of axillary straps. With this combination of components, the orthosis resists extension, flexion, and lateral flexion of the thoracic and lumbar spines (Figure 15-9).[14]

Thermoplastic Spinal Orthoses

Molded thermoplastic orthoses that encase the trunk are prescribed when the therapeutical goal is immobilization of the spine in all three planes of motion. These orthoses are indicated when instability or dysfunction is present at several vertebral levels or for patients with significant instability after a burst vertebral fracture. They are often used in the postoperative care of patients with traumatic thoracic or lumbar vertebral fracture or spinal cord injuries and patients with spinal deformity who have had fusion or instrumented surgeries at the thoracolumbar level. They may be custom fabricated, made to measure from a computer-aided design system, or prefabricated. There is some controversy as to whether the made-to-measure or prefabricated orthoses fit and function as well as the custom fabricated ones.

Rigid thermoplastic spinal orthoses may be necessary for persons whose size, shape, or condition precludes the use of a traditional LSO or TLSO. Some rigid thermoplastic spinal orthoses are custom fit from prefabricated blanks; others are custom molded over a positive model of the person's trunk. Many are made from perforated materials to release body heat that is generated during activity. Some are lined with closed cell foam to increase comfort and to minimize the risk of pressure-related skin problems.

Most patients wear a lightweight T-shirt under the orthosis to wick perspiration away from the skin and minimize friction and the potential for skin irritation. Typically, the superior trimlines of LSO are at the level of the xiphoid process; the superior trimline of a TLSO extends upward to the notch of the sternum.[20] Thermoplastic LSOs and TLSOs are carefully shaped to envelop the pelvis; most have an anterior-inferior trimline at the groin.

Raney Flexion Lumbosacral Orthoses

The custom-fit or molded Raney flexion LSO is the thermoplastic version of the traditional Williams flexion orthosis (see Figure 15-5). Because it encases the pelvis entirely, the Raney is better able to hold the LS spine in a flexed position (posterior tilt) during activity than is its traditional counterpart. The major difference between these two devices is that, although the dynamic design of the Williams LSO allows flexion while preventing extension, the Raney jacket is rigid, holding the pelvis in a static position. More abdominal compression occurs with the semirigid plastic anterior shell of the Raney jacket than is possible with the flexible anterior corset of the Williams LSO. The Raney flexion jacket is often used in the management of spinal instability and pain in patients with spondylosis and spondylolisthesis.[21]

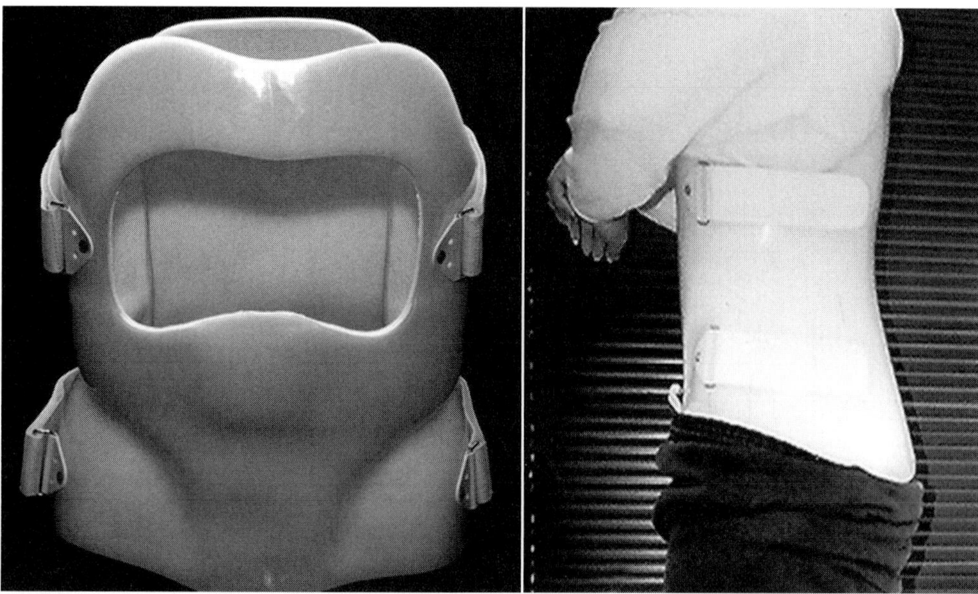

Figure 15-10
The Boston Overlap lumbosacral orthosis brace is used when there is a need to hold the pelvis and low back in a neutral or slight extension (anterior tilt).

Boston Overlap Braces

For patients who require immobilization in a neutral pelvic position or minimal lordosis (lumbar extension), the Boston overlap brace (BOB) is often prescribed (Figure 15-10). Prefabricated shells are custom fit to meet the patient's individual positioning needs. The posterior shell encloses the trunk from the inferior angle of the scapula to the sacrococcygeal level and the anterior shell from the xiphoid process of the sternum to the pubis. These trimlines ensure that the BOB effectively controls motion in the sagittal and coronal planes. The BOB is often used for patients with stable, nondisplaced fractures of the mid and lower lumbar spine, spondylolysis, or spondylolisthesis. Persons with fractures of L1 and L2 are better managed with a molded TLSO.

Custom-Molded Thoracolumbosacral Orthoses

Molded TLSOs are most commonly used in the postsurgical management of patients with fracture or spinal deformity of the thoracic and upper lumbar spine. The total contact design maintains spinal alignment and limits movement of the trunk in all three planes of motion (Figure 15-11).[22] The orthosis can be fabricated as a single piece with an anterior opening or in a bivalve design with anterior and posterior shells. In both versions the superior anterior trimline of the orthosis is just below the clavicle. Shoulder flanges or extensions can be added to enhance motion control of the spine as persons use the upper extremities during daily activities. The superior posterior trimline falls just below the spine of the scapula. The anterior-inferior edge of the orthosis is trimmed at the distal pubis and arches slightly upward laterally to accommodate the thigh in sitting. The inferior edge of the posterior shell is trimmed low at the sacrococcygeal junction.

If a person has upper thoracic instability or significant thoracic kyphosis, it is often necessary to add a cervical component, such as a sternooccipitomandibular immobilizer (SOMI), four-poster, or CD Denison cervical orthosis (CD Denison Orthopaedic Appliance Corp., Baltimore), to the TLSO to achieve the desired control of motion. Similarly, if the goal of orthotic intervention is immobilization at the LS junction, the body jacket LSO or TLSO must be extended, via an orthotic hip joint and thigh cuff, to limit the pelvic motion that normally accompanies extension of the hip.

Thoracolumbarsacral Mechanisms of Action

TLSOs are prescribed when the goal of intervention includes restriction of gross motion of the spine, immobilization of spinal segments, or to hold the spine in hyperextension.

Restriction of Gross Motion

Various orthotic designs are available when limitation of gross trunk motion (flexion/extension, lateral flexion/side bending, and axial rotation) is the primary goal. In a study comparing the effectiveness of four spinal orthoses (the Raney jacket, a custom-molded polypropylene TLSO, a Camp canvas LS corset [Camp International, Inc., Jackson, Mich.], and an elastic corset) in restricting gross motion of the lumbar spine, motion was most effectively limited by the Raney jacket and molded TLSO. The Camp canvas corset was moderately restrictive, and the elastic corset was minimally restrictive. All orthoses restricted lateral flexion/side

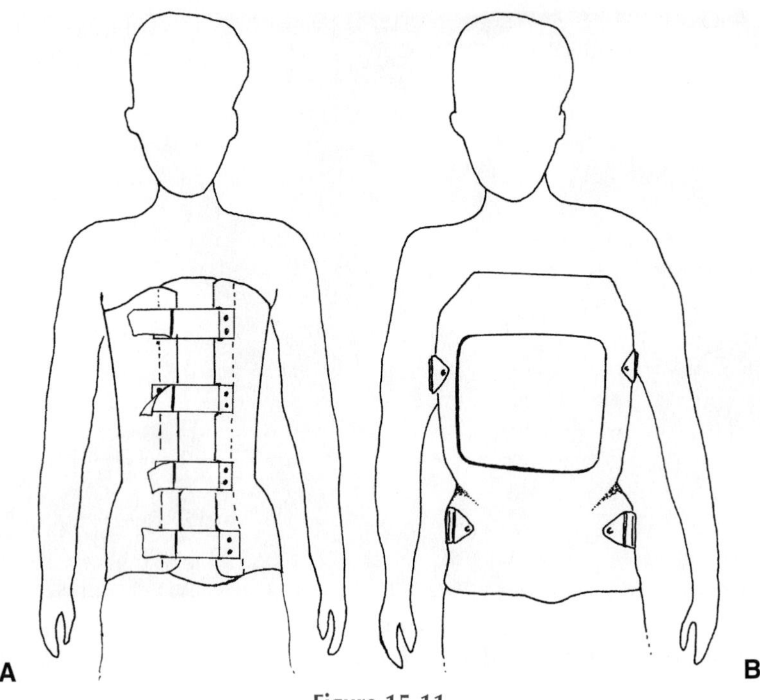

Figure 15-11
*Molded thermoplastic thoracolumbosacral orthoses (body jackets) use a total contact design to control flexion/extension in the sagittal plane, lateral flexion/side bending in the frontal plane, and trunk rotation in the transverse plane. They can be fabricated as a single unit **(A)** with an anterior opening, or in a bivalve design similar to the Boston Overlap Brace **(B)** with an anterior and posterior shell and lateral Velcro closures.*

bending more effectively than lumbar flexion/extension.[23]

Lantz and Schultz[24] compared restriction of gross body motion (flexion and extension, lateral bending, and torsion and rotation) during sitting and standing in patients using an LS corset, a chairback orthosis, and a custom-molded TLSO. As might be anticipated, the custom-molded TLSO restricted motion most effectively, and the LS corset was least effective, especially for upper trunk and body motion.

Segmental Immobilization

Nagel and coworkers[25] investigated the ability of three orthoses (a three-point hyperextension orthosis, a Taylor-Knight TLSO, and a body cast) to provide segmental immobilization by evaluating the effect of a seat belt–type injury at L1-2 of the spines of human cadavers. Joint space range of motion was measured in flexion and extension, lateral bending, and axial rotation before and after orthotic intervention. The three-point hypertension orthosis was able to limit flexion and extension motion but did not prevent vertebral motion in lateral bending or axial rotation. The Taylor-Knight orthosis was effective in limiting vertebral motion in lateral bending and, to a lesser extent, in flexion and extension but had little effect on limiting axial rotation. The body cast was able to limit segmental motion in all three motions.

Norton and Brown[26] evaluated the ability of an orthosis to limit motion at different vertebral levels. None of the orthoses they evaluated was particularly effective in limiting segmental motion; most were better able to reduce motion at upper rather than lower levels. At times increased motion was observed at the LS joint. Lumsden and Morris[27] confirmed this observation for axial rotation at the LS joint, noting that a chairback orthosis was more effective than a corset and that the orthoses in general were most effective at immobilizing upper levels and least effective at the LS joint.

Fidler and Plasmans[23] compared the effectiveness of the canvas corset, Raney jacket, baycast, and baycast spica on limiting segmental motion in flexion in normal adults. In their study, segmental motion at midlumbar levels was reduced by one third when subjects wore a canvas corset and by two thirds when subjects wore a Raney jacket or baycast. Only the baycast with spica limited motion at the lower lumbar levels.

Hyperextension of the Spine

Patwardhan and coworkers[28] studied the effectiveness of the Jewett hyperextension orthosis for patients with single- and two-level injuries of the spine. For single-level injuries with a 50% loss of segmental stiffness, the Jewett orthosis effectively restored stability under normal gravitational load and when large flexion loads were imposed. For persons with severe two-level injuries with loss of stiffness between 50% and 85% of normal, the Jewett orthosis restored stability as long as the person's activity level was restricted. For patients with more than 85% loss in segmental stiffness, the orthosis alone was not effective in preventing progression of deformity.

ORTHOTICS FOR TREATMENT OF TRAUMATIC SPINAL FRACTURES

When using an orthosis for spinal injury, it is best to thoroughly understand the pattern of instability. This leads to better understanding the mechanisms of action of an orthosis for the inoperative or postoperative orthosis. Denis[29] categorized the different types of traumatic fractures of the thoracolumbar spine as to how many columns (anterior, middle, posterior) of the spine are disrupted and to the mechanisms of each specific injury (Box 15-1 and Figure 15-12).

The primary function of orthoses in the management of persons with spinal fracture is to provide biomechanical stability. The orthoses is used to increase the magnitude of axial load the spine can withstand without increasing the deformity associated with the instability.[30]

Compression Fractures

When there is a compression fracture involving the anterior column of the spine, the middle column must provide enough structural integrity to ensure stability (Figure 15-13, *A*).[29] Some severe compression fractures may progress post-traumatically toward increasing kyphosis. Ferguson and Allen[31] found that anterior compression fractures of more than 50% of original vertebral body height are more likely to result in progressive lesions despite an intact middle

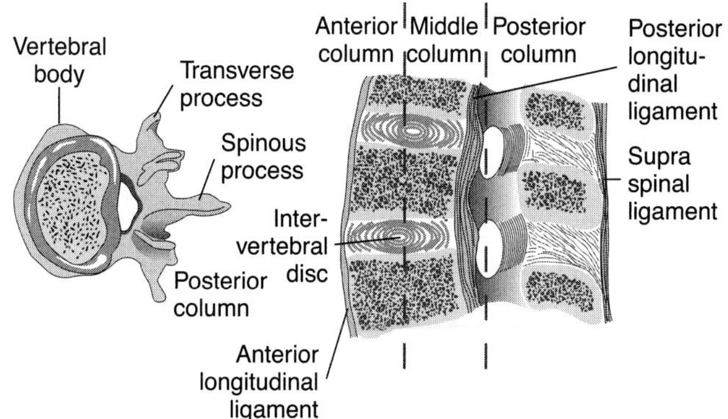

Figure 15-12
*Horizontal (**A**) and lateral (**B**) views of the functional columns of the spine, the basis for Denis classifications of vertebral fractures. When only the anterior column is fractured, and the middle and posterior columns are intact, the spine is "stable" and can be managed with nonoperative orthotic intervention until bony healing occurs. Fractures of the middle and posterior columns result in an unstable spine and often require surgical repair, followed by orthotic intervention to protect the surgical construct.*

Box 15-1 *Classification System for Traumatic Fractures of the Thoracolumbar Spine*

COMPRESSION FRACTURES (DENIS TYPE 1)

Mechanism of injury: spinal flexion with compression

Subtype	I-A	Anterior fracture only
	I-B	Anterior fracture with lateral components

BURST FRACTURES (DENIS TYPE II)

Mechanism of injury: spinal compression with flexion

Subtype	II-A	Fracture of both end plates or retropulsion, or both, of the posterior wall as a free fragment
	II-B	Fracture of the superior end plate, occasional retropulsion of inferior wall as a free fragment
	II-C	Fracture of the inferior end plate
	II-D	Burst fracture with rotational injury
	II-E	Burst fracture with lateral flexion injury

SEAT BELT INJURIES (DENIS TYPE III)

Mechanism of injury: spinal flexion with distraction

Subtype	III-A	(Chance fracture) single segment, posterior or middle column opening
	III-B	(Slice fracture) single segment, posterior and middle column opening through soft and bony tissue
	III-C	Two segments, posterior and middle column opening through soft and bony tissue
	III-D	Two segments, posterior and middle column opening through soft tissue only

FRACTURE DISLOCATIONS (DENIS TYPE IV)

Mechanism of injury: translation, flexion, rotation, with shear

Subtype	IV-A	Flexion and rotation injury with disruption through bone or intervertebral disk, or both
	IV-B	Due to shear (anterior-posterior or posterior-anterior) with fracture and dislocation of facet joints
	IV-C	Ligamentous injury to posterior and middle column, with failure (marked instability) of the anterior column
	IV-D	Oblique shear forces resulting in significant instability of involved segment (bone or disk)

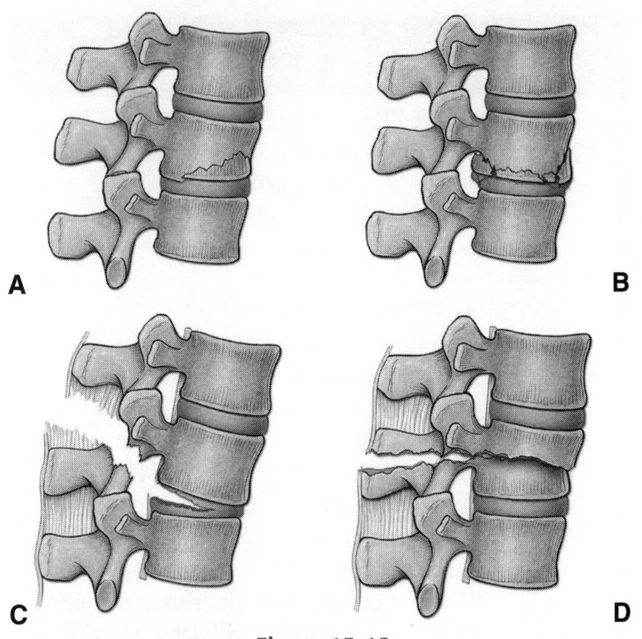

Figure 15-13

Traumatic spinal fractures. ***A,*** *Compression fractures may result in a wedge-shaped vertebral body in the anterior column of the spine.* ***B,*** *In burst vertebral fractures there is damage to both anterior and middle columns of the spine, with or without displacement of fragments.* ***C,*** *In a chance or lap belt fracture, the posterior column (pedicles and posterior soft tissue structures) are damaged.* ***D,*** *Fracture dislocations are often horizontal, damaging all three columns of the involved vertebra.*

column, because of compressive forces on the segment in upright posture. They describe this type of compression fracture as a *compressive flexion fracture.* Ferguson and Allen[31] also stress the importance of the flexion mechanism that Daffner and coworkers[32] have found to be the cause of 85% of thoracolumbar fractures. This flexion occurs on an axis at the level of the middle column that has been left intact and may cause posterior ligamentous damage. The posterior ligamentous injury is the main factor that destabilizes compression fractures (mainly at the thoracic level). This concept has been liberally reported in the literature.[33-35] An isolated body fracture carries few hazards for worsening and can resist to loads similar to those of an intact vertebral body. When increased sagittal deformity develops, it will occur at the level of the disks adjacent to the injured vertebra. Displacement within the disks is usually due to a major disruption of the posterior ligamentous structures.

When type I fractures are treated, both the anterior compression and the posterior ligamentous injury must be evaluated by assessing the interspinous process space on the lateral radiograph or the magnetic resonance imaging (MRI) scan.[36] In subtype I-A, there is an anterior fracture of the vertebral body. In subtype I-B, there is an anterior fracture with a lateral component. I-B fractures are more likely to develop into a progressive disruption because of injury to intervertebral disks both above and below the fractured vertebra. The fracture line for this injury is in the posterior of the midportion of the vertebral body; at times (rarely) it can lead to vertebral body pseudoarthrosis.[37]

The flexion axis for spines with compression fractures is the middle column, and there is a direct relationship between the amount of anterior column compression and severity of posterior ligamentous damage. If the anterior wall compression is equal to or greater than 50% of vertebral body height, there are usually associated ligamentous injuries in the posterior column. Most compression fractures can be managed conservatively (nonoperatively). Conservative management of a Denis type I compression fracture positions the spine in hyperextension (as tolerated by the wearer) while limiting or preventing spinal flexion (movement toward kyphosis). The orthoses that can be used to accomplish this include the CASH orthosis, the Jewett orthosis, a molded or prefabricated hyperextension TLSO, or a Knight-Taylor TLSO in hyperextension. A lumbosacral corset is sometimes used for minor or mild compression fractures.

Burst Fractures

Denis type II burst fractures typically result from excessive spinal compression coupled with spinal flexion, resulting in injury of both anterior and middle columns of the spine (see Box 15-1 and Figure 15-13, *B*). According to Holdsworth,[38] the posterior column typically remains intact, although a green stick-type fracture of the lamina may be evident on a radiograph.

The compression component of the injury results from a large perpendicular load applied axially to the end plate. Because of the thoracolumbar spine's contour, compression forces are associated with a flexion moment, and at the lumbar level, the force is usually more posterior, causing bony injury at the level of the posterior elements with a vertical fracture line.[39]

Middle-column injuries are typical for these fractures. Decreased height of the posterior body wall and adjacent disks is apparent on the radiograph and MRI. There may also be retropulsion of bone fragments from the posterior or inferior walls, resulting in bone fragments. The most severe burst fractures (subtypes II-D and II-E) often behave more like fracture/dislocations (Denis type IV) than like burst fractures because they include posterior articular injuries and some degree of dislocation. In types II, III, and IV, there may be comminution of the vertebral body.[40]

The inability to categorize instability in terms of "burst" is controversial.[41] Although Denis evaluates instability as it relates to the integrity of the medial column, others base their evaluation of instability on the presence of injury to the posterior elements.[38,42,43] Kilcoyne and coworkers,[44] however, report unstable fractures with intact posterior elements. The criterion for instability at the level of the middle column depends on the structural integrity of both the bony and ligamentous structures.[36,45,46]

There is some disagreement in the orthopedic surgery literature about the most appropriate approach to management of burst fractures. Two-column instabilities are most often managed conservatively with an orthosis. More severe burst fractures with posterior element instability most often require surgical stabilization or fusion, although Knight reported successful management with conservative treatment.[56]

The most frequent conservative strategies to manage burst fractures include a body cast, a custom-molded TLSO, or a custom-fit prefabricated TLSO. Each of these are designed to stabilize the spine in hyperextension so that appropriate bony remodeling can occur. A Jewett orthosis is sometime used for less severe injuries. Currently, the efficacy of custom-molded hyperextension TLSO is comparable to surgical intervention.[4-6,48,49]

Seat Belt Injuries

Although Denis type III fractures are often caused by seat belt restraint in high velocity, sudden impact motor vehicle accidents, they also occur in other situations that involve excessive spinal flexion with distraction. They can best be thought of as an "opening" of the posterior and middle columns of the spine, whether seat belt related or otherwise (see Box 15-1, and Figure 15-13, *C*). The mechanism for this injury is forced flexion, and the axis of rotation is on the anterior column of the spine. These types of vertebral fractures are also referred to as a "chance" or "slice" fracture.

The most frequent *chance* fracture, comprising 50% of all seat belt injuries, is a Denis type III-A fracture, with damage to a single segment and posterior and middle column opening through bony tissue.[50] Bony instability in chance fractures lasts only the amount of time required for the bone to heal. Conservative treatment in a hyperextension TLSO or body cast usually enables predictable healing. A Jewett orthosis is sometimes used when bony injury is mild.

A *slice* fracture occurs when the fracture line passes through the discoligamentous space. After this type of fracture, a long-lasting instability may be anticipated, as the soft tissues do not heal as predictably as the bony injury. These injuries (Denis III-B, III-C, and III-D) most often require surgical intervention because of the extent of soft tissue damage.

Fracture/Dislocations

Denis type IV injuries occur when there is a combination of excessive translatory, flexion, and rotary forces that result in significant shearing of soft and bony tissue (see Box 15-1 and Figure 15-13, *D*). Most are catastrophic fractures, frequently resulting in paraplegia. They require surgery for fusion and stabilization and are often followed by postoperative use of a TLSO or body cast for several months, to immobilize the spine and protect the surgical construct while the fusion heals.

Denis identifies three subtypes of fracture dislocations, which are defined by a three-column stability disruption. Type IV-A flexion-rotation injuries are most frequent and can be classified further as disruption through bone or intervertebral disk, or both. Type IV-B shear injuries can be either anterior-posterior or posterior-anterior, following the dislocation. They are rarely true dislocations at the thoracolumbar level but are associated with facet joint fracture/dislocation. Type IV-C flexion and distraction injuries can be confused with Denis III-B fractures, because they are similar mechanisms of injury and present similar ligamentous injuries to the posterior and middle columns of the spine. In this injury the anterior column failure creates a major instability. Finally, type IV-D injuries often result from excessive, obliquely applied force to the vertebrae. All Denis type IV fracture-dislocations are unstable; clinically, they can be considered pure dislocations of either bony nature or discoligamentous nature.

Clinical Considerations

Compression fracture involves failure of the anterior column with the middle and posterior columns remaining intact. The burst fracture involves failure of both the anterior and middle columns. The seat belt–type injuries represent failure of the middle and posterior columns. Finally, the fracture dislocation injury represents failure of all three columns and always requires surgical reduction and stabilization. The number of mechanical columns disrupted influences the extent of the instability on the load-carrying capacity of the spine.

Disruption of a single column such as the anterior column due to a compression fracture results in minimal loss of load carrying capacity.[25] The instability associated with a two-column disruption such as that caused by a burst fracture or a flexion-distraction seat belt injury is more severe.[51] Mild injuries such as those that affect only a single level and single column are at low risk of progression and require minimally immobilizing orthoses. More severe two-level and two-column injuries with marginal stability do not require surgery but do require orthoses that offer maximal stabilization and resistance to further progression of the deformity.

For nonoperative management of spinal fractures with an orthosis, the primary role of the orthosis is to change the alignment of the spine from the pathological "gibbus" or "kyphos" toward a more normal shape. The orthosis is used to position the spine in an alignment of inherent internal stability to allow for healing (Figure 15-14). If an orthosis is misaligned, there is risk of progression of the injury, as well as onset or progression of neurological symptoms, because the spine is essentially unstable within the orthosis. For compression, burst, and chance fractures, maximal or excessive hyperextension can create an environment of inherent stability.

Fracture dislocations are too unstable to manage nonoperatively in an orthosis. Slice fractures do not heal properly when managed in an orthosis, as they are primarily soft tissue injuries.

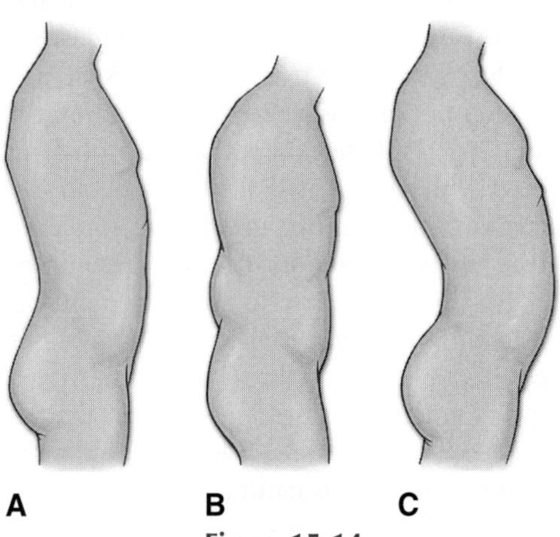

Figure 15-14

*A, In the neutral position there is slight lumbar lordosis and thoracic kyphosis. **B,** When the torso is held in pelvic flexion (posterior tilt), the lumbar spine is flattened and there tends to be increased thoracic kyphosis and a forward head. **C,** In a hyperextended spine, the pelvis is in excessive anterior tilt. The nonoperative management of spinal fractures that cause abnormal spinal alignment employs a lumbosacral orthosis or thoracolumbosacral orthosis to hold the spine in a neutral position until adequate healing has occurred. (Courtesy BioConcepts Orthotic Prosthetic Center, Burr Ridge, Ill.)*

CASE EXAMPLE 1

An Individual with Traumatic Compression Fracture of the Spine

J. Z., 32, is a mother of twins who was injured in a car accident when she suddenly braked to avoid a deer in her lane. She was thrown forcefully forward, "curling" around her seatbelt as it stopped her motion (there were no airbags in her older car). She felt immediate significant mid to low back pain that made her afraid to get out of the car. Paramedics immobilized her on a spine board, and she was flown by helicopter to the regional trauma center. Radiographs of her spine in the emergency department reveal T12 compression fracture, with moderate angulation of the anterior vertebral body. There is tenderness and some ecchymosis on her sternum and anterior chest, most likely from the seatbelt, but no other musculoskeletal or cardiopulmonary injuries and no neurological deficit. J. Z. is a former professional theatrical dancer who continues to work out regularly and reports that she is healthy. She is 5'7" tall and 130 lb.

Questions to Consider

- What columns of the spine are typically damaged in a traumatic compression fracture? What soft tissue structures may also be damaged? How does this type of injury affect the stability and alignment of the spinal column?
- What is the typical mechanism of injury in thoracic compression fractures? Are thoracic compression fractures likely or unlikely to result in neurological deficit? Why or why not? Where in the thoracic spine would a compression fracture carry the greatest risk of associated neurological deficit? Are you concerned about J. Z.'s risk of developing neurological signs and symptoms? Why or why not?
- After reviewing the radiographs, the orthopedic surgeon recommends that J. Z. be placed on bed rest for the next 48 hours and that a decision about the need for spinal surgery or orthosis be made afterward. Why is he recommending 48 hours of bed rest? What does he anticipate will happen to the compressed vertebral body in this time period?
- After 48 hours of bed rest, a second radiograph is taken. What does the orthopedist look for when he examines the image of the damaged T-12 vertebral body? What criteria does he use to decide if a spinal orthosis is indicated?
- The second radiograph reveals a vertebral body height loss of 35%. The orthopedist decides that surgical stabilization is unnecessary and requests that the orthotic/prosthetic department be called in to provide an appropriate spinal orthosis. What type of spinal orthosis is likely to be prescribed? What are the primary goals of an orthosis used in the conservative management of compression fractures?
- How will the use of an extension orthosis affect functional mobility? Would a referral for rehabilitation (physical therapy or occupational therapy, or both) be appropriate before discharge? Why or why not? Should J. Z. be encouraged to ambulate and use an assistive device? Why or why not? What types of activity restrictions are typically recommended for individuals with compression fractures who are being managed conservatively with an extension orthosis?
- What type of wearing schedule would likely be recommended for this individual? How many weeks or months is she likely to have to use the orthosis? What is the anticipated prognosis for individuals with traumatic compression fractures of the spine?
- What type of follow-up care with her physician, orthotist, and therapists is appropriate for J. Z. while she wears her orthosis? What strategy can be used to "wean" her from the orthosis once her fracture has healed? What type of follow-up or rehabilitation is necessary once she is no longer required to use the orthosis?

CASE EXAMPLE 2

An Individual with Traumatic "Burst" Spinal Fracture

M. P., 55, is an auto mechanic whose motor vehicle accident resulted in an L2 burst fracture, a ruptured spleen, a comminuted fracture of the femoral head, a punctured lung, and a pneumothorax. The trauma and internal medicine services have stabilized M. P.'s medical condition, and the next priority is for the orthopedic service to perform a total joint arthroplasty on the fractured right hip. Extension/flexion films of the spine determined that there is an intact anterior longitudinal ligament. Computed tomography scans demonstrated a 90% obliteration of the vertebral canal with bone fragments retropulsed from the associated gibbus. There are some signs of mild lower limb neurological deficit (dorsiflexors 4/5, quadriceps 4/5).

M. P. is now in the intensive care unit with chest tubes, intubation, hip traction, and monitors. He is anxious and is taking pain medication. When awake, he follows instructions and commands. He is 6′4″ tall and 300 lb. Surgery for the hip is scheduled for tomorrow morning, and the spine surgeon is consulting with the joint surgeon about operating on the hip without spinal support.

Questions to Consider

- What is a burst fracture? Which columns of the spine are involved? What impact does this type of fracture have on the stability and alignment of the spine? What is the typical mechanism of injury for this type of fracture?
- Are burst fractures likely or unlikely to present with a neurological deficit? Why is neurological function so important to monitor when this type of fracture has occurred?
- What concerns does the trauma team have about M. P.'s functional status in the period before his spinal surgery? How will the team examine and evaluate his status during this time?
- Does M. P. need spinal immobilization during his hip surgery, which is scheduled before surgical stabilization of his spine? What type of orthosis or cast do you suggest? Why do you recommend this orthosis?
- Can the orthotist measure, fabricate, and fit a hyperextension TLSO that fits with enough pelvic openness that the joint surgeon can operate on the hip without removing the orthosis?
- Surgical repair of M. P.'s spinal column is scheduled a few days following his total hip arthroplasty. Does M. P. require a different spinal orthosis for immobilization of his repaired spine? Why or why not? What are the primary goals of postoperative orthotic intervention for M.P.? What spinal segments must be protected or immobilized? What planes of motion must be limited to protect his surgical construct?
- What impact does M. P.'s size and weight have on the fitting of the orthosis? Given the nature of his spinal injury and repair, what do you expect to see on a lateral radiograph when M. P. wears the orthosis?
- How long do you anticipate M. P. must wear the orthosis? What is a typical daily wearing schedule?
- Do you expect M. P.'s mild neurological deficit to resolve following his spinal stabilization and immobilization in a TLSO? Why or why not?
- What impact does the orthosis, total hip arthroplasty, and pneumothorax have on M. P.'s functional mobility and activities of daily living (ADLs)? Would M. P. benefit from referral to rehabilitation services? Why or why not?

ORTHOTICS IN THE MANAGEMENT OF LOW BACK PAIN

Low back pain can result from mechanical stress, protrusion or degeneration of an intervertebral disk (nonspecific, discogenic-mechanical pain), or from spinal stenosis or spondylolisthesis (neurocompressive pain). Corsets and spinal orthosis may be used in conjunction with other conservative and pharmacological interventions for patients with disabling pain or following surgical intervention aimed at relieving pain or stabilizing the spinal column.

The prevalence of low back pain in the United States is extremely high: 80% to 85% of the population will experience significant low back pain at some time in their lives. The *Annual Survey of Occupational Injuries and Illnesses* conducted by the Bureau of Labor Statistics indicated that in 1998 overexertion caused 279,507 back injuries resulting in lost work days.[52]

The primary goal of an orthosis in the management of low back pain is to decrease pain. Most designs accomplish this by (1) limiting motion of the lumbar spine and (2) providing greater abdominal support.[21] Optimal lumbar posture has been identified as an important contributor to pain reduction. An orthosis that supports the lumbar spine in optimal posture may be an effective conservative treatment modality for low back pain. For patients with nonspecific-mechanical chronic back pain, effective pain relief is often accomplished by positioning the spine in lumbar extension.[13] For patients with neurocompressive disorders (stenosis or spondylolisthesis), pain relief is usually accomplished when orthosis is oriented toward lumbar flexion.[13] A wide variety of orthotic designs, ranging from lumbosacral corsets to rigid thermoplastic thoracolumbosacral orthoses (TLSOs), meet this goal. For back pain with discogenic-mechanical etiology, useful orthoses include lumbosacral or dorsolumbar corsets, chairback or Knight LSOs, various commercially produced prefabricated LSOs (e.g., those from Aspen Medical

Products, Inc.; DeRoyal Industries, Inc.; OrthoAmerica Products, Inc.), or custom-molded LSOs. For individuals with pain from stenosis or spondylolisthesis, the most commonly prescribed orthoses include lumbosacral corsets chairback or Knight LSOs, prefabricated LSOs, Raney or Williams Flexion LSOs, or custom-molded LSOs.

Assessing Effectiveness of Orthotic Intervention: The Wiss Test Orthosis

An important study reported by Willner[53] found that a rigid orthosis prescribed randomly and independently of diagnosis for persons with chronic low back pain was effective approximately 50% of the time. In a subsequent study Willner[54] predicted the likelihood that a rigid orthosis would be a successful intervention for low back pain with reasonable accuracy on the basis of pain relief provided by a testing orthosis that stabilized the spine. On the basis of his findings, a program for management of chronic low back pain with Willner's instrument for spinal stabilization (WISS) test orthosis has been developed. The WISS is an adjustable TLSO that can either extend or flex the lumbar spine, depending on the initial setting of the posterior pad in extension, neutral, or flexion (Figure 15-15). The anterior panel is also adjustable and provides abdominal support while helping to keep the orthosis in place.

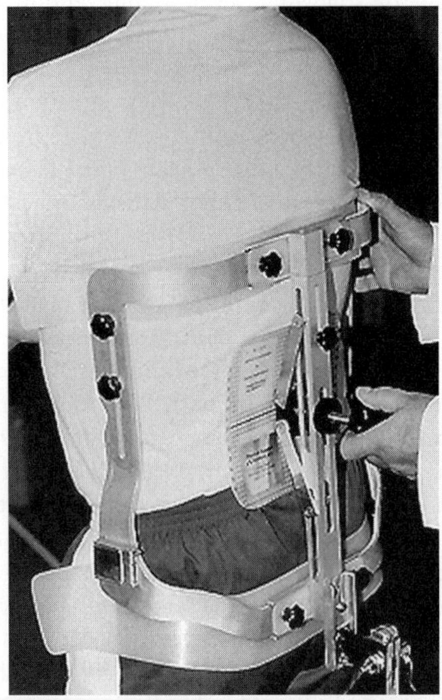

Figure 15-15
The Willner's instrument for spinal stabilization (WISS) test orthosis is used to determine optimal spinal position for pain relief in managing chronic low back pain of various etiologies. If symptoms are reduced after a trial period in the WISS orthosis, a custom-fit or molded orthosis can be fabricated for longer-term use.

Gavin and coworkers[13] conducted a prospective study to determine whether a 5-day trial wearing of the WISS orthosis would predict the outcome of orthotic treatment for chronic low back pain. Persons enrolled in the study had back pain that had not been relieved by conventional treatment for at least 6 months. For patients with disk herniation, multiple-level disk bulging, degenerative disk disease (excluding those with L5-S1 pathologies), the WISS orthosis was set at maximum lumbar extension. For those with spondylolisthesis, lumbar stenosis, or facet syndrome, the WISS orthosis was set in maximum lumbar flexion. Patients who reported moderate to good relief in the test orthosis then opted to proceed with an LSO in the same sagittal angulation found to be optimal in the WISS or discontinue orthotic treatment. They wore the LSO for 3 to 6 months. Then they were weaned from the device and proceeded with physical therapy. Persons with long-standing low back pain unrelieved by conventional treatment obtained pain relief from orthotic treatment when prescribed after a successful 5-day trial with the WISS orthosis.

Use of the WISS orthosis or a similar trial extension device allows the orthotist and individual who will wear the orthosis to ascertain (1) the most effective spinal position for pain relief to be incorporated into the orthosis, (2) whether the device can relieve enough pain to make it worthwhile for daily wearing, (3) whether ADLs might be compromised while wearing the device, and (4) whether the patient can don and remove this device properly at home.

Clinical Considerations

For patients with mild lumbosacral pain, a lumbosacral corset may provide enough immobilization to effectively manage the pain. This used in conjunction with physical therapy and medical management may provide significant relief. When a corset fails to provide significant pain relief, it is important to assess whether another orthotic intervention may be warranted. Although many patients abandon orthotic management, a more rigid orthosis capable of increasing or decreasing lumbar lordosis may be able to provide pain relief.

For patients with pain from either a herniated disk or degenerative disk disease, lumbar extension relieves most of the pain. For patients with spinal stenosis or pain from spondylolisthesis, a lumbar flexion orthosis relieves most of the pain. If a patient with a symptom indicating that extension is the most optimal sagittal geometry is fitted with a device that flexes the lumbar spine contrary to what is indicated, the pain will usually be exacerbated. Similarly, if someone with painful lumbar stenosis, which is best managed by alignment in lumbar flexion, is fitted with an orthosis that holds the spine in extension, symptoms are likely to worsen.

An orthosis may be a low-cost alternative for back pain management when other conservative modalities have failed. Clinical evaluation must be thorough to determine who will or will not benefit from an orthosis. If a person's symptom increases while sitting and decreases while standing, he or she will probably benefit from an extension orthosis. If the inverse is true, the patient will probably benefit from a flexion orthosis. Someone with acute symptoms and spinal muscle spasms is not likely to benefit from an orthosis. However, someone with sciatica radiculopathy, or other chronic symptoms, usually gains some relief from the symptom while in the orthosis. It is unlikely that a patient with stenosis or spondylolisthesis would maintain symptom relief indefinitely once the orthosis were removed; however, the person with mechanical or nonspecific pain may find an orthosis an acceptable modality for definitive treatment.

CASE EXAMPLE 3

An Individual with Prior Spinal Cord Injury Who Develops Low Back Pain

T. L., 34, is an elementary school teacher who sustained an L2 burst fracture with incomplete L2 paraplegia in a motor vehicle accident 10 years ago. Currently she uses a lightweight, solid-frame wheelchair for mobility at work and at home. She lives independently in a single-story home that has been adapted (in the kitchen and bathroom) for ease of function from a wheelchair and drives a Volkswagen Beetle with hand controls. On examination her lower extremity strengths are hip extensors 2/5 bilaterally, knee extensors 3/5 on right, 2/5 on left, dorsiflexors 3/5 bilaterally, plantar flexors 4/5 bilaterally. She has spotty sensation in her lower limbs with multiple paresthesias. Patellar and Achilles reflexes are weak and symmetrical. Immediately following her injury 10 years ago, she underwent surgical fusion of L1-L4 for the fracture with a variable slot plate pedicle screw construct.

One year ago T. L. began experiencing low back pain, which she describes as intermittent, beginning at the lateral aspect of the sacral area and radiating laterally to the gluteus medius region. After prolonged sitting in her wheelchair, during humid weather, and any time she lifts an object from the floor or table height, T. L. feels an exacerbation of the symptom. On the visual analog scale (0-10) she rates the symptom average 8. Recently she noticed that her symptom "radiated" down her right leg along the sciatic route. No radiculopathy is apparent. T. L. reports that she can usually reduce her back pain by rolling onto her stomach and propping on her elbows and by "bridging" (raising her hips up) when lying on her back with her knees bent. She is not taking pain medication. She has had physical therapy and an epidural steroid injection without any resolution of pain. Her chronic low back pain is decreasing her functional level and causing depression.

Questions to Consider

- Given her signs and symptoms, what do you suspect is the underlying cause of T. L.'s low back pain? Is this pain likely to be discogenic, due to spinal instability, or is it likely to be related to her previous surgical fusion? Why or why not?
- Does T. L. demonstrate any ergonomic positional relief? Biomechanically, why are these positions effective in reducing her symptoms?
- Would a trial in the WISS orthosis (for sagittal angular optimization) or similar extension test device be beneficial before deciding what type of orthosis should be prescribed? What information would a trial in the WISS provide?
- What orthotic design do you think an orthotist would recommend for T. L.? How would the orthosis help to minimize or control her symptoms?
- What is the long-term prognosis for someone with back pain similar to T. L.? What kind of follow-up care might you recommend from the orthotist, physical therapist, or physician?
- What recommendations can the team make to T. L. about when and how long to wear her new orthosis? Will this change over time? What other interventions (exercise, modalities) might be warranted at this time?
- How can you assess whether the orthosis is effective in the management of her current signs and symptoms and the long-term outcome of the orthosis in managing her low back pain?

CASE EXAMPLE 4

A Young Construction Worker with Significant Low Back Pain and Spondylolisthesis

J. R., 24, is a male construction worker who is currently unable to work because of recurrent, severe back pain. He is referred to the orthotist practice with a prescription for a "back brace." The radiograph he brings to his appointment reveals an L5 on S1 isthmic spondylolisthesis of a grade II + with a minimal slip angle. J. R. has a feeling of "needles and pins" in his legs and spotty sensation in his feet. He feels burning in his feet and rates his pain a 6 on the 0-10 visual analog scale. He feels uncomfortable with standing and prefers to sit. Despite signs of lumbar stenosis, his physician does not recommend surgery in the near future.

J. R. demonstrates no back pain and some mild pain near the sciatic notch, which he calls his "bad hips." An MRI depicts compression of the cauda equina, and his electromyogram signals are asymmetrical. All motor function, joint range of motion, and muscle strength are normal. He has slow Achilles and Babinski reflexes, but all other reflexes are normal.

Questions to Consider

- What is the prognosis for individuals with isthmic spondylolisthesis and lumbar stenosis? What are the roles of orthotic intervention, rehabilitation, and surgery in the long-term management of this condition? How does the age of the individual (prepuberty vs. postpuberty) influence efficacy of intervention?
- Would you recommend an orthosis for this patient? Why or why not? Would you choose an orthosis that holds the spine in flexion, neutral, or hyperextended position? Why?
- Describe the protocol and wearing schedule you would recommend for an individual new to spinal orthotic use. What would you recommend as optimal time in orthosis for J. R.? Would it be different if he were an adolescent?
- How often will J.R. return to his orthotist and his physician for follow-up? How will outcome/efficacy of the intervention be assessed?

ORTHOSES FOR THE OSTEOPOROTIC SPINE

Osteoporosis is a significant health problem, especially for postmenopausal older women. The number of individuals living with osteoporosis is significantly greater than the number of individuals with traumatic spinal injuries and idiopathic scoliosis combined. The risk of pathological compression fractures of the thoracic and lumbar spine, occurring without significant trauma, increases exponentially with the severity and duration of osteoporosis. Typically, a person with the diagnosis of a pathological thoracic or thoracolumbar compression fracture from osteoporosis is prescribed either a dorsolumbar corset, a CASH orthosis, or a Jewett orthosis.[16] If the orthosis is unable to reduce pain or improve the quality of life, it is usually discarded, and orthotic management is abandoned. Although tradition suggests that orthoses for persons with spinal fractures secondary to osteoporosis are burdensome and not well liked by the affected people and the health care workers alike, the appropriately designed and fit orthosis can be a valuable intervention.

For patients with an osteoporotic spinal fracture, the main objective is to improve the quality of life and reduce pain, *not* to stabilize a fracture as is the case for orthotic management of traumatic fractures. The mechanisms of pain and pain relief must be considered. Many individuals with osteoporotic fracture lose normal lordosis as a consequence of the fracture. This results in a sagittal plane malalignment: the head and shoulders are abnormally anterior to the sacrum. A simple clinical measurement of this is to use a plumb line at the acromion and measure the distance of this line to the greater trochanter. Frequently there is an anterior displacement of the plumb line of several centimeters. In this abnormal posture the erector spinae muscle group is also lengthened abnormally. Theoretically, restoration of some lumbar lordosis to realign the head and upper trunk over the sacrum should reduce pain and minimize progression of postfracture kyphosis.

A dorsolumbar corset cannot provide enough postural realignment to bring the plumb line displacement to any point posterior to the trochanter. A CASH or Jewett orthosis is excellent at applying anteriorly directed shear force at the fracture itself but does little to induce lordosis and reduce the length of the erector spinae, thereby positioning the head and shoulders above or posterior to the sacrum. It may be argued that a posteriorly directed force to realign the thoraco-lumbar spine on the sagittal plane by inducing lordosis and retracting the upper torso into the "righted" position may make more sense.

Although preliminary, the authors have designed and fitted several hundred such devices with promising success. The posterior shell TLSO is an excellent device to gradually "right" these people on the sagittal plane (Figure 15-16). Other than kyphoplasty and physical therapy, older adults with pathological osteoporotic fractures do not have

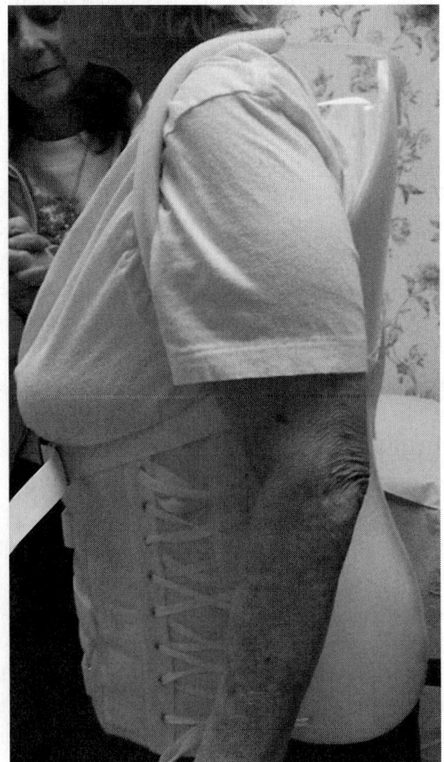

Figure 15-16
The posterior shell thoracolumbosacral orthosis in hyperextension realigns the spine in lumbar lordosis and supports the upper torso over the pelvis for individuals with pathological osteoporotic fractures. It is used to reduce pain, enhance functional ability, and minimize progression of kyphosis. This orthosis may be better tolerated than a CASH or Jewett orthosis.

recourse to effective management of their problem. Kyphoplasty may realign the fractured vertebra but does little to restore lordosis. The posterior shell TLSO, combined with physical therapy for strengthening and endurance training, holds promise for older patients and their families as an effective alternative to manage the osteoporotic spine. Once the orthosis is fabricated and fitted, the caregivers are instructed to increase the shoulder strap tightness daily over 1 month to achieve this goal. Usually, once the person is realigned, he or he can ambulate without a walker and for a significantly longer time period. Although clinical studies are forthcoming, experience suggests that most of those who have been successfully "repositioned" in the first month of treatment will continue to wear the posterior shell during daily activities.

CASE EXAMPLE 5

An Older Woman with Pathological Osteoporotic Fractures of the Thoracic Spine

E. P., 84, is a generally healthy, independently living woman with known osteoporosis who reports a sudden onset of midback pain while opening a "stubborn" window at her summer home. She has a history of previous pathological fracture at T-8, which occurred 2 years ago when she lifted a box of winter clothing up to the top shelf in her closet. Her initial fracture was managed conservatively with a CASH orthosis, which she disliked a great deal but wore as recommended. After she healed sufficiently to tolerate activity, she began a pool-based exercise program to become stronger and improve her posture, increased her intake of calcium, began a daily walking program, and started taking Fosamax. She has "no intention of becoming a frail old lady" and leads an active lifestyle, maintaining her apartment in the city and her summer lake house with little help.

She now presents with a moderately kyphotic posture and notable loss of lumbar lordosis. Although she reports her height as 5 feet, 2 inches, she currently measures 4 feet,11½ inches when standing as erect as possible. Her weight has been steady at 105 lb for the past 2 years, and her wrist circumference is 5 inches. A radiograph reveals a new wedge compression fracture of the anterior column at T-7, and a healed wedge compression fracture of the anterior column at T-8.

Questions to Consider

- In what ways are pathological spinal fractures similar to or different from traumatic spinal fractures in terms of etiology, spinal columns, and spinal segments most likely to be involved; conservative or surgical management; and prognosis for recovery or recurrence?
- What are the options for conservative management of pathological osteoporotic fracture involving the anterior column? What impact does this type of fracture have on stability and the health of the spine?
- What are the goals of orthotic intervention for persons with pathological osteoporotic fracture? What are the advantages and limitations of each? What type of orthosis would you recommend for E. P.? Why have you chosen this orthosis from among available options?
- What is E. P.'s prognosis for recovery from this fracture? How might this episode affect her daily function and independence during the acute recovery phase, as well as in the months ahead? What are her risks of future fractures? What type of follow-up might she require?

POSTOPERATIVE ORTHOSES FOR THE THORACOLUMBAR SPINE

Postoperative orthoses act to restrict motion, protecting injured segments from motion and theoretically reducing loads on the surgical constructs until solid fusion occurs. Evidence indicates that the Milwaukee brace and body cast worn postoperatively in patients with idiopathic scoliosis reduce axial force on the Harrington rod (spinal instrumentation) during standing and walking.[55] With advances in surgical instrumentation, however, the actual effectiveness of postoperative orthoses in reducing stresses on any particular implant is not well documented. The role of an orthosis for postoperative immobilization after spinal fusion for low back pain remains controversial. A custom-molded TLSO in neutral sagittal alignment is standard postoperative immobilization for persons with significant thoracolumbar injuries. In these cases, the goal of surgery (with instrumentation, bone graft, or fusion) is to restore segmental stability; the role of a postoperative orthosis is to protect the surgical construct from the planes of motion that make it vulnerable to failure. Typically, motions to be guarded against in the immediate postoperative period are trunk flexion and trunk torsion/rotation.

To be effective, the TLSO must have enough anterior height to resist forward bending at the sternum as well as firm end point stabilization of the pelvis. The distal trimlines often must extend into the groin to capture the pelvis firmly, which may interfere somewhat with the patient's ability to sit comfortably and perform lower extremity ADLs. Although this may make rehabilitation challenging for a short period, the goal of spinal stabilization takes precedent in the postoperative period. The orthotist is also careful with upright alignment to ensure that the orthosis holds the trunk in a neutral position, avoiding the application of a flexion or extension load to the torso to minimize the translation of stresses onto surgical instruments.

Although custom-molded TLSOs are excellent at reducing motion in most of the lumbar spine,[22] a thigh extension with an orthotic hip joint is added to the postoperative custom-molded TLSO of patients with spinal fusion at L5-S1 to immobilize the LS joint effectively (see Figure 15-4).[56] A TLSO without this thigh extension may have no effect or may actually increase lumbosacral motion. For patients with midthoracic to upper thoracic injury or injury at multiple levels, an orthosis designed to immobilize the cervical spine can be added to the TLSO to better stabilize the repaired spinal segments.

A design of the spinal orthosis for thoracolumbar injury is based on understanding its biomechanical mechanism of action, clinical intuition, and clinical assessment. Use of a brace that provides too much or too little stabilization compromises desired surgical and functional outcomes. Many trauma centers have established criteria for selection of an orthosis. Patient and caregiver education about the purpose and design of the orthosis and the consequences of noncompliance is another important component to ensure that the best outcome is achieved.

ORTHOTICS IN CERVICAL SPINE INSTABILITY

Cervical orthoses can be classified or grouped in several ways. One strategy is to divide orthoses into two groups: skin contact orthoses and skeletal devices. Another is to classify orthoses by the magnitude of motion control that they provide into a minimum control group and an intermediate control group. This chapter refers to Nachemson's classification of cervical and cervicothoracic orthoses, which has three groups (soft collars, reinforced collars, and rigid orthoses) based on material construct.[17]

Biomechanics

The cervical spine is complex, and knowledge of its anatomy and kinematics provides the foundation for understanding the role of the many orthoses designed to manage cervical spine instability. The seven cervical vertebrae and their surrounding soft tissues constitute the most mobile segment of the spine. Anatomically unique, the atlantoaxial complex (occiput, C1, C2) can be considered and examined separately from the rest of the cervical spine. The cervical spine rotates in the transverse plane for a total excursion of 160 degrees. Approximately one half of this rotation occurs at the C1 and C2 level, with the remainder occurring across the joints below this level. Although movements of flexion and extension occur at all cervical levels, the greatest range of these motions happens at the C5-6 level. Lateral flexion occurs in the more caudal (C3-7) levels of the cervical spine.

Examination of the complete cervical spine requires several strategies. Anterior surfaces of the first and second vertebrae (C1, C2) are best viewed through an open mouth. Palpation of the Adam's apple (thyroid cartilage) approximates the levels of C4-6. Maximal forward flexion of the head and neck exposes the bony spinous processes of the C7 and T1 vertebrae.

Cervical and cervicothoracic orthoses are designed to minimize the physiological loads and motions between the head and thorax. Several studies have assessed the ability of different orthoses to restrict motion of the cervical spine, enabling the orthotist to classify orthoses from least to most restrictive. Control of flexion/extension motion in the sagittal plane is the most easily accomplished; restriction of rotation and lateral tilt is much more challenging. This discussion begins with orthoses that provide the least restriction of motion, moving to those that provide the most motion control of the cervical spine.

The primary mechanisms of action of cervical collars and cervical thoracic orthoses (CTOs) are to immobilize specific levels and specific planes of movement. Cervical orthoses must address not only bending flexion and extension but also translational flexion and extension. Lateral bending and transverse rotation are also important to immobilize for many injuries.

Gavin and coworkers[57] measured the efficacy of two cervical collars (Aspen, Miami J) and two CTOs (Aspen 2-post, Aspen 4-post) in reducing cervical intervertebral and gross range of motion in flexion and extension in 20 normal volunteer subjects. The gross sagittal motion of the head and neck was measured relative to the horizon using an optoelectronic motion measurement system. Simultaneous measurement of intervertebral motion was performed using a video fluoroscopic (VF) machine. Surface electromyographic data were used during data analysis to control for subject effort. There were no statistically significant differences between the Miami J and Aspen collars. Both CTOs provided significantly more restriction of gross flexion and extension motion as compared with the two collars. The Aspen 2-post CTO and 4-post CTO performed similarly in flexion, but the Aspen 4-post CTO provided significantly more restriction of extension motion. The CTOs as a group were significantly better at restricting both flexion and extension than the collars as a group.

Cervical Orthoses

The most commonly used cervical orthoses include prefabricated soft collars (which provide minimal support or immobilization) and prefabricated adjustable or custom-fit reinforced collars (which provide intermediate support or immobilization).

Soft Collars

Although patients find a soft collar quite comfortable to wear, this type of cervical orthosis does little to restrict cervical motion in any plane (Figure 15-17). This device is used primarily as a kinesthetic reminder for patients with mild whiplash injury or neck pain to restrict their cervical motion. Because this orthosis is not stabilized against the upper trunk or occiput, wearing it does not guarantee optimal cervical alignment and may actually contribute to

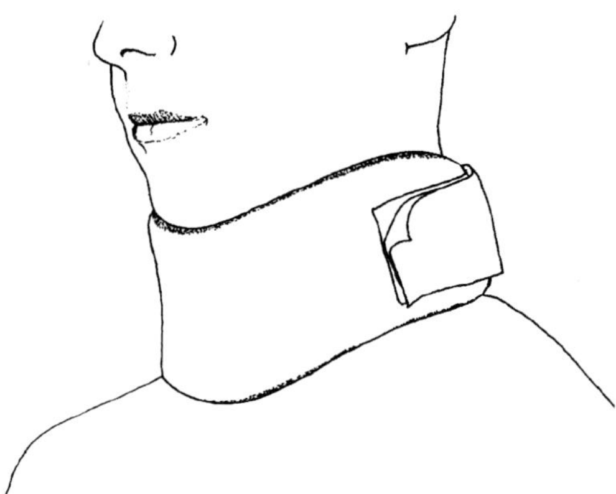

Figure 15-17
A soft collar reminds the wearer to limit motion of the neck but provides little stability for the cervical spine.

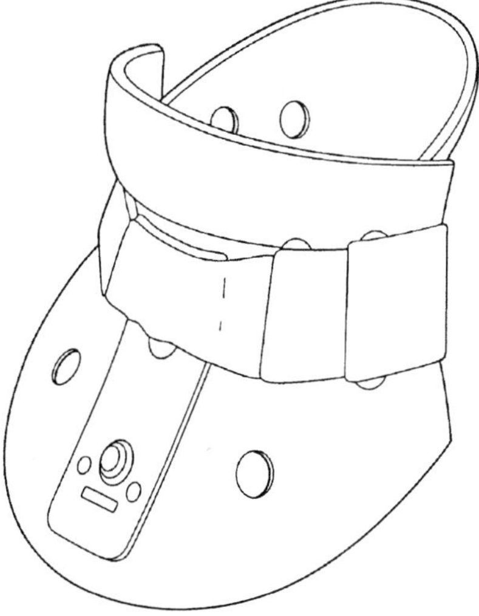

Figure 15-18
The Philadelphia collar, with an anterior opening for tracheostomy care. (From Shurr DG. Prosthetics, orthotics and orthopaedic rehabilitation. In Clark CR, Bonfiglio M [eds], Orthopaedics: Essentials of Diagnosis and Treatment. *New York: Churchill Livingstone, 1994. p. 340.)*

development of a forward head position if the wearer rests his chin on the collar. Patient education about maintaining optimal alignment of the head and neck is essential whenever a soft collar is provided. The collar is usually a narrow block of foam rubber material covered with stockinet or knitted material, and it is closed around the neck with Velcro.

Reinforced Cervical Collars

To provide more stability than is possible in a soft cervical collar, various commercially manufactured reinforced collars are available. A reinforced collar has an outer plastic, semirigid frame and an inner soft pad or closed cell foam shell that interfaces with the skin. Many have anterior openings to accommodate respiratory apparatus fixation. The Philadelphia collar is the most recognized reinforced collar (Figure 15-18). Most reinforced collars have an anterior shell that supports the chin and a posterior shell that supports the occiput of the skull, attached firmly together by Velcro closure. Although the Philadelphia collar provides some support for the weight of the head in the sagittal plane, its low trimlines prevent it from effectively immobilizing the cervical spine enough to prevent lateral bending or rotation.[58,59]

Other reinforced collars (e.g., the Newport, Miami J, or Aspen collars) are designed with higher trimlines in an attempt to provide more motion control (Figure 15-19). The semirigid frame of these orthoses tends to be longer than that of the Philadelphia collar. The distal trimline and padding typically lie against the manubrium of the sternum anteriorly and the spinous processes of the first several thoracic vertebrae posteriorly. The proximal trimline and padding encompass the lateral surface and underside of the mandible anteriorly and fit snugly against the lateral and posterior surface of the skull. Like the Philadelphia collar, these cervical orthoses are held in place by Velcro closures.

Cervicothoracic Orthoses

At times nonoperative and postoperative care of cervical spine injuries requires more stability or better immobilization than is possible with reinforced cervical collars. To provide greater motion control, the distal end point control must encompass at least the upper thoracic spine and trunk. Various "poster" orthotic designs that have thoracic components are connected to occipital and mandibular pieces by two or four uprights or posts. Various thermoplastic bivalve designs encase the upper trunk, neck, chin, and occiput. Control of sagittal plane flexion and extension is enhanced by the stabilizing effect of the thoracic extension in both CTO designs. Although control of lateral flexion and rotation is often better than that achieved by a reinforced collar, these motions cannot be completely limited by poster-style or rigid cervicothoracic orthoses. The only orthosis that maximizes cervical immobilization is a "halo" cervical device.[58,59]

Sternooccipitomandibular Immobilizers

The SOMI is a metal and thermoplastic orthosis that is most often chosen for patients with instability at or above the C4 vertebral level (Figure 15-20).[60] The SOMI has a T-shaped yoke worn over the shoulders and anterior chest that connects to the occipital support with a U-shaped metal rod. The distal end of the yoke is anchored by a strap that wraps around the patient's midtrunk. The mandibular support is attached to the yoke by a single flat post and to the occipital support by lateral straps.

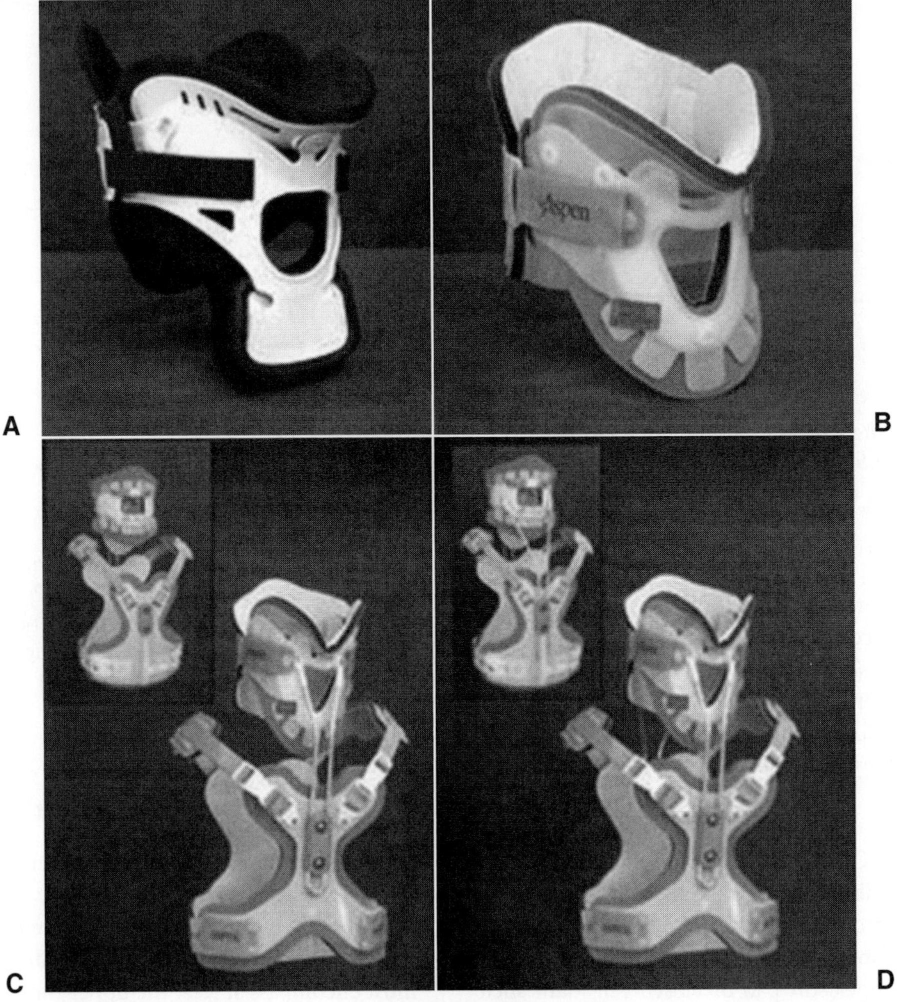

Figure 15-19
*The longer trimlines of the Miami J Collar (**A**) and the Aspen Collar (**B**) provide more aggressive motion control of the cervical spine than the Philadelphia collar. The Aspen 2-post cervicothoracic orthosis (**C**), and 4-post cervicothoracic orthosis (**D**) control cervical and upper thoracic spinal motion.*

An alternate configuration uses a headband to stabilize the head in the device rather than the mandibular support, which makes feeding and oral care less problematic. The SOMI is especially effective in controlling flexion. The metal support rods can be adjusted to a neutral, extended, or flexed neck position given the nature of the person's injury or surgical repair. The device is relatively simple to fit and can be easily donned and doffed when the person is supine.

Yale Cervicothoracic Orthoses

The Yale CTO, a thermoplastic device designed to stabilize the lower cervical spine, is used in patients with spinal instability or injury below the C4 vertebral level (Figure 15-21). The Yale orthosis is basically a snugly fit reinforced cervical collar with anterior and posterior extensions attached to a thoracic band. The extensions and thoracic band create a longer lever arm for more effective control of spinal motions. Although the device effectively limits flexion/extension, patients are able to rotate through a limited range of motion.

Minerva Cervicothoracic Orthoses

The Yale CTO was designed as a lighter-weight and less care-intensive version of the Minerva CTO. The Minerva is a custom-molded thermoplastic orthosis with anterior and posterior shells (bivalve design) encasing the person's neck and upper chest from jaw to umbilicus on the anterior surface and from occiput to midback on the posterior surface (Figure 15-22). The shells of the Minerva are held snugly in place around the neck and trunk by Velcro closures. Although this rigid orthosis provides more aggressive control of gross and intersegmental motion of the cervical and upper thoracic spine than is possible with other CTO

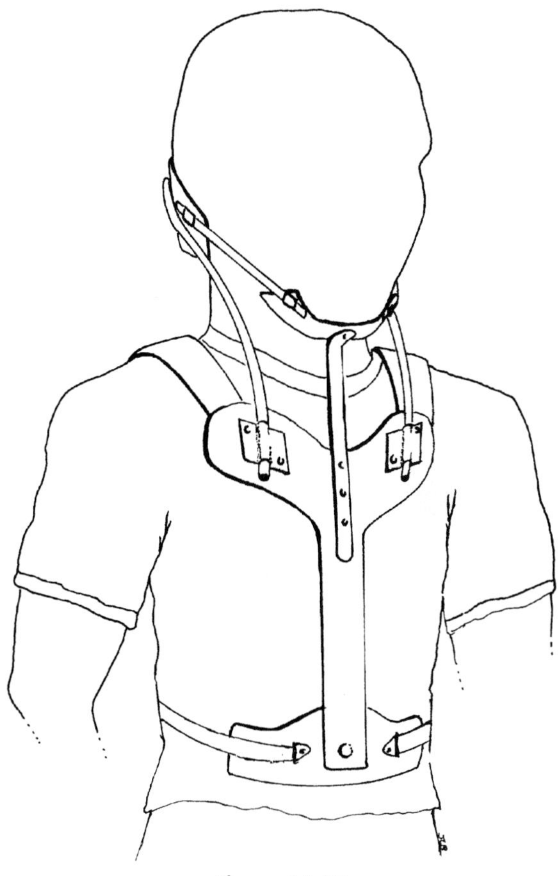

Figure 15-20
The sterno-occipito-mandibular immobilizer is used to stabilize the upper cervical spine. The U-shaped metal support rod, connecting the anterior chest and occiput, can be adjusted to match the specific needs of a patient's condition.

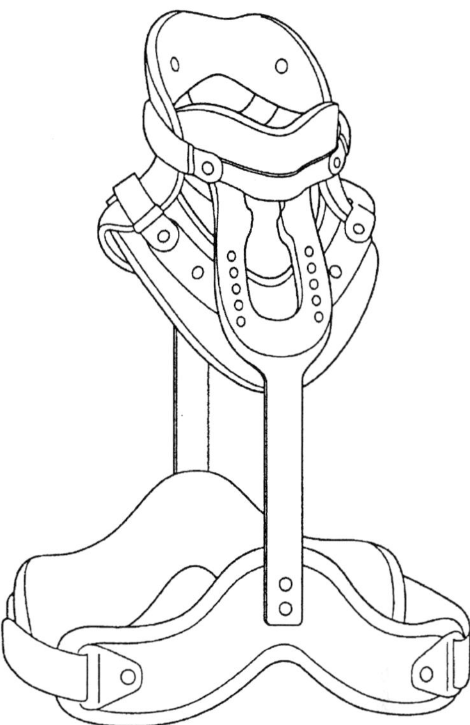

Figure 15-21
The chest extensions of a Yale cervical thoracic orthosis provide leverage for better control of lower cervical and upper lumbar vertebral motion. (From Shurr DG. Prosthetics, orthotics, and orthopaedic rehabilitation. In Clark CR, Bonfiglio M [eds], Orthopaedics: Essentials of Diagnosis and Treatment. *New York: Churchill Livingstone, 1994. p. 341.)*

designs, several disadvantages must be considered. The Minerva can be difficult to apply and remove. It is hot to wear and is not well tolerated by persons in warm climates. It is also associated with a higher incidence of skin irritation and pressure sores compared with other CTO designs.[60]

Other Cervicothoracic Orthoses

A number of other poster CTO designs are available for patients with serious spinal injuries or surgeries. The CD Denison design uses an anterior and posterior bar placed at the midline to support the weight of the head on a yoked thoracic component. In four-poster designs, two anterior and two posterior posts connect the lateral undersurface of the mandibular support and occipital support to the thoracic component.

These orthoses are more restrictive than reinforced cervical collars but may not restrict motion as well as the Yale CTO or Minerva design. These designs are often incorporated into a TLSO for persons with multiple injuries or extensive spinal surgery that require protection of the cervical, thoracic, and lumbar spine.

Cervical Halo

When complete control of the cervical and upper thoracic spine in all three planes of motion is required, the orthosis of choice is the halo (Figure 15-23).[61] The halo was first used as an extension of a body jacket for immobilization of patients with severe poliomyelitis and paralysis of the cervical musculature.[62] In current practice, the halo is used in three ways. If applied before surgery, it minimizes movement and protects the spinal cord during surgical procedures. If applied immediately after open reduction–internal fixation or fusion surgery, the halo controls cervical motion until adequate healing and bony union have been achieved at the surgical site. The halo is also used in conservative nonoperative management of nondisplaced upper cervical vertebral fractures.

The halo has three primary components: the ring and skull pins that surround the skull, a vest worn around the thorax, and the superstructure that fixates the ring to the vest.

Ring and Skull Pins

The ring of the halo is positioned approximately 1 cm above the eyebrow and the tip of the ears, with at least 1 cm

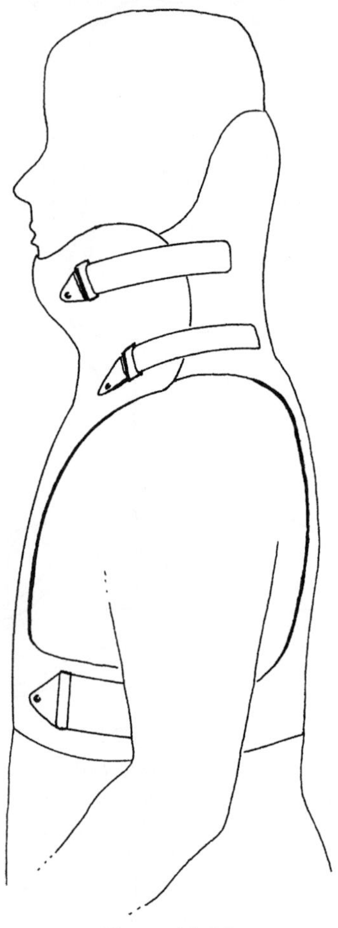

Figure 15-22
The Minerva cervical thoracic orthosis encases the cervical and upper thoracic spine to limit motion in all three planes.

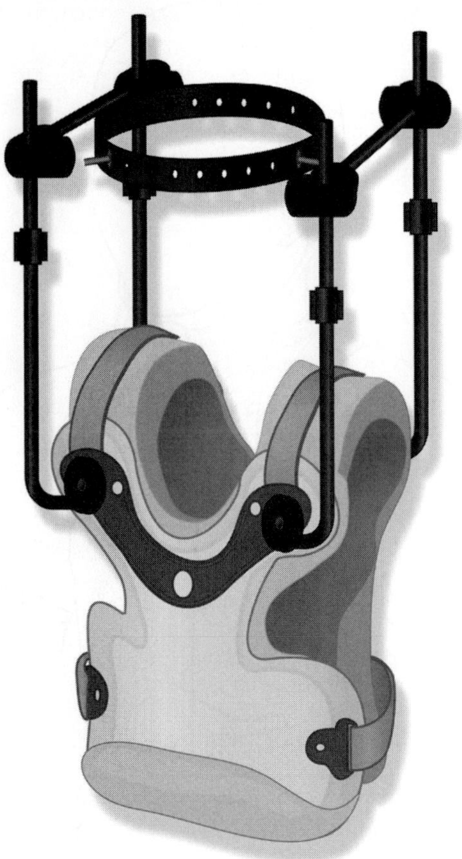

Figure 15-23
The halo orthosis is the only device that immobilizes the cervical spine in all three planes of motion. The head is stabilized within an open or a closed ring by a set of pressure pins. The halo is anchored to the stabilizing thoracic vest by the halo's metal suprastructure (Courtesy BioConcepts Orthotic Prosthetic Center, Burr Ridge, Ill.)

clearance between the ring and skin surface. Four pins are inserted ⅛ inch into the outer bony layer (table) of the skull with 6 to 8 lb/in of torque.[63] The anterior pins are placed in the lateral one third of the eyebrow to avoid the frontal sinus, supraorbital and subtrochlear nerves, and temporalis muscle. Posteriorly, pins are placed 1 to 2 cm posterior to the ear in diagonal opposition to the anterior pin site. This arrangement places the ring below the greater equator of the skull, in areas that are most likely to have the thickest bone mass.[63]

Optimally, pins are inserted perpendicularly to the skull to maximize the ultimate load and minimize deformation of the pin bone complex to reduce the risk of failure.[64,65] Additional pins inserted with less torque are used for children with incompletely developed skulls, for patients with skull fractures, for those with sloping brows, and for patients who are in traction before application of the halo. Halo rings are available in open and closed configurations. Although open rings can facilitate fitting, increased pain and pin problems can occur when an open ring is used.[66]

Halo Superstructure

The superstructure of the halo orthosis is available in several designs. In one design, two anterior and two posterior metal rods rigidly link the ring apparatus to the vest. In another, two lateral rods rise toward the ring from a metal yoke that arches over the shoulders and is anchored to the vest. The purpose of the superstructure is to fixate the ring to the vest. Most superstructures can be adjusted so that the patient's head and neck can be held in the position or plane necessary for the particular injury or surgical procedure that warrants a period of immobilization.

Vest

The vest is the foundation and point of stability for the halo system. A halo vest is usually fabricated from flexible thermoplastic and has a removable liner made from lamb's wool or a similar material. With the patient supine, the anterior shell of the vest can be opened without compromising stability for hygiene. This feature is also important if emergency respiratory access is needed. In most halo vests, the distal trimline is at or slightly above the inferior costal margin of the last rib; extending it beyond this provides no additional cervical stability.[61]

Avoiding Halo Complications

A number of potentially serious problems are associated with the halo orthosis, including loosening of pins, pin site infection, pin discomfort, ring migration, pressure sores, nerve injury, prolonged bleeding at pin sites, and puncture of the dura.[64] Caregivers and health care providers who work with patients in a halo during rehabilitation must watch for signs of these problems and notify the physician or orthotist promptly to ensure appropriate intervention or adjustment. The risk of problem development is minimized when a routine of halo care is in place.

Daily pin care requires cleansing of each pin site with its own cotton swab soaked in one-half strength peroxide and normal saline solution, followed by an application of povidone-iodine (Betadine) solution. Two important signs of impending infection are soreness or oozing at a pin site and extreme sensitivity to touch during routine care. Pin site or headache pain that persists beyond the third day "in halo" should also be reported to the physician.

A well-fit vest should not create undue pressure over any body prominence. Complaints about point pressure, tightness, or irritation over the scapulae, ribs, clavicles, or other areas covered by the vest often suggest that vest adjustment is necessary. It is not unusual for patients to complain of itchiness under the vest. Using lotion or massaging gently with a blunt object gently should relieve this itch.

Halo in Rehabilitation

The added mass of a halo orthosis changes the position of the center of gravity within the trunk. Initially, patients may experience this extra mass as being top-heavy. For patients without neurological deficit who are able to ambulate while in the halo, a posture that accommodates this added mass is slight forward flexion of the trunk. Some patients might require a cane or walker until postural control adapts to the halo. Patients with cervical spinal cord injury who begin their rehabilitation with a halo may have to readjust their postural control strategies in sitting when the halo is discontinued later in their rehabilitation, because their center of mass shifts back to its normal position.

If a patient in a halo has a fall, pin sites should be examined for loosening or bleeding. If the apparatus appears to be less stable after a fall, it is best to have the patient remain supine until the physician or orthotist evaluates and adjusts the device.

CASE EXAMPLE 5

An Individual with a Nondisplaced Odontoid Fracture

T. S., 27, is at the emergency department after falling backwards from a nearly vertical surface while rock climbing with friends. Although his safety harness stopped his fall, he reports that his neck "snapped hard" and he felt an "electric shock" as the harness checked his fall. He regained control despite considerable neck pain and descended the rockface without assistance. Because of his pain, his companions called 911 and made him lie down until the paramedics arrived. Although he had no neurological deficits, the paramedics immobilized T. S. on a backboard and transported him to the trauma center.

He is alert and oriented, although anxious. His neurological examination is normal. A radiograph reveals nondisplaced fracture of the odontoid process of C-2 vertebrae. The orthopedic surgeon on call recommends conservative management with immediate orthotic immobilization.

Questions to Consider

- Given the location of his fracture, what motions of the cervical spine must be limited or controlled to allow for bony healing?
- Use your understanding of the cervical spine to decide which cervical or cervicothoracic orthosis the team will choose to immobilize T. S.'s spine. Why would the team choose this orthosis from among all the other options?
- What possible complications might occur as a result of his fracture? How will the team screen or monitor his motor and sensory status?
- What are the possible complications or limitations of the immobilization strategy you have recommended? How might the risk of complications or impact of limitations imposed by the immobilization strategy be minimized?
- How will the immobilization strategy you have recommended affect mobility and ADLs? Why (or why not) would referral to rehabilitation services be appropriate?
- What is T. S.'s prognosis for recovery? How long might the immobilization strategy be necessary? What kind of follow-up care might you recommend?

Clinical Considerations

Several important points should be remembered if a reinforced collar or a CTO is to be as effective as possible during rehabilitation: a snug fit, pressure relief and skin care, and neutral alignment. The keys to success are understanding the purpose of the collar and consistently wearing the device.

It is often tempting to loosen the straps of the collar in an effort to be more comfortable. The effectiveness of the collar worn less tightly closed than in the original fitting, however, is equivalent to being out of the collar completely.[66] The superior edge of a well-fit collar is in total contact against the mandible and occipital areas; the inferior edge rests against the sternum, muscle belly of the upper trapezius, and upper thoracic spine. When adjusted correctly, neck motion within the collar is at a minimum.

Because of the firm fit and total contact of reinforced cervical collars on the mandible, posterior skull, and superior trunk surfaces, patients who wear them are at risk of skin irritation or breakdown, especially if the contact pressure of the orthosis reaches or exceeds the amount of pressure that would cause capillary closure.

Plaisier and coworkers[67] compared craniofacial pressures exerted by four different reinforced collars. The Stifneck extraction collar, often used by emergency medical technicians as a means of immobilization when cervical spinal cord injury is suspected, exceeded capillary closing pressure at most contact points. This suggests that extraction-type collars are best used for a short duration and are not appropriate for long-term use during rehabilitation. It is also important to have a routine for skin care and shaving and keep the mandibular and chin support of the anterior shell clean and free of food or debris that can become entrapped at mealtime.

Most reinforced cervical collars are designed to hold the head and neck in as close to a neutral position as possible. A patient who wears the collar when supine in bed must maintain a neutral position. Optimally, only a single pillow placed under the upper back (scapula), neck, and head is used for sleeping. When several pillows are placed under the person's head and neck, a large flexion moment is created, which, in turn, creates areas of high-pressure contact with the skin, increasing discomfort and the risk of skin breakdown. The Philadelphia collar, for example, exerts acceptable pressures in the upright position but greater than capillary closure pressure when the patient is supine, even if no pillows are used.[60] It is equally important to limit exercises that cause cervical motion while the collar is worn so that neutral alignment is not inadvertently compromised.

PROPER USE OF SPINAL ORTHOSES

When the spine is vertical, it bears approximately three times the weight of the torso section it is maintaining in the erect posture.[68] For example, if the weight of a torso on the sacrum is 80 lb, the muscle coactivation required to keep the spine erect triples the load to approximately 240 lb. Since spinal orthoses are designed and fitted to reduce deformity, increase stability (maximum amount of axial load that may be carried without an increase in deformity), or protect an implant, it is best to measure and don an orthosis while the person is horizontal. This reduces the axial load to near the value of weight, minimizes the amount of force necessary to correct a pathological deformity, and reduces strains on implants while vertical. The measurable result of this mechanism is that the person should be significantly taller when vertical in a spinal orthosis. If an orthosis is measured and donned on a vertical person, this result is minimized.

This mechanism is thought to influence load sharing in the spinal orthosis, a function yet to be measured in the laboratory but well known in knee orthoses and spinal implants. Since this effect has not been quantified, it is still unknown. However, if the amount of load sharing suggested by the in-orthosis height increase is significant, this may be the most important mechanism of action of all spinal orthoses. This is currently a major point of contention and debate as many clinicians still advocate the measurement and donning of an orthosis while vertical.

It is noteworthy that the spine will undergo a major viscoelastic creep within the first 15 minutes of wearing the orthosis. This means that a retightening of the orthosis is necessary before the person wearing the orthosis changes from a supine position into sitting or standing postures. This concept may be analogous to the need to occasionally retighten an orthodontic apparatus.

In addition, most patients requiring a spinal orthosis are usually injured and in pain. Therefore ensuring proper social care of people wearing spinal orthoses may be beneficial. They are at a mechanical disadvantage for tightening their own device and may not possess the strength to do so. Many people will eventually be able to apply and tighten their orthoses properly, but not in the initial weeks of wearing. If patients do not have the social support at home to ensure proper donning, a home health nurse may be required for a few weeks to assist the donning process. Since the patient should wear the orthosis whenever vertical, possibly from waking until nighttime, the caregiver may only need to visit once a day for 15 minutes in the morning.

In conclusion, a spinal orthosis must be properly measured, fabricated, donned, and retightened to maximize the function.

SUMMARY

Selection of an appropriate spinal orthosis for a given patient is based on various objective and clinically informed subjective factors. These include the type and severity of the disorder, the age and size of the patient, the availability of assistance and support in the home and community, and the desired mechanisms of action of the orthosis. These factors are best evaluated and orthotic decisions are most effectively made in the context of a multidisciplinary team. Effective teams share information about the nature of a patient's condition, the reason that an orthosis is necessary, and the factors (positive and negative) that will influence the eventual outcome of the orthotic intervention. Communication is the foundation for effective teaming.

The orthotist is responsible for recommending and providing the ideal orthosis to treat a patient's spinal condition. A properly fitted spinal orthosis does not inflect pain or cause skin breakdown. Patients and caregivers using these orthoses, as members of the team, must clearly understand why an orthosis is being prescribed and what impact the orthosis will have on daily function and mobility. Regularly scheduled follow-up appointments are necessary so that the orthotist can adjust the orthosis should technical errors come to light or the patient's status change over time. Recognition of potential problems before they develop can only enhance outcome.

Rehabilitation professionals who work with patients using spinal orthoses are responsible for creating rehabilitative programs that respect and facilitate the use of spinal orthoses. To accomplish this, therapists must understand how the orthosis is designed to stabilize or support the spine. Open communication between rehabilitation professionals and the orthotist is essential so that the goals of the orthosis and rehabilitation are supportive and any problems or questions are quickly addressed.

Consistent clinical evidence has shown that spinal orthoses are effective in the nonsurgical and postoperative care of many types of spinal disorders. Research in biomechanical design and engineering has advanced understanding of how spinal orthoses work, why they work, and how their use can be optimized. Comparative studies have begun to identify differences in efficacy and outcomes of various LSO, TLSO, cervical orthotic, and CTO devices. The design of spinal orthoses will be refined and improved as research continues in this important area.

The natural history of many spinal disorders managed with orthoses is not well understood and warrants further epidemiological study. The impact of orthoses on the progression or resolution of the disorder also requires further clinical study. The results of these types of studies can only enhance the clinical team's confidence in their recommendations and their ability to predict outcomes of orthotic treatment. Clinicians should be aware that, among the many orthoses that are currently produced and mass marketed, some devices are not well supported by scientific research. Rehabilitation professionals, as advocates for their patients, should be informed and critical consumers.

This chapter has provided an overview of the major types of spinal orthoses that may be encountered by health professionals who work in acute care and various rehabilitation settings. We have also discussed many factors that facilitate and inhibit successful orthotic outcome. Recognition of the importance of fit, proper donning technique, the need for follow-up and maintenance, and the importance of education and compliance can only enhance the success of orthotic intervention. Failure to recognize and act on these issues compromises the rehabilitation process and can lead to serious secondary problems, complications, or surgical failure, as if the patient with spinal disorder or injury had no orthosis at all.

REFERENCES

1. American Academy of Orthopaedic Surgeons. *Atlas of Orthopaedic Appliances.* Ann Arbor, MI: Edwards Bros., 1952. pp. 180-187.
2. Andry N. *Orthopaedia.* Philadelphia: J.B. Lippincott, 1961 (facsimile reproduction 1st ed in English, London: 1743).
3. Havey R, Gavin TM, Patwardhan AG, et al. A reliable and accurate method of measuring orthosis wearing time. *Spine* 2002;27(2):211-214.
4. Cantor JB, Lebwohl NH, Garvey T, Eismont FJ. Nonoperative management of stable thoracolumbar burst fractures with early ambulation and bracing. *Spine* 1993;18(8):971-976.
5. Chow GH, Nelson BJ, Gebhard JS, et al. Functional outcome of thoracolumbar burst fractures managed with hyperextension casting or bracing and early mobilization. *Spine* 1996;21(18):2170-2175.
6. Mumford J, Weinstein JN, Spratt KF, Goel VK. Thoracolumbar burst fractures. The clinical efficacy and outcome of nonoperative management. *Spine* 1993;18(8): 955-970.
7. Tropiano P, Huang RC, Louis CA, et al. Functional and radiographic outcome of thoracolumbar and lumbar burst fractures managed by closed orthopaedic reduction and casting. *Spine* 2003;28(21):2459-2465.
8. Reid DC, Hu R, Davis LA, Saboe LA. The nonoperative treatment of burst fractures of the thoracolumbar junction. *J Trauma* 1988;28(8):1188-1194.
9. Weinstein JN, Collalto P, Lehmann TR. Thoracolumbar "burst" fractures treated conservatively: a long-term follow-up. *Spine* 1988;13(1):33-38.
10. Andersson GB, Brown MD, Dvorak J, et al. Consensus summary of the diagnosis and treatment of lumbar disc herniation. *Spine* 1996;21(24 Suppl):75S-78S.
11. Rohlmann A, Bergmann G, Graichen F, Neff G. Braces do not reduce loads on internal spinal fixation devices. *Clin Biomech* 1999;14(2):97-102.
12. Buchalter D, Kahanovitz N, Viola K, et al. Three-dimensional spinal motion measurements. Part 2: a noninvasive assessment of lumbar brace immobilization of the spine. *J Spinal Disord* 1988;1(4):284-286.
13. Gavin TM, Boscardin JB, Patwardhan AG, et al. Preliminary results of orthotic treatment for chronic low back pain. *J Prosthet Orthot* 1993;5(1):5-9.
14. Gavin TM, Patwardhan AG, Bunch WH, et al. Principles and components of spinal orthoses. In American Academy of Orthopaedic Surgeons (eds), *Atlas of Orthoses and Assistive Devices,* 3rd ed. St Louis: Mosby-Yearbook, 1993. pp. 155-194.
15. Norton PL, Brown T. The immobilizing efficiency of back braces; their effect on the posture and motion of the lumbosacral spine. *J Bone Joint Surg Am* 1957;39A:111-139.
16. Fishman S, Berger N, Edelstein JE, Springer W. Spinal orthoses. In American Academy of Orthopedic Surgeons (eds), *Atlas of Orthotics, Biomechanical Principles and Applications,* 2nd ed. St. Louis: Mosby, 1985.
17. Nachemson AL. Orthotic treatment for injuries and diseases of the spinal column. *Phys Med Rehabil Clin N Am* 1987; 1:22-24.
18. Williams PC. Lesions of the lumbosacral spine—lordosis brace. *J Bone Joint Surg Am* 1937;19:702.

19. Jewett EL. Hyperextension back brace. *J Bone Joint Surg Am* 1937;19:1128.
20. Patwardhan AG, Gavin TM, Slosar P, Lorenz MA. Stabilization of fractures of the thoracolumbar spine. In Lorenz MA, Akbarnia B (eds), *Spine: State of the Art Reviews: Fracture-Dislocation,* 1993;7(2):203-222.
21. Perry J. The use of external support in the treatment of low back pain. *J Bone Joint Surg Am* 1970;52-A(7):1440-1442.
22. Vander Kooi D, Abad G, Basford JR, et al. Lumbar spine stabilization with a thoracolumbosacral orthosis: evaluation with video fluoroscopy. *Spine* 2004;29(1):100-104.
23. Fidler MW, Plasmans CM. The effect of four types of support on the segmental mobility of the lumbosacral spine. *J Bone Joint Surg* 1983;65(7):943-947.
24. Lantz SA, Schultz AB. Lumbar spine orthosis wearing—I. Restriction of gross body motions. *Spine* 1986;11(8):834-837.
25. Nagel DA, Koogle TA, Piziali RL, Perkash I. Stability of the upper lumbar spine following progressive disruptions and the application of individual internal and external fixation devices. *J Bone Joint Surg Am* 1981;63(1):62-70.
26. Norton PL, Brown T. The immobilizing efficiency of back braces; their effect on the posture and motion of the lumbosacral spine. *J Bone Joint Surg* 1957;39A:111-139.
27. Lumsden RM, Morris JM. An in vivo study of axial rotation and immobilization at the lumbosacral joint. *J Bone Joint Surg* 1968;50(8):1591-1602.
28. Patwardhan AG, Li S, Gavin TM, et al. Orthotic stabilization of thoracolumbar injuries—a biomechanical analysis of the Jewett hyperextension orthosis. *Spine* 1990;15(7):654-661.
29. Denis F. The three-column spine and its significance in the classification of acute thoracolumbar spinal injuries. *Spine* 1983;8(8):817-831.
30. Gavin TM, Shurr D, Patwardhan AG. Orthotic treatment of spinal disorders. In Weinstein SL (ed), *The Pediatric Spine,* vol 2. New York: Raven Press, 2000. pp. 1795-1828.
31. Ferguson RL, Allen BL. An algorithm for the treatment of unstable thoracolumbar fractures. *Orthop Clin North Am* 1986;17(1):105-112.
32. Daffner RH, Deeb ZL, Goldberg AL, et al. The radiologic assessment of post-traumatic vertebral stability. *Skeletal Radiol* 1990;19(2):103-108.
33. Whitesides TE. Traumatic kyphosis of the thoracolumbar spine. *Clin Orthop* 1977;Oct(128):78-92.
34. White AA, Panjabi MM. *Clinical Biomechanics of the Spine,* 2nd ed. Philadelphia: J.B. Lippincott, 1990.
35. Lindahl S, Willen J, Nordwall A, Irstam L. The crush-cleavage fracture: a "new" thoracolumbar unstable fracture. *Spine* 1983;8(6):559-569.
36. Farcy JP, Weidenbaum M, Glassman SD. Sagittal index in management of thoracolumbar burst fractures. *Spine* 1990;15(9):958-965.
37. Roy-Camille R, Lelievre JF. Pseudarthrosis of the dorso-lumbar vertebrae. *Rev Chir Orthop Reparatrice Appar Mot* 1975;61(3):249-257.
38. Holdsworth F. Fractures, dislocations, and fracture-dislocations of the spine. *J Bone Joint Surg* 1970;52(8):1534-1551.
39. Willen J, Anderson J, Toomoka K, Singer K. The natural history of burst fractures at the thoracolumbar junction. *J Spinal Disord* 1990;3(1):39-46.
40. Gertzbein SD, Crowe PJ, Fazl M, et al. Canal clearance in burst fractures using the AO internal fixator. *Spine* 1992;17(5):558-560.
41. McEvoy RD, Bradford DS. The management of burst fractures of the thoracic and lumbar spine. Experience in 53 patients. *Spine* 1985;10(7):631-637.
42. McAfee PC, Yuan HA, Lasda NA. The unstable burst fracture. *Spine* 1982;7(4):365-373.
43. Slosar PJ, Patwardhan AG, Lorenz M, et al. Instability of the lumbar burst fracture and limitations of transpedicular instrumentation. *Spine* 1995;20(13):1452-1461.
44. Kilcoyne RF, Mack LA, King HA, et al. Thoracolumbar spine injuries associated with vertical plunges: reappraisal with computed tomography. *Radiology* 1983;146(1):137-140.
45. Argenson C, de Peretti F. Injury of the spine; diagnosis, development, prognosis. *Rev Prat* 1993;43(1):105-12.
46. Argenson C, Dintimille H. Unstable fractures of the spine. III. Instability. B. Experimental instability. Experimental traumatic lesions of the spine in monkeys. *Rev Chir Orthop Reparatrice Appar Mot* 1977;63(5):430-431.
47. Knight RQ. Comparison of operative versus nonoperative treatment of lumbar burst fractures. *Clin Orthop* 1993;Aug(293):112-121.
48. Shen WJ, Liu TJ, Shen YS. Nonoperative treatment versus posterior fixation for thoracolumbar junction burst fractures without neurologic deficit. *Spine* 2001;26(9):1038-1045.
49. Wood K, Butterman G, Mehbod A, et al. Operative compared with nonoperative treatment of a thoracolumbar burst fracture without neurological deficit. A prospective, randomized study. *J Bone Joint Surg* 2003;85-A(5):773-781.
50. Chance GQ. Note on a type of flexion fracture of the spine. *Br J Radiol* 1948;2:452.
51. Ferguson RL, Tencer AF, Woodard P, Allen BL. Biomechanical comparisons of spinal fracture models and the stabilizing effects of posterior instrumentations. *Spine* 1988;13(5): 453-460.
52. U.S. Department of Labor Bureau of Labor Statistics. Table R32. *Number of nonfatal occupational injuries and illnesses involving days away from work by event or exposure leading to injury or illness and selected parts of body affected by injury or illness.* Washington, DC: U.S. Department of Labor Bureau of Labor Statistics, 1998.
53. Willner S. Effect of a rigid brace on back pain. *Acta Orthop Scand* 1985;56(1):40-42.
54. Willner S. Test instrument for predicting the effect of rigid braces in chronic low back pain. *Prosthet Orthot Int* 1990;14(1):22-26.
55. Nachemson A, Elfstrom G. In vivo wireless telemetry of axial forces in Harrington distraction rods in patients with idiopathic scoliosis. *J Bone Joint Surg* 1971;53A(3):445-465.
56. Schimandle JH, Weigel M, Edwards CC. Indications for thigh cuff bracing following instrumented lumbosacral fusions. Presented at the eighth annual meeting of the North American Spine Society, San Diego, October 1993.
57. Gavin TM, Carandang G, Havey R, et al. Biomechanical analysis of cervical orthoses in flexion and extension: a comparison of cervical collars and cervical thoracic orthoses. *J Rehab Res Dev* 2003;40(6):527-538.
58. Johnson RM, Hart DL, Simmons EF, et al. Cervical orthoses: a study comparing their effectiveness in restricting cervical

motion in normal subjects. *J Bone Joint Surg* 1977;59(3): 332-339.

59. Askins V, Eismont FJ. Efficacy of five cervical orthoses in restricting cervical motion: a comparison study. *Spine* 1997;22(11):1193-1198.
60. King A. Spinal column trauma. In Myers MH (ed), *The Multiply Injured Patient with Complex Fractures.* Philadelphia: Lea & Febiger, 1984.
61. Wang GJ, Moskal JT, Albert T, et al. The effect of halo-vest length on stability of the cervical spine. *J Bone Joint Surg* 1988;70(3):357-360.
62. Perry JP, Nickel VL. Total cervical spine fusion for neck paralysis. *J Bone Joint Surg* 1959;41A:37-60.
63. Garfin SR, Botte MJ, Centeno RS, Nickel VL. Osteology of the skull as it affects halo pin placement. *Spine* 1985;10(8): 696-698.
64. Botte MJ, Byrne TP, Abrams RA, Garfin SR. The halo skeletal fixator: current concepts of application and maintenance. *Orthopedics* 1995;18(5):463-471.
65. Triggs KJ, Ballock RT, Lee TQ, et al. The effect of angled insertion on halo pin fixation. *Spine* 1989;14(8):781-783.
66. Wetzel FT, Dunsieth NW, Kuhlengel KR, Paul EM. The effectiveness of the cervical halo: open versus closed ring, a preliminary report. *Paraplegia* 1995;33(2):110-115.
67. Fisher SV. Proper fitting of the cervical orthosis. *Arch Phys Med Rehab* 1978;59(11):505-507.
68. Plaisier B, Gabram SG, Schwartz RJ, Jacobs LM. Prospective evaluation of craniofacial pressure in four different cervical orthoses. *J Trauma* 1994;37(5):714-720.
69. Patwardhan AG, Havey RM, Meade KP, et al. A follower load increases the load-carrying capacity of the lumbar spine in compression. *Spine* 1999;24(10):1003-1009.

16

Orthotics and Therapeutic Interventions in the Management of Scoliosis

THOMAS M. HARRIGAN

LEARNING OBJECTIVES

On completion of this chapter, the reader will be able to do the following:

1. Demonstrate an understanding of the terminology and classification system for describing scoliosis.
2. Understand the natural history of idiopathic scoliosis.
3. Understand the treatment options available to address the impairments resulting from scoliosis.
4. Describe the biomechanics that lead to scoliotic deformity.
5. State the goals for orthotic intervention for both idiopathic and neuromuscular scoliosis.
6. Describe and demonstrate the clinical evaluation of the scoliotic patient.
7. Describe the role of exercise and formulate goals in the treatment of any impairments resulting from scoliosis.

This chapter provides insight into the diagnosis and treatment of idiopathic and neuromuscular scoliosis. Thorough knowledge of the natural history of this disease is critical to fully understanding the process of orthotic prescription for persons with scoliosis. The roles of the orthotist and therapist, as well as the goals of bracing and exercise, are discussed. The chapter also explores the evaluation process and the options for conservative and surgical management of individuals with scoliosis.

HISTORY OF SPINAL TRACTION AND BRACING

With all the advances in medical technology, people may forget that many of today's most common ailments have been treated for thousands of years. Hippocrates (born in 460 BC) first described the signs and symptoms of scoliosis 2400 years ago and noted that curvature of the spine occurred even in individuals who were apparently in good health.[1] Hippocrates also described the use of spinal traction to straighten the spine in scoliosis, a concept that may have its roots in ancient Egypt. Using traction for spinal problems led to numerous surgical and nonsurgical treatment approaches. Galen (131-200 AD) first used the terms *scoliosis, kyphosis,* and *lordosis*; he also used traction in the treatment of this deformity.

In 1874 Sayre first applied a cast to a patient with spinal deformity who was under traction. In 1895 Brackett and Bradford developed a distraction frame that was the precursor to the currently used Risser casting frame.[2,3] Hibbs and Risser developed and used hinged or turnbuckle casts in the 1920s.[4]

Milwaukee Brace

In 1944 the Milwaukee brace was developed by Blount and Schmidt. The Milwaukee brace, a cervicothoracolumbosacral orthosis (CTLSO), was initially employed as a postoperative modality but soon found a more important role. Since 1954 it has been used in the nonoperative treatment of idiopathic scoliosis.[5] The brace consists of a pelvic section, which helps to reduce lumbar lordosis, and an attached "superstructure." The superstructure comprises three metal uprights that are attached to a neck ring superiorly. It provides an end point of control to make the spine structurally more rigid and better aligned and, importantly, a means of attachment for the spinal pads (Figure 16-1). This style is considered a full-time brace; in other words, it is prescribed to be worn 23 hours a day. The initial design incorporated distraction; however, this has since been modified secondary to problems with malocclusion of the jaw. Subsequent to the Milwaukee brace, various low-profile thoracolumbosacral orthoses (TLSOs) have been introduced. Most of these spinal orthoses are named for the city where they were developed (e.g., Boston brace, Miami orthosis, Wilmington brace, Lyon brace). These spinal orthoses share one characteristic: All

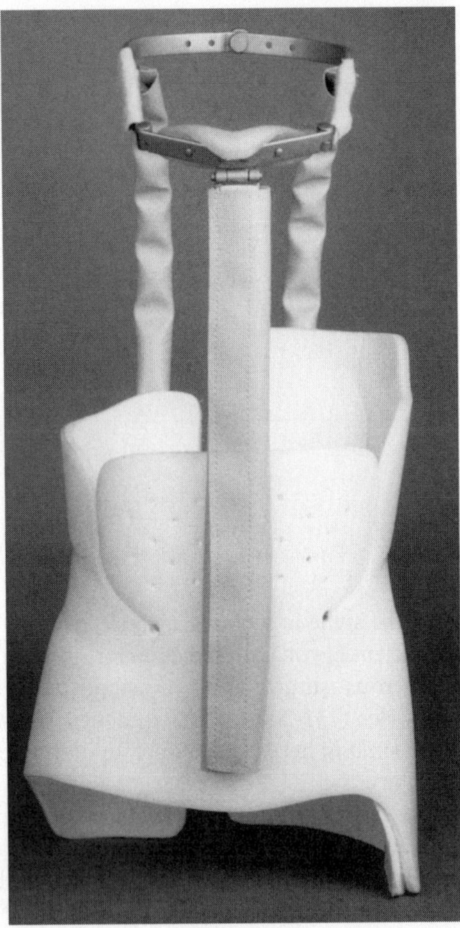

Figure 16-1
Milwaukee brace. Note the tightly fitting pelvic section and the superstructure with its ringlike chin and occipital supports.

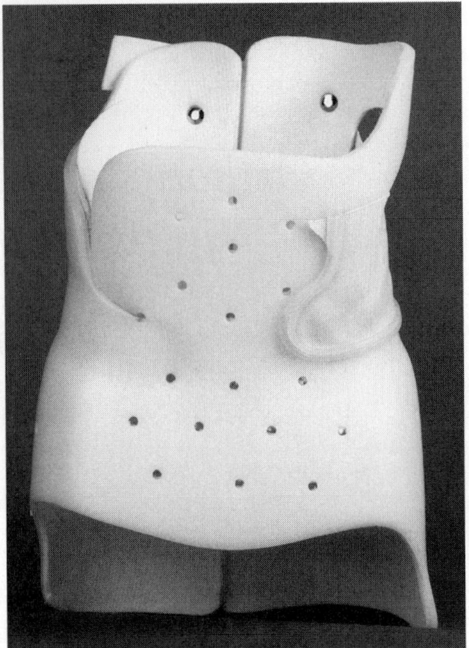

Figure 16-2
An example of the Boston brace, designed for patients with a thoracic curve.

control the alignment of the thoracolumbosacral spine but have no superstructure.

Boston Brace

The Boston brace was developed in the 1970s by Hall and Miller.[7] Like the Milwaukee brace, the Boston brace is prescribed in most treatment centers to be worn full time. Although other biomechanically sound brace systems function well in controlling curve progression, the Boston brace system is more globally accepted (Figure 16-2). As a result of its frequent use, much more long-term data are available to substantiate the merits of the Boston brace than are available for other orthoses.[8-10] Despite the differences in brace name and style, most TLSOs designed for individuals with scoliosis follow similar principles of prescription, wearing schedules, and discontinuance.

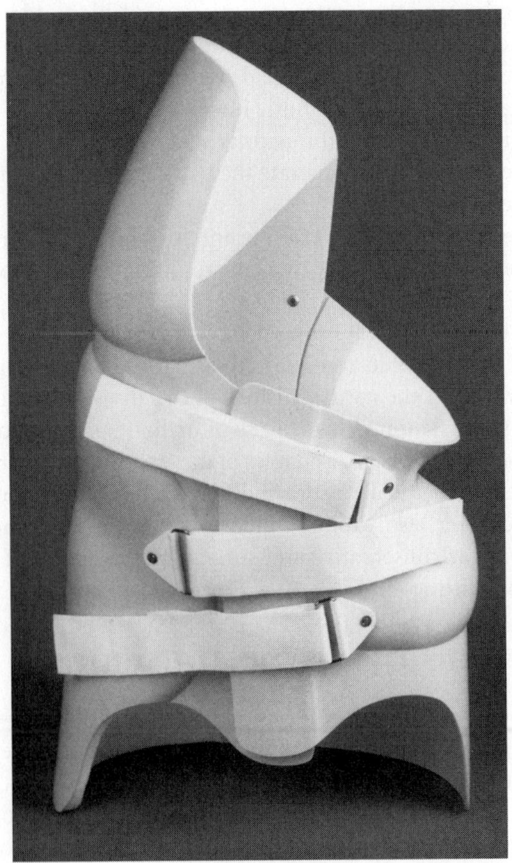

Figure 16-3
An example of the Charleston bending brace, designed for nocturnal use only.

Nocturnal Orthoses for Scoliosis

Another type of TLSO, which is prescribed to address idiopathic scoliosis, is the nocturnal orthosis. As the name

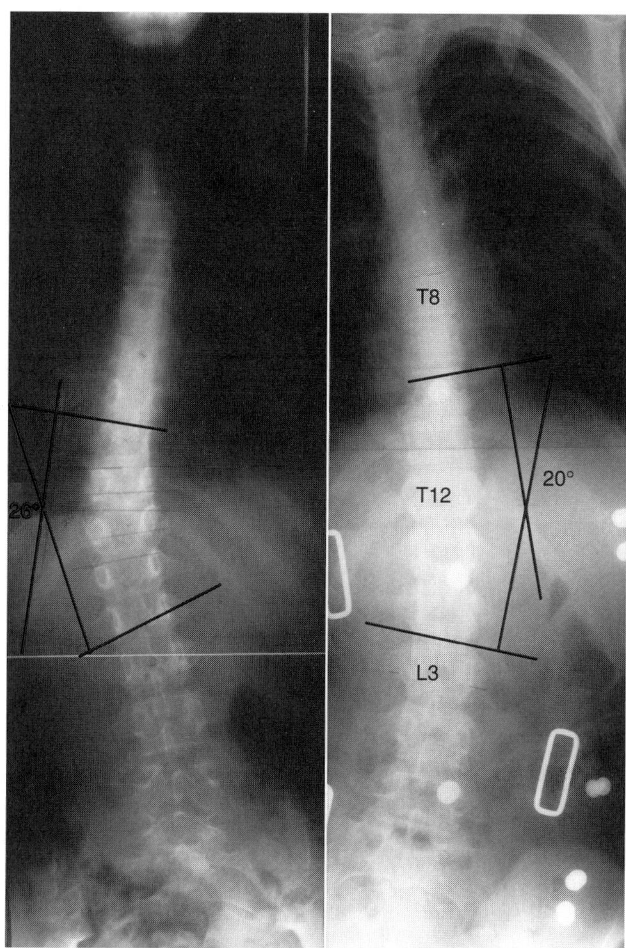

Figure 16-4
*The Charleston bending brace uses the mechanics of long lever arms to unbend a curve; this is possible only in a brace worn solely in a recumbent position. This radiograph shows a 26-degree left thoracolumbar curve (**A**) that is reversed entirely in the brace (**B**). In this case the brace produces a highly effective result; it induces a 20-degree right thoracolumbar curve.*

implies, it is worn only during sleep hours. Two popular nocturnal-only designs are the Providence and the Charleston braces (Figure 16-3). The Charleston bending brace is designed to reverse or unbend the curvature. The most recent literature suggests that the efficacy of this brace can alter curve progression in individuals with single-curve patterns with a magnitude of 36 degrees or less.[11-13] The Charleston orthosis seeks to reverse the curve by positioning the individual in a position of maximum side bending. In most cases the brace can reduce a single curve to 0 degrees or even induce a curve in the opposite direction (Figure 16-4).

TERMINOLOGY AND CLASSIFICATION OF SCOLIOSIS

The Scoliosis Research Society has adopted a set of terms and definitions to describe the multitude of spinal conditions that can lead to scoliosis.[14-16] Curves can be described either by etiology of the structural changes (Box 16-1) or by the spinal level of the anatomical apex of the curve. In a cervical scoliosis, the apex of the curve is at or between the vertebral body of C1 and C6. In a cervicothoracic curve, the apex is at C7, C8, or T1. A thoracic curve has an apex at or between T2 and T11. A thoracolumbar curve reaches its apex at the T12 or L1 vertebral body. A lumbar curve occurs at L2, L3, or L4, whereas a lumbosacral curve reaches its apex at L5 or S1. Numerous descriptive terms are also used in the diagnosis, evaluation, and management of scoliosis

Box 16-1 *Classification System for Idiopathic and Neuromuscular Structural Scoliosis*

IDIOPATHIC
Infantile (0-3 years)
Resolving
Progressive

Juvenile (3-10 years)

Adolescent (older than 10 years)

NEUROMUSCULAR
Neuropathic
Upper motor neuron
- Cerebral palsy
- Spinocerebellar degeneration
- Friedreich's ataxia
- Charcot-Marie-Tooth disease
- Roussy-Lévy disease
- Syringomyelia
- Spinal cord tumor
- Spinal cord trauma
- Other

Lower motor neuron
- Poliomyelitis
- Other viral myelitides
- Trauma
- Spinal muscular atrophy
- Werdnig-Hoffmann disease
- Kugelberg-Welander disease
- Myelomeningocele (paralytic)
- Dysautonomia (Riley-Day syndrome)
- Other

Myopathic
Arthrogryposis
Muscular dystrophy
- Duchenne's (pseudohypertrophy)
- Limb-girdle
- Fiber-type disproportion

Congenital hypotonia
Myotonic dystrophica
Other

(Table 16-1). These standards and definitions are used throughout this chapter.

Scoliosis can also be described by etiology. A child or adolescent who develops scoliosis after relatively typical growth and development is diagnosed as having *idiopathic scoliosis.* An individual who develops scoliosis as a secondary complication of nervous system or muscle disease is described as having *neuromuscular scoliosis.*

Table 16-1
Glossary and Definitions of Terms in Scoliosis

Term	*Definition*
Adolescent scoliosis	Spinal curvature presenting at or about the onset of puberty and before maturity
Adult scoliosis	Spinal curvature that develops after skeletal maturity
Angle of thoracic	The angle between the horizontal plane and inclination plane across the posterior rib cage at the greatest prominence of a rib hump, assessed with the trunk flexed 90 degrees at the hips
Apical vertebra	The most rotated vertebra in a curve; the most deviated vertebra from the vertical axis of the patient
Body alignment	1. Alignment of the midpoint of the occiput over the sacrum in the same vertical plane as the shoulders over the hips
	2. In radiography, when the sum of the angular deviations of the spine in one direction is equal to that in the opposite direction (also described as balance or compensation)
Café au lait spots	Light-brown, irregular areas of skin pigmentation; if they are sufficient in number and have smooth margins, they suggest neurofibromatosis
Cobb angle or method	On radiograph, the uppermost and lowermost vertebrae in the curve are identified; a perpendicular line (curve measurement) is drawn from the transverse axes of these vertebrae, and the angle formed at their intersection (Cobb angle) measures the severity of the curve; if vertebral end plates are poorly visualized, a line through the bottom or top of the pedicles can be used
Compensatory curve	A curve, which can be structural, above or below the major curve that tends to maintain normal body alignment
Congenital scoliosis	Scoliosis due to congenitally anomalous vertebral development
Double major scoliosis	Scoliosis with two structural curves
Double thoracic curves	Two structural curves within the thoracic spine
End vertebra	1. Uppermost vertebra of a curve, the superior surface of which tilts maximally toward the concavity of the curve
	2. The most caudal vertebra, the inferior surface of which tilts maximally toward the concavity of the curve
Fractional curve	Compensatory curve that is incomplete because it returns to the erect; its only horizontal vertebra is its caudad or cephalad one
Full curve	Curve in which the only horizontal vertebra is at the apex
Gibbus	Sharply angular kyphos
Hyperkyphosis	Sagittal alignment of the thoracic spine in which more than the normal amount of kyphosis is present (a kyphos)
Hypokyphosis	Sagittal alignment of the thoracic spine in which less than the normal amount of kyphosis is present but not so severe as to be lordotic

Continued

Table 16-1
Glossary and Definitions of Terms in Scoliosis—cont'd

Term	*Definition*
Hysterical scoliosis	Nonstructural deformity of the spine that develops as a manifestation of a conversion reaction
Idiopathic scoliosis	Structural spinal curvature for which no cause is established
Iliac epiphysis or apophysis	Epiphysis along the wing of an ilium
Inclinometer	Instrument used to measure the angle of thoracic inclination or rib hump
Infantile scoliosis	Spinal curvature that develops during the first 3 yrs of life
Juvenile scoliosis	Spinal curvature that develops between the skeletal age of 3 yrs and the onset of puberty (10 yrs)
Kyphos	Change in alignment of a segment of the spine in the sagittal plane that increases the posterior convex angulation; an abnormally increased kyphosis
Kyphoscoliosis	Spine with scoliosis and a true hyperkyphosis; a rotatory deformity with only apparent kyphosis should not be described by this term
Kyphosing scoliosis	Scoliosis with marked rotation such that lateral bending of the rotated spine mimics kyphosis
Lordoscoliosis	Scoliosis associated with an abnormal anterior angulation in the sagittal plane
Major curve	Term used to designate the largest structural curve
Minor curve	Term used to refer to the smallest curve, which is always more flexible than the major curve
Nonstructural curve	Curve that has no structural component and that corrects or overcorrects on recumbent side-bending radiographs
Pelvic obliquity	Deviation of the pelvis from the horizontal in the frontal plane; fixed pelvic obliquities can be attributable to contractures either above or below the pelvis
Primary curve	First or earliest of several curves to appear, if identifiable
Risser sign	Rating system used to indicate skeletal maturity, based on degree of ossification of the iliac epiphysis
Rotational prominence	In the forward-bending position, the thoracic prominence on one side is usually due to vertebral rotation, causing rib prominence; in the lumbar spine, the prominence is usually due to rotation of the lumbar vertebrae
Skeletal age (bone age)	Age obtained by comparing an anteroposterior radiograph of the left hand and wrist with the standards of Greulich and Pyle's atlas
Structural curve	Segment of the spine with a lateral curvature that lacks normal flexibility; radiographically, it is identified by the complete lack of a curve on a supine film or by the failure to demonstrate complete segmental mobility on supine side-bending films
Vertebral end plates	Superior and inferior plates of cortical bone of the vertebral body adjacent to the intervertebral disk
Vertebral growth plate	Cartilaginous surface covering the top and bottom of a vertebral body, which is responsible for linear growth of the vertebra
Vertebral ring apophyses	Most reliable index of vertebral immaturity, seen best in lateral radiographs or in the lumbar region in side-bending anteroposterior views

TESTS AND MEASURES USED IN THE CLINICAL EXAMINATION

Clinical examination of individuals with scoliosis begins with a careful assessment of posture and key anthropometric characteristics. With the patient standing in a relaxed or typical posture, the orthotist or therapist notes frontal plane symmetry or asymmetry and alignment of the trunk, typical head and neck position, shoulder height, and scapular alignment. The fullness or relative muscle bulk in the muscles of the shoulder girdle and of the paraspinal muscle groups is noted, as is the shape of the chest wall. Symmetry or asymmetry of the pelvis is indicated by comparing positions of the height of the posterior-superior iliac spine (PSIS) and iliac crest. Leg length is assessed by observing symmetry of left and right popliteal creases while both knees are fully extended and the feet are flat on the floor. Postural assessment in the sagittal plane includes observation and measurement of cervical and lumbar lordosis as well as thoracic and sacral kyphosis.

Truncal decompensation (trunk balance) describes the relative position of the head with respect to the sacrum: the horizontal distance between a plumb line dropped from the center of the occiput and a plumb line dropped from the spinous process of the first sacral vertebra (Figure 16-5). The Adams test, which assesses rotation deformity, is an important component of the examination. In this functional test, the patient stands with the knees straight, feet together, and hands together with palms and fingers in opposition and then bends forward from the waist (Figure 16-6). The examiner views the spine from anterior, posterior, and lateral points of view so that symmetry or asymmetry and rotation of the cervical, thoracic, and lumbar spine can be fully assessed. A scoliometer is a tool that, when placed at the point of maximal prominence, measures the degree of rotational deformity when it is placed at the position of maximal prominence (Figure 16-7).

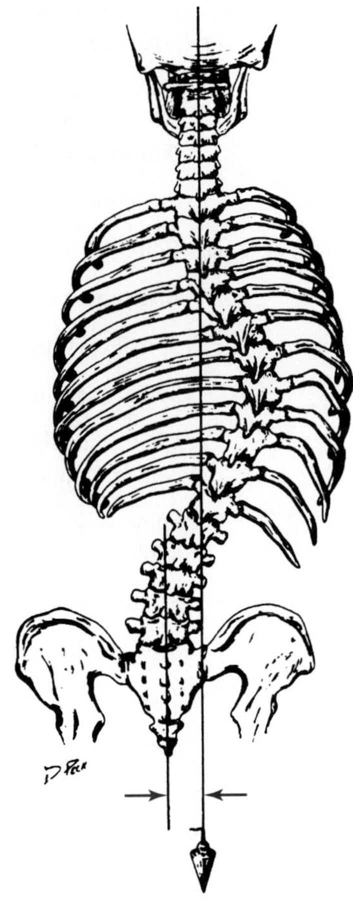

Figure 16-5
In this diagram of a right thoracic curve, the occiput is aligned well to the right of the first sacral spinous process. Because of its relative position to the right with respect to S1, the patient would be described as being decompensated to the right.

The flexibility of the spinal deformity is also assessed in the Adams test maximum trunk flexion position. The examiner stabilizes the patient's pelvis and then asks the patient to side bend to the left and then to the right, applying a gentle passive force at the end of the active range. This provides information about the extent of unbending and derotation that may be possible for the patient's particular curve. The relative stiffness of the curve provides information about the structural features of the deformity.

The accuracy of the forward bend test can be influenced by limitations in muscle length, especially if hamstring or erector spinae tightness is present.[17] An assessment of lower extremity ROM as part of the evaluation, including special tests (e.g., the Thomas test for hip flexion tightness or contracture and straight leg raise testing for hamstring length), is important. Limitations in normal ROM of the lower extremities often influence brace wear and comfort. For example, the pelvic modules for the Milwaukee or Boston braces are fabricated with 16 degrees of lordosis. While wearing the brace, the patient's pelvis is positioned in a posterior pelvic tilt. If significant tightness of the iliopsoas muscle is present, individuals may not be able to achieve the desired pelvic position with a comfortable erect standing posture. Instead, they will stand with slight knee flexion to relieve tension on the hip flexor group and then attempt to align their center of mass by extending their trunk over the superior-posterior edge of the brace. In addition to being uncomfortable, this posture within the orthosis may induce hypokyphosis.[18]

Other measurements taken during the initial evaluation include leg length, muscle girth, muscle strength of the trunk and lower extremities, and neurological assessment, including a check of abdominal reflexes. Absent or diminished reflexes may be a sign of intraspinal pathology.[19] Evaluation of the

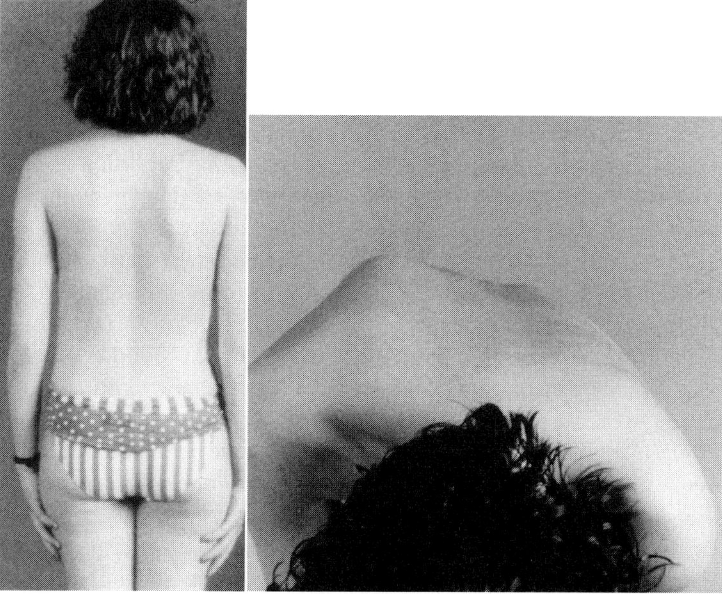

Figure 16-6
In the Adams test of maximum trunk flexion, the patient bends forward from the waist, keeping the knees straight and feet flat on the floor. A spine that appears relatively symmetric in quiet standing is obviously asymmetric once the patient with idiopathic scoliosis bends forward. Rib hump is a consequence of abnormal rotation of the involved vertebral bodies. The examiner determines the point of maximum prominence by observing from the front, from behind, and from each side.

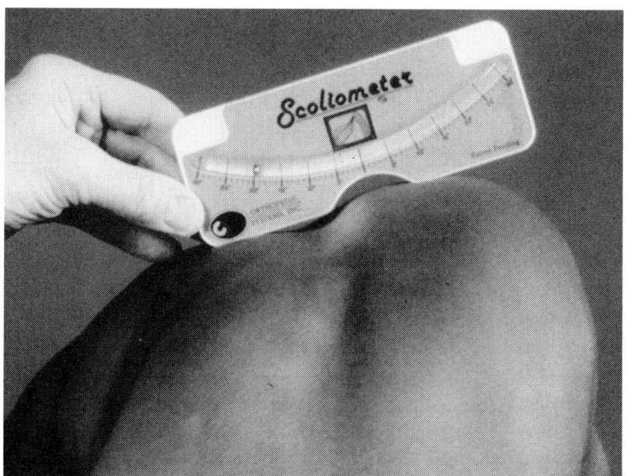

Figure 16-7
A scoliometer can be used to measure the degree of rotation of thoracic or lumbar curves. The device is placed on the most rotated part of the curve, as determined by observation in the Adams test of maximum trunk flexion. The scoliometer is a gauged device that functions like a builder's level.

skin and soft tissue is also necessary to determine if underlying neurological conditions such as neurofibromatosis or myelodysplasia, which present with various skin irregularities (e.g., café au lait skin pigmentation, hair patches over the spine), are present. Box 16-2 presents a summary of the clinical evaluation.

Box 16-2 *Summary of Clinical Examination*

- Postural assessment
- Flexibility of spinal deformity
- Range of motion of trunk and lower extremities
- Strength assessment of trunk and lower extremities
- Neurological assessment
- Skin/soft tissue assessment

IDIOPATHIC SCOLIOSIS

Factors that lead to the development of idiopathic scoliosis are not well understood. The possible role of genetic factors, growth velocity, musculoskeletal irregularities such as ligamentous imbalances across vertebral segments, muscle strength imbalances, vestibular and central nervous system dysfunction, and biochemical factors have all been explored, but no explanatory model has evolved.[20-28] Lonstein[19] suggested that the etiology of scoliosis must be multifactorial, with two underlying mechanisms at work—one related to curve development and the other related to curve progression. Each potential contributor that has been investigated (e.g., genetic, chemical, biomechanical, neuromuscular) may be involved, and the interrelationship of these factors determines whether a curve is progressive or nonprogressive.[19]

Prevalence and Natural History

Effective intervention and management of scoliosis are founded on understanding the prevalence and the natural history of the disease. Idiopathic scoliosis has been studied and documented for many years. Epidemiological studies have documented that, with few exceptions, the prevalence of scoliosis is constant worldwide.[29] Prevalence does vary by age group, type of scoliosis, and magnitude of curve. In their examination of school-aged children, Lonstein and colleagues[30] identified structural scoliosis in 1.1% of subjects. In studying the distribution of idiopathic scoliosis in a group of individuals categorized by age at onset, Risenborough and Wynne-Davies[31] reported that 0.5% were classified as having infantile scoliosis, 10.5% had juvenile onset, and 89% had onset in adolescence. The juvenile group is likely underrepresented, because many children are not carefully evaluated until they become adolescents. The distribution of curve magnitude also varies: The prevalence of "small" curves (between 10 and 20 degrees) is 20 to 30 per 1000, the prevalence of moderate curves (between 20 and 30 degrees) is 3 to 5 per 1000, and the prevalence of large curves (more than 30 degrees) is 2 to 3 per 1000 people.[27]

Studies of the *infantile idiopathic scoliosis* population (with onset between birth and 3 years of age) suggest a genetic tendency in the development of scoliosis. A gender difference is also seen in infantile scoliosis, with a greater incidence among male than female infants. The most common pattern is a left thoracic curve. Fortunately, the condition is quite rare and is usually self limiting, with 80% to 90% of the infantile scoliosis curves resolving spontaneously.[32,33] Infantile scoliosis can be divided into two types of curves: resolving or progressive. In 1972 Mehta[34] observed that progressive and resolving curves could be differentiated by examining the rib vertebral angle difference (RVAD). In a normal spine no difference is found between the left and right angles, and the relationship between rib and vertebra is symmetric. A child with scoliosis has asymmetry, and the RVAD is measured as the difference between the rib vertebral angle of the concave and convex ribs of the apical vertebra. Mehta also describes two phases of rib deformity. In phase I the convex rib head does not overlap the vertebral body, whereas in phase II an overlap can be seen. Resolving curves have a phase I configuration and an RVAD of less than 20 degrees.

Juvenile idiopathic scoliosis manifests between 4 and 10 years of age and accounts for between 11% and 16% of all idiopathic scoliosis. Prevalence varies by gender across age subgroups: Distribution is fairly equal among male and female children between 4 and 6 years, whereas it is more frequent in girls between 7 and 10 years of age. The most commonly observed pattern in juvenile idiopathic scoliosis is a right thoracic curve.[35]

In *adolescent idiopathic scoliosis,* the curve manifests after the age of 10 years. This is a fairly common condition, affecting approximately 1% of all children.[27,30] The prevalence of curves increases progressively in girls as the curve magnitude increases. The overall female/male ratio within this group is 3.6:1, but it increases to 6.4:1 when curve magnitude is 20 degrees or more.[29] The single right thoracic curve is the most common pattern among adolescents with idiopathic scoliosis.[36]

The most important predictors for curve progression identified to date include curve pattern, age, menarche status, and a positive Risser sign.[37-39] Curve flexibility and decompensation may be important, although the evidence is not conclusive. Lonstein and Carlson's work[37] examining the natural history of this condition has furthered the ability to predict the likelihood of progression (Tables 16-2 and 16-3).

Four factors are known to increase the risk for curve progression: a younger age at diagnosis, the occurrence of the initial curve before the onset of menstruation, an increase in the magnitude of the curve, and the presence of a double curve pattern. Individuals whose curves measure less than 30 degrees at skeletal maturity tend not to progress regardless of curve pattern. The amount of vertebral rotation appears to be related to further progression into adulthood. Curves of more than 30 degrees with apical vertebral rotation greater than 25% are twice as likely to progress. Thoracic curves that

Table 16-2
Incidence of Progression as It Relates to the Magnitude of the Curve and Risser Sign

Risser Sign	*Percentage of Curves That Progressed*	
	5- to 19-Degree Curves	*20- to 29-Degree Curves*
Grade 0 or 1	22	68
Grade 2, 3, or 4	1.6	23

From Lonstein JE, Carlson M. Prediction of curve progression in untreated scoliosis during growth. *J Bone Joint Surg Am* 1984;66A(7):1061-1071.

Table 16-3
Incidence of Progression as Related to Magnitude of the Curve and the Age of the Patient When First Seen

	*Percentage of Curves That Progressed**	
Age When First Seen (yr)	*5- to 19-Degree Curves*	*20- to 29-Degree Curves*
10 and younger	45 (38)	100 (10)†
11–12	23 (147)	61 (61)
13–14	8 (201)	37 (119)
16 and older	4 (67)	16 (84)

*Numbers in parentheses indicate the number of individuals in each group.
†This figure of 100% is on the basis of only 10 individuals.
From Lonstein JE, Carlson M. Prediction of curve progression in untreated scoliosis during growth. *J Bone Joint Surg Am* 1984;66A(7):1061-1071.

measure between 50 and 75 degrees progress the most rapidly, at rates of between 0.75% and 1% per year.[40]

Patient/Client Management

When a patient with scoliosis or other curvatures of the spine (ICD-9-CM codes: 737.1, kyphosis-acquired; 737.2, lordosis-acquired; or 737.3, kyphoscoliosis and scoliosis) is referred to an orthotist or physical therapist, the first step in the evaluation process is obtaining a *thorough* patient history. In addition to obtaining information such as general demographics (e.g., age, gender, education), social history (family and social support resources), school and leisure activities, growth and development (spinal maturity), living environment, general health status and overall health history, and current functional status, questions specific to spinal health should be posed. These include the following:

1. When was the curve first noticed (onset of the curve)?
2. Who made the initial diagnosis and what circumstances led to its diagnosis?
3. What are the results of any tests or measures that have already been performed?
4. What is the family's health history, especially related to spinal dysfunction?
5. What previous interventions (orthotic, exercise, or surgical) were performed and what were their outcomes?
6. Is pain present? If so, what is its nature and location?
7. What is the efficacy of pain management strategies?

A systems review for individuals with idiopathic scoliosis must include screening for impairments of cardiorespiratory, musculoskeletal, neuromuscular, and integumentary systems, as well as assessment of learning style, cognitive status, and overall affective/emotional function.

Use of Radiographs in Diagnosis and Treatment

Radiographs are essential clinical tools in diagnosis and treatment of idiopathic scoliosis. They are used to determine specifically the type and location of the curve and quantify its magnitude and the degree of rotation. Radiographs are also used to assess trunk balance or decompensation and determine skeletal age on the basis of either the Risser sign or wrist and hand bone age. Congenital spinal malformations are detected by close inspection of the films. Radiographs taken while the patient is in the orthosis allow the clinician to determine immediately the appropriateness of pad positions and overall efficacy in terms of curve reduction.

Several important prognostic indicators for curve progression in scoliosis are based on radiographs. The Risser sign describes skeletal maturity based on the degree of ossification of the epiphysis of the iliac crest. Ossification begins at the anterosuperior iliac spine and progresses posteriorly. The iliac crest is divided into four quarters, and the excursion or stage of maturity is designated as the amount of progression from the anterosuperior to the posterosuperior iliac spine. The curve magnitude is often measured using the Cobb technique (Figure 16-8). Bone age can be accurately determined by comparing the left wrist/hand radiograph with that of Greulich and Pyle's atlas,[41] and vertebral rota-

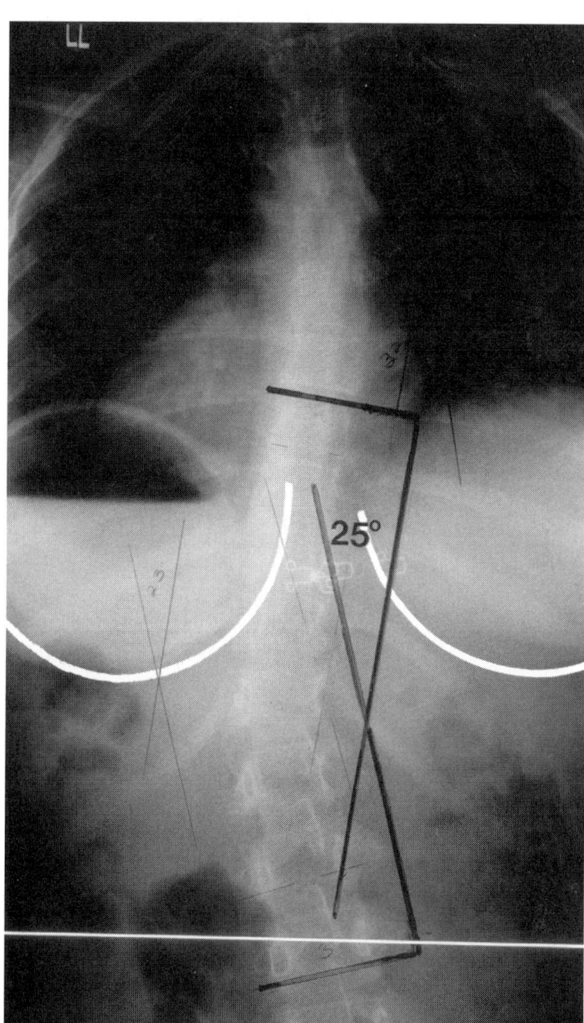

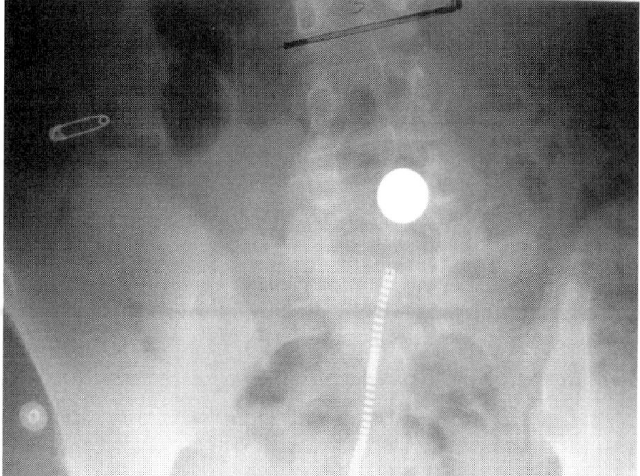

Figure 16-8

In the Cobb method of measuring curvature, a perpendicular line is drawn from the upper edge of the topmost vertebra that inclines most toward the concavity. A similar line is drawn from the inferior edge of the lowest vertebra with the most angulation toward the concavity. The angle at which these perpendicular lines intersect forms the Cobb angle. The apical vertebra does not enter into the measurement. The Cobb angle is usually measured directly on the radiograph.

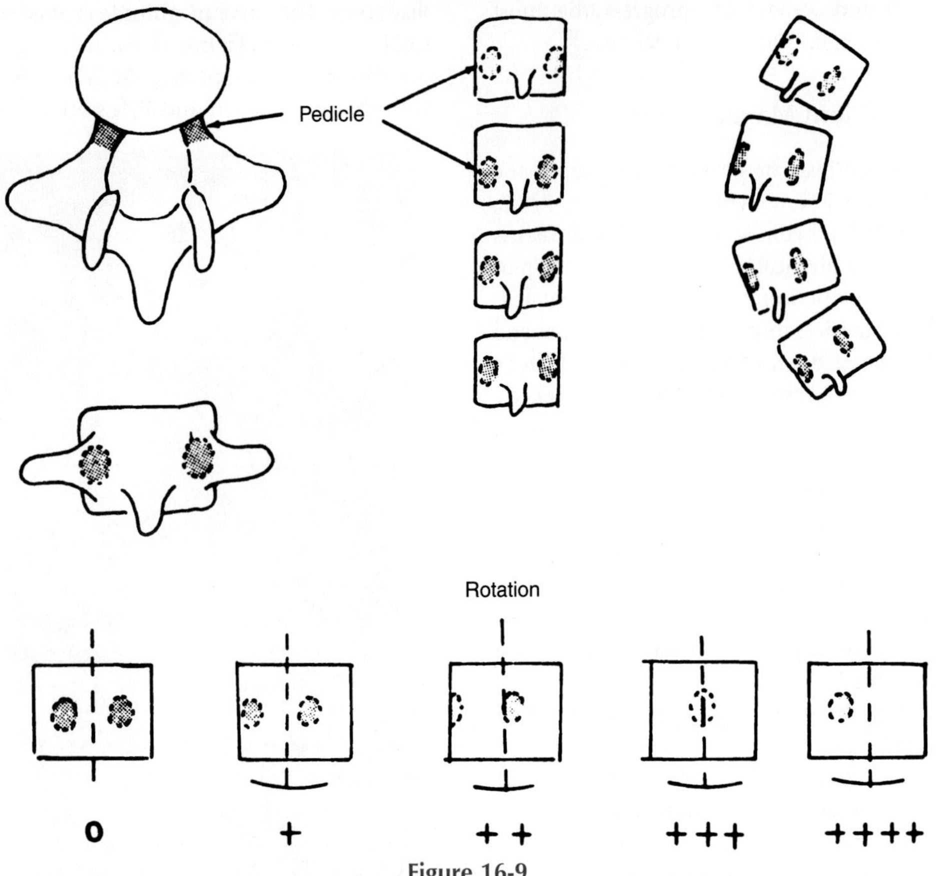

Figure 16-9

Radiographs are also used to measure vertebral rotation. The pedicles are visualized, and their relationship to the midline is rated on a scale of 0 (normal position) to ++++ (rotated past the midline position). Although this scale has not been standardized and is not used in all scoliosis clinics, it does provide a means of tracking relative curve progression over subsequent examinations. (From Calliet R. Scoliosis: Diagnosis and Management. *Philadelphia: F.A. Davis, 1975. p. 29.)*

tion can be graded using a system described by Nash and Moe[42] (Figure 16-9).

Other tests such as magnetic resonance imaging (MRI) are not routinely used in the assessment of scoliosis unless evaluative findings are inconsistent or complex. One indication for MRI or other special testing is a finding of asymmetric or diminished lower extremity and abdominal reflexes, and another is a suspicious or unusual curve pattern. Individuals with left thoracic curve patterns may be referred for MRI, because this group has a 20% incidence of intraspinal pathology (e.g., Arnold-Chiari malformation).[43]

NONSURGICAL INTERVENTIONS FOR IDIOPATHIC SCOLIOSIS

Information about the natural history of scoliosis assists the clinician in answering two important questions:

1. Is the curve likely to progress in a patient who has not yet reached skeletal maturity?
2. If a patient has reached skeletal maturity, will the curve progress into adulthood?

On the basis of the answers to these questions, the physician, orthotist, and therapist can choose one of three options:

1. Observe the curve's status carefully over time
2. Manage the patient's scoliosis nonoperatively with a spinal orthosis and exercise
3. Intervene surgically to correct the curve

Careful observation is most often the strategy chosen for individuals with curves of less than 25 degrees. Reevaluation is typically scheduled every 6 months. The tests and measures most often used include accurate recording of height and weight, radiography to assess curve progression, and an estimation of when skeletal maturity might be reached.

When a patient's curve progresses beyond 25 degrees or if the curve has increased 5 degrees or more over the 6-month interval, a spinal orthosis is prescribed and an exercise program is implemented. All skeletally immature children who initially present with a curve between 30 and 45 degrees are managed with an orthosis and exercise. Bracing is usually contraindicated for skeletally mature individuals, as well as for those who present with curves of more than 45 degrees or less than 25 degrees without documented progression. Use of an orthosis is also contraindicated in the presence of thoracic lordosis.[26] Depending on the location of the curve, the clinician will recommend either a Milwaukee brace (CTLSO) or a low-profile TLSO-style orthosis such as the Boston brace.

Although the efficacy of orthoses in the management of idiopathic scoliosis has been controversial, long-term and multicenter studies suggest that bracing is an effective intervention. In 1994 an important report by Lonstein and Winter[44] documented their experience in treating adolescent idiopathic scoliosis with Milwaukee bracing and compared their orthoses-based outcome with those of previously published natural history studies. Unsuccessful orthotic outcome (rate of failure) was defined as a curve progression of 5 degrees or more at final follow-up, or progression to surgery. In Lonstein and Winter's sample, 40% of individuals with initial curves of less than 30 degrees and Risser signs of 0 and 1 "failed," compared with 68% in the natural history studies. For individuals with Risser signs of 2 or more, the failure rate with the Milwaukee brace was 10%, compared with 23% in the natural history studies. Rates of failure were found to be less in the 30- to 39-degree group as well.[44]

In 1997 the Scoliosis Research Society published a meta-analysis of the efficacy of nonoperative treatment of idiopathic scoliosis.[45] They concluded that bracing alters the curve progression of scoliosis and electrical stimulation did not significantly improve outcomes in groups treated with observation only. They also suggested that full-time brace wear with either a CTLSO or TLSO was more effective than part-time wear.

Nachemson and associates[9] reported the results of a multicenter prospective study of brace efficacy that compared the effect of treatment with observation only versus underarm TLSO on skeletally immature girls with adolescent idiopathic scoliosis. Individuals in the study had right thoracic or thoracolumbar curves of 25 to 35 degrees. The rate of failure for those who wore the orthosis was 19% versus 50% in the observation-only group. Overall, the use of the orthosis was 40% more effective than treatment with observation alone. Nachemson's multicenter study also examined transcutaneous electrical stimulation versus observation only and found that the curves treated with transcutaneous electrical stimulation only progressed to surgery at a rate equal to those who were observed only.[9] The brace wear group was the only group that demonstrated a significant change from the natural history.

Montgomery and Willner[39] reported an almost 300% greater risk of failure among individuals when orthotic intervention was initiated after the curve had progressed 45 degrees or more, compared with interventions initiated when curves measured between 25 and 35 degrees. No other nonoperative treatment beside bracing has altered the curve progression of idiopathic scoliosis.

Orthoses

The risk of curve progression is best understood from a biomechanical perspective. The spine functions as a flexible column. All flexible structures have an upper load limit; when this limit is exceeded, plastic deformation begins to occur. Unlike a straight or rigid column that quickly reaches the point of failure and rapidly collapses when overloaded, the spine slowly bends as it collapses (i.e., plastic deformation of the spinal column occurs). Critical load is the point at which the spine begins to bend and deformation commences. As curve magnitude increases, magnitude of critical loading is reduced and deformation becomes more likely. Critical load rapidly drops as curves progress past 25 degrees; as a result, the rate of curve progression increases as the magnitude of the curve increases. An orthosis is designed to stiffen the spine artificially, reducing the curve, raising the critical load, and substantially reducing the likelihood of additional plastic deformation. Consider a curve with an initial deformity of 30 degrees: With orthotic correction (reduction) of this curve to 20 degrees, critical load increases from 50% to 80% of normal (erect stance) (Figure 16-10). For those with large and less correctable curves, however, critical load is not sufficiently influenced by the orthosis. In curves of 45 degrees, critical load is approximately 20% of normal. Unless wearing the orthosis can reduce the curve by

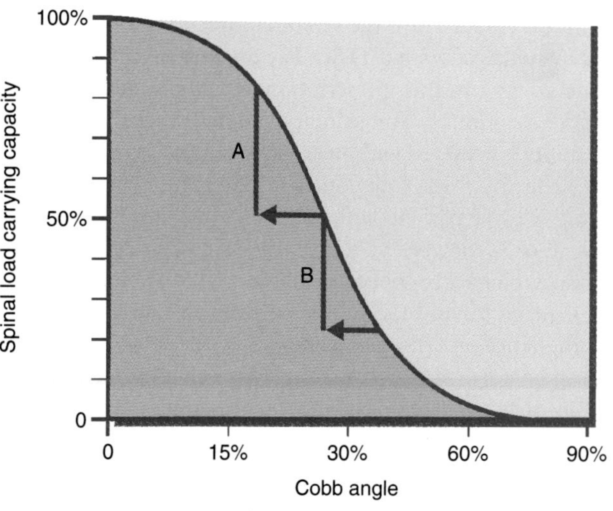

Figure 16-10

Effect of bracing on increasing critical load. A, *Indication that reducing a curve from 30 degrees to 20 degrees increases the stability of the curve 50% to 80%.* B, *Indication that critical load is increased 20% to 50% of normal if an orthosis can reduce a 45-degree curve to 30 degrees. (From Gavin TM, Patwardhan AG, Bunch WH: Principles and components of spinal orthosis. In Goldberg B, Hsu JD [eds]:* Atlas of Orthoses and Assistive Devices. *St. Louis: Mosby, 1997.)*

at least 50%, the minimal improvement in critical load is insufficient to forestall further deformation and progression of the curve.[46]

Goals

The primary goal of orthotic intervention in idiopathic scoliosis is prevention, or at least minimization, of further progression for individuals with skeletal immaturity, throughout the entire growth period until skeletal maturity can be documented. Orthotic intervention does not result in permanent correction of spinal alignment. The orthosis is designed to stabilize the curve through growth until skeletal maturity is reached. Most studies report that the curve magnitude after bracing is approximately the same as the prebracing curve; the important outcome is arresting or forestalling progression of the curve.[8,47-49]

The Milwaukee brace and most low-profile orthoses used to treat idiopathic scoliosis (e.g., Boston or Miami braces) use similar biomechanical principles to achieve the goals of end point control, curve correction, and continuous transverse support.[50] The degree of correction depends on four factors: the positioning of the pad, the magnitude of the corrective force applied by the pad, the direction of the applied force, and the duration that these forces are applied. The effectiveness of the pads is limited by the physical characteristics of the underlying tissue, specifically the tissue's ability to transmit and tolerate forces that are necessary for curve correction. The location of the apex of the curve is the critical determinant of which style of orthosis is prescribed. Curves with an apex at or above the seventh thoracic vertebra most often require the Milwaukee style CTLSO, whereas curves below the seventh thoracic vertebra are effectively managed with a TLSO. Factors that must also be considered in orthotic prescription include skeletal age and curve magnitude. For primary thoracic curves, maximum stability is achieved with the CTLSO; the TLSO is up to 25% less effective.[50] For individuals at high risk of curve progression (e.g., a patient with an idiopathic juvenile scoliosis curve of 40 degrees or more), the CTLSO is often a better choice than a TLSO because of the CTLSO's biomechanical advantage for in-brace curve correction. The likelihood of compliance or orthotic acceptance by the child and parents must be weighed against optimal biomechanics: A Milwaukee brace that achieves excellent correction but is worn sporadically because of compromised cosmesis will not be an effective intervention. In this case the slightly less efficient TLSO may be preferable if it will be worn consistently.

In-Brace Curve Correction

Most orthotists strive to fabricate an orthosis that achieves as much curve correction as possible while being worn, a goal based on premises that passive curve reduction lessens abnormal forces acting on the spine and that this external stability minimizes the likelihood of curve progression. Ideally the goal is 100% correction within the brace. In reality, factors such as inflexibility of the curve and skin tolerance to pad pressure limit complete correction. An important predictive factor for successful orthotic outcome is degree of initial in-brace correction.[51,52] An initial in-brace correction of 50% appears to be the minimum necessary to achieve the desired long-term orthotic outcome.[8,48]

Spinal Balance

Little clinical evidence exists to support the need to achieve complete spinal balance or compensation while the brace is being worn. However, bending movements apparently decrease when the head and mass of the body are centered over the pelvis. Biomechanical modeling demonstrates that decompensation does have a destabilizing effect.[49] For this reason, attention to spinal balance is important in brace design and fitting. Additional components, such as an axillary sling on a Milwaukee brace or an axillary extension on a Boston brace, may effectively address this issue.

Derotation

Correction of the abnormal rotation of spinal segments is an additional goal of orthotic intervention in scoliosis. The relationship of lateral curvature to rotation is not 1:1. However, because of the three-dimensional nature of scoliosis deformity, when lateral curvature is reduced, the magnitude of the rotation deformity is also reduced. The goal of orthotic intervention is to reduce the rotational deformity to zero while the patient wears the brace. The Boston brace system that is used to manage thoracic curves may incorporate posterolaterally positioned derotational pads to provide sagittal and coronal plane corrective forces. Such forces act to reduce lateral curvature and abnormal rotation of the vertebrae.

One problem associated with idiopathic scoliosis is hypokyphosis, which evidence indicates may be exacerbated by an orthosis.[18,53] Because of the risk of further loss of kyphosis in the spine that is already hypokyphotic, the posterior component of the thoracic pad has been eliminated in most brace designs. Although forces aim at achieving lateral correction, any decrease in Cobb angle also results in a decrease in the rotational deformity.[49] Because spinal rotation is so difficult to measure, however, the efficacy of these techniques cannot be fully evaluated. One method that approximates measurement of vertebral rotation is assessment of trunk shape. Rib hump deformity associated with vertebral rotation is apparently not greatly influenced by the brace, although cosmetic appearance can be improved.[54,55]

Delaying Surgical Spinal Fusion

For children and adolescents with significant or large curves, the goals of orthotic intervention are to minimize the risk of rapid curve progression and delay the need for surgical intervention. This delay is important so that the child can achieve as much trunk height as possible before spinal fusion. Because only 80% of trunk stature is achieved by age

10, this delay is especially important in younger individuals so that skeletal growth can continue as long as possible.[56] Orthotic intervention is important, even when future surgical correction is predicted; efficacy of surgical correction of the curve may be enhanced when less soft tissue contracture and vertebral deformity are present in small presurgical curves.

Exercise

Exercise programs have long been used and recommended in the treatment of idiopathic scoliosis.[57] Historically, exercise has had an important role as an adjunct to the prescription of the Milwaukee brace as a form of nonsurgical management of scoliosis.[46,47,58] Treatment with the Boston brace and other low-profile TLSOs such as the Wilmington, Miami, or Cuxhaven also use exercise protocols.[8,18,59-61] Although exercise programs vary among institutions and the types of braces, exercise alone does not significantly influence the curve progression of idiopathic scoliosis.[62,63] Because no conclusive studies have justified the efficacy of exercise, some physicians believe that ordering exercise programs as part of a routine protocol is unnecessary. Underlying this approach are beliefs that compliance to prescribed exercise protocols is usually poor, and that muscle strength, ROM, and respiratory capacity can be maintained without specific exercise with the encouragement of a high-level activity for out-of-brace time. Many physicians, therapists, and orthotists recognize the importance of exercise as an adjunct to nonoperative treatment with an orthosis in managing individuals with scoliosis. Typically, a physical therapist performs a comprehensive evaluation of muscle function, posture, respiratory function, and daily activities and, on the basis of findings, identifies existing and potential problems, establishes functional and preventive goals, and formulates a plan of care. The exercise program is created to target impairments or functional limitations for individual patients with scoliosis. For example, an individual may present with tight hip flexors. Because the brace is designed to reduce lordosis, this impairment will be counterproductive; a postural response of forward flexion and knee and hip flexion is likely to be induced. Stretching exercises for the hip flexor muscle group will make the patient more comfortable while wearing the brace and improve its function (Figure 16-11).

Exercise programs must be concise, reasonable, and simple to perform so that the potential for noncompliance is minimized. Typically, the physical therapist sees individuals and their families for initial instruction and then for follow-up visits scheduled over a longer time period so that progress and compliance can be more easily ascertained. Box 16-3 summarizes the overall goals of an exercise program for individuals with scoliosis.

Exercise enhances the efficacy of nonsurgical management of scoliosis by focusing attention on building the patient's awareness of posture and alignment. Instruction in postural self-correction exercises is an important part of the treatment plan. Structural curves often create asymmetric postures, resulting in decompensation of the trunk. Individuals must understand their particular curve pattern and how it changes their normal postural alignment. On the basis of this understanding, they learn which "self-correcting" movements enhance symmetry. Often, use of a mirror for visual feedback helps the patient to self-correct in the early stages of learning these exercises.

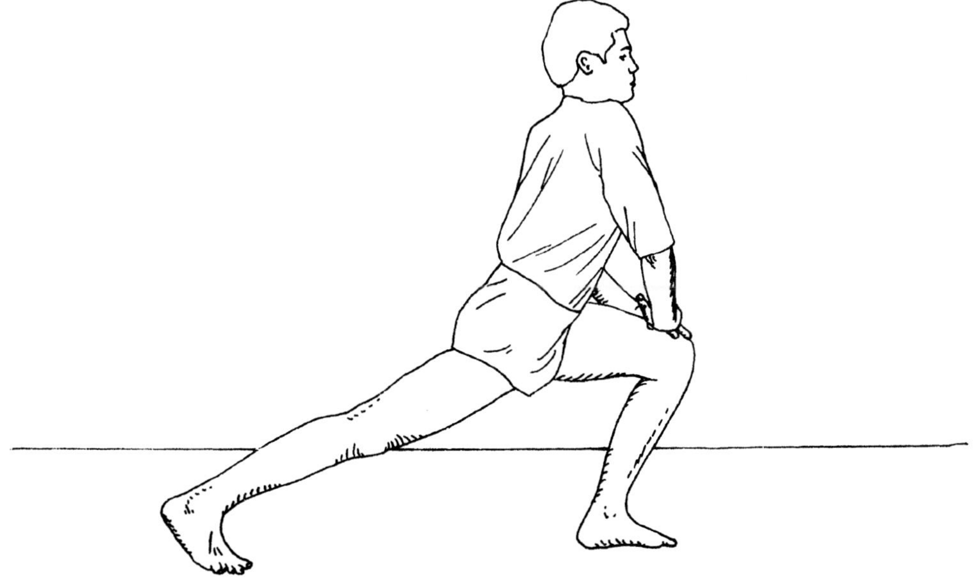

Figure 16-11
One position for stretching the hip flexors. Before initiating the stretch, an individual should perform a posterior pelvic tilt and maintain it.

Box 16-3 *Goals of Exercise Programs for Individuals with Scoliosis*

- Develop or enhance the patient's awareness of his or her posture
- Augment the function of the orthosis through active exercise while in the brace
- Enhance respiratory function and chest mobility
- Improve trunk muscle strength and function
- Improve or prevent further loss of range of motion of the spine and lower extremities
- Enhance proper body mechanics and activities of daily living while wearing the orthosis

Box 16-4 *Sample Exercises for Individuals with Scoliosis*

- Exercises to address muscle function and flexibility of the trunk and pelvis
- Posterior pelvic tilts, in multiple functional positions
- Abdominal exercises for upper, lower, and oblique muscle groups
- Anterior chest wall stretches
- Spinal stabilization and stretching into the curve convexity
- Exercises to address the lumbopelvic relationship and lower extremity musculature
- Hip flexor stretches and strengthening
- Hamstring stretches and strengthening
- Iliotibial/tensor fascia latae stretches and strengthening
- Erector spinae stretches and strengthening

Box 16-5 *Surgical Goals*

- Reduce maximum curve
- Achieve spinal balance postoperatively
- Provide spinal stabilization by arthrodesis
- Arrest further curve progression at the fusion site

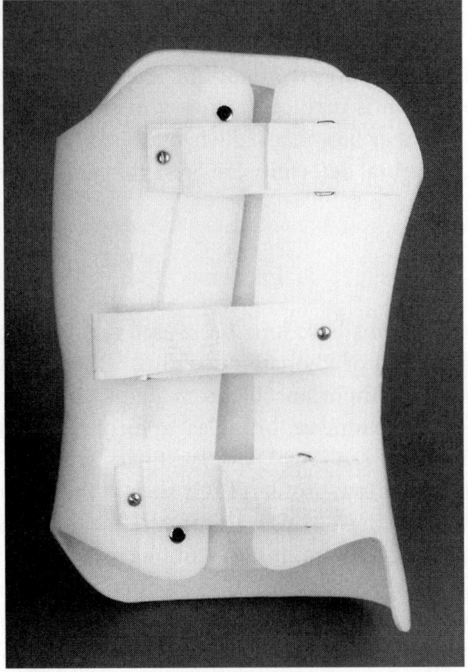

Figure 16-12
Example of a postoperative, anterior-opening, total contact thoracolumbosacral orthosis. The shell of this particular orthosis is polyethylene, with a foam lining. This type of orthosis is prescribed when passive rigid control is desired.

Brace design dictates whether in-brace exercise should be performed. For the best results, patients fitted with active orthotic designs, which have relief areas incorporated, should perform self-correcting exercises programs while out of the orthosis *and* while wearing it. Consider the design of the Boston brace: Its most important biomechanical corrective feature is pelvic control. When the pelvis is stabilized, pads placed strategically within the orthosis can deliver effective derotation and lateral corrective forces on this stable base. The function of this orthosis is enhanced when the patient learns to actively correct the lateral and rotatory deformity. These active exercises also serve to maintain strength and ROM of the trunk and pelvis. Individuals who are fitted with passive orthotic designs typically perform self-correcting exercises only during out-of-brace times. Exercises that target muscle function, soft tissue excursion and flexibility, and postural alignment are added to the self-correcting movements as well (Box 16-4).

The long-term effects orthosis use on trunk muscle strength, ROM, chest mobility, and respiratory capacity are not well documented. Prolonged use of an orthosis that encompasses much of the trunk would seemingly induce dysfunction. Although some degree of pulmonary limitation occurs even with mild to moderate curves,[64-67] decreased maximum oxygen uptake appears to be the consequence of deconditioning and lack of regular aerobic exercise and not necessarily of the orthosis or the scoliosis itself.[68,69] Poor perception of health and body image, as well as fear of injury, may contribute to inactivity and the resultant decrease in aerobic capacity.[70,71] Refsum and colleagues[72] suggest that, although some loss of respiratory capacity occurs while the patient is in brace in the early weeks of orthotic wear, adjustment to the orthosis appears to occur: At 6 months no significant differences were seen in cardiopulmonary function when in-brace and out-of-brace tests were compared. The lack of adequate normative data for children and adolescents describing normal ventilatory response to hypercapnia and hypoxia is problematic.

SURGICAL MANAGEMENT OF IDIOPATHIC SCOLIOSIS

For many individuals with scoliosis, the curve progresses despite compliant brace wear. When nonoperative treatment has been unsuccessful, surgical management of the curve must be considered. Curves that progress beyond 40 degrees in skeletally immature individuals and beyond 50 degrees in those who have reached full skeletal maturity typically require surgery.[40] Surgery for scoliosis has four goals: (1) to achieve the maximally prudent curve reduction, (2) to achieve spinal balance postoperatively, (3) to provide spinal stabilization by arthrodesis, and (4) to arrest further curve progression at the fusion site. The first successful spine surgery for scoliosis was performed by Hibbs in 1911. Since then, surgical technique and instrumentation have advanced significantly. Harrington distraction and compression rods, first used in 1962, became the standard for operative intervention for individuals with scoliosis. Other surgical techniques and procedures can also be used in surgical management of scoliosis, such as the Luque segmental, Cotrel and Dubousset, and Texas Scottish-Rite techniques. A study by McMaster[73] compared the Harrington and Luque techniques and found frontal correction to be similar in the two groups, but those who received Luque segmental instrumentation demonstrated better sagittal contouring and less loss of correction. These newer types of instruments, combined with increased attention to the improvement of sagittal contouring, have resulted in better postoperative outcomes. Box 16-5 summarizes surgical goals.

Many children are managed postoperatively with custom-fit, total-contact TLSOs (Figure 16-12). These orthoses have a protective function; their goal is to limit gross movement of the trunk, thereby reducing stress on the new surgical hardware and bony implants. The orthotist usually measures or casts the patient for the orthosis on the first or second postoperative day. Unless significant asymmetries are present in the trunk and pelvis, a TLSO can be fabricated from accurate circumferential and length measurements of the patient's trunk. In the presence of significant asymmetry, however, the patient must be molded with plaster of Paris to achieve a comfortable and well-functioning orthosis.

A complete preoperative assessment of posture, range of motion (ROM), strength, and respiratory function by a physical therapist is helpful. Preoperative review of breathing exercises, postural drainage positions, effective coughing techniques, and use of proper body mechanics can be helpful in lessening postoperative morbidity. In many settings, however, referral to physical therapy occurs after surgery, and the therapist becomes involved in the early postoperative care. Instruction in breathing exercises, effective coughing, and (if necessary) postural drainage, as well as practice of proper body mechanics and mobility training, is typically part of early postoperative physical therapy management. In many settings, individuals begin to get out of bed and resume limited functional activities within 2 to 3 days after surgery, and discharge occurs within a week after operation. Physical and occupational therapists also assess the need for adaptive equipment, potential architectural barriers to mobility, and the need for additional services at home.

CASE EXAMPLE 1

An Adolescent with Idiopathic Scoliosis

H. S., nearly 15, has been referred to the scoliosis clinic after a curve was detected during a school sports physical. Her medical history is unremarkable. Radiographs reveal a 26-degree right thoracic and a 13-degree left lumbar curve. She is 11 months postmenarchal and demonstrates a Risser sign of 2. Initially, no treatment other than close observation is recommended.

At a follow-up appointment 6 months later, another series of radiographs reveal that the right thoracic curve has progressed to 35 degrees and the left lumbar to 20 degrees. Additionally, H. S. still presents as a Risser 2/3 (Figure 16-13, *A*). The orthopedist recommends treatment with a Boston-style scoliosis orthosis, to be worn 23 hours a day, and orders a physical therapy evaluation.

Questions to Consider

- Given this patient's history and current presentation, what additional tests and measures would provide helpful information to use in your evaluation process?
- What is your movement dysfunction–related diagnosis for this patient?
- What might the prognosis be for this patient? What are your patient's goals for intervention? What are your rehabilitation goals? How long do you think it will take to achieve the goals that you and the patient agree upon?
- On the basis of your patient's goals and expectations, as well as your understanding of the underlying disease process, what recommendations would you make for intervention at this point? What "evidence" from the clinical research literature supports your recommendations? What have you chosen as possible interventions and how have you prioritized them?
- How will you assess whether the patient's and the rehabilitation goals have been met?
- What type of follow-up do you recommend for this patient?

Recommendations for a Patient with Idiopathic Scoliosis

The certified orthotist on the scoliosis clinic team measures and fits H. S. with a Boston-style orthosis that has a thoracic pad and lumbar pad. The in-brace correction is adequate; H. S. is reduced to 14 degrees in the thoracic and 11 degrees in the lumbar (see Figure 16-13, *B*). After approximately 2 weeks of progressively longer periods of wearing the orthosis, H. S. can wear the brace 23 hours a day, as prescribed.

The physical therapy examination and evaluation reveals the following impairments:

- Decreased hip flexor ROM (15-degree contracture bilaterally) and tightness in iliopsoas and hamstring musculature (straight leg raise 65 degrees bilaterally)
- Muscle tightness in erector spinae and quadratus lumborum on the concave side of the curve
- Weakened rectus abdominis and internal and external obliques (3+ on manual muscle testing)
- Poor postural awareness

H. S. also demonstrates functional limitations in advanced mobility and difficulty with activities of daily living (ADLs) while wearing the orthosis.

Physical therapy intervention consists of a home exercise program to address the impairments noted on evaluation, including (1) stretching and flexibility exercises to address her hip flexors and hamstring tightness, (2) a strengthening

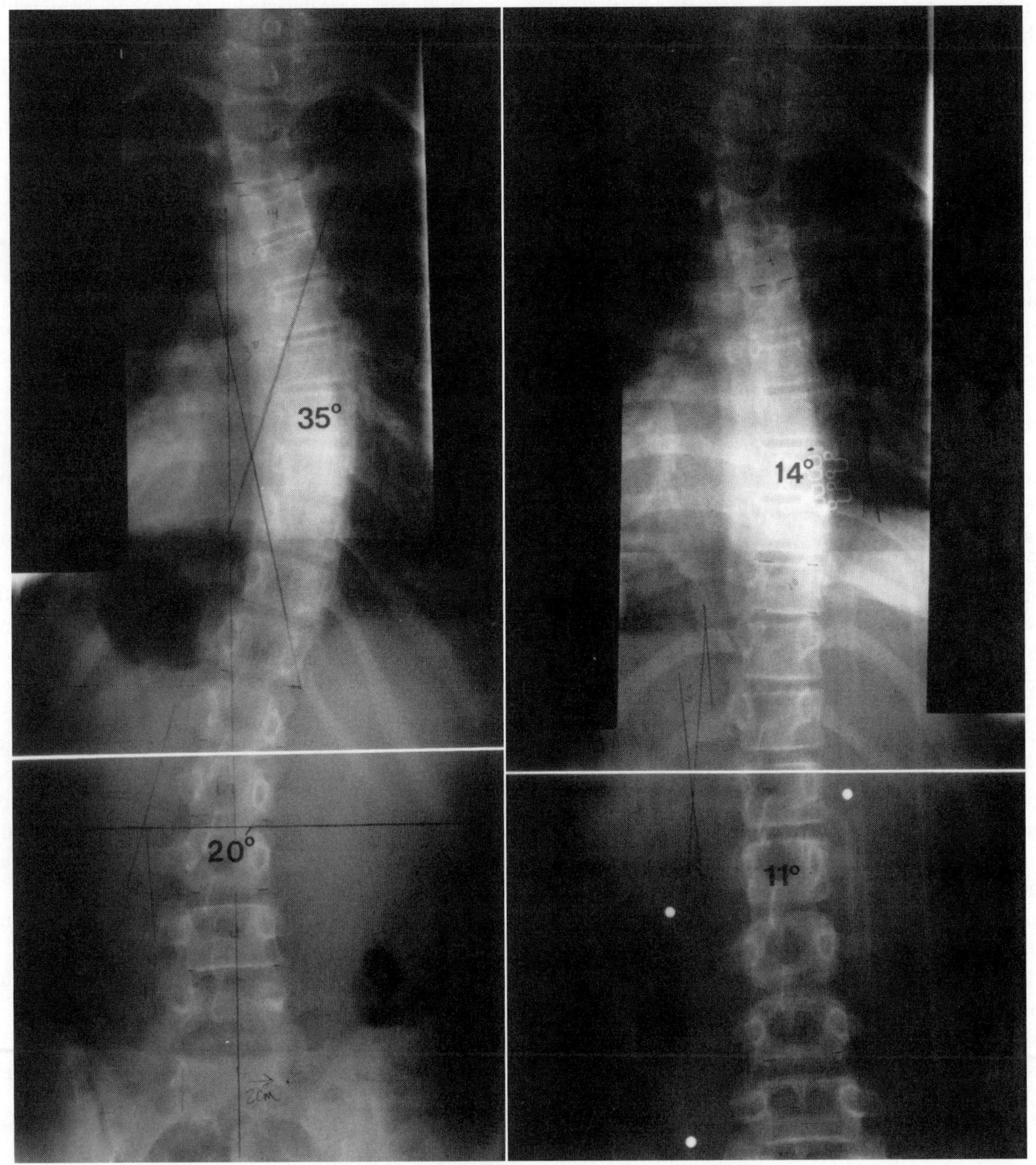

Figure 16-13

Case study radiographs. ***A,*** *Curves have progressed to a 35-degree right thoracic and a 20-degree left lumbar scoliosis.* ***B,*** *Initial in-brace curve correction 14-degree right thoracic and 11-degree left lumbar curvature.*

program for targeting abdominal muscle strength and endurance, (3) active exercise while wearing the orthosis, and (4) stretching to erector spinae and quadratus concavity of curve (Figure 16-14). The therapist also helps H. S. recognize kinesthetic clues and other postural reeducation strategies to enhance her awareness of posture and spinal alignment and recommends altering ADLs to compensate for restrictions imposed by the brace.

H. S. has regular 6-month follow-up appointments. The physical therapist and orthotist reassess her status at each appointment and change her exercise program or brace as needed.

At 16 years and 2 months of age, H. S. reports that she has not worn her orthosis for 3 weeks because of growth and fit issues; her curve is stable in the brace, and after almost 18 months of brace wear she has a Risser score of 5. The orthopedist discontinues the use of the orthosis because H. S. has reached full skeletal maturity and her curve has demonstrated stability. Plans are made to continue monitoring H. S. for the next 2 years to confirm that progression is under control.

NEUROMUSCULAR SCOLIOSIS

The underlying conditions that contribute to the progressive nature of most neuromuscular curves are vastly different from those of idiopathic curves. Neuromuscular curves result from either muscle or neurological disease that affects the function of the muscles supporting the trunk and pelvis. Flaccidity, hypotonicity, hypertonicity, rigidity, or athetosis can create asymmetry or compromise postural stability. The prevalence of neuromuscular scoliosis varies depending on the underlying etiology (Table 16-4). Unlike idiopathic scoliosis, which typically presents in adolescence, neuromuscular scoliosis often develops at an early age, because underlying neurological or muscular diseases are present in early childhood. Also unlike idiopathic scoliosis, most neuromuscular curves, even small ones, are progressive in nature, often increasing in severity throughout adulthood.[49,74] Younger individuals with truncal and pelvic muscle tone asymmetries or with severe paralysis of trunk musculature, tend to have more rapidly progressive and difficult to manage curves.

Table 16-4
Prevalence of Spinal Deformities in Various Neuromuscular Disorders

Neuromuscular Disorder	*Percentage with Spinal Disorder*
Cerebral palsy	25
Myelomeningocele	60
Infantile quadriplegia	100
Preadolescent quadriplegia	90
Duchenne's muscular dystrophy	95
Spinal muscular atrophy: types I, II, III	100
Friedreich's ataxia	95

From Lonstein JE, Renshaw TS. Neuromuscular spine deformities. *Instructional course lectures. Am Acad Orthop Surg* 1987;36:285-304.

Etiology

Stiffness and length are the most important biomechanical factors that influence progression of neuromuscular curves. The load-carrying capacity of a scoliotic spine decreases as stiffness of the spine decreases and length of the curve increases. The normal passive and active stiffening that affects muscles, ligaments, and disks on the spine is absent, diminished, or asymmetric in neuromuscular disorders.

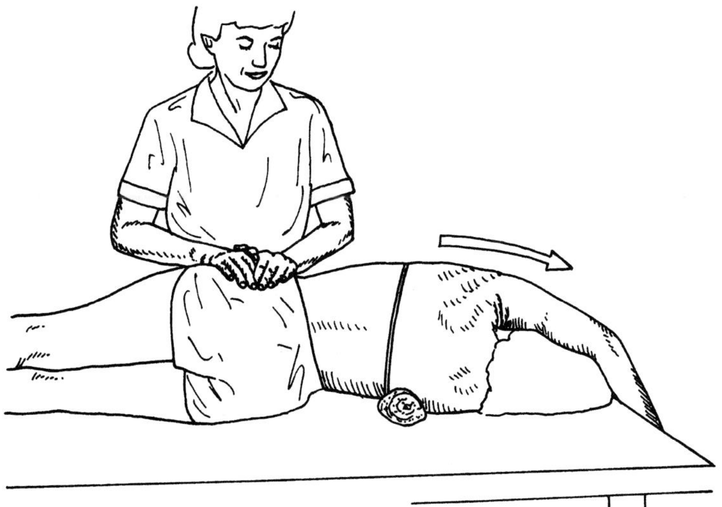

Figure 16-14
Stretching tight musculature on the concave side of the curve. The lumbar spine is stabilized with manual contacts on the pelvis.

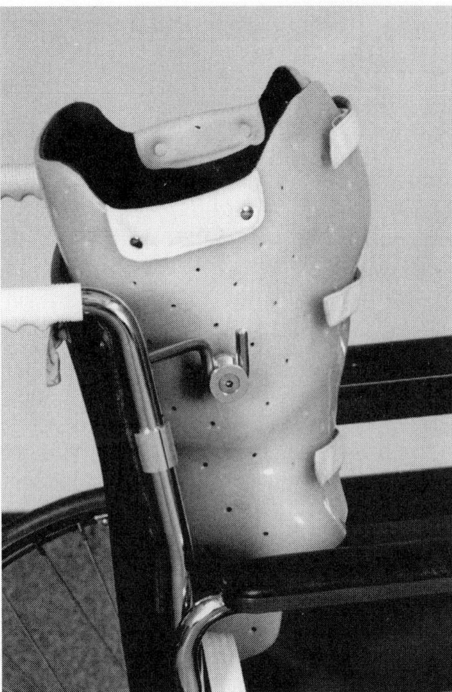

Figure 16-15
A thoracic suspension orthosis is suspended on this wheelchair by lateral posts, which rest on hooks attached to the wheelchair. This suspension unweights the ischial tuberosities and sacrum and distracts the spine, resulting in improved sitting and breathing in children with little or no trunk function secondary to their underlying neuromuscular disease.

Consequently, these less stiff spines are more susceptible to curvature and curve progression. As curve magnitude increases beyond 30 degrees, loss of stability is even more rapid. The combination of factors, such as increasing curve magnitude, trunk height, and loss of stiffness, create a situation in which curves can quickly progress.[56]

Nonsurgical Interventions for Neuromuscular Scoliosis

The management of a person with neuromuscular scoliosis is, in many respects, similar to that of individuals with idiopathic scoliosis, including careful observation and monitoring of curve status. Changes in curve magnitude beyond 30 degrees or changes in function indicate the need for orthotic or surgical intervention. Two important functional indicators of progression of spinal deformity are changes in the patient's ability to walk or sit upright during functional activities.[74] Orthoses are often indicated for all neuromuscular curves that have progressed to 30 degrees or beyond. The goal of orthotic treatment is to slow the progression of the deformity and allow for continued maximal trunk height growth until surgical stabilization is indicated.

The degree of volitional trunk control is one determinant of orthotic design. Individuals with poor trunk control most often benefit from a passive supportive orthosis, whereas those with better trunk control may benefit from an active orthosis. The passive orthosis is a total contact orthosis; it has a three-point force system in which the walls of the orthosis provide forces that act on the spine (see Figure 16-12). These orthoses can be more or less flexible depending on the patient's skin tolerance and weight, as well as the flexibility and degree of deformity of the spine. An alternative approach is a thoracic suspension orthosis, a TLSO suspended by hooks from a seating system (Figure 16-15). This suspension creates a distractive effect on the spine as well as an unweighting of the ischial tuberosities and sacrum. This type of orthosis is most often prescribed for individuals with recurrent or nonhealing sacral or ischial decubitus ulcers or for people with significant respiratory compromise because of their underlying neuromuscular disease. Use of this style of orthosis is limited; individuals who weigh more than 40 lb are often unable to tolerate the skin pressures associated with suspension. Chapter 19 includes more information about seating systems used in the treatment of scoliosis.

An active orthosis induces curve correction by passive and active forces; the walls of the orthosis act in conjunction with the individual's own muscle contractions to effect correction. Reliefs are provided in the orthosis opposite to the convexity so that rib excursion and resultant curve reduction are possible. Children with neuromuscular scoliosis are prescribed the same Boston and Milwaukee orthoses worn by those with idiopathic scoliosis if trunk function permits active correction as a component of nonsurgical management of their curves (see Figures 16-1 and 16-2).

Custom-molded seating is an orthotic alternative for individuals with neuromuscular pathoses who demonstrate poor or absent sitting and head control and for those who may be at high risk for skin breakdown. Many individuals can be effectively fit into a prefabricated, custom-fit system. Seating is often augmented by use of a TLSO: Curve management is addressed by the TLSO, and function issues are addressed by the seating. In many seating clinics, a multidisciplinary team of physical and occupational therapists, physicians, orthotists, and wheelchair vendors work with the family to create the most functional and beneficial seating arrangement. Postures assumed in the wheelchair must be analyzed carefully. Consideration of weight distribution is also important to prevent skin irritation and pressure ulcer formation. Weight distribution in supported sitting is affected by footrest position, seat depth, chair back angulation, and altered alignment or positions when an orthosis is worn. Many children who require custom-fit or custom-molded seating use joystick or microswitch systems for independent mobility; joystick or microswitch position can also improve sitting posture. Box 16-6 summarizes the orthotic goals in treating individuals with neuromuscular scoliosis.

Box 16-6 *Goals of Orthotic Treatment of Neuromuscular Scoliosis*

- Slow curve progression
- Allow for continued growth
- Allow individual to achieve maximal truncal height before surgical stabilization

Surgical Management for Neuromuscular Scoliosis

The goal of surgery is to achieve a stable, well-balanced spine. The need for spinal surgery varies with the underlying neuromuscular pathology. For example, many factors influence the decision to operate on children with cerebral palsy. These children who have normal or mildly impaired cognitive function can be managed with orthotic and exercise protocols similar to those of children with idiopathic curves. Children with spastic quadriplegic cerebral palsy can be evaluated for spinal surgery when their curve impairs their ability to be functional in sitting. The nature of the curve determines surgical indications and technique (e.g., the extent of spinal fusion and the use of internal fixation devices). Postoperatively, many children are placed in casts until the fusion mass solidifies. After their cast is removed, most children use a TLSO for up to 1 year to protect the spine during functional activity. Early mobilization by the physical therapy team is crucial because in many cases the preoperative health and vitality of these individuals is already precarious.

CASE EXAMPLE 2

A Child with Neuropathic Scoliosis

K. L. is a 6½-year-old female with an underlying diagnosis of diplegic cerebral palsy. She has been followed in a cerebral palsy clinic since 9 months of age to address her evolving needs. At her latest visit she is diagnosed with a 20-degree right thoracolumbar scoliosis. The interdisciplinary team involved in K. L.'s care advises her mother to continue K. L.'s ongoing therapy for gross and fine motor development and have her observed at 6-month intervals.

Over the next 12 months the curve remains stable, but at 18 months after the initial diagnosis radiographs reveal that it has progressed to 27 degrees. The orthopedist now recommends a TLSO scoliosis brace to address the impairment; additionally, she recommends that K. L.'s existing physical therapy program address this new impairment.

Questions to Consider

- Given this patient's history and current presentation, what additional tests and measures would provide helpful information to use in your evaluation process?
- What is your movement dysfunction–related diagnosis for this patient?
- What might the prognosis be for this patient? What are your patient's goals for intervention? What are your rehabilitation goals? How long do you think it will take to achieve the goals that you and the patient agree upon? How are the goals for this patient with neuromuscular scoliosis similar to or different from those for the patient with idiopathic scoliosis?
- On the basis of your patient's goals and expectations, as well as your understanding of the underlying disease process, what do you recommend for intervention at this point? What "evidence" from the clinical research literature supports your recommendations? What have you chosen as possible interventions and how have you prioritized them?
- How will you assess whether patient and rehabilitation goals have been met?
- What type of follow-up do you recommend for this patient?

The certified orthotist on the clinic team fits K. L. with a Boston-style TLSO. Within 3 weeks she can tolerate full-time brace wear (23 hours/day).

K. L. returns to the scoliosis clinic at 6-month intervals. At age 10+, despite consistent brace wear, the curve continues to progress—her original curve of 20 degrees now measures 45 degrees. The orthopedist recommends continued use of the orthosis in an effort to slow progression and says surgical stabilization is likely required. Now the goals are to reduce speed of progression and stabilize the curve as much as possible in an effort to reach maximal trunk stature before arthrodesis.

Over the next year, the curve continues to progress; it now measures 51 degrees. The orthopedist asks a surgeon to explain the surgical procedure; he is satisfied that K. L. has attained most of her adult trunk stature and the curve is still flexible enough to attain reasonable correction.

She is admitted on a Monday, and the open reduction with internal fixation (ORIF) is performed that day. On Wednesday a staff orthotist sees her for casting and measurement of a postoperative TLSO. On Friday the orthotist delivered and fit the total contact orthosis, and the surgeon referred K. L. to rehabilitation services.

Occupational and physical therapists evaluate the patient together, assessing all impairments and functional limitations. The spinal body jacket allows them to begin work on mobility skills and ambulation with K. L. Before surgery, K. L. was independent with all mobility and did not use assistive devices for ambulation. The primary goals at the early stage of treatment are mobility: bed mobility, transfers and ambulation, independence of family/patient to manage TLSO donning and doffing, maintenance of skin integrity, and improved respiratory function.

After 2 weeks she is discharged home with services. She is now independent with bed mobility and transfers and is ambulating with a walker, requiring only contact guard. Her mother is independent with donning and doffing and skin inspection, and K. L. is independent with the use of spirometer and breathing exercises to address decline in pulmonary function. She is monitored at home for another 10 weeks until discharged by therapy. She is now independently ambulating with bilateral Lofstrand crutches, donning and doffing the TLSO, and performing all ADLs. The plan is to return to school and continue therapy in that setting. Goals continue to be mobility oriented until K. L. progresses fully back to independence without assistive devices.

SUMMARY

This chapter has explored the etiology of idiopathic and neuromuscular scoliosis and the biomechanical factors that contribute to curve progression. It has also described a strategy for evaluation of curve severity and the special tests and measurements used to assess individuals with scoliosis. This discussion includes the use of orthoses in the nonoperative management of scoliosis and differentiates between orthoses that incorporate the cervical spine, such as the Milwaukee brace, and those that have a low-profile TLSO design, such as the Boston or Miami brace. Exercise is identified as an important adjunct to orthotic management, with the goal of facilitating self-correction of the curve and improved postural awareness, as well as prevention of secondary functional and cardiopulmonary impairments related to inactivity imposed by long-term orthotic wear. An overview of indications for surgery and the roles of orthoses, exercise, and functional training that may be required during postoperative care is provided. In conclusion, optimal management is best achieved when a multidisciplinary team of health professionals who understand the complexities of scoliosis contribute their special skills to individuals' care.

REFERENCES

1. Hippocrates. *The Genuine Works of Hippocrates* (translated by Francis Adams). New York: WM Wood, 1849.
2. Bradford EH, Brackett EG. Treatment of lateral curvature by means of pressure correction. *Boston Med Surg J* 1893;128:463.
3. Risser J. The application of body casts for the correction of scoliosis. American Academy of Orthopaedic Surgeons. *Instr Course Lect* 1955;12:255.
4. Hibbs RA, Risser JC, Ferguson AB. Scoliosis treated by fusion method. An end result study of 360 cases. *J Bone Joint Surg Am* 1931;13:91.
5. Blount WP, Schmidt AC, Keever ED, Leonard ET. Milwaukee brace in the operative treatment of scoliosis. *J Bone Joint Surg* 1958;40A:511.
6. Logan WR. The effect of Milwaukee brace on the developing dentition. In *Transaction of the British Society for the Study of Orthodontics.* London: the Society; 1962. pp. 1-8.
7. Hall J, Schumann W, Stanish W. A refined concept in the orthotic management of scoliosis: a preliminary report. *Prosthet Orthot Int* 1975;29:7-13.
8. Emans JB, Kaelin A, Bancel P, Hall JE. Boston brace treatment of idiopathic scoliosis. Follow up results in 295 patients. *Spine* 1986;11(8):792-801.
9. Nachemson AL, Peterson LE, Brace Study Group SRS. Effectiveness of treatment with a brace in girls who have adolescent idiopathic scoliosis. *J Bone Joint Surg* 1995;77A(6):816-821.
10. Weinstein SL, Ponseti IV. Curve progression in idiopathic scoliosis. *J Bone Joint Surg* 1983;65A(4):447-455.
11. Katz DE, Richard S, Browne RH, et al. A comparison between the Boston brace and the Charleston bending brace in adolescent idiopathic scoliosis. *Spine* 1997;22:1302-1312.
12. Trivedi JM, Thompson JD. Results of Charleston bracing in skeletally immature patients with IS. *J Pediatr Orthop* 2001;21:277-280.
13. Howard A, Wright JG, Hedden D. A comparative study of TLSO, Charleston and Milwaukee braces for IS. *Spine* 1998;23:2404-2411.
14. Goldstein LA, Waugh TR. Classification and terminology of scoliosis. *Clin Orthop* 1973;June(93):10-22.
15. McAlister WH, Shackelford GD. Classification of spinal curvatures. *Radiol Clin North Am* 1975;13(1):93-112.
16. Terminology Committee, Scoliosis Research Society. A glossary of scoliosis terms. *Spine* 1976;1:57-58.
17. Kendall FP, McCreary EK, Provance PG. *Muscles, Testing and Function,* 4th ed. Baltimore: Williams & Wilkins, 1993.
18. Emans JB, Cassella MC. *Boston Brace Instructional Course.* Avon, MA: Boston Brace International, 1996.
19. Lonstein J. Idiopathic scoliosis. In Lonstein JE, Bradford DS, Winter RB, Ogilvie JW (eds), *Moe's Textbook of Scoliosis and Other Spinal Deformities.* Philadelphia: Saunders, 1995.
20. Cowell HR, Hall JN, MacEwen GD. Genetic aspects of idiopathic scoliosis. *Clin Orthop* 1972;86:121-131.
21. Willner S. A study of height, weight, and menarche in girls with idiopathic structural scoliosis. *Acta Orthop Scand* 1975;46(1):71-78.
22. Waters RL, Morris JM. An in vitro study of normal and scoliotic interspinous ligaments. *J Biomech* 1973;6(4): 343-348.
23. Riddle HV, Roaf R. Muscle imbalance in the causation of scoliosis. *Lancet* 1975;1:1245-1247.
24. Yekutiel M, Robin GC, Yarom R. Proprioceptive function in children with adolescent idiopathic scoliosis. *Spine* 1981;6(6):560-566.
25. Herman R, Mixon J, Fisher A, et al. Idiopathic scoliosis and the central nervous system: am otor control problem. *Spine* 1985;10(1):1-14.
26. Sahlstrand T, Petruson B. A study of labyrinth function in patients with adolescent idiopathic scoliosis. *Acta Orthop Scand* 1979;50(6):759-769.
27. Willner S, Uden A. Prospective prevalence study of scoliosis in southern Sweden. *Acta Orthop Scand* 1982;53(2):233-237.
28. Hagglund G, Karlberg J, Willner S. Growth in girls with adolescent idiopathic scoliosis. *Spine* 1992;17(1):108-111.

29. Weinstein SL. Natural history. *Spine Surg* 1999;24(24): 2592-2600.
30. Lonstein JE, Bjorkland S, Wanninger MH, Nelson R. Voluntary school screening for scoliosis in Minnesota. *J Bone Joint Surg* 1982;64A(4):481-488.
31. Risenborough EJ, Wynne-Davies R. A genetic survey of idiopathic scoliosis in Boston, Massachusetts. *J Bone Joint Surg* 1973;55A(5):974-982.
32. Wynne-Davies R. Infantile idiopathic scoliosis. Causative factors, particularly in the fist six months. *J Bone Joint Surg Br* 1975;57(2):138-141.
33. Scott JC, Morgan TH. The natural history and prognosis of infantile idiopathic scoliosis. *J Bone Joint Surg* 1955;37B: 400-413.
34. Mehta MH. The rib vertebral angle in the early diagnosis between resolving and progressive infantile scoliosis. *J Bone Joint Surg* 1972;54B(2):230-243.
35. Figueiredo UM, James JIP. Juvenile idiopathic scoliosis. *J Bone Joint Surg* 1981;63B(1):61-66.
36. Duval-Beaupere G, Lamireau T. Scoliosis at less than 30 degrees. Properties of the evolutivity (risk of progression). *Spine* 1985;10(5):421-424.
37. Lonstein JE, Carlson JM. Prediction of curve progression in untreated idiopathic scoliosis during growth. *J Bone Joint Surg* 1984;66A(7):1061-1071.
38. Weinstein SL. Adolescent idiopathic scoliosis: Prevalence and natural history. *Instr Course Lect* 1989;38:115-128.
39. Montgomery F, Willner S. Prognosis of brace treated scoliosis; comparison of the Boston and Milwaukee method in 244 girls. *Acta Orthop Scand* 1989;60(4):383-385.
40. Kehl DK, Morrissy RT. Brace treatment in adolescent idiopathic scoliosis. An update on concepts and technique. *Clin Orthop* 1988;229:34-43.
41. Greulich WW, Pyle SI. *Radiographic Atlas of Skeletal Development of the Hand and Wrist,* 2nd ed. Stanford, CA: Stanford University Press, 1959.
42. Nash C, Moe J. A study of vertebral rotation. *J Bone Joint Surg* 1969;51A(2):223-229.
43. Winter RB, Lonstein JE, Denis F. The prevalence of spinal canal or cord abnormalities in idiopathic, congenital, or neuromuscular scoliosis. *Orthop Trans* 1992;16:135.
44. Lonstein JE, Winter RB. The Milwaukee brace for treatment of adolescent idiopathic scoliosis. A review of 1020 patients. *J Bone Joint Surg Am* 1994;76(8):1207-1221.
45. Rowe DE, Bernstein SM, Riddick MF, et al. A meta-analysis of the efficacy of nonoperative treatments for IS. *J Bone Joint Surg* 1995;79A:664-674.
46. Bradford DS, Hu SS. Neuromuscular spinal deformity. In Lonstein JE, Bradford DS, Winter RB, Ogilvie JW (eds), *Moe's Textbook of Scoliosis and Other Spinal Deformities.* Philadelphia: Saunders, 1995.
47. Moe JH, Kettleson DN. Idiopathic scoliosis. *J Bone Joint Surg* 1970;52A(8):1609-1633.
48. Keiser RP, Shufflebarger HL. The Milwaukee brace in idiopathic scoliosis. *Clin Orthop* 1976;July/August(118):19-24.
49. Willers U, Normelli H, Aaro S, et al. Long term results of the Boston brace treatment on vertebral rotation in idiopathic scoliosis. *Spine* 1993;18(4):432-435.
50. Patwardhan AG, Gavin TM, Bunch WH, et al. Biomechanical comparison of the Milwaukee brace (CTLSO) and the TLSO for the treatment of idiopathic scoliosis. *J Prosthet Orthot* 1996;8(4):116-122.
51. Olafsson Y, Saraste H, Soderlund V, Hoffsten M. Boston brace in the treatment of idiopathic scoliosis. *J Pediatr Orthop* 1995;16(4):524-527.
52. Carr WA, Moe JH, Winter RB, Lonstein JE. The treatment of idiopathic scoliosis in the Milwaukee brace. *J Bone Joint Surg* 1980;62A(4):599-612.
53. Tanner JM, Whitehouse RH. Clinical longitudinal standards for height, weight, height velocity, and stages of puberty. *Arch Dis Child* 1976;51(3):170-179.
54. Weisz I, Jefferson RJ, Carr AJ, et al. Back shape in the treatment of idiopathic scoliosis. *Clin Orthop* 1989; March(240):167-163.
55. Raso VJ, Russell GG, Hill DL, et al. Thoracic lordosis in idiopathic scoliosis. *J Pediatr Orthop* 1991;11(5): 599-602.
56. Bunch WH, Patwardhan AG. *Scoliosis: Making Clinical Decisions.* St Louis: Mosby, 1989. pp. 50-65.
57. Lovett RW. *Lateral Curvature of the Spine and Round Shoulders.* Philadelphia: P Blakiston's Son and Co, 1907.
58. Moe JH. The Milwaukee brace in the treatment of scoliosis. *Clin Orthop* 1971;77:18-31.
59. Faraday J. Current principles in the nonoperative management of structural adolescent idiopathic scoliosis. *Phys Ther* 1983;63(4):512-523.
60. Bassett GS, Bunnell WP, MacEwen GD. Treatment of idiopathic scoliosis with the Wilmington brace. Results in patients with twenty to thirty-nine degree curve. *J Bone Joint Surg* 1986;68A(4):602-605.
61. Edelmann P. Brace treatment in idiopathic scoliosis. *Acta Orthop Belg* 1992;58(suppl 1):85-90.
62. Hungerford DS. Spinal deformity in adolescence. Early detection and nonoperative management. *Med Clin North Am* 1975;59(6):1617-1625.
63. Stone B, Beekman C, Hall V, et al. The effect of an exercise program on change in curve in adolescents with minimal idiopathic scoliosis. A preliminary study. *Phys Ther* 1979;59(6):759-763.
64. Kearon C, Viviani GR, Killian KJ. Factors influencing work capacity in adolescent idiopathic scoliosis. *Am Rev Respir Dis* 1993;148(2):295-303.
65. DiRoccoc PJ, Vaccaro P. Cardiopulmonary functioning. I. Adolescent patients with mild idiopathic scoliosis. *Arch Phys Med Rehabil* 1988;69(3):198-203.
66. Smyth RJ, Chapman KR, Wright TA, et al. Ventilatory patterns during hypoxia, hypercapnia, and exercise in adolescents with mild scoliosis. *Pediatrics* 1986;77(5):692-697.
67. Kennedy JD, Robertson CF, Hudson I, Phelan P. Effect of bracing on respiratory mechanics in mild idiopathic scoliosis. *Thorax* 1989;44(7):548-553.
68. Kesten S, Garfinkel SK, Wright T, Rebuck AS. Impaired exercise capacity in adults with moderate exercise. *Chest* 1991;99(3):663-666.
69. MacLean WE, Green NE, Pierre CB, Ray DC. Stress and coping with scoliosis: psychological effects on adolescents and their families. *J Pediatr Orthop* 1989;9(3):257-261.
70. Goldberg MS, Mayo NE, Poitras B, et al. The Ste-Justine Adolescent Idiopathic Scoliosis Cohort Study. *Spine* 1994;19(14):1662-1672.

71. Valentine LE. *Alteration of Body Image of Adolescent Females Braced as a Treatment for Adolescent Idiopathic Scoliosis* [thesis]. Washington, DC: Catholic University; 1991.
72. Refsum HE, Naess-Anderson CF, Lange JE. Pulmonary function and gas exchange at rest and exercise in adolescent girls with mild idiopathic scoliosis during treatment with Boston thoracic brace. *Spine* 1990;16(5):420-423.
73. McMaster M. Luque rod instrumentation in the treatment of adolescent idiopathic scoliosis; a comparative study with Harrington instrumentation. *J Bone Joint Surg* 1991;73B(6):982-989.
74. Lonstein JE, Renshaw TS. Neuromuscular spine deformities. *Instr Course Lect* 1987;36:285-304.

17

Orthotics in the Management of Hand Dysfunction

NOELLE M. AUSTIN AND MARYLYNN JACOBS

LEARNING OBJECTIVES

On completion of this chapter, the reader will be able to do the following:

1. Define immobilization, mobilization, and restriction splinting and give examples of splints in each category.
2. Explain the differences among static, dynamic, serial static, and static progressive splinting and discuss which may be appropriate at each of the three wound healing stages.
3. Identify the three arches of the hand and discuss their significance.
4. Identify a 90-degree angle of pull and explain its importance to application of force.
5. Describe the various handling and physical characteristics of thermoplastic materials and discuss how they affect splint fabrication.
6. Understand the importance of patient education related to proper splint wear, care, and precautions.

He who works with his hands is a laborer,
He who works with his hands and his mind is a craftsman,
He who works with his mind and his heart is an artist.
UNKNOWN

The hand is the body's tool to interact with the surrounding environment. A hand afflicted with disease or injury greatly impairs the ability to function, even if normal functioning elbow and shoulder joints and muscles are present. The therapist's ability to provide clinical intervention can positively affect the use of the hand and therefore overall function. One therapeutic tool at a therapist's disposal is splinting. The appropriate use of splints during specific phases of tissue healing, depending on the diagnosis, can be an effective adjunct to traditional therapy techniques for restoring use of the limb. Treatment decisions must be based on an integration of knowledge and clinical experience along with information specific to the individual patient, including diagnosis, general medical status, and the physician's prescription. Clinicians need to understand the principles associated with splint design and fabrication.

This chapter focuses on splinting for the hand and upper extremity and includes discussion of nomenclature, materials, mechanical and anatomical principles, and case studies to provide examples of splinting intervention with emphasis on critical thinking.

SPLINT NOMENCLATURE

In the medical literature, the terms *splint, brace, support,* and *orthotic* have similar definitions.[1,2] This is often puzzling to physicians, therapists, students, insurance companies, and even those who fabricate these devices. Are splints made by a therapist? Is an orthosis made by an orthotist? In 1989, the American Society of Hand Therapists put together a task force to address issues such as proper nomenclature and redefinition of splints in an attempt to enhance and clarify communication among all disciplines.[1] The task force developed a Splint Classification System (SCS) and addressed the similarity in definitions of the words *splint, brace, support,* and *orthosis* (Figure 17-1). The task force's review confirmed that these words were so similar in nature that they were used interchangeably in the hand therapy literature. Another key issue that challenged the task force was how to define splints to provide universal comprehension and approval.

Traditionally, splints have generally been described according to their form (e.g., thumb spica splint, wrist cock-up splint, ulnar gutter splint).[3] This form-based nomenclature, however, can often lead to confusion and misunderstanding regarding the actual splint requested. The SCS painstakingly describes most universally used splints according to their specific function (e.g., thumb immobilization splint, wrist/hand extension mobilization splint). By following this

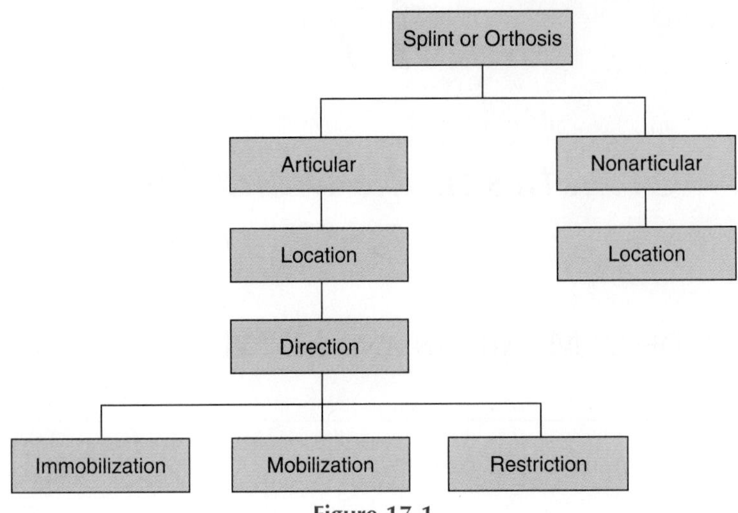

Figure 17-1
The American Society of Hand Therapists SCS.

functional-based description of splints, clinicians will have a clear concept of what the splint must look like and what its function should be. The specific splint categories described by the SCS are outlined in Table 17-1.

Articular and Nonarticular Splints

Splints are classified into two broad categories: articular and nonarticular. *Articular splints*, the most common type of fabricated splint, are those that cross a joint or series of joints. Examples of articular splints include a wrist immobilization splint, proximal interphalangeal (PIP) joint extension mobilization splint, and elbow flexion restriction splint. The word *articular* is implied in the splint's description and is not necessary in the title of the splint.

Nonarticular splints do not cross a joint; instead, they stabilize the body segment to which they are applied. The American Society of Hand Therapists recommends that

Table 17-1
Characteristics of Thermoplastic Splinting Materials

Company Name	*Stretch Resistance*		
	Minimum	*Moderate*	*Maximal*
AliMed	Polyform Multiform	Orthoplast II Polyflex II Multiform Clear	Ezeform Orthoplast
DeRoyal	LMB Drape	LMB Blend LMB Flex	LMB Royal
North Coast Medical	NCM Clinic Prism NCM Preferred Orfilight	Encore Orfit NCM Spectrum Omega Max	Orifbrace Omega Plus Solaris Orthoplast
Sammons Preston Rolyan	Polyform Kay-Splint I Aquaplast ProDrape-T	Polyflex II Kay-Splint II Aquaplast-T Aquaplast Original Aquaplast Watercolors	Ezeform Kay-Splint IV Aquaplast Resilient-T Aquaplast Original Resilient Synergy San-Splint
WFR Corporation	Reveal XS	Reveal MS	Reveal LS

clinicians include the term *nonarticular* before a splint's description; a splint used to stabilize the humerus would be called a nonarticular humerus splint, and a splint designed to stabilize a metacarpal would be called a nonarticular metacarpal splint. Without this designation, the splint maker may not know whether to include or exclude proximal or distal joints in the splint design.

Location

Location refers to the specific body part or joint levels acted on by the splint. The primary joint is the target joint. The secondary joints are included for protection, stabilization, or comfort. When several primary joints are involved (e.g., crush injury to the hand), the description of the splint can be simplified by grouping all the joints together, such as "hand splint" or "digit splint."

Direction

Direction refers to the primary direction of the force applied when the splint is worn. This includes flexion, extension, radial or ulnar deviation, supination, pronation, abduction, and adduction. Information regarding direction is essential because it tells the clinician the desired joint positioning. Direction notation is also critical when fabricating a mobilization splint; accurate application of the direction of force is essential to achieve the goal of joint or soft tissue mobility.

Purpose of Splint

The purpose of the splint is the single most important aspect documented in the splint's description. The purpose of the splint can be to (1) immobilize a structure, (2) mobilize a tissue, or (3) restrict an aspect of joint motion.

Immobilization

The purpose of an *immobilization splint* is simply to place a structure in its anatomical or most comfortable resting position. Immobilization splinting is perhaps the most popular and simple form of splinting, although it can be used for complex injuries. Immobilization splints are either articular or nonarticular, immobilizing the joints they cross (articular) or stabilizing a structure to which they are applied, as in the case of a nonarticular forearm splint.

Mobilization

Mobilization refers to moving or stretching specific soft tissues or joints to create change. The benefits of using *mobilization splinting* as a treatment modality have been well documented in the literature.[4,5] The effectiveness of mobilization splinting does not rely on stretching tissue but rather on the facilitation of cell growth. The target tissue will lengthen when the living cells of the contracted tissues are stimulated (by force) to grow. The stimulation occurs when steady tension is applied through the splint over a specific period. The living cells recognize the tension applied and permit the older collagen cells to be actively absorbed and replaced with new collagen cells oriented in the direction of tension.[6-13] Tissue growth has been clearly demonstrated in certain cultures in which elongating certain body parts, such as earlobes and lips, is popular. In these cultures, dowels are used to serially increase the diameter of the intended structure, slowing allowing it to expand and accommodate to the new tension and diameter. Splints that mobilize tissue include serial static, static progressive, and dynamic splints.

Restriction

Restriction splints restrict or block an aspect of joint motion. These are generally simple splints applied in such a way that they limit desired motion. Static splints, dynamic splints, and forms of taping are considered types of restrictive splints because they can be made to restrict some portion of joint motion while allowing the rest of the joints to move freely.

An example of three PIP splints demonstrates the critical impact that the words *immobilization, mobilization,* and *restriction* can have when describing a splint. Within the PIP extension immobilization splint, the PIP joint is immobi-

A

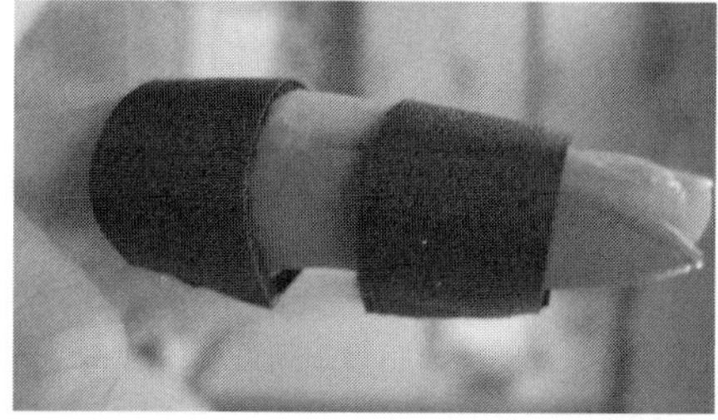

B

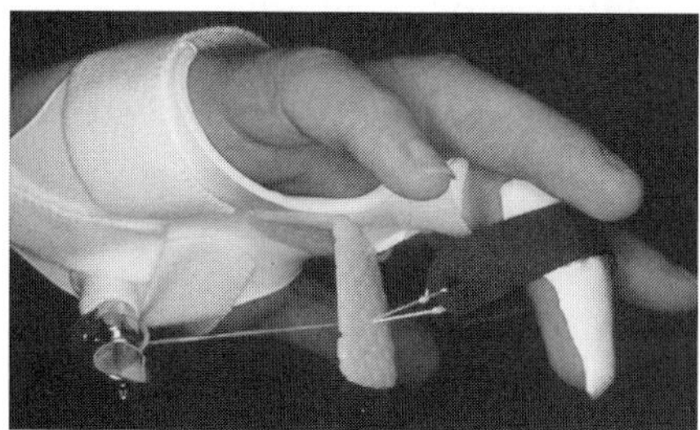

C

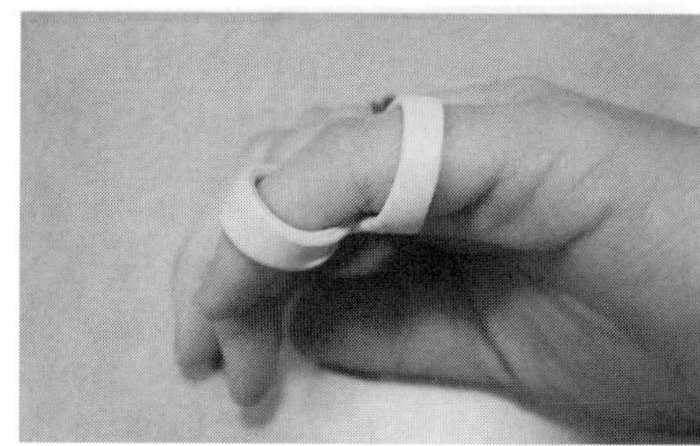

Figure 17-2
Three different PIP joint splints. ***A,*** *A PIP immobilization splint;* ***B,*** *a PIP flexion mobilization splint;* ***C,*** *a PIP extension restriction splint.*

Box 17-1 *Splint Design Descriptors*

Digit-based	Originating from the digit, allowing MP joint motion
Hand-based	Originating from the hand, allowing wrist motion
Thumb-based	Originating from the thenar eminence or thumb, incorporating one or more joints of the thumb
Forearm-based	Originating from the forearm, allowing full elbow motion
Circumferential	Encompassing the entire circumference of the involved body part or limb segment
Gutter	Inclusion of only the radial or the ulnar portion of the limb
Radial	Incorporation of the radial aspect of the limb
Ulnar	Incorporation of the ulnar aspect of the limb
Dorsal	Traverses the dorsal (posterior) aspect of the hand or forearm
Volar	Traverses the volar (palmar, anterior) aspect of the hand or forearm
Anterior	Traverses the anterior aspect of the body part
Posterior	Traverses the posterior aspect of the body part

lized in a comfortably extended resting position to allow the involved structures to heal (Figure 17-2). This PIP flexion mobilization splint gently mobilizes the PIP joint into flexion to address a PIP extension contracture (see Figure 17-2, *B*). The PIP joint is restricted from full extension but allowed to flex fully within the boundaries of this PIP extension restriction splint (see Figure 17-2, *C*).

Design Descriptors

Design descriptors are used to increase clarity of the specific splint request and provide detail in notes or during correspondence to physicians or reimbursement sources. The design descriptors are non-SCS nomenclature but are commonly used by the hand therapy and surgery community.[14] The most commonly used descriptors are summarized in Box 17-1.

Choices of Splint Designs

The choices of splint design include familiar terminology: static, serial static, dynamic, and static progressive splinting. A splint design should be chosen to achieve the goals of immobilization, mobilization, or restriction of a specific tissue.

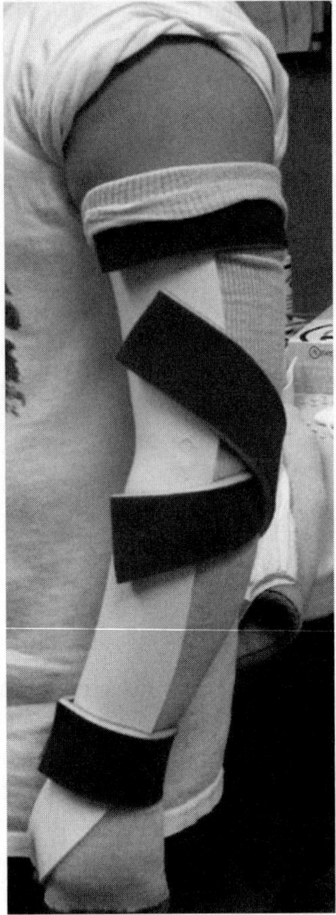

Figure 17-3
This anterior elbow mobilization splint, including the wrist, is used to prevent forearm rotation.

Static Splint

Static splints have a rigid base, immobilizing the joints they traverse (Figure 17-3). A static splint may also be considered a nonarticular splint, having no direct influence on joint mobility but providing stabilization, protection, and support to a body segment such as the wrist or metacarpal. Static splints are perhaps the most common splints made. They can be used as an adjunct to treatment by blocking a distal or proximal joint to increase glide of another joint or improve tendon excursion.

Serial Static Splint

Serial static splints or casts are applied with the joints, soft tissue, or musculotendinous units they cross in a lengthened position (near maximum) and are worn for extended periods (Figure 17-4). Tissue held in this end-range position should react and accommodate by stretching into the desired direction of correction. Serial static splints are often removed during therapy and exercise sessions so that the clinician and patient can work on the involved structures with modalities such as heat, ultrasound, joint mobilization, and range of motion (ROM). The splint is then remolded to maintain the gains made during the exercise session. This

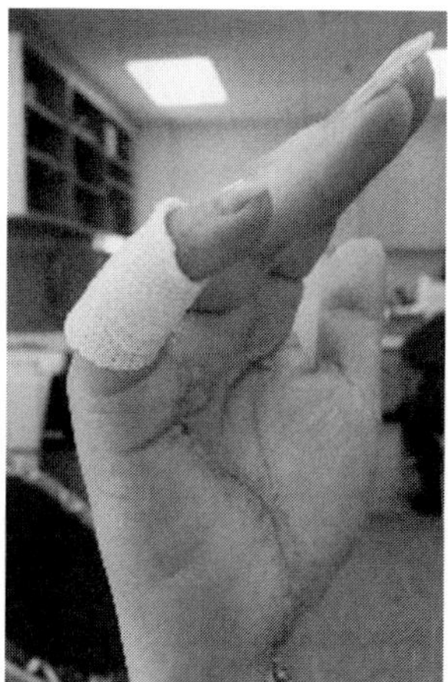

Figure 17-4
This PIP extension mobilization splint is designed to address a fixed flexion deformity with a serial static approach.

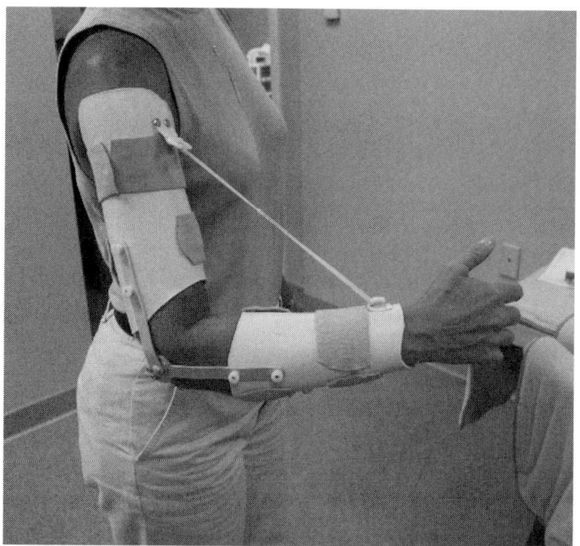

Figure 17-5
An elbow flexion mobilization splint uses a rubber band to apply a mobilization force.

design may provide greater patient compliance and ensures therapists and physicians that the tissue is being continually stressed without the risk of the tissue rebounding if the splint were removed. Nonremovable serial static splints may also be a better choice for patients who are young, who have cognitive or behavioral issues, or who have fluctuating tone and spasticity.

Dynamic Splint

Dynamic splints use an elastic-type force to mobilize specific tissues to achieve increases in ROM (Figure 17-5). Most dynamic splints have a base that permits the attachment of various outriggers and components. The mobilizing forces applied through a dynamic splint are elastic (dynamic) in nature, such as rubber bands, springs, or wrapped elastic cord. The dynamic force applied continues as long as the elastic component can contract, even when the tissue reaches the end of its elastic boundary.[15]

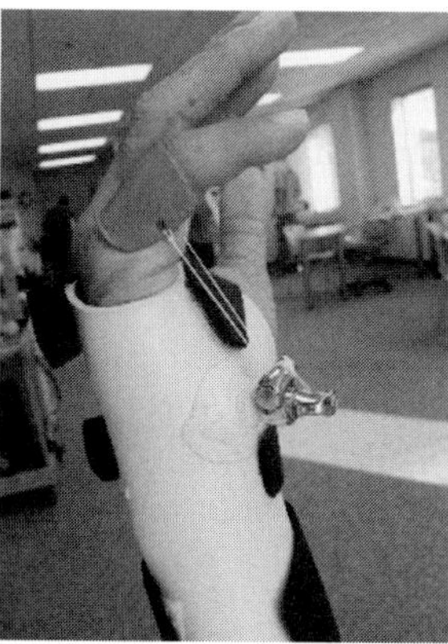

Figure 17-6
This MP splint uses a static line and a static progressive component to apply a mobilization force.

Static Progressive Splint

Static progressive splints achieve tissue mobilization by applying low-load force to the tissue's end range in one direction (Figure 17-6).[4] The goal is that the tissue will eventually accommodate to this position. The fabrication of a static progressive splint is similar to a dynamic splint, but with the force applied being static or nonelastic. The mobilization force can be generated through nylon cord, nonelastic strapping materials, screws, hinges, turnbuckles, and various types of inelastic tape. When the joint position is achieved and the tension on the static progressive component is set, the splint will not continue to stress the tissue beyond its elastic limit.[15] Force can be altered by the patient or therapist through progressive splint adjustments. Some patients may tolerate static progressive splinting better than dynamic splinting. One reason may be that the joint position is constant while the tissue accommodates gently and gradually to the tension, without the influences of gravity and motion.[15,16]

Objectives for Splinting

The key objective for splint fabrication may not always be straightforward. The objectives for splinting intervention may be multiple, as in a wrist and hand immobilization splint (resting hand splint) used on a patient with rheumatoid arthritis. The splint may be constructed to immobilize inflamed arthritic joints, yet place the metacarpophalangeal (MP) joints serially in a gently extended and radially deviated position to minimize ulnar drift and periarticular deformity.

Critical thinking is a necessary process when fabricating splints; multiple injuries, wound status, age, and lifestyle must be taken into consideration. More skilled clinicians can appreciate that there can be several purposes for one splint; therefore, creative problem solving must be used when splinting the more involved, complex injury.

Immobilization Splints

Splints designed to hold or immobilize a joint or limb segment can be used to do the following[14]:

- Provide symptom relief
- Protect and position edematous structures
- Aid in maximizing functional use
- Maintain tissue length
- Protect healing structures and surgical procedures
- Provide support and protection for soft tissue healing
- Maintain and protect reduction of fracture
- Improve and preserve joint alignment
- Block and transfer muscle and tendon forces
- Influence a spastic muscle
- Prevent possible contracture development

Mobilization Splinting

Splints designed to change or mobilize tissues or structures are used to do the following[14]:

- Remodel long-standing, dense, mature scar
- Elongate soft tissue contractures, adhesions, and musculotendinous tightness
- Increase passive joint ROM
- Realign or maintain joint and ligament profile
- Substitute for weak or absent motion
- Maintain reduction of an intraarticular fracture with preservation of joint mobility

Restriction Splinting

Splints designed to restrict or limit motion may be used to do the following[14]:

- Limit motion after nerve injury or repair
- Limit motion after tendon injury or repair
- Limit motion after bone or ligament injury or repair
- Provide and improve joint stability and alignment
- Assist in functional use of the hand

ANATOMY-RELATED PRINCIPLES

Therapists treating the upper extremity need to have a thorough understanding of the complex anatomical features of the hand and arm to manage patients with dysfunction effectively. Disturbance of the delicate relations among the bones, muscles, nerves, and other soft tissue structures, either by disease or trauma, can result in disruption of normal function. Knowledge of normal anatomical features and how pathological conditions affect them is important for therapists to make appropriate clinical decisions regarding treatment interventions.[8,17-19]

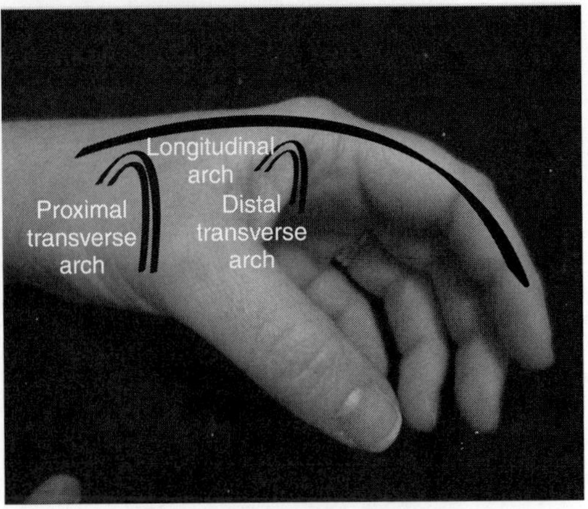

Figure 17-7
The fixed proximal transverse arch, the flexible distal transverse arch, and the longitudinal arch of the hand.

Arches of the Hand

The configuration of the bones in the hand, along with the tension of the muscles and ligaments in this region, contribute to the creation of an arch system composed of the proximal transverse, distal transverse, and longitudinal arches (Figure 17-7).[20,21] This arch system is vital for positioning the hand to allow for normal function related to grasp and prehension.[21,22] Incorporating these arches within a splint is essential to allow maximal function within the splint.

The fixed *proximal transverse arch* is created by the configuration of the distal row of the carpal bones and the taut volar carpal ligament. This region is also referred to as the carpal tunnel, through which the long flexors and median nerve pass en route to the hand.[23] This fixed structure provides mechanical advantage to the flexors, maximizing grasp function.

The mobile *distal transverse arch* is located at the level of the metacarpal heads. This arch is adaptive by the mobile ulnar fourth and fifth carpometacarpal (CMC) joints and highly mobile thumb trapeziometacarpal joint.[24] This increased mobility of the peripheral digits allows for optimal grasping abilities.

The *longitudinal arch* spans the length from the metacarpal to the distal phalanx. A disruption of this arch occurs in patients who have sustained an ulnar nerve injury with resulting loss of intrinsic muscle function. In this situation, the hand takes on an intrinsic minus position with the MP joints hyperextended and the PIP and distal interphalangeal joints flexed.[20]

Palmar Creases

The regular arrangement of creases is easily visible on the volar surface of the hand (Figure 17-8). The thick palmar skin is fixed to the underlying structures by fibrous connections that aid in formation of these creases.[24] Therapists need to appreciate the location of these creases and how they

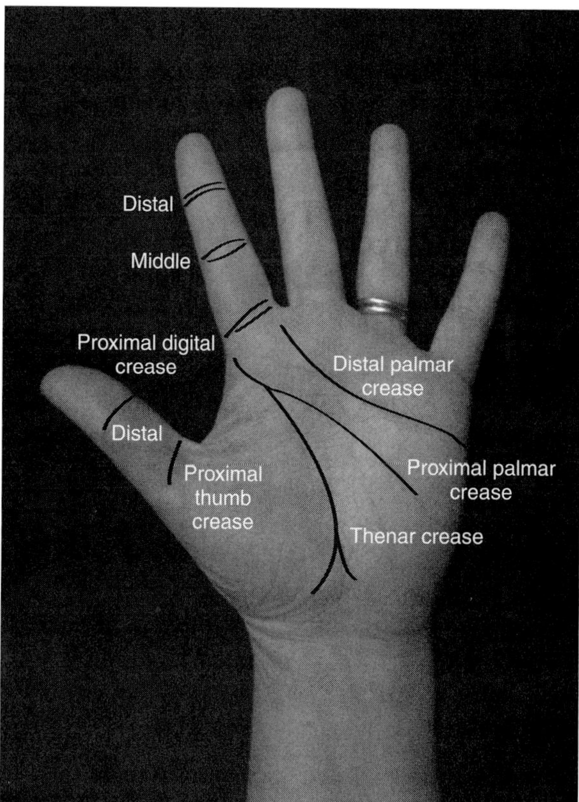

Figure 17-8
Creases of the hand can be helpful guidelines during the splint fabrication process.

correlate with the underlying anatomy. Commonly, these creases are used by therapists as an anatomical guide when creating splint patterns. For example, the distal palmar crease and proximal palmar crease must be fully cleared when fabricating a wrist immobilization splint to allow for unrestricted ROM at the MP joints.

Metacarpal Length and Mobility

Dual obliquity is a concept relating to the anatomy of the metacarpals.[20,22] Because of the differing lengths of the metacarpals (radial side of hand longer than ulnar), when an object is held in the hand, an oblique angle is formed compared with the distal ends of the radius and ulna (Figure 17-9, *A*). In addition, the object is angled in accordance with the distal transverse arch and increasing mobility of the ulnar metacarpals (Figure 17-9, *B*). This dual obliquity should be incorporated into the splint to provide a comfortable and functional splint that resists migration because of the incorporation of the arches.

Positioning the Hand

When deciding how to position the hand within a splint, many factors must be considered, including the patient's diagnosis, healing time frame, and splinting goals. Proper positioning within a splint can help prevent future joint and soft tissue contractures. The two most common positions described in the literature include the *position of function* and the *position of rest*,[14,25] See Figure 17-10 for the general joint angles described for each position.

A

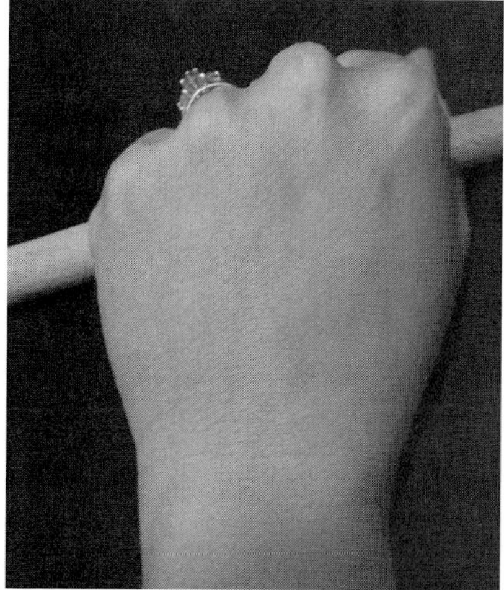

B

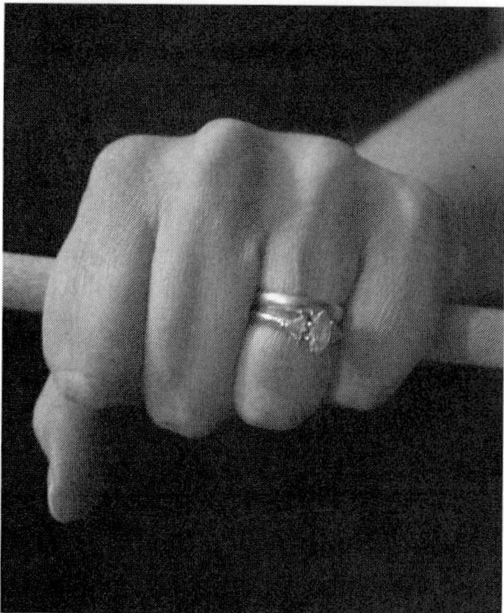

Figure 17-9
*The dual obliquity of the hand, from the dorsal (**A**) and transverse (**B**) perspective.*

The *antideformity position* considers the unique anatomical characteristics of the MP and PIP joints worth highlighting here. The length of the collateral ligaments at the MP joint varies according to the position of the MP joint (Figure 17-11).[26] The collateral ligaments are slack with MP joint extension, whereas tension in the collateral ligaments increases with greater amounts of MP joint flexion. Placing the joints in flexion within a splint helps prevent MP joint extension contractures (limited flexion). If the joints were placed in extension with resulting MP contractures, the disruption of the longitudinal arch would greatly impair grasping abilities.

Similarly at the PIP joint level, the volar plate is placed on tension with PIP joint extension, whereas flexion at the PIP

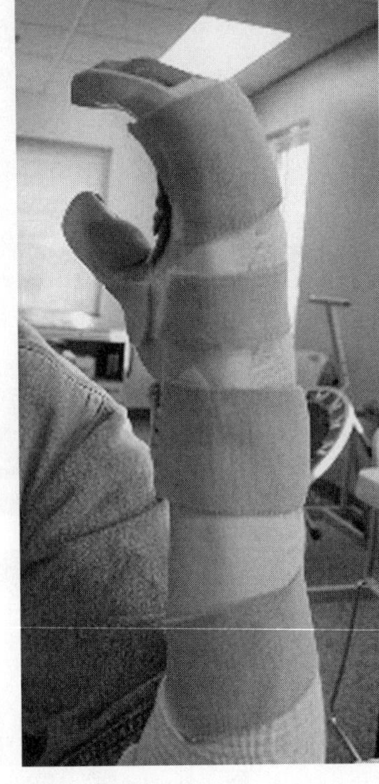

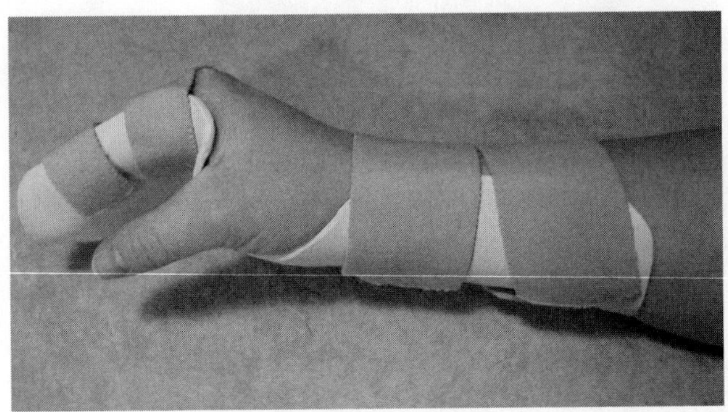

Figure 17-10

*The functional position of the hand (**A**) places the wrist in 20 to 30 degrees of extension, the MP joints in 35 to 45 degrees of flexion, the PIP joints in 45 degrees of flexion, the distal interphalangeal joints in a relaxed flexed position, and the thumb in palmar abduction. The antideformity position of the hand (**B**) places the wrist in 30 to 40 degrees of extension, the MP joints in 60 to 90 degrees of flexion, the PIP and distal interphalangeal joints in extension, and the thumb in palmar abduction.*

joint places the volar plate at risk for shortening (see Figure 17-11, *A* and *B*).[26] Shortening of the volar plate could result in debilitating PIP joint flexion contractures, which can significantly affect the ability to grasp and especially release objects. Therefore, careful positioning of the PIP joint in extension is crucial to maintain the length of the volar plate.

Tissue Precautions

In the upper extremity, a number of areas exist where bony protuberances or superficial nerves are highly susceptible to compression from splints (Box 17-2).[27] If these areas are not accounted for in the fabrication process, the splint will likely be uncomfortable for the patient and therefore possibly not worn. Special consideration must be given to the patient with impaired sensation (those with peripheral nerve injury, neuropathy, nerve root compression, or central nervous system pathosis). Those with limited or absent sensation do not have the normal ability to feel or detect areas of pressure; instead, they must rely on visual inspection to determine integrity of skin and soft tissue.

Because superficial bony prominences have minimal soft tissue coverage, they are vulnerable to compression. Excessive external pressure can place the tissue at risk for irritation and eventual breakdown (necrosis). Older adults may be at most risk because they commonly have minimal subcutaneous fat combined with extremely fragile skin, making the bony areas more apparent. Patients may report pain, redness, and irritation over the bone area. To prevent such occurrences, these at-risk areas on the splint can either be padded with foam or gel or flared away during the molding process (Figure 17-12).[14]

Box 17-2 *Superficial Structures Vulnerable to Pressure*

BONY PROMINENCES

Olecranon process at the elbow
Lateral and medial epicondyles of the humerus
Ulnar and radial styloid processes at the wrist
Base of the first metacarpal
Dorsal thumb and digit MP and interphalangeal joints
Pisiform bone

SUPERFICIAL NERVES

Radial nerve at the radial groove of the humerus
Ulnar nerve at the cubital tunnel
Superficial branch of the ulnar nerve at the distal forearm
Median nerve at the carpal tunnel
Digital nerves at the volar aspect

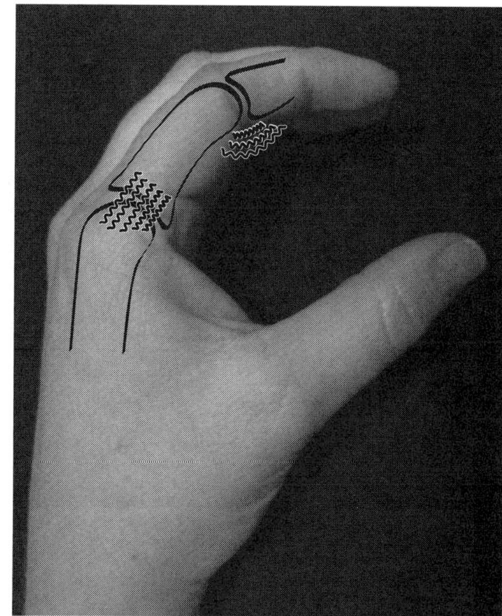

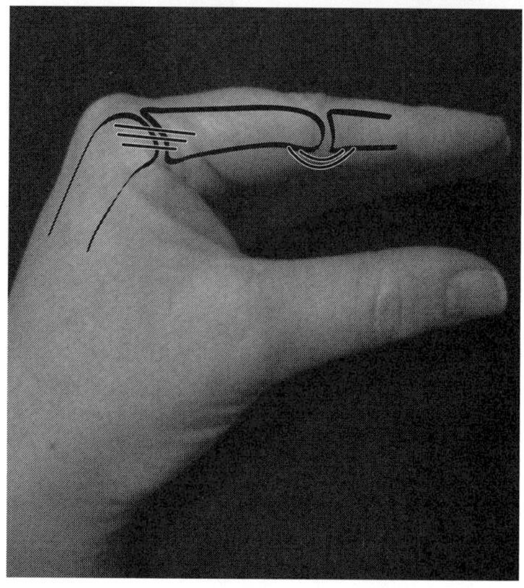

Figure 17-11
Soft tissue length changes associated with joint positioning. ***A,*** *Placing the MP joint in extension will cause the MP collateral ligaments and the PIP volar plate to become "slack" and at risk of becoming shortened.* ***B,*** *Placing the MP joint in flexion elongates both the MP collateral ligaments and the volar plate of the PIP joint to minimize risk of shortening of these structures.*

Therapists must also appreciate peripheral nerve anatomy and how splints and strapping may place undue pressure over these regions, potentially leading to nerve compression.[28] Patients may report pain, redness, paresthesias (tingling), and numbness in that nerve's distribution. Timely modification of the splint is necessary to prevent long-term nerve irritation. Splinting over gel or the use of wider straps to disperse the pressure better are two techniques that may be useful to address this issue.[14]

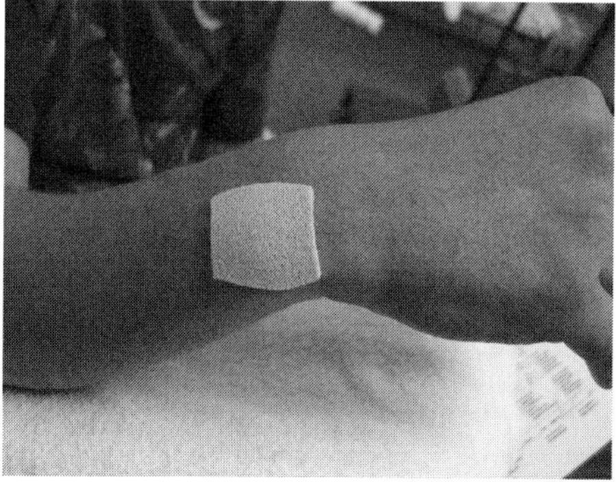

Figure 17-12
Padding bony prominences, such as the ulnar styloid, before molding of the splint can decrease the risk of high-pressure areas and potential for skin irritation or breakdown.

Also of note is the potential for compression of vascular structures when a splint is worn.[29] Symptoms of throbbing, color changes, temperature changes, and pain should immediately be dealt with. These symptoms are all consistent with vascular compromise. Reporting these side effects is especially important if any surgical reconstruction of vascular structures was performed. Wide straps and slings to distribute pressure maximally along with the appropriate use of elasticized wraps can aid in preventing this problem.[21] Most important, educating the patient regarding these potential signs and symptoms of bony and neurovascular compromise is key to preventing any long-term problems caused by splint application.

TISSUE HEALING

The phases of specific tissue healing (e.g., bone, nerve, tendon, ligament) aid in directing appropriate splint selection, fabrication, and wearing schedule.[30,31] Appreciation of what role a splint can play during each phase is a critical step in the therapeutic process (i.e., knowing when to rest tissue versus mobilize tissue). Clinicians must recognize that although the stages of tissue healing are described as chronological, overlap in their incidence can occur. Take, for example, a patient after a traumatic snow blower injury who has sustained soft tissue, bone, tendon, and nerve damage. Depending on the severity of each of these injuries, healing rates of each specific tissue may be different even though it is the same hand. As the healing stages overlap, so may the time frames for using specific splint designs.

Stages of Tissue Healing

Therapists must understand how each specific injury affects the surrounding tissues. For example, immobilization splints may be indicated throughout the length of the healing process but are most commonly used during the inflammatory stage. The three main phases of tissue healing are the

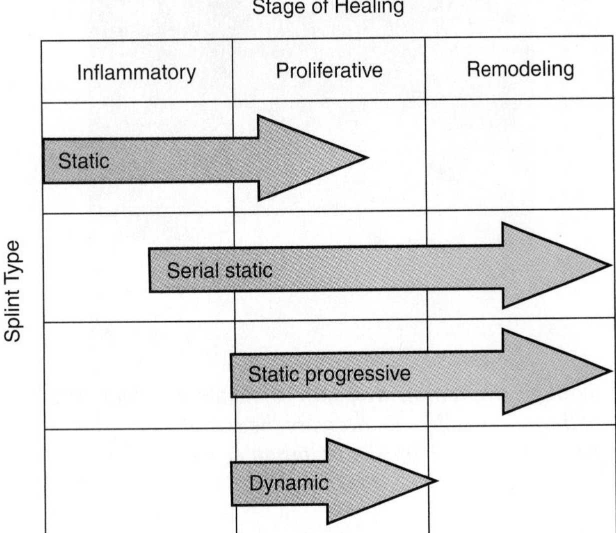

Figure 17-13
An algorithm for the uses of various types of splints according to the stages of healing.

inflammatory, proliferative (fibroplasia), and remodeling (chronic) phases (Figure 17-13).

During the *inflammatory phase*, an influx of white blood cells occurs to cleanse the area (edema).[32,33] Clinically the tissue feels soft, boggy, and easy to mobilize. This stage typically lasts for 1 week or less. Rest is normally more important than exercise during the inflammatory stage, so immobilization splints are appropriate in the days immediately after tissue injury.[21]

During the *proliferative phase*, collagen is laid down and the wound gains strength. The clinician begins to see and feel more tissue resistance (scar adherence), although the tissue is still soft and "movable" with tension. This phase lasts from 1 to 6 weeks. Dynamic-type splints that mobilize tissue can be effective during this time frame. They provide gentle stress that can facilitate tissue growth, resulting in tissue lengthening.[1,10]

The last phase of tissue healing is referred to as the *remodeling phase*. During this stage the tensile strength of the tissue is enhanced. Clinically, the tissues involved feel dense, hard, and inelastic. Tissues may actually shorten because of a decrease in elasticity; therefore, stretching is a valuable tool to prevent unwanted contractures. Superficial scars also begin to soften during this stage. This stage begins as early as 6 weeks and can last up to 12 to 24 months. Serial static and static progressive approaches to mobilize tissue during this phase are most appropriate.[4]

Factors That Influence Tissue Healing

Tissue healing is influenced by several factors. For example, tissue that is deprived of oxygen requires a longer healing time and also influences the splint wearing time. Therapists must thoroughly discuss medical history and lifestyle habits with the patient to determine any factors that may delay or impair tissue healing. Tobacco, for example, diminishes the body's ability to heal, decreasing blood flow and nutrition.[34] Excessive alcohol intake can impair the immune system, leading to malnourishment and liver damage.[35] The most common factors that influence the rate of tissue healing include the following[14]:

- Age
- Nutritional status
- Tobacco use
- Diabetes
- Edema
- Infection
- Rheumatoid arthritis
- Alcohol use
- Sickle cell disease
- Steroids
- Radiation therapy
- Peripheral vascular disease
- Raynaud's disease
- Systemic lupus erythematosus

MECHANICAL PRINCIPLES

Before fabricating a splint, therapists need to know basic mechanical principles and be able to integrate this information into the splint design and construction process.[14,21,30,36,37] This section briefly reviews the most common principles to consider. Careful attention to the following principles will improve the fabrication, function, and fit of a splint.

Levers

Levers are rigid structures through which a force can be applied to produce rotational motion about a fixed axis.[14] A lever system is composed of a fulcrum, or fixed axis, and two arms: the effort arm and resistance arm. The effort arm, also referred to as the force arm, is the segment of the lever between the fulcrum and the effort force that is attempting to stabilize or mobilize a structure. In a splint design, the fulcrum corresponds with the anatomical axis of the target joint, the effort arm is the segment of the splint that applies the effort force, and the resistance arm is the segment of the limb that resists the effort force. Ideally, the effort and resistance forces work in concert to create opposing torques about the fulcrum. However, cases occur in which the axis of rotation (fulcrum) has been interrupted from disease or injury (e.g., fracture, rheumatoid arthritis).

Most splints are categorized as first-class levers in which the fulcrum is between the effort and resistance arms (Figure 17-14). Common examples of first-class lever systems are a seesaw, a pair of scissors, and a pair of pliers. The goal when designing a splint is to create the most efficient work. The length of the resistance arm greatly influences the mechanical advantage of the force applied. The effort arm of the splint can also influence mechanical advantage by how carefully it is molded about the body part.

Both the effort and resistance arms should be vigilantly formed, incorporating arches, clearing for creases, and allowing adequate surface area for maximal distribution of pressure. As forces actively influence a joint, a balance-counterbalance effect must occur. If the opposing force (effort arm) is not distributed well to counterbalance the distal forces (resistance arm), the splint may not sit flush with the body part. This may create high-pressure areas, shear stress, and an unproductive application of force. Clinicians can generate "mechanical advantages" through careful application of splinting principles and meticulous attention to detail while molding. Clinically, splints tend to be most comfortable when well molded, incorporating adequate length and depth. Short, narrow, and shallow splints can cause increases in localized pressure and overall discomfort.

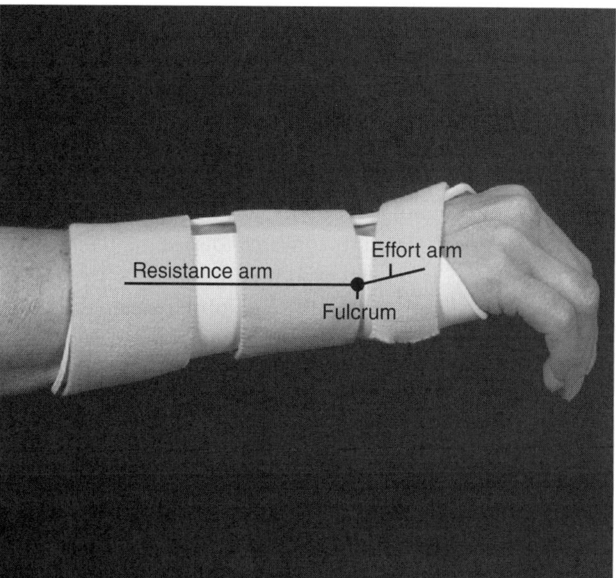

Figure 17-14
The fulcrum of a splint is placed at the axis of joint motion. The resistance arm is applied by the proximal segment of the splint; the effort arm is applied by the distal segment of the splint.

Stress

Stress can occur in various forms. The most common types that relate directly to splinting are compression, shear, tension, bending, and torsion.[14] *Compressive stress* (also referred to as pressure) is defined as force per unit area. In the process of creating and planning a splint design, therapists must understand the various forms of stress that can be produced by the external forces of a splint. For example, compression can be minimized by increasing the surface area (designing the splint base wider and longer) over which the force can be maximally distributed. Optimizing the conformity of materials to the shape of the body part being splinted can minimize compressive stress.

A number of factors can result in areas of high pressure. Narrow strap width, especially in conjunction with "shallow" splints, can produce high compressive stress on the soft tissue. Splint borders should lie flush with the skin surface that the strap traverses. The strap should not bridge the two borders of the splint; it should come in contact with the skin.

The slings used in mobilization splints are another possible source of compression stress that should be considered, especially if edema or neurovascular issues are evident in the patient's limb. Compression to the lateral, dorsal, or volar aspects of the digit can be avoided by using several techniques. The splint line can be attached to each side of a sling (two pieces of line), then joined after they pass through the pulley. This design prevents the circumferential compression created when one line is threaded through both ends of the sling. Alternatively, a custom-fabricated thermoplastic "pan" can be placed under the sling as a support. The digital "pan" disperses the compressive forces applied through the sling by lifting the borders away from the skin and increasing the area of force application (see Figure 17-2, *B*).

Shear stress results from a parallel force applied to the surface and produces a tendency for an object to either deform or slide along the surface.[14] When fabricating mobilization splints, the mobilizing force, which is attached to the proximal splint base, usually traverses the length of the splint and terminates distally at the body segment. If the proximal portion (base) of the splint is not adequately secured to the limb with appropriate strapping, there will be an undesirable migration or dragging and shearing of the proximal base over the skin when the mobilization force is distally applied (Figure 17-15). Being mindful of incorporating the arches of the hand as well and obtaining a well-contoured splint during the molding process aid in preventing this migration. In some cases, a nonskid material such Dycem (Dycem Technologies Limited, Bristol, England) or foam tape to line the splint can also help keep the splint stable on the extremity.

Angle of Force Application

The angle of force application is critical to the proper design and fabrication of mobilization splints. Ideally, the force should be applied 90 degrees to the body segment being mobilized (Figure 17-16), which maximizes the therapeutic effect of the force being applied. With a pure 90-degree orientation to the part being mobilized, there are virtually no forces disseminated in other directions. However, if the angle is other than 90 degrees, a portion of the force is dissipated elsewhere, thereby diminishing the therapeutic effect and causing potentially harmful compression or shear stress.

Clinically, the use of custom-made or prefabricated line guides or pulleys can be helpful to achieve a 90-degree angle of application. The therapist must view the splint from all angles to ensure that the line of application is directed centrally over the segment and oriented properly in all planes. To improve flexion of the digits with a mobilization splint, the anatomical configuration of the hand necessitates the line of force application to converge toward the scaphoid. If this orientation is not incorporated into the splint design, excessive stress is placed on the MP joints, causing discomfort and potential harm. Occasionally, a force applied in either a radial or ulnar direction is indicated, as with postoperative MP joint arthroplasties or sagittal band repairs.

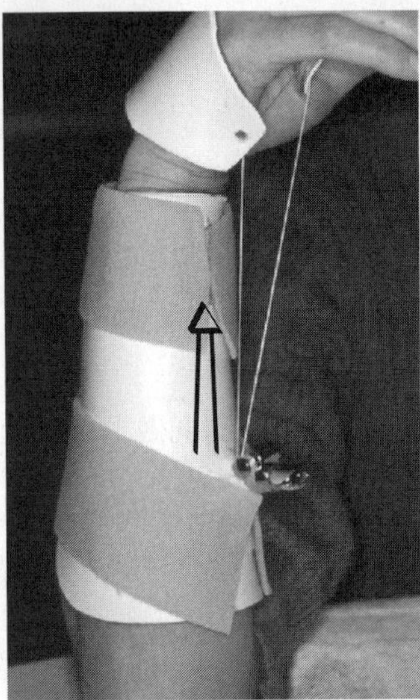

Figure 17-15
When tension is applied to this wrist flexion mobilization splint, shear stress is created as the proximal splint migrates distally on the forearm.

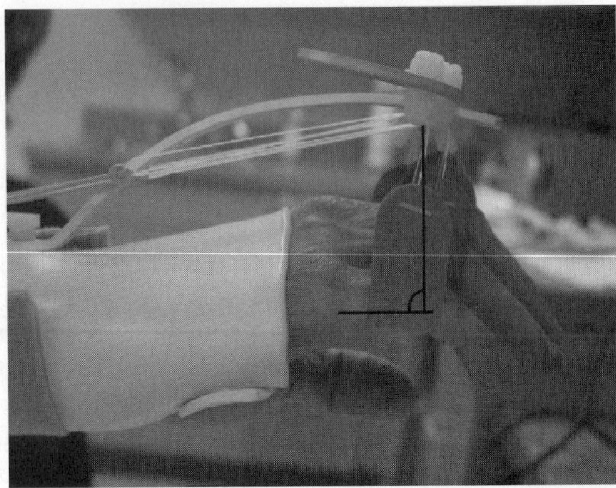

Figure 17-16
Notice the optimal 90-degree angle formed by the proximal phalanx and the monofilament line in this dynamic splint.

Except for special circumstances such as these, the line of application should be centrally located over the longitudinal axis of the bone being mobilized.

Force Application

When using elastic force to mobilize stiff structures, therapists must consider the therapeutic objectives.[38-40] Is the goal mobilization of a mature, dense joint contracture, or is it stabilization of the MP joints in extension after MP joint arthroplasty? Both situations may require an elastic force; however, both the amount of force and the materials used to achieve these goals vary considerably.[41] The amount of force necessary to mobilize various tissues depends on such factors as individual tolerance, diagnosis, stage of tissue healing, chronicity of problem, severity of contracture, density of contracture, age, smoking, alcohol use, and other health-related issues. Ranges of 100 to 300 g have been suggested for mobilization of the small joints of the hand, whereas higher parameters (350+ g) may be more effective for larger structures.[1,21] This 300 g of force is based on what is tolerated per unit of surface area of the skin, not the tolerance of the contracted tissue to tension. In most cases skin tolerance becomes the limiting factor in determining appropriate splint tension, not the risk of injury to the specific targeted tissue. The therapist can almost always rely on the tissue's response to the tension to help determine the effectiveness of the mobilizing forces. Signs of too much stress include edema, skin blanching, vascular changes, and pain. The amount of time the force is applied is another factor to consider with mobilization splinting.[42] In general, the force should be applied with the goal of providing a low load but prolonged stress to the tissue.

MATERIAL AND EQUIPMENT

Numerous companies market and distribute splinting supplies (Box 17-3), which include many types of thermoplastic material, strapping, component systems, and equipment. The best way to become educated regarding what is on the market is by spending time reviewing the catalogs and contacting local sales representatives to request samples. In addition, attending splinting workshops and hand therapy conferences can be a helpful means to gain knowledge and practice skills that can be used in the clinical setting.

Thermoplastic Materials

Low-temperature thermoplastics are the most commonly used material by therapists to fabricating custom splints. The material is sold in sheets or precut designs also known as sling banks. The material is softened in warm water before application to the body part. Once on the body part, the material cools and hardens into shape. Therapists can select from a wide range of thermoplastic material, making the

Box 17-3 *Distributors of Splinting Products*

AliMed
297 High Street, Dedham, MA 02026
Phone: 800-225-2610
Fax: 800-437-2966
www.alimed.com

DeRoyal/LMB
200 DeBusk Lane, Powell, TN 37849
Phone: 800-938-7828
Fax: 865-362-1230
www.deroyal.com

North Coast Medical
18305 Sutter Blvd, Morgan Hill, CA 95037
Phone: 800-821-9319
Fax: 877-213-9300
www.ncmedical.com

Sammons Preston Rolyan
PO Box 5071, Bolingbrook, IL 60440
Phone: 800-323-5547
Fax: 800-547-4333
www.sammonspreston.com

UE Tech
PO Box 2145, Edwards, CO 81632
Phone: 800-736-1894
Fax: 970-926-8870
www.uetech.com

WFR Corporation
30 Lawlins Park, Wyckoff, NJ 07481
Phone: 800-526-5274
Fax: 800-831-8174
www.reveals.com

3-Point Products
1610 Pincay Court, Annapolis, MD 21401
Phone: 888-378-7763
Fax: 410-349-2648
www.3pointproducts.com

choice of which to use for a specific patient confusing for novice practitioners. The splint maker must have a sound understanding of the differences to be able to make an informed decision, taking into account the purpose of the splint and the specifics of a particular patient's diagnosis. In addition to considering the patient's needs, other factors therapists must consider include level of splinting experience, availability of materials, and cost constraints.

Few studies have examined the characteristics of thermoplastic materials in an attempt to categorize their differences.[43-45] However, a knowledge of handling and physical characteristics and the different categories of thermoplastic materials can help therapists make informed selections.

Handling Characteristics

Handling characteristics refer to the way a material behaves during the molding process. The three most important characteristics of splinting materials that must be considered are conformability and resistance to stretch, memory, and bonding characteristics.

Conformability and Resistance to Stretch

The ability for a material to conform to a body part is related to its level of resistance to stretch (Figure 17-17).[46,47] A helpful system for organizing thermoplastic materials is to group them into categories according to their degree of resistance to stretch (see Table 17-1).[46,47] Materials with minimal resistance to stretch are highly conforming and may be the best choice when a splint is to be applied by an experienced therapist. The less hands-on the better during the fabrication process because this material tends to contour well without much assistance. Gravity-assisted positioning during the molding process is essential. These materials may be appropriate for the patient who has a high level of pain and would not tolerate hands-on molding or for those splints for which achieving an intimate fit is crucial to maximize comfort. Smaller splints such as finger or hand-based splints are best made with these highly conforming materials.

Materials with maximal resistance to stretch are minimally conforming and demand more hands-on work from the splint maker to obtain an intimate fit. Therapists with nominal splinting experience may do better with these materials because they tolerate more aggressive handling. These materials are appropriate for use when fabricating larger splints such as elbow splints or in situations in which splinting against gravity is not an option. Because this material does not contour as precisely, it may be the best choice when splinting over wound dressings when the dimensions are altered with each dressing change.

Memory

Memory refers to a material's ability to revert to its original shape once heated, ranging from 0% to 100% memory.[46,47] Materials with this property are good choices for splints that need to be frequently remolded, such as when fabricating a serial static splint that needs to be reheated and reformed to the body part as ROM increases. Caution must be used when removing the splint from the body part after molding to be sure the material is completely cool, or the material may shrink and the fit achieved within the splint lost. Also, spot heating is not advised with this material because of the possibility of altering adjacent regions.

Bonding

Bonding is the ability of a material to adhere to itself (Figure 17-18).[46,47] The presence of a protective coating prevents this occurrence, and material with coating is recommended for the beginner therapist. Without a coating, the material may stick to a wound dressing, the patient's body hair, or itself.

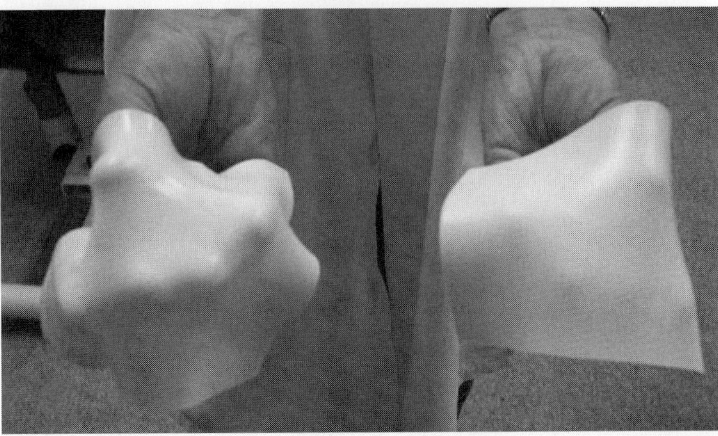

Figure 17-17
The drape, or contouring of the material, placed over the left hand indicates a low resistance to stretch, whereas the less moldable material over the right hand is more resistant to stretch.

The coating can allow two pieces of material to be popped apart after the splint is formed, which can be particularly helpful when applying a circumferential design such as around the thumb. The coating must be removed with solvent or disrupted by scratching the surface to allow for adherence, which is commonly required for attaching mobilization components. The coating may make the splint easier to clean. When using material without a coating, apply a barrier between the two pieces such as a wet paper towel or hand lotion to prevent adherence.

Physical Characteristics

Physical characteristics are evident on visual inspection. The most relevant include the material's thickness, the presence of perforations, and the color of the material.[14]

Thickness

Low temperature thermoplastics are available in a variety of thicknesses, including $^1/_{16}$, $^3/_{32}$, $^1/_8$, and $^3/_{16}$ inches.[46,47] The appropriate thickness for a splint depends on the body part, diagnosis, and required rigidity of the splint. For example, an elbow immobilization splint for a patient with a large arm who sustained a fracture and underwent surgical fixation would best be made from a thick $^1/_8$-inch material for a more rigid support. On the contrary, a hand-based thumb splint for an elderly patient with arthritis might be better served with a thinner $^1/_{16}$-inch splint to achieve a light support. The goal should be to provide the least bulky, lightest weight splint possible that still performs its intended function. Thinner materials are generally quicker to heat and harden faster than their thicker counterparts.

Perforations

Thermoplastic materials with perforations allow for air exchange and produce a lighter-weight splint compared with splints made with solid materials.[46,47] Materials with a high density of perforations create a splint that is flexible (less rigid), which may not be appropriate for specific diagnoses. Caution must be used to ensure that the edges of the splint, cut-through perforations, are smoothed to prevent irritation to the patient's skin.

Colors

A wide array of colors is available, making the splint fabrication process even more creative.[45,46] Choices in splint and strap colors can improve compliance with splint wear in children. Providing splint straps in a color other than white can be helpful for patients to prevent loss within bed linens. Be sure to ask for requests from patients to make them feel they have contributed in the construction of the splint and hopefully improve their acceptance for wear.

Categories of Splint Materials

Thermoplastic materials can be categorized according to their chemical composition.[43-45] This composition determines the way the material behaves during the fabrication process and affects how the finished splint functions. Thermoplastic materials may be made of plastics (e.g., Polyform [Sammons Preston Rolyan, Bolingbrook, Ill.] or Multiform [AliMed, Dedham, Mass.]), rubber or rubberlike materials (e.g., Ezeform [Sammons] or Orthoplast [AliMed]), combination plastic and rubberlike materials (e.g., Tailorsplint, PolyFlex II [Sammons], or Encore [North Coast Medical, Morgan Hill, Calif.), and elastic materials (e.g., Aquaplast [Sammons] or Reveal [WFR Corporation, Wyckoff, N.J.]).

Plastic materials typically have a low resistance to stretch, allowing a highly contoured finished splint. Rubber or rubberlike materials are highly resistant to stretch but offer more control during the fabrication process. Combination plastic and rubberlike materials offer the best of both worlds in terms of conformability and control during the molding process. Elastic materials possess memory and may be suitable for the beginner splint maker who wishes to have the ability to remold the splint if necessary.

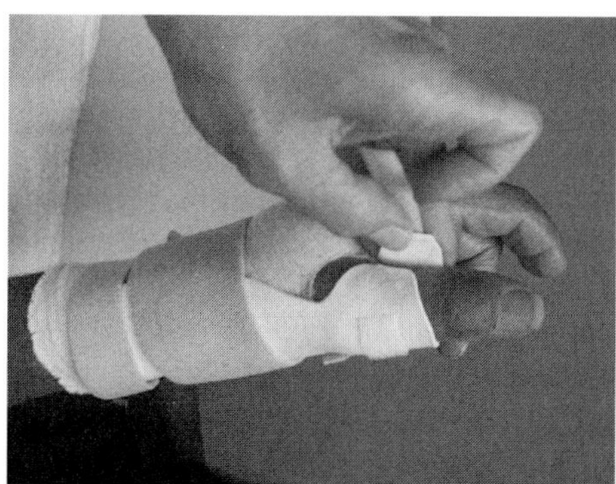

Figure 17-18
The presence of coating on this material allows the circumferential segment around the thumb to be pulled apart to form a "trap door" on this wrist and thumb mobilization splint.

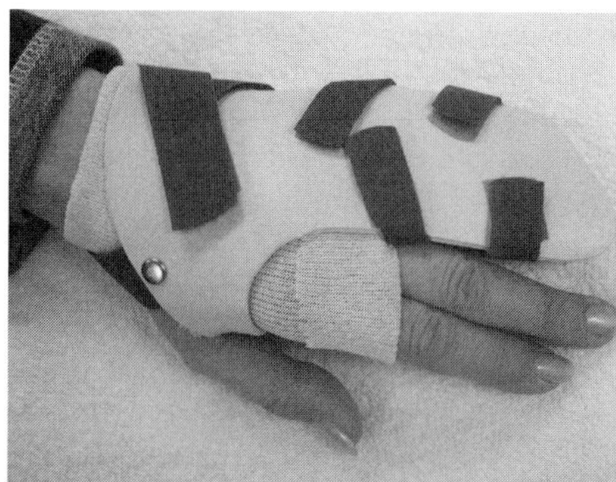

Figure 17-19
A rivet can be applied to secure strapping to the splint by forming holes in the thermoplastic material and the strap with a hole punch; pliers are used to set it in place.

Splints may also be fabricated from alternative materials.[14,46,47] These materials include lined materials (e.g., Rolyan AirThru [Sammons], Silon-LTS [Sammons], or Multiform Soft [Alimed]), mesh-type materials (e.g., X-Lite [Sammons]), casting materials (e.g., plaster of Paris or QuickCast [Sammons]), and soft materials (e.g., Neoprene or Kinesio Tape [Sammons]).

Strapping

Many different strapping systems are offered through distributors.[46,47] The choice of appropriate strapping depends on the patient diagnosis and splint design and availability in the same way that the choice of the appropriate thermoplastic material does. Strapping is essential to secure the splint to the body part properly. If the strapping is not adequate, the splint will likely be uncomfortable or ineffective in achieving its desired goals. Generally, adhesive hook-and-loop material (e.g., Velcro; Velcro USA, Manchester, N.H.) is applied to the splint base, and strapping material secures the segment within the splint. The most commonly used strapping mechanisms consist of traditional loop, foam, neoprene, or elasticized straps. In small areas where adhesive hooks may continue to pull off, rivets may be used to secure the loop material (Figure 17-19).

Other adjuncts to strapping include D-rings that offer the ability to easily adjust the tension on the straps or circumferential wrapping for those patients with significant edema. Straps should be wide and conforming to distribute the pressure maximally, but not so wide that they inhibit ROM of adjacent joints.[14,21] The patient should be educated in how to apply the straps snugly enough to secure the splint in place without compromising the neurovascular system.

Padding and Lining

Padding and lining products are available in a wide variety of thicknesses, textures, and materials.[46,47] Therapists may use padding in specific regions during the splinting process to accommodate bony prominences or superficial nerves. Ideally, this padding should be applied to the target area before molding the splint so that the splint can contour to its proportions. Attaching the padding after the splint is made can potentially cause a shift in pressure distribution and lead to problematic areas of high stress. Foam padding can also be adhered to straps at strategic places to improve joint position and prevent migration within the splint.

Lining a splint with an adhesive product may be indicated in rare cases, such as when the patient has very fragile skin. Application of these adhesive liners should be used sparingly because of hygienic concerns; they are not easily cleaned or removed. As an alternative, disposable liners on the body part can be a way to improve comfort within a splint by placing a barrier between the skin and the plastic (see Figure 17-19). Cotton or elasticized stockinettes are the most commonly used products.

Components

Various component systems exist that are an important element of mobilization splinting.[46,47] Current rehabilitation catalogs help therapists keep abreast of what is available. In general, outrigger systems are designed to help provide optimal force application to a body part. These devices are usually highly adjustable to allow the therapist to maintain the crucial 90-degree angle of force application. If the commercial systems are not accessible, therapists can fabricate homemade ones with wire and scrap pieces of thermoplastic material. Four basic elements of an outrigger system are used in a digit mobilization splint: the proximal attachment device, mobilization force, pulley system, and finger loops or slings (Figure 17-20).

The *proximal attachment device* provides the means to secure the mobilization force to the splint. The *mobilization force*, whether it be static line (static progressive approach) or elastic (dynamic approach), traverses through a *pulley system* to maintain the 90-degree angle of force application. Distally, the force is imparted to the body part, in this example the finger, by a *sling* or *loop*.

Mobilization splints can be challenging to fabricate for a new therapist. Learning through practicing and obtaining feedback from more experienced colleagues are important ways to improve fabrication skills. Patients must consistently receive follow-up in the clinic to assess and modify the splint to achieve a positive outcome; the splints need frequent adjustments as the tissue responds to the stress.

Equipment

Quality tools in the clinic can help make the splinting process easier for the therapist. Sharp scissors designated for thermoplastic use only are essential; if the scissors are used for all products, most notably adhesive products, the blades can retain the residue and make cutting the thermoplastic difficult. Scissors with a nonstick coating are now available and are quite effective when cutting adhesive-backed products. Dull scissors do not provide a clean cut, which can lead to frustration and unsightly splints. Other tools helpful to keep on hand include a hole punch, blunt nose pliers, hand drill, and heat gun.

OVERVIEW OF SPLINTING PROCESS

A comprehensive prescription from the referring physician is essential for appropriate splint application and therapeutic intervention. In addition to the patient's name, the prescription must contain the following information:

- Diagnosis, including surgical procedures if applicable
- Date of injury and surgery
- Any precautions that must be followed
- Splint goals, including purpose, joint positions, and wearing schedule

Radiographs and the patient's surgical report can assist the therapist in gaining a clear understanding of the tissue involvement. As always, good communication with the physician is key in terms of gathering and sharing information regarding a patient's status.

After obtaining all the essential information regarding the patient's diagnosis and the physician's orders, the therapist should perform a comprehensive evaluation. The evaluation begins with a patient interview for gathering subjective information and continues with a review of systems and a detailed physical examination.[6,19] The therapist uses the results of the history and examination to form a clinical judgment and movement dysfunction diagnosis, including a list of problems. From these problems the therapist determines the prognosis for improvement of function and formulates an appropriate plan of care.

To prepare a comprehensive therapeutic plan of care, therapists must use critical thinking skills to integrate all their knowledge with the information obtained from physicians and patients. The therapist has many modalities that can be used to treat the patient, only one of which is splinting. Not all patients are appropriate for splinting; determining if and when splinting may be appropriate is the challenge of the therapist.

If splinting is deemed appropriate, the patient must be thoroughly educated regarding its use. This education must always include a written handout outlining the specifics of wear, care, and precautions. The key points to stress include the following:

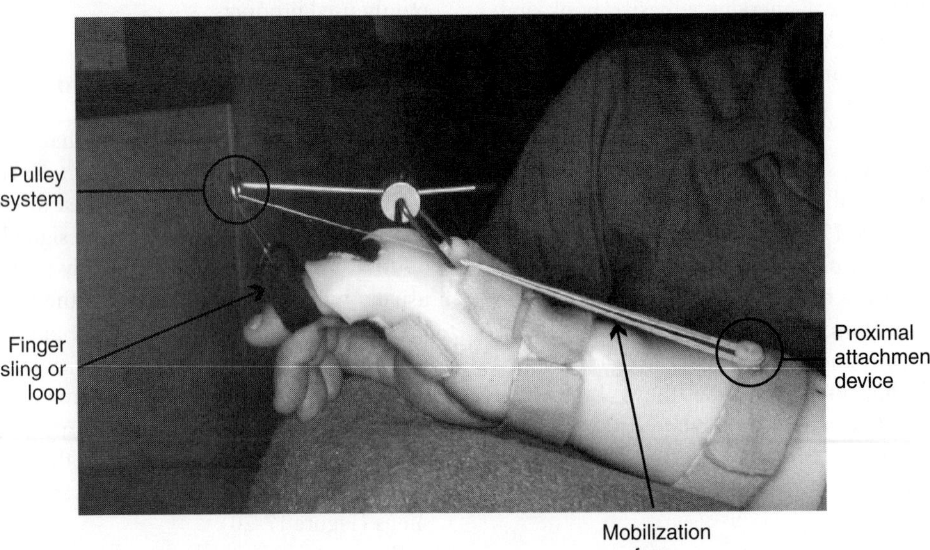

Figure 17-20
Elements of this forearm-based PIP joint extension mobilization splint include a proximal attachment device, a mobilization force through a pulley system, and a finger sling or loop.

- The purpose of splint, specific to the patient's diagnosis
- Key indicators of problems that might occur and information about what to do if they occur
- Any functional limitations that might result from wearing the splint and suggestions of how to compensate for such limitations
- The wearing schedule
- Information about washing or cleaning the splint
- Information or diagrams about how to properly don and doff the splint (if applicable)
- Precautions related to the patient's diagnosis and indicators of tissue tolerance (signs and symptoms of neurovascular compromise or bony irritation)
- Avoidance of heat to prevent loss of splint shape
- Contact information (the therapist's name and clinic phone number) with encouragement to call if any questions or problems should arise.

CASE EXAMPLE 1

A Patient with Osteoarthritis of the Carpometacarpal Joints

M. F. presents to the hand surgeon with progressive onset of thumb pain. Symptoms of aching and tenderness are exacerbated by activities such as turning keys, opening jars, and writing. Deformity from joint subluxation at the first carpometacarpal (trapeziometacarpal) joint and osteoarthritis (OA) are evident (Figure 17-21). The patient also has a positive grind test—the manual application of longitudinal compression force of the first metacarpal into the trapezium. (This test is positive for carpometacarpal OA when pain and crepitation are present.) M. F. receives a steroid injection into the joint space to decrease local inflammation and a prescription for therapy.

Questions to Consider

- Given this patient's current presentation, what additional tests and measures might be important in the evaluation process?
- What is your movement dysfunction–related diagnosis for this patient?
- What do you think the prognosis will be for this patient? What are the patient's goals for intervention? What are your rehabilitation goals? How long do you think it will take to achieve the goals that you and the patient agree on?
- On the basis of the patient's goals and expectations as well as your understanding of the underlying disease process, what recommendations would you make for intervention at this point in time? What evidence from the clinical research literature supports your recommendations? What have you chosen or prioritized from these possible interventions?

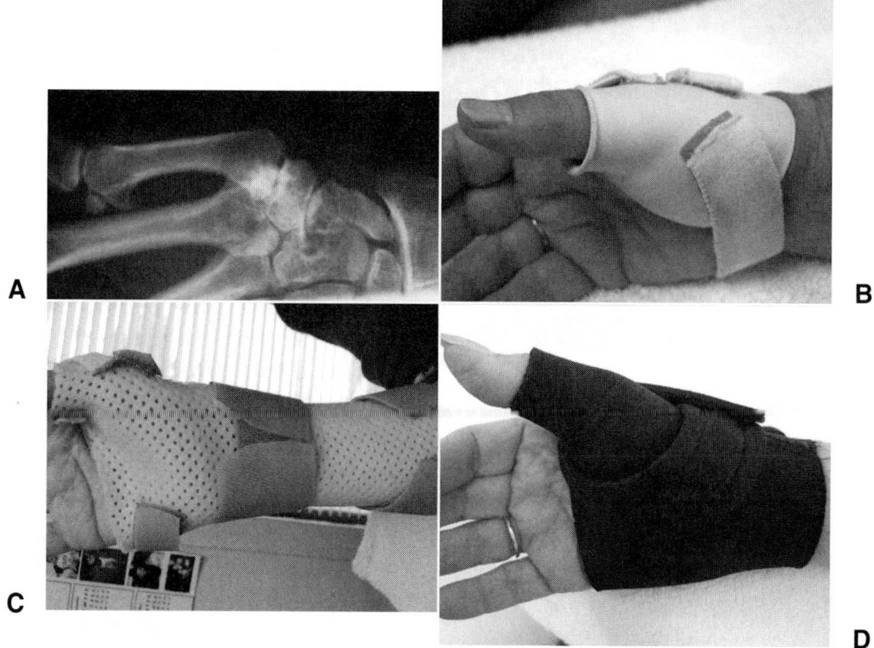

Figure 17-21

A, *A radiograph indicating osteoarthritis at the CMC joint of the thumb.* ***B,*** *A custom thumb splint designed to reduce stress on the CMC joint during activities of daily living.* ***C,*** *After ligament reconstruction and arthroplasty, a forearm immobilization splint is used during the proliferative stage of healing.* ***D,*** *When adequate healing and fixation have occurred, a neoprene sleeve is used to support the thumb during activities of daily living.*

- What type of follow-up would you recommend? How might the goals and interventions change as the patient progresses through the stages of tissue healing? How would you assess the outcomes of your interventions?

Recommendations for a Patient with OA of the Carpometacarpal Joint

A custom thumb splint is fabricated from a lightweight thermoplastic material (thickness: $\frac{1}{16}$ inch) (see Figure 17-21, *B*). M. F. is instructed to use this during the day to decrease stress on the joint during activities of daily living. She is also educated in activity modification and joint protection principles. Some of the strategies include avoiding forceful, repetitive, and sustained pinching along with using pens and kitchen utensils with larger handles.

Despite these interventions, M. F. continues to have symptoms and returns to the physician to discuss her treatment options. M. F. undergoes a ligament reconstruction with tendon interposition arthroplasty, which includes a trapezium excision with a slip of the flexor carpi radialis interposed between the scaphoid and the first metacarpal.[23] For the initial 3-week postoperative period, during the initial inflammatory stage of healing when resting the tissue is important, a cast is used to immobilize the region. As healing progresses into the proliferative stage at 3 weeks, the patient is placed in a removable forearm-based wrist/thumb immobilization splint that is removed for periodic range of motion exercises (see Figure 17-21, *C*).

At approximately 6 weeks after surgery, as the healing continues to progress, the patient uses a custom neoprene thumb splint to aid in the transition from the rigid thermoplastic splint (see Figure 17-21, *D*). The neoprene material offers a restrictive splint combining warmth and gentle support for use during activities of daily living. At 12 weeks, all splints are discontinued and M. F. returns to normal use without pain.

CASE EXAMPLE 2

A Patient with a Wrist Fracture

V. A. presents to the hand surgeon's office after a fall onto an outstretched hand. The radiograph reveals a comminuted wrist fracture requiring surgical fixation. The surgeon performs an open reduction internal fixation with a plate and screws (Figure 17-22). At 5 days after surgery, the patient is referred to therapy for protective splinting and an early range of motion program.

Questions to Consider

- Given this patient's current presentation, what additional tests and measures might be important in the evaluation process?
- What is your movement dysfunction–related diagnosis for this patient?
- What do you think the prognosis will be for this patient? What are the patient's goals for intervention? What are your rehabilitation goals? How long do you think it will take to achieve the goals that you and the patient agree on?
- On the basis of the patient's goals and expectations, as well as your understanding of the underlying disease process, what recommendations would you make for intervention at this point in time? What "evidence" from the clinical research literature supports your recommendations? What have you chosen or prioritized from these possible interventions?
- What type of follow-up would you recommend? How do you anticipate your intervention will need to be modified as the patient progresses through the phases of tissue healing? How would you assess the outcomes of your interventions?

Recommendations for a Patient with Open Reduction and Internal Fixation of Wrist Fracture

A forearm-based wrist immobilization splint is fabricated with a precut zipper design with $\frac{1}{8}$-inch material to obtain a rigid support to be used during this initial stage of healing (see Figure 17-22, *B*). The patient is instructed to remove the splint six times a day for gentle range of motion of the wrist and digits. As expected, all wrist motions are significantly limited. He is encouraged to move the digits frequently while in the splint between exercise sessions and incorporate the hand in light activities of daily living.

At 4 weeks after surgery, because the radiograph revealed adequate healing along with the stable fixation provided by the plate and screws, the wrist splint is discontinued and therapy progresses with the addition of gentle passive range of motion. All movements of the wrist improve except wrist extension and forearm supination, which are significantly restricted passively. At 6 weeks, these limitations continue to be problematic and the physician recommends the addition of a wrist extension mobilization splint (see Figure 17-22, *C*) and a forearm supination mobilization splint (see Figure 17-22, *D*).

The wrist extension mobilization splint is fabricated with a standard hook and loop material to provide the mobilization force by a static progressive approach. This method is chosen because of the high degree of wrist stiffness. The supination mobilization splint is fabricated with a tubing mechanism to provide the stretching force. The patient is instructed to wear each device four times a day for 30 minutes, increasing the passive stretch on the tissue as tolerated. The previously used wrist immobilization splint continues to be used at night as a serial static device, by remolding to position the wrist at maximal

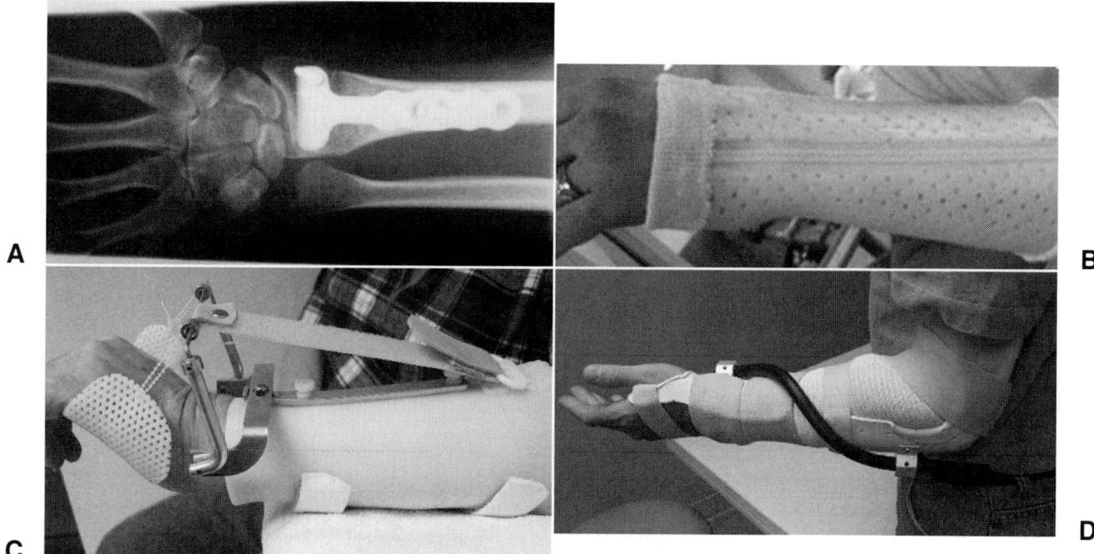

Figure 17-22

A, *A radiograph of open reduction and internal fixation of a comminuted wrist fracture.* ***B,*** *A forearm-based wrist immobilization splint used during the initial stages of healing. When adequate healing had occurred, a wrist extension mobilization splint (**C**) and a forearm supination mobilization splint (**D**) are fabricated to help increase functional ROM.*

extension to maintain all the gains made throughout the day.

After 4 weeks of use, V. A. begins to plateau at 55 degrees of wrist extension and 70 degrees of supination, which is functional and, because of the severity of the injury, quite acceptable.

SUMMARY

Splinting is a commonly used intervention for clinicians treating the upper extremity. Gaining an appreciation for how different splints can be created for specific purposes aids in obtaining maximal patient outcome. This chapter has reviewed many aspects of splinting, including nomenclature, tissue healing, anatomical and mechanical principles, and has provided an overview of the various splinting products on the market. Through comprehensive study and practice, splinting can be another tool used successfully in the clinic.

REFERENCES

1. American Society of Hand Therapists. *Splint Classification System.* Garner, NC: The American Society of Hand Therapists, 1992.
2. Fess EE. A history of splinting: to understand the present, view the past. *J Hand Ther* 2002;15(2):97-132.
3. Tenney CG, Lisak JM. *Atlas of Hand Splinting.* Boston: Little, Brown, 1986.
4. Schultz-Johnson K. Static progressive splinting. *J Hand Ther* 2002;15(2):163-178.
5. Raphael J, Skirven T. Contractures and splinting. In *Atlas of Hand Clinics,* Vol. 6(1), Philadelphia: Saunders, 2001.
6. Bell-Krotoski JA. Plaster cylinder casting for contractures of the interphalangeal joints. In: Mackin EJ, Callahan AD, Osterman AL, et al (eds). *Rehabilitation of the Hand and Upper Extremity,* 5th ed. St. Louis: Mosby, 2002. pp. 1839-1845.
7. Bell-Krotoski JA, Figarola F. Biomechanics of soft tissue growth and remodeling with plaster casting. *J Hand Ther* 1995;8(2):131-137.
8. Brand P, Hollister A. *Clinical Mechanics of the Hand,* 3rd ed. St. Louis: Mosby–Year Book, 1999.
9. Colditz JC. Therapist's management of the stiff hand. In Mackin EJ, Callahan AD, Osterman AL, et al (eds). *Rehabilitation of the Hand and Upper Extremity,* 5th ed. St. Louis: Mosby, 2002. pp. 1021-1049.
10. Flowers KR, LaStayo P. Effect of total end range time on improving passive range of motion. *J Hand Ther* 1994;7(3):150-157.
11. Gyovai JE, Wright Howell J. Validation of spring forces applied in dynamic outrigger splinting. *J Hand Ther* 1992;5(1):8-15.
12. Prosser R. Splinting in the management of proximal interphalangeal joint flexion contracture. *J Hand Ther* 1996;9(4):378-386.
13. Tribuzi SM. Serial plaster splinting. In Mackin EJ, Callahan AD, Osterman AL, et al (eds). *Rehabilitation of the Hand and Upper Extremity,* 5th ed. St. Louis: Mosby, 2002. pp. 1828-1838.
14. Jacobs M, Austin NM. *Splinting the Hand and Upper Extremity: Principles and Process.* Baltimore: Lippincott Williams & Wilkins, 2003.
15. Schultz-Johnson KS. Splinting: a problem solving approach. In Stanley BG, Tribuzi SM (eds). *Concepts in Hand Rehabilitation.* Philadelphia: F.A. Davis, 1992. pp. 238-271.

16. Schultz-Johnson K. Splinting the wrist: mobilization and protection. *J Hand Ther* 1996;9(2):165-175.
17. Mackin EJ, Callahan AD, Osterman AL, et al (eds). *Rehabilitation of the Hand and Upper Extremity,* 5th ed, St. Louis: Mosby, 2002.
18. Green DP, Hotchkiss RN, Pederson WC, et al. *Operative Hand Surgery,* 4th ed. New York: Churchill Livingstone, 1999.
19. Stanley BG, Tribuzi SM (eds). *Concepts in Hand Rehabilitation.* Philadelphia: F.A. Davis, 1992.
20. Tubiana R, Thomine JM, Mackin E. *Examination of the Hand and Wrist,* 2nd ed. St. Louis: Mosby, 1996.
21. Fess EE, Philips C. *Hand Splinting: Principles and Methods,* 2nd ed. St. Louis: Mosby–Year Book, 1987.
22. Kiel J. *Basic Hand Splinting: A Pattern Designing Approach.* Boston: Little, Brown, 1983.
23. Rotman MB, Donovan JP. Practical anatomy of the carpal tunnel. *Hand Clin* 2002;18(2):219-230.
24. Chase AE. Anatomy and kinesiology of the hand. In Mackin EJ, Callahan AD, Osterman AL, et al (eds), *Rehabilitation of the Hand and Upper Extremity,* 5th ed. St. Louis: Mosby, 2002. pp. 60-76.
25. Coppard BM, Lohman H. *Introduction to Splinting: A Critical-Thinking & Problem-Solving Approach,* 2nd ed. St. Louis: Mosby, 2001.
26. Austin N. The wrist and hand complex. In Levangie PK, Norkin CC. *Joint Structure and Function: A Comprehensive Analysis,* 4th ed. Philadelphia: F.A. Davis, 2005.
27. Fess EE. Splints: mechanics versus convention. *J Hand Ther* 1995;8(2):124-130.
28. Cannon NM, Foltz RW, Koepfer J, et al. *Manual of Hand Splinting.* New York: Churchill Livingstone, 1985.
29. Bell-Krotoski JA, Breger-Stanton DE. Biomechanics and evaluation of the hand. In Mackin EJ, Callahan AD, Osterman AL, et al (eds). *Rehabilitation of the Hand and Upper Extremity,* 5th ed. St. Louis: Mosby, 2002. pp. 240-262.
30. Van Lede P, van Veldhoven G. *Therapeutic Hand Splints: A Rational Approach.* Antwerp, Belgium: Provan, 1998.
31. Fess EE, McCollum M. The influence of splinting on healing tissue. *J Hand Ther* 1998;11(2):157-161.
32. Strickland JW. Biologic basis for hand splinting. In Fess EW, Phillips C. *Hand Splinting: Principles and Methods,* 2nd ed. St. Louis: Mosby, 1987. pp. 43-70.
33. Smith KL, Dean SJ. Tissue repair of the epidermis and dermis. *J Hand Ther* 1998;11(2):95-104.
34. Smith J, Feske N. Cutaneous manifestations and consequences of smoking. *J Am Acad Dermatol* 1996;34(5 pt 1):717-726.
35. Rund C. Postoperative care of skin graft, donor sites, and myocutaneous flaps. In Krasner D, Kane D. *Chronic Wound Care: A Clinical Source Book for Healthcare Professionals,* 2nd ed. Wayne, NJ: Health Management Publication, 1997.
36. Wilton JC. *Hand Splinting: Principles of Design and Fabrication.* Philadelphia: Saunders, 1997.
37. McKee P, Morgan L. *Orthotics in Rehabilitation.* Philadelphia: F.A. Davis, 1998.
38. Brand PW. The forces of dynamic splinting: ten questions before applying a dynamic splint to the hand. In Mackin EJ, Callahan AD, Osterman AL, et al (eds). *Rehabilitation of the Hand and Upper Extremity,* 5th ed. St. Louis: Mosby, 2002. pp. 1811-1817.
39. Flowers KR. A proposed decision hierarchy for splinting the stiff joint, with an emphasis on force application parameters. *J Hand Ther* 2002;15(2):158-162.
40. McClure PW, Blackburn LG, Dusold C. The use of splints in the treatment of joint stiffness: biological rationale and an algorithm for making clinical decisions. *Phys Ther* 1994;74(12):1101-1107.
41. Mildenberger LA, Amadio PC, An KN. Dynamic splinting: a systematic approach to the selection of elastic traction. *Arch Phys Med* 1986;67(4):241-244.
42. Glasgow C, Wilton J, Tooth L. Optimal daily total end range time for contracture: resolution in hand splinting. *J Hand Ther* 2003;16(3):207-218.
43. Lee DB. Objective and subjective observations of low-temperature thermoplastic materials. *J Hand Ther* 1995;8(2):138-143.
44. Breger Lee DE, Buford WL. Properties of thermoplastic splinting materials. *J Hand Ther* 1992;5(3):202-211.
45. Breger Lee DE, Buford WL. Update in splinting materials and methods. *Hand Clin* 1991;7(1):569-585.
46. Sammons Preston Rolyan Catalog. Bolingbrook, IL, 2004.
47. North Coast Medical Inc. Hand Therapy Catalog. San Jose, CA, 2003-2004.

18

Splinting, Orthotics, and Prosthetics in the Management of Burns

R. SCOTT WARD

LEARNING OBJECTIVES

On completion of this chapter, the reader will be able to do the following:

1. Describe the elements of burn injury that contribute to decision making regarding splints, orthotics, and prosthetics.
2. Describe how wound care may affect the use and application of splints, orthotics, and prosthetics.
3. Describe components of rehabilitation intervention that may incorporate or affect the use of splints, orthotics, and prosthetics.
4. Describe the use of splints and orthotics in the care of patients with burn injuries.
5. Describe the use of prosthetics for patients with amputations associated with burn injuries.

Rehabilitation of a patient with burns involves programs that focus on restoring functions compromised by the burn injury.[1] Treatment strategies used by therapists address five important goals:

1. Improve or promote wound healing by reducing wound infection
2. Prevent or reduce deformity
3. Increase mobility and strength to achieve maximal function
4. Reduce effects of hypertrophic scarring
5. Educate the patient about recuperation

The rehabilitation plan for patients with burns centers on wound care, positioning, range of motion exercises, splinting, strengthening exercises, endurance and functional exercises, gait training, and scar control. Modern burn care emphasizes the need for a comprehensive team approach to achieve maximal clinical results.[1,2]

BURN INJURY

Each year, more than 730,000 people sustain burn injuries that require emergency room visits. Of these, more than 300,000 are seriously injured directly by fire, and almost 8000 die as a result of the injury.[3,4] The American Burn Association has outlined criteria for determining the severity of burn injury, which include cause of the injury, burn depth, total body surface area burned, location of the burn, and patient age.[5] A burn injury of any given size is more severe for patients who are very young or very old. The deeper the injury, the more serious is the burn. Involvement of the face, eyes, ears, perineum, hands, and feet make the injury more critical. Associated trauma, smoke inhalation injury, and poor preinjury health status are factors that increase severity of the injury. An appropriate understanding of the nature of burn injury and the location and depth of the burn wound is important in understanding and anticipating the possible problems a patient may face during rehabilitation.

Causes of Burns

Types of burn injury include flame, scald, flash (radiant heat explosions), contact, chemical, electrical, and other (e.g., irradiation, radioactivity) burns.[6]

Flame and scald burns are the most common causes of burn injury.[6-8] The elderly and preschool age children are at the highest risk of receiving scald injuries.[9-11] Chemical and electrical burns present differently than other burn injuries. Burns resulting from chemical agents require identification of the causative agent so that proper neutralization of the chemical can take place. Assessment of the depth of chemical burns is difficult at first, but these wounds are predictably deep.[12] An electrical injury may have areas of significant surface burn; however, these areas are often the result of associated flash burns. Small, deep wounds where the current enters or exits the body are more typical.[6,13] The major complication with rehabilitative consequence of electrical injury is musculoskeletal necrosis, which frequently results in amputation.[14]

Burn Depth

Thomsen[15] has studied Indian writings dating back to approximately 600 BC that describe four levels or degrees of burn depth and declare that deep burns heal slowly and with scarring.[15] There are two methods to describe burn depth: by *degree* (first, second, or third degree) or *thickness* (superficial, partial thickness, and full thickness).[16,17] The thickness terminology is more commonly used in clinical practice. A superficial injury corresponds to a first-degree injury, a partial thickness to a second-degree injury, and a full thickness to a third-degree injury (Figure 18-1).

Clinical characteristics associated with the injury thickness are helpful in identification of the depth of burn. *Superficial* (first degree) injuries involve only the epidermis. They are often painful, erythematous, and mildly edematous. Superficial burn injuries usually heal in 3 to 7 days and they rarely result in scarring. *Superficial partial-thickness* burns (superficial second degree) compromise the epidermis and upper dermis. These burns are very painful, very red, and often have blisters or weeping wounds. Superficial partial-thickness burns usually heal in 14 to 21 days and rarely develop scar. In *deep partial-thickness* burns (deep second degree), deeper layers of the dermis are damaged. The wound may or may not be painful, it may be cherry red or pale, and the skin is still pliable. Deep partial-thickness burns require more than 21 days to heal spontaneously and will scar. In *full-thickness* burns (third degree) all layers of the skin are destroyed. The wound generally has a tan or brown appearance and exhibits a leathery texture. Full-thickness wounds are painless and will need several weeks to heal without surgical intervention. Deep partial-thickness burns are often managed by skin grafting; full-thickness injuries require skin grafting. A deeper burn generally correlates with an increased severity of injury.

Surgical Management of Burns

Small burn wounds may be excised and primarily closed; however, most burn wounds require excision of the burn followed by coverage of the site with a skin graft.[18] Excision of the burn wound is ordinarily performed tangentially; that is, thin layers of the burn are removed until viable tissue is reached.[19] Autografts (*split-thickness grafts*) are harvested from undamaged areas of the body for coverage of the excised wound.[20] Skin grafts placed on tangentially excised wounds demonstrate good long-term functional results.[21] Full-thickness skin grafts can also be used. Interestingly, split-thickness grafts scar more than full-thickness grafts.[21]

Progress has been made in the use of skin substitutes and

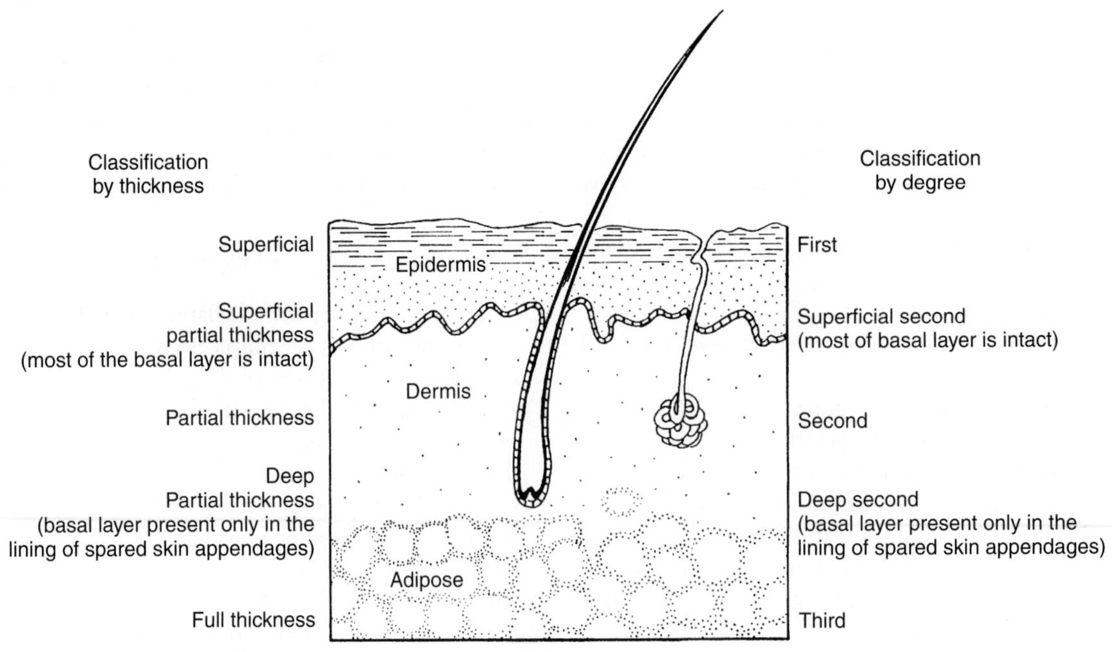

Figure 18-1

The depths of burn injury, referencing both the contemporary thickness classification with the more traditional degree terminology. (From Ward RS. The rehabilitation of burn patients. CRC Crit Rev Phys Med Rehabil *1991;2[3]:121-138.)*

cultured skin for the coverage of the excised burn.[22-25] Areas treated in this fashion tend to be fragile and susceptible to breakdown.[26] Wounds treated with cultured epithelium do not aggressively scar; however, little information is available about the rehabilitative ramifications of this treatment approach.[27]

Burn Size

Burn wound size is reported as a percentage of the total body surface area (TBSA) that is injured. Lund and Browder[28] describe a method for estimating percent TBSA. Variations in body part ratios during development and diversified proportions of individual anatomical parts are considered in the estimation (Figure 18-2). A burn injury increases in severity as the percentage of TBSA burn increases. Large burns usually require longer convalescence, which in turn increases the rehabilitative needs of the patient.

Location of the Burn

Burns of the face, perineum, hands, or feet create special problems. Burns of the face are distressing because of cosmetic disfigurement, the potential for visual impairment, and compromised nutrition (intake of food). Injuries of the face are often accompanied by inhalation injuries. Hands and feet have broad functional importance that can be substantially compromised after burn injury. Severity of injury is significantly magnified as the total surface area of the hand or foot encompassed by the burn increases. Any burn that crosses a joint increases the risk of functional compromise and creates challenges in rehabilitation.

WOUND CARE

The time it takes to heal a burn wound is directly related to depth of the injury. The more superficial a wound, the faster it heals. Surgical intervention, such as skin grafting, is often used to reduce healing time for deep wounds. Wound infection can significantly delay healing.

Topical Agents and Wound Dressing

In intact skin, the outermost layer of epidermis (stratum comeum) is too dry to support microbial growth and serves as an effective barrier to microbial penetration. As a result, skin infections seldom occur unless the skin is opened.[29] Because this protective barrier is compromised or destroyed in burn injury, the risk of infection is greatly increased. Topical agents may be applied to these open wounds after each cleansing and debridement to prevent or manage infections. Topical agents are particularly important for ischemic wounds in which systemic delivery of natural substrates to fight infection is compromised.[30] A well-applied dressing minimizes discomfort and allows mobility.

Mild lotions are important in relieving dryness and itching in maturing healed wounds.[29] The use of moisturizers helps prevent healed wounds from cracking or splitting. Because alcohol is a desiccant to the skin and exacerbates dryness, lotions that contain alcohol should be avoided. Fragrance-free moisturizers are recommended; most hypersensitivity reactions are triggered by perfumes. Moisturizers can also be beneficial when applying a splint, orthotic, or prosthetic device to a patient with healed burns or scar because they help protect the skin from desiccation and shear.

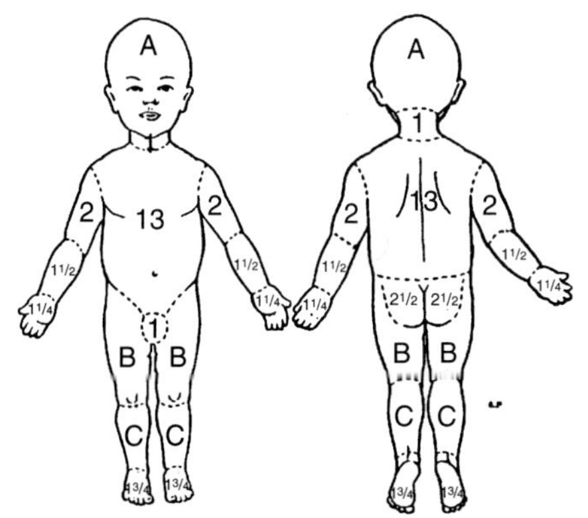

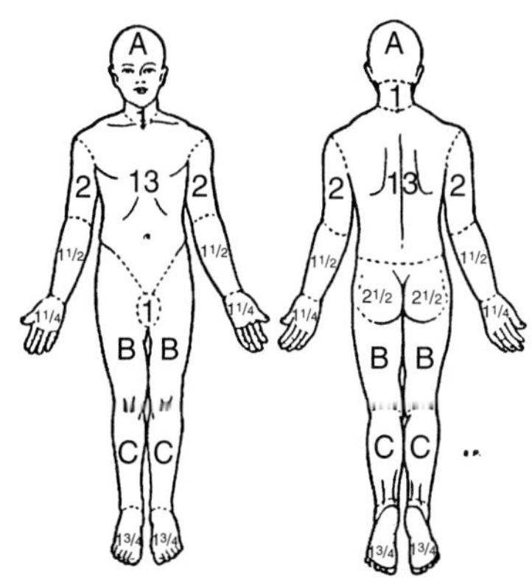

Relative Percentages of Areas Affected by Growth

Area	Age 0	1	5
A = 1/2 of head	9 1/2	8 1/2	6 1/2
B = 1/2 of one thigh	2 3/4	3 1/4	4
C = 1/2 of one leg	2 1/2	2 1/2	2 3/4

Area	Age 10	15	Adult
A = 1/2 of head	5 1/2	4 1/2	3 1/2
B = 1/2 of one thigh	4 1/4	4 1/2	4 3/4
C = 1/2 of one leg	3	3 1/4	3 1/2

Figure 18-2

The original Lund and Browder chart outlines the accepted method for determining the TBSA of a burn injury. (From Lund CC, Browder NC. The estimation of areas of burns. Surg Gynecol Obstet *1944;79:352-358.)*

Rehabilitative personnel often take an active role in the wound care of a patient with burns. Involvement in wound care provides a better understanding of the reasons for discomfort. Familiarity with wound care procedures is often necessary for outpatient therapy sessions.[31,32] Adjustments in the treatment plan are often necessary as the wound heals and tolerance of certain rehabilitative procedures changes. Consideration of the effects of pressure, shear, and friction on a healing wound or newly healed, fragile skin is especially important when splints, orthotics, prosthetics, or other external devices are being used.

PSYCHOLOGY OF BURN INJURY

An acute burn injury creates emotional distress. Treatment of the burns is often traumatic as well; stress and anxiety continue during the period of recovery. The psychological consequences of burn trauma in the adult include depression, intrusive avoidance and regressive behavior, despair, fear, anxiety, and guilt.[33-38] Malt[38] estimates that 30% of adults with burns will have psychological problems. Children often feel more guilt than adults and often manifest loss of interest in play, unpredictable sadness, avoidance, and regression.[39-41] Even with similar support mechanisms and preexisting psychological status, psychiatric prognosis is less hopeful for children than for adults.[42]

Psychological adaptation in early phases after burn injury includes denial (often manifest by a feeling of calmness), and concern about prognosis, pain, personal issues, and dependence on staff (depression).[34,39,43] Individuals who become actively involved in the process of rehabilitation and self-care often are more encouraged and optimistic about the future.[39,43]

Rehabilitation professionals can facilitate psychological function and recovery of patients with burns in several ways. Encouraging independence by allowing individuals as much control over medical procedures as possible helps them focus on recovery and empowers them to a certain degree.[43,44] Patients feel more comfortable with caregivers if they have the opportunity to get to know one other outside painful treatment settings.[34,39,44,45] Support and understanding demonstrate a caring attitude. Tactful but honest answers to questions about prognosis, cosmesis, and functional outcome help establish trust.[39] Ongoing education about the recovery process is important because it helps the patient develop realistic expectations about recovery.

REHABILITATION INTERVENTION

Early surgical intervention, availability of nutritional support, and pharmaceutical advances have improved survival after burn injury.[46] This improvement, in turn, has increased the emphasis on and need for rehabilitation of patients with burns. Physical therapists and occupational therapists are important members of the burn care team.

After examination and evaluation, the team establishes goals and designs and implements an appropriate plan of care. Important rehabilitation goals for patients with burns include the following[31,47]:

1. Minimizing the occurrence and adverse consequences of hypertrophic scar formation
2. Minimizing contracture formation and maintaining full joint range of motion
3. Preserving motor skill function
4. Improving strength and endurance

Burn rehabilitation interventions emphasize patient independence through achievement of maximal functional recovery.

Wound Healing and Scar Formation

Unhealed burn wounds can create challenges during rehabilitation. Most problems in burn rehabilitation are caused by the ceaseless contraction and hypertrophy of immature burn scars.[48] Scar contracture leads to visible cosmetic deformity of body parts, especially in the face and hands. Functional limitations are common when the scar crosses a joint. The contraction of scar has been classically associated with a type of fibroblast called myofibroblasts, which have contractile properties.[49]

Burn wound healing encompasses three phases: the inflammatory phase, the proliferative phase, and the maturation, or remodeling, phase.[50] The *inflammatory phase* is characterized by the formation of new blood vessels, an initial defense against infection, and migration of fibroblast and epithelial cells into the injured area. Treatment focuses on proper wound care to encourage vascular regrowth and retard contamination of the site. The *proliferative phase* is marked by continued revascularization, rebuilding and strengthening the wound site as a result of vigorous synthesis of collagen by fibroblasts, and reepithelialization. Treatment is directed toward promoting epithelialization and encouraging proper alignment of newly deposited collagen fibers. During the *maturation phase*, the wound site is further strengthened by protracted deposition of collagen fibers by active fibroblasts. Treatment during maturation stresses lengthening the scar, reconditioning the patient, and returning the patient to preburn functional levels. Activity and rehabilitation interventions aimed at opposing wound and scar tightness and education about the process of recovery are critical in all phases of healing.

While fibroblasts deposit collagen during the proliferative phase, macrophages and endothelial cells release enzymes that degrade collagen. The severity of scar formation is determined by the balance between collagen synthesis and lysis: the more that collagen deposition exceeds its breakdown, the more likely a significant scar will form. A hypertrophic scar is raised above the normal surface of skin (Figure 18-3).[51,52] A keloid occurs when the scar extends beyond the initial boundaries of the wound.[51,52]

An immature scar is raised, red, leathery, and stiff. As the scar matures, it becomes pale, relatively soft and flattened, and more yielding.[53-55] The process of scar maturation requires 6 to 18 months after wound closure; scars actively contract during maturation.[53,54] Contraction is most vigorous in the early months of maturation but continues throughout this period of remodeling.

Superficial and partial-thickness burns usually do not scar; full-thickness burns almost always do. Full-thickness wounds closed by a skin graft scar significantly less than a similar wound allowed to heal spontaneously. Very dark-skinned or very fair-skinned individuals and those with familial history of susceptibility to scarring are more likely to form hypertrophic scar.[56-58] The larger the burn, the greater the likelihood of scar formation.[57-59] A contracture occurs when a portion or distortion of the shortening scar becomes fixed or semifixed. The face, neck, axilla, and hand are the most common and most problematic sites of scar contracture formation.[56,58] One of the most important goals of burn rehabilitation is to prevent, counteract, and minimize the adverse affects of scar contraction.

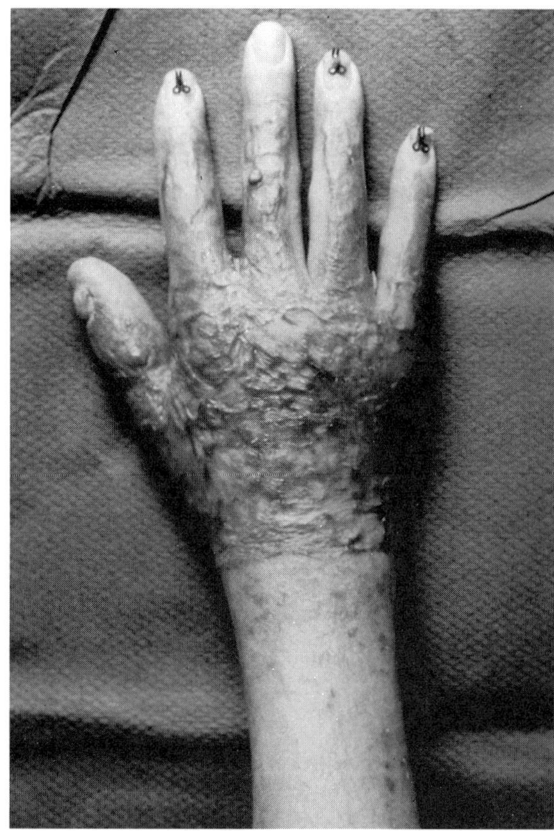

Figure 18-3
The dorsum of this patient's hand exhibits hypertrophic scarring. (From Ward RS. Pressure therapy for the control of hypertrophic scar formation after burn injury: a history and review. J Burn Care Rehabil *1991;12[3]:257-262.)*

Operative Scar Management

Surgery is used to correct scar contractures that have created specific functional deficits or deformities.[58] Surgical techniques used to release scar contracture include split-thickness or full-thickness skin grafts, skin flaps, Z-plasties, and tissue expansion.[58,60] Most surgeries are deferred until at least 6 months after the burn or until the scar is sufficiently mature.[58,61,62] Although surgery alleviates contracture-related problems, it also creates a new wound with its own subsequent scar maturation process. Rehabilitation is necessary after a majority of reconstructive surgeries to again avert the affects of contraction.

Nonoperative Scar Management

The nonoperative control of hypertrophic scarring involves pressure therapy and the application of silicone gel sheeting. The use of continuous pressure for the treatment of burn scars was described in 1971 and is still well accepted.[63-65] Pressure has also been shown to relieve other aggravating discomforts of the healing burn wound, such as itching and blistering.[66,67] Range of motion is not significantly impeded with pressure garments despite the restriction felt by patients (particularly initially) when fit with pressure garments.[68] The use of silicone gel sheets has shown some success in controlling hypertrophy.[69-71] This treatment is typically used over small scars or over areas where ample pressure cannot be attained. The mechanisms of the effects of pressure and silicone gel are not known.

Pressure therapy is indicated when healing requires more than 14 days or if skin grafting has been performed. There are several strategies to assess burn scar condition. The Vancouver Scar Scale developed by Sullivan and colleagues describes severity of the scar by rating pigmentation, vascularity, pliability, and height of the scar tissue (Box 18-1).

Early pressure therapy is used to control edema in a wound even if there is no ensuing scar formation. Some of the most common elastic materials used on newly healing, still fragile wounds include elastic bandages, Coban self-adherent wrap (3M Medical, St. Paul, Minn.), or elasticized cotton tubular bandages such as Tubigrip (SePro Healthcare, Inc., Montgomeryville, Pa.). These materials are useful while the patient is waiting for the arrival of custom-fit, antiburn scar supports.[73]

Individuals with scars are commonly fitted with custom-fit pressure garments for the duration of the maturation phase of healing. Custom-fit, antiburn scar supports are available from manufacturers such as Bio-Concepts (Phoenix, Ariz.), Barton-Carey Medical Products (Perrysburg, Ohio), and Gottfried Medical (Toledo, Ohio). Although the measuring procedure varies by manufacturer, most require measurements approximately every 1 to 1.5 inches along each extremity, with special guidelines for the torso, face, and hands. Burn scar supports can be fabricated to fit almost any body part,

Box 18-1 *Vancouver Scar Scale Ratings for Assessing Burn Scar*

PIGMENTATION
0 = Normal (scar color closely resembles that of the rest of the body)
1 = Hypopigmentation
2 = Hyperpigmentation

VASCULARITY
0 = Normal (scar color closely resembles that of the rest of the body)
1 = Pink
2 = Red
3 = Purple

PLIABILITY
0 = Normal
1 = Supple (flexible with minimum resistance)
2 = Yielding (gives way to pressure)
3 = Firm (inflexible, not easily moved, resistant to manual pressure)
4 = Banding (ropelike tissue that blanches with extension on the scar)
5 = Contracture (permanent shortening of scar, producing deformity or distortion)

HEIGHT
0 = Normal (flat)
1 = Raised less than 2 mm
2 = Raised less than 5 mm
3 = Raised more than 5 mm

Modified from Sullivan T, Smith J, Kernoda J, et al. Rating the burn scar. *J Burn Care Rehabil* 1990;11(3):256-260.

including the face, torso, upper extremity, hand, and lower extremity. Some burn centers fabricate rigid or semirigid face masks (essentially orthotics) in an attempt to gain a better match with facial contours.

Pressure garments and devices are worn through the entire process of scar maturation, to be discontinued only when the scar has completely matured.[1] Fit of pressure garments is regularly reassessed to ensure the desired therapeutic effect. Regular follow-up provides an opportunity for the patient to discuss other ongoing rehabilitative problems associated with the burn.

BURN REHABILITATION INTERVENTIONS

Many different types of rehabilitation interventions are appropriate in the care of patients with burns. Although many interventions are briefly described in the following section, the emphasis is on the use of splints, orthoses, and prosthetic devices.

Therapeutic Exercise

Exercise helps minimize outcomes of burn scar formation by improving mobility and function.[74] As important and effective as exercise is in burn rehabilitation, some individuals may be reluctant to exercise (and some therapists may be reluctant to encourage them) because of the anticipation of increased pain or anxiety about damaging newly healing tissue. Exercise programs for patients with burns are principally directed at the prevention of burn scar contractures and the side effects of inactivity and disuse. Additional consequences of immobilization in these patients can include progressive contracture of the joint capsule and pericapsular structures, atrophy and contracture of muscle, deleterious effects on articular cartilage, and possible decrease in bone strength. Exercise is a significant health promotion and disability prevention component in the rehabilitation of patients with burns.

Assessment of location and depth of burn injury identifies those areas most at risk of burn scar contracture. This assessment also guides design of an exercise program to improve mobility, strength, and functional status. Past and present medical conditions influence rehabilitative expectations; a previous orthopedic injury may have already reduced range of motion of a particular joint whereas a concomitant inhalation injury may limit exercise tolerance.

Active Exercise

After a burn, exercise may be difficult because of edema, pain (particularly over areas of partial-thickness burns), the loss of skin elasticity in the burned tissue, and wound contraction.[60] Early on, edema is a major contributor to stiffness of joints; active exercise is valuable in reducing the edema.[31,75] Positioning and compressive wraps or devices are used for edema control in addition to exercise. Pain tolerance varies widely among individuals. The therapist is challenged to help the patient understand the importance of activity despite the pain involved. Many individuals have relief of their pain and stiffness after exercise periods, which may encourage them to participate in the subsequent therapy sessions. Persons who understand the advantages of exercise may be asked to confer with, and encourage, newly injured individuals or those having difficulty with their exercises.

General stiffness from the loss of skin elasticity and wound contracture is a short-term problem but often persists during the process of scar maturation, especially for those who form a hypertrophic scar. Exercise targeting those areas most vulnerable to scar formation identified in the initial evaluation must begin as early as possible after admission.[47,76] Early presentation of an exercise routine aids edema control, relieves stiffness, and prevents loss of strength and range of motion. The early introduction of active exercise reinforces the importance of exercise to the individual, who will incorporate daily exercise as a important contributor to overall recovery. Because of the wide scope of benefits derived from active exercises, they are the preferred form of range-of-motion (ROM) exercises for patients with burns.

Patients are also encouraged to perform independent activities of daily living.[47,75] Self-reliance is important after burn injury, and independence can increase the patient's self-confidence.[75] It is likely that the more patients can do, particularly in directing their exercise programs, the more compliant they will become.[76] Independence in an exercise program is therefore an important goal for those recovering from burn injury.

The primary goal of active exercise for patients with acute burns is opposition of tissue contraction; the secondary goal is strengthening. For an individual with a burn crossing the antecubital fossa and weakness of the biceps brachii, exercise is primarily focused on preservation of elbow-extension ROM. If a patient with a burn encompassing the lower leg and ankle also has weakness and atrophy of the triceps surae, appropriate strengthening exercises may be performed, but not at the sacrifice of active ankle ROM.

Conditioning exercises are often used to improve the cardiovascular status of the patient. Occupation-specific training programs may be a part of the long-term rehabilitation plan as patients plan to return to their jobs. This type of activity may be directed at one or a few specific functions or may incorporate a traditional work-hardening program.

Gait Training

The functional nature of ambulation makes it the most important exercise for burned lower extremities.[77] Ambulation assists with edema control, ROM, and strengthening in all lower extremity joints. Ambulation also helps with the function of other physiological systems such as the cardiovascular, gastrointestinal, and renal systems. Individuals with lower extremity burns exhibit gait deviations related to compromised joint function, such as incomplete hip and knee flexion in initial swing and incomplete knee extension in terminal swing. Initial contact may be made with the entire foot (foot flat) instead of the heel, and loading response may be compromised by lack of plantar flexion ROM or an unwillingness to perform the controlled knee flexion necessary for shock absorption. Excessive knee flexion in midstance, poor or absent heel off and weight shift in terminal stance, and inadequate knee flexion in preswing are often present.[32] Differences in individual gait deviations in gait phases are generally based on variations in the location, size, and depth of the burn injury and levels of pain. Any gait deviation caused by the burn may accentuate the need for vigilant gait training of a patient with burns who also has a lower extremity prosthesis. Exercise is an important adjunct to gait training because it can address specific movement limitations of the lower limbs.

Passive Exercise and Stretching

Passive exercise is included in therapy regimens if patients are unable to move on their own or cannot actively complete normal ROMs. Passive ROM and slow, gentle stretching exercises that elongate healing soft tissues are used to preserve and improve joint ROM.[78,79] Blanching of the scar indicates an appropriate amount of stretch. Although the scar should be stretched to the point of tolerance, joint movement should not be forced because of possible tissue damage and the potential for heterotopic ossification.[80-82]

Positioning or splints are used after a stretching session to maintain the achieved ROM. Suitable stretching positions must also consider scars that cross multiple joints and therefore affect a broad kinematic chain. Techniques such as contract-relax or hold-relax have been found to be beneficial stretching approaches.[31]

Most of the exercise equipment typically found in rehabilitation settings is appropriate for patients with burns. The therapist must decide when certain equipment will be most beneficial and incorporate the use of this resource into the plan of care. The use of latex rubber tubing for strengthening and overhead reciprocal pulleys for increasing ROM are a few examples of simple equipment that have been described in the literature.[83-85] Bicycle ergometers for either the upper or lower extremities assist with motion, provide resistance, and allow for some cardiovascular workout.

Physical Agents

Because of the variety of treatment goals important for burn rehabilitation, many different types of modalities are used for appropriate intervention. Hydrotherapy, functional electrical stimulation (neuromuscular electrical stimulation), transcutaneous electrical stimulation, ultrasound, continuous passive motion (CPM), and paraffin are physical agents that have been effectively used in burn care. Hydrotherapy is most often used for wound care but may also be used for dressing removal and exercise. If hydrotherapy is chosen as a thermal modality, precautions similar to those used for any open wound care are necessary to reduce the chance of cross-contamination.

Functional electrical stimulation has been successfully used to treat hands that have responded poorly to typical treatment.[86] Burn pain has been altered by transcutaneous electrical stimulation in some cases.[87] Ultrasound has been used to treat pain and ROM impairments in patients with burns; however, the efficacy of ultrasound in either decreasing pain or improving motion is still a matter of some debate.[88-90] More than half the major burn treatment centers have used CPM as an adjunct to treatment.[91] Successful use of CPM has been specifically reported for hand burns and lower extremity burns at the knee.[92,93] The gentle heat provided by paraffin, as well as the potential skin softening from the mineral oil in the paraffin, may be reasons for the use of this modality in burn care.[94]

Healing skin and recently healed skin are often very sensitive. Scar tissue has varying levels of sensory deficit.[95,96] Accordingly, heat, cold, coupling agents, and electrode adhesives may lead to skin breakdown. Caution must be exercised when applying any modality; thorough pretreatment and posttreatment inspection of the site is warranted.

Positioning

Positioning is an important component of any burn rehabilitation program. Positioning is used for acute burn and postsurgical edema control and to prevent or treat scar contractures. The initial burn therapy evaluation identifies sites at risk for contracture formation; appropriate counteractive positions become part of the therapy plan. Contracture prevention is more successful when a program of positioning and activity is instituted as soon after burn as possible.[47,58]

Postexercise positioning extends the effects of activity; positioning is also fundamental for individuals who cannot move or exercise. Manufactured positioning devices, such as arm boards that attach to the side of the bed, are available to assist in proper positioning of extremities. Positioning need not be expensive or require intricate equipment. Avoiding the use of a pillow behind the head is a simple way of decreasing neck flexion and facilitating a neutral alignment of the head and neck. A pillow or several folded blankets placed under the arms can effectively elevate the burned limb while keeping the elbows extended and supporting the hands. At least some horizontal flexion of the shoulders is indicated to minimize prolonged stretch of the brachial plexus.[97,98] A washcloth, towel, or gauze roll placed in the palm helps hold the hand in a functional position. Pillows, high-top tennis shoes, towels, blankets, and foot boards help position the foot with a neutral ankle.[47] Positions of choice for a patient with burns are shown in Box 18-2.

Box 18-2 *Preferred Positions for Patients with Burns*

Neck	Extension, no rotation
Shoulder	Abduction (90 degrees) External rotation Horizontal flexion (10 degrees)
Elbow and forearm	Extension with supination
Wrist	Neutral or slight extension
Hand	Functional position (dorsal burn) Finger and thumb extension (palmar burn)
Trunk	Straight postural alignment
Hip	Neutral extension/flexion Neutral rotation Slight abduction
Knee	Extension
Ankle	Neutral or slight dorsiflexion No inversion Neutral toe extension/flexion

SPLINTING AND ORTHOTICS

Hippocrates described burn scars as "tetanus," and Wilhelm Fabry illustrated a splint to treat a hand for hyperextension scar contractures.[15] In the early to mid-1900s, patients with burns were placed in splints immediately on admission to the hospital in an effort to prevent contraction; splints were removed for brief periods to permit wound care. Most burns were not covered by skin graft until at least 5 weeks after

Box 18-3 *Advantages, Disadvantages, Indications, and Contraindications of Therapist-Fabricated Splints in Burn Care*

ADVANTAGES
Maintains or increases (serial or dynamic) joint position
Can be used during any phase of healing
Custom formed for each individual
Adjustable
May protect tissue (e.g., exposed tissues such as tendon or joint capsule, or skin from pressure)

DISADVANTAGES
Potential for skin breakdown
Shearing may occur if not properly fit or fixed over a joint
May be difficult for nontherapist to apply

INDICATIONS
Need for positioning specific joints
Wound or scar contraction
Decreased joint range of motion
Need for safeguarding anatomical structures
Need for conforming scar tissue
Uncommunicative or nonresponsive patient

CONTRAINDICATIONS
Direct application onto fragile tissue
Constrictive fixation strapping or wraps

injury. The advent of surgical excision and grafting in the mid-1900s decreased the time required for a burn to heal. As a result, prophylactic splinting became a less common procedure, and in the late 1970s and early 1980s active exercise became the primary treatment method used by burn therapists.[47] The use of splints has, however, become a critical adjunct to active exercise and positioning of individuals with burns. The term *splint* is used in burn care more often than *orthotic*, even though the terms and the devices they represent are nearly synonymous.

Splinting is often used to protect fragile wounds or newly grafted burn wounds. Splints are also used to position joints to maintain achieved ROM or as dynamic devices to apply gentle prolonged stretch to increase ROM. Splints cannot replace active exercise; contractures will form even in desirable positions if a patient is constantly splinted in a particular position. Static splints are designed to maintain a position of choice by immobilizing the joint.[99,100] Dynamic splints are designed to exercise or mobilize a joint.[100] A splint may also enhance the pressure applied to a scar by a pressure support. If unusual pain (other than from gentle tissue elongation or stretch), sensory impairment, or wound maceration occurs at the site of the splint, it must be removed and the fit adjusted.[101]

A splint should be fabricated with a proper, secure fit to minimize friction injuries or skin breakdown at pressure points. Pressure points over bony prominences are particularly vulnerable in this regard. Large, broad surface contact areas better distribute forces and reduce the likelihood of pressure-related tissue injury. The splint is worn only when it will not impede the functional activities or requisite exercises of the patient; splints are often donned during rest periods and at night when the patient is sleeping. The corners and edges of the splint are rounded and sometimes padded to avoid shear stresses. The design of the splint may also need to be adapted for orthopedic hardware such as surgical pins or for intravenous line sites. The splint design should, whenever possible, allow for ease of application and removal to enhance compliance among staff and family members who otherwise might struggle while maneuvering the splint.

Material used in fabricating splints include thermoplastics, Supracor (Supracor Inc., San Jose, Calif.), Hexalite (Reebok International, Canton, Mass.), plaster, and elastomer compounds. Hexalite and plaster are most often used to make temporary splints. Thermoplastic material, which can be remolded to adjust fit, make it an ideal splinting material for patients with burns. The amount of material to be used is determined by measuring the area to be splinted and the design of the splint. The splint is then molded to the individual. When the splinting material is set, or hardened, the splint should be inspected for correct fit to avoid pressure- and shear-related problems. Splints are often padded with gauze or any of the numerous cushion or foam materials available. For areas where fragile skin is problematic, foam is a soft alternative splinting material; however, it does not provide the same resistance to force that more rigid materials do. The advantages and disadvantages, as well as indications and contraindications of therapist-fabricated splinting and burn care, are summarized in Box 18-3. Although a number of appropriate splint designs for each anatomical site are possible, some are chosen more commonly than others.

Neck

The possible consequences of anterior neck burns include flexion contracture, facial disfiguration, loss of cosmetic contours of the neck, and difficulty with mastication.[101,102] A molded neck conformer splint helps prevent neck flexion contracture and provides compression on the forming scar. A rectangular piece of low-temperature thermoplastic splinting material is cut to span the distance from ear to ear along the jaw line and from below the lower lip to the sternoclavicular notch. After heating, the splint is molded directly on the patient's neck. Padding is added to protect vulnerable areas, and a hook-and-loop material strap is attached over the back of the neck to secure the splint.[101] Because this type of splint is occlusive and covers many bony prominences, the splint must be frequently removed to inspect the skin for any areas of irritation or breakdown.

For wounds that do not involve much of the chin, soft cervical collars have also been successful in providing positioning, pressure, and contour.[101,102] Although soft collars are more comfortable to wear, they do not extend over the chin for increased moment arm resistance. Commercially available Philadelphia collars may be an alternative. Watusi splints can also be designed to assist with conforming neck scarring and maintaining neck position.[103]

Axilla and Shoulder

Burns involving the axilla and shoulder may lead to adduction contracture and webbing of the axillary folds. This type of deformity contributes to difficulty in reaching and overhead use of the arm, components of many functional activities. A custom-fit conforming splint is often used to inhibit development of such contracture and webbing. Conforming splints for axillary burns support the entire arm, from the wrist through the axilla, and extend down the trunk to at least waist level.[104] The splint wraps around the trunk from umbilicus to spine, one third of the circumference of the chest, at the axilla around both folds, and one half of the circumference of the arm at the brachium, elbow, and wrist.[101,105,106] The splint is molded directly to the patient (flaring at the iliac crest may be necessary) and appropriate padding is applied. Hook-and-loop material strapping or other wraps around the trunk, shoulder, arm, and wrist secure the splint. A more traditional airplane splint may also be used to counteract the problems at the shoulder (Figure 18-4). Clavicle straps or soft foam may also be used to help conform the axillae.

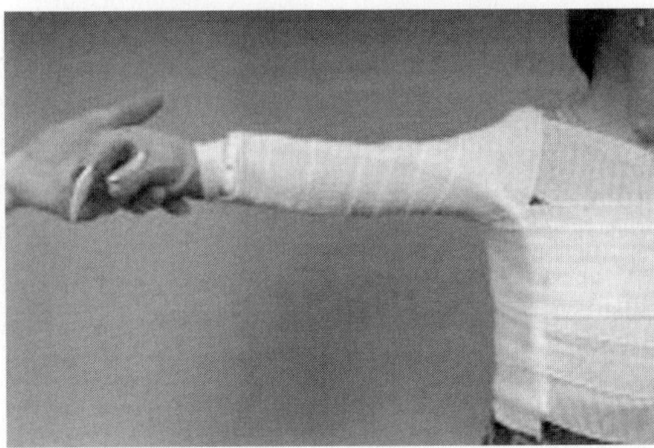

Figure 18-4
An example of a thermoplastic airplane splint designed to reduce the likelihood of development of an axillary contracture during burn healing. (Courtesy Shriners Hospitals for Children, Cincinnati Burn Hospital, Cincinnati, Ohio.)

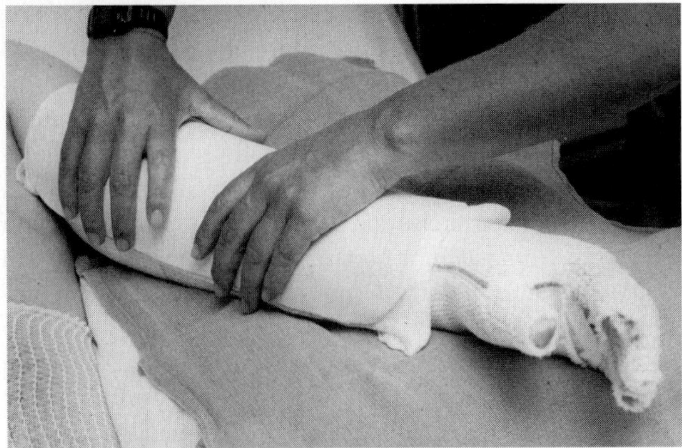

Figure 18-5
A thermoplastic anterior elbow gutter splint being custom fit for a patient with burns of the antecubital fossa.

Elbow and Forearm

The most common deformities caused by burns involving the elbow and forearm are elbow flexion and pronation contractures. The elbow joint is most often fit with a conformer splint designed as either an anterior or posterior gutter or trough (Figure 18-5).[101,102,105] The splint is fit to the arm from the proximal third of the brachium to the distal third of the forearm. Partial circumference measurements are taken at the proximal and distal sites and the elbow. The splint is molded directly on the patient, with padding added. The splint should be flared or "bubbled" at the bony prominences of the elbow. The splint is held in place by hook-and-loop material straps or by circular gauze or elastic wrapping. Commercially available three-point extension or air splints may also be used.

Wrist and Hand

Burns of the wrist may lead to contractures in extension or flexion or ulnar or radial deviation, depending on the location of the burn. The prevention of flexion or extension contractures of the hand and fingers is important, as is maintenance of the web space of the thumb. Many different designs of wrists and hand splints exist; the best option for a particular individual is based on the anticontracture position of the joint or joint complex that is involved.

The most common splint used at the wrist and the hand is the antideformity splint.[101,102,105,107-109] This splint is designed to position the wrist and hand in the functional position. A modification of this splint, the pan splint, positions all finger joints in extension (Figure 18-6). Splints that conform to the thumb, thumb web space, and the index finger can help preserve the thumb web space.[101,102,105] Dorsal- or palmar-resting extension splints, used when the wrist has been burned but the hand is not damaged, may be custom molded or are commercially available. Finger gutter or trough splints are used to treat individual fingers, on the basis of the same principles used in elbow conformer splints.

Another easily fabricated splint that is useful to minimize formation of either flexion or extension contractures when multiple joints of the fingers have been burned is the sandwich splint.[102,108] Foam padding is attached to two pieces of splinting material that have been cut large enough to cover the hand. The burned hand is "sandwiched" between these two padded supports, which are held in place with a circumferential wrap (Figure 18-7).[110]

Trunk and Pelvis

Patients with burns involving the anterior trunk are at risk of developing kyphosis. Clavicular straps in a figure-of-eight design have been used to position the shoulders in retraction and counteract the flexion forces in healing upper trunk burns.[101,102] Commercially available corsets or thoracolumbar spinal orthotics may be prescribed to help maintain posture for individuals with burns of the mid and lower trunk if it is being compromised by scar contracture.

For burns of the pelvis, groin, and hip, the problem is the likelihood of hip flexion and adduction contractures. Hip abduction splints reinforced with a spreader bar or an anterior hip spica splint may be necessary for some patients.[102]

Lower Extremity

At the knee, flexion contracture is an important concern. Splinting of the knee is similar to that of the elbow, adjusted to fit the longer segments of the lower extremity.[101,102,105,111] Although knee conformer splints are most often chosen for

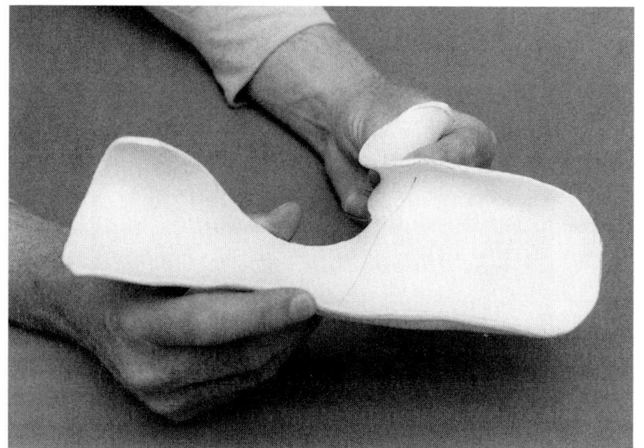

Figure 18-6
A thermoplastic pan splint that been molded to support the wrist in a functional position, with fingers in full extension.

patients with burns involving the knee, three-point extension splints or air splints have also been used to reduce risk of flexion contracture as the burn scar matures.

Because of the complexity of structure and arthrokinematics, burns of the ankles and feet often present challenges for splinting similar to those of the wrist and hand. The location of the burn dictates whether the patient is at risk for contracture in either a plantar flexion or dorsiflexion direction (or both). Posterior foot drop splints, or anterior or posterior ankle conformers, are the most commonly fabricated ankle splints.[101,102,105] The distance from toes to calf is measured, and limb half-circumferences determine the width of the splint. After the desired splint pattern is cut from thermoplastic material, the splint is molded directly on the patient. Necessary padding is applied and the splint is flared at the malleoli and often on the posterior heel. Successful treatment of burns to the dorsum of feet can be difficult.

Another important consideration is the extrapolation of splint designs for other anatomical areas to a seemingly unrelated location. In 2001, Guild[112] reported an application of the designs from various splints for dorsal hand burns to a splint for the treatment of burns of the dorsal foot. The splint has a base and a dorsal thermoplastic piece that fits over the toes and is secured with a hook-and-loop material strap. This splint is intended to minimize or prevent contractures of the dorsal foot during scar maturation. "Bunny boots" and other commercial foot drop splints can also be used for positioning ankles that have been burned.[101] Molded leather shoes can be useful in positioning both the ankles and toes of involved feet.[102] High-top gym shoes provide a less expensive but similar option for foot splinting.[39,102] Toe conformer splints can be fabricated for the dorsal surface of the foot to prevent toe extension contracture.

A

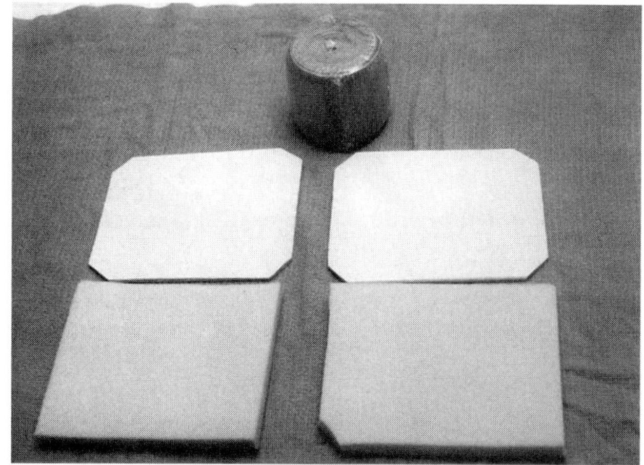

B

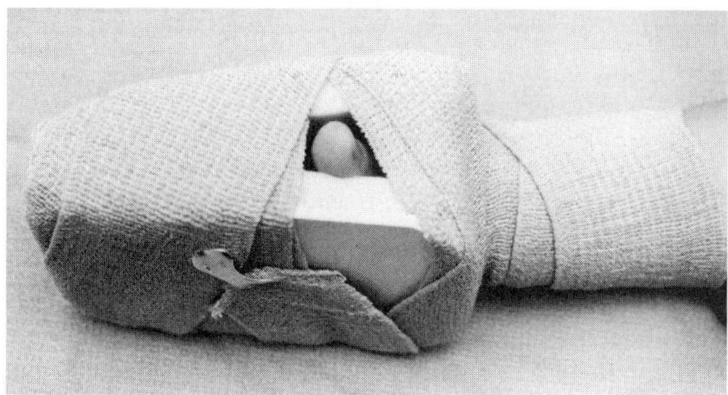

Figure 18-7
A, *Materials used for a sandwich splint include thermoplastic splinting material, foam, and a compression wrap.* ***B,*** *A sandwich splint applied to the hand with burns. (From Ward RS, Schnebly WA, Kravitz M, et al. Have you tried the sandwich splint? A method of preventing hand deformities in children.* J Burn Care Rehabil *1989;10[1]:83-85.)*

Face and Mouth

Burns of the face can affect the eyes and eyelids, the contours of the face, and the soft tissue around the mouth.[113-115] Contracture of the mouth (microstomia) is particularly troublesome because it interferes with feeding (and subsequently nutrition), speaking, and dental care.[116] Splints designed to support the functional contours of specific areas of the face are often fabricated (Figure 18-8). This type of splint helps decrease scar hypertrophy and minimize or prevent ectropion (eversion) deformity of the lower eyelids and the lips.

Microstomia prevention splints, designed to apply pressure or stretch to commissures and fibrotic oral muscles, are commercially available or may be custom made (Figure 18-9).[113-115] This type of splint or appliance is worn at all times when the patient is not eating or receiving oral care or is speaking.[114] In cases in which contracture affects the actual opening of the mouth, cone-shaped splints of thermoplastic material can be used to increase the opening of the mouth

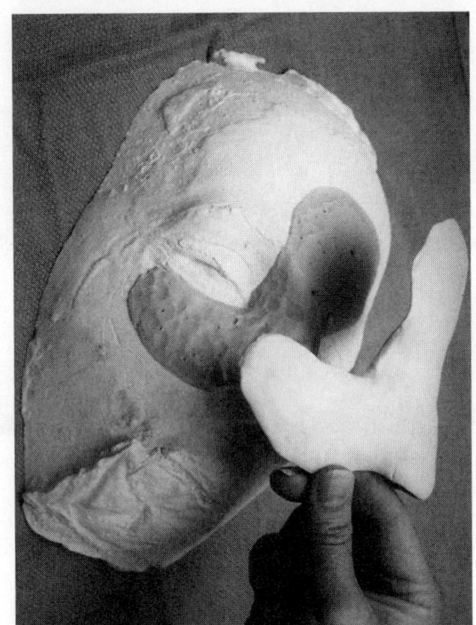

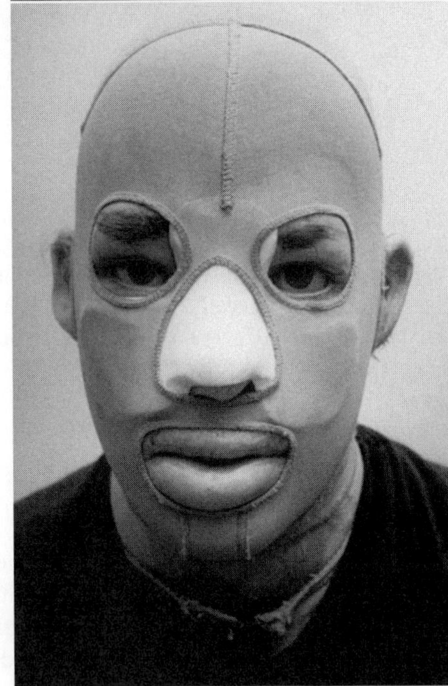

Figure 18-8

A, *This elasmer mold of the patient's nose and cheeks will be reinforced with rigid thermoplastic material.* ***B,*** *When worn under a compression garment, the insert will deliver pressure more effectively to areas of the face than the compression garment alone. Splint inserts may help minimize ectropion (eversion) of the lower eyelids. Both would be worn during the maturation phase of healing to prevent excessive contracture and hypertrophic scarring. (From Ward RS. The rehabilitation of burn patients.* CRC Crit Rev Phys Med Rehabil *1991;2[3]:121-138.)*

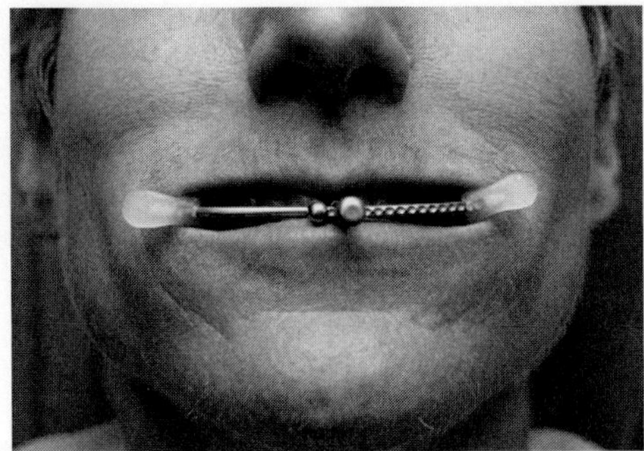

Figure 18-9

A microstomia prevention appliance is used to preserve the oral opening.

progressively. The cone is placed between the teeth after the mouth is opened. As the mouth is able to open wider, the narrower portions of the cone are cut off and the patient progresses to a wider part of the splint to widen the opening of the mouth.

Additional Considerations

Simple materials such as tongue depressors secured with gauze wrapping at various joints have been described as "splints."[117] Elastic wraps have also been used to increase range of motion much like dynamic splints.[118,119] These methods may be useful as temporary devices but are not effective substitutes for more stable splinting materials.[118]

For patients with existing contractures, a serial splinting protocol is often used to assist in stretching the deformity. Plaster casts, thermoplastic materials, and Dynasplints (Dynasplint Systems Inc., Severna Park, Md.) have been successfully used in this manner.[120,121] Individually fabricated dynamic splints are also helpful for individuals with contracture after burns.

Any splint worn over an open wound may be a transfer agent for microorganisms from the burn. In fact, organisms can be cultured from splint surfaces 50% of the time.[122] Effective strategies for cleaning burn splints are imperative. Simple washing and drying of the splint is not always effective in eliminating all organisms. The use of quaternary ammonia (1 oz per gallon of water) has been found to be 100% effective as a cleaning agent and is the recommend splint-cleaning strategy.[122]

Occasionally, special rehabilitative complications arise after burn injury, especially in patients who have sustained deep thermal wounds or an electrical injury. The most commonly encountered complications are exposed tendons and peripheral neuropathy with motor or sensory deficit. Splints can be useful in protecting or supporting these areas. Exposed tendons must be kept moist with an ointment-based gauze or biological dressing. The limb is splinted in a position where the tendon is slack, and exercise is avoided.[78] Idiopathic neuropathy occurs most often in patients with 20% or more TBSA burn involvement.[1,22] Secondary neuropathies may be caused by overelongation or compression of a peripheral nerve; such problems can be prevented by careful systematic monitoring of a patient's position, tightness of dressings, and the fit of splints.[78] Splints may also be fit to overcome a temporary or long-term neurological deficit such as a drop foot.

CASE EXAMPLE 1

A Patient with Burns of Both Upper Extremities

M. J. is a 17-year-old woman who was injured in a house fire 3 weeks ago and sustained 11% total body surface area burns to her face and both upper extremities. Facial burns were partial thickness in depth and spontaneously healed within 2 weeks. The burn injuries affecting both arms from mid-brachium down each forearm and the dorsum of each hand were full thickness and required skin grafting for wound closure. Skin grafting procedures were completed during the first 2 weeks of hospitalization in a series of three surgeries.

Questions to Consider

- What tests and measures would be most appropriate to document and track changes in M. J.'s range of motion (ROM), strength, endurance, and functional status? How might they need to be modified or adapted because of the severity of her burns?
- How will the medical care of her healing partial-thickness facial burns, and her full-thickness, grafted upper extremity burns be similar or different in terms of pain control, likelihood of scarring, and wound care? What factors might influence maturation of burn scars in this young woman?
- At this point in time, what are the primary rehabilitation goals for this young woman? How do rehabilitation goals change over the stages of wound healing (inflammatory, proliferative, and maturation)?
- What joints are most at risk of developing contracture in the early phases of healing? What positions would be optimal to reduce risk of contracture development? What type of orthosis might you recommend at this time? What other interventions would be important to consider as she progresses through the stages of wound healing?
- What passive and active exercise strategies might you recommend to enhance ROM, flexibility of healing tissues, strength, and endurance?
- What education and supportive strategies might be necessary?
- How long would you expect M. J. to be involved in rehabilitation activities? How will you assess if your interventions are accomplishing the rehabilitation goals?

Interventions and Outcomes

When M. J. is not immobilized after surgery, she is involved in a treatment program that includes upper extremity mobility exercises and strengthening exercises and an aerobic conditioning exercise program. Early ROM is generally mildly limited because of edema and wound contraction. After the skin-grafting procedures, ROM at all affected joints is improving, with the exception of declines in left elbow extension and left hand metacarpophalangeal flexion (digits 2 through 5). An anterior elbow-conforming splint is fabricated for the left arm and a functional position splint with approximately 40 degrees of metacarpophalangeal flexion is made for the left hand. Both splints are made of thermoplastic material and secured with hook-and-loop material strapping. These splints are applied during rest periods, naps, and during the night to prevent further loss of ROM. When awake, M. J. participates in therapy sessions and a home program of passive stretching and active exercise of all the affected joints, with emphasis on the troublesome left elbow and hand. Use of the splints is discontinued after 2 weeks because the range of motion has improved to normal.

AMPUTATION AND PROSTHETICS IN BURN REHABILITATION

Electrical burn injuries are more likely to lead to amputation than any other types of burns. Significant damage occurs as electrical current passes through nerve tissue, vascular tissue, and other deep structures. The current can cause destruction of cells, coagulation of tissues, thrombosis of blood vessels, neuropathies, and tissue necrosis. Other types of burn injuries may necessitate amputation if the wound is very deep or has associated tissue trauma. Some amputations, however, can be the consequence of an unrelenting infection.

Patients with burns who require limb amputation may have complications that delay prosthetic fitting and training as a result of multiple wound or scar sites, skin grafting on the residual limb, repeated surgical procedures (not necessarily associated with the residual limb), and burn-induced catabolic atrophy. Individuals with burns are also susceptible to the same postoperative complications faced by any patient with a new amputation: edema, phantom pain, and formation of neuroma or bone spur. Patients with amputation as a result of electrical injury may be susceptible to the formation of bone spurs.[129] Otherwise, heterotopic bone formation does not appear to be more prevalent in a burn population. Edema after burn injury is generally a short-term problem and seldom creates long-term delays in prosthetic training. There are no reports that suggest individuals with burns with amputations are more likely to develop phantom limb pain than other patients with amputation.

Any of these complications may intensify discomfort or the amount of work and time required for prosthetic training, which can be reasons for limited use or rejection of the prosthesis. Despite these concerns, patients with burn-related amputations are successfully rehabilitated with standard protocols.[124-126]

Skin Condition

For individuals with skin graft sites on the residual limb, fragility of skin (its tolerance of pressure and shear forces) is an important concern. Blisters or small open wounds may appear where a skin graft or a fragile scar breaks down as a result of forces on the residual limb during gait. Wearing of the prosthesis is often discontinued until the new wound is adequately healed. Wounds or skin grafts on areas associated with the prosthesis use, such as the shoulder or scapula under an upper extremity prosthesis harness, may demonstrate these same initial problems with wound breakdown. Even though the presence of a skin graft or fragile scar may delay or prolong prosthetic training, most patients with burn-related amputation are eventually successful in using their prostheses on skin-grafted limbs.[124-128] New "antishear" prosthetic socket suspension and lining materials may be especially helpful for individuals with burn-related amputation.

Contracture

The typical postamputation contracture in patients with burns is a result of muscle and soft tissue shortening related to a decreased moment arm of the affected extremity. When there is a maturing burn scar or graft site over the joint of the residual limb, the risk of contracture significantly increases (Figure 18-10). Such contractures may form more rapidly with the additional shortening force of the contracting scar tissue (Figure 18-11). The prevention of joint contracture after amputation requires vigilant positioning and stretching, which may be augmented by knee extension splints for individuals with transtibial amputation.

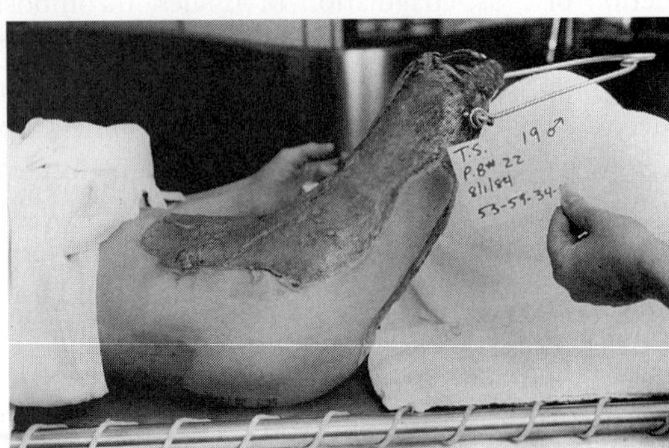

Figure 18-10
This patient with burn-related transfemoral amputation has increased risk of flexion contracture caused by scarring of the graft sites over the anterior surface of the hip. (From Ward RS, Hayes-Lundy C, Schnebly WS, et al. Rehabilitation of burn patients with concomitant limb amputation: Case reports. Burns *1990;16[5]:390-392.)*

Delayed Fitting

For patients with large TBSA burns, repeated surgical skin-grafting procedures are often necessary to cover the burn wound adequately. Repeated surgical procedures often delay prosthetic fitting and training. Individuals may be placed on postoperative bed rest for up to 7 days to ensure initial healing of the grafted area. To protect the new graft site and promote healing, the limb may be temporarily positioned in a less than optimal position for prosthetic use. Continued monitoring by the therapist, along with conscientious wrapping of the residual limb, can help overcome some of the problems caused by successive surgeries.

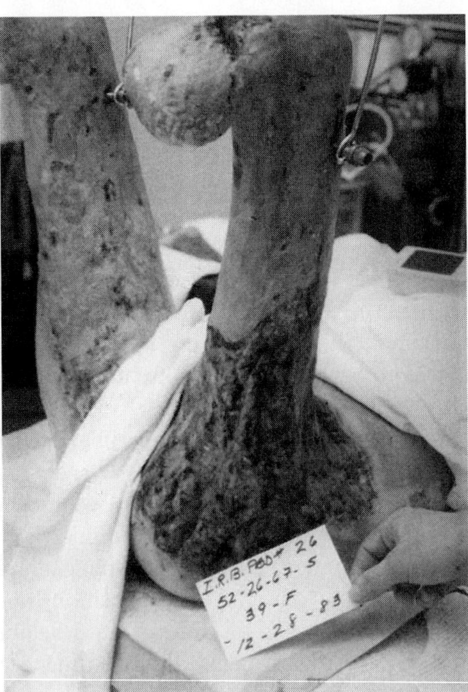

Figure 18-11
This patient has sustained bilateral transtibial amputation as a result of severe burn injury. She is at risk of significant knee flexion contracture because of the positioning required for her burn care and the inevitable contraction and scarring of her extensive graft sites. The areas of skin graft in her distal residual limbs may not initially tolerate the pressure and shear forces associated with prosthetic use, leading to delays in prosthetic fit and training.

Stabilization of Body Weight

It is common for patients with burns to lose weight because of hypermetabolism. A large burn can nearly double the body's metabolic requirements. Although individuals with significant burns receive nutritional supplementation, this often slows but does not prevent catabolic weight loss. Most individuals regain the weight lost in the catabolic process; this may require a series of revisions or refabrications of temporary sockets until weight stabilizes enough to fit a permanent prosthesis.

CASE EXAMPLE 2

A Patient with Amputation After Electrical Burns

C. T. is a 32-year-old man who was injured when a metal ladder he was using to trim tree branches made contact with overhead electrical wires. He sustained 35% total body surface area burns to his face, trunk, both upper extremities (including the right axilla), and his right lower leg. A right transhumeral amputation and a right transtibial amputation were required because of significant tissue damage from the electrical current. The amputations were performed on the third day after the burn; both residual limbs required several revisions of the amputation sites. Both residual limbs were successfully covered with a skin graft by the sixth day after the initial amputation.

Questions to Consider

- What tests and measures would be most appropriate to document and track changes in C. T.'s range of motion (ROM), strength, endurance, and functional status? How might they need to be modified or adapted because of the severity of his burns?
- Given the cause of his burns, what are the possible issues related to wound healing, contracture formation, and preprosthetic care that will influence your clinical decision making? What are the most pressing rehabilitation goals considering both his burns and his amputations in this early period of rehabilitation? In the months ahead?
- What will pain management and wound healing be like for someone like C. T., who has undergone amputation after electrocution, compared with someone with thermal burns who has had skin grafting?
- What factors will influence C. T.'s readiness for prosthetic fitting for this transtibial limb? For his transhumeral limb? What is C. T.'s prognosis for prosthetic use at both transtibial and transhumeral levels? How might the presence of skin grafts influence the prosthetist's recommendation for socket type and suspension of the prostheses? How will maturation of the residual limb and likely changes in body weight over time influence prosthetic fit and function?
- What are the key components in your preprosthetic plan of care for C. T.'s residual limbs? How might tissue healing influence his progression through prosthetic training? What passive and active exercise strategies might you recommend to enhance ROM, flexibility of healing tissues, strength, and endurance?
- What education and supportive strategies might be necessary for this young man with serious burns and amputation?
- How long would you expect C. T. to be involved in rehabilitation activities? How will you assess if your interventions are accomplishing the rehabilitation goals?

Interventions and Outcomes

Although C. T. was fitted with a transtibial prosthesis within 3 weeks of skin grafting, the fitting of C. T.'s initial upper extremity prosthesis must be postponed because of the time required to obtain closure of the remaining burn wounds on the right upper extremity (6 weeks). Given the extent of his burns, signal sites for a myoelectric (externally powered) prosthesis are difficult to identify; thus, C. T. is fit with a conventional body-powered transhumeral prosthesis with a hook as a terminal device. (See Chapters 33 and 34 for more information about prosthetic options and rehabilitation for individuals with upper extremity amputation.) Deep burns on both shoulders and the left trunk further delay (10 weeks) this fitting because of intolerance of the newly healed skin to the prosthetic harness.

C. T. quickly becomes functional with his transtibial prosthesis although susceptibility to pressure requires a special antishear, pressure-distributing liner. (See Chapters 26 and 27 for more information on prosthetic options and rehabilitation for patients with transtibial amputation.) During the fitting and training delays for his transhumeral prosthesis, an aggressive treatment program, including mobility exercises and strengthening exercises, is directed at the right upper extremity. The residual limb is also shaped with compression wraps and stockinet. C. T. also participates in similar mobility and strengthening exercises for other affected areas as well as an aerobic exercise program aimed at improving his endurance.

Twelve weeks after injury, C. T. is fit for and begins formal training with his prosthesis (dual-control cable system). There is one incident of skin breakdown under the harness over the left scapula. This area is dressed and padded with dense foam. There are no further incidences of skin breakdown. C. T. is discharged from physical therapy associated with the amputation 15 weeks after injury.

During his episode of care for rehabilitation and prosthetic training, C. T. endured several delays in management of his amputations as a result of the care related to other burn injuries, particularly those in strategic anatomical regions. It was important to maintain focus on preparation of the transtibial residual limb for containment within and functional use of the prosthesis and to prepare his transhumeral residual limb and opposite arms for the figure-of-eight harness and control system. Much of C. T.'s rehabilitation care concentrated on mobility ROM, and strength (especially of his upper extremities and the shoulder girdle) and endurance training.

EDUCATION

The patient with burns is the most important member of the rehabilitative burn care team. Family members and any others who will be caregivers outside the hospital must be included as early as possible to learn about the process of burn recovery and rehabilitation. Effectiveness of education is reflected by the individual's and caregiver's ability to demonstrate knowledge and understanding of the rehabilitation program.[35] Skin care, exercise programs, use of pressure supports, positioning techniques, and splint protocols are the obvious items that need to be taught to the patient.[130,131] Reinforcement, reasoning, and reassurance are key words to remember when designing an educational process.

SUMMARY

Optimal care of individuals recovering from burn injury taps the knowledge and skills of many different health care providers. Rehabilitation professionals are actively involved in many facets of postburn care, such as wound care and surgical grafting procedures; education about the burn rehabilitation process; and preventive care to minimize risk of hypertrophic scarring, contractures, deformity, and subsequent disability. Postburn rehabilitation care requires knowledge of and expertise in splint design and fabrication, exercise prescription (stretching and flexibility, strengthening, endurance), adaptive and assistive devices for gait and activities of daily living, and often prosthetic prescription and training.

REFERENCES

1. Petro JA, Salisbury RE. Rehabilitation of the burn patient. *Clin Plastic Surg* 1986;13(1):145-150.
2. Helm PA, Head MD, Pullium G, et al. Burn rehabilitation: a team approach. *Surg Clin North Am* 1978;58(6):1263-1278.
3. Frank HA, Berry C, Wachtel TL, et al. The impact of thermal injury. *J Burn Care Rehabil* 1987;8(4):260-262.
4. Silverstein P, Lack B. Epidemiology and prevention. In Boswick (ed), *The Art and Science of Burn Care.* Rockville, MD: Aspen, 1987. pp. 11-12.
5. American Burn Association Guidelines for service standards and severity classification in the treatment of burn injury. *Am Coll Surg Bull* 1984;69(10):24-26.
6. Van Rijin OJL, Bouter LM, Meertens RM. The aetiology of burns in developed countries: review of the literature. *Burns* 1989;15(4):217-221.
7. Lyngdorf P, Sorenson B, Thomsen M. The total number of burn injuries in a Scandinavian population—a prospective analysis. *Burns* 1986;12(8):567-571.
8. Brodzka W, Thornhill HL, Howard S. Burns: causes and risk factors. *Arch Phys Med Rehabil* 1985;66(11):746-751.
9. Jay MJ, Bartlett RH, Danet R, et al. Burn epidemiology: a basis for burn prevention. *J Trauma* 1977;17(12):943-947.
10. Murray JP. A study of the prevention of hot tap water burns. *Burns* 1988;14(3):185-193.
11. Baptiste MS, Feck G. Preventing tap water burns. *Am J Public Health* 1980;70(7):727-729.
12. Herbert K, Lawrence JC. Chemical burns. *Burns* 1989;15(6):381-384.
13. Monafo WW, Freedman BM. Electrical and lightning injury. In Boswick JA (ed), *The Art and Science of Burn Care.* Rockville, MD: Aspen, 1987. pp. 241-253.
14. Haberal M. Electrical burns: a five years experience. *J Trauma* 1986;26(2):103-109.
15. Thomsen M. It all began with Aristotle: the history of the treatment of burns. *Burns Incl Therm Inj* 1988;suppl:S1-S46.
16. Solem LD. Classification. In Fisher SV, Helm PA (eds), *Comprehensive Rehabilitation of Burns.* Baltimore: Williams and Wilkins, 1984. pp. 9-15.
17. Choctaw WT, Eisner ME, Wachtel TL. Causes, prevention, prehospital care, evaluation, emergency treatment, and prognosis. In Achauer BM (ed), *Management of the Burned Patient.* Norwalk, CT: Appleton & Lange, 1987. pp. 3-19.
18. Klasen HJ. Early excision and grafting. In Settle JAD (ed), *Principles and Practice of Burns Management.* New York: Churchill Livingstone, 1996. pp. 275-288.
19. Janzekovic Z. A new concept in the early excision and immediate grafting of burns. *J Trauma* 1970;10(12): 1103-1108.
20. Achauer BM. Treating the burn wound. In Achauer BM (ed), *Management of the Burned Patient.* Norwalk, CT: Appleton & Lange, 1987. pp. 93-108.
21. Jones T, McDonald S, Deitch EA. Effect of graft bed on long-term functional results of extremity skin grafts. *J Burn Care Rehabil* 1988;9(1):72-74.
22. Burke JF, Yannas IV, Quinby WC, et al. Successful use of physiological acceptable skin in the treatment of extensive burn injury. *Ann Surg* 1981;194(4):413-428.
23. Jaksic T, Burke JF. The use of artificial skin for burns. *Ann Rev Med* 1987;38:107-117.
24. Wainwright D, Madden M, Luterman A, et al. Clinical evaluation of an acellular allograft dermal matrix in full-thickness burns. *J Burn Care Rehabil* 1996;17(2):124-136.
25. Rennekampf HO, Hansbrough JF, Woods V, et al. Integrin and matrix molecule expression in cultured skin replacements. *J Burn Care Rehabil* 1996;17(3):213-221.
26. Desai MH, Mlakar JM, McCauley RL, et al. Lack of long-term durability of cultured keratinocyte burn-wound coverage: a case report. *J Burn Care Rehabil* 1991;12(6): 540-545.

27. Stern R, McPherson M, Longaker MT. Histologic study of artificial skin used in the treatment of full-thickness thermal injury. *J Burn Care Rehabil* 1990;11(1):7-13.
28. Lund CC, Browder NC. The estimation of areas of burns. *Surg Gynecol Obstet* 1944;79:352-358.
29. Ward RS, Saffle JR. Topical agents in burn and wound care. *Phys Ther* 1995;75(6):526-538.
30. Saffle JR, Schnebly WA. Burn wound care. In Richard RL, Staley, MJ (eds), *Burn Care and Rehabilitation: Principles and Practice.* Philadelphia: F.A. Davis, 1994. pp. 19-176.
31. Wright PC. Fundamentals of acute burn care and physical therapy management. *Phys Ther* 1984(8);64:1217-1231.
32. Ward RS. The rehabilitation of burn patients. *CRC Crit Rev Phys Med Rehabil* 1991;2(3):121-138.
33. Steiner H, Clark WR. Psychiatric complications of burned adults: a classification. *J Trauma* 1977;17(2):134-143.
34. West DA, Shuck JM. Emotional problems of the severely burned patient. *Surg Clin North Am* 1978;58(6):1189-1204.
35. Wallace LM, Lees J. A psychological follow-up study of adult patients discharged from a British burn unit. *Burns* 1988;14(1):39-45.
36. Chang FC, Herzog B. Burn morbidity: a follow-up study of physical and psychological disability. *Ann Surg* 1976;183(1):34-37.
37. Tempereau CE, Grossman AR, Brones MF. Psychological regression and marital status: determinants in psychiatric management of burn victims. *J Burn Care Rehabil* 1987;8(4):286-291.
38. Malt U. Long term psychological follow-up studies of burned adults: review of the literature. *Burns* 1980;6(3): 190-197.
39. Goodstein RK. Burns: an overview of clinical consequences affecting patient, staff, and family. *Comp Psychiatry* 1985;26(1):43-57.
40. Stoddard FJ. Body image development in the burned child. *J Am Acad Child Psychiatry* 1982;21(5):502-507.
41. Mahaney MB. Restoration of play in a severely burned three-year-old child. *J Burn Care Rehabil* 1990;11(1):57-63.
42. Andreason NJC. Neuropsychiatric complications in burn patients. *Int J Psychiatry Med* 1974;5(2):161-171.
43. Watkins PN, Cook EL, May SR, et al. Psychological stages of adaptation following burn injury: a method for facilitating psychological recovery of burn victims. *J Burn Care Rehabil* 1988;9(4):376-384.
44. Tollison CD, Still JM, Tollison JW. The seriously burned adult: psychologic reactions, recovery and management. *J Med Assoc Ga* 1980;69(2):121-124.
45. Peeling B. One day at a time on a burn unit. *Can Nurse* 1978;74(10):38-43.
46. Feller I, Tholen MS, Comell RG. Improvements in burn care, 1965 to 1979. *JAMA* 1980;244(18):2074-2078.
47. Schnebly WA, Ward RS, Warden GD, et al. A nonsplinting approach to the care of the thermally injured patient. *J Burn Care Rehabil* 1989;10(3):263-266.
48. Ward RS. Pressure therapy for the control of hypertrophic scar formation after burn injury: a history and review. *J Burn Care Rehabil* 1991;12(3):257-262.
49. Gabbiani G, Ryan G, Majeno G. Presence of modified fibroblasts in granulation tissue and their possible role in wound contraction. *Experientia* 1971;27(5):549-550.
50. Hardy MA. The biology of scar formation. *Phys Ther* 1989;69(12):1014-1024.
51. Ketchum LD. Hypertrophic scars and keloids. *Clin Plast Surg* 1977;4(2):301-310.
52. Rockwell WB, Cohen IK, Erlich JP. Keloids and hypertrophic scars: a comprehensive report. *Plast Reconstr Surg* 1989;84(5):827-837.
53. Hunt TK. Disorders of wound healing. *World J Surg* 1980;4(3):289-295.
54. Clark JA, Cheng JCY, Leung KS, et al. Mechanical characterization of human postburn hypertrophic skin during pressure therapy. *J Biomech* 1987;20(4):397-406.
55. Rudolf R. Wide spread scars, hypertrophic scars, and keloids. *Clin Plast Surg* 1987;14(2):253-260.
56. Davies D. Scars, hypertrophic scars, and keloids. *Br Med J* 1985;290(6474):1056-1058.
57. Deitch EA, Wheelahan TM, Rose MP. Hypertrophic burn scars: analysis of variables. *J Trauma* 1983;23(10):895-898.
58. Rudolf R. Construction and the control of contraction. *World J Surg* 1980;4(2):279-287.
59. Stern PJ, Law EJ, Benedict FE, et al. Surgical treatment of elbow contractures in postburn children. *Plast Reconstr Surg* 1985;76(3):441-446.
60. Parry SW. Reconstruction of the burned hand. *Clin Plast Surg* 1989;16(3):577-586.
61. Alexander JW, MacMillan BG, Martel L, et al. Surgical correction of postburn flexion contractures of the fingers of children. *Plast Reconstr Surg* 1981;68(2):218-224.
62. Huang TT, Blackwell SJ, Lewis SR. Ten years experience in managing patients with burn contractures of axilla, elbow, wrist, and knee joints. *Plast Reconstr Surg* 1978; 61(1):70-76.
63. Larson DL, Abston S, Evans EB, et al. Techniques for decreasing scar formation and contractures in the burned patient. *J Trauma* 1971;11(10):807-823.
64. Kischer CW, Shetlar MR, Shetlar CL. Alteration of hypertrophic scars induced by mechanical pressure. *Arch Dermatol* 1975;111(1):60-64.
65. Ward RS. Pressure therapy for the control of hypertrophic scar formation after burn injury: a history and review. *J Burn Care Rehabil* 1991;12(1):257-262.
66. Torring S. Our routine in pressure treatment of hypertrophic scars. *Scand J Plast Reconstr Surg* 1984;18(1):135-137.
67. Robertson JC, Druett JE, Hodgson B, et al. Pressure therapy for hypertrophic scarring: preliminary communication. *J R Soc Med* 1980;73(5):348-354.
68. Ward RS, Hayes-Lundy C, Reddy R, et al. Influence of pressure supports on joint range of motion. *Burns* 1992;18(1):60-62.
69. Gold HM. A controlled clinical trial of topical silicone gel sheeting in the treatment of hypertrophic scars and keloids. *J Am Acad Dermatol* 1994;30(3):506-507.
70. Perkins K, Davey RB, Wallis KA. Silicone gel: a new treatment for burn scars and contractures. *Burns* 1982;9(3):201-204.
71. Ahn ST, Monafo WW, Mustoe TA. Topical silicone gel: a new treatment for hypertrophic scars. *Surgery* 1989;106(4): 781-787.
72. Sullivan T, Smith J, Kerrnode J, et al. Rating the burn scar. *J Burn Care Rehabil* 1990;11(3):256-260.

73. Kealey GP, Jensen KT. Aggressive approach to physical therapy management of the burned hand. *Phys Ther* 1988;68(5):683-685.
74. Dobbs ER, Curreri PW. Burns: analysis of results of physical therapy in 681 patients. *J Trauma* 1972;12(3):242-248.
75. Howell JW. Management of the acutely burned hand for the nonspecialized clinician. *Phys Ther* 1989;12(12):1077-1089.
76. Parrot M, Ryan R, Parks DH, et al. Structured exercise circuit program for burn patients. *J Burn Care Rehabil* 1988;9(6):666-668.
77. Johnson CL, Cain VJ. Burn care—the rehab guide. *Am J Nurs* 1985;85(1):48-50.
78. Helm PA, Kevorkian CG, Lushbaugh M, et al. Burn injury: rehabilitation management in 1982. *Arch Phys Med Rehabil* 1982;63(1):6-16.
79. Humphrey C, Richard RL, Staley MJ. Soft tissue management and exercise. In Richard RL, Staley MJ (eds), *Burn Care and Rehabilitation Principles and Practice.* Philadelphia: F.A. Davis, 1994. pp. 331-336.
80. Tepperman PS, Hilbert L, Peters WJ, et al. Heterotopic ossification in burns. *J Burn Care Rehabil* 1984;5(4):283-287.
81. Crawford CM, Vaeghese G, Mani M, et al. Heterotopic ossification: are range of motion exercises contraindicated? *J Burn Care Rehabil* 1986;6(4):323-327.
82. VanLaeken N, Snelling CFT, Meek RN, et al. Heterotopic bone formation in the patient with burn injuries: a retrospective assessment of contributing factors and methods of investigation. *J Burn Care Rehabil* 1989;10(4):331-335.
83. Tafel JA, Thacker JG, Hagemann JM, et al: Mechanical performance of exertubing for isotonic hand exercise. *J Burn Care Rehabil* 1987;8(4):333-335.
84. Johnson CL. Physical therapists as scar modifiers. *Phys Ther* 1984;64(9):1381-1387.
85. Richard RL, Miller SF, Finley RK, et al. Home exercise kit for the shoulder. *J Burn Care Rehabil* 1987;8(2):144-145.
86. Apfel LM, Wachtel TL, Frank DH, et al. Functional electrical stimulation in intrinsic/extrinsic imbalanced burned hands. *J Burn Care Rehabil* 1987;8(2):97-102.
87. Lewis SM. Clelland JA, Knowles CJ, et al. Effects of auricular acupuncture-like transcutaneous nerve stimulation on pain levels following wound care in patients with burns: a pilot study. *J Burn Care Rehabil* 1990;11(4):322-329.
88. Bierman W. Ultrasound in the treatment of scars. *Arch Phys Med Rehabil* 1954;35:209-214.
89. Baryza MJ. Ultrasound in the treatment of postburn skin graft contracture: a single case study. *Phys Ther* 1996;76:S54.
90. Ward RS, Hayes-Lundy C, Reddy R, et al. Evaluation of therapeutic ultrasound to improve response to physical therapy and lessen scar contracture after burn injury. *J Burn Care Rehabil* 1994;15(1):74-79.
91. Johnson CL. PT/OT Forum [editorial]. *J Burn Care Rehabil* 1988;9(4):396.
92. Covey MH, Dutcher K, Marvin JA, et al: Efficacy of continuous passive motion (CPM) devices with hand burns. *J Burn Care Rehabil* 1988;9(4):397-400.
93. McAllister LP, Salazar CA. Case report on the use of CPM on an electrical burn. *J Burn Care Rehabil* 1988;9(4):401.
94. Head M, Helm P. Paraffin and sustained stretching in treatment of burn contracture. *Burns* 1977;4(2):136-139.
95 Ward RS, Saffle JR, Schnebly WA, et al. Sensory loss over grafted areas in patients with burns. *J Burn Care Rehabil* 1989;10(6):536-538.
96. Ward RS, Tuckett RP. Quantitative threshold changes in cutaneous sensation of patients with burns. *J Burn Care Rehabil* 1991;12(6):569-575.
97. Cooper S, Paul EO. An effective method of positioning the burn patient. *J Burn Care Rehabil* 1988;9(3):288-289.
98. Heeter PK, Brown R. Arm hammock for elevation of the thermally injured upper extremity. *J Burn Care Rehabil* 1986;7(2):144-147.
99. Waymack JP, Fidler J, Warden GD. Surgical correction of burn scar contractures of the foot in children. *Burns* 1988;4(2):156-160.
100. Duncan RM. Basic principles of splinting the hand. *Phys Ther* 1989;69(12):1104-1116.
101. Malick MH, Carr JA. *Manual on Management of the Burn Patient.* Pittsburgh: Harnarville Rehabilitation Center, 1982. pp. 32-62.
102. Daugherty MB, Carr-Collins JA. Splinting techniques for the burn patient. In Richard RL, Staley MJ (eds), *Burn Care and Rehabilitation Principles and Practice.* Philadelphia: F.A. Davis, 1994. pp. 242-317.
103. Mathew Jose R, Varghese S, Nandakumar UR. Modified Watusi splint: a simple and economical device. *Br J Plast Surg* 2002;55(3):270.
104. Manigandan C, Gupta AK, Venugopal K, et al. The wrist in axillary burns—a forgotten focus of concern. *Burns* 2003;29(5):497-498.
105. Walters C. *Splinting the Burn Patient.* Laurel, MD: RAMSCO, 1987. pp. 9-97.
106. Manigandan C, Gupta AK, Venugopal K, et al. A multi-purpose, self-adjustable aeroplane splint for the splinting of axillary burns. *Burns* 2003;29(3):276-279.
107. Kwan MW, Ha KW. Splinting programme for patients with burnt hand. *Hand Surg* 2002;7(2):231-241.
108. Van Straten O, Sagi A. "Supersplint": a new dynamic combination splint for the burned hand. *J Burn Care Rehabil* 2000;2:71-73.
109. Tilley W, McMahon S, Shukalak B. Rehabilitation of the burned upper extremity. *Hand Clin* 2000;16(2):303-318.
110. Ward RS, Schnebly WA, Kravitz M, et al. Have you tried the sandwich splint? A method of preventing hand deformities in children. *J Burn Care Rehabil* 1989;10(1):83-85.
111. Yildirim S, Avci G, Akan M, et al. Anterolateral thigh flap in the treatment of postburn flexion contractures of the knee. *Plast Reconstr Surg* 2003;19(4):225-233.
112. Guild S. A new splinting approach for dorsal foot burns. *J Burn Care Rehabil* 2001;22:454-456.
113. Heinle JA, Kealey GP, Cram AE, et al. The microstomia prevention appliance: 14 years of clinical experience. *J Burn Care Rehabil* 1988;9(1):90-91.
114. Sela M, Tubiana L. A mouth splint for severe burns of the head and neck. *J Prosthet Dent* 1989;62(6):679-681.
115. Lehman CJ. Splints and accessories following burn reconstruction. *Clin Plast Surg* 1992;19(3):721-731.
116. Moore DJ. The role of the maxillofacial prosthetist in support of the burn patient. *J Prosthet Dent* 1970;24(1):68-76.
117. Kaufman T, Newman RA, Weinberg A, et al. The kerlix tongue depressor splint for skin-grafted areas in burned children. *J Burn Care Rehabil* 1989;10(5):462-463.

118. Wilder RP, Doctor A, Paley RJ, et al. Evaluation of cohesive and elastic bandages for joint immobilization. *J Burn Care Rehabil* 1989;10(3):258-262.
119. Richard RL, Miller SF, Finley RK Jr, et al. Comparison of the effect of passive exercise vs static wrapping on finger range of motion of the hand. *J Burn Care Rehabil* 1987;8(6): 576-578.
120. Richard RL. Use of the Dynasplint to correct elbow flexion burn contracture: a case report. *J Burn Care Rehabil* 1986;7(2):151-152.
121. Bennett GB, Helm P, Purdue GF, et al. Serial casting: a method for treating burn contractures. *J Burn Care Rehabil* 1989;10(6):543-545.
122. Wright MP, Taddonio TE, Prasad JK, et al. The microbiology and cleaning of thermoplastic splints in burn care. *J Burn Care Rehabil* 1989;10(1):79-83.
123. Helm PA. Peripheral neurological problems in acute burn patients. *Burns* 1977;3(2):123-125.
124. Ward RS, Hayes-Lundy C, Schnebly WS, et al. Rehabilitation of burn patients with concomitant limb amputation: case reports. *Burns* 1990;16(5):390-392.
125. Ward RS, Hayes-Lundy C, Schnebly WS, et al. Prosthetic use in patients with burns and associated limb amputation. *J Burn Care Rehabil* 1990;11(4):361-364.
126. Meier RH. Amputations and prosthetic fitting. In Fisher SA, Helm PA (eds), *Comprehensive Rehabilitation of Burns.* Baltimore: Williams & Wilkins, 1984. pp. 267-310.
127. Rosenfelder R. The below-knee amputee with skin grafts. *Phys Ther* 1970;50(9):1338-1346.
128. Wood MR, Hunter GA, Millstein SG. The value of stump split skin grafting following amputation for trauma in adult upper and lower limb amputees. *Prosthet Orthot Int* 1987;11(2):71-74.
129. Helm PA, Walker SC. New bone formation at amputation sites in electrically burn-injured patients. *Arch Phys Med Rehabil* 1987;68(5 part 1):284-286.
130. Kaplan SH. Patient education techniques used at burn centers. *Am J Occup Ther* 1985;39(10):655-658.
131. Neville C, Walker S, Brown B, et al. Discharge planning for burn patients. *J Burn Care Rehabil* 1988;9(4):414-418.

19

Adaptive Seating in the Management of Neuromuscular and Musculoskeletal Impairment

Barbara Crane

LEARNING OBJECTIVES

On completion of this chapter, the reader will be able to do the following:

1. Describe the population of individuals who use wheelchairs and adaptive seating.
2. Identify the elements of a basic wheelchair and seating evaluation.
3. List potential outcomes for adaptive seating and mobility intervention.
4. Summarize biomechanical principles related to adaptive seating and wheeled mobility.
5. Rank the major types of wheelchair technologies in order from lowest technical sophistication to highest technical sophistication.
6. Explain various factors related to development of pressure ulcers for wheelchair users with a spinal cord injury.
7. Specify which of the current technologies for postural control in seating would be most effective in the management of severe spasticity in a patient with cerebral palsy.
8. Recommend an appropriate wheeled mobility base and adaptive seating system for a patient after a cerebrovascular accident.

Neuromuscular and musculoskeletal impairments often limit a person's functional gait potential. When this occurs, adaptive seating support and wheeled mobility interventions are essential in returning a person to a maximal level of independent function. Individuals use their wheeled mobility device for many hours each day. People who use wheeled mobility devices (wheelchairs or scooters) for some or all of their mobility often require adaptive seating support. Additionally, individuals who use wheeled mobility devices often require assistance for other activities of daily living and may require postural support and balance in a seated position. Individuals with neuromuscular impairments typically require specialized seating support to attain a maximal level of independent function, comfort, safety, and quality of life. Individuals with musculoskeletal impairment in the absence of neurological deficits may also require postural support because of the amount of time they spend in a seated posture or, in some cases, because of the inability to either stand or walk.

Individuals who use wheelchairs and adaptive seating systems are of all age groups and races. They use their wheelchairs in many different environments and for many different reasons. Some are full-time wheelchair users because they cannot stand or walk. Others spend part of their day in the wheelchair to augment their mobility over long distances or on uneven surfaces. Some use wheelchairs for short-term conditions that resolve within weeks or months, such as lower extremity fractures or joint replacement surgeries. Others use wheelchairs long term because of permanent disabling conditions.

There are approximately 1.7 million community-dwelling people in the United States who use wheelchairs or powered scooters to assist them with mobility.[1] Of these, approximately 1.5 million use manual wheelchairs, 155,000 use electric-powered wheelchairs, and 142,000 use electric-powered scooters. In addition to these permanent users, there are likely to be several million part-time or temporary wheeled mobility device users at any given time in the United States, not including individuals residing in institutional settings. The National Medical Expenditure Survey conducted in 1987 indicated there were 2.5 million individuals residing in long-term care facilities, and of these, more than 50% use wheelchairs for mobility.[3,4] Individuals who use wheelchairs range from very young children who never attain the ability to walk to very old adults who have lost this ability because of various disabling conditions and processes.

Among all age groups, the leading condition associated with wheelchair use is cerebrovascular disease. Among individuals aged 18 to 64 years, the leading condition associated with wheelchair use is multiple sclerosis.[1] Other conditions commonly associated with wheelchair use include osteoarthritis and rheumatoid arthritis, congenital absence or amputation of lower extremities, tetraplegia and paraplegia, cardiopulmonary diseases and disorders (e.g., emphysema) that limit endurance, cerebral palsy, diabetes, and orthopedic impairment of the lower extremities.[1]

Individuals who use adaptive seating and wheeled mobility live in many different environments. Many live in the community independently or with assistance or support. Others live in long-term care settings or in assisted-living environments. Individuals use wheelchairs at home, school, work, and outdoors. People rely on their wheeled mobility devices to allow them to work, learn, play, care for themselves, and meet their personal goals. Therefore the assessment for and recommendation of a wheeled mobility device and seating support system is an important responsibility typically undertaken by a team of trained individuals.

WHAT IS A WHEELCHAIR?

A wheelchair, or wheeled mobility device, is a complex piece of assistive technology. In addition to providing a means for mobility, this device provides the foundation for all other function, that is, activities of daily living such as bathing and dressing, work activities, and recreation. To do this, several interrelated components of the wheeled mobility device must work together to meet the needs of the individual user. The three major components of a wheelchair are the seating system (the postural support component), the wheelchair frame (the supporting structure), and the propelling structure (Figure 19-1).[5] All three components provide different functions but must form an integrated unit for efficient and safe wheeled mobility. Successful integration is critical to the function of the wheelchair user.

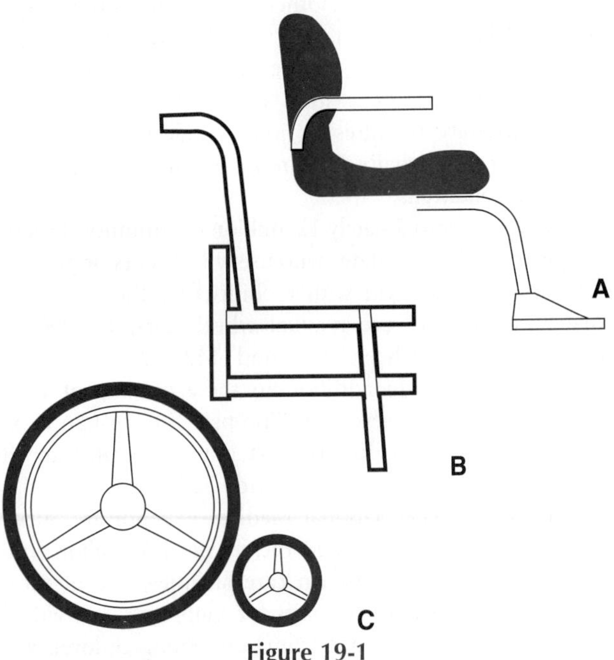

Figure 19-1

*The three components of a wheelchair include the postural support (**A**), the supporting structure (**B**), and the propelling structure (**C**).*

Seating System

The seating system, or adaptive seating component, of the wheeled mobility device is primarily responsible for support and positioning of the wheelchair user or wheelchair rider. This component can be thought of as an orthotic intervention in wheeled mobility prescription. Adaptive seating is used to promote postural support and positioning so that the user may function optimally.[6] To do this, it must accomplish the following five goals:

1. Provide effective postural support and positioning for the pelvis, trunk, lower body, and sometimes extremities and head
2. Provide optimal soft tissue loading by pressure redistribution to minimize the risk of pressure ulcer development
3. Provide optimal comfort so that the seating system may be tolerated for long periods
4. Facilitate distal extremity function by providing a stable base of support for the user
5. Permit optimal access to the mobility interface component (e.g., the wheel rims of a manual chair or the power controller of a powered wheelchair) of the wheelchair

Although all these goals are critical to the optimal function of any wheeled mobility device, goals must be prioritized on the basis of personal needs of each user. For example, a wheeled mobility device user with a spinal cord injury who has good overall posture but lacks sensory function requires greater emphasis on pressure management goals than on postural support.

The seating system is often divided into several components, each with responsibility for supporting different body segments. A summary of indications for each type of seating component is found in Table 19-1.

Support Frame and Mobility Components

The support frame is integrated with the seating component and is closely linked with the propelling structure. The main purpose of the support frame is to provide a smooth integration or connection of the seating support system and the mobility component of the wheeled mobility device. Many styles of frames are available; some provide specialty purposes, such as tilt, recline or standing frames, but the majority are configured to allow attachment of adaptive seating systems and facilitate access to the mobility structures of the device by the user.

Table 19-1
Postural Support Components and Indications for Use

Postural Support Component	*Indications for Use*
Seat cushion	Wheelchair use for any amount of time (see Table 19-6 for detailed descriptions of types of seat cushions)
Solid seat support	Wheelchair use for any amount of time, particularly a folding wheelchair with sling seat upholstery
Solid back support	Wheelchair use of 4 hours or more per day Impaired sitting balance or trunk control Scoliosis or any need for lateral and posterior spinal support
Lateral thoracic supports	Impaired sitting balance or trunk control Flexible or fixed spinal scoliosis Need for additional lateral support for safe or efficient activities of daily living (e.g., driving)
Lateral pelvic supports	Impaired pelvic and lower trunk control Flexible or fixed scoliosis
Medial knee supports	Lower extremity adduction while sitting Hypertonicity (spasticity) of lower extremities Windswept deformities of lower extremities
Knee blocks	Impaired anterior stability of pelvis in wheelchair If the patient slides out of wheelchair on a regular basis Severe extensor spasticity in lower extremities
Head support	Impaired head control from weakness or abnormal muscle tone
Anterior pelvic support	Anterior/posterior instability of pelvis while sitting (e.g., falling into posterior pelvic tilt or excessive anterior tilt, sliding out of chair)
Anterior trunk support	Anterior trunk instability If additional support is needed for safe and efficient functional activities (e.g., wheelchair propulsion, mobility over rough terrain, driving activities, or transportation needs)

The mobility base, or propelling structure, of the wheelchair is composed of the drive wheels, caster wheels, tires, and some type of user interface component. Goals for the mobility base focus on the facilitation of mobility within the user's environment and can include the following:

1. Independent mobility in all environments encountered by the individual
2. Safe access to mobility and the prevention of injuries, such as overuse or secondary injuries
3. Maximum efficiency in mobility
4. Facilitation of overall function within the person's environment

In Cook and Hussey's Human Activity Assistive Technology model, wheeled mobility devices and seating systems are defined as "extrinsic enablers."[5] These devices facilitate or allow the user to perform many functions. A seating support system is referred to as a "general-purpose extrinsic enabler"[5] because it facilitates many different functions for the user, such as self-care, recreation, or mobility. The wheeled mobility device is a "specific purpose extrinsic enabler," meaning it specifically allows users to be mobile within their environment.

SEATING AND MOBILITY ASSESSMENT

Seating and mobility assessment is a highly complex process involving multiple component evaluations and tests.[7] Seating and mobility assessments have many similarities to physical therapy and occupational therapy assessments but are more specific to the seating and wheeled mobility needs of the patient. The major difference in the outcome between more traditional therapy assessment and seating and mobility assessment is the intervention. The intervention plan in a seating and mobility assessment involves recommending a particular wheeled mobility device and adaptive seating system. As with any therapeutic intervention, the first step is an examination of the patient.[8] This examination allows the therapist to collect all appropriate information to evaluate the patient's needs and determine the most appropriate intervention plan.

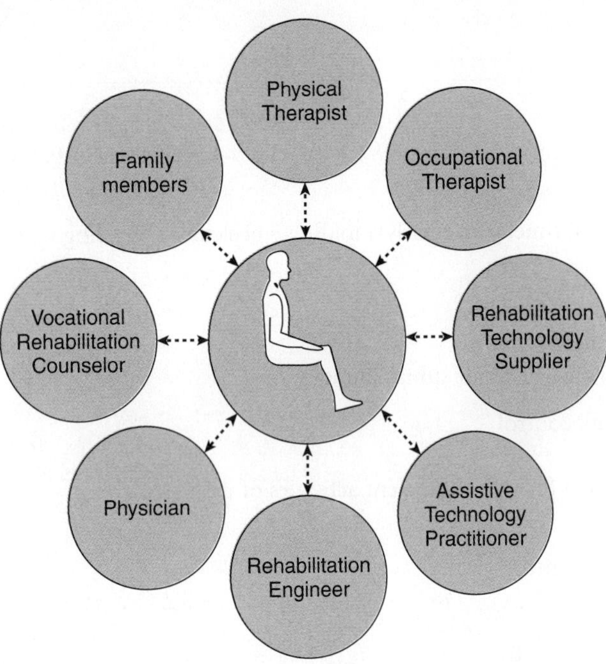

Figure 19-2

The interdisciplinary seating and mobility assessment team is most successful if it is consumer focused.

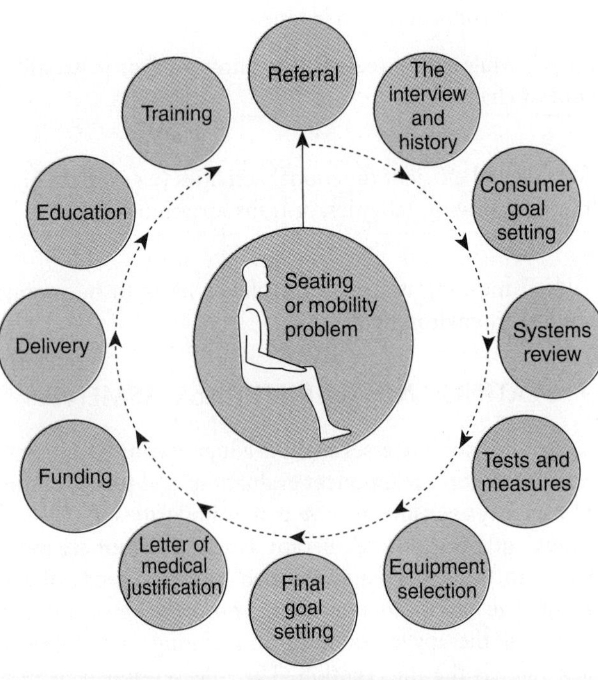

Figure 19-3

When a patient is referred to the team, the first steps in the process involve collecting relevant information and examination, including specific tests and measures. The team uses this information to select appropriate components on the basis of prognosis and the patient's functional needs. Once ordered and delivered, the team works with the patient on mobility, safety, and maintenance issues.

Members of the Assessment Team

Specially trained clinicians, organized in a team structure, are usually responsible for performing seating and mobility assessments (Figure 19-2). This team may consist of physical or occupational therapists with specialized training in wheelchair seating and mobility, physicians, rehabilitation technology suppliers, orthotists, and other health care professionals. The rehabilitation technology supplier is the team member who will ultimately be responsible for providing the equipment to the patient. The rehabilitation technology supplier participates in the assessment process, compiles an equipment quotation and cost estimate, orders the equipment from the manufacturer, submits the justification and billing information to the equipment funding source(s), and then assembles the components in preparation for delivery of the wheeled mobility system. When an individual with seating or mobility problem is referred to the team, a multistep process of assessment, prescription, and training begins (Figure 19-3). The team must carefully document its findings and recommendations.

History

As with most therapeutic examinations, a detailed history is an essential component of a seating and mobility assessment. This history typically includes information related to diagnosis, nature of the disabling condition, related health problems, current and past assistive technology use, description of the home environment and other environments in which the equipment will be used, transportation needs of the patient, and funding source information for the equipment. All these elements are critical to the selection of an appropriate seating and wheeled mobility device.

The diagnosis of the patient is a critical component of the history—particularly diagnoses related to why he or she requires a wheeled mobility device. If a patient has a gait disability, the cause of the disability must be described both to evaluate the most effective intervention and to justify the need for the equipment to the funding source. Important questions to ask include the following:

1. When was the onset of the disability?
2. Was it sudden or slow?
3. Is the disability progressive or nonprogressive?

In addition to the major diagnosis, information about associated health problems is also important. Related health problems may include breathing problems, cardiovascular or circulatory problems, seizure disorders, bowel and bladder continence problems, nutrition and digestion, medications the individual takes, surgeries in the past or planned surgeries, orthopedic concerns such as subluxation or dislocation of the hip or shoulder, osteoporosis, other orthotic interventions (including any leg or foot orthoses or trunk orthoses), skin condition problems or concerns, sensation, pain problems, visual deficits, hearing deficits, and cognitive and behavioral problems.[9] Diagnostic information and related health concerns have a direct impact on the selection of appropriate equipment.

The history must also include elements related to the patient's equipment use and the environmental demands. Gathering information about current and past assistive technology use is important. Knowing what the individual has tried and the outcomes of these interventions helps avoid the repetition of mistakes. Also, knowledge of previously used assistive technology is important for interfacing any new devices with already existing devices, such as alternative communication systems. Also, knowledge of the mode of transportation (e.g., car, adapted van, public transportation, school-provided transportation) is critical because equipment must be chosen to meet these transportation needs. The demands of the patient's home environment or other environments in which the equipment will be used must be understood, including school or workplace environment and recreational activities.[7] Last, but certainly not least, the funding source or sources for the equipment must be discerned. Different funding sources have different requirements for evidence documented in support of patient needs and benefits of selected devices and for medical necessity to justify reimbursement for the equipment.

Systems Review

Once this detailed history is gathered, the therapist may move on to a systems review.[8] A systems review includes a limited examination of the major systems affecting the selection of the assistive device (Table 19-2), including the cardiovascular and pulmonary system, the integumentary system, the musculoskeletal system, the neuromuscular system, and the communication and cognitive abilities of the individual.[8] During the systems review, additional questions may arise related to the history of the patient, particularly related to past equipment use; these questions should be incorporated into the remainder of the examination and the responses integrated with the history already recorded.

If an individual is already using a wheeled mobility device, the systems review must include an assessment of the patient's use of the current equipment. The make and model of any devices currently used should be recorded, along with the sizes of all items and their present condition. In addition to the condition of the equipment, the patient's posture and function while using this equipment should be noted. Determining why the person needs an assessment for new equipment is extremely important. Questions to ask include the following:

- Did the patient "outgrow" the equipment or did the equipment exceed its expected lifespan?
- Did the patient's needs change because of a change in medical condition or functional status?

Specific details of how the current equipment is used and whether such use is appropriate and effective help with

Table 19-2
Components of the Systems Review for Seating and Wheelchair Assessment

System	*Issue to Assess*

Musculoskeletal	Range of motion
	Strength of all muscles
	Postural asymmetry
	  Pelvic obliquity
	  Pelvic rotation
	  Pelvic tilt (anterior/posterior)
	  Scoliosis
	  Excessive kyphosis
	  Lordosis
	Flexibility of any noted asymmetries

Integumentary	History of skin breakdown Surgeries performed Skin inspection to identify current problems Performance of active pressure reliefs Condition of pressure management equipment Success/failure of technologies in the past
Neurological	Motor control Abnormal muscle tone Abnormal primitive reflexes
Cardiovascular	Heart rate Blood pressure (at rest and with activity) Edema
Pulmonary	Respiratory rate Shortness of breath (dyspnea) Blood oxygenation (pulse oximetry) Change in pulmonary status with activity Change in pulmonary status with position

Communication	Verbal and nonverbal
	Use of alternative or augmentative systems
	Effectiveness of communication
	  With family or familiar individuals
	  With unknown or unfamiliar individuals

Cognitive status	Type of cognitive impairments present Developmental delay Progressive dementia Overall mental health and judgment Ability to learn Understanding of wheeled mobility function

setting goals and determining the most effective equipment intervention for the future.

The reason for the seating and wheeled mobility assessment often translates into the justification for the recommended equipment, so this information is critical to ascertain during the examination. If the patient has not used any device in the past, why is one needed now? What change has triggered the referral for an evaluation? During this review, the specific, patient-centered, functional goals related to wheeled mobility device use should also be determined. These goals are incorporated into the intervention after all the data are collected and the evaluation is made.

Cardiovascular and pulmonary assessment, including blood pressure, heart rate, pulse oximetry, respiratory rate, and edema are also important. Skin condition must be assessed, particularly over all seating contact areas. Gross musculoskeletal status should be assessed and the patient's height and weight recorded. General assessments of function and movement ability in the current wheeled mobility system and the patient's communication skills and abilities and cognition should also be performed.

Tests and Measures Used in Seating and Mobility Assessment

The systems review helps determine which areas require a more comprehensive assessment in the form of specific tests and measures, including seated and supine mat evaluation, seating simulation, equipment simulation, and pressure mapping (Table 19-3). If a patient has a cardiovascular condition, such as postural hypotension, then more extensive testing of different seated positions and interventions along with detailed tracking of changes in blood pressure are necessary during the mat evaluation and the seating simulation. Many tests and measures are used during the seating and wheeled mobility examination process. Some are necessary for all patients requiring adaptive seating, and some are used only in particular instances. Tests and measures for adaptive seating and mobility intervention can be classified according to postural and technical or instrumentation requirements, such as mat table or seat simulator.

Mat Evaluation

Many of the tests and measures used are incorporated into the mat evaluation, which consists of an evaluation with the patient in both seated and supine postures.[7] During a seated mat evaluation, the therapist measures or determines a person's unsupported seated posture, postural asymmetries, sitting balance, joint flexibility (particularly of the spine and pelvis) and functional abilities in terms of transfers and seated function, such as reaching ability. A supine mat evaluation is essential for measuring specific joint range of motion, strength, coordination, and abnormal muscle tone and reflexes. Particular attention must be paid to true hip joint mobility, orthopedic deformities such as pelvic asymmetries, hip joint subluxations or dislocations, and flexibility of spinal postures.[7] The supine mat evaluation is critical in determining the flexibility of postural deformities because of the change in the effects of the gravitational pull on the body. If a postural deformity is present during the sitting assessment and then disappears during the supine mat evaluation, that deformity is "flexible" in nature and may be correctible in the adaptive seating system. If, on the other hand, the postural asymmetry is present in both seated and supine postures, in spite of any attempt at repositioning, then this asymmetry is described as a "fixed" posture.

SIMULATION TECHNIQUES AND EQUIPMENT

The other tests and measures of a seating and mobility assessment are performed by using simulation techniques or equipment. Three primary simulation techniques are used: hand simulation, simulation with a commercial seated simulator, and simulation with commercial seating and mobility products similar to those likely to be selected.[9,10]

Hand simulation is often performed with the patient seated on the mat. During this simulation the therapist uses his or her hands to simulate or mimic forces applied by various components of an adaptive seating system. In this manner, the therapist can determine if external supports are capable of providing the desired effect on the patient's posture and how much force is required or what the optimal application point on the body will be.[7]

After hand simulation, a *seating simulator* may be used to verify the manual data. A seating simulator is a highly adjustable wheelchair frame with many interchangeable components.[10] This device is first preset to provide the desired supports; then the patient sits in it so the therapist can determine if the settings actually produce the desired postural or functional outcomes.

The third simulation method involves assembling actual commercial products into a system similar to that being recommended to assess its effect. This may be done if a commercial simulator is not available as an additional component after performing the other types of simulation. This final simulation provides evidence of the effectiveness of actual products in meeting the desired goals of the seating and mobility assessment and may be an excellent way of providing the funding source with information regarding why specific equipment is being recommended.

Other tests and measures used for seating and mobility assessment include pressure mapping (Figure 19-4),[11] custom contour seat simulation, pulse oximetry during simulation, specific circulatory assessments during simulation, and functional wheelchair propulsion testing.[12] These specific measures may not be used in all seating and mobility assessments but can be mixed and matched according to the needs of the patient. All these tests and measures provide the therapist with necessary information required for evaluation and determination of final equipment selections.

Table 19-3
Tests and Measures Used in Seating and Wheelchair Assessment

Component of Evaluation	*Measures or Task Analysis*

Seated mat evaluation	Unsupported seated posture
	Sitting balance
	Postural flexibility
	Functional abilities
	  Transfers
	  Reaching
	  Activities of daily living simulation

Supine mat evaluation	Seating angles
	  Thigh to trunk angle
	  True hip flexion range of motion
	  Thigh to lower leg angle
	  Hamstring tightness
	  Lower leg to foot angle
	Pelvic flexibility
	Abnormal muscle tone
	Mobility skills and abilities
	  Supine to/from sitting transition

Mat (hand) simulation	Position of supports required Amount of force required Ability to reduce flexible asymmetries

Seated simulation testing	Desired seating dimensions
	Desired seating angles
	  Seat tilt or orientation
	  Seat to back angle support
	  Need for biangular back support
	Other simulated supports and effects
	  Lateral pelvic supports
	  Lateral trunk supports
	  Arm supports
	  Leg and foot supports
	  Head support

Equipment simulation	What equipment was used Results of mobility assessment in mock-up Consumer comfort Ability to meet goals with simulated system Photos to include with justification documents

Pressure mapping	Note cushions used during testing
	Results of cushions tested
	  Pressure distribution patterns
	Consumer education
	  Importance of proper seat cushion use
	  Optimal pressure relief methods

Other	Custom molding simulation Pulse oximetry Circulatory testing Functional wheelchair propulsion testing

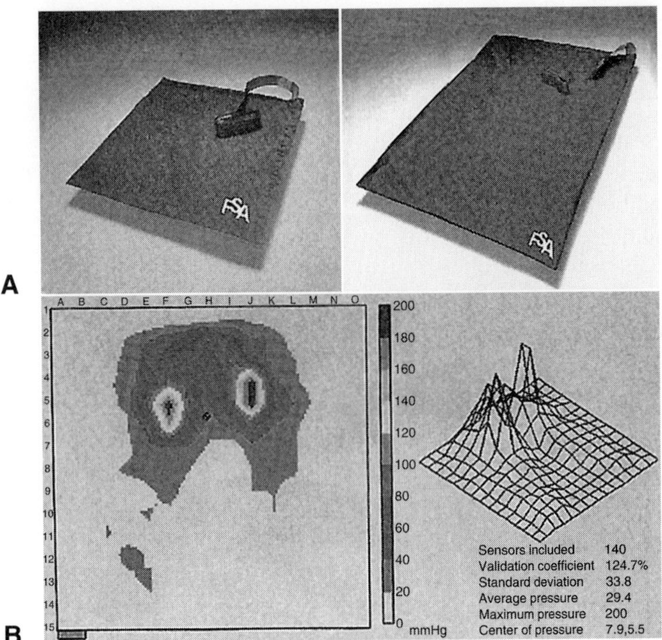

Figure 19-4

*An example of a pressure measurement system. The pressure-sensitive mat that the patient sits on is connected to a computer (**A**). The computer generates a two-dimensional (**B**) or three-dimensional (**C**) display of seating pressures. (From Cook AM, Hussey SM [eds].* Assistive Technologies: Principles and Practice, *vol 1, 2nd ed. St. Louis: Mosby, 2002. p. 196.)*

Plan of Care and Equipment Prescription

The evaluation of all this information will lead to a diagnosis related to the patient's level of function and a plan to address specific adaptive seating and wheeled mobility device needs that have been identified (Table 19-4). The clinician and patient also set specific goals for use of the equipment within various environments. The actual intervention process in seating and wheeled mobility is often called the equipment recommendation or equipment prescription. During this process a specific mobility base is selected and adaptive seating equipment is specified.

Other major components of adaptive seating and mobility intervention involve coordination, communication, and documentation. The physical or occupational therapist typically has the primary responsibility of coordinating the seating team and assuring that all team members are working together to assist in the attainment of the patient's goals. Communication with all team members is essential during this process. All team members must be made aware of the results of the examination and the ultimate goals involved. Each team member may have some responsibilities in this process; the rehabilitation technology supplier, for example, has a primary responsibility to provide specific manufacturer's specifications for the equipment needed. These specifications will then be used to prepare the letter of medical justification.

In addition to all the typical documentation of the history and physical assessment, the therapist also has a primary responsibility, in the case of adaptive seating intervention, to prepare the letter of medical justification. The letter is critical because it is the primary means of communication with all funding sources involved to obtain necessary funding for the seating and wheeled mobility system.

Documentation: The Letter of Medical Justification

The intention of the letter of medical justification is to provide the funding source with a clear picture of the patient with a disability and the equipment being recommended, with a focus on why the specific equipment being prescribed is required. This letter must contain several elements. The introductory paragraph should describe the person with a disability. This description includes the diagnoses, onset dates, prognosis, and a summary of the history and the systems review.

Next, detailed information is provided about the specific tests and measures used during the examination and outcomes of the evaluation. These include, but are not limited to, the individual's functional status, strength, range of motion, orthopedic deformities, motor coordination, abnormal tone or reflex findings, and the results of the equipment simulation. This information can be organized and reported on a standardized form or in a narrative style.

Specific measurable, functional goals for the adaptive seating and wheeled mobility system should be clearly stated. All the specifications of the selected equipment must be included, and the reason for each item must be effectively justified as to why the person requires this specific piece of equipment (Box 19-1). The funding source sometimes also requires a description of other possible lower cost options and an explanation of why these options are not effective for the patient. Finally, a summary of the patient information and contact information for the primary therapist and the prescribing physician should be provided so that the funding source may contact these individuals if any questions arise during the review process.

Meticulous preparation of the letter of medical justification may mean the difference between efficient funding of the seating and mobility system and a long, drawn-out review process that may delay the delivery of equipment by several months.

When the Seating and Mobility System Is Delivered

After approval by the funding source and after the adaptive seating equipment is ordered and obtained, the rehabilitation technology supplier notifies the therapist that the seating and mobility system is ready for delivery. The patient then returns to the seating clinic and the adaptive seating and

Table 19-4
Components Included in Final Recommendations

Category	*Details*
Wheelchair propulsion ability	Distance Speed Safety In recommended wheelchair In less expensive options

Final equipment selection	Mobility base
	  Access method
	  Postural support components

Goals of the seating system	Based on consumer's stated goals
	  Objective
	  Measurable
	  Related to recommended equipment

Wheelchair and seating fitting and delivery needs	Is preliminary fitting required? How many visits will be necessary? Estimated time to delivery

Training and education plans	When will the training begin?
	Who will carry out the training?
	  Referral for additional training?
	Written materials to be provided
	  Product manuals
	  Care and maintenance instructions
	  Safety recommendations and concerns
	  Guidelines for proper and effective use

Plan for follow-up care	When will follow-up occur? Scheduled visits or as needed? Frequency of reevaluation?

mobility device is delivered and adjusted to ensure proper fit and efficient function. Delivery of the wheelchair or seating system is a critical element in the intervention process and directly affects the outcomes related to use of the equipment.

Delivery of equipment typically occurs several months after the examination and prescription process. The therapist is responsible for ensuring that the status and needs of the patient have not changed since the initial seating and mobility assessment. If the needs have changed, then recommended modifications to the equipment must be specified at this time. The equipment must then be verified to ensure it meets all the recommended specifications. Finally, the equipment must be adjusted for proper fit and the patient must be trained in its safe use, adjustment, maintenance, and care.

The patient should have the opportunity to function in and use the equipment during the initial delivery to ensure that the goals set during the examination can be effectively attained. This may require a period of training and further rehabilitation intervention as an outpatient or in the patient's living environment. In addition, the patient and caregivers are instructed in routine maintenance and cleaning of the equipment, by verbal instruction, demonstration, and in written format, such as review of the owner's manuals provided by the equipment manufacturers. The patient and caregivers also need to learn when they should return to the clinic for adjustment or modification of the equipment.

Assessment of Seating and Mobility Outcomes

The final critical component of an adaptive seating evaluation is reexamination, or follow-up and follow-along. Adaptive seating equipment needs are fluid over time. Fixed orthopedic deformities may change or progress, and functional abilities often change. Equipment needs must be reevaluated when the patient's needs are no longer met by the equipment. This may happen as equipment ages and falls into disrepair, or as the patient's functional or physical status changes over time. Most adaptive seating equipment has a usable life span of 3 to 5 years. If a person is particularly active or if the equipment is used in harsh and demanding

Box 19-1 *Examples of Adaptive Seating and Wheeled Mobility Interventions and Goals*

EXAMPLE 1

Reason for referral:	Frequent falls in the home
Evaluation finding:	Only able to ambulate for 20 feet and unsteady; high risk of falling
Goals:	Safe and independent mobility for functional distances, at least 200 feet for indoor environments
Equipment feature:	Manual, power assist, or power wheeled mobility device
Justification:	Patient able to safely and independently propel the selected wheeled mobility device for functional distances in his or her environment

EXAMPLE 2

Reason for referral:	Having problems sitting upright in wheelchair; falls to the left and has difficulty propelling chair
Evaluation findings:	Impaired sitting balance noted during mat evaluation, poor trunk muscle strength resulting in poor trunk control, no ability to react to sitting balance challenges
Goals:	Able to maintain upright sitting posture and perform all functional activities without falling, such as wheelchair propulsion, activities of daily living
Equipment feature:	Solid seat cushion and back support, possible lateral trunk supports, seat tilt posterior or open seat to back angle if simulation shows increased stability in these postures without compromising function
Justification:	Patient able to sit upright with adequate support for pelvis and spine to allow maximal function of upper body for activities of daily living or other functional activities (e.g., access to propulsion)

EXAMPLE 3

Reason for referral:	Impaired endurance; fatigues easily and cannot go into community
Evaluation findings:	Unable to tolerate wheelchair propulsion farther than 100 feet and becomes quite short of breath with indoor manual propulsion, even in lightweight wheelchair
Goals:	Ability to tolerate mobility for functional distances in all desired environments, in home and community
Equipment feature:	Powered wheelchair or powered scooter
Justification:	Patient independent for all mobility with selected device for functional distances for his or her home environment

EXAMPLE 4

Reason for referral:	Pressure ulcer under the left ischial tuberosity
Evaluative findings:	Stage 2 pressure ulcer under left ischial tuberosity observed during mat evaluation skin inspection; pelvic obliquity noted in sitting, disappears in supine (flexible)
Goals:	Improve pressure distribution and correct pelvic obliquity to minimize pressure under left ischial tuberosity; provide equipment and training for active pressure relief while seated in wheelchair
Equipment features:	Skin protection and positioning seat cushion that redistributes pressure, minimizing pressure under the ischial tuberosities, and supports pelvis in a neutral position; may also require increased trunk support, possibly lateral supports for correcting pelvic obliquity posture
Justification:	Equipment will provide safe seating for up to 4-hour intervals without worsening of pressure ulcer and will facilitate healing of current ulcer over time; seating will correct pelvic obliquity and minimize weight bearing under left ischial tuberosity, to be verified with pressure mapping

EXAMPLE 5

Reason for referral:	Right shoulder pain and weakness; difficulty with transfers and manual wheelchair propulsion
Evaluative findings:	Right shoulder rotator cuff tear with resulting pain and muscle weakness
Goals:	Maximize functional abilities while minimizing pain and decreasing stress on right shoulder
Equipment features:	Powered wheelchair with access method that minimizes stress on right shoulder; sliding board and training for transfers that minimize stress on right shoulder
Justification:	Patient will function independently with minimal pain in right upper extremity and will be independent for all mobility and transfer activities

environments, the equipment may have a shorter functional lifespan. Periodic reexamination of equipment and patient needs is essential to maintain optimal function. Although planning reexamination appointments is important, the patient needs to understand when and why contacting the therapist and requesting a reexamination between scheduled visits might be necessary. The patient is the most knowledgeable person regarding the adequacy of the equipment and whether goals are being met.

BIOMECHANICAL PRINCIPLES IN SEATING AND MOBILITY

Adaptive seating for persons who use wheelchairs involves the strategic application of forces to provide postural support and stability for optimal function. All applications of forces in this context are governed by the laws of physics and described in the field of biomechanics, the study of body position and movement.[5] All adaptive seating components exert forces or torques on the body that ultimately affect changes in posture and static or dynamic equilibrium. Improperly applied forces or improper fit of components can lead to a variety of seating and mobility problems. The most commonly encountered problems are summarized in Table 19-5.

Propulsion of a wheeled mobility device, particularly manual propulsion, depends on the forces and torques applied by the user. These forces must be understood because of their possible long-term effects on the body; wheelchair users are at risk of repetitive motion and overuse injuries.[13] Understanding basic biomechanical principles and how they affect the design of adaptive seating and wheeled mobility is

Table 19-5
Potential Problems Resulting from Improper Biomechanics in Support or Propulsion

Support or Access Problem	*Possible Resultant Biomechanical Problem*	*Potential Equipment Solutions*
Seat too long	Posterior pelvic tilt Sliding out of wheelchair	Shorten seat or provide additional back support (effectively shortening seat)
Seat too short	Pressure ulcer, lack of support under femurs Sliding out of seat	Increase seat depth of wheelchair or add longer seat cushion with solid support underneath
Seat too wide	Lateral shift of pelvis in chair Pelvic obliquity Trunk scoliosis Feeling of instability	Narrow wheelchair seat or add lateral pelvic supports to properly center pelvis in wheelchair
Seat too narrow	Pressure ulcers over greater trochanters Difficulty transferring in and out of wheelchair	Widen wheelchair seat
Back too wide	Flexible scoliosis Lateral trunk leaning Pelvic obliquity Feeling of instability	Narrower back support Lateral thoracic supports Lateral pelvic supports
Back too narrow	Lack of movement needed for function Skin breakdown on lateral trunk Discomfort caused by inability to move	Widen wheelchair back support
Back too low	Upper trunk instability; limited function Excessive thoracic kyphosis Posterior pelvic tilt	Higher back support Solid back support (if current back is sling)
Back too high	Falling forward in wheelchair Inability to propel wheelchair optimally	Lower back height Narrower upper back support to allow increased scapular excursion
Rear wheels too far back	Shoulder pain; impingement Inability to optimally propel wheelchair	Move rear wheels forward
Rear wheels too far forward	Wheelchair tipping backwards; user unable to control	Move rear wheels back on frame

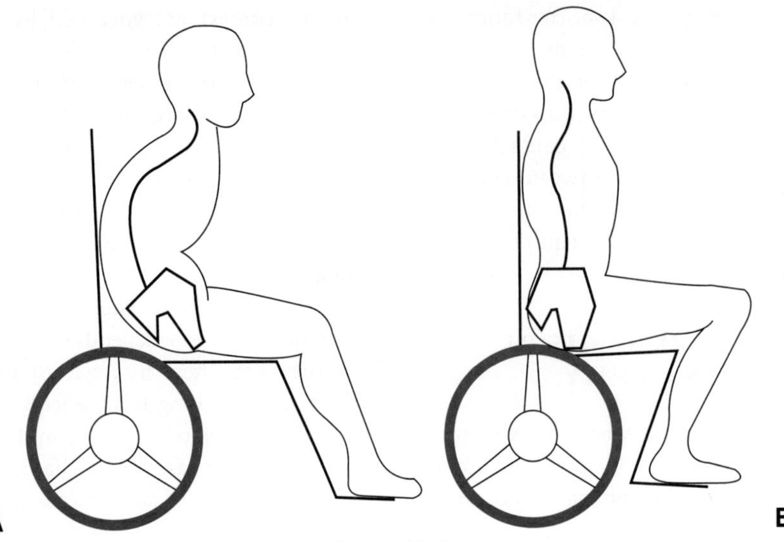

Figure 19-5

***A,** In the presence of hamstring tightness, if knees are relatively extended, the pelvis falls into a position of posterior rotation, with a decrease in lumbar lordosis, an increase in thoracic kyphosis, and cervical lordosis. **B,** One strategy to achieve optimal alignment of pelvis and spine in the presence of hamstring tightness is to reduce seat depth and position slightly under the seat.*

critical to the strategic application of forces to maximize function and minimize risk of injury for the wheeled mobility device user.

No single strategy, or even a small set of strategies, works for every wheelchair user. Each wheelchair user is unique, with a unique set of problems and goals, and each therefore requires an individualized approach to adaptive seating.[14] Many biomechanical and ergonomic principles govern the application of forces in adaptive seating, but all center on basic principles, as outlined by Engstrom.[14] These include the following:

1. Providing a stable base of support for the pelvis
2. Providing adequate pressure distribution
3. Allowing an individual to move into an active position (e.g., to lean forward)
4. Allowing variations in positions
5. Providing support for the back
6. Allowing free movement of the feet and legs if possible
7. Providing the user with a feeling of safety, security, and comfort

Providing adaptive seating that meets all these requirements is often quite challenging.

Stability of the Pelvis

One of the basic challenges inherent in seated posture is achieving pelvic stability. Although the base of support is larger and the body's center of gravity is lower when sitting than standing,[15] the pelvis is actually more unstable when seated. In standing, ligamentous tension and balanced muscle activity contribute to stability of the pelvis. When sitting, many of the ligaments become slack, and the flexed hip position alters the line of pull and efficiency of muscles around the hip. If, in addition, the patient who is sitting demonstrates a lack of flexibility (shortening or tightness) in the hamstring muscles, the pelvis rotates posteriorly and the spine adopts a more flexed posture than in standing (Figure 19-5).[15] This flexed posture has been implicated in muscle fatigue and abnormally high disk pressures, both of which contribute to discomfort and pain in prolonged sitting.

Forces exerted in an adaptive seating system must overcome these natural tendencies as well as any postural asymmetries caused by abnormally high muscle tone or other disability-related impairments. To do this, forces to the body must be applied as strategically as possible by considering both the lever arm and the surface area through which the force will be applied.

When a *torque* is applied to control or influence the position of a body part, the force necessary is inversely related to the lever arm, the distance from the axis of rotation of the body part, and the point of application of the force. As the distance away from the point of rotation increases, the force required to achieved the desired outcome decreases.[5] This principle is very important for adaptive seating, because in dealing with application of forces on the surface of the body, decreasing the force necessary is critical to a person being able to tolerate that force. One way to accomplish this is to apply the force as far from the part to be controlled as reasonably possible.

Pressure is directly related to the force applied but inversely related to the area over which the force is distributed. This means that, if high forces are necessary to achieve the desired outcome, providing a larger area of contact will decrease the pressure exerted on the body.[5] Applying forces over as large an area as possible is critical to avoiding pressure-related skin ulcers as well as increasing comfort and tolerance for the wheelchair user.

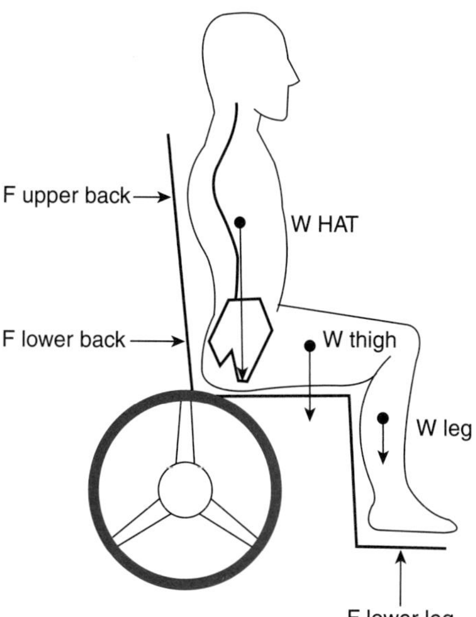

Figure 19-6
Each body segment has its own center of mass (W HAT, W thigh, W leg). *These downward forces must be counterbalanced by opposing forces from support surfaces (seat, upper back, sacral, foot).* W, *weight = gravity acting on center of mass;* F, *opposition forces.*

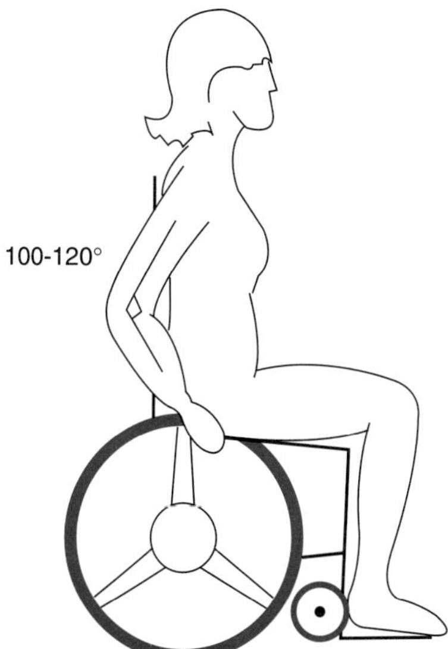

Figure 19-7
For maximum biomechanical efficiency in manual wheelchair propulsion, the elbow should be flexed between 100 and 120 degrees when the hand is resting on top of the push rim.

Understanding and applying these two biomechanical principles assists the clinician in designing adaptive seating systems that accomplish the goals of postural support and positioning for function while being comfortable and well tolerated by the patient.

One of the main forces that adaptive seating systems must balance is the force of *gravity* (Figure 19-6). Gravity is a constant force exerted on the body that must be counteracted for an individual to remain in an upright-seated posture. The adaptive seating components must provide enough external support so that, combined with the internal muscular forces generated by the wheelchair user, an individual can sit in a desired position for long periods of time and perform all desired functional activities. This can be quite challenging, depending on the ability of the wheelchair user to generate muscular forces that work in opposition to the force of gravity. Body positions should allow gravity to facilitate desired postures or functions if an individual has severe weakness or muscle fatigue. This is often a main reason for using tilt or recline seating systems. These systems allow the person's body to be reoriented in space, allowing the force of gravity to facilitate desired postures or functions rather than requiring the user to generate muscular forces to counteract the force of gravity at all times.

Propulsion

Biomechanical principles are also extremely important in the propulsion of manual wheelchairs.[13] Manual wheelchair users have many problems associated with shoulder and wrist pain and injuries.[16] Understanding wheelchair propulsion biomechanics and the importance of wheelchair configuration and wheelchair propulsion training is critical to minimizing or preventing these overuse injuries. The weight of the wheelchair user should be distributed rearward (with the seat moved back in relation to the rear wheels) to decrease rolling resistance and make the wheelchair easier to propel.[17] This will also make the wheelchair easier to tip backward, so the skill of the user in controlling this tipping must be carefully considered.

The seat surface should be low enough to allow a 100- to 120-degree bend in the elbow when the user's hand is placed at the top of the wheel rim (Figure 19-7). This position tends to minimize impact on the shoulders and maximize efficiency in propulsion.[17,18]

Individuals who self-propel manual wheelchairs must master and consistently use proper propulsion techniques.[19] Long, smooth strokes limit excessive forces on upper extremity joints and soft tissue and decrease the rate of loading on the push rims. In contrast, short, choppy pushes are associated with higher energy expenditure and the development of repetitive use syndromes. Allowing the hands to drop below the rims during the "recovery," or nonpropulsion part of the stroke, aids in smooth motion and protects the shoulders from injury.[17]

SEATING CLASSIFICATION AND MATERIALS

Many new wheeled mobility and adaptive seating technologies have been developed over the last 20 years.[7] Technological development has helped meet the challenges involved in two major wheelchair seating objectives: postural support and pressure management. Individuals with neuromuscular impairments leading to wheelchair use for significant portions of their day require critical support for maintaining optimal postures that maximize function and minimize fatigue and discomfort while still attending to pressure build-up issues that might cause local tissue damage.

Seating support surfaces, often referred to as "wheelchair cushions," are actually far more complex. Seating components can be classified in many different ways, such as by their shape and contour or their component materials. Garber[20] divides wheelchair seating into two basic categories based on purpose: seating for positioning and seating for pressure management. Many patients require seating that optimizes both positioning and pressure management. Although this classification helps us understand the basic functional division in seating products, it is too simplistic for most seating devices. Many seating support surfaces are designed to address both positioning and pressure management needs, especially for individuals with neuromuscular impairments (Figure 19-8). Those who use a wheelchair on a part-time basis generally do not rely on external support for positioning and may sit on a "general use" foam cushion to enhance comfort. The advantages and disadvantages of wheelchair cushions, are summarized on the basis of purpose in Table 19-6.

Passive and Active Seating Systems

Seating surfaces can also be described or classified as active or passive devices.[21] Most support surfaces discuss in this chapter are passive in nature; they react to pressure exerted by the body but do not actively exert or change any forces. Recently, however, active cushion technologies have led to the development of various pressure management devices. These cushions have an active (mechanical) mechanism, such as a battery-powered pump system, that actually causes the cushion to change in some way to systematically alter pressure distribution. Although active cushions may be highly effective at pressure management for certain individuals, they are quite expensive and rely on a pumping system and a battery pack that make them heavier than typical seat cushions. They also are subject to malfunction and require more maintenance to be effective.

Table 19-6
Wheelchair Seat Cushions: Advantages and Disadvantages

Primary Purpose of Seat Cushion	*Features of Seat Cushions*	*Typical Client Problems Addressed*
General use (comfort)	Composed of foam, flexible material, air, fluid, gel, or a combination of materials	General wheelchair use: fewer than 4 hours per day May be for temporary or intermittent use Individual has protective sensation Individual has good posture and sitting balance
Pressure management (skin protection)	Composed of two or more materials that may include foam, flexible material, air, fluid, gel	Wheelchair use greater than 4 hours per day Individual with limited sensation
	Deeper contour when loaded than general use cushion	Individual with limited ability to shift or reposition his or her body
	Design must enhance pressure redistribution	Individual at high risk for skin breakdown
Postural support and positioning	Composed of same materials as skin protection; includes additional postural supports that may include preischial bar (antithrust seat), lateral pelvic support, medial thigh support, lateral thigh supports	Wheelchair use greater than 4 hours per day User with abnormal muscle tone User with flexible postural asymmetries User with poor sitting balance or pelvic/lower extremity control in sitting
Pressure management, postural support, and positioning	Combination of properties found in both skin protection and postural support cushion above	User who sits more than 4 hours per day User has impaired sensation or high risk for skin breakdown User has postural support needs as listed above

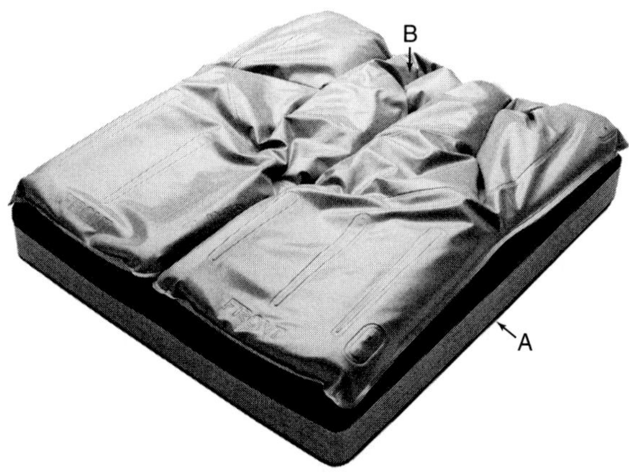

Figure 19-8
The J2 cushion is an example of a passive seat cushion with two objectives. Its firm contoured foam base provides postural support (A), and its fluid-filled bladder provides increased contact area so that weight-bearing pressures are reduced (B). (Courtesy Sunrise Medical, Longmont, Colo.)

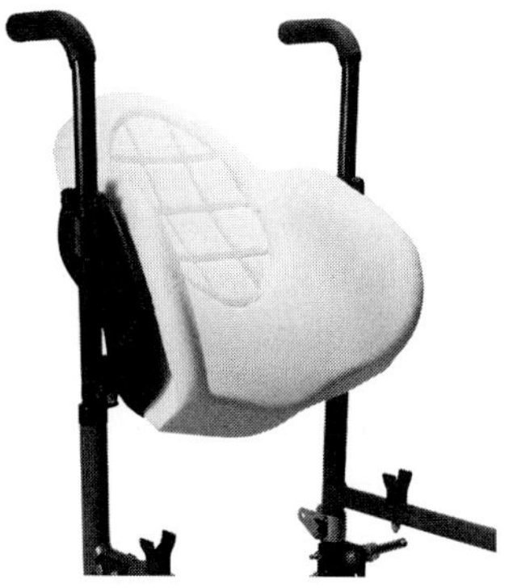

Figure 19-9
The Jay Care Back is an example of a precontoured back support. The back can be tilted as necessary, and the crosshatched foam distributes pressures away from spinous processes for patients with pronounced thoracic kyphosis. (Courtesy Sunrise Medical, Longmont, Colo.)

Noncontoured and Contoured Seating Systems

Regardless of the specific purpose of the cushion, seating surfaces can be classified according to their shape or amount of contour.[22] The most basic surfaces are planar or noncontoured. These surfaces are most easily manufactured. They are also most readily modified to allow for growth or other changes in the patient's needs. The drawback for noncontoured seating surfaces is their inability to accommodate the many body surfaces that are not flat in nature; the result is a less than optimal surface area for contact with the body, creating areas of relatively high pressure under bony prominences and soft tissues that contact the seating surface. To increase the amount of contact area and better distribute pressures, increasing the surface's contour is typically necessary to match the shape of the body more closely.[22]

Two levels of contoured surfaces exist: precontoured (generically contoured) seating surfaces and custom-contoured seating surfaces. Precontoured seating surfaces are designed around generic molds intended to match the body's shapes more precisely than planar components. Many are available in a number of sizes. Precontoured surfaces are available as seat components designed to match the shape of the pelvis better and as trunk support components to match alignment of the spinal column better (Figure 19-9). The effectiveness of these surfaces for either postural support or pressure management depends on the precision of fit. The clinician determines precision of fit at the time of the initial assessment and prescription.

Custom-contoured surfaces are constructed directly from the shape of the patient. Many technologies are available to assist measurement for custom seating surfaces, including hand-shaping foam, computer-assisted design/computer-assisted manufacturing systems, and "foam in place" technologies, among others.[23] All these systems have the same general purpose: to record the shape of a person's body as precisely as possible to manufacture a support surface that precisely matches the contours of the person.

Material

Another method of classifying seat cushions or other postural supports is according to the component materials included in the support device. A variety of materials are being used to create postural support devices. The most commonly used materials include various foams, air, gel materials, water-based materials, or a combination of these. The properties and characteristics (including advantages and disadvantages) of the each material must be carefully considered to select the seating system that will best meet a patient's seating needs and minimize the major risk factors for the development of pressure ulcers, such as pressure over bony prominences, shear and friction forces, temperature, and moisture.[24]

Foams are the most common component material used in making support surfaces. Two major categories of foam are available: *elastic* (available as either a closed-cell or open-cell material) and *viscoelastic*. Both types have advantages that make them well suited for use in postural supports as well as disadvantages that must be considered. Elastic foams deform in proportion to the applied load, which helps them reduce peak pressure over bony prominences.[24] They do not, however, provide good envelopment characteristics and they tend to insulate heat and keep it near the body. *Viscoelastic foams* are temperature sensitive, meaning they become softer and more compliant at higher temperatures.[24] This characteristic helps them provide even better pressure distribution than elastic foams, but it depends on the heating effect of being positioned near the body.

Fluid-filled cushions are often composed of materials such as air, water, or viscous fluids contained in one or more containers, either large or small.[24] Most of these products provide greater immersion into the cushion, thus distributing pressure over larger areas of the body and reducing pressures at bony prominences (see Figure 19-8). The type of material used in the cushion influences both skin temperature and the moisture build-up where the body makes contact with the support surface.[25] Understanding the different kinds of material helps the clinician select an appropriate seat cushion for pressure management and support or positioning in wheelchair seating.

Covering material is important to the function of postural support devices, especially seat cushions and back cushions. Regardless of the materials comprising the support itself, the covering material alters the performance characteristics of the support.[25] For example, an inflexible covering material prevents a cushion from providing optimal envelopment for the user. Also, if a covering material with a high coefficient of friction encloses a material selected for its low coefficient of friction, the advantage of the selected cushion material is lost. Covering material also needs to be resilient, easy to clean, in some cases moisture repellent, and aesthetically pleasing to the user.

CASE EXAMPLE 1

Patient with a C5/C6 Complete Spinal Cord Injury

J. J. is a 24-year-old man who sustained an injury to his spine at the C5 vertebral level in a motor vehicle accident 8 weeks ago. He has total loss of motor function on his right side below the level of the C5 nerve root and on his left side below the C6 nerve root level. He was referred to the clinic for an evaluation for his first wheelchair after his in-patient rehabilitation.

J. J.'s sensation is severely impaired below the level of his shoulders, although he has some ability to feel in localized areas of his body. At the time of his visit to the seating clinic, he was using a cervical orthosis for stabilization of his surgically repaired cervical spinal column. He has undergone surgery consisting of a spinal fusion from C4 through T1 vertebrae. J. J. will be returning home to live with his wife and 2-year-old child. He is an architect and works in an office approximately 20 miles from his home. His job responsibilities include visiting construction sites involved in his design projects.

During his rehabilitation, J. J. has been propelling a fully adjustable manual wheelchair with specialty wheelchair propulsion gloves and plastic-coated wheel rims. He is able to propel his wheelchair on indoor surfaces for 300 feet at a time but still has problems with fatigue and neck pain. He requires assistance for outdoor surfaces and for propelling up or down ramps. J. J. lives in a home with 3 steps to enter, but his neighbors are building him a ramp that will be ready by the time he returns home. He has wall-to-wall carpeting throughout his home with the exception of the kitchen and bathroom floors.

J. J.'s stated goals include the following:

- Being as independent as possible in his home and workplace
- Being able to transport his wheelchair in a car
- Returning to work as soon as possible
- Helping care for his 2-year-old-son and his home
- Improving his endurance and reducing his level of neck pain so that he can sit up and function for a full day

Questions to Consider

- Given his history and stated goals, what should the systems review include?
- What specific tests and measures will likely be used in the examination?
- How might his current functional status and his prognosis for recovery or accommodation of impairments and associated functional limitations influence the assessment of his needs?

Evaluation and Prognosis

J. J. has no active movement in his legs or trunk. He has good strength in elbow flexion on the left side, fair strength in elbow flexion on the right side, good strength in both of his shoulders, but no evidence of triceps activity on either side. His range of motion is normal with the exception of his neck range, which cannot be tested because of the cervical orthosis. His conscious sensation is spotty, and he has no sensation in his buttock region. He requires assistance for all transfers and other mobility and for activities of daily living, such as bathing and dressing. J. J. has a healed pressure sore in the region of his coccyx; it developed during his acute hospitalization but is now healed, and he is able to sit for 6 to 8 hours per day. He has been using an ultra-lightweight, folding-frame, manual wheelchair and a foam and gel seat cushion.

Questions to Consider

- What will the team's priorities be for J. J.'s seating and mobility system? How are these priorities similar or different from J. J.'s priorities? What compromises might be necessary?
- What options might be considered for J. J. in terms of seating system (noncontoured, contoured, or custom)? Support frame (lightweight, heavy duty)? Mobility component (manual or powered chair)?
- What recommendations should be made for managing pressure in J. J.'s seating system (active, rotational, reclined, or passive)? Why?

Recommendations

General recommendations for J. J. include a manual wheelchair with a power assist add-on component to allow him more independent mobility and access to all his environments while minimizing stress on his shoulders and neck and accomplishing his goal of transportability by car. Seating will consist of a gel and foam seat cushion contoured to match the shape of his buttocks and manage pressure distribution as evenly as possible. J. J. requires a solid back support with generic contour and angle adjustability to allow appropriate upright posture to maximize his function and balance and minimize future development of spinal deformities. Plastic-coated wheel rims and specialty gloves will maximize his wheel/rim interface, allowing him optimal propulsion as well.

ACCESSING THE MOBILITY UNIT

For wheelchair users to be independent in mobility in their environment, they must be able to perform some movement that can be translated into wheel movement of the mobility base. This movement is called the *access method* for wheeled mobility.[5] Access method can be entirely manual, entirely powered, or manual with power assistance. Access method for a manually propelled chair is different from that needed for an electrically powered chair. Advantages, disadvantages, and indicators for the various wheeled technologies are summarized in Table 19-7. The best access method and frame characteristics are those that allow wheelchair users to obtain the most efficient mobility from their access method (Figure 19-10).

Whether ordering a manual or powered wheelchair, the team must also carefully consider the need for back support, support of extremities, and type of locking mechanism that will be most appropriate for each patient's needs. An overview of the advantages and disadvantages of various limb support and locking mechanisms is found in Table 19-8.

MANUAL WHEELCHAIRS

Manual wheelchairs typically have one large pair of wheels, most often at the rear, that cause the wheelchair to move when pushed. These are sometimes called the drive wheels. The diameter of these wheels is typically between 20 and 26 inches. The wheels are most often equipped with *push rims* that are slightly smaller in diameter, attached to the outside of the wheel itself. The push rims, rather than the wheel, are the access point for most manual wheelchair users. By pushing the wheel rims, the user has control over both the speed and direction of the wheelchair depending on how he or she pushes each of the wheels.

The axle position of these drive wheels is critical for optimal wheel rim access for the user as well as for maximal efficiency in manual propulsion. Standard wheelchairs do not have adjustable axle attachment points and are therefore quite difficult to optimize for efficient mobility. Many ultralightweight and maximally adjustable wheelchairs do have adjustability of this axle location, allowing for adjustment of the wheelchair to the user's needs (Figure 19-11).

Although the majority (90%) of manual wheelchair users propel in a traditional push rim propulsion method with both upper extremities,[26] this is not the only method for wheelchair propulsion and may not be the best in light of problems such as repetitive strain injuries. Some wheelchair

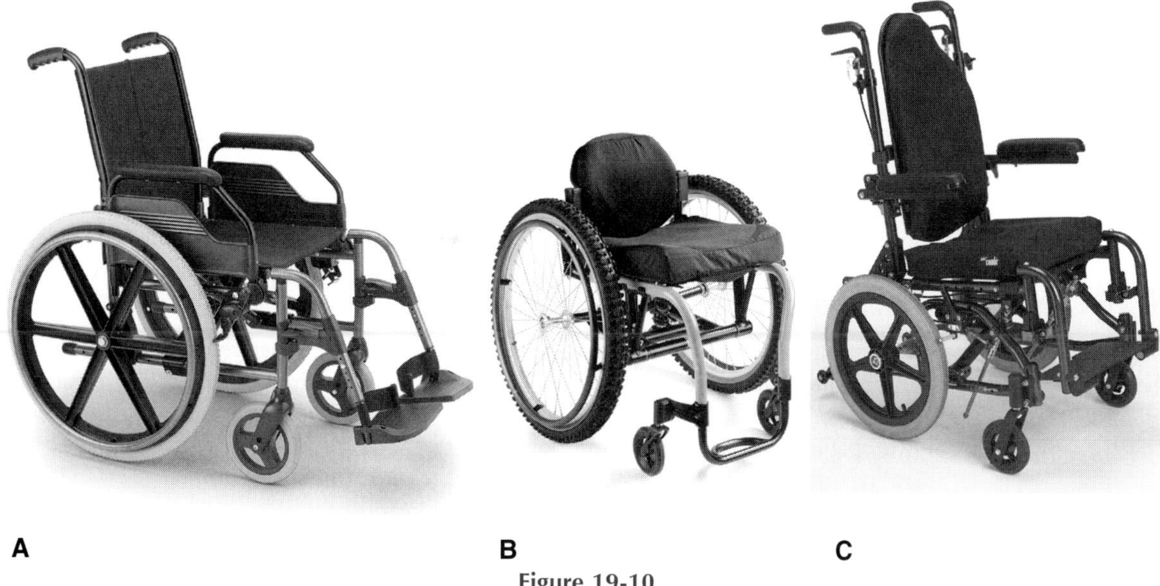

Figure 19-10

Examples of wheelchair support structure and mobility base options. ***A,*** *A standard lightweight, semiadjustable wheelchair with arm support and swing-away leg rests.* ***B,*** *An ultra-lightweight wheelchair with rigid frame, precontoured seat and back support, and shock-absorbing mechanism.* ***C,*** *A pediatric wheelchair with reclining back and precontoured seating system. (Courtesy Sunrise Medical, Longmont, Colo.)*

Table 19-7
Advantages, Disadvantages and Possible Applications of Various Wheeled Mobility Technologies

Wheeled Mobility Device	*Advantages*	*Disadvantages*	*Possible Application*
Semiadjustable manual wheelchair (lightweight)	Simple to use Folds for transportation Lighter weight than standard wheelchair Partial adjustability Easier to propel Durable Will accommodate custom seating	Not custom fit Lack of axle adjustability may limit manual propulsion by user Still may be too heavy for many users	Intermittent or temporary use Possible use for in-home applications if environment tolerates
Fully adjustable manual wheelchair with a folding frame (ultra-lightweight)	Very light frame Maximal adjustability, especially of rear axle position Custom fit to user Accommodates custom seating Accommodates to uneven ground by flexing Folds side to side for easy transportation	Many adjustable or removable parts More complex design, requires more maintenance Some propulsion energy lost in flex of frame	Full-time wheelchair user with permanent disability User wants to transport in trunk of vehicle Environment includes travel over uneven surfaces
Fully adjustable manual wheelchair with a rigid frame (ultra-lightweight)	Very light frame Maximal adjustability, especially of rear axle position Custom fit to user Fewer removable or adjustable parts than folding frame Accommodates custom seating	Does not accommodate to uneven terrain as easily as folding frame May be more difficult to transport in trunk of car (less compact when folded)	Full-time wheelchair user with permanent disability User wants most efficient system for propulsion Used mainly indoors or on even terrains
Power assist manual wheelchair	Light frame Maneuvers like manual wheelchair Minimizes stress on shoulders	Heavier than non-power assist More difficult to disassemble for transport	Lightweight manual wheelchair user with limited endurance or shoulder limitations Manual wheelchair user with long-distance ambulation needs or difficulty managing outdoor terrain independently
Tilt-in-space frame wheelchair	Allows rotation in space for pressure management or other benefits Available for both manual and powered wheelchairs	Frame often heavier and bulkier Usually does not fold for transportation If on manual wheelchair, typically has small rear wheels, requiring an attendant to propel	Wheelchair user requires rotation in space for pressure management or other medical reason, such as respiratory disease

Continued

Table 19-7
Advantages, Disadvantages and Possible Applications of Various Wheeled Mobility Technologies—cont'd

Wheeled Mobility Device	*Advantages*	*Disadvantages*	*Possible Application*
Reclining frame wheelchair	Allows for change in seat-to-back angle, often to full supine position Available for both manual and powered wheelchairs	Frame often heavier and bulkier Rear wheels set further back to provide larger base of support when in recline position Difficult to propel if used with manual wheelchair	Used when a need for change in seat to back angle is required Used for pressure management May be used for self-care in wheelchair May be used when supine bed transfers are required Often used when building sitting tolerance during initial rehabilitation
Powered scooter	Allows simple to learn powered mobility Good outdoor access Swivel seat for ease of transfers Baskets and other accessories for function, such as shopping	Only one access method Large turning radius; difficult to use in many homes Does not accommodate custom seating; few seating support options	Used with individuals who have limited endurance Often used for primarily outdoor mobility purposes
Powered wheelchair	Full access to powered mobility for both indoor and outdoor use Multiple access methods possible Accommodates custom seating supports Accommodates power seating options, such as tilt or recline	Heavy Requires van for transportation Less maneuverable than manual wheelchair Requires more initial training for optimal safety and function	Individuals who cannot propel manual wheelchair effectively Used for indoor and outdoor mobility for long distances May be used in work or school applications for part-time manual wheelchair users

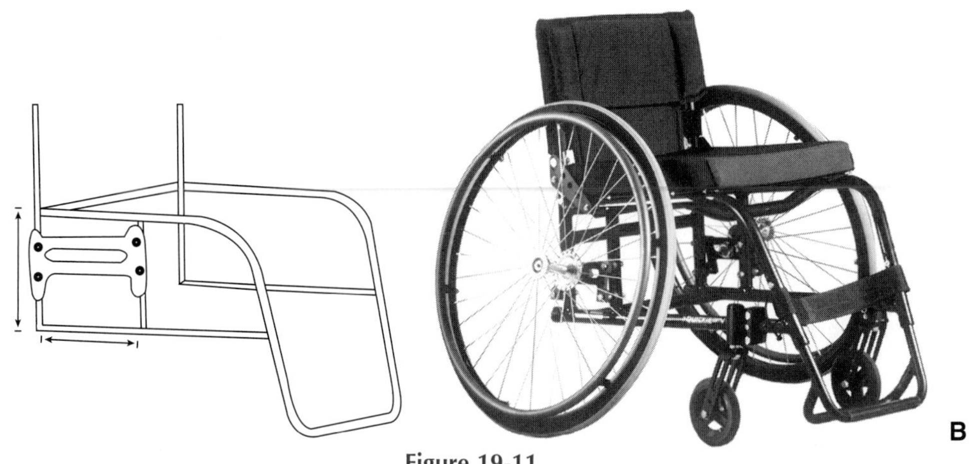

Figure 19-11
In maximally adjustable wheelchair frames, wheel position can be tailored to meet the user's specific needs by adjusting the location of the wheel axis in an anteroposterior slide and vertical position on the frame. ***A,*** *A rigid frame in which the wheel bracket can be positioned as needed on the frame.* ***B,*** *An actual chair. (Courtesy Sunrise Medical, Longmont, Colo.)*

Table 19-8
Advantages and Disadvantages of Various Wheelchair Components

Wheelchair Component	*Options*	*Advantages*	*Disadvantages*
Leg and foot supports	Swing-away foot rests	Lightweight Support for lower extremities Removable for transfers	Add to weight of wheelchair (vs. platform) Require maintenance Require management by wheelchair user
	Flip-up foot platform	Lightweight Few moving parts Very stable Often allows increased knee flexion angle; more comfortable and compact for user	Very little adjustability Both lower extremities supported at same angle Unable to accommodate moderate or severe ankle contractures Not removable; may interfere with transfers for some users
	Manual elevating leg rests	Allows multiple leg positions May prevent some dependent edema (true edema management also requires recline or tilt to elevate the legs above heart level) May increase lower extremity comfort	Heavier than standard leg supports Many moving and adjustable parts; higher maintenance needs More strength and dexterity needed to manage
Arm supports	Flip-back arm rests	Stable arm support Typically lightweight Easy to manage	Multiple moving parts Require maintenance to work properly May not be adjustable enough for all individuals
	Tubular swing-away arm rest	Extremely lightweight Easy for wheelchair user to manage Requires very little hand dexterity and strength	May not feel stable to user May not tolerate extreme or repeated stresses Attachment hardware requires maintenance
	Detachable, adjustable-height arm rest	Support upper extremities in multiple positions Removable for transfers	Heavier More moving parts; higher maintenance requirement May be difficult for users to manage; especially to replace on the wheelchair
	Desk-length arm rest	Allow wheelchair user to approach tables, sinks, desks for improved function Lighter in weight than full-length arm supports	May not provide adequate support during transfers Do not provide full arm support
	Full-length arm rest	Provide full arm support Provide improved support during transfers	Heavier than desk-length arm Do not allow close approach to tables, sinks, or desks
Wheel locks	Pull-to lock	Allow closer access for transfers to surfaces Move away from wheels so hands do not hit with propulsion	May be more difficult to lock
	Push-to lock	Lock easily and securely	May interfere with propulsion May interfere with transfers
	Under-seat or scissor locks	Complete clearance for hands during propulsion No interference in transfers	Significantly better balance and coordination required for locking and unlocking More difficult to adjust

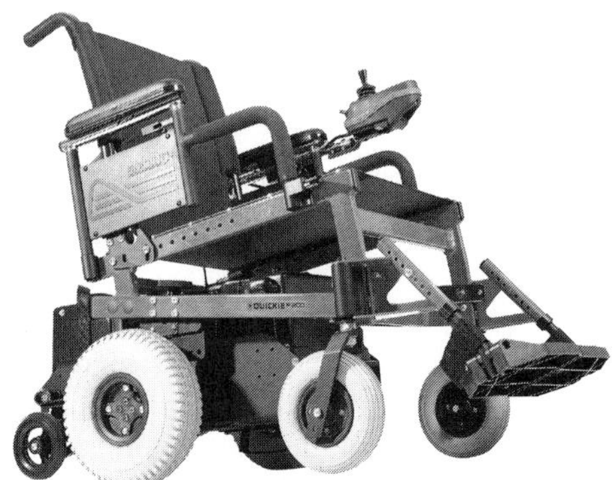

Figure 19-12

In this powered wheelchair, the mobility component includes the wheel base as well as the joystick (or alternative access method) used to control the movement of the chair. Note that anterior-posterior wheel base dimension is longer to accommodate the weight of the batteries and motors of the chair. (Courtesy Sunrise Medical, Longmont, Colo.)

and head-controlled devices, among others. These options make it more likely that an effective control system can be designed for powered wheelchair users with various and significant impairments and functional limitations. The decision making process, however, is more complex for clinicians who must evaluate and assist in the selection of an access method.

The best method of powered wheelchair access allows the wheelchair user optimal control and function in the environment over the long term. Sometimes the simplest method to learn may not ultimately be the best for the user over the long term. Some input methods, such as head control systems, require a longer training period, but the ultimate function of the user may be superior to a simpler joystick system. A thorough evaluation with multiple episodes of training may be required before an ultimate access method is selected. To select appropriate power access options and effectively train a wheelchair user in the proper use of these devices, clinicians must be aware of the different types of equipment and how each works to stop and start, turn or change direction, lock and unlock, and alter velocity of movement. Ideally, clinicians also must know how to adjust the control mechanism to allow the user to be most energy efficient and effective. These skills may take many years of training to develop, most often when the clinician functions as a specialist who works with individuals with highly complex access needs on a regular basis.

TRAINING STRATEGIES

Regardless of the type of wheelchair selected or the access method chosen, intensive training of the person using the wheelchair is necessary. Training takes place across settings and over time. Wheelchair skills are typically introduced during inpatient rehabilitation but training usually continues either in home care or outpatient settings until the new user gains independence with advanced skills. Initial training may actually be accomplished with loaner or temporary equipment used to assess options and designs that will allow optimal mobility before a wheelchair prescription is finalized. Additional training is typically necessary once the permanent wheelchair and associated equipment have been delivered.

Functional manual wheelchair users are well trained in the safe use of equipment, are able to effectively manage obstacles in the home environment and community (work and leisure settings), are able to perform or direct basic maintenance of the equipment (including cleaning procedures and maintaining moving parts), and know when and whom to contact if something out of the ordinary occurs with the wheelchair.

Wheelchair users often require more extensive periods of training than manual chair users to achieve optimal mobility and function. This training must include management of indoor terrain and obstacles such as turning in tight spaces, managing door frames and transitions between flooring surfaces, and negotiating other indoor obstacles such as elevators. Training should also include outdoor terrain and obstacles, such as ramps, curbs, side slopes, grassy surf[illegible] gravel surfaces, and safe operation on crowded sidewa[illegible] when crossing streets. If a powered seating system is [illegible]scribed, the user must be educated regarding the proper a[illegible] safe use of this powered seating system, including how ofte[illegible] to use it, under what conditions it should (and should not) be used, and whom to contact if the powered seating system is not functioning properly.

Although the assessment and prescription for a wheelchair usually takes place in a specialty clinic, functional training after delivery of the equipment is typically provided by outpatient or home care therapy services. A therapist who has questions about a particular piece of equipment that a patient is learning to use should contact the seating clinician and work on a training protocol that will be most effective.

CASE EXAMPLE 2

Patient with Cerebral Palsy

S. W. is a 35-year-old woman with spastic tetraplegia attributable to cerebral palsy. She has been using a fully adjustable manual wheelchair for most of her life with good success. Her current wheelchair is 10 years old and she reports that it is falling apart (her rehabilitation technology supplier confirms the extensive repair history of this wheelchair). She came to the seating clinic for an assessment for a replacement wheelchair and seating system.

S. W. has no functional movement in her lower extremities and has severe extensor tone in both legs. She has impaired motor control in her arms but is able to users have only one functional upper extremity or one upper extremity and one lower extremity, often on the same side of the body (such as individuals with hemiplegia). Still others have severely weakened upper extremities but somewhat stronger lower extremities. For individuals with these different skills, alternative access for manual wheelchairs exists.[26]

Wheelchair users with only one strong upper extremity may use a one arm drive or lever drive system on their wheelchairs. These systems connect the axles of both drive wheels (either with a dual push rim or a lever system) so that the user can control both wheels and have effective directional control from one side of the chair. Wheelchair users with one functional arm and leg often propel their wheelchairs by pushing on one wheel rim and using their functional lower extremity on the ground to assist in directional control and to increase their speed or power of propulsion. Likewise, wheelchair users with stronger lower extremities and weaker upper extremities often "foot propel" their wheelchairs by using both lower extremities on the ground, bypassing the typical wheel rim input and controlling the movement of the chair by interfacing with the ground and indirectly causing the wheels of the chair to react to these forces.

Regardless of the method used for manual wheelchair propulsion, maximal efficiency is critical to functional mobility.[13] Upper extremity musculature is poorly suited to providing the body with ambulation, and without efficiency obtained through the technology, manual propulsion may be highly stressful and fatiguing for the wheelchair user. The environments in which most wheelchair users must function are much better suited to bipedal mobility, making it even more difficult for wheeled mobility to be an adequate substitute when an individual loses the ability to walk.

Many risks are associated with the use of a manual wheelchair. Some of these risks are manageable through other therapeutic interventions (e.g., training) or technological modifications. Others are more serious and must be carefully considered when a manual mobility system is prescribed for a user. Short-term risks include the potential for injury for a new user who is not fully able to control the balance of a wheelchair. This may lead to tipping a wheelchair over (most often falling backwards) when maneuvering up or down ramps or curbs. Other common injuries include trauma involving fingers and hands inadvertently caught in the wheel spokes or wheel lock mechanisms, injuries to lower extremities that are not properly supported, and injuries to limbs that fall off their supports during propulsion. Most of these risks can be minimized by adequate training and safety mechanisms added to a wheelchair during the initial training period. The most common of these strategies is the use of rear anti-tip tubes until a new wheelchair user gains enough strength and postural control to master the "wheelie" maneuver and managing steep inclines or steps.

Other risks associated with manual wheelchair propulsion are less well understood and are the focus of much current research. These risks include long-term risks of manual wheelchair user for repetitive use strain injuries, leading to impairment in function or pain in the shoulders and upper extremities.[16] The two main areas of focus are the shoulders (e.g., rotator cuff tears) and wrists (e.g., carpal tunnel syndrome).[27] These risks may be much larger than previously thought, particularly for individuals who have depended on wheeled mobility use over long periods. Because of the increased longevity of persons with different types of disabilities who have relied on manual wheeled mobility for 20 years or more, these injuries are becoming much more prevalent and may be extremely detrimental to continued independent function.

WHEN IS A POWERED CHAIR APPROPRIATE?

The choice of manual or powered mobility is straightforward for many wheelchair users. For example, an individual with tetraplegia who has little movement in the upper extremities benefits most from powered mobility. Likewise, persons with minimal trunk and upper body impairment are obvious manual wheelchair candidates. The problem arises when individuals have skills and abilities that are not so clearly indicative of a particular variety of mobility, or when the environmental demands placed on the individual really require use of powered mobility in spite of the individual's basic ability to propel a manual mobility device.

One of the most important decisions for any wheelchair user is that of manual versus powered mobility. Both types of mobility have advantages and disadvantages, and overall function is greatly affected by this basic selection. Conditions and impairments that often indicate need for powered mobility include the following:

1. Severe upper extremity or upper trunk weakness leading to an inability to propel any type of manual wheelchair
2. Ataxic or uncoordinated movement of the upper extremities
3. Endurance limitations, whether from muscular or cardiopulmonary impairment
4. Progressive conditions that will likely lead to loss of upper extremity strength or poor endurance (particularly a rapidly progressing condition)
5. Orthopedic problems in the upper extremity joints (e.g., arthritis or preexisting rotator cuff or carpal tunnel impairments)
6. Environments that require long-distance travel on a regular basis or travel over rough terrain

Once a determination has been made that powered mobility is necessary, one of the next decisions is the access method for control of the device. If the powered mobility device is a powered scooter, this decision is uncomplicated; a tiller mechanism is the most efficient and effective choice. If, however, the device under consideration is a powered wheelchair (Figure 19-12), the access methods available are far more complex. Powered wheelchair access methods include standard joysticks, switch arrays, sip and puff input devices, propel her manual wheelchair with some difficulty. She transports her wheelchair in her car with some assistance from others for disassembling the seating and folding the wheelchair for stowing. The muscle tone in her trunk and arms fluctuates, but she has significant intermittent extensor tone.

S. W. works independently in an office as an administrative assistant. Her home is wheelchair accessible and her office setting does not require long-distance propulsion. When she shops or goes to the mall, her friends assist her with her mobility or she borrows a powered scooter from the grocery store.

Susan's goals include the following:

- Maintaining or improving her current level of mobility
- Improving her perception of postural stability in her wheelchair
- Being able to transport her wheelchair in her car with no more difficulty than she currently has
- Having a wheelchair that is easy to manage and maintain (fewer moving parts to break)

Questions to Consider

- Given her history and her stated goals, what should the systems review include?
- What specific tests and measures would likely be used in the examination?
- How might her current functional status and the chronic nature of her neuromuscular condition (coupled with the aging process), with its associated impairments and functional limitations, influence the assessment of her needs?

Evaluation and Prognosis

S. W. has severely impaired strength in her legs and trunk, poor unsupported sitting balance, severe extensor spasticity in both legs, hip flexion limited to a 100-degree pelvis-to-thigh angle, moderate weakness in her arms with poor motor control, and fluctuating muscle tone. S. W. also has a severe scoliosis and a pelvic rotation and pelvic obliquity. With moderate trunk support she is able to use her arms functionally and feels secure.

Questions to Consider

- What will the team's priorities be for S. W.'s seating and mobility system? How are the team's priorities similar to or different than S. W.'s priorities? What compromises might be necessary?
- What options might be considered for S. W. in terms of seating system (noncontoured, contoured, or custom)? Support frame (lightweight, heavy duty)? Mobility component (manual or powered chair)?
- What recommendations should be made for managing pressure in S. W.'s seating system (active, rotational, or passive)? Why?

Recommendations

General recommendations for S. W. may include a new custom manual wheelchair with a folding titanium frame with a fixed-axle position specified to her particular needs, a custom-contoured seat and back cushion to support and position her, spring-loaded foot rests with elevating leg rests for her lower extremities, a push-button pelvic belt with special loops so that she can fasten and secure it around her hips, and a hook-and-loop material chest belt to stabilize her upper body. The combination of custom-contoured seating and anterior support devices that she can tighten herself will improve her feeling of stability and the overall fit of the wheelchair seating. This wheelchair will be more durable with fewer moving parts and will meet her mobility needs.

SEATING SYSTEMS FOR PRESSURE MANAGEMENT

Selection of the wheeled mobility device itself is only part of the equation when working with individuals who use wheelchairs for much or all of their mobility. The seating system or postural support system is as important as the wheeled mobility base and access method. The seating system is critical to integrating the person and the wheeled mobility system, and several major issues must be considered in its selection.

One of the major issues for many wheelchairs users is pressure management. Any person who sits for more than 4 hours per day is at increased risk for pressure-related damage to the skin.[28] This risk is exacerbated by many factors, including impaired sensation, increased heat or moisture build-up near the skin, inadequate nutrition or hydration status, and atrophy of muscle tissue leading to decreased soft tissue protection for bony prominences.[29]

The major problem associated with pressure sustained over long durations is skin breakdown. This problem has been the focus of a great deal of research for more than 30 years and is better understood than it used to be, but still mysterious. The individual and interactive effects of pressure, friction, and shear are the current focus of research regarding skin breakdown, its causes, and ways to prevent it. Skin breakdown is an extremely costly and debilitating problem for many wheelchair users.[30,31] Treatment for skin breakdown often involves costly surgical interventions and prolonged hospital and rehabilitation stays. Skin breakdown may also be responsible for ultimately reducing the life expectancy for individuals with disabilities who use wheelchairs for mobility.[30]

Active and Passive Strategies

Many technologies have been developed to provide pressure management. Recognizing that low pressure exerted over

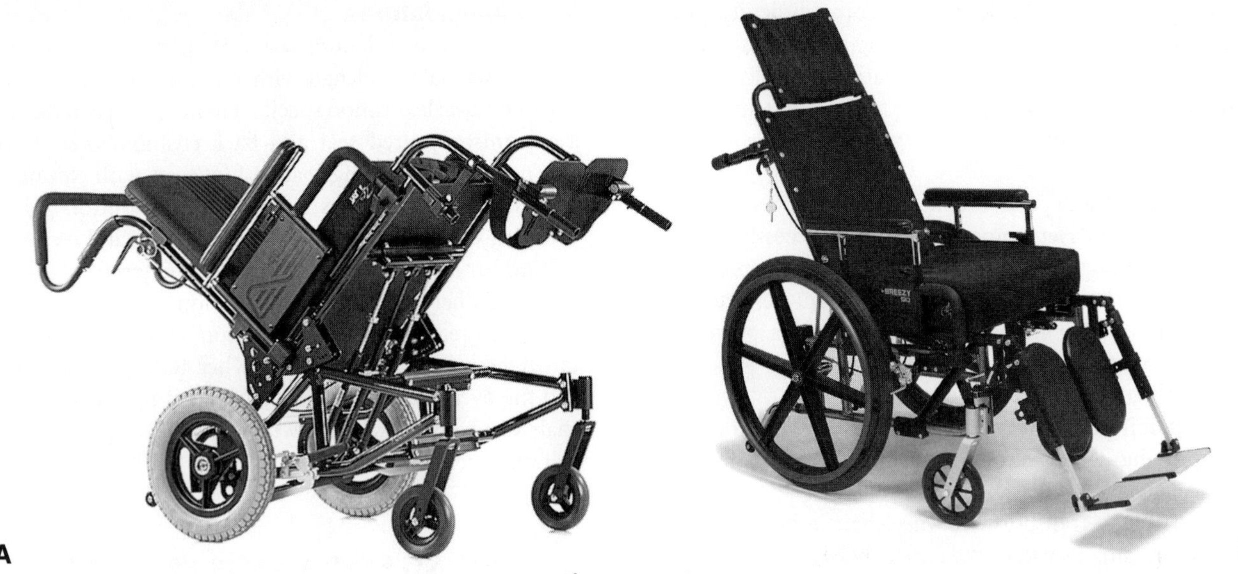

Figure 19-13
*Rotational pressure management strategies include tilt, in which hip angle doesn't change **(A)**, and reclining **(B)**, in which hip angle (extension) is opened (increased). Rotational pressure management systems are available for both manual and powered wheelchairs. (Courtesy Sunrise Medical, Longmont, Colo.)*

long periods can be as dangerous for skin as high pressures exerted over short periods, pressure management technologies provide options either to distribute pressure over as wide a surface area as possible or to change position so that the forces exerted on weight-bearing surfaces vary over time. Most rely on good user training and use of the systems for optimal function and outcome; no pressure management system can entirely prevent skin breakdown if used improperly or inconsistently.

Technologies can be grouped into three general categories on the basis of whether they use an active, rotational, or passive strategy to provide pressure relief. *Active technologies*, such as active or dynamic seat cushions, are designed to relieve areas of high pressure periodically. Dynamic seat cushions are often divided into a series of alternating chambers. A motor pumps air or fluid through chambers to change the configuration of the support surface gently and continuously (much like an alternating-pressure mattress used in hospital beds for patients who are unable to change position). *Rotational seating systems* include those with a powered tilt or recline mechanism, a manual tilt or recline system, or a standing system (Figure 19-13). *Passive technologies* for pressure management focus on increasing seating surface area, usually by increasing envelopment or compliance of the seating surface or by shifting pressure from traditionally high-risk areas, such as ischial tuberosities, to lower risk areas, such as distal femurs. Some passive technologies completely off-load areas such as the ischial tuberosities, and others simply aim to reduce pressure in these areas by using more compliant materials in certain zones of the cushion (see Figure 19-8).

Some supports can cause skin "hammocking," or stretching the skin and soft tissues across bony surfaces such as the coccyx, when unloading other regions such as the ischial tuberosities. This effect can cause skin breakdown even in the absence of direct external tissue loading.

Size and Setup

In addition to the technological development of products for pressure management, clinicians have learned a great deal about seating intervention to manage pressure as effectively as possible. Proper size and setup of wheelchairs is often critical in appropriately managing pressure.[21] The strategic use of contoured surfaces, different types of materials and coverings, and a well-planned mobility system and any active seating choices, such as tilting or reclining seating systems (also known as rotational systems) must be integrated in a holistic approach to protect wheelchair users from skin breakdown.[28]

Training

In addition to choices of technologies, proper training and education of wheelchair users is essential to the effective application of this technology. Most of the technologies developed rely on proper use, either through correct positioning on the wheelchair and proper maintenance and adjustment, or schedules by the user. Sometimes an apparent failure of a particular technology has more to do with how it was used or in what combinations different technologies were used than the actual failure of the technology itself.

Seating for Function and Comfort

Although pressure management in seating often dominates research and technological development, maximal function and optimal comfort are equally important.[7] Wheelchair users who are not able to function optimally or become uncomfortable when seated will probably not reach their full potential. Individuals who have discomfort when seated also have problems with satisfaction with their equipment, which may cause equipment abandonment.[32] To function optimally individuals must be comfortable and secure in their seating systems.

The priorities of a seating system depend on the problems and goals identified during the assessment process. If a patient has a lack of sensation and a history of skin breakdown problems, then seating for pressure management will most likely be the highest priority. However, if the problems identified focus on a lack of optimal function or feelings of discomfort when using the equipment, then goals for enhanced function and comfort may be more critical. For some patients all three issues are priorities, and equipment must be carefully selected that will balance all needs and allow the individual to meet all goals of seating.

The determination of these priorities is often quite challenging. For a health care team, the primary medical concern might be pressure management or improving comfort, but the user may be focused on a particular functional goal that he or she believes is more critical than pressure management. Occasionally, equipment selection will be difficult because some needs may have to be compromised to meet other needs optimally. An air fluid cushion, for example, may provide the maximal pressure management desired by the team but might feel unstable to the wheelchair user, disrupting comfort, function, or both.

When compromises must be made, a conflict can occur between the health care or seating team and the wheelchair user. The best way to resolve conflicts is to find a technology intervention that meets all the stated needs. If this is not possible, then the wheelchair user must be properly educated regarding the risks and benefits of the equipment selected and ultimately make an informed choice. Health professionals should remember that the user is the only one who can decide what will be best for his or her circumstances. Forcing choices on an individual often has very negative consequences in terms of equipment abandonment or improper use and can also negatively affect the individual's satisfaction with the process and equipment provided. The best solution is one that meets all the needs to the greatest extent possible and that yields optimal consumer satisfaction.

CASE EXAMPLE 3

A Patient with Cerebrovascular Accident

M. L. is an 80-year-old woman who has been referred for an assessment for wheeled mobility because of a recent decline in her ability to walk. M. L. had a stroke 10 years ago that impaired the strength on the left side of her body. Although she regained the ability to walk and can do so with a quad cane, she has begun to fall more frequently and currently is severely limited by her mobility impairment. She can walk only a distance of 10 feet and must have assistance from another person to do so safely. Because of this limitation, she spends most of her time sitting in a recliner chair in her living room and is becoming quite depressed. She has always been an active woman and would like to be able to participate in activities outside her home as well as move around inside her home by herself.

Questions to Consider

- Given her history and her stated goals, what should the systems review include?
- What specific tests and measures should be used in the examination?
- How might her current functional status and the chronic nature of her neuromuscular condition (coupled with the aging process), with its associated impairments and functional limitations, influence the assessment of her needs?
- What will the team's priorities be for M. L.'s seating and mobility system? How are the team's priorities similar or different from M. L.'s priorities? What compromises might be necessary?
- What options should be considered for M. L. in terms of seating system (noncontoured, contoured, or custom)? Support frame (lightweight, heavy duty)? Mobility component (manual or powered chair)?
- What recommendations should be made for managing pressure in M. L.'s seating system (active, rotational, reclined, or passive)? Why?

Recommendations

M. L. was evaluated in the seating and mobility clinic. The team arranged for her to borrow a semiadjustable, lightweight manual wheelchair and a powered wheelchair for a week so that she could assess which might best meet her needs. She was only able to propel the manual wheelchair on smooth indoor surfaces and could not move the chair up an incline without great difficulty. She was fully independent in operating the powered wheelchair but was discouraged by its large size.

The rehabilitation technology supplier obtained a smaller powered wheelchair considered transportable and that more closely resembles a manual wheelchair in overall size and shape. M. L. evaluated this wheelchair in her home environment and was pleased with her increased independence and access to all areas of her home and immediate outdoor environment. For seating, M. L. was prescribed a generically contoured foam seat cushion and a solid, adjustable back support. With this equipment, her posture was improved and she felt comfortable and secure.

SUMMARY

The science associated with adaptive seating and mobility for persons with disabilities is still in its infancy. Significant research in this field only began in the 1960s, and serious growth of this research has only been happening for the last 10 to 20 years.[33] Recent work has focused on the development of wheeled mobility that allows individuals to participate in a variety of leisure and competitive sport activities (Figure 19-14). In spite of this, several important research findings related to wheelchair seating and mobility are now beginning to be applied to the practice of wheelchair mobility seating.

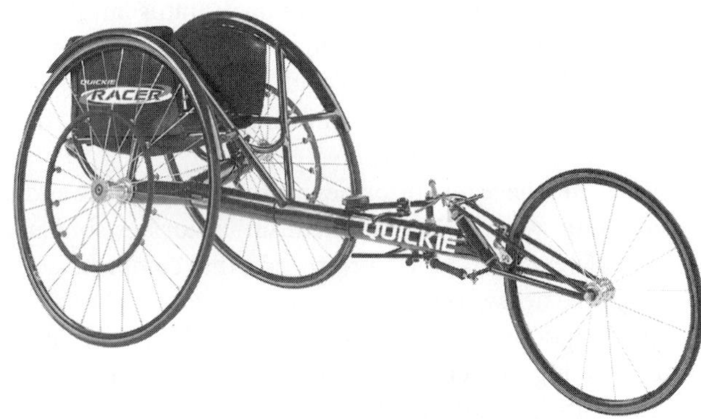

A

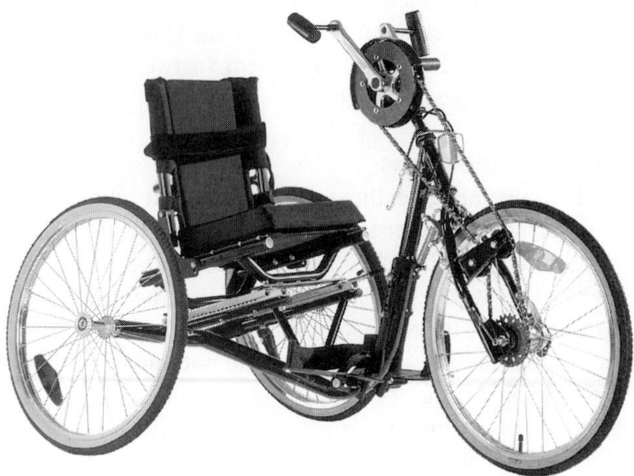

B

Figure 19-14
*Examples of wheelchairs designed for wheelchair racing **(A)** and upper extremity–powered bicycling **(B)**. (Courtesy Sunrise Medical, Longmont, Colo.)*

A great deal of research has contributed to and resulted from the development of international and national seating and wheelchair standards. The Rehabilitation Engineering and Assistive Technology Society of North America has been actively working toward the development of wheelchair seating standards since 1979.[34] These standards are intended to provide objective information to consumers about the safety and performance of wheelchairs.[34] In addition to this, wheelchair standards have facilitated improvements in quality and performance of wheeled mobility equipment.[35] Standards development has also provided a platform for research into characteristics of wheelchairs that are most beneficial to consumers and allowed the justification of higher-quality products based on ultimate cost effectiveness.[36-39] Wheelchair seating standards regarding the strength, efficacy, and safety of postural support devices are currently under development to provide many of these same benefits to the development and research related to adaptive seating products.

In addition to the research being performed in the standards arena, a great deal of interest and research in evidence-based practice exist for wheelchair seating and mobility. Although many seating clinicians prefer to practice with an evidence-based model, little research exists to support the efficacy of either the intervention process used or the equipment prescribed.[40,41] Several researchers are developing and validating outcomes measures to facilitate development of evidence-based practice in this field.[6,12,42-45] Once appropriate seating and wheeled mobility outcomes measures are developed, applying these outcomes in clinical and research settings and building the evidence so desperately needed in this field will be possible. Few randomized, controlled clinical trials assessing efficacy of seating and mobility intervention have been performed.[46,47] They have primarily focused on preventing pressure ulcers as an outcome of seat cushion intervention. More research regarding the many other possible outcomes of wheelchair seating and mobility intervention is still needed.

REFERENCES

1. Kaye HS, Kang T, LaPlante MP. *Mobility Device Use in the United States.* Washington, DC: U.S. Department of Education, National Institute on Disability and Rehabilitation, 2000. pp. 1-60.
2. Jones ML, Sanford JA. People with mobility impairments in the United States today and in 2010. *Assist Technol* 1996;8(1):43-53.
3. Schoenman JA. Description of the US working age disabled populations living in institutions and in the community. *Disabil Rehabil* 1995;17(5):231-238.
4. Simmons SF, Schnelle JF, MacRae PG, et al. Wheelchairs as mobility restraints: predictors of wheelchair activity in nonambulatory nursing home residents. *J Am Geriatr Soc* 1995;43(4):384-388.

5. Cook AM, Hussey SM. Seating systems as extrinsic enablers for assistive technologies. In Cook AM, Hussey SM (eds), *Assistive Technologies: Principles and Practice,* vol 1, 2nd ed. St. Louis: Mosby, 2002. pp. 165-211.
6. Pedersen JP, Lange ML, Griebel C. Seating intervention and postural control. In Olson DA, DeRuyter F (eds), *Clinician's Guide to Assistive Technology.* St. Louis: Mosby, 2002. pp. 209-236.
7. Minkel JL. Seating and mobility considerations for people with spinal cord injury. *Phys Ther* 2000;80(7):701-709.
8. American Physical Therapy Association. Guide to Physical Therapist Practice. *Phys Ther* 2001;81(1):21-138.
9. Zollars JA, Knezevich J. Special seating: an illustrated guide. Minneapolis: Otto Bock Orthopedic Industry, 1996.
10. Trefler E. Then and now. *Team Rehab Report* 1999;10(2):32-36.
11. Ferguson-Pell M, Cardi MD. Prototype development and comparative evaluation of wheelchair pressure mapping system. *Assist Technol* 1993;5(2):78-91.
12. Kirby RL, Swuste J, Dupuis DJ, et al. The Wheelchair Skills Test: a pilot study of a new outcome measure. *Arch Phys Med Rehabil* 2002;83(1):10-18.
13. McLaurin CA, Brubaker CE. Biomechanics and the wheelchair. *Prosthet Orthot Int* 1991;15(1):24-37.
14. Engstrom B. *Seating and Mobility for the Physically Challenged, Risks and Possibilities When Using Wheelchairs,* vol 1, 2nd ed. Sweden: Posturalis Books, 2002.
15. Zacharkow D. *Posture: Sitting, Standing, Chair Design and Exercise.* Springfield, IL: Charles C. Thomas, 1988.
16. Curtis KA, Drysdale GA, Lama D, et al. Shoulder pain in wheelchair users with tetraplegia and paraplegia. *Arch Phys Med Rehabil* 1999;80(4):453-457.
17. Koontz AM, Boninger ML. Proper propulsion. *Rehab Management* 2003;16(6):18-22.
18. van der Woude LH, Veeger DJ, Rosendal RH, et al. Seat height in hand rim wheelchair propulsion. *J Rehab Res Dev* 1989;26(4):31-50.
19. van der Woude LH, Veeger HE, Rozendal RH. Propulsion technique in hand rim wheelchair ambulation. *J Med Eng Technol* 1989;13(1-2):136-141.
20. Garber SL. Wheelchair cushions: a historical review. *Am J Occup Ther* 1985;39(7):453-459.
21. Ham R, Aldersea P, Porter D. *Wheelchair Users and Postural Seating: A Clinical Approach,* vol 1. New York: Churchill Livingstone, 1998.
22. Hobson DA. Seating and mobility for the severely disabled: Technology overview and classification. In Leslie J (ed), *Rehabilitation Engineering.* Boca Raton, FL: CRC Press, 1988. pp. 201-218.
23. St-Georges M, Valiquette C, Drouin G. Computer-aided design in wheelchair seating. *J Rehabil Res Dev* 1989;26(4):23-30.
24. Brienza DM, Geyer MJ. Understanding support surface technologies. *Adv Skin Wound Care* 2000;13(5):237-244.
25. Stewart SFC, Palmieri V, Cochran GVB. Wheelchair cushion effect on skin temperature, heat flux, and relative humidity. *Arch Phys Med Rehabil* 1980;61(5):229-233.
26. van der Woude LH, Dallmeijer AJ, Janssen TWJ, et al. Alternative modes of manual wheelchair ambulation: an overview. *Am J Phys Med Rehabil* 2001;80(10):765-777.
27. Boninger ML, Cooper RA, Roberson RN, et al. Wrist biomechanics during two speeds of wheelchair propulsion: an analysis using a local coordinate system. *Arch Phys Med Rehabil* 1997;78(4):364-372.
28. Bergman-Evans B, Cuddigan J, Bergstrom N. Clinical practice guidelines: prediction and prevention of pressure ulcers. *J Gerontol Nurs* 1994;20(9):19-26.
29. Bergstrom N, Braden BJ, Laguzza A, et al. The Braden Scale for predicting pressure sore risk. *Nursing Res* 1987;36(4): 205-210.
30. Allman RM. Pressure ulcer prevalence, incidence, risk factors, and impact. *Clin Geriatr Med* 1997;13(3):421-436.
31. Cuddigan J, Berlowitz DR, Ayello AE. Pressure ulcers in America: prevalence, incidence, and implications for the future. *Adv Skin Wound Care* 2001;14(4):208-215.
32. Weiss-Lambrou R. Satisfaction and comfort. In Scherer MJ (ed), *Assistive Technology: Matching Device and Consumer for Successful Rehabilitation.* Washington, DC: America Psychological Association, 2002. pp. 77-94.
33. McLaurin CA. Current directions in wheelchair research. *J Rehabil Res Dev*1990(suppl 2):88-99.
34. Axelson P, Minkel J, Chesney D. *A Guide to Wheelchair Selection: How to Use the ANSI/RESNA Standards to Buy a Wheelchair.* Washington, DC: Paralyzed Veterans of America, 1994.
35. Hartridge M, Seeger BR. International wheelchair standards: a study of costs and benefits. *Assist Technol* 1990;2(4):117-123.
36. Cooper RA, Boninger ML, Rentschler A. Evaluation of selected ultralight manual wheelchairs using ANSI/RESNA standards. *Arch Phys Med Rehabil* 1999;80(4):462-467.
37. Cooper RA, DiGiovine CP, Rentschler A, et al. Fatigue-life of two manual wheelchair cross-brace designs. *Arch Phys Med Rehabil* 1999;80(9):1078-1081.
38. Cooper RA, Gonzalez J, Lawrence B, et al. Performance of selected lightweight wheelchairs on ANSI/RESNA tests. *Arch Phys Med Rehabil* 1997;78(10):1138-1144.
39. Cooper RA, Robertson RN, Lawrence B, et al. Life-cycle analysis of depot versus rehabilitation manual wheelchairs. *J Rehabil Res Dev* 1996;33(1):45-55.
40. Rader JD, Jones D, Miller L. The importance of individualized wheelchair seating for frail older adults. *J Gerontol Nursing* 2000;26(11):24-32, 46-7.
41. Scherer MJ. Outcomes of assistive technology use on quality of life. *Disabil Rehabil* 1996;18(9):439-448.
42. Aissaoui R, Boucher C, Bourbonnais D, et al. Effect of seat cushion on dynamic stability in sitting during a reaching task in wheelchair users with paraplegia. *Arch Phys Med Rehabil* 2001;82(2):274-281.
43. Demers L, Wessels R, Weiss-Lambrou R, et al. Key dimensions of client satisfaction with assistive technology: a cross-validation of a Canadian measure in The Netherlands. *J Rehabil Med* 2001;33(4):187-191.
44. Hobson D, Crane B. State of the science white paper on wheelchair seat comfort. In *Wheelchair Seating: A State of the Science Conference on Seating Issues for Persons with Disabilities.* Orlando, FL: Rehabilitation Engineering Center on Wheeled Mobility and the School of Health and Rehabilitation Sciences at the University of Pittsburgh, 2001. pp. 29-33.
45. May LA, Butt C, Minor L, et al. Measurement reliability of functional tasks for persons who self-propel a manual wheelchair. *Arch Phys Med Rehabil* 2003;84(4):578-583.

46. Conine TA, Hershler C, Daechsel D, et al. Pressure ulcer prophylaxis in elderly patients using polyurethane foam or Jay wheelchair cushions. *Int J Rehabil Res* 1994;17(2):123-137.

47. Geyer MJ, Brienza DM, Karg P, et al. A randomized control trial to evaluate pressure-reducing seat cushions for elderly wheelchair users. *Adv Skin Wound Care* 2001;14(3):120-129.

III

Prosthetics in Rehabilitation

20

Etiology of Amputation

Caroline C. Nielsen

LEARNING OBJECTIVES

On completion of this chapter, the reader will be able to do the following:

1. Describe the purpose of the field of epidemiology.
2. Describe how physical therapists and prosthetists use "evidence" from epidemiological studies to rehabilitate persons with amputation.
3. Compare and contrast the four major causes of amputation and address their etiology, incidence, and prevalence.
4. Describe the interrelationships of the major risk factors for dysvascular/neuropathic-related amputation.
5. Explain the differences in risk factors of amputation among various racial and ethnic groups.
6. Identify key issues considered by the rehabilitation team when caring for older adults with amputation.

Throughout the history of medicine, amputation has been a relatively frequently performed medical procedure and has often been the only available alternative for complex fractures or infections of the extremities. The earliest amputations were generally undertaken to save lives; however, their outcomes were often unsuccessful—many resulted in death from shock due to blood loss or onset of infection and septicemia in those who survived the operation. In these early amputations, removal of the compromised limb segment as quickly as possible was essential. With the advent of antisepsis, asepsis, and anesthesia in the midnineteenth century, physicians focused increasingly on the surgical procedure and conservation of tissue.[1] The development of modern medical treatment has provided alternatives to amputation. Today, when amputation is necessary, surgery is undertaken with consideration for the functional aspects of the residual limb. This chapter defines the causes for amputation, describes the incidence and outcome expectations for particular populations, and discusses approaches to rehabilitation.

INCIDENCE OF AMPUTATION SURGERY

Amputation is a complex problem for patients, the health care system, and the country. In 2003 approximately 2 million persons had amputations in North America. Every year an additional 150,000 people lose a limb as a result of an accident or disease.[2] In addition to immense personal suffering, the costs to the health care system for the care of a patient with an ischemic limb, including wound care, vascular reconstruction, and amputation, are enormous. The more than 50,000 lower extremity amputations performed in the United States in 1985 contributed approximately $500 million per year in direct medical costs.[3] Currently 80,000 to 100,000 amputations are performed in the United States at a cost of more than $50,000 per patient.[4] In past years the incidence of amputation in the United States reflected the effects of war injuries. Today a higher percentage of adults are living longer and requiring amputations due to disease.

Current information on the incidence of amputations, particularly lower extremity amputations, is limited by the lack of a standardized approach to gathering data. Differences among studies in case definition, level of ascertainment, and population structure often make meaningful comparisons difficult.[5] The two major resources for data are the National Health Interview Survey (NHIS) and the National Hospital Discharge Survey (NHDS). The NHIS is an annual household survey of a probability sample of the U.S. population. Rates for the incidence of particular diseases and disabilities are drawn from these annual surveys. A limitation of this survey is that it may underreport the actual incidence of some disabilities, diseases, and impairments. Respondents may also underreport the use of orthotic or prosthetic devices. The NHDS collects data on a sample of short-stay, nonfederal hospitals in the United States. The survey generally samples less than 1% of discharges. A limitation of this survey is that it may underrepresent the incidence of some diseases, disabilities, and impairments. Federal hospitals, particularly those serviced by the Veterans' Administration, are frequently a primary source of care for persons with amputations. Despite the limitations of data sources, data from various sources can be coordinated to obtain current information on rates of amputation and disabilities requiring orthotic or prosthetic intervention.

More amputations occur among men than women, and amputation rates increase steeply with age.[6,7] Dysvascular disease accounts for about 82% of all limb loss hospital discharges (Figure 20-1). Between 1988 and 1996 the estimated increase in the rate of dysvascular amputations was 27%, with the highest percentage of disease-related amputations occurring in persons 65 years of age and older.[8] Most of these were lower extremity amputations, which are performed 11 times more frequently than upper extremity amputations.[9] The disease most frequently related to amputation is peripheral vascular disease (PVD) complicated by neuropathy. Although PVD and neuropathy are frequently associated with long-term, adult-onset (type 2) diabetes, vascular disease also occurs independently of diabetes. The increased frequency of amputation for PVD likely reflects increased growth in the older population. This increase is likely to continue with current population projections. The population in the age group 45 to 64 years is projected to increase 23.8% between 2002 and 2020, and the population at greatest risk for amputation, those 65 to 85 years and older, is expected to increase by 71%.[10] The population of individuals older than 85 years of age is projected to increase at the highest rate. Because the prevalence of PVD increases with age, these demographic changes will likely have a large impact on the amount of vascular reconstruction and amputation that will be performed.

The second leading cause of amputation is trauma, accounting for 5.86% of amputations in 1996. Traumatic

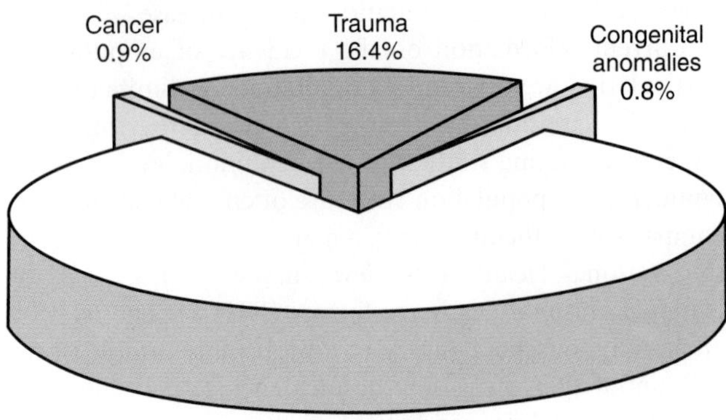

Figure 20-1

Causes of amputation by percent. The majority of amputations result from a disease process. (From Dillingham TR, Pezzin LE, Mackenzie EJ. Limb amputation and limb deficiency: epidemiology and recent trends in the United States. South Med J *2002;95[8]:875-883.)*

amputation is most common in the young adult age group. The leading causes of trauma-related amputation are injuries involving machinery (40.1%), power tools and appliances (27.8%), firearms (8.5%), and motor vehicle crashes (8%).[8] The incidence of trauma-related major amputation has continued to decrease over time. This reduction in traumatic amputation can be attributed to implementation of new safety regulations, the development of safer farm and industrial machinery, improved safety in work conditions, and medical advancement in techniques for salvaging traumatized limbs. Whenever there is a period of significant armed conflict, the number of veterans with traumatic amputation increases.

Amputations related to tumors accounted for 4.5% of amputations in 1974.[1] The tumor most commonly associated with amputation is osteosarcoma, which primarily affects children and adolescents in the 11- to 20-year age group. Currently amputation is no longer the primary intervention for osteosarcoma, and the current rate of amputation for this disease is less than 1%.[5] With development of new surgical techniques, including bone graft and joint replacement, and advancement in chemotherapy and radiation, the incidence of amputation due to osteosarcoma has decreased significantly.

Congenital limb deficiencies, as well as the amputations used to adjust or correct them, are relatively rare, and little has changed over time in the birth prevalence of congenital limb deficiencies. Rates have been reported ranging from 3.8 per 10,000 births to 5.3 per 10,000 births.[8] This percentage has remained relatively stable and is less than 1% of all amputations.

LEVELS OF AMPUTATION

Amputation can be performed as a disarticulation of a joint or as a transection through a long bone. The level of amputation is usually named by the joint or major bone through which the amputation has been made (Table 20-1).[9] An amputation that involves the lower extremity can affect an individual's ability to stand and walk, requiring the use of prosthetics and, often, an assistive device for mobility. Amputation involving the upper extremity can affect other activities of daily living, such as feeding, grooming, dressing, and a host of activities that require manipulative skills. Because of the complex nature of skilled hand function, prosthetic substitution for upper limb amputation does not typically restore function to the same degree that lower extremity prosthetics do.

The levels of amputation surgery that are most commonly performed today involve the lower extremity below the knee (including transtibial, foot, and toe amputations), accounting for 97% of all dysvascular limb loss discharges (Table 20-2). This high percentage reflects the prevalence of peripheral arterial vascular disease of the lower extremities. Transfemoral amputations account for approximately 26%

Table 20-1
Terminology Used to Describe the Site of Lower Extremity Amputation

Site	*Terminology*
Toe	Phalangeal
Forefoot	Ray resection (one or more complete metatarsal) Transmetatarsal (across the metatarsal shaft)
Midfoot	Partial foot (e.g., Chopart's, Boyd's, Pirogoff's)
At the ankle	Syme's
Below the knee	Transtibial (long, standard, short)
At the knee	Knee disarticulation
Above the knee	Transfemoral (long, standard, short)
At the hip	Hip disarticulation
At the pelvis	Hemipelvectomy

Table 20-2
Incidence of Lower Limb Amputation: Average Annual Number and Percent of Hospital Discharges after Lower Extremity Amputation, 1988-1996

Level of Amputation	*Number*	*Percent*
Toe	338,288	33.11
Foot and ankle	116,302	11.38
Transtibial	287,295	28.12
Knee disarticulation	5291	0.52
Transfemoral	266,465	26.08
Hip and pelvis	6588	0.64
Bilateral amputations	1504	0.15
Total	1,021,733	100

From Dillingham TR, Pezzin LE, Mackenzie EJ. Limb amputation and limb deficiency. Epidemiology and recent trends in the United States. *South Med J* 2002;95(8):875-883.

of all dysvascular amputations.[8] In general the proportion of lower limb amputations in relation to upper limb amputations is increasing. This most likely reflects an increase in the number of older persons with lower extremity amputations rather than an actual decrease in the number of upper extremity amputations.

Because PVD typically affects both lower extremities, a significant number of individuals eventually undergo amputation of both lower extremities. Approximately 50% of persons undergoing diabetes-related amputation will have contralateral amputation within 3 to 5 years. Between 25% and 45% of persons with amputations have had amputations of both lower extremities, most often at the transtibial level in both limbs, or a combination of transtibial amputation of one limb and transfemoral amputation of the other.[11]

Today the majority of transtibial and transfemoral amputations are performed with an understanding of wound healing and the functional needs and constraints of prosthetic fitting so that rehabilitation outcomes are usually positive. Other levels of amputation, although less commonly performed procedures, continue to pose challenges for the surgeon, prosthetist, physical therapist, and patient during prosthetic fitting and rehabilitation.

CAUSES OF AMPUTATION

Currently the most likely reasons for amputation are (1) complications of peripheral neuropathy and PVD, (2) trauma, or (3) cancer (generally osteosarcoma). Children with congenital limb deficiencies are a special population group and may require surgical revision during or after periods of significant growth or after conversion to a more functional level for prosthetic fitting.

Peripheral Vascular Disease

PVD is the most common contributing factor for lower extremity amputations. In epidemiological studies, two symptoms are classic indicators of vascular insufficiency: intermittent claudication and loss of one or more lower extremity pulses. Intermittent claudication is a significant cramping pain, usually in the calf, that is induced by walking or other prolonged muscle contraction and relieved by a short period of rest. In arteriosclerosis obliterans, at least one major arterial pulse (at the dorsal pedis artery at the ankle, popliteal artery at the knee, or femoral artery in the groin) is often absent or markedly impaired (Figure 20-2).[3]

The major risk factors for development of PVD are the same as those for cardiovascular and cerebrovascular disease, most notably poorly managed hypertension, high serum cholesterol and triglyceride levels, and a history of tobacco use and smoking. Peripheral neuropathy and PVD are the major predisposing factors for lower extremity amputation in individuals with diabetes.[12]

According to the NHDS, the number of hospital discharges that listed diagnoses of amputation and diabetes increased 27% from 1988 to 1996.[8] The prevalence of PVD among persons with diabetes, whether men or women, is significantly greater than in those without diabetes. The Framingham Heart Study found a four to five times greater relative risk of intermittent claudication in persons with diabetes, even when controlling for blood pressure, cholesterol, and smoking.[13] The age-adjusted rate of lower extremity

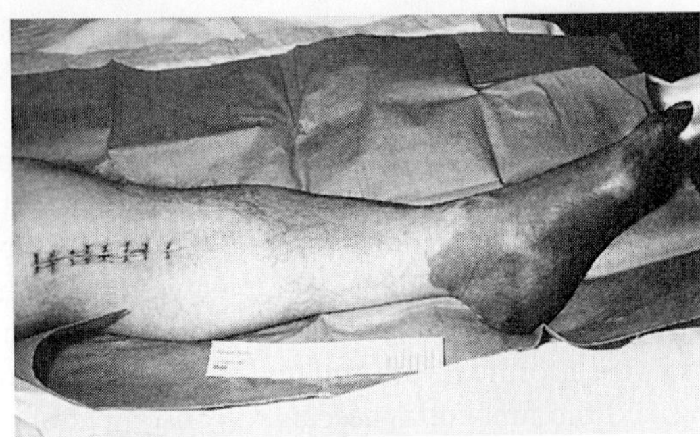

Figure 20-2
This patient with atherosclerosis obliterans underwent a femoral-distal popliteal bypass in an attempt to revascularize the foot. The demarcation indicating ischemia at the ankle and foot is clear. Transtibial amputation is necessary when revascularization is unsuccessful. (From Robinson KP. The dilemma: amputation or revascularization. In Murdock G, Wilson AB [eds], Amputation: Surgical Practice and Patient Management. *Oxford, UK: Butterworth-Heinemann, 1996. p. 169.)*

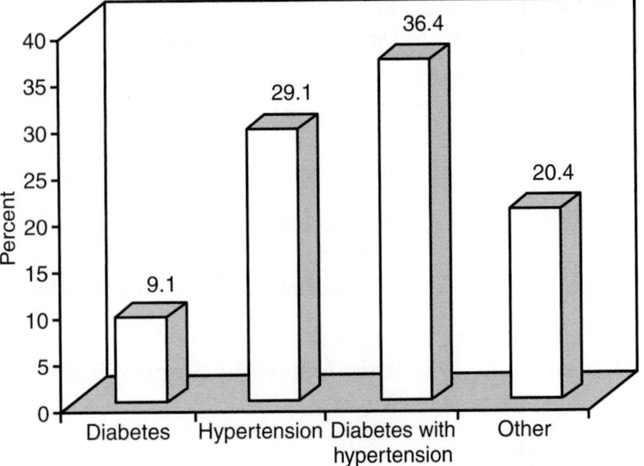

Figure 20-3
Lower extremity amputations, classified by predisposing factors. Hypertension, especially in the presence of diabetes, is a powerful risk factor. "Other" includes a combination of risk factors including race, gender, cigarette smoking, and previous vascular surgery. (Based on data reported by Lee CS, Sariego J, Matsumoto T. Changing patterns in the predisposition for amputation of the lower extremities. Am Surg *1992;5[8]:474-477.)*

amputation among persons with diabetes in the United States is approximately 28 times that of the nondiabetic population. More than 50% of the lower limb amputations in the United States are diabetes related, although persons diagnosed with diabetes represent only 3% of the population.[14] A study in Rochester, Minn., compared non–insulin-dependent persons with diabetes with the general population. The risk of any first lower extremity amputation in non–insulin-dependent persons with diabetes was nearly 17 times higher than that of the general population.[15] Although major improvements have been made in noninvasive diagnosis, surgical revascularization procedures, and wound-healing techniques, between 2% and 5% of individuals with PVD and without diabetes and between 6% and 25% of those with diabetes eventually undergo an amputation.[15-17]

The three most common predisposing factors for lower extremity amputation appear to be (1) concurrent diabetes and hypertension, (2) hypertension without diabetes, and (3) diabetes without hypertension (Figure 20-3). Other predisposing factors include race, gender, history of smoking, and previous vascular surgery. The incidence of lower extremity amputation among persons with diabetes is almost 50% higher for men than for women.[8] The most frequently cited criteria for amputation among persons with diabetes include gangrene, infection, nonhealing neuropathic ulcer, severe ischemic pain, absent or decreased pulses, local necrosis, osteomyelitis, systemic toxicity, acute embolic disease, or severe venous thrombosis.[15,17,18]

In individuals with diabetes, the prevalence and severity of PVD increase significantly with age and the duration of diabetes, particularly in men. Initial amputation may involve a toe or foot; subsequent revision to transtibial or transfemoral levels is likely to occur with progression of the underlying disease.[11] In individuals with diabetes, a diagnosis of PVD increases the risk of a nonhealing neuropathic ulcer, infection, or gangrene, all of which increase the likelihood of amputation. An epidemiological study examined the relationship between the diagnoses of diabetes and PVD.[15] On initial diagnosis of diabetes, 8% of subjects had clinical evidence of arteriosclerosis obliterans. As the duration of diabetes lengthened, the prevalence of PVD increased to 15% at 10 years and 45% at 20 years. Today, patients with diabetes who are 65 years old or older account for most diabetes-related lower extremity amputations. In 1996 the estimated amputation rate was 1.4 times higher for persons with diabetes who were 65 to 74 years old and 2.4 times higher for those 75 years of age or older, compared with those 0 to 64 years of age.[19]

Peripheral neuropathy is a common complication of diabetes. Neuropathy is as important and powerful as PVD as a predisposing factor for lower extremity amputation. Peripheral neuropathy is suspected when one or more of the following clinical signs are present: deficits of sensation (loss of Achilles and patellar reflexes, decreased vibratory sensation, and loss of protective sensation), motor impairments (weakness and atrophy of the intrinsic muscles of the foot), or autonomic dysfunction (inadequate or abnormal hemodynamic mechanism, tropic changes of the skin, and distal loss of hair).[3] The resulting loss of thermal, pain, and protective sensation increases the vulnerability of the foot to acute, high-pressure and repetitive, low-pressure trauma. Patients may also experience significant numbness or painful paresthesia of the foot and lower leg. Individuals with peripheral neuropathy may not be aware of minor trauma,

pressure from poorly fitting shoes along the sides and tops of their feet, or pressure from thickening plantar callus, all of which contribute to the risk of ulceration, infection, and gangrene. Motor neuropathy and associated weakness and atrophy contribute to development of bony deformity of the foot. The bony prominences and malalignments that are associated with foot deformity change weight-bearing pressure dynamics during walking, further increasing the risk of ulceration. Peripheral neuropathy is one of the most crucial precursors of foot ulceration, especially in the presence of PVD. Nonhealing or infected neuropathic ulcers precede approximately 85% of nontraumatic lower extremity amputations in individuals with diabetes.[14] Chapter 21 discusses conservative management of patients who are vulnerable to nonhealing neuropathic ulcers due to peripheral neuropathy and peripheral vascular disease.

CASE EXAMPLE 1

A Patient with Dysvascular Disease–Related Amputation

T. S., 67, is an African-American man with a 10-year history of type 2 (adult onset) diabetes mellitus. Until 2 years ago, he smoked one pack daily, but he "quit" after coronary artery bypass grafting (CABG × 4) following acute myocardial infarction (MI). He became insulin dependent at the time of his MI and CABG surgery. Comorbid medical problems include hypertension, managed pharmaceutically with a beta blocker, and moderate vision loss secondary to diabetic retinopathy.

T. S. underwent complete transmetatarsal amputation of the left foot 6 months ago because of a nonhealing plantar ulcer under the second and third metatarsal heads that had progressed to osteomyelitis. Three weeks ago, intermittent claudication of the right calf became severe enough to warrant medical attention. On evaluation T. S. was noted to have a neuropathic ulcer under his first metatarsal head, probing to bone. Doppler studies were monophasic, suggesting inadequate vascular supply for healing. Arteriography indicated markedly diminished distal arterial flow to his foot but adequate arterial supply to midtibial levels.

After an interdisciplinary meeting involving his internist (who helps him manage his diabetes), cardiologist (who helps him manage his hypertension and heart disease, vascular surgeon (who oversaw this evaluation), physical therapist and prosthetist (who explained the process of rehabilitation), social worker (who explained services and support available to those with amputation), and family, T. S. concurred with the recommendation for an "elective" transtibial amputation. His surgery occurred 2 weeks ago, and he is impatiently waiting for his wound to heal sufficiently to begin prosthetic training.

Questions to Consider

- What possible medical and physiological factors have contributed to this patient's loss of limb?
- What impact will his current health status and comorbid conditions have on his prognosis for rehabilitation, both in terms of eventual outcome and in duration of this episode of care?

Lower extremity amputation continues to be a major health problem for the diabetic population. For this group of patients, amputation is associated with significant morbidity, functional limitation and disability, mortality, and high health care costs. Approximately 130,000 lower extremity amputations are performed on individuals with diabetes in the United States each year.[2] The average cost for a patient per hospitalization for amputation is about $50,000, and the direct medical care costs for all amputations, excluding the cost of rehabilitation, in the U.S. diabetic population is more than $600 million.[20] According to the U.S. Public Health Service, reducing the incidence of lower extremity amputations in persons with diabetes is a key health care objective in terms of quality of life and containment of health care costs. Current projections indicate there will be about 22 million people in the United States with diabetes in 2025. Planned health promotion efforts will hopefully reduce the risk of diabetes and amputation, minimizing the impact of risk factors and increasing access to care by multidisciplinary health care teams.

Incidence Among Minority Populations

Evidence indicates that certain racial and ethnic groups are at increased risk for lower extremity amputation. This increased risk appears to be linked to a higher prevalence of diabetes complicated by PVD. Minority groups with the highest incidence of diabetes and greatest risk of lower extremity amputation are Native Americans, African-Americans, and Hispanic Americans. Native Americans are 3.5 times more likely to have lower extremity amputation than their non-Hispanic white counterparts.[21] African-Americans are two to four times more likely to lose a limb as a result of diabetes complications.[22] Hispanic Americans are diagnosed with diabetes at twice the rate of whites and are 1.5 times more likely to have an amputation.[23]

Native Americans have a two to five times higher prevalence of diabetes than the overall population in the United States. This high prevalence is directly reflected in increased amputation rates. Among Pima Indians with diabetes, the rate of amputation is 3.7 times higher than the rate of other persons with diabetes.[24] A survey of lower extremity amputations among patients in the areas served by the Indian Health Service in 1982 to 1987 found that the age-adjusted incidence rates of all lower extremity amputations among Native Americans with diabetes were substantially higher than the overall rate for the United States.[25] This increased

risk was found in the Navajo Nation even in 1997.[5] Why these populations have a significantly higher rate of lower extremity amputation is unclear. Potential contributors include a genetic or familial predisposition to diabetes, a higher prevalence of hypertension and smoking, or both. Health promotion and education efforts that target this high-risk population (including programs aimed at effective management of diabetes, minimization of other risk factors, and special foot care programs for early detection of neuropathic and traumatic lesions) are effective strategies to reduce the likelihood of amputation. Further research is necessary to better understand the causes of racial differences in amputation rates and to identify and promote health initiatives that will alleviate this excess risk among minority populations.

Outcome of Vascular-Related Amputation

The morbidity and mortality risks associated with systemic diseases, such as diabetes and vascular disease, continue after amputation. As a result, death in the years immediately after amputation is not uncommon. The 3-year survival rate after initial lower extremity amputation for persons with diabetes is only approximately 50%; the 5-year survival rate ranges in various studies from 39% to 68%.[14] Because neuropathy and PVD occur in a symmetric distribution, the risk of subsequent amputation of the contralateral lower extremity is high. Even with successful healing of the primary amputation site, amputation of part of the contralateral limb occurs in 50% of patients within 2 to 5 years.[11] The most common causes of death in persons with amputation include complications of diabetes, cardiovascular disease, and renal disease.

Evidence is growing that the incidence of lower extremity amputation in persons with diabetes can be significantly reduced through particular kinds of preventive care. Large clinical centers have demonstrated the effect of early intervention for the diabetic population, using an interdisciplinary team approach to preventive care. Interventions to prevent neuropathy and PVD target smoking reduction programs, as well as dietary, exercise, and pharmaceutical interventions, to obtain better control of hypertension, hyperlipidemia, and hyperglycemia. Reduction of these predisposing factors is likely to further reduce the incidence of amputation, heart disease, and stroke among people with diabetes. For those with existing diabetic neuropathy or PVD, intensive foot care programs should focus on prevention of ulceration and early intervention to prevent expansion, infection, or gangrene of small lesions. Foot care programs are most effective if they develop in a team setting and focus on patient education.

The decision to undergo amputation often follows a long struggle to care for an increasingly frail foot by the patient, the family, and health care providers. In this circumstance, elective amputation is often perceived by the patient and family as a positive step toward a more active and less stressful life. The multidisciplinary team approach best addresses the complex needs of the individual with diabetes, including clinical evaluation, determination of risk status, patient education, footwear selection, decision making about amputation, and rehabilitation after surgery.

Traumatic Amputation

Traumatic loss of a limb, the second most common cause of amputation, occurs most frequently in vehicle- or work-related accidents, as a result of violence such as gunshots or warfare, or after severe burns and electrocution (Figure 20-4). Trauma-related amputation occurs most commonly in young adult men but can happen at any age to men or women. Because the mechanism of injury in traumatic amputation is quite variable, this type of amputation is usually classified or categorized according to the severity of tissue damage. The extent of injury to the musculoskeletal system depends on three interacting factors: (1) movement of the object that causes the injury; (2) direction, magnitude, and speed of the energy vector; and (3) the particular body tissue involved.

In partial traumatic amputations, at least one half the diameter of the injured extremity is severed or damaged significantly. This kind of injury can incur extensive bleeding, because all of the blood vessels involved may not be vasoconstrictive. A second type of traumatic amputation occurs when the limb becomes completely detached from the body. As much as 1 liter of blood may be lost before the arteries spasm and become vasoconstrictive.[27]

For optimal outcome, surgical intervention is usually necessary within the first 12 hours after the accident for revascularization or for treatment of the amputated site. When replantation is considered, the window of opportu-

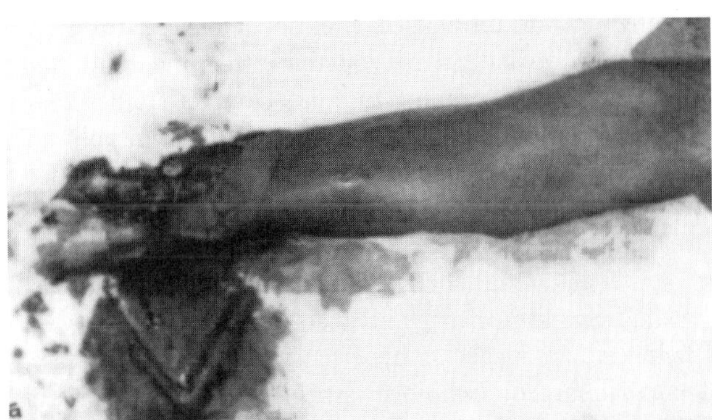

Figure 20-4

This patient sustained a traumatic amputation of his left foot and distal tibia when he stepped on a buried land mine. (From Coupland RM, Korver A. Injuries from antipersonnel mines: the experience of the International Committee of the Red Cross. BMJ *1991;303[14]:1509. Reprinted from the BMJ Publishing Group.)*

nity is much narrower. The decision to replant is a difficult one and is influenced by the patient's age and overall health status, the level of extremity injury, and the condition of the amputated part. Replantation has been most successful in the distal upper extremity. The goal of upper extremity replantation is to provide a mechanism for functional grasp rather than cosmetic restoration of the limb. The period of recovery and rehabilitation after replantation is often significantly longer than that after amputation.

Persons with trauma-related amputation undergo extreme physiological changes, as well as psychological trauma. With the sudden loss of a body part, the patient may experience an extended period of grieving. Addressing the patient's psychological needs as well as physical needs is important for optimal outcome. An interdisciplinary team approach to rehabilitation is the most effective means of addressing the comprehensive needs of a patient who has unexpectedly lost a limb to trauma.[27]

CASE EXAMPLE 2

A Patient with Traumatic Amputation

C. J., 20, is a national guardsman on active duty overseas as a result of a conflict in the Middle East. He sustains significant shrapnel injury to both lower extremities when a rocket-propelled grenade is fired at the convoy in which he is riding. After emergency care on the ground, C. J.'s condition is considered critical enough to warrant immediate transport to a military hospital in Europe. Trauma surgeons at the center determine his wounds are severe enough to require midlength transtibial amputation on the right and a long transfemoral amputation on the left. Because of wound contamination from shrapnel and debris and a resulting high risk of infection, C. J.'s surgical wounds are initially left "open" (unsutured) while local and intravenous antimicrobials are administered. After several days of care, C. J. is returned to the operating room for revision and closure of his residual limbs. He now has significant edema and serosanguineous drainage on the right limb with a small area of dehiscence in the middle of the suture line. Although the left residual limb is not as edematous, the suture line is inflamed and ecchymotic, with more than a dozen healing puncture wounds from shrapnel fragments over the anterior and lateral thigh. When medically stable, C. J. will be moved to a military rehabilitation hospital in the United States for preprosthetic care and rehabilitation.

Questions to Consider

- Given the circumstances of these traumatic amputations, how does this patient's prognosis differ from the previous patient with dysvascular-neuropathic amputation?
- How might the rehabilitation of this patient be similar to or different from the previous patient with dysvascular-neuropathic amputation, in terms of eventual outcome and duration of care?

Cancer

Amputation due to a primary cancer generally results from osteogenic sarcoma (osteosarcoma) (Figure 20-5). This type of cancer occurs predominantly in late childhood, adolescence, or the early young adult years. The incidence is slightly higher among young males than females. Osteosarcoma typically occurs at or near the epiphyses of long bones during times of rapid growth, especially the distal femur, proximal tibia, or proximal humerus. Most patients have a history of worsening, increasingly deep-seated pain, sometimes accompanied by localized swelling. Children with osteosarcoma are vulnerable to pathological fracture, an event that often prompts diagnosis. Since the early 1990s, the need for amputation in osteosarcoma has been greatly reduced by advances in early detection, improved imaging techniques, more effective chemotherapy regimens, and better limb resectioning and salvage procedures. Tumor resection followed by limb reconstruction frequently provides a functional extremity. Weight bearing is limited, and the limb is protected by an orthosis early in rehabilitation. Once satisfactory healing occurs, full weight bearing and near normal activity can be resumed. With new techniques, 5-year survival rates for individuals with osteosarcoma increased from approximately 20% in the 1970s to 80% in the 1990s.[28]

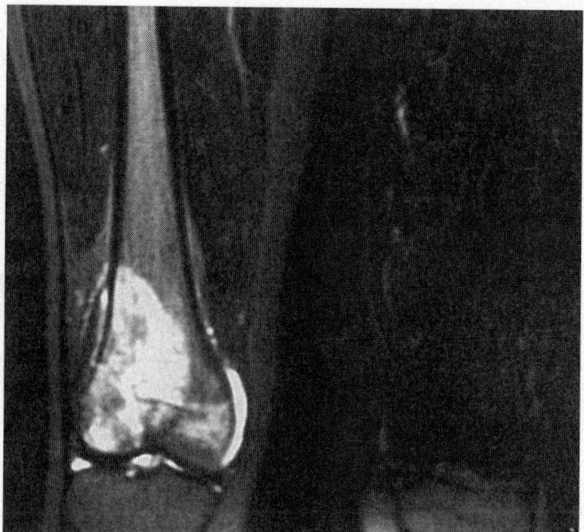

Figure 20-5
Magnetic resonance image of the distal femur of a patient with an osteosarcoma of the bone and marrow canal. The bright signal beyond the bone indicates invasion of surrounding soft tissue. (From Lundon K. Orthopedic Rehabilitation Science: Principles for Clinical Management of Bone. *Boston: Butterworth-Heinemann, 2000. p. 147.)*

CASE EXAMPLE 3

A Patient with Osteosarcoma

R. K., 16, sustained an unexpected fracture of the distal femur in a collision during playoffs for the state soccer title. He experienced increasing lateral knee pain for the previous 4 weeks but did not complain to his coaches and parents for fear he would have to "sit out." Examination in the emergency department reveals a swollen and tender distal femur and knee. A radiograph reveals a fracture just proximal to a radio-dense lesion of the medial femoral condyle, including articular surfaces of the knee. Magnetic resonance imaging reveals that the tumor extends posteriorly, close to the neurovascular bundle in the popliteal fossa. Biopsy confirmed osteosarcoma. The orthopedic surgeon and oncologist review options for limb salvage and amputation with R. K. and his parents, recommending amputation because the location of the tumor precludes the wide clear margins at the knee required for endoprosthetic knee replacement or cadaver allograft salvage strategies. His fractured limb is stabilized in a knee orthosis while a preoperative course of chemotherapy is undertaken and the possibility of metastasis to the lungs is evaluated by further testing. Resection of the tumor to a midlength transfemoral level of amputation will occur once the initial course of chemotherapy is completed and will be followed by a second course of chemotherapy. R. K. and his family have been encouraged by visits from a survivor of osteosarcoma who had transfemoral amputation 7 years ago and is now a competitive runner at the national and Paralympic level.

Questions to Consider

- How does the diagnosis of a serious cancer affect the rehabilitation of young people with medically necessary amputations? What psychological and physiological factors must be considered?
- What are the similarities and differences in the prognosis and plan of care for this patient with cancer-related amputation, as compared with the previous patients with dysvascular-neuropathic and trauma-related etiology, in terms of eventual outcome, and duration of this episode of care?

Congenital Limb Deficiencies

The incidence of congenital limb deficiency has remained relatively stable over time, accounting for only about 0.8% of all limb loss–related hospital discharges. The rate in 1996 was 25.64 per 100,000 live births. A slight male preponderance in the incidence of limb reductions has been reported, as well as a slightly higher incidence of upper limb reductions among newborns with limb deficiencies.[8]

The actual incidence of congenital limb deficiencies is difficult to determine because of lack of a common definition and reporting mechanisms. Six categories of limb deficiencies have been recognized[29]:

1. *Failure of formation* of parts, indicating a partial or complete arrest in limb development
2. *Failure of differentiation* or separation of parts, when the basic structures have developed but the final form is not completed
3. Duplication of parts, such as *polydactyly*
4. Skeletal overgrowth, also called *gigantism*
5. Congenital *constriction band syndrome,* characterized by constriction bands, which may compromise circulation to the distal part
6. Generalized skeletal abnormalities

Upper limb deficiencies in children vary from minor abnormalities of the fingers to major limb absences. Embryological differentiation of the upper limbs occurs most rapidly at 5 to 8 weeks after gestation, often before pregnancy has been recognized or confirmed. During this period the upper limbs are particularly vulnerable to malformation. The etiology of limb malformation is unclear. Potential contributing factors cited in the research literature include (1) exposure to chemical agents or drugs, (2) fetal position or constriction, (3) endocrine disorders, (4) exposure to radiation, (5) immune reactions, (6) occult infections and other diseases, (7) single gene disorders, (8) chromosomal disorders, and (9) other syndromes with unknown causes.[29] For many children, an upper limb deficiency is their only

Table 20-3
Classification of Longitudinal Congenital Limb Deficiencies

Limb Segment	*Upper Extremity Bone Segment**	*Lower Extremity Bone Segment**
Proximal	Humeral	Femoral
Distal	Radial Central Carpal Metacarpal Phalangeal	Tibial Central Tarsal Metatarsal Phalangeal
Combined (indicated by the bone segments that remain)	Partial or complete	Partial or complete
	Specific carpal, ray, or phalanx remaining	Specific carpal, ray, or phalanx remaining

Modified from May BJ. *Amputations and Prosthetics: A Case Study Approach.* Philadelphia: F.A. Davis, 1996. p. 221.
*May be partial or complete.

anomaly. However, as many as 12% of these children have coexisting nonlimb malformations.

Limb deficiencies present at birth are classified according to an international standard based on skeletal elements (Table 20-3). These deficiencies are referred to as *transverse* or *longitudinal.* Transverse deficiencies are described by the level at which the limb terminates. In longitudinal deficiencies, a reduction or absence occurs within the long axis of the limb, but normal skeletal components are present distal to the affected bones (Figure 20-6).[29,30]

The use of prosthetics is a common intervention for children with congenital limb deficiencies. Sometimes surgery is necessary to prepare the existing limb for the most effective use of a prosthesis, especially after periods of rapid growth. The goals of prosthetic training for the child should be to enhance the function of the limb and provide a cosmetic replacement for a missing limb. Rehabilitation efforts (discussed in Chapter 32) are designed with the child's cognitive, motor, and psychological development in mind.

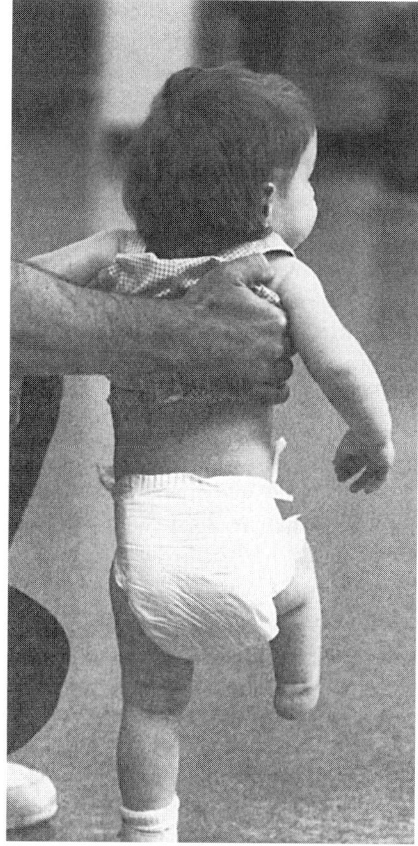

Figure 20-6
This child was born with a unilateral proximal focal deficiency of the right lower extremity. In order to facilitate prosthetic use, she has undergone an elective amputation of her foot at the ankle. Note the popliteal crease near the diaper line, indicating where her knee is located. (From Campbell SK, Vanderlinden DW, Palisano RJ [eds]. Physical Therapy for Children, *2nd ed. Philadelphia: Saunders, 2000. p. 380.)*

REHABILITATION ISSUES FOR THE PERSON WITH AN AMPUTATION

Several factors influence the success of rehabilitation after amputation. These include age, health status, cognitive status, sequence of onset of disability, concurrent disease and comorbidity, and the level of amputation.[31] With anticipated growth in segments of the population most vulnerable to PVD, amputation in the U.S. geriatric population will probably double from 28,000 to 58,000 per year by 2030, requiring considerable rehabilitation resources.[32]

Progression in rehabilitation has been measured in different ways. Traditionally, physical therapists have focused on the ability to perform functional activities such as walking, turning, and managing ramps and other uneven or unpredictable surfaces safely, independently, and efficiently with and without a prosthesis. Physical therapists assist physicians and prosthetists in determining an individual's readiness for prosthetic fitting and are often involved in decisions about prosthetic components. After initial fitting, physical therapists coordinate prosthetic training, consulting with prosthetists if problems with prosthetic alignment arise. Once these basic mobility activities are mastered, the therapist can serve as a consultant to assist the person with amputation in returning to preamputation employment and leisure activities. Treatment programs, predictors of outcome, and measures of success or failure are often based on these functional activities.

In one study of progression through rehabilitation (n = 459), between 85% and 89% of persons with lower extremity amputations mastered basic functional activities, such as moving about the bed, moving from supine into sitting position, and sitting balance, within the second postoperative week. Between 65% and 75% of persons with amputation demonstrated independence in transfers and dressing of upper and lower limbs in the third to fifth postoperative week. Although steady gains were made in the ability to doff and don the prosthesis and to walk indoors and outside during the fifth to the twelfth postoperative weeks, just one third of people in the study achieved independence within this time frame.[33] Optimal rehabilitation outcome, achievement of the highest functional level of which the person with amputation is capable, requires ongoing contact with and support of a multidisciplinary rehabilitation team.

As many as 70% of persons with a lower extremity amputation report using their prosthesis on a full-time basis: putting it on in the early morning, wearing it all day, and taking it off in the evening.[34] Two major reasons for limited use or nonuse are generally cited—physical discomfort when walking with the prosthesis and psychological discomfort. The wide variation reported in the success of functional ambulation with a prosthesis after below-knee amputation appears to be related to age and concurrent disease.[4] Healing time, indicated by time between surgery and fitting for the first prosthesis, correlates with age but not with the cause of amputation. Age is also more important than the etiology of amputation in predicting the total length of time in rehabilitation and achievement of functional ambulation: Older adults with amputation are likely to require a longer rehabilitation period to accomplish an ambulatory status equal to that of the younger group.[35] Although most people recovering from amputation achieve some level of upright mobility, a smaller percentage of older persons with concurrent chronic disease become functional ambulators when compared with younger persons who had amputations because of trauma or osteomyelitis.

The typical age at the time of initial lower limb amputation is between 51 and 69 years; therefore consideration must be given to the special rehabilitation needs of the older patient. The complexity of issues during rehabilitation of the older adult who is undergoing an amputation is often compounded by comorbidity, fragile social supports, and limited resources.[4] In patients with PVD, concomitant cerebrovascular disease can complicate rehabilitation: A preamputation history of stroke or occurrence of stroke during the course of rehabilitation is not uncommon. Similarly, cardiovascular disease can limit endurance and exercise tolerance; endurance training becomes a critical component of the post-amputation, preprosthetic rehabilitation program. Optimal rehabilitation care begins with consultation and patient and family education efforts before surgery. A specialized multidisciplinary team most effectively provides this presurgical and perisurgical care (Table 20-4). Team members often include a surgeon, physical therapist, certified prosthetist, occupational therapist, nurse or nurse practitioner, recreational therapist, psychologist, and social worker.[31] The patient and family members are active and essential members of the team as well. Effective communication provides the team with the necessary information to develop a tentative treatment plan from the time of amputation to discharge home.

With a specialized treatment team and the use of new lightweight and dynamic prosthetic designs, the potential for rehabilitation of the older patient has increased significantly in the past decade. At the time of surgery, special consideration is given to the optimal level of amputation. This is a particularly important concern for the older patient. The selection of the surgical level of amputation is probably one of the most important decisions to be made for the patient undergoing an amputation. A lower limb prosthesis ideally becomes a full body-weight–bearing device. However, bony prominences, adhesions of the suture line scar, fragile skin and open areas, shearing forces at the skin/socket interface, and perspiration can complicate this function.[31] The energy cost of ambulation must be considered, especially for older patients with significant deconditioning or comorbid conditions. The higher the level of amputation and loss of joints, long bone length, and muscle insertion, the greater the impairment of normal locomotor mechanisms. This leads to increased energy costs in prosthetic control and functional ambulation and a greater likelihood of functional limitation and disability.

Preservation of the knee joint seems to be a key determinant in determining the potential for functional ambulation and successful rehabilitation outcome. Persons with transtibial amputation, who have an intact anatomical knee joint, demonstrate a more energy-efficient prosthetic gait pattern and postural responses and are more likely to ambulate without additional assistive devices (walkers, crutches, or canes). They are also more likely to be full-time prosthetic wearers than are persons with transfemoral amputation. The benefits of preserving the knee, particularly among older adults, are so crucial that a transtibial amputation may be attempted even with the risk of inadequate healing; this may necessitate later revision to a higher level.[31]

The patient with a bilateral transfemoral amputation faces additional rehabilitation challenges. The significant increase in energy consumption that is required can prevent long-distance ambulation. Many older patients, as well as younger persons with bilateral transfemoral amputation, may choose wheelchair mobility as a more energy-efficient and effective means of locomotion. Ambulation potential depends on cardiac function, strength, balance, and endurance.[31]

Options for prosthetic components for the older person with an amputation have increased dramatically in the past 20 years. Selecting the most appropriate components for the individual requires the input of the complete rehabilitation team, in close communication with the patient and the family members.

REHABILITATION ENVIRONMENT

Traditionally, preprosthetic and early prosthetic programs have been housed in rehabilitation departments of acute care hospitals. In this environment, the care may not be specialized for the older person with an amputation. A specialized treatment team is best able to address the complex needs of this group of patients. However, in today's health care environment, it may not be possible for older patients with an amputation to stay in the acute care hospital until they are ready for prosthetic fitting. For patients with multiple medical complications, rehabilitation may be continued in a subacute setting or skilled nursing facility. For patients without complications and with a strong social support network, an outpatient rehabilitation program may be preferable. This plan allows them to reintegrate into home and community while maintaining support of the treatment team. The most effective care and rehabilitation for individuals undergoing an amputation require the skills and ongoing support of an integrated treatment team.[36]

Table 20-4
Members and Roles of the Multidisciplinary Team for Rehabilitation after Amputation

Team Member	*Role*
Physician	Often serves as coordinator of the team
	Assesses need for amputation, performs surgery, monitors healing of suture line
	Monitors and manages patient's overall medical care and health status
	Monitors condition of remaining extremity for patients with peripheral vascular disease (PVD), neuropathy, or diabetes
Physical therapist	Provides preoperative education about the rehabilitation process and instruction in single limb mobility
	Designs and manages a preprosthetic rehabilitation program that focuses on mobility and preparation for prosthetic training
	Evaluates patient's readiness for prosthetic fitting; can make recommendations for prosthetic fitting
	Designs and manages a prosthetic training program that focuses on functional ambulation and prosthetic management
	Monitors condition of the remaining extremity for patients with PVD, neuropathy, or diabetes
Prosthetist	Designs, fabricates, and fits the prosthesis
	Adapts the prosthesis to individuals, adjusts alignment, repairs/replaces components when necessary
	Monitors fit, function, and comfort of the prosthesis
	Monitors condition of the remaining extremity for patients with PVD, neuropathy, or diabetes
Occupational therapist	Assesses and treats patients with upper extremity amputation, monitors readiness for prosthetic fitting, recommends components
	Assists with problem solving in activities of daily living for patients with upper or lower limb amputations
	Makes recommendations for environmental modification and assistive/adaptive equipment to facilitate functional independence
Social worker	Provides financial counseling and coordination of support services
	Acts as liaison with third-party payers and community agencies
	Assists with patient's and family's social, psychological, and financial issues
Dietitian	Evaluates nutritional status and provides nutritional counseling, especially for patients with diabetes or heart disease or those who are on chemotherapy or are recovering from trauma
Nurse/Nurse practitioner	Monitors patient's health and functional status during rehabilitation
	Provides ongoing patient education on comorbid and chronic health issues
	Monitors condition of remaining extremity for patients with PVD, neuropathy, or diabetes
Vocational counselor	Assesses patient's employment status and potential
	Assists with education, training, and placement

Modified from May B. Assessment and treatment of individuals following lower extremity amputation. In O'Sullivan SB, Schmitz TJ (eds), *Physical Rehabilitation: Assessment and Treatment.* Philadelphia: F.A. Davis, 1994. p. 379.

SUMMARY

Although the rehabilitation process after amputation presents many challenges for patients, their families, and the professionals involved in their care, it also allows many opportunities for success and rewards. Understanding the risk factors for amputation and the influence of comorbid disease and age on progression of rehabilitation is important. Optimal outcome after amputation is best achieved through the interaction of a patient-centered, multidisciplinary health care team.[36] With effective rehabilitation and prosthetic care, most individuals with amputation can return to a level of activity and lifestyle similar to their preamputation status.

REFERENCES

1. Sanders GT, May BJ. *Lower Limb Amputations: A Guide to Rehabilitation.* Philadelphia: F.A. Davis, 1988. pp. 12-53.
2. Limb Loss Research and Statistics Program, Summer 2000;1(1):1-5.
3. Bild DE, Selby JV, Sinnock P, et al. Lower extremity amputation in people with diabetes: epidemiology and prevention. *Diabetes Care* 1989;12(1):24-31.
4. Green GV, Short K, Easley M. Transtibial amputation. Prosthetic use and functional outcome. *Foot Ankle Clin* 2001;6(2):315-327.
5. Ephraim PL, Dillingham TR, Sector M, et al. Epidemiology of limb loss and congenital limb deficiency: a review of the literature. *Arch Phys Med Rehabil* 2003;84:747-761.
6. Group TG. Epidemiology of lower extremity amputation in centers in Europe, North America, and East Asia. The global lower extremity amputation group. *Br J Surg* 2000;87(3): 328-337.
7. Unwin N. Global lower extremity amputation study. Progress report. Retrieved September 7, 2003, at http://www.ncl.ac.uk/hopst/hopst_gleas.htm.
8. Dillingham TR, Pezzin LE, Mackenzie EJ. Limb amputation and limb deficiency: epidemiology and recent trends in the United States. *South Med J* 2002;95(8):875-883.
9. Shurr DG, Michael JW. Introduction to prosthetics and orthotics. In *Prosthetics and Orthotics,* 2nd ed. Norwalk, CT: Appleton & Lange, 2000. pp. 1-19.
10. US Department of Congress, Bureau of the Census. *Projection of the Total Resident Population by Five Year Age Groups, and Sex with Special Age Categories. Middle Series.* Washington, DC: US Department of Congress, Bureau of the Census, 2000.
11. Meltzer DD, Pels S, Payne WG, et al. Decreasing amputation rates in patients with diabetes mellitus. An outcome study. *J Am Podiatr Med Assoc* 2002;92(8):425-428.
12. Centers for Disease Control. Hospital discharge rates for non-traumatic lower extremity amputation by diabetes status-United States, 1997. *Mor Mortal Wkly Rep CDC Surveill Summ* 2001;50(43);954-958.
13. Kannel WB, McGee DL. Diabetes and glucose tolerance as risk factors for cardiovascular disease: the Framingham study. *Diabetes Care* 1979;2(2):120-126.
14. Reiber GE, Boyko EJ, Smith DG. Lower extremity foot ulcers and amputations in diabetes. In Harris MI, Cowie CC, Stern MP, et al (eds). *Diabetes in America,* 2nd ed. Washington, DC: U.S. Dept of Health and Human Services, NIH, DHHS Pub No. 95-1468, 1995. pp. 409-427.
15. Humphry LL, Palumbo PJ, Butters MA, et al. The contribution of non-insulin dependent diabetes to lower-extremity amputation in the community. *Arch Intern Med* 1994;154(8): 885-892.
16. May B. Assessment and treatment of individuals following lower extremity amputation. In O'Sullivan SB, Schmitz TJ (eds), *Physical Rehabilitation: Assessment and Treatment,* 4th ed. Philadelphia: F.A. Davis, 2001. pp. 619-644.
17. Centers for Disease Control. Lower extremity amputations among persons with diabetes mellitus—Washington, 1988. *Mor Mortal Wkly Rep CDC Surveill Summ* 1991;40(43): 737-739.
18. Fylling CP, Knighton DR. Amputation in the diabetic population: incidence, causes, cost, treatment, and prevention. *J Enterostom Ther* 1989;16(6):247-255.
19. Centers for Disease Control and Prevention. *Diabetes Surveillance, 1993.* Atlanta: US Department of Health and Human Services, 1993. pp. 87-93.
20. Mast BA. Epidemiology of diabetic amputations, Division of Plastic and Reconstructive Surgery, Department of Surgery, University of Florida, Gainesville. Available at http:/www.medinfo.utl.edu/cme/grounds/mast/slide37.html.
21. Centers for Disease Control. Lower extremity amputation episodes among persons with diabetes—New Mexico, 2000. *Mor Mortal Wkly Rep CDC Surveill Summ* 2003;52(4);66-68.
22. Dillingham TR, Pezzin LE, Mackenzie EJ. Racial differences in the incidence of limb loss secondary to peripheral vascular disease: a population-based study. *Arch Phys Med Rehabil* 2002;83:1252-1257.
23. Centers for Disease Control. *CDC Reports that Hispanics Are Diagnosed with Diabetes at Twice the Rate of Whites.* Atlanta: National Center for Chronic Disease Prevention and Health, Division of Media Relations, January 15, 1999.
24. Nelson RG, Ghodes DM, Everhart JE, et al. Lower extremity amputation in NIDDM: 12-year follow-up study in Pima Indians. *Diabetes Care* 1988;11(1):8-16.
25. Valway SE, Linkins RW, Gohdes DM. Epidemiology of lower-extremity amputations in the Indian Health Service, 1982-1987. *Diabetes Care* 1993;16(1):349-353.
26. Coleman PG. Lower limb amputation and diabetes: the key is prevention. *MJA* 2000;173:341-342.
27. Brown LW. Traumatic amputation. *AAOHN J* 1990;38(10):483-486.
28. LaQuaglia MP. Osteosarcoma: specific tumor management and results. *Chest Surg Clin N Am* 1998;8(1):77-95.
29. Gover AM, McIvor J. Upper limb deficiencies in infants and young children. *Inf Young Child* 992;5(1):58-72.
30. May BJ. The child with amputation. In *Amputations and Prosthetics: A Case Study Approach,* 2nd ed, Philadelphia: F.A. Davis, 2002. pp. 255-268.
31. Esquenazi A. Geriatric amputee rehabilitation. *Clin Geriatr Med* 1993;9(4):731-743.
32. Fletcher DD, Andrews KL, Hallett JW, et al. Trends in rehabilitation after amputation for geriatric patients with vascular disease: implications for future health resource allocation. *Arch Phys Med Rehabil* 2002;83(10):1389-1393.

33. Ham R, de Trafford J, Van de Ven C. Patterns of recovery for lower limb amputations. *Clin Rehabil* 1994;8(4):320-328.
34. Dillingham TR, Pezzin LE, Mackenzie EJ, Burgess AR. Use and satisfaction with prosthetic devices among persons with trauma-related amputations: a long-term outcome study. *Am J Phys Med Rehabil* 2001;80(8):563-71.
35. Scremin AM, Tapia JI, Vichick DA, et al. Effect of age on progression through temporary prostheses after below-knee amputation. *Am J Phys Med Rehabil* 1993;72(6):350-354.
36. Osterman H. The process of amputation and rehabilitation. *Clin Podiatr Med Surg* 1997;14(4):585-97.

21

Conservative Management of the High-Risk Foot

Carolyn B. Kelly

LEARNING OBJECTIVES

At the conclusion of this chapter the reader will be able to do the following:

1. Explain the relationship between diabetes and foot ulceration.
2. Identify the interactive factors that contribute to ulceration in the high-risk foot.
3. Describe the components of an effective high-risk foot examination.
4. Compare and contrast the efficacy and drawbacks of the most commonly used options for reducing pressure to promote ulcer healing and prevention.
5. Appreciate the impact that diabetic neuropathy has on balance and gait.
6. Apply one's understanding of risk category to formulate an effective plan of care to prevent foot ulceration.

Treatment of foot wounds is not new to rehabilitation professionals. For many years, clients with such problems have been referred for traditional physical therapy treatment, including whirlpool, debridement, and dressing changes. Originally, many of these patients were instructed in crutch walking or asked to limit ambulation to protect their vulnerable feet. Although some of their wounds healed, many recurred when the patient returned to function under the same conditions that caused the original problem. Unfortunately, some patients were referred for treatment of wounds so advanced that conservative intervention was unlikely to make a difference. Physical therapists began asking, "Couldn't something have been done earlier in the process to prevent this foot from getting so bad?" When whirlpool treatments resulted in little progress, physical therapists raised the question, "Can't something more effective be done?" The answer to both questions is *yes,* and such interventions are the focus of this chapter.

HIGH-RISK FOOT

A patient with a high-risk foot has an underlying disease process that places the soft tissues of the foot at greater than normal risk for damage. The smallest opening in the skin becomes a potential portal of entry for bacteria, which can lead to deep infection and ultimately amputation.

Diabetes mellitus, although not the only cause, is the diagnosis most frequently associated with foot ulceration and lower extremity amputation. A reported 6% of hospital discharges between 1983 and 1990 in persons with diabetes were associated with a foot ulcer problem.[1] Individuals with diabetes have a 15% risk of developing a foot ulcer sometime in their lives,[1] with foot ulcers preceding an estimated 85% of lower extremity amputations in diabetic patients.[2] The Centers for Disease Control and Prevention reported that of the total number of nontraumatic lower amputations in the United States in 2001, approximately 60% (82,000) were performed on patients with diabetes and accounted for 924,000 hospital days.[3] If the high cost of medical care is considered, the impact on the health care dollar is tremendous.[1] Just as important, however, is the impact on the quality of life of the patient with diabetes, who may be left with compromised function, permanent disability, and an increased risk of mortality.

A physical therapist's role in treating patients with high-risk feet is to manage their functional rehabilitation programs and participate in the examination, evaluation, treatment, and prevention of foot ulcerations that tend to occur in this population. Before one can establish an appropriate plan of care for a patient with a foot ulcer, one must have a basic understanding of the disease processes that cause them. The two disease processes most commonly linked to foot wounds are peripheral vascular disease (PVD) and peripheral neuropathy.[1,2,4]

Many individuals, health care practitioners included, erroneously assume that all patients with diabetes have poor circulation and that most diabetic foot problems are due to vascular compromise. Similarly, many patients with diabetes, when questioned about their circulation, report that it is poor. When asked how they know this, they may answer, "because I am diabetic" or "because my feet feel cold." Patients with diabetes do have a much greater than normal risk for development of vascular disease, and vascular disease alone can cause tissue breakdown or impair wound healing.[5] Therefore vascular screening is an important part of a high-risk foot examination. However, poor circulation, though a common complicating factor, is not the *primary* cause of most diabetic foot ulcers. Most can be attributed to a combination of increased mechanical stress on the foot and sensory loss due to neuropathy.[2,6,7]

Mechanical Stress

Plantar ulceration has been associated with lower extremity peripheral neuropathy and excessive plantar pressures.[8-11] Pressure on the soft tissues of the foot is related to three variables: the magnitude of the force applied to the foot, the amount of surface over which the force is applied, and the length of time over which the force is sustained.[6] Because much of the focus in treating and preventing foot ulcers is on reducing pressure, one must understand the relationship of pressure to these three variables. The following formula should be considered:

$$\text{Pressure} = \text{Force/Area}$$

As indicated, anything that increases the magnitude of the force applied to the foot or decreases the area over which the force is applied increases pressure and makes tissue damage more likely. Immediate injury can occur from extremely high force applied over a small area, as when a patient steps on a tack or piece of glass. Injury occurs because tremendously high pressure exceeds the tensile strength of the skin. Pressure on the foot can also become excessive when a moderate amount of force is repeatedly applied over a small surface area—when bony deformities cause small localized areas of weight bearing or when partial foot amputations decrease the patient's weight-bearing surface. The force applied to the foot (body weight) remains essentially the same, but the actual pressure on the tissues is greater because of reduction of the surface area. In patients with diabetes, factors such as limited joint mobility,[12-16] structural abnormalities,[17-19] and previous amputation[20,21] can lead to increased force or decreased surface area. All of these have been associated with increased plantar pressures and ulceration.

Further complicating this picture is the time factor. In looking at tissue ischemia and resultant ulceration, Kosiak[22] found an inverse relationship between the amount of pressure applied to tissues and length of time that the pressure was sustained (Figure 21-1). Low pressures sustained over long periods of time caused tissue necrosis. This is the mechanism of tissue injury when decubitus ulceration occurs in bedridden, poorly mobile patients. Tissue necrosis also occurs along the medial or lateral borders of the feet or tops of hammer toes when patients wear shoes that are too tight. Kosiak found that as the magnitude of pressure increased, fewer hours were necessary to induce injury.

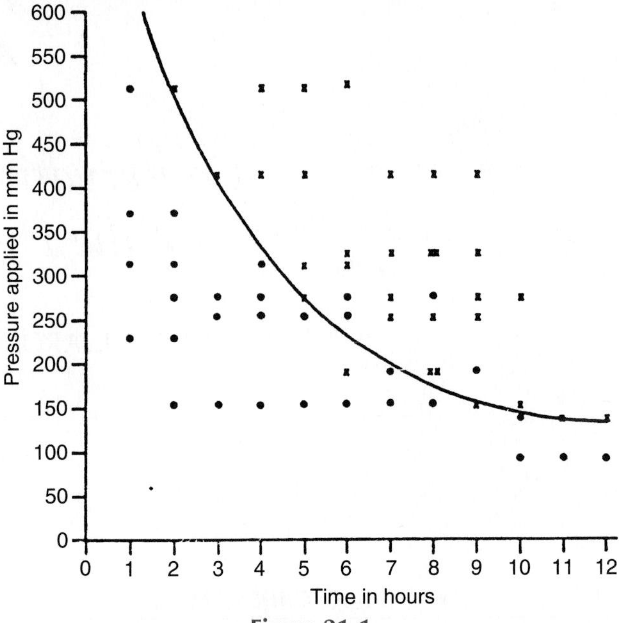

Figure 21-1
Results of Kosiak's experiments on dogs show an inverse relationship between the amount of pressure applied and the time that it takes to cause ischemic necrosis. x, *ulceration;* •, *no ulceration. (From Kosiak M. Etiology and pathology of ischemic ulcers.* Arch Phys Med Rehabil *1959;40[2]:62-69.)*

The most common cause of skin breakdown in the neuropathic foot is repeated bouts of moderate pressure during everyday walking.[23] This was demonstrated by Brand[6]: Using foot pads of anesthetized rats, he demonstrated that repeated bouts of moderate pressure caused inflammatory changes. With continued repetition, this inflammation progressed to ulceration. For health professionals who care for patients with diabetic foot problems, two facts from this research hold particular significance. First, when the inflammatory changes (heat and swelling) began to persist from one day to the next, breakdown of the tissue was prevented by discontinuing the repeated stress. Second, breakdown was prevented by either decreasing the amount of pressure per repetition or by reducing the number of repetitions. The findings of Brand and Kosiak suggest that the variables of force, area, and time and repetition contribute to tissue breakdown and that changing one or more of these variables must be considered in the treatment plan for patients with a high-risk foot.

Neuropathy

Peripheral neuropathy has many causes and types.[24,25] Although peripheral neuropathy is frequently related to patients with diabetes, Box 21-1 demonstrates the numerous diagnoses that can result in a neuropathic limb. This chapter refers frequently to the patient with diabetes, yet the rehabilitation practitioner should remember that nondiabetic patients with neuropathic feet are likely to be seen in any setting. A foot that does not feel, regardless of the etiology of sensory impairment, is a foot at risk and needs to be managed as such. In diabetes the most common type of neuropathy is a distal symmetric polyneuropathy.[24] Although there is agreement that the etiology of diabetic neuropathy is multifactorial, diabetic neuropathy is not fully understood and further delineation of causes is still needed.[26,27] Its clinical manifestations often include *sensory, motor,* and *autonomic* components that affect the feet.[25-27]

Sensory Dysfunction in Neuropathy

Patients with neuropathy often experience sensory changes as their initial symptoms. Common subjective complaints are "numbness" and "cold feet" (however, on clinical examination, the feet are often warm to the touch and well perfused). Pain descriptors may include "stabbing," "pins and needles," "shooting," "electric shock," or "lancinating." Muscular complaints described as "night cramps," "spasms," or "aching" may also be present. Pain is often worse at rest, particularly at night.

The pain of neuropathy must be distinguished from the pain associated with arterial disease. *Intermittent claudication* is a cramping or aching pain that occurs most commonly in the calves of patients with peripheral arterial disease. It occurs in response to walking and is relieved when the patient stops. In contrast, walking often improves or diminishes *neuropathic pain.* Patients with more significant arterial disease may experience rest pain, usually worse at night. Elevation makes the pain worse, although placing the foot in a dependent position brings relief. Elevation or dependent positioning has little impact on neuropathic pain.

The patient with neuropathy often has objective signs of sensory loss in addition to subjective symptoms. These are of particular concern, because patients with such sensory deficits may not perceive dangerous conditions that are injuring their feet. Individuals with normal sensation immediately take action to relieve the source of discomfort, sustaining only minor, if any, skin damage. The patient with sensory loss, on the other hand, is not aware of the need to take action and unknowingly walks a significant wound into the foot. Patients with a foot ulcer often report, "I didn't know anything was wrong until I saw a blood stain on my sock."

Many objective tests can assist in the diagnosis of diabetic neuropathy.[26] These include electrodiagnostic tests (nerve conduction velocities and electromyography) and quantitative sensory measures (current, thermal, and vibratory perception

Box 21-1 *Diseases and Processes That Result in a Neuropathic Foot*

NEUROPATHY ASSOCIATED WITH SYSTEMIC DISEASES
Diabetes mellitus
Uremia
Amyloidosis

NEUROPATHY ASSOCIATED WITH NUTRITIONAL DISTURBANCES
Alcoholism
Pernicious anemia

NEUROPATHY ASSOCIATED WITH INFECTIOUS DISEASE
Leprosy
Syphilis
Poliomyelitis

NEUROPATHY ON A VASCULAR BASIS
Cerebrovascular accident
Spinal cord infarction
Diabetic mononeuropathy
Arteritis
Peripheral vascular disease

HEREDITARY MOTOR AND SENSORY NEUROPATHY
Roussy-Lévy syndrome
Charcot-Marie-Tooth disease

HEREDITARY SENSORY AND AUTONOMIC NEUROPATHY
Hereditary sensory neuropathy
Congenital sensory neuropathy
Dysautonomia (Riley-Day syndrome)

CEREBELLAR DEGENERATION
Friedreich's ataxia

MOTOR NEURON DISEASE
Amyotrophic lateral sclerosis

DISEASES OF THE SPINAL CORD
Spina bifida
Syringomyelia

TRAUMA
Spinal cord injury
Peripheral nerve injury
Spinal root trauma

COMPRESSIVE NEUROPATHY
Spinal cord tumor
Peripheral nerve compression

TOXIC NEUROPATHY
Lead poisoning

OTHER CAUSES
Cerebral palsy

From Heartherington VJ. The neuropathic foot. In McGlamry ED, Banks AS, Downey MS (eds), *Comprehensive Textbook of Foot Surgery,* 2nd ed. Baltimore: Williams & Wilkins, 1992.

threshold testing and quantitative esthesiometry). Physical therapists who focus on treating and preventing foot wounds in the high-risk population use sensory testing to identify patients whose sensory deficits correlate with risk for ulceration. Of the sensory modalities, increased vibratory perception thresholds[11,28-32] and loss of protective sensation[4,13,30-34] are strong indicators of risk for ulceration in the neuropathic foot.

An instrument used to measure vibratory perception thresholds is the biothesiometer (Biomedical Instrument Co., Newbury, Ohio), an electronic device that delivers varying degrees of vibration to the foot. The point at which the patient begins to feel the vibration is his or her vibratory perception threshold.

The term *protective sensation* describes the amount of sensation necessary for individuals to protect themselves from tissue trauma. In 1986 Birke and Sims[33] used Semmes-Weinstein sensory monofilaments to define quantitatively protective sensation in a group of patients diagnosed with Hansen's disease or with diabetes who had a history of foot ulcers. Semmes-Weinstein filaments are a set of progressively thicker nylon filaments (much like those of a nylon hairbrush), with one end embedded into a handle. When sufficient pressure is applied against the tip of the filament, the filament bends (Figure 21-2). Each test probe in the set is calibrated so that a different and defined amount of force is necessary to bend the filament. The thinner the nylon is, the lower the amount of pressure is necessary to make it bend.

Using a set of three monofilaments, labeled by the manufacturer as 4.17, 5.07, and 6.1 and equal to a buckling force of 1 g, 10 g, and 75 g, respectively, Birke and Sims tested 100 patients (72 with Hansen's disease, 28 with diabetes) with the presence or history of plantar ulceration. No patient sensed the 5.07 (10 g) monofilament. The authors concluded that the ability to perceive the 5.07 monofilament was consistent with the presence of protective sensation. Similar studies in patients with diabetes have confirmed this definition.[4,13,30-35] Overall, research using the Semmes-Weinstein monofilaments has determined that they are a valid and reliable tool for identifying patients who are at risk for foot ulceration.[36] The fact that they are inexpensive, quite portable, and easy to use makes them ideal for use in the clinic.

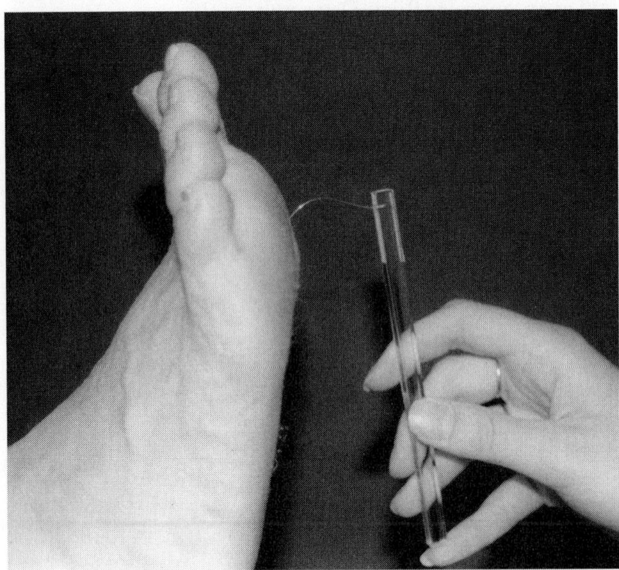

Figure 21-2
A monofilament is used to test protective sensation on the sole of the foot. The filament is held perpendicularly to the skin surface, and pressure is applied until the monofilament buckles. The number associated with the smallest-diameter filament perceived at each site is recorded.

Motor Dysfunction in Neuropathy

The second component of polyneuropathy is damage to the motor nerves. Motor neuropathy causes weakness of the muscles of the foot and leg, which alters the pattern of force on the foot during walking.[7] At times such weakness is obvious by observing the patient's gait. For instance, in a peroneal neuropathy, weakness of ankle dorsiflexors causes the foot to contact the ground in a plantar-flexed position. The result is increased pressure on the plantar forefoot. Stretching tight plantar flexors and using an ankle foot orthosis to reestablish a more normal force pattern are appropriate interventions.

More commonly, motor neuropathy in the patient with diabetes leads to foot deformities caused by muscle imbalances. Such deformities are associated with high plantar pressures. The most common deformity is clawing of the toes. These deformities are result from weakness of intrinsic foot muscles. The classic "intrinsic-minus" foot is characterized by cocked-up toes, prominent extensor tendons, a high arch, and prominent metatarsal heads. The skin underlying the metatarsal heads is vulnerable because it sustains great pressure from plantar flexion of the metatarsals (Figure 21-3),[37] distal migration of the plantar fat pad,[38] and

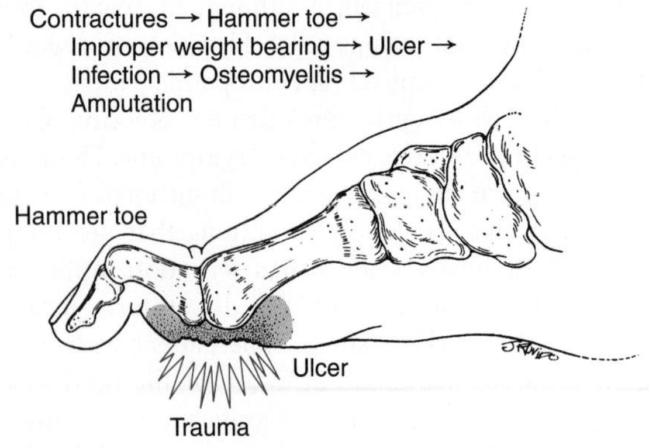

Figure 21-3
Progression of motor neuropathy and development of an intrinsic minus foot eventually leading to ulceration under the metatarsal heads. (Courtesy Michigan Diabetes Research and Training Center, University of Michigan Hospital, Ann Arbor, 1983.)

changes in the underlying soft tissues.[39-41] The dorsal surfaces of the proximal interphalangeal joint (which may rub against the shoe's toe box) and the distal tips of the toes (which do not tolerate the increased weight-bearing forces) are also vulnerable to breakdown.

Autonomic Dysfunction in Neuropathy

Polyneuropathy may also involve autonomic nerves. Damage to sympathetic nerves causes impairment in sweat gland function and results in reduced hydration of the tissues. The skin of the foot becomes dry, less pliable, and much more prone to fissuring. Fissures can prove devastating to the vulnerable foot because they enable entry of bacteria that can lead to serious infection (Figure 21-4).

Autonomic neuropathy also affects vasomotor regulation in the lower extremities. Loss of sympathetic control causes dilation of the arterioles of the foot, with resulting hyperemia of the soft tissues and bone. Increased bone blood flow and arteriovenous shunting due to autonomic neuropathy are factors in the development of Charcot's arthropathy,[42] a condition that can cause severe bony destruction and leave the patient at high risk for ulceration.

EXAMINATION OF THE NEUROPATHIC FOOT

Numerous factors in addition to those mentioned previously are believed to be related to ulceration and amputation in the vulnerable foot.[1,10,43] In evaluating patients, all of these factors should be considered in order to choose the most appropriate education and interventions. The initial examination serves several purposes:

1. Identify factors that have led to or may lead to soft tissue injury
2. Obtain objective data on which to base a diagnosis, prognosis, and plan of care
3. Establish a baseline with which to compare later data

Patient History

The first component of the examination is a review of the patient's overall medical and surgical history. The patient interview reveals much information, yet not all patients are accurate historians or have a thorough understanding of their medical problems. Information should be verified by the referring clinician or medical record. Questions that are particularly important to consider include the following:

1. Does the patient have diabetes? If so, when was the diabetes diagnosed? How well is blood sugar controlled? How much does it fluctuate? Unexplained, unusually high blood sugars may signal the presence of infection. Patients with diabetes must understand that they are at risk for development of neuropathy and PVD and that these risks increase with the duration of diabetes.[4] A large multicenter study of patients with insulin-dependent diabetes mellitus indicated that patients whose blood glucose levels were intensely and accurately controlled demonstrated significantly less risk of developing the complications of nephropathy, retinopathy, and neuropathy.[45] Patients with foot wounds should be taught that control of blood glucose levels provides a better environment for wound healing.

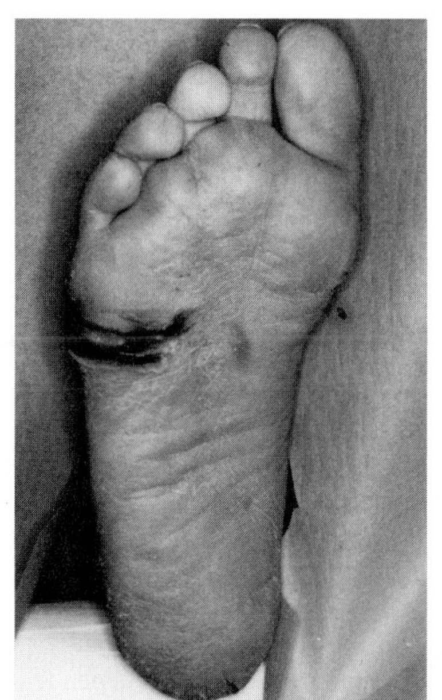
A

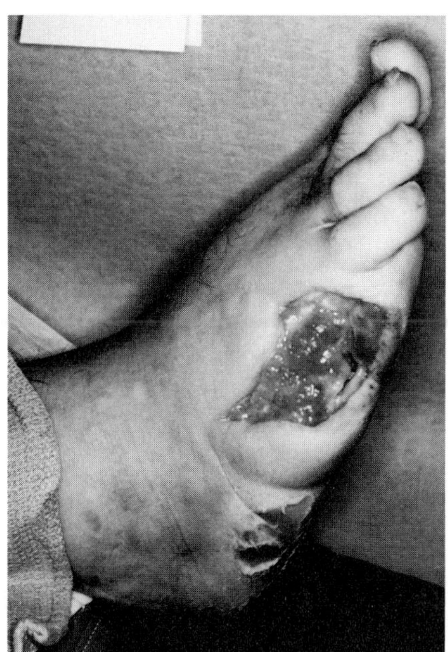
B

Figure 21-4
*What began as a dry fissure (**A**) turned into significant infection that resulted in loss of soft tissue and bone (**B**).*

2. What other systemic diseases are present? How might these contribute to the patient's lower extremity signs and symptoms?
3. What is the patient's foot health history? Has the patient had previous fractures, foot surgeries, ulcerations, or vascular procedures? If a foot ulcer is present, how long has it been there? How has it been treated? Many patients have been appropriately treated with wound debridement and dressings but have failed to heal because pressure relief was not addressed.
4. What diagnostic testing has been done (radiographs, bone scans, vascular studies, and others)? What have the tests revealed?
5. Does the patient complain of pain? How is the pain described? What makes it better or worse? Answers to these questions may help distinguish between neuropathic, vascular, and musculoskeletal causes.
6. What medication is the patient currently taking? Some medication may affect healing or contribute to current symptoms.
7. Does the patient have visual deficits? Patients with a history of neuropathic ulceration may have insufficient visual acuity to examine their feet correctly or to recognize early signs of ulceration.[46]
8. Does neuropathy also affect the hands? If so, patients may be unable to perform their own dressing changes or all parts of a foot self-examination. They may require modifications to footwear to allow for independent donning, making compliance with footwear more likely.
9. What has the patient been using for footwear? Could this be contributing to foot problems? Previous studies have recognized poorly fitting footwear as a precipitating factor in diabetic foot ulceration.[47,48] If the patient has protective footwear, is it being worn both inside and outside of the home?[49]
10. What is the patient's occupation or level of activity? Is it compatible with what the patient's feet will tolerate?
11. Does the patient have a history of falls or note problems with balance or gait that warrant intervention?

Physical Examination

Peripheral arterial disease, sensory neuropathy, foot deformity, prior ulceration,[50] limited range of motion, previous amputation, and poorly fitting footwear are predisposing factors in the development of foot ulceration. With this understanding, certain tests and measures should be undertaken to help recognize the presence of risk factors in patients (Figure 21-5).

Vascular Examination

The combination of sensory loss and mechanical stress is accepted as the most common cause of ulceration in those with high-risk feet. However, since inadequate circulation can both impair healing and be the primary cause of ulceration, it is imperative that vascular screening be part of the high-risk foot examination. Before clinical vascular screening procedures are performed, a number of observations are necessary. If present, they may signal vascular compromise and indicate a need for further workup (Box 21-2).

The vascular examination begins by checking for pulses in the foot. Pulses are palpated at the dorsalis pedis artery on the dorsum of the foot and at the posterior tibial artery located just behind the medial malleolus. If pulses are palpable, the patient likely has adequate blood flow to the foot.

Although lack of palpable pulses is often a sign of peripheral vascular disease, inability to palpate a pulse in the foot does not always mean inadequate blood flow. The extremity may demonstrate reasonably good circulation when further evaluated by Doppler examination or other noninvasive methods. The Doppler examination uses a Doppler stethoscope to auscultate over the dorsalis pedis and posterior tibial arteries. Assessment of blood flow is based on the number of sounds heard with each pulsation. When audible, sounds are triphasic, biphasic, or monophasic (having three sounds, two sounds, or one sound). Triphasic or biphasic sounds are generally indicative of adequate flow. Monophasic sounds indicate compromised circulation and warrant referral of the patient for further noninvasive tests.

Several noninvasive procedures provide general information about the patient's arterial status. The first is the use of *segmental systolic pressures* (Figure 21-6). Systolic blood pressure is measured at various levels along the lower extremities (proximal and distal thigh, upper calf, ankle, and great toe) and at the brachial artery using a standard pneumatic cuff and Doppler probe. The ankle/arm or *ankle/brachial index* (ABI) is defined as the ankle systolic pressure divided by the brachial systolic pressure. The ABI has been used as a general measure of arterial insufficiency. In a normal situation the brachial and ankle systolic pressures are approximately equal so that a normal value for ABI is 1. As blood flow in the lower extremity decreases with arterial insufficiency, ankle pressure decreases. An ABI of less than 0.9 is considered abnormal—the lower the number, the greater the arterial insufficiency. Wound healing is unlikely with ABIs of less than 0.45.[51,52]

Box 21-2 *Clinical Signs of Peripheral Vascular Disease*

- Absent pulses
- Cold feet
- Dependent rubor
- Shiny skin
- Intermittent claudication
- Loss of hair on leg and foot
- Atrophy of subcutaneous fat
- Rest pain relieved with dependency
- Delayed capillary filling time
- Ischemic lesions

OCHSNER FOOT CARE PROGRAM
DIABETIC PATIENT PHYSICAL EXAM

DATE____________________
NAME____ PATIENT NUMBER_____________________________

PHYSICAL APPEARANCE: Foot type________________________________Color________________________

Nails____

Plantarflexed 1st ray R___ L___ Plantarflexed lesser metatarsal R______ L______

LIMITATION OF ANKLE DORSIFLEXION: knee ext. R=___ L=___ knee flex. R=___ L= ___
SUBTALAR JOINT ROM: R____________________ L____________________
REARFOOT:_________________________ FOREFOOT:__________________________

Manual Muscle Test:

Anterior tibial	R____ L____	Drop Foot R_____ L_____
Extensor hallucis longus	R____ L____	
Flexor hallucis longus	R____ L____	Intrinsics R_____ L_____
Posterior tibial	R____ L____	
Peroneus longus	R____ L____	
Gastoc/Soleus	R____ L____	

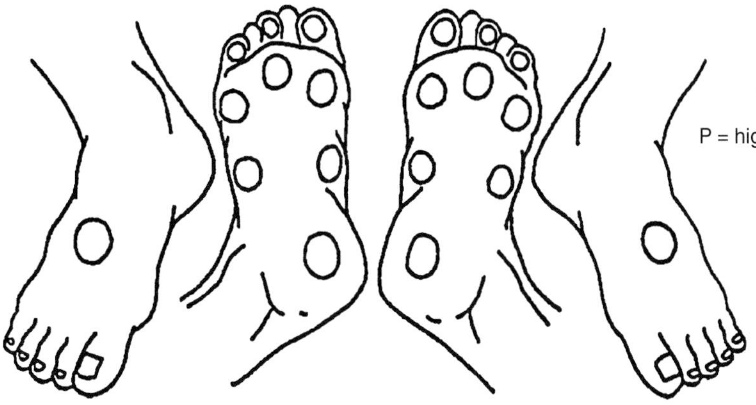

D = dryness
S = swelling
R = redness
n = temp. deg. C
callous
P = high pressure point

H = Hammered M = Mallet C = Clawed PU = Previous ulcer site

Sensory Test (Semmes-Weinstein): 1 = 1 gram 2 = 10 grams 3 = 75 grams 4 = No perception 75 grams
Toes L___ R___ Forefoot L___ R___ Heel L___ R___ Ankle L___ R___
Biothesiometer: R________________________ L________________________

PEDAL PULSES: Right: DP___ PT___ Left: DP___ PT___
Ankle/brachial index: R____ L____ After one-minute excercise: R_____ L_____
Footwear: Describe____

Figure 21-5

A foot evaluation form helps to structure the foot examination and allows for easy recording of data. (From Coleman WC, Birke JA. The initial foot examination of the patient with diabetes. In Kominsky SJ [ed], Medical and Surgical Management of the Diabetic Foot. *St. Louis: Mosby-Year Book, 1994. p. 12.)*

Patients with diabetes often have stiff lower extremity vessels because of calcification of the medial arterial walls. Because of this stiffness, greater pressure from the blood pressure cuff is necessary to compress the arteries. Systolic pressure measurements may then be artificially elevated and the ABI inaccurate.[51,53] Because of this, additional measurements are included in the noninvasive examination.

The *pulse volume recorder* measures variations in the arterial volume at a particular limb segment during each cardiac cycle.[54] These variations are represented by the waveforms that they produce (Figure 21-7). As blood flow deteriorates, the wave forms begin to flatten. For a patient with diabetes and arterial insufficiency, the ABI could be read as normal as a result of vessel calcification, but flattening of the pulse volume recorder tracing would identify abnormal flow. Because medial arterial calcinosis is less likely to affect the digital arteries, toe systolic pressure is considered a more accurate measure than ankle systolic pressure in patients with diabetes.[53,55]

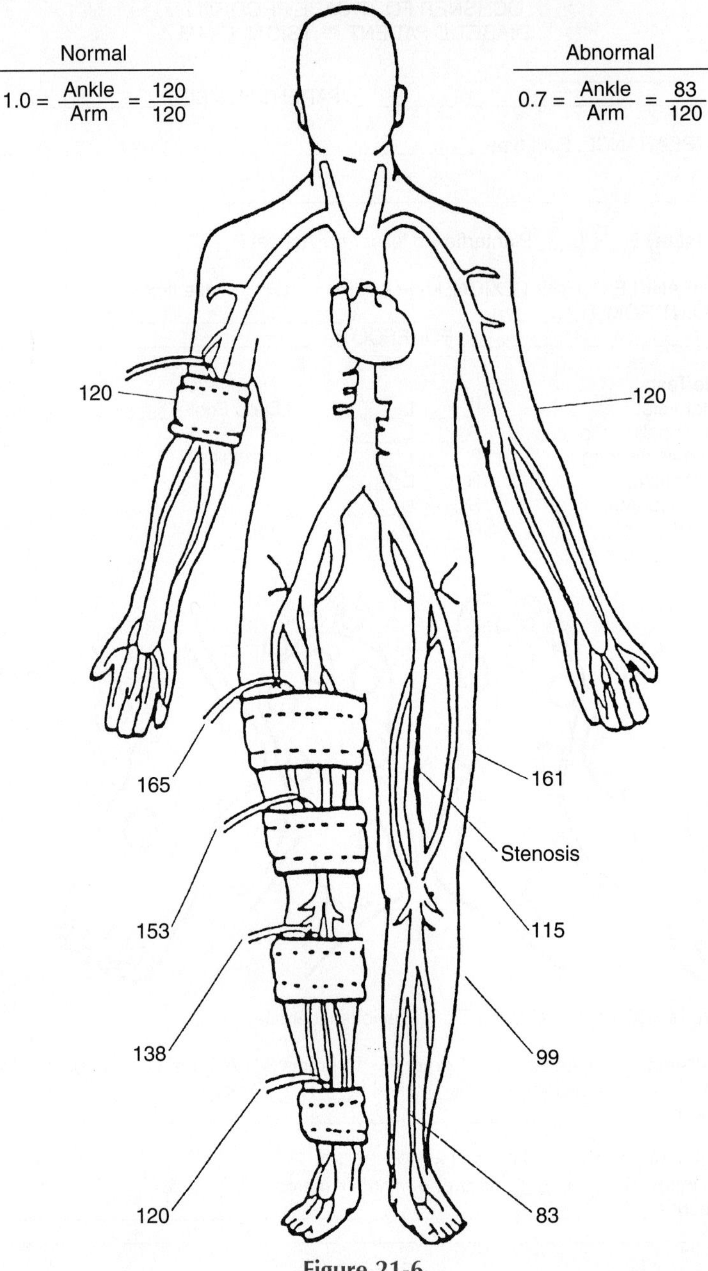

Figure 21-6

Segmental systolic pressures show a normal condition on the left. A 0.7 ankle/brachial index on the right indicates a reduction in flow. Also of note is the greater than 30 mm Hg drop in pressure between two successive thigh cuffs, which indicates stenosis or occlusion of the segment. (From Hoffman AF. Evaluation of arterial blood flow in the lower extremity. In Robbins J [ed], Clinics in Podiatric Medicine, Surgery, and Peripheral Vascular Disease. *Philadelphia: Saunders, 1999. p. 42.)*

Low *transcutaneous oxygen pressure measurement* ($TcPO_2$), a measurement of skin perfusion, has been shown to be a predictor of ulceration[4] and healing.[56] In 1999 the American Diabetes Association's Consensus Development Conference on Diabetic Foot Wound Care recommended use of abnormal toe systolic pressures and $TcPO_2$ measurements to predict poor outcomes.[57] Generally, no single noninvasive test provides enough information to make decisions about vascular intervention. Analysis is usually done by a vascular specialist who interprets the results of a combination of tests.

If signs of arterial insufficiency are present and the patient has a foot wound, or if the patient has none of the typical symptoms of ischemia but has a nonhealing wound despite adequate control of infection and external pressure, referral for further vascular evaluation is warranted. Many patients have significant arterial disease but few clinical signs, such as

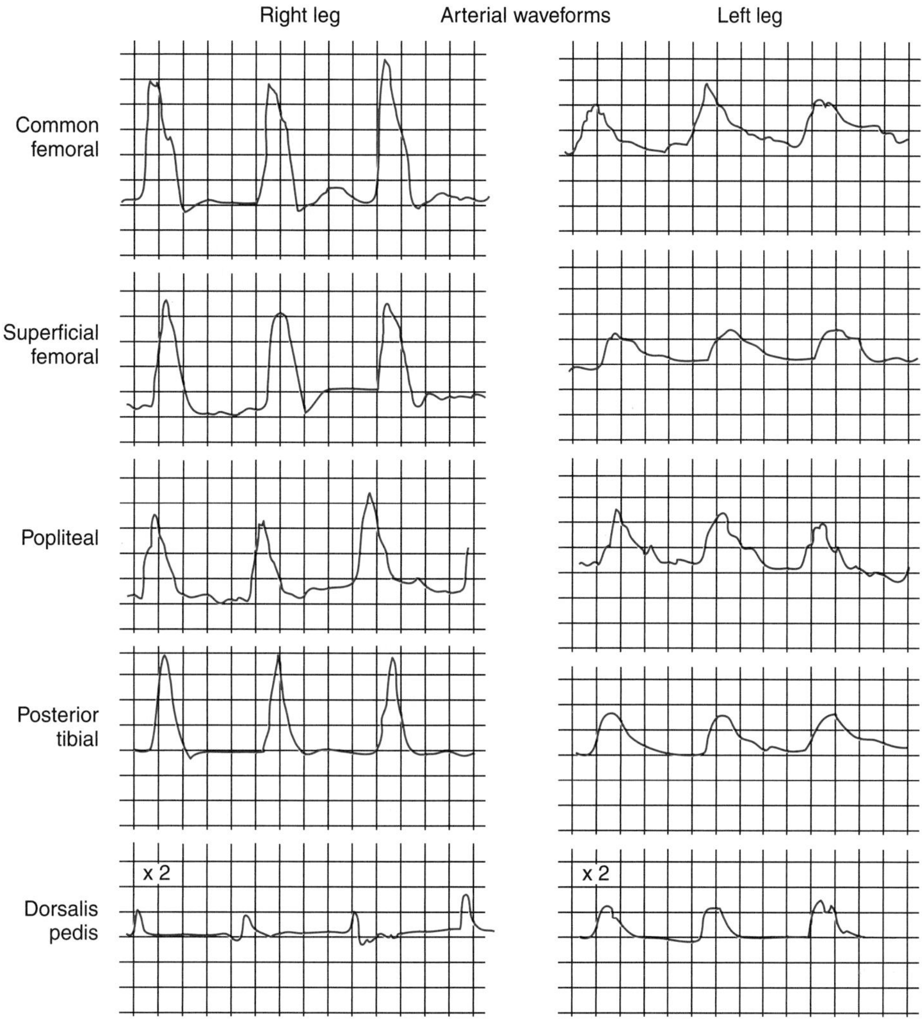

Figure 21-7

Doppler waveform analysis. The right leg waveforms show normal triphasic Doppler flow signals. The left leg, with pronounced occlusive peripheral vascular disease, shows monophasic waves that are diminished in amplitude. (From Jarrett F. Vascular Surgery of the Lower Extremity, *St. Louis: Mosby, 1985. p. 14.)*

pain or open wounds, that warrant the risks involved with an invasive vascular procedure. They should still be educated in foot care and proper shoe fit. Because better circulation may be necessary to heal an open wound than to keep unbroken skin intact, the goal for patients with arterial insufficiency is to prevent foot wounds from occurring.

Sensory Examination

Commonly, patients with significant ulcerations on the plantar surfaces of the feet walk into the clinic without any discomfort. Specialized tests are unnecessary to determine that sensory impairment is present. Many of these individuals are completely unaware of their sensory deficits. Sensory neuropathy does not affect all forms of sensation equally. The ability to feel something touch or brush against the foot may be retained while protective sensation is lost. Because a patient can feel the touch of a hand on his or her foot or the friction of a sock being pulled on, he or she may assume that sensation is normal. Standard tests of light touch and pressure do not reflect the actual risk for ulceration. The sensory examination must include those sensory measures that indicate risk.

Increased vibratory perception thresholds and the absence of protective sensation are the neurological impairments most highly correlated with the development of foot ulcers. Quantitative assessment of at least one of these functions is an essential part of the physical examination.

Vibratory perception thresholds are assessed with a biothesiometer, a hand-held device with a rubber tractor that vibrates at 100 Hz. The patient is positioned prone with the dorsum of the feet supported and the plantar surfaces facing up. The tractor is balanced vertically against the plantar surface of the hallux. The voltage is increased until the patient feels the vibration, and the corresponding number on the unit scale

(0 to 50) is recorded. Three trials are performed, with the speed of voltage increase varied with each trial. The average of the three trials is considered the vibratory perception threshold at that site. Risk of ulceration has been associated with a threshold of greater than 25 volts and increases as threshold values rise.[11,28,29]

Protective sensation is assessed by the use of Semmes-Weinstein sensory monofilaments.[33,34] Before the test is performed, the patient is shown a monofilament, and the test is demonstrated on an area of the body that is known to have intact sensation. This assures the patient that the monofilament will not puncture the skin and allows him or her to experience the type of stimulus to which he or she is being asked to respond. The test is performed with the patient supine; the eyes are closed or blindfolded. The monofilament is applied perpendicularly to the plantar surface (see Figure 21-2) with enough force to make the filament buckle as follows: 1-second touch, 1-second hold, 1-second lift.[33] Typical test areas include the plantar surfaces of the first, third, and fifth metatarsal heads and tips of the corresponding toes; the medial and lateral midfoot; the heel; and the dorsum of the foot (see Figure 21-5). The patient is instructed to say "yes" each time the touch of the filament is felt but needs not localize the stimulus. If the patient cannot perceive a particular stimulus in four of five of the trials (80%), he or she is retested with the next higher filament. The smallest filament to which the patient responds at least 80% of the time is the threshold value.[13,36] Threshold values can vary across areas of the foot that are being tested.

When using the monofilaments, care must be taken to avoid calluses, which could interfere with the pressure perception. The timing between each stimulus should be randomized to minimize patient guessing based on rhythm. The filament should not be allowed to slide, as many patients can sense this sliding but are unable to feel the filament when it is properly applied. Protective sensation has been described as the ability to perceive the 5.07 monofilament.[4,13,33-35] Using this monofilament is appropriate when screening for the presence of protective sensation. Use of other monofilaments (4.17 and 6.10) allows physical therapists to document improvement or progression of the sensory loss.

Musculoskeletal Examination

Patients with diabetes who have neuropathy tend to have abnormally high plantar pressures compared to diabetic and nondiabetic controls without neuropathy, and those with a previous history of ulceration show these high pressures at the former ulcer sites.[7-9,58] High plantar pressure is considered a risk factor in neuropathic foot ulceration. Limited joint mobility[14,15,59,60] and foot deformity[16-18] contribute to high plantar pressures. Therefore tests that look for abnormalities in strength, range of motion, and biomechanics are important. Higher plantar pressures are also related to the presence of toe or partial foot amputations.[20,21]

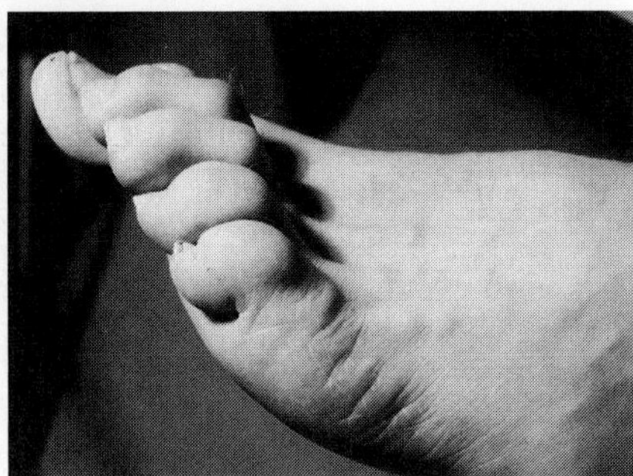

Figure 21-8
Claw toe deformity commonly seen in patients with diabetes.

Numerous deformities should be considered when one performs the musculoskeletal evaluation. These deformities often alter weight-bearing pressure enough to predispose the patient with insensitive or dysvascular feet to soft tissue damage. They include hammer and claw toes, hallux valgus, hallux rigidus, hallux limitus, plantar-flexed first ray, prominent bones on the plantar surface, ankle equinus, partial foot resections and amputations, and deformities due to Charcot's. Hammertoes and claw toes cause localized pressure at the tips of the distal phalanges, at the dorsum of the toes, or under the metatarsal heads (Figure 21-8). It has been generally accepted that in patients with diabetes, these deformities are due to intrinsic muscle weakness associated with motor neuropathy. A recent report suggests disruption of the plantar fascia as a possible cause.[60] In weight bearing, these deformities decrease loading under the toes while increasing loading under the metatarsal heads.[7,58]

Deformities that involve the first metatarsophalangeal (MTP) joint include hallux valgus and hallux limitus. Hallux valgus is characterized by marked lateral drifting of the great toe and prominence of the medial surface of the first metatarsal head. As a result, crowding of the forefoot and hammer toeing or overlapping of the lesser toes occur.[61] Excessive medial metatarsal head pressure from a toe box that is too narrow for the foot is a common problem.

Hallux limitus or hallux rigidus is marked by limited extension of the first MTP joint and is associated with ulceration of the plantar surface of the hallux.[14] With normal walking, this joint must dorsiflex to at least 45 degrees as body weight moves over the forefoot in terminal stance and preswing.[62] Limitation in range of motion causes increased pressure on the plantar surface of the interphalangeal joint. The interphalangeal joint may become overstretched and hyperextended as it compensates for limited MTP motion.

The first ray is considered plantar flexed when limited dorsiflexion of the first metatarsal causes the metatarsal head to sit plantarly in relation to the relative plane of the lesser metatarsal heads (Figure 21-9). This position is related to high pressure and ulceration.[16] Any of the bones of the feet's plantar surface may be prominent in relation to the others and a likely target for future ulceration. In the plantar

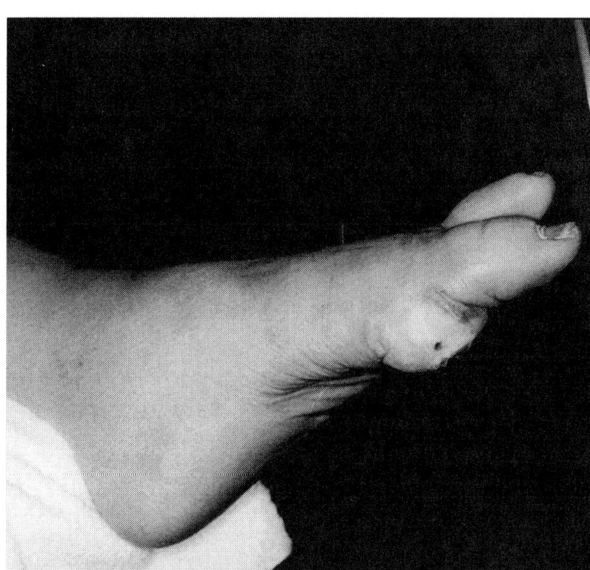

Figure 21-9
This first ray is plantar flexed in relation to the others, causing excessive pressure and leading to ulceration under the first metatarsal head.

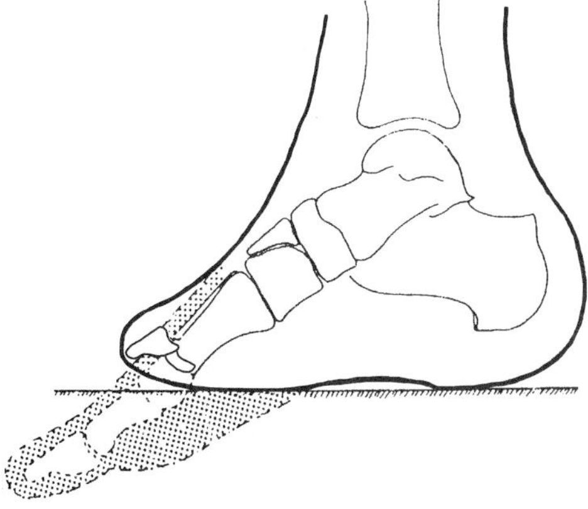

Figure 21-10
Tracings of superimposed radiographs showing hidden equinus in a shortened foot (nonshaded) compared with the contralateral normal foot (shaded). (From Birke JA, Sims DS. The insensitive foot. In Hunt GC [ed], Physical Therapy of the Foot and Ankle. *New York: Churchill Livingstone, 1988. pp. 133-168.)*

forefoot, prominence of the metatarsal heads is common. The joint destruction of Charcot's arthropathy often causes abnormal bony prominences in the midfoot.[63] The plantar prominences that are identified on visual and palpatory examination when patients are not weight bearing are likely high-pressure areas of the foot. However, because various things can influence foot position during gait (e.g., leg length, balance, problems with proximal joints), high-pressure areas actually may be different than those predicted by the non–weight-bearing examination. Soft tissue changes such as localized erythema or callus, plantar pressure measurements, temperature assessment, and wear patterns of shoes and shoe inserts can be helpful in identifying areas of high mechanical stress.

Limited mobility of the ankle and subtalar joint in patients with diabetes is associated with high foot pressures and ulceration.[12,13,15] Mueller and colleagues[17] found that the location of ulcers in patients with diabetes is similar to characteristic patterns of plantar callus formation found in healthy patients with the same foot types. Evaluation to identify these biomechanical abnormalities is an important component to include in the examination.

Ankle equinus is seen frequently in the high-risk population. Motor neuropathy or partial foot amputation can reduce dorsiflexor strength and allow the stronger plantar flexors to dominate, causing the joint to tighten in a plantarflexed position. Nonenzymatic glycosylation of protein that occurs as a result of diabetes has been shown to reduce the elasticity of tissue. This may cause the limitation in dorsiflexion range of motion that has been documented in people with diabetes and plantar ulceration.[13] Inadequate dorsiflexion is defined as a measurement of less than 10 degrees of dorsiflexion measured with a fully extended knee and subtalar neutral ankle position.[64] In patients with partial foot amputation this limitation may be more difficult to recognize because of the loss of the usual bony landmarks for measurement. In such cases a comparison of weight-bearing radiographs of the intact and shortened foot may be helpful (Figure 21-10). With insufficient dorsiflexion, pressure on the distal plantar surface of the foot is increased during the propulsive phase of gait.[59] Pressure problems that arise from ankle equinus may improve with stretching or surgical lengthening of the Achilles tendon.[65]

Partial foot amputation can have numerous effects that alter plantar pressure distribution. Because the surface area to carry the force of body weight is smaller, pressure on the remaining structures increases. Studies that have looked at great toe amputation in patients with diabetes have found an increase in plantar pressure and the development of new deformities and ulcerations after amputation.[20,21] As loss of parts of the foot occurs, the mechanics of the foot change, transferring stresses to new areas with the potential for ulceration.

Diabetic neuropathic osteoarthropathy, also known as *Charcot's foot,* is a highly destructive process that can significantly alter the bony architecture of the foot. The severity of the joint changes often leads to excessive plantar pressures[66] and subsequent ulceration (Figure 21-11). This process was first recognized in the nineteenth century by Jean-Martin Charcot. In working with patients who had neurological changes related to tabes dorsalis, Charcot described sudden, unexpected arthropathies in the lower extremities that were characterized by ligamentous laxity, luxation of the joints, and enormous wear and tear of the heads of the bones that he felt were clearly different from

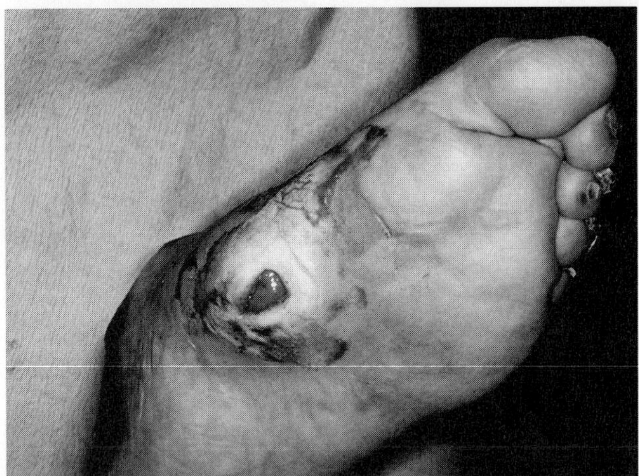

Figure 21-11
Charcot's arthropathy causing collapse of the medial midfoot has led to ulceration underlying the bony prominence in the "arch."

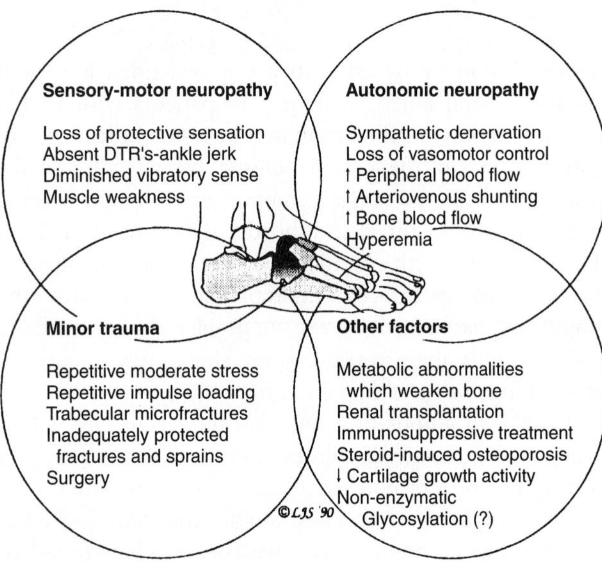

Figure 21-12
Multiple possible contributing factors in the development of Charcot's arthropathy. DTR, deep tendon reflex. (From Sanders LJ, Frykberg RG. Diabetic neuropathic osteoarthropathy: the Charcot foot. In Frykberg RG [ed], The High Risk Foot in Diabetes Mellitus. *New York: Churchill Livingstone, 1991. p. 305.)*

ordinary osteoarthritis.[42] In 1936 W.R. Jordan first associated neuropathic osteoarthropathy of the foot and ankle with diabetes.[42] Although many neurological conditions can lead to Charcot's foot, diabetes is currently the most common disease related to this process.[67]

Charcot's foot is often misdiagnosed because no single diagnostic test can confirm its presence. Medical history, clinical manifestations, and radiographic findings all must be considered (Figure 21-12). Charcot's foot occurs in the

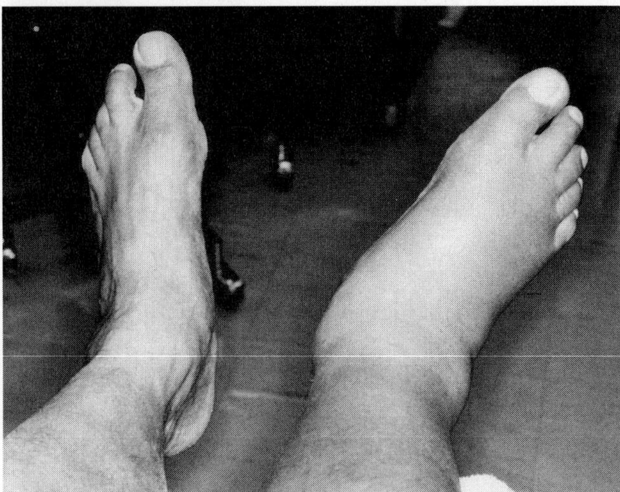

Figure 21-13
Acute Charcot's arthropathy affecting the right midfoot.

presence of neuropathy and most often in patients with adequate circulation. Autonomic neuropathy can contribute to poorly regulated blood flow, including increased bone blood flow and arteriovenous shunting. This abnormal flow pattern coupled with possible metabolic abnormalities[42] leads to weakening of the bones[68] and ligamentous attachments. Supporting structures of the joints are further weakened as excessive stresses during gait cause them to be stretched beyond their normal range of motion. With weakening of the bone and ligamentous attachments, it takes only minor trauma to begin a sequence of events that may include subluxation, dislocation, fragmentation, and fracture.

Clinically, the foot of a patient with an acute Charcot problem shows swelling, erythema, and warmth (Figure 21-13). Because early radiographs are often negative for fracture, patients are frequently misdiagnosed as having a soft tissue injury. Positive findings on a bone scan can be misinterpreted as osteomyelitis. As many clinicians are unfamiliar with Charcot's foot, it is not uncommon for a patient with this problem to go from clinician to clinician (still walking on the foot!) before the problem is correctly diagnosed. By that time, a great deal of destruction to the foot may have occurred (Figure 21-14). Charcot's foot should be suspected if a patient with neuropathy presents with sudden onset of localized swelling, warmth, and erythema in the absence of an open wound. Appropriate treatment for Charcot should be initiated until this condition is ruled out on further testing. During acute Charcot's arthropathy, joint destruction can be minimized by immobilization in a total-contact cast and avoidance of weight bearing until signs of healing become apparent (decreased temperature, decreased swelling, and improved radiographic findings). Both lack of compliance with non–weight bearing and use of orthotic devices in place of cast immobilization have shown prolonged healing times.[69,70] When cast immobilization is discontinued, the use of an orthotic device for continued

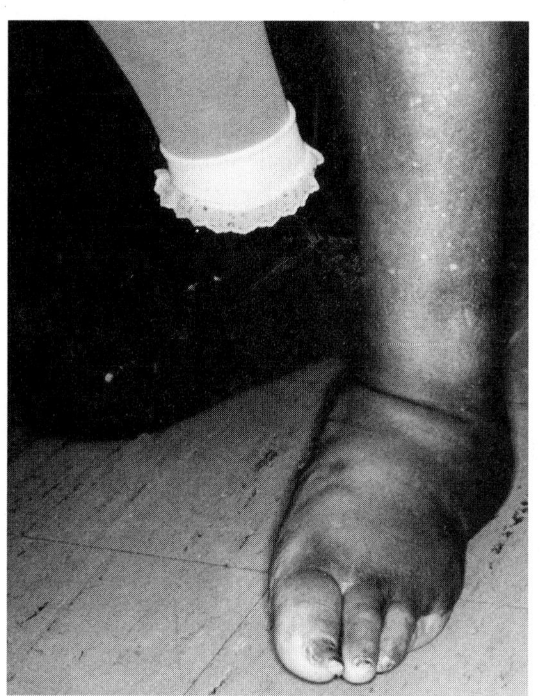

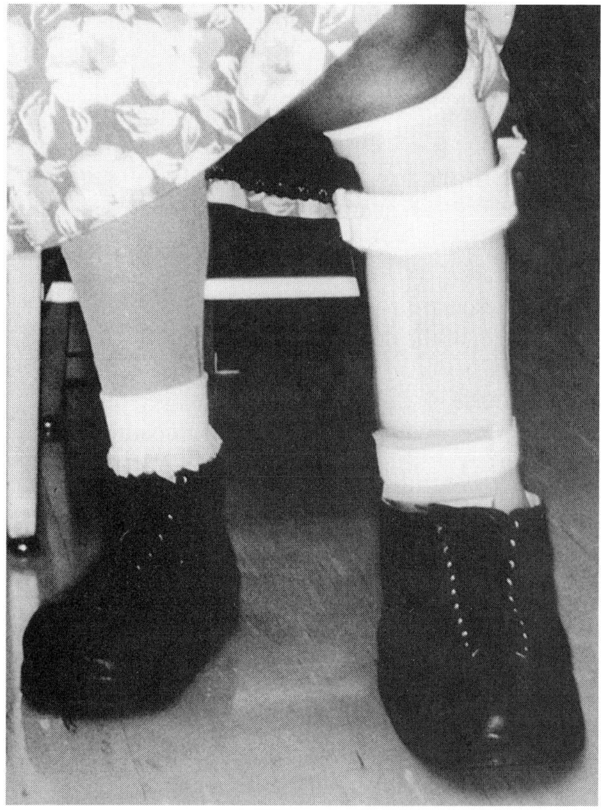

Figure 21-14
A, Patient with significant rear-foot deformity secondary to Charcot's foot, which was untreated during the acute phase. B, Appropriate orthotic intervention has kept this patient from ulcerating.

protection of the joints during the initial return to weight bearing should be considered.[66,70]

The architectural changes that occur in the foot secondary to neuropathic osteoarthropathy result in high-pressure areas.[66] Because of this, following the period of immobilization and limited weight bearing, patients with a history of Charcot's foot must be provided with appropriate footwear to stabilize the foot and reduce plantar pressure.

Surgical intervention may be indicated for unstable or severely malaligned fractures or dislocations, which create problems with recurrent ulceration, fitting of shoes, or ability to ambulate.[71,72] Some of these procedures require months of immobilization and avoidance of weight bearing, which can be difficult for many patients with diabetes and neuropathy. Such surgery is usually advocated only if non-surgical management fails.

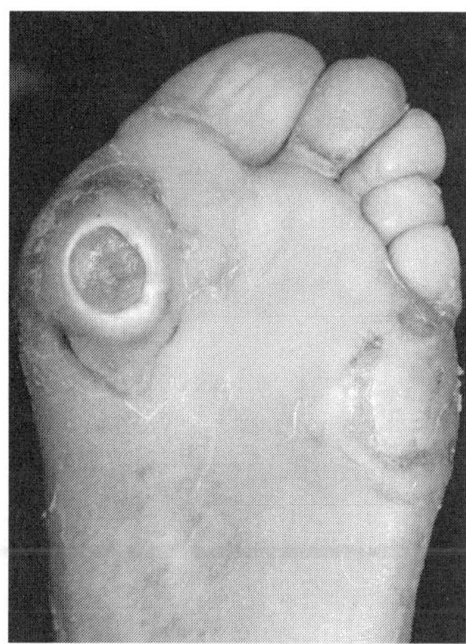

Figure 21-15
A typical neuropathic foot ulcer, under the first metatarsal head.

Soft Tissue Examination

Several abnormal characteristics of soft tissue are associated with problems in the vulnerable foot. These characteristics include loss of fat pad; presence of edema; changes in skin color, temperature, and texture; and the presence and appearance of open wounds.

Distinct characteristics help to differentiate neuropathic from vascular lesions. Neuropathic lesions are most often located on the plantar surface of the foot in areas of high pressure (Figure 21-15).[7,17] The body responds to the localized pressure by forming a protective callus. With repetitive pressure from walking, the callus continues to thicken and becomes a source of additional pressure.[50,73] Signs of inflammation (i.e., heat, erythema) begin to appear. If localized pressure is not reduced, the inflammatory symptoms progress to tissue damage marked by blistering or hemorrhage and, ultimately, ulceration. The end result is commonly a relatively circular wound with a raised callus border, often under a bony prominence. Unless there is infection or ischemia, these wounds usually have a clean, pink base and are painless due to sensory neuropathy. Because vascular disease often coexists with neuropathy and can compromise the healing of neuropathic ulcers, vascular screening is important to include.

Lesions that result from arterial insufficiency are more commonly located on the dorsum of the foot and toes and in the interdigital spaces.[76] They are not associated with callus formation. The base of the wound is often necrotic or pale and, unless there is significant sensory neuropathy, it is painful. Early signs may include blue discoloration or mottling of the skin, which may progress to necrosis. Because circulation is compromised, the skin may be cool to the touch. Temperature assessment is performed by using the back of the hand or the first dorsal web space to feel the skin of the foot and ankle. Although some specialized clinics use hand-held infrared thermometers to measure temperatures,[64] the experienced hand can usually detect temperature differences. Localized temperature increases, particularly if accompanied by redness and warmth, indicate inflammation and possibly infection. Temperature decreases may suggest arterial insufficiency.

While inspecting the skin of the foot for changes in color, it is important to note patterns of change. Erythema under or over a bony prominence in the absence of a wound often indicates inflammation caused by local stresses. If the erythema persists for 30 to 60 minutes after the stress is removed, intervention is warranted. Some degree of redness is associated with new open wounds. Redness around the perimeter of a wound may be a normal inflammatory response. If the redness is extensive or extends some distance away from the wound edges, infection is likely.[74] Lymphangitis is marked by a red streak that runs proximally from a wound site.[75] It indicates ascending infection and requires immediate attention by a physician. Redness of dependency (dependent rubor), blue discoloration, and pallor are commonly associated with arterial insufficiency.

Evaluation of limb volume or edema includes comparison with the other leg. Bilateral lower extremity edema suggests a systemic etiology rather than a localized foot or ankle problem. Control of the edema is desirable to avoid problems with venous ulceration and shoe fit. Unilateral swelling of the foot and ankle that is unrelated to venous incompetence indicates a more localized problem. If the patient has neuropathy and no open wounds are present, Charcot's arthropathy must be considered.

The skin of the normal foot is well hydrated, soft, and compliant. With aging, vascular disease, or diabetes, the skin is likely to be dry and prone to cracking. Daily moisturizing is an important part of skin care for these patients. Taut, shiny, hairless skin is characteristic of patients with significant peripheral arterial disease.[24] Changes in collagen associated with aging[76] and diabetes[75] reduce tissue compliance and increase the risk of soft tissue injury. Palpation of the plantar surface of the foot may reveal reduced soft tissue padding under bony prominences at the forefoot and heel. Studies using ultrasound have found loss of foot pad thickness in patients with diabetes and neuropathy,[39,41,77] and these areas of loss correspond with high plantar pressure.[39,41] One study using computed tomography found that a decrease in soft tissue thickness under the metatarsal heads correlated with age rather than diabetes.[18] Localized callus correlates with higher plantar pressure[41,50,73] and risk for ulceration.[50] Thick callus should be trimmed during the examination because unrecognized preulcerative signs or ulcers may be present underneath.

Preulcerative signs include localized heat, erythema, and calluses possibly with underlying hemorrhage or fluid. Blisters are the result of shearing forces and are commonly found in areas where a shoe has been rubbing or there has been too much movement in the shoe. A poorly fitting shoe can cause blisters and wounds that appear along the sides of the foot or dorsum of the toes. Preulcerative areas on the plantar surfaces of the feet of patients with sensory neuropathy are usually sites of high pressure during gait. Pressure relief techniques prevent these from advancing to ulcerations. Plantar wounds caused by a skin tear or other trauma sometimes fail to heal because of continued pressure during walking. Any open wound found on examination requires correlation with other parts of the history and examination; only then can the most appropriate intervention strategy be selected.

Footwear

Poorly fitting shoes can be a precipitating factor in foot ulceration.[48,78] Examination of the patient's footwear provides important information. A well-fit shoe accommodates the shape and size of the patient's foot, as well as any protective insole materials. Many patients arrive at the clinic wearing shoes that are too narrow in the toe box. Although rounded or squared toe boxes better match the contours of the foot, many patients find them unfashionable. A patient's shoe style preference may affect compliance if special footwear is necessary for his or her particular foot problem.[79]

Gait and Balance

Motor neuropathy causes weakness of foot and ankle musculature that may result in gait deviations that change plantar pressure patterns or contribute to instability. The use of ankle-foot orthoses or shoe modifications may help restore a more normal gait, stabilize joints, or improve balance. Studies have found that patients with peripheral neuropathy secondary to diabetes have problems with gait and postural stability.[80-84] In examining a patient with a high-risk foot, physical therapists must include not only the patients' foot problems but also their overall functional status. Recommendations that address safety and function should be included in the treatment plan.

Evaluation

Evaluation involves using the data collected in the neuropathic foot examination to establish a diagnosis, prognosis, and plan of care.[85] The patient with a high-risk foot will either be at risk for or already have impaired skin integrity. As discussed earlier, this may be caused by impairments in circulation, sensory perception, muscle strength, joint limitations, and biomechanics. Although goals may be related to improved functional mobility, healing an existing foot wound is the primary goal for patients who present with foot ulcers. Once healed or identified as "at risk," prevention becomes the focus.

CASE EXAMPLE 1A

Examination and Evaluation of a Patient with Diabetic Neuropathy, Vascular Insufficiency, and Charcot's Arthropathy

L. M., 68, presents to a neuropathic foot clinic with a nonhealing ulceration on the plantar surface of her left midfoot. Her wound had been managed for the past 2 months with wound debridement and dressing changes.

L. M.'s past medical history includes insulin-dependent type 2 diabetes for 12 years, peripheral vascular disease, a right transtibial amputation 2 years ago, and Charcot's arthropathy of the left midfoot 1 year ago.

L. M. is a retired factory worker and the primary caregiver for her debilitated 93-year-old mother, who lives with her. L. M.'s husband lives at home, but problems with alcohol abuse make him unreliable in assisting the patient or her mother.

On physical examination, L. M. cannot accurately perceive the 5.07 Semmes-Weinstein monofilament at any location of the plantar foot surface. Vibratory perception threshold level is greater than 50 volts. Significant midfoot collapse exists secondary to Charcot's arthropathy, resulting in plantarly prominent medial cuneiform.

Dorsal pedis and posterior tibial pulses are nonpalpable. Noninvasive vascular studies done 2 months before the current clinic visit demonstrated diminished arterial supply but potential for healing.

The ulcer underlying the medial cuneiform measures 1.5 × 1.5 cm at the surface and is 0.2 cm deep. The wound base has 100% red granulation.

L. M. ambulates independently without an assistive device, using her right prosthesis for long functional distances. Her gait pattern is wide based with increased postural sway. L. M. does not want to use an assistive device, believing it would make her daily activities more difficult. Currently she wears standard, soft leather shoes with the manufacturer's insole.

Questions to Consider

- On the basis of your evaluation of information collected in the history and examination, what diagnostic label would you give L. M.'s wound?
- What two major reasons (etiological factors) led to this wound?
- What concurrent conditions probably also contributed to development and nonhealing of her wound?
- On the basis of her vascular study results and your understanding of wound healing, what do you think the prognosis for wound healing might be? How long do you think healing may require?

CASE EXAMPLE 2

Examination and Evaluation of a Patient with Recurrent Foot Ulcer

E. P., 76, presents at a neuropathic foot clinic with a recurrent ulceration underlying the second metatarsal head of her left foot.

E. P.'s past medical history includes type 2 diabetes mellitus for 30 years, coronary artery disease, and neuropathic ulceration underlying the second metatarsal head of her left foot with multiple recurrences. All ulcers have healed rapidly with double-layered felted foam relief pads.

On physical examination, the team finds that E. P. cannot perceive the 5.07 monofilament on any area of her left foot. Her vibratory perception threshold is 42 volts. She demonstrates a "classic" intrinsic-minus foot with claw toe deformities, most severe at the second metatarsophalangeal joint. The team also notes a plantarly prominent second metatarsal head. Minimal fat pad underlies the metatarsal heads.

The ulcer underlying her left second metatarsal head measures 1.2 × 0.6 × 0.1 cm, with 100% granulation of the wound base.

Distal pulses are palpable but weak. On palpation, her forefoot and toes are slightly cooler than her rearfoot.

E. P. wears extra-depth inlay shoes with rocker soles and molded inserts that have been modified to increase weight bearing through the midfoot. E. P. reports that she wears her shoes at all times, except for the several trips to the bathroom at night when she is in stocking feet.

Questions to Consider

- On the basis of your evaluation of information collected in the history and examination, what diagnostic label would you give E. P.'s wound?
- What physiological, mechanical, and behavioral factors have led to the recurrence of this wound?

- On the basis of your understanding of wound healing, what do you think the prognosis for wound healing might be? How long do you think healing may require? What might reduce the risk of recurrence of a similar wound?

Once the ulcer healed with the use of a relief pad, the patient was instructed to keep her shoes at the bedside and slip them on each time she got up to go to the bathroom. At her 4-week check-up the patient reported compliance with these instructions and her foot showed no signs of excessive pressure as it had in the past at this time interval.

INTERVENTION

The plan of care for patients with neuropathic ulceration has three components:

1. Effective management of the wound to facilitate healing
2. Interventions aimed at reducing abnormal pressures on the vulnerable area
3. The establishment of an appropriate plan for follow-up care

Wound Management

A thorough wound assessment includes documentation of surface area, depth, appearance of the wound bed, quantity and quality of the wound drainage, and condition of the tissue surrounding the wound. The surface area can be evaluated in several ways.[86] If a wound is circular, measurements of diameter may be adequate in tracking progress toward healing. If the wound has a more irregular shape, tracing the wound perimeter onto transparent film and placing the tracing over metric graph paper provides a more accurate record. Color photographs that include rulers held adjacent to the wound help to provide both a quantitative and qualitative record. Successive color photographs allow for comparisons as treatment progresses. Undermining of the wound is carefully measured using a blunt sterile probe and then added to the documentation for a more accurate description of the wound size.

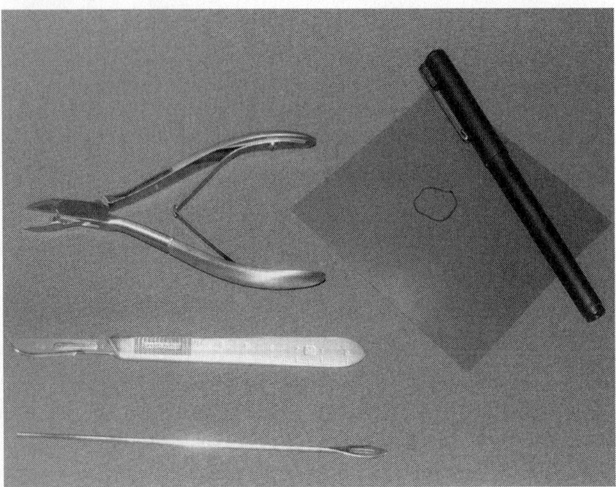

Figure 21-16
Instruments used in wound care include tissue nipper, scalpel, probe, transparent film, and marking pen.

Wound depth is also assessed by gentle use of a probe. Some wounds may track to the tendon, bone, or joint. Bubbly fluid released during probing near a joint is most often joint fluid. Bone has a hard, scratchy feel when probed. This is felt much more readily with a metal probe than with a cotton-tipped applicator. If probing contacts bone, the presence of underlying osteomyelitis is a strong probability.[87] Infections, particularly those that involve tendon or bone, tend to prevent wound healing and require referral to a physician for further care and management. The presence of pus or a foul odor from a wound is a clear clinical sign of infection. Absence of granulation tissue or a pale or gray color to the wound bed is abnormal and could be related to ischemia or infection.

Wounds are commonly described using a classification system. Such systems allow for standardization of terms and provide a means of assigning treatment algorithms or tracking outcomes. A number of classification systems for diabetic foot wounds have been developed, but no one system has been universally accepted.[57]

A comprehensive assessment based on the patient history, physical examination, and wound characteristics should be made before an ulcer management plan is established. Many factors can alter a wound's ability to heal, but the most common are the presence of infection, insufficient circulation, and inadequate relief of pressure. If the findings point to arterial insufficiency, referral to a vascular specialist is necessary. In such cases, identifying and removing sources of excessive pressure that compound tissue ischemia are also important. If the wound is infected, referral to the physician for local cultures, biopsies, or radiographic studies is necessary. Medical management of wound infection can range from oral antibiotics to surgical removal of infected bone. Once issues involving circulation and infection have been addressed, the focus turns to local wound care and management of pressure.

Wounds should be debrided of necrotic tissue before dressings and pressure relief devices are applied. Thick callus around the perimeter of neuropathic foot ulcers is debrided back to healthy epithelium. Local sharp debridement can be performed efficiently with the use of forceps and scalpel or with a tissue nipper (Figure 21-16).[88] For wounds that are deeper than they are wide, it may be necessary to open them wider to prevent superficial closing with trapping of underlying fluid. Special caution should be exercised when dealing with patients who have a secondary diagnosis of PVD or who are taking anticoagulants. Because whirlpool treatment causes dependent edema and tissue maceration, it has not been advocated for the treatment of neuropathic foot ulcers.[24] The use of more efficient wound debridement techniques is preferred.

After debridement, the wound is cleaned and an appropriate dressing is applied. Although a discussion of topical wound cleansers, antibiotics, and wound dressings is beyond the scope of this chapter, several points should be made. A moist wound environment favors wound healing.[89] Wounds are dynamic, and their needs may change over time. If the wound becomes too wet or too dry, a different dressing is necessary. The wound dressing must also be compatible with the appropriate pressure relief device (i.e., if the dressing must be changed daily, it should not be used with a total contact cast that remains in place for up to 2 weeks). Many wound cleansers and topical agents have ingredients that are cytotoxic to healing tissues.[89,90] This means that the risks and benefits for the individual patient should be weighed before wound cleansers and topical agents are applied. Finally, because mechanical stress is often the major cause of ulceration in a neuropathic foot, pressure relief is often the most important component of the treatment plan. The best wound dressing is unlikely to heal a wound if the pressure remains excessive.

Pressure Reduction

Numerous strategies can effectively reduce pressures on the neuropathic foot. No single plan works for all patients. The most appropriate strategy is determined by the patient's coexisting medical and functional problems, the condition of the wound and its surrounding tissue, and the significance of the deformity. The patient's home environment, economic situation, and likely compliance with the instructions associated with the intervention must also be considered. Choosing the most appropriate strategy is a process of weighing the advantages and disadvantages as they relate to the individual patient.

Non–Weight Bearing

Placing a patient on bed rest eliminates all force from the plantar surface of the foot. Historically, patients with foot wounds were admitted to the hospital for the purpose of providing local wound care and keeping them off their feet. In today's health care environment, this occurs only in the case of uncontrolled infection or acute ischemia when other medical or surgical intervention is necessary. Where long-term bed rest may benefit the soft tissues of the feet, it can contribute to osteoporosis, increase risk of developing pressure ulcers, and cause general deconditioning of the patient. At home, the patient must be concerned with remaining non–weight bearing while moving short distances from the bed to the bathroom or to the kitchen. For some patients, this is physically impossible or so difficult that it puts them at risk for falls. For others, the absence of pain may tempt them to get out of bed and walk with the foot unprotected for short distances, thinking that just a few steps will do no harm. Depending on the condition of the tissues and the degree of deformity, a few steps can undo the progress that many hours of non–weight bearing provided.

Total Contact Casting

Total contact casts (Figure 21-17) have been shown to reduce vertical and shear forces that act on the foot.[91,92] Dr. Paul Brand is credited with bringing the total contact cast to the United States after he experienced success with its use on the ulcerated feet of patients with Hansen's disease in India.[93] The total contact cast differs from a conventional cast because little padding is present except over the bony prominences and around the toes. The total contact cast is designed to reduce pressure at the ulcer site by distributing weight bearing over all areas of the foot and leg. Immobilization of the ankle in the cast eliminates the push-off phase of gait, which is often associated with high peak pressure. Total contact with the foot and leg prevents movement of the foot, thus reducing the potential for shear. As the cast loosens with the reduction of edema, it must be changed to ensure that total contact is maintained.

Numerous studies report favorable results in healing diabetic foot ulcers with the use of the total contact cast.[91-97] Particularly interesting are the results of a prospective,

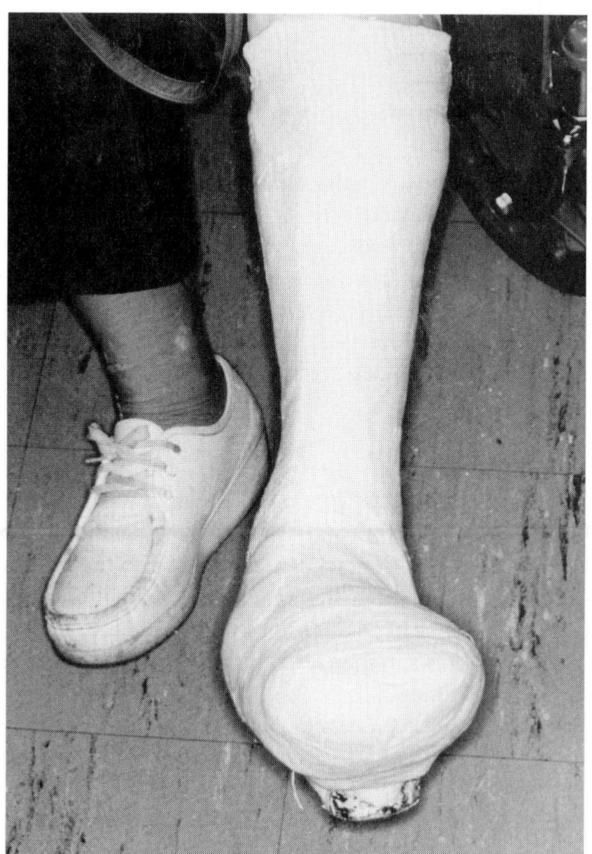

Figure 21-17
Total contact cast.

randomized, controlled clinical trial done by Mueller and colleagues[96] that compared the effectiveness of total contact casting and reduced weight bearing with traditional treatment (debridement, daily dressing changes, the use of accommodative footwear, and instruction to avoid weight bearing through the use of assistive devices). Of 21 ulcers in the total contact cast group, 19 healed, compared to 6 of 19 in the traditional treatment group. Ulcers treated by total contact casting healed in 42 ± 29 days, whereas the traditionally treated ulcers healed in 65 ± 29 days. Five of 19 patients in the traditional treatment group required hospitalization for infection, versus no one in the total contact cast group.

One study showed that although some removable cast walkers were as effective as total contact casts in relieving pressure from ulcer sites,[98] the total contact cast still healed a higher number of foot ulcers in a shorter time period.[97] Average healing time in the total contact cast has been reported to be 36 to 43 days.[99] Standard orthopedic casts are also effective in reducing plantar pressures.[100] The traditional total contact cast was made of plaster material, which required the patient to be non–weight bearing for at least 24 hours. Many clinics now do a combination of plaster and fiberglass or all fiberglass casts to allow patients to return to weight bearing more quickly. Use of a walking heel on total contact casts has been shown to reduce postural stability.[101] Eliminating the walking heel and using a cast boot is recommended.

Because the condition of the foot cannot be monitored while it is enclosed in a cast, the patient must be able to recognize the warning signs indicating the need to have the cast changed. These signs include excessive swelling of the leg that causes the cast to become too tight, loosening of the cast that allows the foot and leg to move within the cast, a sudden increase in body temperature or of blood glucose level that might indicate infection, staining and drainage through the cast, excessive odor from the cast, new complaints of pain, or damage to the cast. Box 21-3 summarizes the advantages and disadvantages of the use of the total contact cast.

Box 21-3 *Advantages and Disadvantages of Total Contact Casting*

ADVANTAGES

- Faster healing times than with traditional treatment
- Reduction in edema
- Decreased opportunity for infection
- No need for daily dressing changes
- Protective weight bearing maintained
- Ambulation maintained

DISADVANTAGES

- Skill necessary to apply cast
- Time consuming to remove and reapply cast
- Cannot monitor condition of wound
- Possible abrasions of other areas due to rubbing from cast
- Cast must be kept dry when bathing/showering
- Too cumbersome for some patients to manage
- Patient must not bear weight until cast is dry
- Difficult to drive if casted foot needed

CONTRAINDICATIONS

- Uncontrolled infection
- Fluctuating edema
- Highly fragile skin
- Significant peripheral vascular disease

Walking Splints

An alternative to the total contact cast is the walking splint (Figure 21-18).[102] Fabrication of a walking splint is much like that of the total contact cast; however, with the anterior portion removed, the splint requires more reinforcement posteriorly. Elastic bandages are used to secure it to the foot and leg. Box 21-4 summarizes the advantages and disadvantages of the walking splint.

Clinical expertise, access to materials, and administrative support are necessary for effective clinical programs that use splinting and casting techniques. Some patients may not accept splinting or casting or may not be candidates for the use of these devices. Other methods of pressure reduction, though less evidence based,[103] may better suit the needs and resources of the patient and clinic.

Box 21-4 *Advantages and Disadvantages of the Walking Splint*

ADVANTAGES

- Can be removed for dressing changes, skin inspection, showering
- Can be removed for sleeping (increased comfort)
- Can be used in most cases in which the total contact cast is contraindicated
- Does not require the frequent refabrication of total contact casting

DISADVANTAGES

- Skill necessary to fabricate
- Time consuming to fabricate
- Can be removed, making unprotected weight bearing more likely
- Difficult to drive if splinted foot needed
- Too cumbersome for some patients to manage

Box 21-5 *Advantages and Disadvantages of the Removable Cast Walker*

ADVANTAGES
- Easy to apply
- Can be removed for dressing changes, showering, sleeping
- Minimal risk if properly fit
- Can be used when total contact cast is contraindicated

DISADVANTAGES
- Too cumbersome for some patients to manage
- Can be removed, making unprotected weight bearing more likely
- Difficulty in accommodating some midfoot deformities
- Difficult to drive with

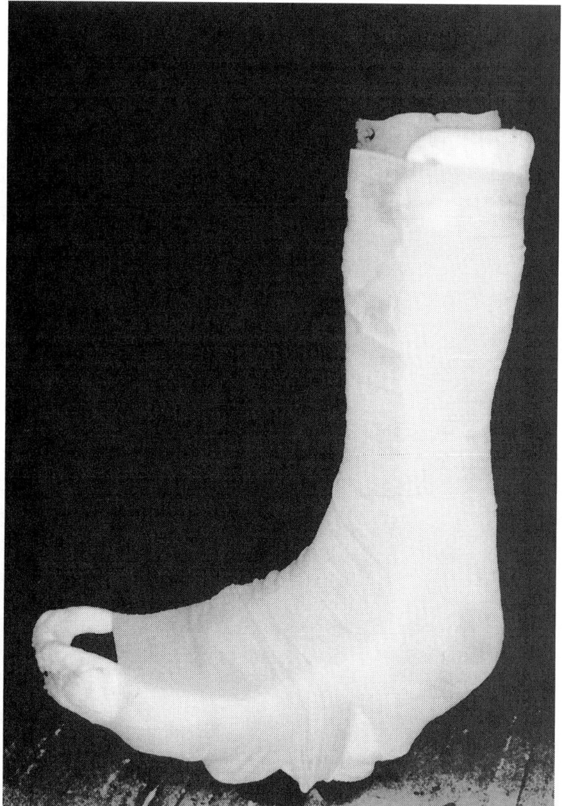

Figure 21-18
The walking splint (an alternative to a total contact cast) is held on the wearer's limb with an elastic wrap.

Removable Cast Walkers

The removable cast walker is an orthotic device with double uprights fixed at a 90-degree angle to a rocker-soled walking platform (Figure 21-19). The use of this walking device has been shown to reduce plantar pressures.[98,104,105] As with the total contact cast and walking splint, the fixed position of the ankle prevents propulsion at the forefoot, where the greatest pressures tend to occur. Removable cast walkers are available from various manufacturers. Because they are not custom made for each patient, care must be taken when fitting the device to ensure that it accommodates the contours of the patient's foot and ankle, particularly in the area of the uprights. A custom-molded insert can be added to most manufactured walkers.

One variation of the removable cast walker, the DH Pressure Relief Walker (Royce Medical/Center Orthopaedics, Camarillo, Calif.), has a removable, multidensity padded insole made up of individual plugs. This insole can be modified by removing plugs to create a relief area for the ulcer site (Figure 21-20).[98,105] Studies show this walker to be more effective in reducing plantar pressures than other offloading devices. Box 21-5 summarizes the advantages and disadvantages of removable cast walkers.

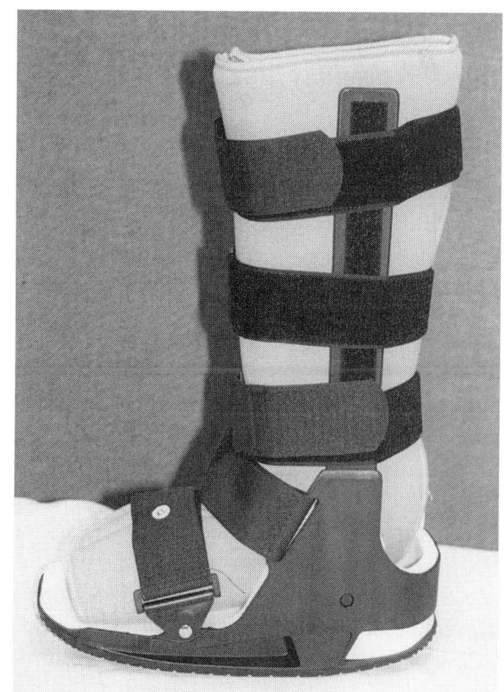

Figure 21-19
Example of a removable cast walker.

Half-shoes

The half-shoe is used for problems that involve the forefoot. Modification of the sole with a wedge causes the body weight to shift back toward the heel, decreasing forces at the forefoot. In one type of this shoe, the sole ends proximal to the metatarsal heads, leaving the forefoot hanging free. Although this removes all pressure from the forefoot, the forefoot is unprotected and more susceptible to trauma. For the vulnerable foot, the half-shoe with an extended sole (Figure 21-21) offers support and protection for the forefoot while shifting weight bearing toward the heel. If the ulcer is

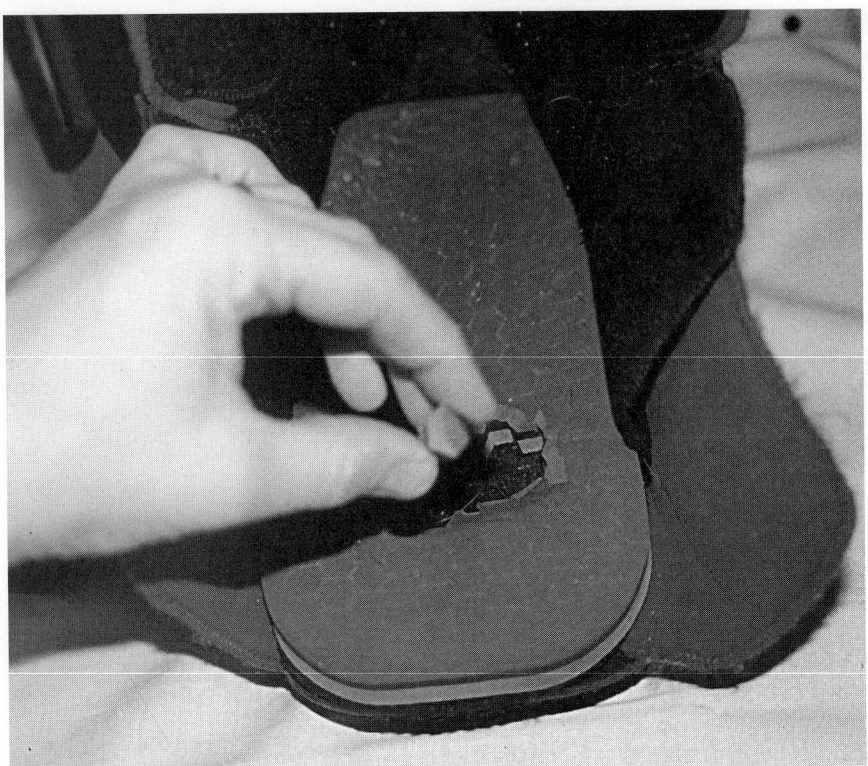

Figure 21-20
Pressure is reduced by removing plugs from the insole of the DH Pressure Relief Walker.

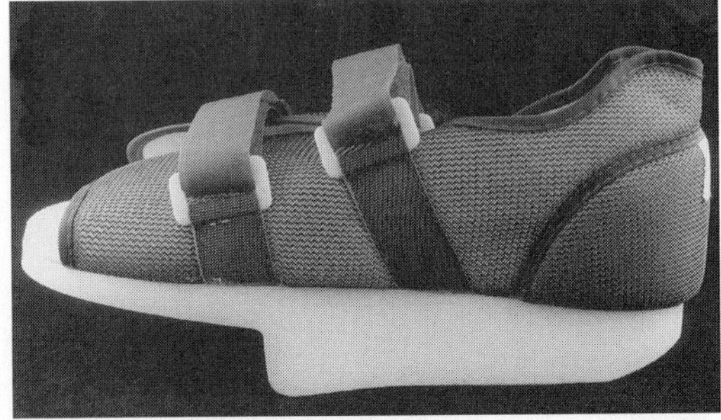

Figure 21-21
An example of a half-shoe, used to unweight the forefoot (Darco Orthowedge).

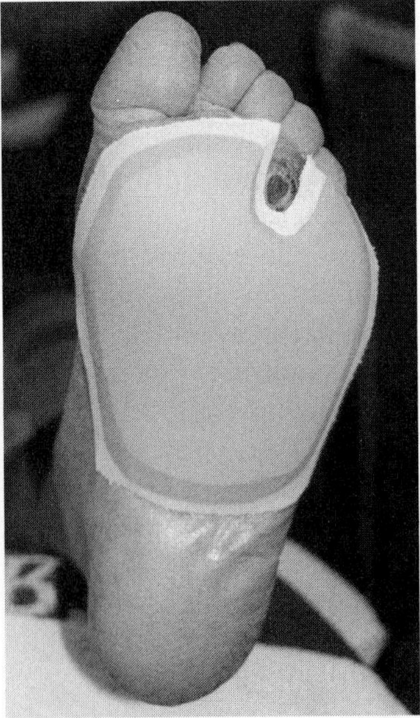

Figure 21-22
Felted foam pressure relief pad applied to the plantar surface of the foot, with a U-shape cutout around the ulcer under the fourth metatarsal head. The foam pad has beveled edges.

under a metatarsal head, one must sure that the distal end of the wedge remains proximal to the metatarsal heads. To maximize pressure reduction, patients should be instructed to take short steps with the contralateral leg. This assures that they do not propel over the wedge causing contact between the distal end of the shoe and the ground. Half-shoes are difficult for patients with limited dorsiflexion. In addition, they may cause gait instability and should not be dispensed without evaluating the need for an appropriate assistive device. The Darco OrthoWedge Shoe (Darco International Inc., Huntington, W. Va.) is effective in reducing forefoot pressures but less effective than the total

Box 21-6 *Advantages and Disadvantages of the Half-Shoe*

ADVANTAGES

- Easy to apply
- Accommodates a bulky dressing, swelling
- Can be used when a cast, splint, or foam is contraindicated
- Can be removed for showering, dressing changes, sleeping

DISADVANTAGES

- Unstable for some patients to walk with
- Can be removed, making unprotected weight bearing more likely
- Difficult to drive with
- Difficult for some patients to maintain the proper gait pattern
- Mobility easier, making excessive activity more likely
- Can bottom out, reducing effectiveness

Box 21-7 *Advantages and Disadvantages of Felted Foam*

ADVANTAGES

- Easy to apply
- Can be used when the total contact cast is contraindicated
- Well accepted by patient
- Minimal risk
- Easier mobility than with cast or splint
- Adhered to foot, so some pressure protection afforded when not in shoe

DISADVANTAGES

- Must be kept dry—foam shifts when wet
- Mobility easier, making excessive activity more likely
- Contraindicated with adhesive allergy or if adjacent tissue too fragile
- Athlete's foot occasionally develops under the pad

contact cast or DH walker.[98] Box 21-6 summarizes the advantages and disadvantages of the half-shoe.

Felted Foam Relief Pads

The felted foam relief pad is an alternative method of pressure reduction (Figure 21-22).[106,107] A custom-fit piece of $\frac{1}{4}$-inch felt-backed foam is adhered to the plantar surface of the foot. A U-shaped aperture is cut in the foam to reduce pressure around the ulcer. The margins of the aperture are positioned close to but not overlapping the wound edge, extending distally beyond the wound. The entire plantar surface of the foot must be examined to identify all vulnerable spots that need accommodation before the pad is applied. The pad is adhered to the foot with rubber cement and reinforced with paper tape or elasticized gauze. For forefoot ulcers, the pad extends proximally along the midfoot to increase the weight carriage in this area. All edges of the foam pad should be beveled to minimize chances of skin breakdown from edge pressure. When a bony deformity is particularly prominent, an additional layer of foam can be used to relieve pressure adequately from the ulcer site. A thin dressing is placed flatly over the ulcer. A healing sandal is used for ambulation. If the area is preulcerative or postulcerative, an extra-depth shoe can be worn. *The pressure relief provided by the foam pad decreases significantly by the fourth day.*[108] Therefore changing the pad every 3 or 4 days may be beneficial.

Felted foam is generally well accepted by the patient. Because this method allows for easier mobility than a total contact cast or walking splint, patients tend to walk more. This may not be desirable considering the possible effect of cumulative pressure. In a study comparing the effects of various offloading devices on peak plantar pressure, total contact casts, removable cast walkers, and half-shoes were more effective. Box 21-7 summarizes the advantages and disadvantages of felted foam.

CASE EXAMPLE 1B

Intervention for a Patient with Diabetic Neuropathy, Vascular Insufficiency, and Charcot's Arthropathy

On the basis of the physical examination results, as well as consideration of L. M.'s caregiving responsibilities and mobility needs, the team decides to implement a 2-week trial of double-layer felted foam to offload the neuropathic ulcer and better distribute weight bearing over the entire plantar surface of L. M.'s left foot. The team is concerned that, given the amputation of her other limb and prosthetic wear, other offloading devices would likely make her too unstable during daily activities. In addition, the team recommends that L. M. use a standard walker as much as possible for additional offloading of her healing limb.

After 2 weeks with minimal healing progress, L. M. and the team agree that a more intensive program of offloading is necessary for the wound to heal. L. M. agrees to seek outside help to care for her mother so that she can be "off her feet" longer. She is now placed in a total contact cast and agrees to use a walker around the house and a wheelchair for longer distances. L. M. is also instructed in a home exercise program to maintain her strength and endurance during the time of reduced activity necessary to achieve healing of her ulcer. She is scheduled for a cast change every 5 days. The wound is anticipated to close within 4 weeks.

Over the next 2 weeks, the ulcer slowly but steadily begins to heal but then seems to stall, and complete wound closure is not achieved in the anticipated time frame. Because wound cultures are negative for infection, the team becomes concerned about the adequacy of arterial flow to the healing wound. L. M. is referred to her vascular surgeon for reevaluation. Noninvasive testing now suggests deterioration of her circulation since the previous examination. Angiography confirms these findings, and an arterial bypass is performed to improve distal arterial flow. Once the suture line is adequately healed, total contact casting is resumed. The midfoot wound completely heals over the next 6 weeks.

Cutout Sandals

A cutout sandal is another alternative to casting.[102,106] With this technique, the foot bed of a custom-molded Plastazote sandal (Alimed, Inc., Dedham, Mass.) is completely cut out in the area of the ulcer, leaving the outer sole intact. The foot bed must be thick enough so that adequate depth is present to keep the ulcer from contacting the upper surface of the sole after modification. If fabrication of a custom-molded sandal is not feasible, a more practical solution may be to supply the patient with a thick, custom-molded Plastazote insert to be worn inside a manufactured healing sandal. The insert is then cut out for the ulcer (Figure 21-23). As with felted foam, care must be taken to bevel the edges of the foot bed or insole to minimize problems with edge pressure. Because Plastazote tends to "bottom out" with repeated loading, the sandal or insert may need to be modified or replaced to be sure that pressure reduction is being maintained. Box 21-8 summarizes the advantages and disadvantages of cutout sandals.

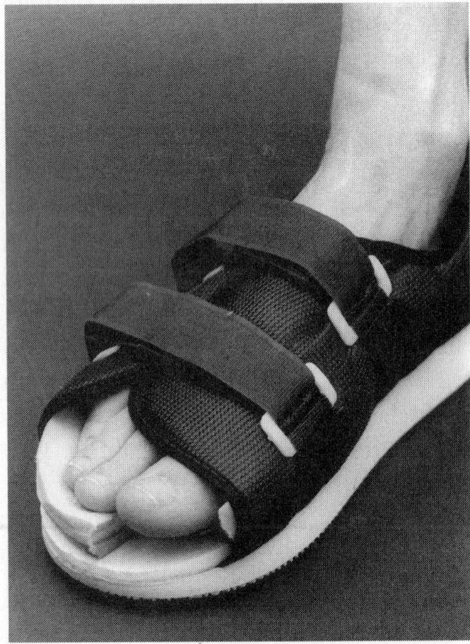

Figure 21-23
This custom-molded insert cutout, designed to relieve pressure on the plantar surface of the hallux, is worn in a healing sandal.

Box 21-8 *Advantages and Disadvantages of the Cutout Sandal*

ADVANTAGES
- Well accepted by patients
- Minimal risk of injury or mobility impairment
- Can be removed for dressing changes, showering, sleeping
- Easier mobility than with cast or splint
- Can be used when total contact cast is contraindicated

DISADVANTAGES
- Can be removed, making unprotected weight bearing more likely
- Mobility easier, making excessive activity more likely
- Can bottom out, reducing effectiveness

Gait Patterns

Although not a primary strategy for healing plantar ulcerations, a change in the gait pattern can help to promote healing by reducing pressures on the foot. A 27% decrease in peak plantar pressures at the forefoot has been demonstrated with a protective gait pattern: The patient can minimize push-off by advancing the leg using hip flexors just before push-off.[109] Healing can also be facilitated if patients purposefully shorten or slow their steps. Studies have found higher plantar pressures with increased cadence or stride length.[110,111] These strategies, as well as the use of assistive gait devices for partial weight bearing, can augment the pressure reduction that is already offered by other pressure relief techniques.

Follow-Up Care

All patients with open wounds require frequent follow-up for reevaluation of the wound and appropriate debridement. Response to treatment may indicate a need to change the type of dressing or the pressure relief technique. With wounds that are slow to respond, consideration may be given to the use of adjunctive therapies such as topical growth factors, vacuum-assisted closure, electrical stimulation, ultrasound, bioengineered tissue, and systemic hyperbaric oxygen. However, none of these adjunctive treatments are likely to be successful if issues of arterial supply, control of infection, and pressure reduction are not adequately addressed.

Once a patient's ulcer has healed, the emphasis of treatment shifts to prevention of recurrent ulceration. Immediately after wound healing, connective tissues are weak and highly vulnerable to stresses on the foot.[6,112] Recurrent ulceration occurs rapidly if a patient with a neuropathic foot wound returns immediately to unprotected weight bearing. For this reason a program of continued protection (e.g., using felted foam or a sandal with a custom-molded foot bed) in combination with an assistive device is recommended for several weeks after initial healing. Patients slowly and progressively increase time and distance of walking, checking their feet often for signs of inflammation. Activity should be limited if signs of inflammation appear.

PREVENTIVE CARE

For all patients with vulnerable feet, whether or not they have a history of ulceration, the primary goal of treatment is prevention. The major components of a preventive program include risk identification, the prescription of appropriate footwear, patient education, and timely follow-up.

Risk Identification

Risk scales classify patients according to their potential for risk of foot injury. Numerous risk scales have been developed, most of which include neuropathy, bony foot deformity, and history of ulceration among the risk factors. The primary criterion for risk of foot injury is the absence of protective sensation. In 1999 a classification system was developed by the International Working Group on the Diabetic Foot (Table 21-1). This system has proven effective in predicting ulceration and amputation.[113] Such a scale can also be used to guide decisions about preventative care. Patients with the highest risk require the most protective footwear and the most frequent follow-up in order to prevent ulceration.

Footwear

A patient assigned to risk category 0 may have a diagnosis of diabetes or PVD and must understand the relationship of the disease process to possible foot damage. Although special footwear is not indicated for this population, the patient must be instructed in proper shoe fit.[114] The contours of the shoe must closely match the contours of the foot. Necessary shoe width varies among individuals and should be measured at the widest part of the forefoot while weight bearing. The widest part of the forefoot should be positioned at the widest part of the shoe. The length of the shoe should include approximately a ½-inch between the end of the longest toe and the end of the shoe. Room within the toe box is also important. Some leather over the dorsum of the forefoot should be able to be pinched between the thumb and index finger if width and depth are adequate.

Patients who lack protective sensation but have no other risk factors (risk category 1) usually do not require specialty footwear. They are instructed in proper shoe fit; encouraged to wear shoes with soft soles; and advised to add a thin, nonmolded, soft insole to cushion high-pressure areas (Figure 21-24, *A*). Running shoes have been shown to decrease plantar pressures compared with standard leather shoes.[115-117] Several shoe styles should be avoided due to their potential to cause increased localized pressure. These include shoes with narrow toes, which can squeeze the sides

Table 21-1
*Diabetic Foot Risk Classifications**

Risk Category	*Definition*
0	No neuropathy
1	With neuropathy, no deformity or PVD
2	With neuropathy and deformity or PVD
3	History of ulceration or amputation

PVD, Peripheral vascular disease.
*Based on consensus of the International Working Group on the Diabetic Foot, 1999.

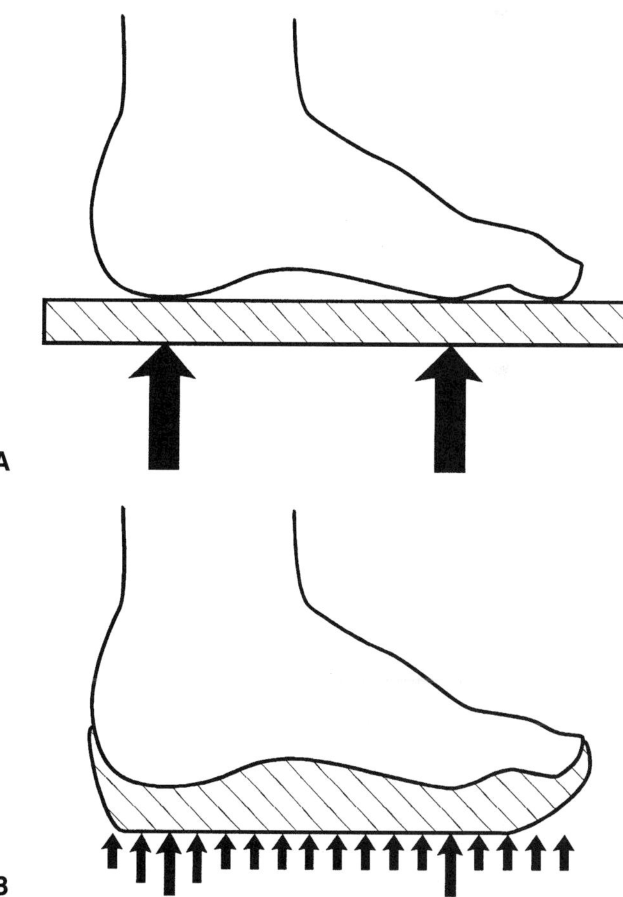

Figure 21-24
A, *A nonmolded insert can cushion high areas of the foot for patients without protective sensation in risk category 1.* ***B,*** *For those in risk categories 2 and 3, a molded insert further decreases pressure at vulnerable locations by increasing the weight-bearing area.*

of the foot; shoes with thongs, which can damage the interdigital space; and high-heeled shoes, which increase the pressures on the plantar forefoot, where ulceration is most common. Because these patients do not have normal sensation, they must understand that although shoes may feel comfortable to them, they still may not fit properly and could place their feet at risk for injury. Objective, rather than subjective, measures must be used when judging fit. Any sense of discomfort is a warning sign to take a closer look at the foot and the shoe fit. Patients sometimes purchase shoes in a larger size to be sure they have plenty of room. A shoe that is too long or too wide, however, allows the foot to slide within the shoe and increases the risk of damage from shear forces.

Patients in the higher-risk categories of 2 to 3 usually require specialty footwear, either in-depth or custom-molded shoes, as well as molded accommodative insoles. Additional modifications to the footwear may also be necessary to further reduce pressure.

The purpose of molded accommodative insoles is to lower plantar pressure by spreading the forces of weight bearing over a greater surface area (see Figure 21-24, *B*). This decreases the localized pressure that is commonly the site of ulceration. Insole materials that demonstrate high dynamic strain deform in response to pressure. Those that have a low dynamic compression set maintain their ability to do this over thousands of steps. Simply stated, the ideal insole material to use when fabricating accommodative insoles is a material that molds and cushions but does not "bottom out" quickly. Because no single material meets all these criteria, inserts are usually made with a combination of materials.[114] Using simulated walking conditions, one study tested some commonly used multidensity materials for their stress and strain properties and their dynamic compression set.[118] They found the better combinations to be Poron (Rogers Corporation, Rogers, Conn.) and Plastazote #2 (Zotefoams, Inc., Hackettstown, N.Y.) or Spenco (Spenco Medical Corp., Waco, Tex.) and Microcel Puff Lite (Acor Orthopaedic, Inc., Cleveland) and recommended these for use as therapeutic orthoses in footwear for diabetic patients. Evidence shows that insert materials lose some of their pressure-relieving properties over time,[118,119] thus monitoring for wear is important. While there is widespread agreement that patients with higher plantar pressures are at greater risk for ulceration,[8,120] no single critical level has been found to identify patients most at risk.

Because of its thickness, a multidensity insole requires the use of an extra-depth shoe. The combination of molded insoles and manufactured extra-depth shoes has proven effective in preventing recurrent ulceration in patients with diabetes.[47,121]

Custom-molded shoes are necessary when the shape of the foot is so abnormal that it cannot be accommodated with a standard extra-depth shoe. Severe hammertoe, hallux valgus, and changes in shape that result from Charcot's arthropathy are common reasons for such a prescription.

For some patients, extra-depth or custom-molded shoes and inserts alone do not adequately protect the foot from damage. Modifications to the shoe or insole may be necessary to further reduce forces in high-pressure areas. Depressions can be incorporated into the insert to protect skin under plantarly prominent sites. This can be done by thinning the insole in the high pressure area, incorporating a soft plug into the midsole of the shoe under the area of concern, or using a firmer material to increase the load in neighboring pressure-tolerant areas to reduce forces at the higher-risk sites. For some patients, biomechanical control of the foot may also be desired. Functional foot orthoses require the use of more rigid materials. Insole modifications and functional orthoses that are aimed at reducing pressure at high-pressure sites do so by increasing pressure in neighboring areas. Careful monitoring is needed ensure that these areas can withstand this additional pressure. Particular caution is advised when rigid materials are used for patients with insensitive feet. If movement occurs between a foot and a rigid orthosis, tissue damage is possible as bony prominences contact areas that were not appropriately relieved for them. Lining the functional orthosis with a softer, more accommodative material reduces this risk.

The rigid rocker sole is a shoe modification used to decrease forefoot pressure during gait (Figure 21-25). The sole of this shoe is rigid to prevent bending at the MTP joints while the rocker allows the center of pressure to roll over the forefoot, minimizing the need for active push-off where peak pressures often occur. Studies of vertical pressures in subjects wearing rigid rocker bottom shoes identified significant reductions in plantar pressures at the forefoot compared with conventional footwear.[122-124] The purpose of one study was to examine the effects of anterior/posterior location of the rocker axis, rocker angle, and shoe height on the pressure distribution under the foot.[124] The authors

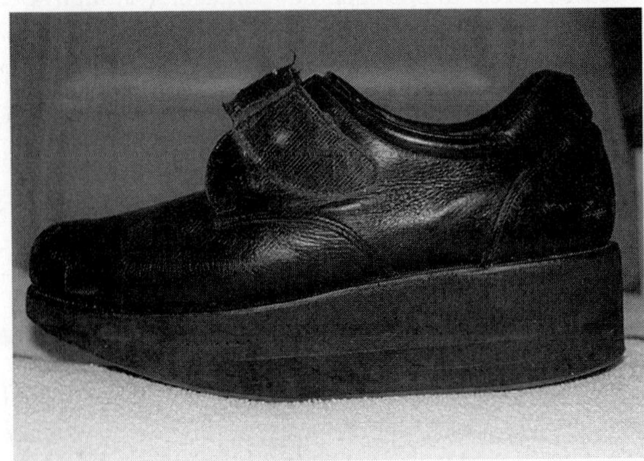

Figure 21-25

Rigid rocker soles added to an extra-depth shoe with a molded insert. Used for treatment of a prominent first metatarsal head with a history of recurrent ulceration.

found that peak pressures were reduced at most forefoot locations but increased at the midfoot and heel. A greater shoe height (thus a greater rocker angle) gave consistently greater pressure relief. On average, the best axis location for reducing pressure was in a region of 55% to 60% of shoe length for the metatarsal heads and 65% for the toes. There was no single placement that was optimal for all subjects at all sites or for all subjects at the same site. Based on this finding, the authors suggested that some form of in-shoe pressure measurement be used while trying different rocker placements for a particular patient.

After transmetatarsal amputation, the shorter foot is at risk for ulceration at its distal end. Two factors that contribute to this risk are increased plantar pressure caused by the equinus deformity, which is common in this population (see Figure 21-10), and the increased torque that is produced when a regular full-length shoe is used on a shortened foot.[106] Mueller and associates[125,126] studied the effects of six different footwear combinations on pressure relief and function in patients with transmetatarsal amputation. The full-length shoe with a total contact insole and rigid rocker bottom sole provided the best pressure reduction for the residuum and contralateral foot. Patients with this footwear combination also displayed faster walking speeds and higher scores on physical performance tests.

One important point must be remembered: A protective shoe only works when the patient is wearing it! If a shoe's appearance is unacceptable to the patient, it is likely to remain in the closet while the patient wears less protective footwear. In situations such as this, a footwear compromise may be necessary. Evidence shows that patients with prescription shoes do not wear them regularly.[49,79] One study dispensed continuous activity monitors and log books to a group of patients. Although 85% of the patients wore their prescribed shoes most or all of the time they were outside their homes, only 15% continued to wear them at home, where they were at least as active. This indicates the importance of more attention to footwear used in the home. Consideration should also be given to protection of the feet when shoes would otherwise not be worn (e.g., when swimming at the pool or beach or during the night when taking short trips to the bathroom).

Patient Education

The goals of a foot care education program are to eliminate poor foot care habits that would otherwise increase the risk of foot injury and replace them with habits that either prevent injuries or allow them to be detected before they become major problems. Such programs have effectively reduced the amputation rate in patients with diabetes.[47,127,128] Instructions to the patient must include issues involving footwear, foot self-inspection, and skin care. Although desirable behaviors must be stressed, avoidable behaviors must also be stressed (Box 21-9).

Professional Foot Care

Patients with high-risk feet frequently do not have the joint mobility or visual acuity to care for their feet adequately.[46] Additionally, impairment in sensation makes it more likely for them to injure themselves while trying to care for their feet. Inadvertent injuries, although most often minor, can be devastating for patients with peripheral vascular disease. Professional follow-up for reevaluation, routine foot care, and check of footwear is advised. Patients who are in risk category 0 require a yearly reevaluation to identify any changes that may alter their risk and thus the plan of care. Those in higher-risk categories require more frequent preventative care. A study that looked at incidence of ulceration, reulceration, and amputation in patients followed in a diabetic foot specialty clinic found that patient noncompliance to routine preventative care was associated with a higher prevalence of ulceration and amputation.[129]

Use of Technology

Technical devices to measure vertical forces under the foot have been used for many years, largely for research purposes. Computerized systems to measure in-shoe pressures have become commercially available.[130,131] Such systems allow visualization of weight-bearing patterns throughout the gait cycle and quantify pressures at specific areas of the foot. They may be of particular use in the clinic to assess change in plantar pressures after surgical intervention, footwear modifications, or changes in gait patterns. Information gathered from these systems may be a useful guide for treatment decisions. Little is known about the contribution of shear stress to ulceration in the foot because of the limited instrumentation available to measure it.[131] Where practical devices for measuring vertical force are available for use in the clinical setting, none currently exist for the measurement of shear.

Specialized Foot Clinics

Specialized foot clinics are effective in reducing the rate of amputation in the high-risk foot population.[44,47,128,129] These multidisciplinary foot clinics involve services that cover various specialties, including vascular, podiatric, orthopedic, and plastic surgeries; infectious disease and endocrinology; physical therapy; nursing; orthotics; prosthetics; and pedorthics. Such programs likely have some relatively costly equipment that allows for quantitative measurements of skin temperature, vibration perception, circulation, or plantar pressures. Often such equipment only verifies what a clinical examination has already revealed.

Specialized clinics with advanced technology are valuable resources but are not the only settings in which effective care for high-risk foot problems occur. Many health care professionals outside of these settings make important contribu-

Box 21-9 *Guidelines for Preventive Foot Care*

SKIN CARE

DO:	Wash feet daily. Dry them well, especially between the toes.
	Apply a thin coat of moisturizer to feet daily, avoiding between the toes.
	Trim toenails after washing and drying feet.
	Cut toenails straight across; smooth any sharp edges with an emery board.
	Have a podiatrist handle any thickened or ingrown toenails.
	Thin thick corns or calluses by gently using a pumice stone or by professional care.
	Check water temperature with a thermometer or elbow before bathing.
	Wear socks at night if feet are cold.
	Use sunscreen on the tops of feet during the summer.
	Ask health care provider to check feet at each visit.
DO NOT:	Soak feet. This can dry them out and cause cracking.
	Use moisturizer between toes. Moisture between the toes allows germs to grow.
	Cut corns and calluses.
	Use chemical agents, corn plasters, strong antiseptics, or adhesive tape on feet, because they can damage skin.
	Use hot water bottles or heating pads because they can burn feet.

FOOT SELF-INSPECTION

DO:	Inspect all surfaces of the feet daily (including between the toes) for signs of injury: reddened areas, blisters, cuts, cracks, or sores.
	Report any injuries to a health care provider immediately.
	Feel for areas of increased temperature.
	Check for tender areas on the bottom of feet.
	Use a mirror if necessary to see the bottom of feet.
	Have a family member, friend, or health care professional check feet if necessary.
DO NOT:	Wait to report problems to a health care provider. Early attention can often prevent small problems from becoming big ones.

FOOTWEAR

DO:	Wear shoes that fit the size and shape of feet and leave room for any necessary insoles.
	Ask a health care provider to recommend the correct type of shoe.
	Break in new shoes slowly, checking feet frequently for signs of irritation. Report signs of irritation to a health care provider.
	Keep shoes and insoles in good repair.
	Always wear socks or stockings with shoes, wearing a clean pair daily.
	Before putting on shoes, check for rough areas, torn linings, or loose objects that can injure a foot.
DO NOT:	Walk barefoot (use slippers at night, special shoes or sandals for the beach).
	Wear socks that are too baggy or have holes or prominent seams.
	Wear socks or stockings that are constricting at the top.
	Use sandals with thongs between the toes.

tions to the care of patients with high-risk feet. If health care providers are interested in this population, understand the principles that surround the evaluation and treatment of high-risk feet, and use other specialists as appropriate, they can make a significant contribution to preserving the quality of life of the patients they serve.

SUMMARY

In this chapter we have explored the interacting factors that contribute to the risk of developing neuropathic wounds and to likelihood of successful healing. Although individuals with diabetes mellitus are most likely to present with the combination of neuropathy and peripheral vascular disease associated with increasing risk of neuropathic ulcer development and delayed healing, the rehabilitation professional must watch for this combination regardless of primary medical diagnosis.

The first step in the management of individuals with vulnerable feet is a careful examination of skin and soft tissue condition, evaluation of musculoskeletal deformity or abnormal foot biomechanics, and assessment of adequacy of distal protective sensation, autonomic function, and vascular supply to the limb. This information, when coupled with inspection of footwear and discussion of usual daily activity level, helps rehabilitation professionals determine tissue tolerance of repeated low-load stress (as encountered in functional ambulation), develop an appropriate plan of care to protect the foot, and, if necessary, adapt activity to allow tissue healing.

Management of a vulnerable foot centers on reducing pressure by distributing weight-bearing forces over as large a surface area as possible, often with an accommodative foot orthosis and an ambulatory assistive device, and reducing the speed and duration of walking activities in an effort to limit stress on the vulnerable tissues. Routinely scheduled visits to podiatrist or interdisciplinary foot clinic to trim callus, inspect foot condition, and reinforce the individual's understanding of how to care for the vulnerable foot are essential for preservation of foot health.

Management of a foot with an existing neuropathic wound often begins with debridement and application of an appropriate dressing and continues with total pressure relief over the wound. This can (ideally) be accomplished by non–weight-bearing ambulation or (more realistically) application of a total contact cast, walking splint, cast walker, felted-foam relief pad, or adaptable insole, in combination with specialized footwear.

For individuals with vulnerable feet, the emphasis must be on prevention of a neuropathic wound; healing a wound in the presence of vascular disease and neuropathy is much more challenging than keeping intact skin relatively healthy. A physical therapist's knowledge of the impact of physical stressors on tissue health and of the physiology of inflammation and of wound healing, in conjunction with the ability to assess alignment and to suggest alternate or accommodative ways of moving to reduce mechanical stressors during functional activities, makes a substantial contribution to the comprehensive care (and as a result, quality of life) for persons coping with vulnerable feet.

ACKNOWLEDGMENTS

The author acknowledges the contribution of those patients served by the Hartford Hospital Neuropathic Foot Program and expresses grateful appreciation to Dr. Larry Suecof, from whom and with whom it has been a pleasure to learn.

REFERENCES

1. Reiber GE. Epidemiology of foot ulcers and amputations in the diabetic foot. In Bowker JH, Pfeifer MA (eds), *Levin and O'Neal's The Diabetic Foot,* 6th ed. St. Louis: Mosby, 2001. pp. 13-32.
2. Pecoraro RE, Reiber GE, Burgess EM. Pathways to diabetic limb amputation: basis for prevention. *Diabetes Care* 1990;13(5):513-521.
3. Centers for Disease Control and Prevention. *Diabetes Surveillance System 2003.* Atlanta: Centers for Disease Control and Prevention, Department of Health and Human Services, 2003.
4. McNeely MJ, Boyko EJ, Ahroni JH, et al. The independent contributions of diabetic neuropathy and vasculopathy in foot ulceration. *Diabetes Care* 1995;18(2):216-219.
5. Hu MY, Allen BT. The role of vascular surgery in the diabetic patient. In Bowker JH, Pfeifer MA (eds), *Levin and O'Neal's The Diabetic Foot,* 6th ed. St Louis: Mosby, 2001. pp. 424-564.
6. Brand PW. The diabetic foot. In Ellenberg M, Rifkin H (eds), *Diabetes Mellitus: Theory and Practice,* 3rd ed. New Hyde Park, NY: Medical Examination, 1983. pp. 829-849.
7. Ctercteko GC, Dhanendran M, Hutton WC, et al. Vertical forces acting on the feet of diabetic patients with neuropathic ulceration. *Br J Surg* 1981;68(9):608-614.
8. Boulton AJ, Hardesty CA, Betts RP, et al. Dynamic foot pressures and other studies as diagnostic and management aids in diabetic neuropathy. *Diabetes Care* 1983;6(1):26-33.
9. Veves A, Murray HJ, Young MJ, et al. The risk of foot ulceration in diabetic patients with high foot pressure: a prospective study. *Diabetologia* 1992;35:660-663.
10. Birke JA, Patout CA, Foto JG. Factors associated with ulceration and amputation in the neuropathic foot. *J Orthop Sports Phys Ther* 2000;30(2):91-97.
11. Kastenbauer T, Sauseng S, Sokol G, et al. A prospective study of predictors for foot ulceration in type 2 diabetes. *J Am Podiatr Med Assoc* 2001;91(7):343-350
12. Delbridge L, Perry P, Marr S, et al. Limited joint mobility in the diabetic foot: relationship to neuropathic ulceration. *Diabet Med* 1988;5(4):333-337.
13. Mueller MJ, Diamond JE, Delitto A, et al. Insensitivity, limited joint mobility, and plantar ulcers in patients with diabetes mellitus. *Phys Ther* 1989;69(6):453-459.
14. Birke JA, Cornwall MW, Jackson M. Relationship between hallux limitus and ulceration of the great toe. *J Orthop Sports Phys Ther* 1988;10(5):172-176.
15. Fernando DJS, Masson EA, Veves A, et al. Relationship of limited joint mobility to abnormal foot pressures and diabetic foot ulceration. *Diabetes Care* 1991;14(1):8-11.
16. Birke JA, Franks BD, Foto JG. First ray joint limitation, pressure and ulceration of the first metatarsal head in diabetes mellitus. *Foot Ankle* 1995;16(5):277-284.
17. Mueller MJ, Minor SD, Diamond JE, et al. Relationship of foot deformity to ulcer location in patients with diabetes mellitus. *Phys Ther* 1990;70(6):356-362.
18. Robertson DD, Mueller MJ, Smith KE, et al. Structural changes in the forefoot of individuals with diabetes and a prior plantar ulcer. *J Bone Joint Surg* 2002;84A(8):1395-1404.
19. Lavery LA, Armstrong DG, Vela SA. Practical criteria for screening patients at high risk for diabetic ulceration. *Arch Intern Med* 1998;158(2):157-162.
20. Quebedeau TL, Lavery LA, Lavery DC. The development of foot deformities and ulcers after great toe amputation in diabetes. *Diabetes Care* 1996;19(2):165-167.
21. Lavery LA, Lavery DC, Quebedeau-Farham TL. Increased foot pressures after great toe amputation in diabetes. *Diabetes Care* 1995;18(11):1460-1462.
22. Kosiak M. Etiology and pathology of ischemic ulcers. *Arch Phys Med Rehabil* 1959;40(2):62-69.

23. Brand PW. Repetitive stress in the development of diabetic foot ulcers. In Levin ME, O'Neal LW (eds), *The Diabetic Foot,* 4th ed. St. Louis: Mosby, 1988. pp. 83-90.
24. Levin ME. Pathogenesis and general management of foot lesions in the diabetic patient. In Bowker JH, Pfeifer MA (eds), *Levin and O'Neal's The Diabetic Foot,* 6th ed. St. Louis: Mosby, 1995. pp. 219-260.
25. Heatherington VJ. The neuropathic foot. In McGlamry ED, Banks AS, Downey MS (eds), *Comprehensive Textbook of Foot Surgery,* 2nd ed. Baltimore: Williams & Wilkins, 1992. pp. 1353.
26. Vinik AI, Holland MT, LeBeau JM, et al. Diabetic neuropathies. *Diabetes Care* 1992;15(12):1926-1975.
27. Tanenberg RJ, Schumer MP, Greene DA, et al. Neuropathic problems of the lower extremities. In Bowker JH, Pfeifer MA (eds), *Levin and O'Neal's The Diabetic Foot,* 6th ed. St. Louis: Mosby, 2001. pp. 13-32.
28. Boulton AJM, Kubrusly DB, Bowker JH, et al. Impaired vibratory perception and diabetic foot ulceration. *Diabet Med* 1986;3(4):335-337.
29. Young MJ, Breddy JL, Veves A, et al. The prediction of diabetic foot ulceration using vibration perception thresholds. *Diabetes Care* 1994;17(6):557-560.
30. Sosenko JM, Kato MK, Soto R, et al. Comparison of quantitative sensory-threshold measures for their association with foot ulceration in diabetic patients. *Diabetes Care* 1990;13(10):261-267.
31. Pham H, Armstrong DG, Harvey C, et al. Screening techniques to identify people at high risk for diabetic foot ulceration. *Diabetes Care* 2000;23(5):606-611.
32. Armstrong DG, Lavery LA, Vela SA, et al. Choosing a practical screening instrument to identify patients at risk for diabetic foot ulceration. *Arch Intern Med* 1998;158(3):289-292.
33. Birke JA, Sims DS. Plantar sensory threshold in the ulcerative foot. *Lepr Rev* 1986;57(3):261-267.
34. Holewski JJ, Stess RM, Graf PM, et al. Aesthesiometry: quantification of cutaneous pressure sensation in diabetic peripheral neuropathy. *J Rehabil Res Dev* 1988;25(2):1-10.
35. Kumar S, Fernando DJS, Veves A, et al. Semmes Weinstein monofilaments: a simple, effective and inexpensive screening device for identifying patients at risk for foot ulceration. *Diabetes Res Clin Pract* 1995;13:63-68.
36. Mueller MJ. Identifying patients with diabetes mellitus who are at risk for lower extremity complications: use of Semmes-Weinstein monofilaments. *Phys Ther* 1996;76(1):68-71.
37. Course Materials, Michigan Diabetes Research and Training Center, University of Michigan Hospital, Ann Arbor, 1983.
38. Habershaw G, Donovan JC: Biomechanical considerations of the diabetic foot. In Kozak GP, Hoar CS, Robatham JL, et al (eds), *Management of Diabetic Foot Problems.* Philadelphia: Saunders, 1984. pp. 32-44.
39. Young MJ, Coffey J, Taylor PM, et al. Weight-bearing ultrasound in diabetic and rheumatoid arthritis patients. *Foot* 1995;5:76-79.
40. Brash PD, Foster J, Vennartt P, et al. Magnetic resonance imaging techniques demonstrate soft tissue damage in the diabetic foot. *Diabet Med* 1999;16:55-61.
41. Abouaesha F, Carine HM, Gareth D, et al. Plantar tissue thickness is related to peak plantar pressure in the high-risk diabetic foot. *Diabetes Care* 2001;24(7):1270-1274.
42. Sanders LJ, Frykberg RG. Charcot neuroarthropathy of the foot. In Bowker JH, Pfeifer MA (eds), *Levin and O'Neal's The Diabetic Foot,* 6th ed. St. Louis: Mosby, 2001. pp. 439-466.
43. Sims DS, Cavanagh PR, Ulbrecht JS. Risk factors in the diabetic foot. *Phys Ther* 1988;68(12):1887-1903.
44. Bild DE, Selby JV, Sinnock P, et al. Lower extremity amputation in people with diabetes: epidemiology and prevention. *Diabetes Care* 1989;12(1):24-31.
45. The Diabetes Control and Complications Trial Research Group. The effect of intensive treatment of diabetes on the development and progression of long-term complications in insulin-dependent diabetes. *N Engl J Med* 1993;329(14):977-986.
46. Crausaz FM, Clavel S, Linger C, et al. Additional factors associated with plantar ulcers in diabetic neuropathy. *Diabet Med* 1988;5(8):771-775.
47. Edmonds ME, Blundell MP, Morris ME, et al. Improved survival of the diabetic foot: the role of the specialized foot clinic. *QJM* 1986;60(232):763-771.
48. Apelqvist J, Larsson J, Ajardh CD. The influence of external precipitating factors and peripheral neuropathy on the development and outcome of diabetic foot ulcers. *J Diabetes Complications* 1990;4(1):21-25.
49. Armstrong DG, Abu-Rumman PL, Nixon BP, et al. Continuous activity monitoring in persons at high risk for diabetes-related lower-extremity amputation. *J Am Podiatr Med Assoc* 2001;91(9):451-455.
50. Murray HJ, Young MJ, Hollis S, et al. The association between callus formation, high pressure and neuropathy in diabetic foot ulceration. *Diabet Med* 1996;13:979-982.
51. Wagner FW. The dysvascular foot: a system for diagnosis and treatment. *Foot Ankle* 1981;2(2):64-122.
52. Reiber GE, Pecoraro RE, Koepsell TD. Risk factors for amputation in patients with diabetes mellitus: a case control study. *Ann Intern Med* 1992;17(2):97-105.
53. Apelqvist J, Castenfors J, Larsson J, et al. Prognostic value of systolic ankle and toe blood pressure levels in outcome of diabetic foot ulcer. *Diabetes Care* 1989;12(6):373-378.
54. Gibbons GW, Campbell DR. Non-invasive diagnostic studies. In Kozak GP, Hoar CS, Rowbotham JL (eds), *Management of Diabetic Foot Problems,* Philadelphia: Saunders, 1984. pp. 91-96.
55. Hurley JJ, Jung, M, Woods JJ, et al. Noninvasive vascular testing: basis, application, and role in evaluating diabetic peripheral arterial disease. In Bowker JH, Pfeifer MA (eds), *Levin and O'Neal's The Diabetic Foot,* 6th ed. St. Louis: Mosby, 2001. pp. 13-32.
56. McMahon JH, Grigg MJ. Predicting healing of lower limb ulcers. *Aust N Z J Surg* 1995;65(3):173-176.
57. American Diabetes Association. Consensus development conference on diabetic foot wound care. *Diabetes Care* 1999;22(8):1354-1360.
58. Boulton AJ, Betts RP, Franks CI, et al. Abnormalities of foot pressure in early diabetic neuropathy. *Diabet Med* 1987;4(3):225-228.
59. Lavery LA, Armstrong DG, Boulton AJ. Ankle equinus deformity and its relationship to high plantar pressure in a large population with diabetes mellitus. *J Am Podiatr Med Assoc* 2002;92(9):479-482.
60. Taylor R, Stainsby GD, Richardson DL. Rupture of the plantar fascia in the diabetic foot leads to toe dorsiflexion deformity (abstract 1071). *Diabetologia* 1998;41(suppl 1):A277.

61. Frykberg RG. Podiatric problems in diabetes. In Kosak GP, Hoar CS, Rowbatham JL, et al (eds), *Management of Diabetic Foot Problems.* Philadelphia: Saunders, 1984. pp. 45-67.
62. Fromherz WA. Examination. In Hunt GC (ed), *Physical Therapy of the Foot and Ankle.* New York: Churchill Livingstone, 1988. pp. 59-90.
63. Johnson JE. Charcot neuropathy of the foot: surgical aspects. In Bowker JH, Pfeifer MA (eds), *Levin and O'Neal's The Diabetic Foot,* 6th ed. St Louis: Mosby, 2001. pp. 587-606.
64. Coleman WC, Birke JA. The initial foot examination of the patient with diabetes. In Kominsky SJ (ed), *Medical and Surgical Management of the Diabetic Foot.* St. Louis: Mosby-Year Book, 1994. pp. 7-28.
65. Armstrong DG, Stacpoole-Shea S, Nguyen H, et al. Lengthening of the Achilles tendon in diabetic patients who are at high risk for ulceration of the foot. *J Bone Joint Surg Am* 1999; 81(4):535-538.
66. Armstrong DG, Lavery LA. Elevated peak plantar pressures in patients who have Charcot arthropathy. *J Bone Joint Surg* 1998;80A(3):365-369.
67. Banks AS. A clinical guide to the Charcot foot. In Kominsky SJ (ed), *Medical and surgical management of the diabetic foot.* St. Louis: Mosby-Year Book, 1994. pp. 115-143.
68. Young MJ, Marshall A, Adams JE, et al. Osteopenia, neurological dysfunction, and the development of Charcot neuroarthropathy. *Diabetes Care* 1995;18(1):34-38.
69. Boninger ML, Leonard JA. Use of bivalved ankle-foot orthosis in neuropathic foot and ankle lesions. *J Rehabil Res Dev* 1996;33(1):16-22.
70. Morgan JM, Biehl WC, Wagner FW. Management of neuropathic arthropathy with the Charcot restraint orthotic walker. *Clin Orthop* 1993;296:58-63.
71. Sammarco GJ, Conti SF. Surgical treatment of neuroarthropathic foot deformity. *Foot Ankle Int* 1998;19(2):102-109.
72. Early JS, Hansen ST. Surgical reconstruction of the diabetic foot: a salvage approach for midfoot collapse. *Foot Ankle Int* 1996;17(6):325-330.
73. Young MJ, Cavanagh PR, Thomas G, et al. The effect of callus removal on dynamic plantar foot pressures in diabetic patients. *Diabet Med* 1992;9(1):55-57.
74. McCulloch JM. Treatment of wounds caused by vascular insufficiency. In McCulloch JM, Kloth LC, Feedar JA (eds), *Wound Healing: Alternatives in Management,* 2nd ed. Philadelphia: F.A. Davis, 1995. pp. 213-228.
75. McCarthy DJ. Cutaneous manifestations of the lower extremities in diabetes mellitus. In Kominsky SJ (ed), *Medical and Surgical Management of the Diabetic Foot.* St. Louis: Mosby-Year Book, 1994. pp. 191-222.
76. Mulder GD, Brazinsky BA, Seeley JE. Factors complicating wound repair. In McCulloch JM, Kloth LC, Feedar JA (eds), *Wound Healing: Alternatives in Management,* 2nd ed. Philadelphia: F.A. Davis, 1995. pp. 47-59.
77. Gooding GAW, Stess RM, Graf PM, et al. Sonography of the sole of the foot: evidence for loss of foot pad thickness in diabetes and its relationship to ulceration of the foot. *Invest Radiol* 1986;21:45-48.
78. Kalker AJ, Kolodny HD, Cavuoto JW. The evaluation and treatment of diabetic foot ulcers. *J Am Podiatr Med Assoc* 1992;72(10):491-496.
79. Knowles EA, Boulton AJM. Do people with diabetes wear their prescribed footwear? *Diabet Med* 1996;13:1064-1068.
80. Cavanagh PR, Derr JA, Ulbrecht JS, et al. Problems with gait and posture in neuropathic patients with insulin-dependent diabetes mellitus. *Diabet Med* 1992;9(5):469-474.
81. Cavanagh PR, Simoneau GG, Ulbrecht JS. Ulceration, unsteadiness, and uncertainty: the biomechanical consequences of diabetes mellitus. *J Biomech* 1993;26(suppl 1):23-40.
82. Simoneau GG, Ulbrecht JS, Derr JA, et al. Postural instability in patients with diabetic sensory neuropathy. *Diabetes Care* 1994;17(12):1411-1421.
83. Uccioli L, Giacomini PG, Monticone G, et al. Body sway in diabetic neuropathy. *Diabetes Care* 1995;18(3):339-344.
84. Courtemanche R, Teasdale N, Boucher P, et al. Gait problems in diabetic neuropathic patients. *Arch Phys Med Rehabil* 1996;77(9):849-855.
85. American Physical Therapy Association. Guide to physical therapist practice. *Phys Ther* 2001;81(1):9-744.
86. Sussman C. Wound measurements. In Sussman C, Bates-Jensen BM (eds), *Wound Care: A Collaborative Practice Manual for Physical Therapists and Nurses.* Gaithersburg, MD: Aspen, 1998. pp. 83-102.
87. Grayson ML, Gibbons GW, Balogh K, et al. Probing to bone in infected pedal ulcer. *JAMA* 1995;273(9):721-723.
88. Armstrong DG, Lavery LA, Vazquez JR, et al. How and why to surgically debride neuropathic diabetic foot wounds. *J Am Podiatr Med Assoc* 2002;92(7):402-404.
89. Feedar JA. Clinical management of chronic wounds. In McCulloch JM, Kloth LC, Feedar JA (eds), *Wound Healing: Alternatives in Management,* 2nd ed. Philadelphia: F.A. Davis, 1995. pp. 137-176.
90. Alvarez OM, Gilson G, Auletta MJ. Local aspects of diabetic foot and ulcer care: assessment, dressings, and topical Agents. In Levin ME, O'Neal LW, Bowker JH (eds), *The Diabetic Foot,* 5th ed. St. Louis: Mosby-Year Book, 1995. pp. 259-281.
91. Pollard JP, LeQuesne LP, Tappin JW. Forces under the foot. *J Biomed Eng* 1983;5(1):37-40.
92. Birke JA, Sims DS, Buford WL. Walking casts: effect on plantar foot pressures. *J Rehabil Res Dev* 1985;22(3):18-22.
93. Coleman WC, Brand PW, Birke JA. The total contact cast: a therapy for plantar ulceration on insensitive feet. *J Am Podiatr Assoc* 1984;74(11)548-552.
94. Helm PA, Walker SC, Pullum G. Total contact casting in diabetic patients with neuropathic ulcerations. *Arch Phys Med Rehabil* 1984;65(11):691-693.
95. Sinacore DR, Mueller MJ, Diamond JE, et al. Diabetic neuropathic plantar ulcers treated by total contact casting. *Phys Ther* 1987;67(10):1543-1549.
96. Mueller MJ, Diamond JE, Sinacore DR, et al. Total contact casting in treatment of diabetic plantar ulcers: controlled clinical trial. *Diabetes Care* 1989;12(6):384-388.
97. Armstrong DG, Nguyen HC, Lavery LA, et al. Offloading the diabetic foot wound: a randomized clinical trial. *Diabetes Care* 2001;24(6):1019-1022.
98. Fleischli JG, Lavery LA, Vela SA, et al. Comparison of strategies for reducing pressure at the site of neuropathic ulcers. *J Am Podiatr Med Assoc* 1997;87(10):466-472.
99. Sinacore DR, Mueller MJ. Total contact casting in the treatment of neuropathic ulcers. In Bowker JH, Pfeifer MA

(eds), *Levin and O'Neal's The Diabetic Foot,* 6th ed. St. Louis: Mosby, 2001. pp. 301-320.

100. Conti SF, Martin RL, Chaytor ER, et al. Plantar pressure measurements during ambulation in weightbearing conventional short leg casts and total contact casts. *Foot Ankle Int* 1996;17(8):464-469.
101. Lavery LA, Fleischli JG, Laughlin TJ, et al. Is postural instability exacerbated by off-loading devices in high-risk diabetics with foot ulcers? *Ostomy/Wound Management* 1998;44(1):26-34.
102. Birke JA, Novick A, Graham SL, et al. Methods of treating plantar ulcers. *Phys Ther* 1991;71:116-122.
103. Armstrong DG, Lavery LA. Evidence-based options for off-loading diabetic wounds. *Clin Podiatr Med Surg* 1998;15(1):95-104.
104. Birke JA, Nawoczenski DA. Orthopedic walkers: effect on plantar pressures. *Clin Prosthet Orthot* 1988;12(2):74-80.
105. Lavery LA, Vela SA, Lavery DC, et al. Reducing dynamic foot pressures in high-risk diabetic subjects with foot ulcerations. *Diabetes Care* 1996;19(8):818-821.
106. Birke JA, Sims DS. The insensitive foot. In Hunt GC (ed), *Physical Therapy of the Foot and Ankle.* New York: Churchill Livingstone, 1988. pp. 133-168.
107. Zimny S, Meyer MF, Schatz H, et al. Applied felted foam for plantar pressure relief is an efficient therapy in neuropathic diabetic foot ulcers. *Exp Clin Endocrinol Diabetes* 2002;110(7):325-328.
108. Zimny S, Reinsch B, Schatz H, et al. Effects of felted foam on plantar pressures in the treatment of neuropathic diabetic foot ulcers. *Diabetes Care* 2001;24(12):2153-2154.
109. Mueller MJ, Sinacore DR, Hoogstrate S, et al. Hip and ankle walking strategies: effect on peak plantar pressures and implications for neuropathic ulceration. *Arch Phys Med Rehabil* 1994;75(11):1196-1200.
110. Hongsheng Z, Wertsch JJ, Harris GF, et al. Walking cadence effect on plantar pressures. *Arch Phys Med Rehabil* 1995;76(11):1000-1005.
111. Soames RW, Richardson RPS. Stride length and cadences: their influence on ground reaction forces during gait. In Winter DA, Norman RW, Wells RP, et al (eds), *Biomechanics IX-A.* Champaign, IL: Human Kinetics, 1978. pp. 406-410.
112. Weiss EL. Connective tissue in wound healing. In McCulloch JM, Kloth LC, Feedar JA (eds), *Wound Healing: Alternatives in Management,* 2nd ed. Philadelphia: F.A. Davis, 1995. pp. 16-31.
113. Peters EJ, Lavery LA. Effectiveness of the diabetic foot risk classification system of the international working group on the diabetic foot. *Diabetes Care* 2001;24(8):1442-1447.
114. Janisse DJ. Pedorthic care of the diabetic foot. In Bowker JH, Pfeifer MA (eds), *Levin and O'Neal's The Diabetic Foot,* 6th ed. St. Louis: Mosby, 2001. pp. 700-726.
115. Perry JE, Ulbrecht JS, Derr JS, et al. The use of running shoes to reduce plantar pressure in patients who have diabetes. *J Bone Joint Surg Am*1995;77(12):1819-1928.
116. Lavery LA, Vela BS, Fleischli JG, et al. Reducing pressure in the neuropathic foot: a comparison of footwear. *Diabetes Care* 1997;20(11):1706-1710.
117. Kastenbauer T, Sokol G, Auinger M. Running shoes for relief of plantar pressure in diabetic patients. *Diabet Med* 1998;15:518-522.
118. Foto JG, Birke JA. Evaluation of multidensity orthotic materials used in footwear for patients with diabetes. *Foot Ankle Int* 1998;19(12):836-841.
119. Lobmann R, Kayser R, Kasten G, et al. Effects of preventative footwear on foot pressure as determined by pedobarography in diabetic patients: a prospective study. *Diabet Med* 2001;18(4):314-319.
120. Armstrong DG, Peters EJ, Athanasiou KA, et al. Is there a critical level of plantar pressure to identify patients at risk for neuropathic foot ulceration? *Foot Ankle Surg* 1998;37(4):303-307.
121. Uccioli L, Faglia E, Monticone G, et al. Manufactured shoes in the prevention of diabetic foot ulcers. *Diabetes Care* 1995;18(10):1376-1378.
122. Nawoczenski DA, Birke JA, Coleman WC. Effect of rocker sole design on plantar foot pressures. *J Am Podiatr Med Assoc* 1988;78(9):455-460.
123. Schaff PS, Cavanagh PR. Shoes for the insensitive foot: the effect of a "rocker bottom" shoe modification on plantar pressure distribution. *Foot Ankle* 1990;11(3):129-140.
124. Van Schie C, Ulbrecht JS, Becker MB, et al. Design criteria for rigid rocker shoes. *Foot Ankle Int* 2000;21(10):833-844.
125. Mueller MJ, Strube MJ, Allen BT. Therapeutic footwear can reduce plantar pressures in patients with diabetes and transmetatarsal amputation. *Diabetes Care* 1997;20(4): 637-641.
126. Mueller MJ, Strube MJ. Therapeutic footwear: enhanced function in people with diabetes and transmetatarsal amputation. *Arch Phys Med Rehabil* 1997;78(9):952-956.
127. Davidson JK, Alonga M, Goldsmith M, et al. Assessment of program effectiveness at Grady Memorial Hospital-Atlanta. In Steiner G, Lawrence PA (eds), *Educating Patients.* New York: Springer-Verlag, 1981. pp. 329-348.
128. Litzelman DK, Slemenda CW, Langefeld CD, et al. Reduction of lower extremity clinical abnormalities in patients with non-insulin dependent diabetes mellitus; a randomized controlled trial. *Ann Intern Med* 1993;119(1):36-41.
129. Armstrong DG, Harkless LB. Outcomes of preventative care in a diabetic foot specialty clinic. *J Foot Ankle Surg* 1998;37(6):460-466.
130. Mueller MJ, Strube MJ. Generalizability of in-shoe peak pressure measures using the F-scan system. *Clin Biomech* 1996;11(3):159-164.
131. Cavanagh PR, Ulbrecht JS, Caputo GM. The biomechanics of the foot in diabetes mellitus. In Bowker JH, Pfeifer MA (eds), *Levin and O'Neal's The Diabetic Foot,* 6th ed. St. Louis: Mosby, 2001. pp. 125-196.

22

Amputation Surgeries for the Lower Limb

JUDITH L. PEPE AND MICHELLE M. LUSARDI

LEARNING OBJECTIVES

On completion of this chapter, the reader will be able to do the following:

1. Compare and contrast the assessments typically used to determine the need for, and optimal level of, amputation surgery for individuals with dysvascular/neuropathic disease, trauma, neoplasm, or congenital limb deficiency.
2. Describe key perioperative concerns and issues for individuals facing lower limb amputation (e.g., complications, hydration/nutrition, pain management, respiratory status, concurrent medical issues for each etiology of amputation).
3. Provide an overview of the most commonly used surgical approaches for each level of amputation (including myodesis, drain position, tissue manipulation, and surgical closures).
4. Apply understanding of biomechanics of surgical approaches and tissue healing to the care of new and maturing residual limbs.

WHEN IS AMPUTATION NECESSARY?

The amputation of a limb is often life altering in terms of self-image and yet can be life saving in the presence of severe trauma or disease. Amputation can be incredibly life improving when burdensome care of a vulnerable or painful dysvascular foot is no longer necessary.[1] Although surgical technique is an important determinant in the "success" of amputation, other factors that are as important include the individual's and family's understanding and acceptance that amputation is the best option of care[2,3]; effective attention to and management of comorbidities during the perioperative period, as well as avoidance of postoperative complications such as pneumonia and wound infection[4,5]; and a promptly implemented rehabilitation plan that the individual, family, surgical team, and rehabilitation team have developed and agreed on.[6]

This chapter provides an overview of the strategies used to determine if amputation is necessary for individuals with dysvascular/neuropathic disease, for those who have sustained significant trauma to their lower limbs, for those with diagnoses of bone or soft tissue neoplasm, and for children who are growing up with congenital limb deficiency. The authors then describe the surgical techniques used in the most commonly performed lower extremity amputation and discuss the rehabilitation implications for each. The goal is to help rehabilitation professionals understand what has happened to soft tissue and bone during surgery and to use this knowledge to better incorporate principles of wound healing and maturation into the preprosthetic and prosthetic care of those who have undergone amputation.

Basic Principles

The decision to amputate a limb, whether because of vascular disease and neuropathy, trauma, or neoplasm, is based on careful consideration of prognosis for survival and for successful rehabilitation. In general, the choice of level of amputation is guided by two principles. First, there must be adequate circulation to ensure successful healing of the incision.[7] Determining an appropriate level can be challenging; surgeons consider factors such as the presence of a palpable pulse at the ankle, posterior knee, or groin; skin color and condition; skin temperature; ankle-brachial index; and the results of transcutaneous oximetry ($TcPO_2$) or of angiography.[8,9] Second, the preservation of as many anatomical joints as possible, especially of the knee, often means more successful functional outcome.[10,11] At times tension occurs between these principles. For individuals with plantar neuropathic ulcers and osteomyelitis, for example, a transmetatarsal amputation has the potential to preserve the ankle joint and permit functional gait without prosthesis and is often less difficult for individuals to accept psychologically.[12] If there is delayed or failed healing, however, the risks of complications associated with limited activity and bed rest (e.g., further deconditioning, pneumonia, deep venous thrombosis, decubitus ulcer) and repeated anesthesia if surgical revisions to more proximal levels become necessary can be significant.[13,14] In these instances an initial surgery at the transtibial level might improve the chances for optimal rehabilitation outcome.

In individuals with traumatic crush injury to the proximal tibia but intact knee joint, an extremely short transtibial residual limb may actually be more difficult to manage prosthetically than a long transfemoral residual limb: the reduced surface area around a short residual tibia and fibula for weight bearing within the socket increases pressure on skin and soft tissue of the residual limb, reducing functional wearing time of the prosthesis despite the advantage of preservation of the anatomical knee joint.[15]

Dysvascular and Neuropathic Disease

The prevalence of peripheral arterial disease (PAD) in the United States is estimated to be between 3% and 6% of the adult population, increasing to as much as 10% in those 65 years and older.[16] Significant morbidity and mortality is associated with PAD: as many as one fourth of those with PAD will likely require amputation, while one third will die within 5 years of diagnosis and three fourths will die within 10 years of diagnosis.[17] Epidemiologists forecast that the incidence and severity of PAD will increase with population aging.[18] PAD is a significant health care issue, affecting the quality of an individual's life, as well as spiraling health care costs.[19]

Three groups of individuals might require revascularization or amputation of the lower limb because of underlying disease processes: those with significant, often acute, occlusive atherosclerotic vascular disease but without neuropathy or diabetes; those without significant vascular disease who have neuropathy-related wounds that may lead to osteomyelitis; and those with diabetes with a combination of vascular disease and sensory, motor, and autonomic neuropathy.[16] The management and prognosis for each of these groups are somewhat different. Vascular bypass surgery or the use of thrombolytic medications may preserve the limbs of those with large vessel vascular disease without neuropathy.[20]

Conservative management with total contact casting or felted foam may be sufficient to heal a neuropathic ulcer (when there are no indications of osteomyelitis), and accommodative orthoses and protective footwear may protect the plantar surface of the foot in those with a healing neuropathic wound.[21] The presence of infection or osteomyelitis, however, often makes amputation necessary.[22] Those with both neuropathy and vascular disease are the most likely to require amputation.[17] Because many of these individuals are older, comorbidities such as cardiovascular and cerebrovascular disease, kidney disease, and visual impairment provide additional challenges for healing, early mobility after amputation, and the prosthetic rehabilitation process.[23]

Because both vascular disease and neuropathic disease are typically symmetrical in distribution, individuals in all of these groups are at risk for compromise of both lower limbs. After amputation of one limb, careful monitoring of vascular status and skin condition and appropriate conservative care of the intact limb and foot are essential. This is especially true in the postoperative/preprosthetic period when there is single limb ambulation with assistive devices, as well as in the months and years following initial amputation.[24-26]

For all of these individuals, clinical decision making must be informed by careful assessment of (1) vascular status to determine whether revascularization or amputation is warranted, (2) cardiovascular and cardiorespiratory function to determine the most appropriate type of anesthesia to use during surgery, and (3) cognitive and psychological status to assure proper perioperative and postoperative care and patient education.

The assessment of an individual with compromised peripheral circulation begins with a careful and detailed health history and review of risk factors, continues with physical examination and routine blood work, and is followed up by additional tests or measures as needed.[27] Cognitive and psychological status is initially assessed by interview and as part of the neurological examination and can be followed up by more formal testing if warranted. Vascular status is first examined using noninvasive methods; if found to be compromised, further assessment with computed tomography arteriography (CTA), magnetic resonance arteriography (MRA), or invasive arteriography may be indicated.[28] The physician's differential diagnosis process focuses on determining which component of the circulatory system is involved (arterial, venous, or lymphatic), if it is an acute problem that requires immediate medical/pharmacological or surgical intervention (e.g., vascular bypass or amputation), or a chronic problem that necessitates conservative medical management (Table 22-1).

Vascular Pain

One of the most common symptoms of chronic arterial vascular insufficiency is *intermittent claudication* (IC). This vascular-related pain has been described as a deep aching, cramping, muscle fatigue, or tightness that develops during physical activity and dissipates with rest. Although most common in the posterior compartment (gastrocnemius and soleus) of the lower leg, claudication can occur in any muscle with compromised blood supply including the muscles of the thigh and hip. Claudication is the result of accumulation of lactic acid as a byproduct of anaerobic metabolism during muscle contraction.[29] Several strategies are used to classify

Table 22-1
Common Peripheral Vascular Disorders

System	*Acute Conditions*	*Chronic Conditions*
Arterial	Arterial thrombosis Embolic occlusion Vasospastic disease (Raynaud's)	Atherosclerosis obliterans Thromboangiitis obliterans Buerger disease Diabetic angiopathy
Venous	Venous thromboembolism	Varicose veins Chronic venous insufficiency
Lymphatic	Lymphangiitis	Primary lymphedema (congenital) Secondary lymphedema (acquired)

severity of PAD and of IC. In 1954 Fontaine first defined four stages of PAD on the basis of the presence and severity of clinical symptoms (Table 22-2).[30,31] More recently, the term *critical limb ischemia* has been used to designate those with severe PAD, when there is pain at rest or ulceration.[32] The time to onset of claudication symptoms during treadmill walking at 120 steps per minute has been used as a strategy to quantify magnitude of vascular insufficiency.[23] Change in the total distance that an individual is able to walk (e.g., number of city blocks or actual measured distance) before onset of symptoms is an alternative means of tracking progression of arterial vascular impairment.[33]

When there is an acute or sudden occlusion of an arterial vessel (and collateral circulation has not yet developed), a much different pattern of pain occurs. Instead of relief with rest, pain is constant and somewhat unrelenting; it may be accompanied by feelings of tingling, numbness, or coldness as peripheral nerves of the lower limb are affected by ischemia.[34] Although a limb with chronic arterial insufficiency demonstrates dependent rubor, the skin of an acutely compromised limb may be quite pale or blanched distal to the site of occlusion (Figure 22-1). Acute occlusion is often an emergent situation, requiring pharmacological or surgical intervention to restore blood flow to the limb, and often necessitates long-term anticoagulation.

Likelihood of PAD increases when there is a history of smoking, significant alcohol use, sedentary lifestyle, and long-term oral contraceptive use.[31,35] Comorbidities associated with PAD include diabetes, hypertension, hyperlipidemia, previous cerebrovascular accident (CVA) or transient ischemic attack (TIA), coronary artery disease and myocardial infarction, angina, syncope, impotence, and varicose veins.[35]

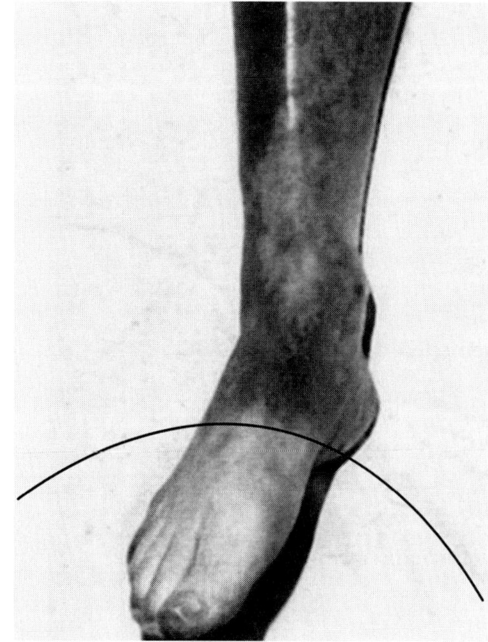

Figure 22-1
A chronically ischemic limb demonstrating rubor of dependency of the distal lower leg and rearfoot and significant pallor suggesting acute ischemia of the forefoot. (Courtesy Carolyn Kelly, Center for Wound Healing and Hyperbaric Medicine, Hartford Hospital, Hartford, Conn.)

Examination of the Ischemic Limb: Skin and Soft Tissue

Assessment begins with visual inspection of the lower extremity and feet, concentrating on skin condition, presence or absence of hair, and nail condition.[36] Open wounds, callus, ecchymosis, dry necrosis and other skin lesions, as well as areas of erythema (redness), mottling, and altered pigmentation are documented on a body chart. Circular wounds that lie under or are surrounded by callus on the plantar or weight-bearing surfaces of the foot are most likely neuropathic ulcers (Figure 22-2, *A*). Dry, blackened, or moist gangrenous wounds in the nail beds and between toes are likely signs of vascular insufficiency (Figure 22-2, *B*). Although many traumatic wounds display clear serosanguineous drainage, any thickened, yellowish, or foul-smelling discharge from a wound suggests soft tissue or bone infection.

Open wounds around ankles or a distal leg surrounded by areas of darkly pigmented skin are typically the result of chronic venous stasis. Progressive circumferential measurements are taken to document the presence of pitting or nonpitting edema resulting from venous or lymphatic insufficiency, localized infection, or as part of an underlying systemic disease of kidney, heart, or lung. Skin temperature is assessed subjectively, using the web space or back of the examiner's hand or objectively using a surface thermometer. Cold areas in particular may have compromised arterial flow, while areas of increased temperature (especially if

Table 22-2
Leriche and Fontaine's Classification of Peripheral Arterial Disease Severity

Stage	*Examination Findings*
I Atherosclerosis without major clinical symptoms	Paresthesia Cold extremities Bruits on auscultation Absent, diminished, or normal pedal pulses ABI < .90 Decreased peak flow (plethysmography)
IIa Atherosclerosis with claudication	As above, with diminished or absent pedal pulses Pain with walking distance > 200 meters, relieved with rest Bruits on auscultation Hair loss Abnormal Doppler sounds Decreased peak flow (plethysmography)
IIb Atherosclerosis with claudication	As above, with more pronounced symptoms or abnormal examination Pain with walking distance < 200 meters, relieved with rest Slight elevation in blood viscosity, fibrinogen, and platelet function
III Atherosclerosis with resting pain (critical limb ischemia)	As above, more pronounced clinical symptoms and abnormal examination Pain most troubling at night (when supine or LE with elevation) Segmental pressure at ankle < 50 mm Hg (in those without DM) Segmental pressure at toe < 30 mm Hg (in those with DM) Diminished TcO_2 Trophic changes in nails Atrophy of intrinsic muscles of the foot
IV Atherosclerosis with tissue damage (critical limb ischemia)	As above, markedly abnormal clinical examination Dry gangrenous wounds, commonly on dorsum of foot Nonhealing plantar neuropathic ulcer in those with diabetes Ulceration with inflammation or infection

ABI, Ankle/brachial index; *DM,* diabetes mellitus; *LE,* lower extremity.

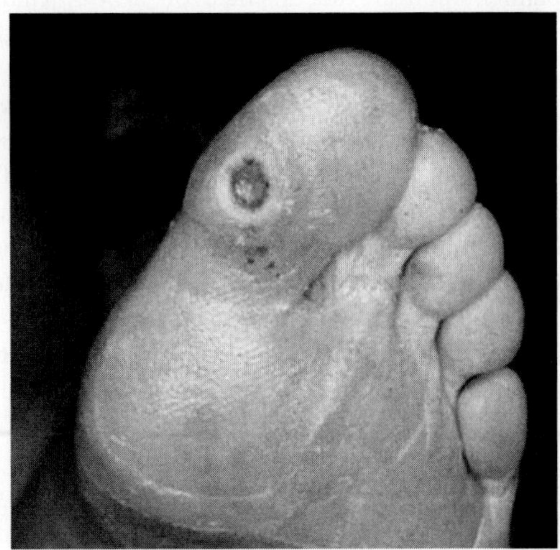

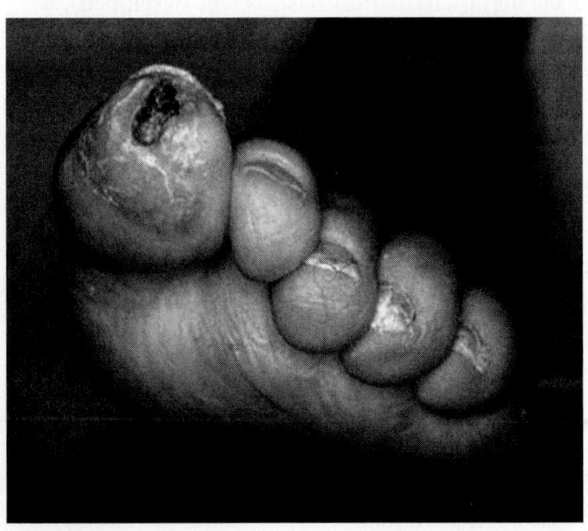

Figure 22-2
A, *Typical round callus-rimmed neuropathic lesion on the plantar surface of the hallux in an individual with diabetic neuropathy.* ***B,*** *Ischemic changes (dry gangrene) on the tip of the hallux in an individual with peripheral arterial disease. (Courtesy Carolyn Kelly, Center for Wound Healing and Hyperbaric Medicine, Hartford Hospital, Hartford, Conn.)*

accompanied by erythema and swelling) often indicate underlying infection.

In the presence of diabetic and other polyneuropathies there is often atrophy or wasting of the intrinsic muscles of the foot with apparent claw toe positioning at rest (see Figure 21-8).[37] Protective sensation (as measured by perception of Semmes-Weinstein 5.07 filament), as well as touch, pressure, vibration, and position sense, are likely to be impaired or inconsistent.[38] Additionally, impairment of the autonomic system often causes dry, tight, shining, easily cracked skin, as well as altered dynamics of blood flowing to the bones of the foot, increasing risk of Charcot's arthopathy.[39]

Vascular Examination: Noninvasive Strategies

The least invasive and simplest strategy used to assess adequacy of vascular supply to the distal limb is palpation of distal lower extremity pulses at the dorsalis pedis and posterior tibial arteries, popliteal pulse at the knee, and femoral pulse at the groin. Strength of pulses at each site is noted as absent (0/4), weak (1/4), normal (2/4), full (3/4), or bounding (4/4).[40] If all pulses are palpable, it is likely that there is adequate circulation to heal a neuropathic ulcer. Absent distal pedal pulses do not, however, confirm vascular insufficiency; it is estimated that pedal pulses are nonpalpable in up to 10% of the general population.[41]

When pedal pulses are not palpable, further assessment might include positional tests of capillary and venous filling time, auscultation with Doppler ultrasound, calculation of an ankle-brachial index (ABI), segmental blood pressure of the limb (see Figure 21-6), transcutaneous oximetry (pulse oximetry), pulse-volume recordings (see Figure 21-7), MRA, computed tomography (CT) angiography, or duplex scanning.[33,40,41] (Readers are referred to Chapter 21 for a detailed description of noninvasive assessment strategies.) Normal values for noninvasive tests are listed in Table 22-3.

Table 22-3
Reference Values for Noninvasive Examination of Peripheral Arterial Circulation

Test/Measure	*Normal Values*	*Abnormal Findings*
Capillary refill time	Elevation of limb 20 sec Return to dependent position Pressure on toe or nail Blanch, then refill in 1-2 sec	Delayed refill or persistent blanching Rubor of dependency
Refill after occlusion	Inflation of BP cuff at thigh for 5 min On release, flush to normal skin color at toes within 10 sec	>10 sec: impaired arterial perfusion
Venous refill time	Elevation of the limb 2 minutes Return to dependent position Veins on dorsum of foot refill in 10 sec	>10 sec: impaired arterial perfusion <10 sec: valvular incompetence of veins
Doppler ultrasound	Triphasic on auscultation	Biphasic: mild vascular impairment Monophasic: significant impairment Absent: complete occlusion
Ankle-brachial index	.9 to 1	<.9 impaired arterial flow <.5 unlikely to heal distal wound
Segmental blood pressure	<15 mm Hg drop in systolic pressure between adjacent sites (groin, thigh, just below knee, and at ankle)	>20 mm Hg decrease: possible occlusion >10 mm Hg: possible vessel calcification
Pulse volume recordings	Sharp peaks at each recorded site Similar across left and right extremities	Flattening on recording: occlusive disease
Transcutaneous oxygen pressures	>40 mm Hg suggest healing of ulcer or surgical incision is likely	<20 mm Hg predict nonhealing of ulcer or surgical incision
Duplex scanning	Low velocity ratio; constant hue and intensity of image	Velocity ratio >4 or peak velocity >400 cm/sec indicates >75% stenosis

BP, Blood pressure.

High-resolution B-mode imaging combined with color and power Doppler and real-time spectral analysis have made duplex scanning one of the most widely used and accurate methods of noninvasive evaluation of arterial disease. Duplex scanning can accurately assess the location and degree of arterial disease from the level of the aorta to the level of the ankle. It provides accurate, objective information that supplements the physical examination. A disadvantage of this modality is the prolonged time it takes to perform an accurate examination of the entire extremity. Screening for arterial disease is done by comparing the signals from the various sites along the peripheral arterial tree and measuring the velocities at points of narrowing and comparing them with velocities in nonnarrowed areas of the arteries. This velocity ratio correlates with a 50% diameter narrowing when it is greater than 2. When the velocity ratio is greater than 4, the corresponding arterial narrowing is greater than 75%. Peak velocities at sites of narrowing can also be used to estimate the degree of narrowing. The sensitivity and specificity of this test is on the order of 90% or greater.[42] Although some surgeons may rely solely on duplex scanning for preoperative peripheral arterial bypass planning, most believe it needs to be supplemented by a more direct method to outline the arterial anatomy.

Two other modalities that are used to outline the specific arterial anatomy in place of standard angiographic mapping are MRA and CTA. Magnetic resonance imaging (MRI) is founded on the ability to detect radiofrequency signals given off by protons within a powerful magnet. Their movement within the studied structures creates a signal or echo that is detectable and can be imaged. Several magnetic resonance techniques are available to image blood within vessels[43]; the use of a contrast agent such as gadolinium injected through a peripheral vein greatly enhances the information gained from the images. MRA studies with contrast are highly specific and 100% sensitive for identification of arterial lesions that require intervention.[44] The advantages of MRA include the ability to create directly acquired images with large fields of view and the avoidance of potentially nephrotoxic contrast agents.

This is particularly important for patients with renal dysfunction. Also, because the magnetic resonance contrast agent is given through a peripheral vein, it avoids the arterial puncture required for angiography, which may precipitate the showering of cholesterol emboli to distal arteries if the artery punctured (often the femoral artery) is diseased with cholesterol-laden atheromatous plaques. The visualization of the distal runoff arterial tree when there are multiple levels of occlusions is much better than that seen with conventional angiography. However, the spatial resolution of MRA images is less than that available through digital subtraction angiography (DSA). Another drawback is that calcium within the artery, which impacts operative planning, cannot be seen in MRA. Other disadvantages include the inability to use this magnet-driven modality in patients with pacemakers, defibrillators, and intracorporeal metallic fragments that might migrate. Although conventional angiography with either film-screen or digital imaging is considered to be the gold standard, Wilkstrom and colleagues[45] showed a sensitivity and specificity of approximately 85% for DSA.

The advent of the helical or spiral CT scanners enabled CT technology to be applied to the diagnosis of peripheral arterial abnormalities due to the markedly reduced time required for scanning. With this technology, large areas of the body can be scanned in 20 or 30 seconds. An iodinated contrast agent is given through a peripheral vein. This avoids potential complications of a direct arterial injection but does not preclude the risk of inducing renal failure. Although less concentrated contrast agents can be used for CTA, the volumes required are larger than those for conventional angiography. Both noncontrast images and postcontrast injection images are taken. One advantage of CTA over MRA is the excellent visualization of vessel wall calcium deposits with CTA. But if there is much calcium, these areas become indistinguishable from the areas opacified after contrast injection. CTA performed for evaluation of the arteries in the lower extremities is beginning to be used more and more in clinical practice. However, its spatial resolution is less than that seen with DSA and small peripheral arteries are not as well visualized.

Vascular Examination: Invasive Strategies

Arteriography is classified as an invasive examination strategy because it involves local surgical placement of a catheter into the femoral artery in the groin (or alternatively, the axillary, radial, or subclavian arteries or the aorta), followed by introduction of radiopaque dye into the arterial tree and exposure to radiation. Because of the risks associated with the procedure, arteriography is typically used before revascularization or amputation surgery to determine specific location and severity of vessel occlusion, as well as the extent of collateral circulation, as a follow-up to noninvasive testing or when MRA imaging is contraindicated for individuals with metal implants such as pacemakers and total joint prostheses. Arteriography is not appropriate for individuals with renal dysfunction, cholesterol emboli syndrome, or allergies to substances containing iodine.[40,41]

An invasive angiography procedure can take 90 minutes or more, depending on what is being imaged and how many images are required. During the procedure the area that is to be punctured is first numbed with a local anesthetic agent. If the person undergoing the procedure is particularly anxious, the physician can administer a sedative agent orally or parenterally before or during the procedure. After the area is adequately anesthetized, an 18-gauge, 2.75-cm needle with a hollow, thin-walled outer cannula and a sharp, beveled inner stylet is inserted into the artery. Once the artery has been punctured, the stylet is removed and replaced with a guide wire that is carefully threaded farther into the vessel;

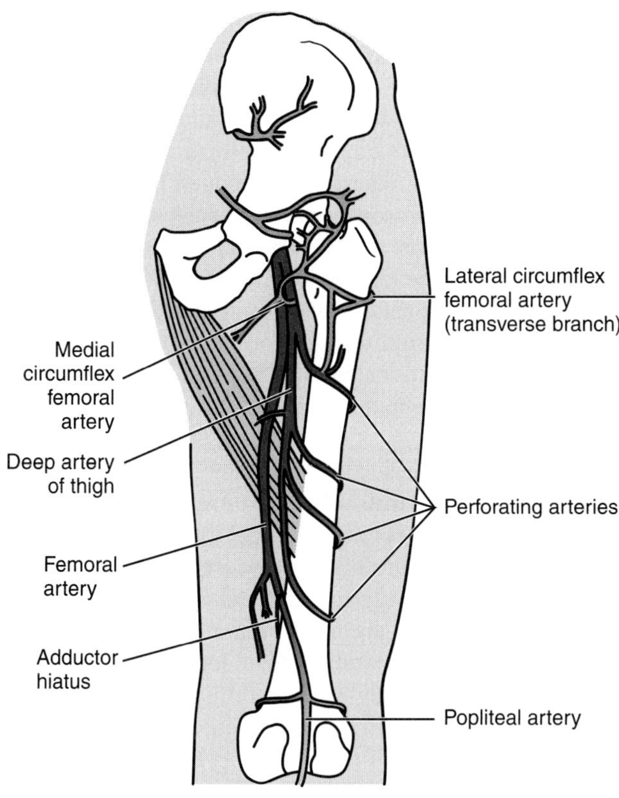

Figure 22-3
Diagram of arterial vessels of the pelvis and femur (posterior view) that can be visualized by MRA, or by invasive arteriography.

this wire then guides placement of the catheter that will deliver contrast medium. Catheters as small as 1-mm outer diameter may be used (3 French), but more commonly, 4 or 5 French catheters are used with outer diameters of 1.32 mm and 1.65 mm, respectively.

Once 40 to 120 ml of contrast medium has been injected, the catheter is flushed with heparinized saline to reduce the risk of clot formation. Successive still or continuous video radiographs record the progression of the dye through the limb's arterial tree (Figure 22-3).[39-41] After the catheter is removed from the femoral artery, manual compression is held locally at the site for several minutes and the patients remain at bed rest for a minimum of 4 hours. To ensure healing of the puncture artery, physical activity (include rehabilitation interventions) is postponed until several hours to a day after the procedure.

Decision Making: Thrombolytic Therapy, Angioplasty, or Amputation?

Intraarterial infusion of thrombolytic agents is used to manage several situations: (1) acute thrombosis of the extremity, (2) following percutaneous angioplasty, (3) after surgical bypass procedure of an extremity, or (4) after acute thrombosis of a diseased native artery.[46-48] The most commonly used thrombolytic agents are streptokinase, urokinase, and tissue plasminogen activator (t-PA). Streptokinase and urokinase are non–fibrin-specific agents that convert circulating plasminogen to plasmin, which subsequently breaks down fibrin, one of the main components of clot. t-PA is a fibrin selective agent. It acts locally by activating plasminogen to form plasmin, which, in turn, breaks up the fibrin in the clot. These agents are typically administered directly at the site of the clot (or as close as possible to it) via a catheter that is threaded through the arterial tree from the initial access site. Because of this, it is not likely that active rehabilitation would be initiated or maintained during this treatment because the person receiving the infusion remains in bed until the infusion is complete, which may require several days.

Frequently, intraarterial infusion of thrombolytic agents is followed by the initiation or continuation of systemic intravenous heparin therapy or warfarin therapy.[49-51] Long-term anticoagulation with warfarin is commonly put into place after acute arterial occlusion of a diseased native artery or an extremity bypass graft. Long-term warfarin therapy, with or without aspirin, may be used for individuals with lower extremity arterial bypass procedures who are determined to be at high risk for graft occlusion. The heparins are a class of agents that bind to antithrombin III to effect anticoagulation. Warfarin blocks the action of the vitamin K–dependent factors in the coagulation cascade. This has implications for the patient undergoing active rehabilitation because these agents increase the risk of bleeding complications, especially with manipulation of the wound in the immediate postoperative period of about 7 to 10 days.

A sudden marked increase in pain at the bypass site or amputation residual limb in any person on anticoagulant therapy is a sign of possible local bleeding; Outward signs of bleeding at the operative site such as swelling, ecchymosis, hematoma, or active bleeding may not be readily apparent early in the course of this complication because the bleeding may begin at the subfascial level. If any of these signs or symptoms occur during rehabilitation, the therapist should stop the therapy session and notify the patient's physician. Sudden onset of increased pain in the wound or extremity, along with recurrence of signs of limb ischemia, may also herald occlusion of the graft or progression of disease in the native vasculature following amputation at any level. It is important to identify signs of the failing graft as early as possible because the limb could possibly be salvaged if intraarterial thrombolytic therapy, as described earlier, is initiated soon enough.

Amputation is the only option for patients with dysvascular or neuropathic limbs in several situations. In the setting of acute or chronic arterial ischemia, amputation is considered the procedure of choice when the patient's arterial anatomy precludes bypass or when the patient presents so late in the course of the ischemia that bypass cannot salvage the tissue, which has become irreversibly ischemic and frankly gangrenous. Arterial bypass may not be an option for individuals with complex medical conditions who are deemed high risk for complications of surgery. Arterial bypass or thrombolytic therapy may be adjuncts to amputation in order to allow amputation at a more distal level, as long as there is no frank infection present (wet gangrene) and the person's arterial anatomy is conducive to bypass. In these cases amputation removes only nonviable skin, and the bypass or thrombolytic therapy improves the chance of healing at the more distal site.

If it is determined that a particular individual has insufficient vascular supply to heal a low-level amputation (transmetatarsal or transtibial) and rehabilitation at a higher level (transfemoral) is unlikely, lower extremity arterial bypass may be indicated in order to salvage a knee joint and maintain potential for ambulation with a prosthesis. Extensive gangrene of the foot, which is complicated by infection, is an indication for an open (guillotine) distal transtibial amputation. Time is given for the infection to be controlled by antibiotics and local wound care of the open surgical construct. The residual limb is then revised more proximally and a formal transtibial or transfemoral amputation with standard closure techniques is done.

Traumatic Injuries

In the United States most traumatic amputations are the result of industrial and farming accidents, motor vehicle accidents, or injury during high-risk sport and leisure activities.[52] In areas of the world where there is current or recent armed conflict, traumatic amputations are more likely to be the result of land mines or grenades, roadside bombs, shrapnel, or direct gunfire.[53] In most of these injuries the wound is likely to be contaminated by weapon fragments and organic materials (dirt, road debris, bits of clothing, vegetation), as well as damaged bone and soft tissue. In both situations the likelihood of infection due to introduced environmental microorganism, ischemia due to vascular damage, and tissue necrosis due to direct damage is high. There may also be significant loss of blood volume and hypovolemic shock, head injury, chest or abdominal injury, and other fractures to contend with.

In emergency care the first priority is to stabilize the medical condition: maintain the airway, support respiration, and ensure adequacy of circulation to the heart and brain.[54] The mangled limb is then carefully cleaned and débrided, a "cocktail" of systemic prophylactic antibiotics (e.g., cephalosporin, gentamicin, and penicillin) is begun, and a tetanus shot is given. Next the trauma team must decide whether the limb can be salvaged or replanted. The team considers many factors in making this difficult decision including severity of fracture and soft tissue injury, likelihood of bony union, adequacy of arterial blood supply, neuromotor and sensory function of the extremity, potential for prosthetic use, recovery time, and anticipated long-term functional status and quality of life.[55] Limb salvage and replantation are associated with high health care costs because of increased likelihood of multiple hospitalizations for successive surgical procedures, complications and delayed healing, and secondary amputation if the salvage attempt failed.[56] With improving microsurgical techniques, long-term outcome (e.g., return to work, perceived health status) is fairly similar when primary amputation and successful limb salvage and reconstruction are compared; however, residual impairment, functional limitation, and disability can have a significant impact on the quality of life in both groups.[56,57] Any severe trauma to the lower extremities, whether salvage is attempted or amputation is the intervention of choice, is life altering.

Decision Making: Limb Salvage or Amputation?

A number of strategies for assessing viability of the severely injured lower extremity have been developed to guide the decision between salvage and amputation[58-63] (Table 22-4). Most of these indices are more accurate in predicting the need for primary amputation than long-term functional outcome of limb salvage.[64] In general, salvage attempts are most likely to demonstrate delayed healing or go on to secondary amputation if there has been high-energy injury, comminuted open fractures of Type IIIC or higher, periosteal stripping, arterial injury with prolonged warm ischemia time, or complete disruption of the tibial nerve.[65,66] Individuals or their family health proxy must be informed of the pros and cons of limb salvage versus amputation including risk of infection and failure, as well as intensity and time frame for rehabilitation and likelihood of returning to premorbid functional levels.

If the decision is made to attempt limb salvage, the individual is taken from the emergency department to the operating room (OR). Arteriography (angiography) may be used to determine the extent of viable arterial perfusion. The next step is precise débridement of the damaged limb; surgeons must be sure that all compromised bone, muscle, and soft tissue are removed to reduce the likelihood of postoperative infection, necrosis, or later development of heterotopic ossification. It can be challenging to determine viability of cortical bone; cancellous bone is more likely to be revascularized. The biomechanical benefit of preserving as much bony length as possible must be weighed against the risk of developing osteomyelitis or delayed healing. Next, fractured fragments are stabilized with appropriate internal fixation, intramedullary rod, or external frame.

Defects in the bone may be filled with antibiotic-impregnated polymethylmethacrylate beads to further reduce the risk of infection and to preserve space for later bone graft. The areas of the limb that were incised during surgery are stitched or stapled closed, while trauma-damaged areas may be temporarily closed with a biological dressing. The reconstructed limb is monitored closely, with sharp débridement of any nonviable tissue in the early post-

Table 22-4
Comparison of Criteria and Grading Systems of the Mangled Extremity Syndrome Index (MESI) and the Mangled Extremity Severity Score (MESS)

MESI		
Component	*Criteria*	*Score*
Injury severity	0-25	1
	25-50	2
	>50	3
Injury type (integumentary)	Guillotine	1
	Crush or burn	2
	Avulsion or degloving	3
Nerve injury	Contusion	1
	Transection	2
	Avulsion	3
Vascular injury	Arterial transection	1
	Arterial thrombosis	2
	Arterial avulsion	3
	Any venous injury	1
Bone injury	Simple fracture	1
	Segmental fracture	2
	Segmental comminuted	3
	Segmental comminuted < 6 cm loss	4
	Segmental fracture involving joint	5
	Segmental fracture at joint < 6 cm	6
	Bone loss	Add 1
	Any bone loss > 6 cm	
Time since injury	Every hour > 6 hr	Add 1
Age	40-50 yr	1
	50-60 yr	2
	60-70 yr	3
Preexisting disease		1
Shock		2
Interpretation	< 20 points total = Limb salvage possible > 20 points total = Amputation recommended	Total

MESS (for Type IIIC Open Tibial Fractures)		
Component	*Criteria*	*Score*
"Energy" type of skeletal/soft tissue injury	Low (stab, closed Fx, sm gunshot)	1
	Medium (open Fx, dislocation, moderate crush)	2
	High (shotgun blast, high velocity gunshot)	3
	Massive crush (logging, railroad, rig accident)	4
Ischemia	None (palpable pulses, normal refill time)	0
	Mild (diminished pulses, near normal refill)	1
	Moderate (no Doppler sounds, paresthesia)	2
	Advanced (no pulse, cool, no movement)	3
Age	< 30 yr	1
	30-50 yr	2
	> 50 yr	3
Shock	Normotensive (stable BP in field and OR)	0
	Initial hypotension (responds to IV fluids in field)	1
	Prolonged hypotension (<90 mm Hg)	2
Interpretation	< 7 points = Limb salvage possible 7 or more points = Amputation recommended	Total

BP, Blood pressure; *Fx,* fracture; *OR,* operating room.

operative period every 24 to 72 hours, as appropriate for the degree of wound contamination on initial injury, until a clean wound bed is obtained. Once the wound bed is consistently clean, the individual whose limb is being salvaged returns to the OR (optimally within 1 week) for definitive closure of the surgical construct. This may be accomplished by delayed primary closure; split-thickness skin graft; local flaps; or, in some cases, vascularized pedicle graft. Subsequent to successful closure, the individual may return to the operating room for bone graft or transplantation or distraction osteogenesis to address osseous defects and limb-length discrepancy.

If the injury is too severe for salvage, a "guillotine" amputation may be performed to remove damaged tissues and restore hemostasis. If there has been significant contamination of the wound, the surgical construct may be left open (without skin closure) until the trauma team is satisfied that no infection has occurred. Once the individual's medical condition has stabilized and the wound is "clean," revision to a definitive level of amputation can be performed. Amputation after severe injuries may require split-thickness skin graft or sometimes even pedicle graft to achieve adequate skin closure. Skin pressure tolerance when wearing a prosthesis can be problematic later in the rehabilitation process when any type of grafting has been necessary.

Traumatic amputation is most likely to occur in young and midlife adults who are otherwise healthy. Once damaged tissue is removed and wound closure is achieved, circulation is often adequate for successful healing. These individuals, however, may be more likely to develop depression in the postoperative period because the injury was so sudden, and amputation so unexpected.[3] The sense of loss and alteration of body image after traumatic amputation can be more substantial than for an older adult with a diseased limb who "elected" to undergo amputation. Similarly, depression is a significant risk in those who are in the midst of limb salvage because of the likelihood of a long period of limited activity and altered appearance of the salvaged limb.

Neoplasm

Various tumors of soft tissue and bone range from slow-growing localized tumors to invasive and aggressive tumors (Box 22-1). Presenting signs and symptoms may include nonpainful enlargement of the limb, persistent pain, and pathological fracture. The incidence of tumors of bone and soft tissue demonstrate two "age peaks"; the first occurs in adolescents and young adults (especially osteosarcoma), with a second peak in adults older than the age of 60 years.[67]

The most frequently diagnosed tumor of the skeletal system is metastatic, usually originating from a primary site in the breast, prostate, lung, or colon.[68] Metastatic cells disrupt and alter the balance of osteoblastic and osteoclastic activity within bone, resulting in higher rates of resorption and lysis of bony structure. Metastatic bone disease is most commonly manifested as a deep pain present at rest and during activity, and it carries an increasing risk of pathological fracture. Metastatic bone disease is typically managed with a combination of radiation and chemotherapy, along with nonsteroidal antiinflammatory or opioid medications, with a primary goal of relieving pain and enhancing function.[69] Some metastatic tumors may require an orthopedic

Box 22-1 *Tumors of Bone and Soft Tissue*

METASTATIC TUMORS OF BONE

Primary site:	Breast Prostate Lung Kidney Melanoma Thyroid
Most common sites:	Rib cage Spine Pelvis Long bones of the extremities Skull
Signs and symptoms:	Pain Hypercalcemia Anemia Pathological fracture

PRIMARY BENIGN TUMORS OF CARTILAGE OR BONE

Osteochondroma (exostoses, bony overgrowths)
Chondroma
Chondroblastoma
Chondromyxoid fibroma
Osteoid osteoma
Osteoblastoma
Giant cell tumor

Signs and symptoms:	Nonpainful unless pathological Fracture occurs

PRIMARY MALIGNANT TUMORS OF BONE, CARTILAGE, OR MARROW

Chondrosarcoma
Osteosarcoma
Ewing's sarcoma
Lymphoma
Myeloma

Signs and symptoms:	Pain, with no history of injury Insidious asymmetry of limbs
Osteosarcoma:	Evidence of osteoblastic activity on radiograph
Chondrosarcoma:	Areas of lysis and of calcification

Once a primary tumor of bone has been typed and staged, the appropriate intervention is initiated. Nonpainful localized benign tumors typically do not require surgical intervention and are followed serially to watch for tumor progression. Symptomatic benign tumors (i.e., those that are painful or interfere with function) are treated by excision with bone graft or cement to fill the resulting bony defect.[87] Localized malignant tumors are excised using limb-sparing and reconstructive strategies. Those with osteosarcoma or Ewing sarcoma almost always have either preoperative or postoperative chemotherapy to minimize the likelihood of recurrence, while those with chondrosarcoma may not require such intervention.[88] For successful limb-saving surgery, the surgeon must first completely remove the tumor, achieving wide, clean margins in the bone above and below the lesion. A tumor in the middle of long bone that does not include epiphyses is often excised en bloc and replaced with an allograft transplant or expandable endoprosthesis.[73] A tumor that crosses the epiphysis or extends into the joint space is also excised en bloc, and a total joint replacement performed to restore function of the limb.[72] When the tumor is large, high grade, and invasive of other soft tissue compartments of the limb, amputation may be the most appropriate strategy.

Following limb-sparing surgery or amputation, appropriate rehabilitation interventions may include exercise to improve strength, range of motion, and endurance; energy conservation strategies; protective weight bearing during gait training with an appropriate assistive device; prosthetic rehabilitation (for those with amputation); functional training for mobility and activities of daily living; pain management (especially for those with metastatic disease); and patient and family education.[88] The therapist's understanding of the biomechanics and tissue manipulation undertaken in the reconstructive or amputation surgery is essential for appropriate exercise prescription and activity planning. Therapists must also be aware of the impact of chemotherapy and radiation treatments on healing soft tissue and bone; on peripheral sensation; and on physiological response to exercise and activity, as well as the individual's overall health status, immune response, prognosis, and level of energy.[68] The most successful rehabilitation programs are individualized and adapt to any adverse effects of concurrent adjuvant oncological interventions.[89] Individuals with recent diagnosis of bone cancer often find significant support in interacting with others who have previously rehabilitated from limb-sparing or amputation surgery.

Congenital Limb Deficiency

The birth of a child with a congenital limb deficiency is initially more distressing and disruptive to the new parents than to the infant. The development of the child's body schema and personality is significantly influenced by the attitudes and expectations of parents and caregivers within the context of the social-cultural environment in which he or she is raised.[90] The rehabilitation, prosthetic, and eventual "elective" surgical management of children with limb deficiency is linked to age-appropriate developmental status with the goal of enhancing function while minimizing deformity.[91,92] The reader is referred to Chapter 31 for in-depth information on developmentally appropriate preprosthetic and prosthetic activities for mobility and skill, as well as discussion of the therapist's and prosthetist's role in counseling and educating the family and child about rehabilitation and prosthetic alternatives.

Orthopedic and surgical management of children with congenital limb deficiency focuses on enhancing appropriate growth of the residual limb, maintaining relatively equal limb length, enhancing joint function, and ensuring appropriate prosthetic fit. This may include custom-fit and fabricated orthoses or prostheses with shoe lifts; surgical and distraction procedures to lengthen bone; rotational osteotomy; simple surgical revisions to optimize shape of the residual limb; surgical correction of terminal overgrowth; and, when the deficiency is complex, conversion to a conventional level of amputation or disarticulation in order to enhance functional use of a prosthesis.[93] School-aged children with a partial longitudinal deficiency of the femur (proximal focal femoral deficiency) may be managed with a Van Ness procedure, a rotation osteotomy that fuses a tibia that has been repositioned 180 degrees to the residual femur (if present) or pelvis so that the foot can function as a knee joint (Figure 22-6) or with an osteotomy without rotation that is subsequently followed by ankle disarticulation to achieve a weight-tolerant residual limb closely resembling "traditional" transfemoral residual limb.[94-97] Deficiencies of the fibula or tibia may be managed, depending on the severity of the defect and resulting deformity, by custom footwear and shoe lift, epiphysiodesis, ankle reconstruction or disarticulation, conversion to "traditional" transtibial amputation and prosthetic fitting, derotation osteotomy, and limb-lengthening procedures.[98-103]

AMPUTATIONS OF THE FOOT AND ANKLE

Amputations of one or more toes (digit, phalanx) or of part of the foot are the most frequently performed surgeries in older individuals, most often secondary to a nonhealing, often infected, neuropathic plantar ulcer. Individuals most vulnerable to development of plantar ulcers usually present with a combination of sensory impairment (loss of protective sensation); autonomic dysfunction (dry and brittle skin); foot deformity resulting from weakness of the intrinsic muscles of the foot; and impaired circulation that, although adequate to sustain an intact limb, is insufficient to allow healing to occur.[104] In these situations it is especially important to determine (before amputation) the point at which limb circulation is sufficient for successful healing of the residual foot.[105]

surgical intervention such as placement of an endoprosthesis, along with orthotic intervention to preserve or restore function, especially if there has been pathological fracture with neuromuscular impairment.[70]

The incidence of primary malignant neoplasm involving bone and soft tissue is quite low when compared with tumors of other systems.[71] Because of this, the management of primary tumors of bone has evolved into a specialty practice, which means that many newly diagnosed individuals are referred to regional centers where national guidelines ensure consistency of care.[72] Although the number of amputations performed as a result of neoplasm is significantly less than those resulting from dysvascular/neuropathic disease, amputations due to neoplasm are more likely to be performed at proximal levels including hip disarticulation. Along with trauma injury, neoplasm is the leading cause of limb loss in children and adolescents.

Decision Making: Limb-Saving Surgery or Amputation?

Until the 1990s most tumors of bone were managed by amputation with adjunctive chemotherapy or radiation. Currently, localized radical resection with bone or joint replacement (cadaver or titanium) and a combination of multiagent chemotherapy, isolated limb perfusion with tumor-necrosis factors, and radiation are being used with increasing frequency, reducing the number of tumor-related amputations performed each year.[73-79] Survival rates and rehabilitation outcomes are surprisingly similar for those with primary bone or soft tissue sarcoma managed by amputation or by limb salvage and reconstruction, although quality of life may be compromised as compared with peers without sarcoma.[80-82] Amputation is often performed when there is large, multifocal, high-grade, proximally positioned sarcoma, especially if there has been pathological fracture or significant involvement of neurovascular structures.[83-85] Amputation is also performed when there is local recurrence following previous limb salvage.[86]

When a tumor of bone or soft tissue is suspected, initial assessment strategies may include a radiograph, bone scan, CT scan, or MRI. In individuals with previous history of cancer who present with bone pain, a radiograph may reveal a "moth-eaten" area within bone, with unclear boundaries or edges (Figure 22-4), demonstrating areas of osteolysis and reactive osteoblastic activity.[68] A whole-body bone scan may be used to determine if there are multiple metastatic sites. A CT scan may be used to assess three-dimensional structural integrity and mineral content of the bone.

An MRI determines which extent of tissue involvement in marrow, bone, and surrounding soft tissue is especially useful in planning surgical intervention for primary malignant tumor of bone or soft tissue (Figure 22-5).[70] Laboratory tests may include blood assays including sedimentation rate, C-reactive protein levels, serum electrophoresis, alkaline and acid phosphate levels, blood calcium levels, blood sugar levels, and hemoglobin concentration. For those with p mary neoplastic bone disease, biopsy is used to determi cell type and contributes to pathological staging of t tumor. Depending on the tumor location, the surgeon m use an open frozen section, cannulated drill, or fine-need aspiration to obtain a biopsy sample.[71,72] For those with pr vious cancers of breast, lung, bone, or colon, biopsy may n be necessary.

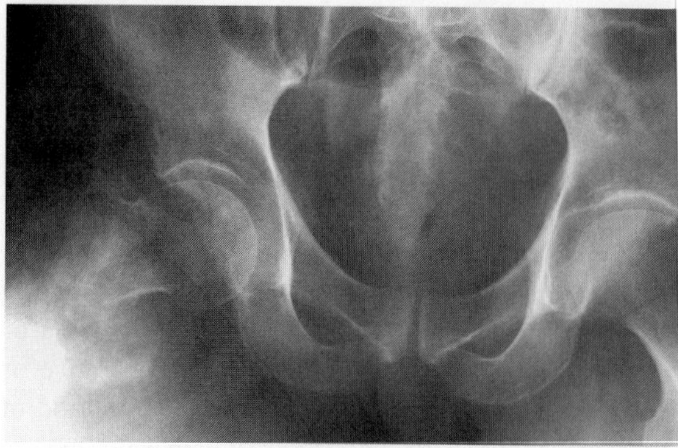

Figure 22-4

Radiograph of the hip joints and pelvis of an individual a metastatic lesion of the right femoral neck and trochan Note the poorly defined edges of the metastatic tumor an differences in appearance of bone when right and left fen are compared. (From Davis AM: Bone neoplasm. In Lun K (ed), Orthopedic Rehabilitation Science: Principles f Clinical Management of Bone. *Boston: Butterworth-Heinemann, 2000.)*

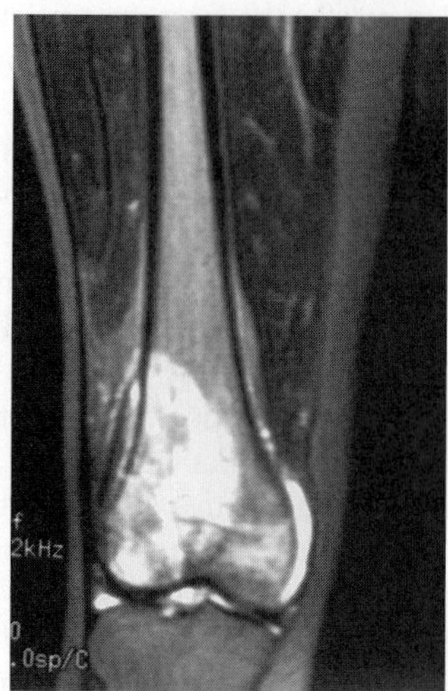

Figure 22-5

A magnetic resonance image of osteosarcoma of the distal femur that extends through both condyles and marrow anc into surrounding soft tissue. (From Davis AM. Bone neoplasm. In Lundon K (ed), Orthopedic Rehabilitation Science: Principles for Clinical Management of Bone. *Boston: Butterworth-Heinemann, 2000. p. 147.)*

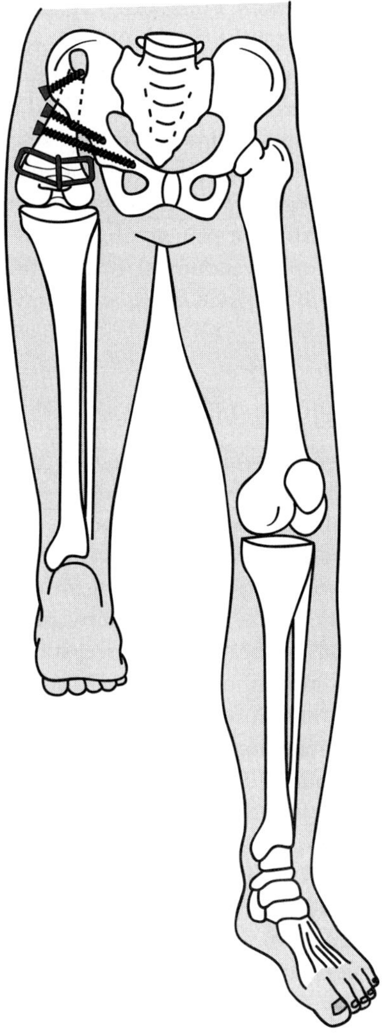

Figure 22-6
A diagram of the surgical resection, rotationplasty, and femoral arthrodesis (modified Van Ness procedure) used to create a functional residual limb that can be fit with a prosthesis for a child with a severe congenital proximal focal femoral deficiency. (Modified from Brown KL. J Bone Joint Surg *2001;83-A(1):81.)*

Physical deconditioning associated with prolonged bed rest (especially problematic in older adults) and increasing likelihood of systemic complications (in persons with cardiac and pulmonary comorbidities) associated with repeated surgical "revisions" of a poorly healing amputation can substantially compromise the rehabilitation process and potential for positive outcome.[106] Amputations of the foot may also be the result of severe crush injury, land mine explosion, shrapnel wounds, or similar acute trauma to the foot. The risk of wound contamination by environmental debris and microorganisms increases the likelihood of infection and may require a two-stage surgical approach.[107] Not all individuals with amputations of the toes are referred for physical therapy and prosthetic rehabilitation, unless they require instruction in non–weight bearing or protected ambulation. Those with partial foot amputation may require adaptive footwear, shoe filler, a passive prosthesis, or accommodative foot orthoses, and may be referred to physical therapy for gait training with an appropriate assistive device.

Amputations of the Toes

Phalangeal (digit) amputations are performed when there is evidence of localized "dry" gangrene on the toe related to vascular insufficiency, when conservative management of a neuropathic ulcer on the plantar toe surface has not been successful, or when there is infection or osteomyelitis of the phalanges.[108] Digit amputation can be performed at the distal, middle, or proximal interphalangeal joints or with removal of the metatarsal head.[109] Adequate circulation for healing of the surgical wound is a prerequisite to amputation surgery at this distal level. Depending on the age, comorbidities, and current medical condition of the individual undergoing surgery, phalangeal amputations can be performed using an ankle block, an epidural, spinal anesthesia, or general anesthesia.[110] The forefoot is thoroughly cleaned, especially between the toes, with an antiseptic solution to reduce the risk of postoperative infection. A tourniquet may be placed around the calf to be inflated to approximately 50 mm Hg above systolic blood pressure as surgery begins in order to minimize bleeding during the procedure.

For removal of digits, sagittal flaps are typically used (Figure 22-7, *A*). If there will also be resection of metatarsal head, the surgeon may opt to use a "racquet" incision. The digits are removed, either by disarticulation through the joint or transection through the shaft of the digit, using a bone cutter or oscillating saw. Transection through the phalanx is the preferred method because of the avascular nature of cartilage, which compromises wound healing. Distal nerves and tendons are cut under tension (to shorten them 5 to 10 mm) and allowed to retract into the foot. Sesamoid bones, if present, are removed, especially when the metatarsal head is resected.

Once the segment being amputated is removed, the tourniquet is deflated to reestablish hemostasis; the surgeon may use ligature or electrocautery to close bleeding vessels as needed. Next, the surgical site is irrigated with sterile saline or an antibiotic solution to remove any tissue debris before closure. Absorbable sutures are placed to close the internal layers of soft tissues, and then the skin is closed with either sutures (for simple digit resection) or staples (for the larger incisions used in resection of a metatarsal head) (Figure 22-7, *B*). A nonadherent dressing (e.g., Adaptic or Xeroform) is placed over the suture line, and several folded 4 × 4 gauze pads are positioned over the wound and around neighboring toes to apply slight pressure over the surgical wound. Kerlix or Ace bandages are then applied in a figure-of-eight

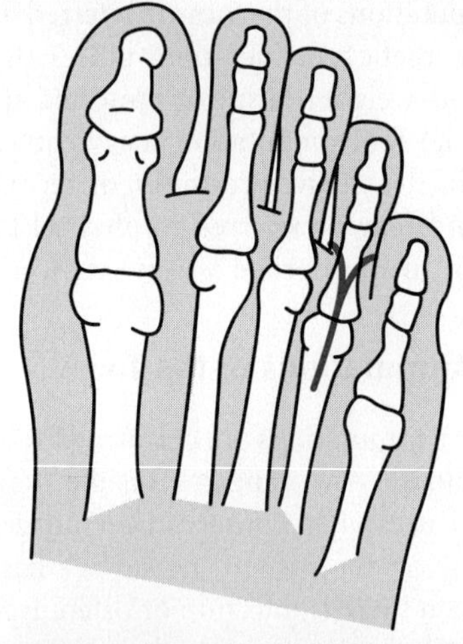

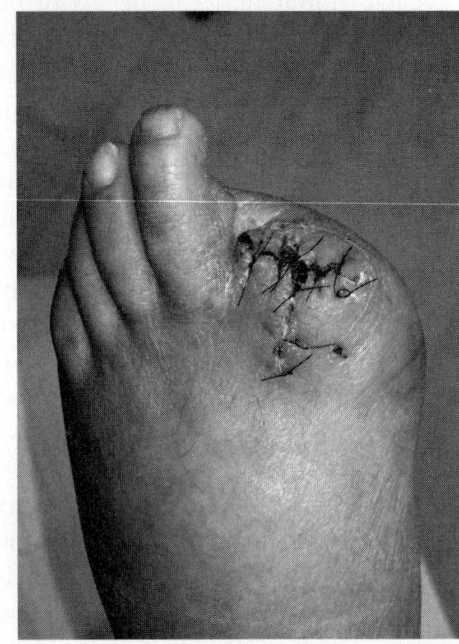

Figure 22-7
A, *Skin incision used for amputation of the fourth toe, with disarticulation at the metatarsal-phalangeal joint.* ***B,*** *Postoperative appearance of the foot after amputation of the hallux. (Courtesy Michael Z. Fein, DPM, Bethel Podiatry, Bethel, Conn.)*

distal toward proximal wrap, leaving remaining toes visible to monitor adequacy of circulation.

The initial dressing typically stays in place up to 5 days unless there are signs of infection (localized pain, excessive or purulent drainage, fever, loss of diabetic control).[109-111] The individual is instructed in non–weight-bearing ambulation using an appropriate assistive device (typically a walker or crutches), on level surfaces, inclines, and stairs. The individual is encouraged to keep the limb elevated as much as possible: education about avoiding prolonged dependency of the limb (i.e., elevating the limb while sitting) is essential.

If the wound heals optimally, many surgeons allow progression to protected partial weight-bearing ambulation after postoperative day 10. Most do not encourage return to weight bearing as tolerated or full weight bearing until all sutures or staples have been removed, often 2 to 3 weeks postoperatively. Many individuals wear a healing sandal for several weeks or months following surgery, before returning to normal footwear. Individuals with dysvascular and neuropathic disease benefit from custom-fabricated accommodative orthosis to distribute plantar pressures and minimize the risk of developing additional neuropathic ulcers on plantar surfaces of the remaining digits and metatarsal heads.

Metatarsal Head Resection

Metatarsal head resections are typically performed when there is a nonhealing plantar ulcer, especially if there is osteomyelitis of the metatarsal head, as long as there is evidence of adequate circulation for postamputation wound healing. The associated digit can be left in place to serve as a "spacer" in the shoe and to minimize the risk of subsequent foot deformity. The methods of anesthesia and preparation are similar to those used in toe amputation. Once again, a tourniquet may be placed to minimize bleeding during surgery.

A longitudinal incision is made along the dorsal shaft of the targeted metatarsal (Figure 22-8, *A*). Soft tissue structures are carefully detached from around the metatarsal head. The metatarsal is transected behind its head using an oscillating saw, and the metatarsal head is dissected from the proximal phalanx. The tourniquet is deflated to reestablish hemostasis, bleeding vessels are ligated or cauterized, and the wound is irrigated with sterile saline or antibiotic solution. Subcutaneous layers are closed with absorbable sutures, and skin closure is achieved with either staples or interrupted fine monofilament sutures (Figure 22-8, *B*). As soft tissue heals, scarring will create a pseudoarthrosis in place of the anatomical metatarsal head. A nonadherent dressing (e.g., Telfa pad) and several 4 × 4 gauze pads are placed over the dorsal incision site. Next, the surgeon turns to the plantar surface of the foot to trim any hypertrophic callus and to débride any plantar ulcer that might be present.

Once cleaned, the ulcer may be packed with gauze soaked in saline or antibiotic solution, and fluff gauze is placed over the plantar wound. The foot is wrapped, in a distal toward proximal progression, with Kerlix gauze or an Ace wrap, or both. Because of the need to monitor and repack any plantar wounds, dressings are typically changed daily. Instruction in non–weight-bearing ambulation with the appropriate assistive device and patient education about avoiding prolonged dependency of the limb should occur as soon as feasible following surgery. Sutures or staples usually remain in place up to 2 weeks postoperatively. Adequate follow-up care must be provided. This usually includes an accommodative orthosis to redistribute plantar pressure to avoid the future development of a "transfer" neuropathic ulcer under remaining metatarsal heads.

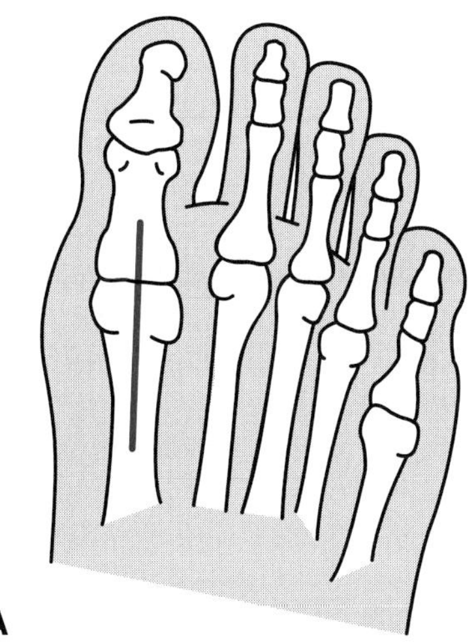

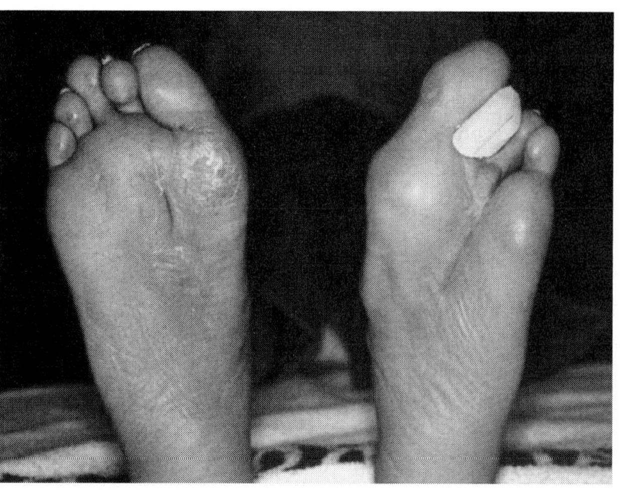

Figure 22-8

A, *Skin incision for excision of the first metatarsal head, when the plan is to leave the hallux intact. Soft tissue scarring will eventually create a pseudarthrosis so that forward progression over the toe in the late stance phase of gait will not be compromised.* ***B,*** *Postoperative appearance of the foot after excision of the second and fourth metatarsal head, with removal of the associated toe. (Courtesy Carolyn Kelly, Center for Wound Healing and Hyperbaric Medicine, Hartford Hospital, Hartford, Conn.)*

Ray Resection

Ray resections may be performed when vascular disease or neuropathic ulcer has compromised one or more "rays" of the forefoot and circulation is compromised enough to make healing unlikely at a more distal level. In this surgery 50% or more of the metatarsal, as well as its associated digits, are removed (Figure 22-9). The residual metatarsal (if any) is beveled at a 30- to 45-degree angle so that there will be no sharp edge to damage tissue during the late stance phase, as body weight rolls over the distal plantar surface of the healed residual limb.[99-101] If multiple rays are resected, skin graft may be required for wound closure.

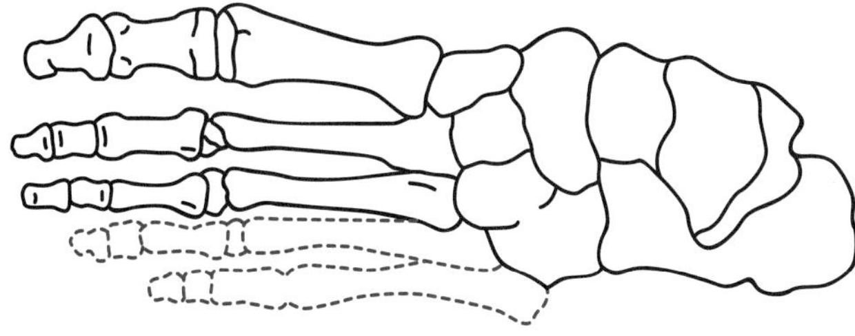

Figure 22-9

In this diagram of a metatarsal ray resection, the fourth and fifth rays (metatarsal and phalanges) have been removed. Surgeons can elect to transect the shaft of the metatarsal and leave the base of the metatarsals in place or to disarticulate through the tarsometatarsal joint.

Ray resection may be the surgery of choice for problems of the fourth and fifth rays: as long as the first through third rays are intact, there is minimum compromise to forward progression in gait on the healed residual limb. When the first and second rays must be removed, however, a complete transmetatarsal amputation managed with custom footwear with a rocker bottom often has better functional outcome than leaving the third through fifth rays intact.

Anesthesia and intraoperative care are similar to those described for toe amputation and metatarsal head resection. The soft dressing applied in the OR is typically changed daily for wound inspection, especially if there has been skin graft or débridement of a plantar ulcer. As soon as feasible, the individual is instructed in non–weight-bearing mobility using a walker or crutches; non–weight-bearing status continues until sutures or staples have been removed. The deformity that results when multiple rays have been amputated may require an accommodative orthosis or a prosthetic "filler" in the shoe, along with adaptive or custom footwear to protect the residual limb from high pressures resulting from altered biomechanics during forward progression and propulsion when walking.

Transmetatarsal Amputation

A complete transmetatarsal amputation is, essentially, ray resection of all five metatarsals proximal to their metatarsal heads. In this surgery the goal is to preserve as much length of the shaft of the metatarsals and healthy plantar skin as possible so that the resulting residual limb will be long enough for an effective biomechanical lever for forward progression over the foot during gait and will have enough plantar surface such that higher shear forces and pressures exerted on the shortened forefoot during the late stance phase of gait will not compromise skin condition.[112] Muscle imbalance between dorsiflexors and plantar flexors increases as the length of a transmetatarsal residual limb decreases, leaving individuals with short transmetatarsal residual limb at risk of developing equinovarus deformity in an already vulnerable foot.

After the limb has been carefully cleaned and draped for surgery, a tourniquet is applied to reduce distal blood flow and a guideline is marked across the dorsal foot just proximal to the metatarsal heads, continuing in a curvilinear arc along the plantar surface almost to the base of the toes (Figure 22-10). This type of incision creates a long posterior flap that will be sutured closed after bony and soft tissue elements have been excised. An oscillating saw is used to transect each of the metatarsals, and then the toes are plantar flexed to allow careful dissection of the soft tissue that will be used as the posterior flap from the bony structures being removed. The tendons and sheaths of extrinsic muscles of the foot, as well as distal attachments of intrinsic muscles, are transected; the plantar surface of residual metatarsals are beveled or rounded (to allow "rollover" in gait without high distal plantar pressures); and any distal nerves are resected under slight tension and allowed to retract into the residual limb. The posterior flap is trimmed and debulked to fit it appropriately to the dorsal incisions for a smooth wound closure. Blood vessels that have been transected are tied off or cauterized, the tourniquet is released, and hemostasis is restored. Just before closure, the surgical wound is thoroughly irrigated with saline and an antibiotic solution. Meticulous attention to hemostasis should preclude the need for placement of a drain; a closed suction drain placed deep to the facial layer of closure would be the preferred choice of drain if it is determined that one is required. The posterior flap is drawn upward to approximate edges of the wound on the dorsal surface. Deep subcutaneous fascia is sutured closed, followed by suturing and stapling of skin.

Once the wound has been closed, a layer of nonadherent dressing (e.g., Adaptic or Xeroform) is placed over the suture/staple line and a bulky dressing of fluffed gauze is placed around the forefoot. Several rolls of gauze bandage are gently wrapped around the entire foot and ankle, and an Ace wrap is applied to provide gentle compression (graded distally toward proximally) and minimize postoperative swelling. Dressings are left in place 3 to 5 days unless there are indications of infection or significant focal pain. Limited mobility and non–weight-bearing ambulation with a walker or crutches are often begun after the first dressing change, although healing is enhanced if the limb is kept elevated when in bed or in sitting in the early postoperative period. Staples and sutures are often left in place from 2 to 3 weeks postoperatively. Once the surgeon is satisfied that adequate wound closure has been achieved, the individual may be placed in a healing sandal and graded partial weight bearing during walking can begin.

Gradual progression to full weight bearing with an assistive device (walker, crutches, single cane) and independent ambulation without an assistive device is determined by skin condition of the residual limb and the individual's previous ambulatory status, postural control, and functional level. Many individuals benefit from wearing a sneaker or oxford with "forefoot filler" and a rocker bottom applied to the sole to dissipate higher weight-bearing forces on the distal plantar residual limb in the late stance phase; those with short residual transmetatarsal limbs may require a custom shoe that encompasses the ankle or a custom thermoplastic ankle-foot orthosis to counteract muscle imbalance leading to equinovarus position during the swing phase of gait and to ensure efficient heel strike at initial contact and appropriate forward progression in stance. (Readers are referred to Chapter 25.) Those with polyneuropathy should be cautioned not to go barefoot, even in their home environment: their ability to detect injury to the plantar (or dorsal) surface of the foot may be significantly compromised. An open wound (neuropathic or traumatic in origin) on a transmetatarsal residual limb that becomes infected or fails to heal often leads to revision to the transtibial amputation level.

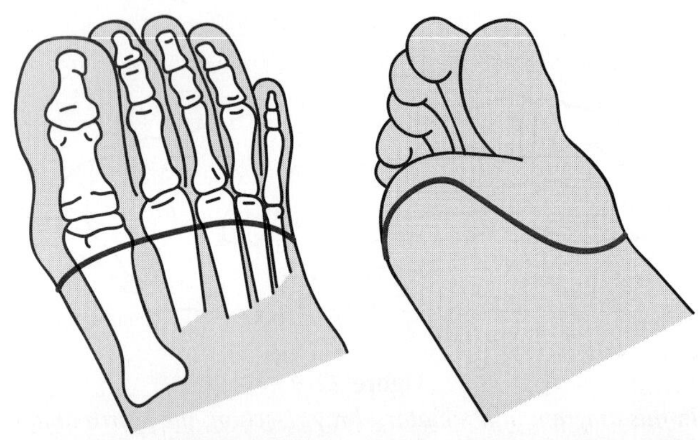

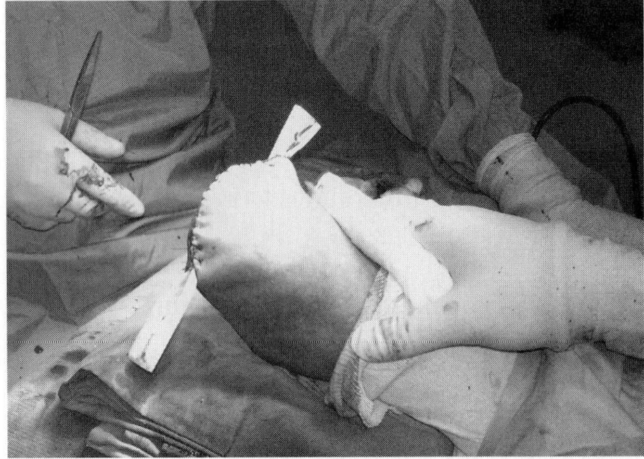

Figure 22-10
Dorsal **(A)** *and plantar* **(B)** *incisions for a complete metatarsal amputation. Each metatarsal will be transected just proximal to its head to preserve as much foot length as possible, and the longer plantar flap will be drawn upward and sutured to close the wound.* **C,** *Postoperative appearance of the foot after transmetatarsal amputation, with surgical drain in place. (Courtesy Michael Z. Fein, DPM, Bethel Podiatry, Bethel, Conn.)*

Amputations and Disarticulations of the Midfoot

The two most commonly performed amputations of the midfoot are tarsometatarsal disarticulation (Lisfranc procedure) and a midtarsal disarticulation (Chopart procedure) (Figure 22-11, see Figure 25-3). The operative approach and postoperative care for both surgeries is similar to that of a transmetatarsal amputation. The surgical incision is made more proximally across the dorsum of the foot, and a long posterior/plantar flap is created to wrap upward toward the dorsal incision when the surgical wound is closed. In a *Lisfranc* procedure, the forefoot is excised from the midfoot through the tarsometatarsal joint, usually leaving the "keystone" base of the second metatarsal in place to maintain a transverse arch of the midfoot. The midtarsal joints may be surgically fused as well to maintain the integrity of the architecture between midfoot and rearfoot.

The distal attachment of the peroneus brevis, peroneus longus, and anterior tibialis may be repositioned during surgery in an attempt to restore some level of equity (power) among muscle groups controlling dorsiflexion/plantar flexion and inversion/eversion positioning of the foot at rest and during walking. In a *Chopart* procedure, the disarticulation takes place in the joints between the talus and navicular bones and the calcaneus and cuboids. Both approaches may also include lengthening of the heel cord to ensure adequate dorsiflexion excursion for rollover during the stance phase of gait. A bulky dressing with an Ace wrap or a slightly dorsiflexed plaster cast is applied in the operating room.[113] Non–weight-bearing mobility with a walker or crutches begins several days after surgery, and protected weight bearing starts once adequate wound closure has been achieved and sutures or stables have been removed.

Lisfranc and Chopart surgeries may be used for individuals with significant traumatic injury or bone or soft tissue tumor in the forefoot; they are rarely used for individuals with dysvascular/neuropathic limbs. Although both approaches preserve the ability to bear weight through the calcaneus, there is even greater likelihood of development of the equinovarus deformity and prosthetic fitting can be challenging. Persons with a midfoot-level residual limbs typically require custom footwear and orthoses to protect the residual limb during functional activities and to ensure biomechanically sound, safe ambulation.[114] Those who develop significant equinovarus with pain and tissue damage during ambulation may opt return to the operating room after maturation of the residual limb, for surgical modification and subtalar arthrodesis of the residual limb, to achieve more comfortable and functional ambulation ability.

Syme Amputation

The most commonly performed amputation involving the rearfoot is the Syme procedure, a surgical technique that disarticulates the talocrural, trims the malleoli to create a "flat" weight-bearing surface, and repositions the fat pad and soft tissue of the heel under the distal tibia and fibula. Although the Syme procedure reduces leg length because the calcaneus and talus have been removed, the well-healed distal residual limb is pressure tolerant for ambulation with a prosthesis and, if necessary, for short distances (e.g., emergencies, getting to the bathroom at night) without a prosthesis.[115-117] Variations of the Syme procedure retain the weight-bearing portion of the calcaneus, fusing it to the distal tibia and fibula.

When the limb has been scrubbed and prepared for surgery and a tourniquet is in place, guidelines for incision are drawn on the anterior ankle from medial to lateral malleoli and then downward around the plantar (posterior calcaneus) surface to outline what will be the distal pad of the residual limb (Figure 22-12, *A, B*). After sharp incision through skin and subcutaneous tissue, toe extensor and dorsiflexor tendons are cut and the anterior capsule of the ankle is exposed. The foot is passively plantar flexed in order to access and open the joint capsule medially to laterally (with care to preserve the posterior tibialis artery going to tissue that will be the pad of the residual limb) and to disarticulate the talus. The posterior joint capsule, posterior tibialis tendon, and flexor hallucis longus tendon are transected. The periosteum of the calcaneus is carefully stripped and preserved for use in attaching the posterior flap/fat pad to the tibia later in the procedure. The Achilles tendon and plantar soft tissue are then dissected from the calcaneus, and the amputated foot completely removed. Plantar tendons and any remaining intrinsic muscle tissue are excised from the posterior flap/fat pad. The distal tips of the medial and lateral malleoli are removed using an oscillating saw, level with the articulating surface of the tibia. The flares of the

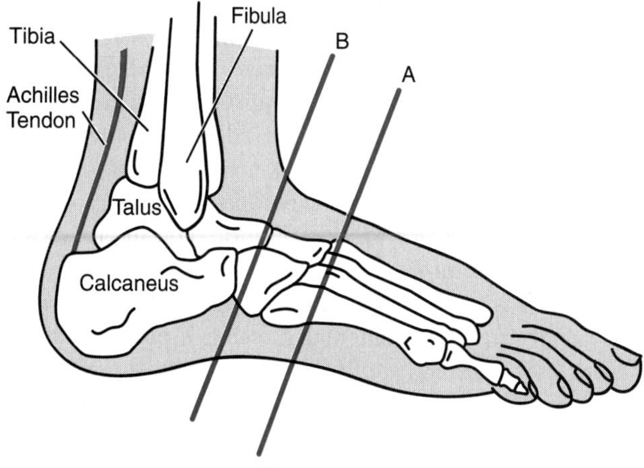

Figure 22-11
Diagram of the levels of amputation or disarticulation for a Lisfranc (**A**) *procedure at the tarsal metatarsal joint and a Chopart procedure* (**B**) *at the midtarsal (talonavicular and calcaneocuboid) joints. In both surgeries a longer plantar flap is left in place and used to close the wound.*

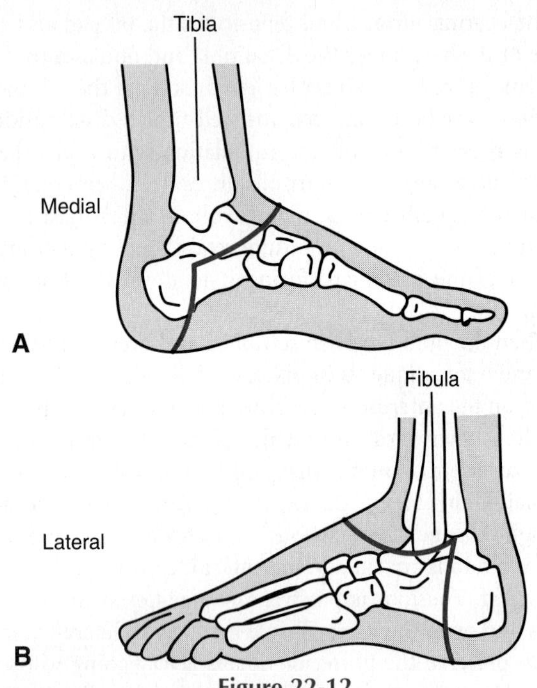

Figure 22-12
*Medial (**A**) and lateral (**B**) views of the incision for a Syme ankle disarticulation. After the talus is removed from its mortise, the distal points of malleoli are trimmed to create a flat surface and the posterior heel pad is drawn upward to close the wound.*

malleoli are trimmed parallel to the long axis of the tibia and fibula in order to create a less bulbous residual limb.

The tourniquet is deflated, and vessels are tied off or cauterized to restore hemostasis. The surgical construct is irrigated with a sterile saline antibiotic solution. Several obliquely oriented holes are drilled in the medial, lateral, and anterior edges of the tibia and fibula to be used as anchors for suturing the preserved periosteum and posterior flap/fat pad in place. A tubular drain is placed through the anterolateral skin to drain the wound as it heals, minimizing the risk of postoperative hematoma between bone and posterior flap. The flap is drawn up into position, and the preserved periosteum is sutured to bone, followed by suturing of the subcutaneous tissue and then stapling of the skin. After wound closure, a nonadherent dressing is placed over the suture line, followed by a fluffed-gauze, bulky dressing, and the limb is wrapped distally toward proximally toward the knee. Depending on surgeon preference, the limb may then be wrapped with a slightly compressive Ace bandage dressing; Unna paste, which will dry into a semirigid dressing; or plaster of Paris cast.

The drain is typically pulled and removed by postoperative day 2, leaving the dressing in place. The initial dressing change may wait until between postoperative days 5 and 7 unless there are clinical signs of infection or necrosis, to assist adherence of the fat pad to the distal surface of the tibia and fibula. Non–weight-bearing ambulation with a walker or crutches begins 2 to 3 days after surgery and continues for up to 8 weeks. This non–weight-bearing status is essential to ensure that the fat pad is not disrupted until it is firmly healed in place. Staples are typically removed after 3 weeks, and a program of gentle compression with Ace wraps or shrinker garment is initiated. Depending on the condition of the residual limb, the individual may be ready for initial prosthetic fitting by 6 to 8 weeks following amputation. Initial prosthetic training must be with careful partial weight bearing and an appropriate assistive device, with frequent inspection of the integrity and positioning of the distal pad. Progression to full weight bearing follows over the next several weeks.

TRANSTIBIAL AMPUTATION

Transtibial amputation typically has positive surgical and rehabilitative outcomes, as long as there is sufficient circulation for healing of the residual limb.[118,119] In the mid 1960s the "ideal" transtibial surgery preserved 15 cm (approximately 6 inches) of residual tibia to allow for effective knee extension power to control the prosthesis and to minimize discomfort and skin problems in the thermosetting hard sockets that were commonly in use at that time.[120,121] As residual tibial length decreases toward the tibial tubercle, mechanical advantage of knee flexors exceeds that of knee extensors, making it difficult to extend the knee enough to advance a prosthesis during swing and for controlled (eccentric) knee extension for stability in the early stance phase (Figure 22-13).

As the surface area for weight bearing within the socket decreases with limb length, the likelihood of discomfort, skin irritation, and limited use of a prosthesis increases. Conversely, in long residual limbs, the larger total surface area to distribute pressures within the socket and long lever arm potentially enhance prosthetic control, although there is a risk of chronic skin irritation and discomfort along the sharp edge of the distal-anterior tibial crest. Recent advances in prosthetic materials and design can accommodate, to some degree, for the biomechanical and prosthetic fitting challenges of slightly increased (more than 66%) or decreased (approaching only 33%) residual tibial length. Comfort in the prosthesis, quality of gait, and energy cost of ambulation seem to be best balanced when the level of amputation preserves 40% to 50% of the tibia.[122]

The type of anesthesia chosen for transtibial amputation surgery is determined by the individual's overall health and comorbid conditions and consideration of potential adverse outcomes of each method. Options include general anesthesia, spinal anesthesia or epidural, regional nerve blocks, and in some cases careful local anesthesia at the site of the incision and underlying tissues.[122] In older individuals

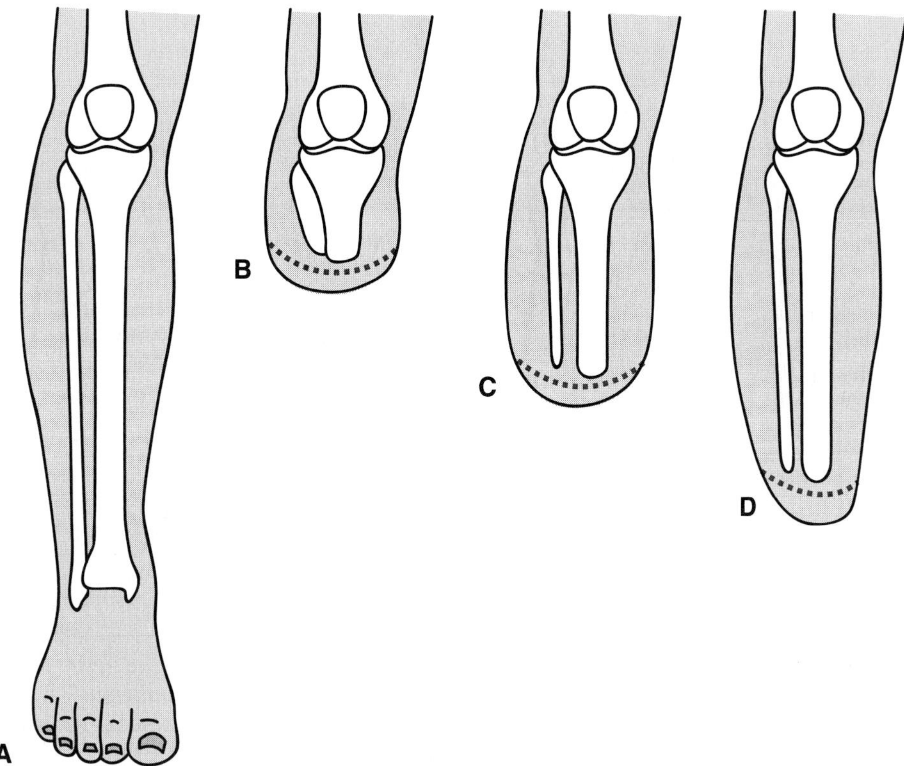

Figure 22-13
*Anatomical diagram of the tibia and fibula (**A**) and of short (**B**), midlength, standard (**C**), and long (**D**) residual limbs after transtibial amputation.* Dotted line *represents the suture line when a posterior flap approach has been used.*

likelihood of postoperative delirium and risks associated with concurrent cardiac disease may lead the anesthesiologist to use spinal anesthesia or regional blocks. In those with multiple traumatic injury, general anesthesia may allow for optimal physiological control during the surgery.

Depending on the condition of the skin and soft tissue, as well as the circumstances that have led to the decision to amputate, the surgeon selects from a number of surgical approaches (Figure 22-14). The most commonly used approach is the long posterior (myofasciocutaneous) flap: this technique preserves the highly vascular gastrocnemius muscle beyond the residual tibia, brings the flap up and forward, and positions the suture line across the distal anterior residual limb below the cut surface of the tibia. The next most common approach creates equal anterior-posterior skin flaps in which the incision runs in a U shape medially to laterally across the bottom of the residual limb. At times the surgeon may opt for equal mediolateral flaps, in which the incision runs in a U anteriorly to posteriorly across the bottom of the residual limb. The surgeon may even use a long medial or a long lateral flap that positions the incision on the distal opposite side of the limb. In all approaches the surgeon seeks to retain enough soft tissue so that there is little or no tension across the closed incision, but not so much that there will be redundant skin and tissue that might challenge prosthetic fitting. The posterior flap approach is discussed next as an example of surgical technique.[123]

The limb is cleansed, prepped, and draped for surgery, and a tourniquet is applied at midthigh level. A guideline for tibial length and for anterior incision sweeping into a distally curved posterior flap is drawn on the leg. The anterior incision is made through skin and then soft tissue to the periosteum of the tibia, and subcutaneous blood vessels are clamped. Next, muscles in the anterior compartment are incised so that the anterior tibial artery, vein, and deep peroneal nerve can be identified, clamped, transected, and ligated. Soft tissue is carefully removed from around the fibula about 2 cm (3/4 inch) shorter than the residual tibia. An oscillating saw or double-action bone cutter is used to transect the fibula. The surgeon then bevels the anterior tibia at an approximate 45-degree angle with an oscillating saw and repositions the saw to complete the transection in the transverse plane, controlling the wedge to be removed with a clamp. The skin and subcutaneous incision are now continued along what will become the posterior flap.

The transected lower tibia and fibula are pulled up and forward to allow access to structures in the posterior compartment and carefully beveled following the line of the posterior incision to create the posterior flap. Once the amputated limb has been removed, the posterior tibial and

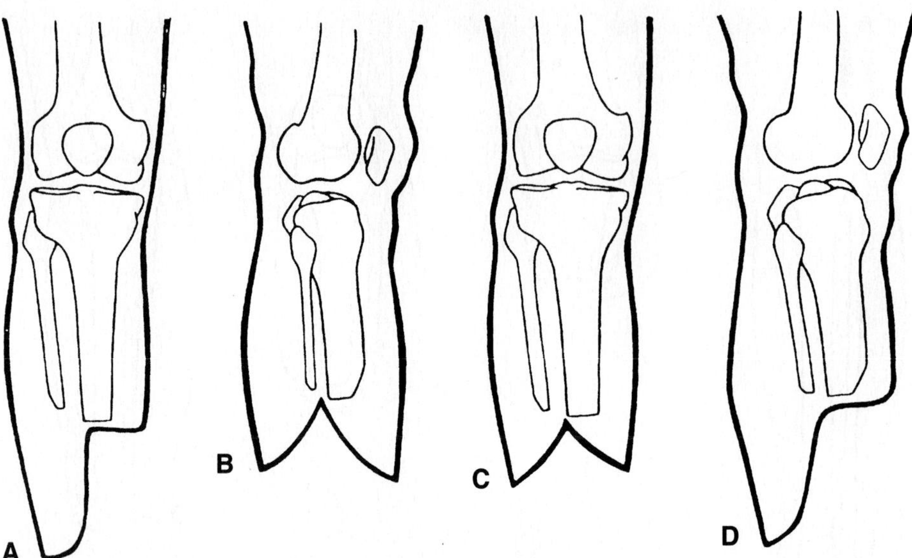

Figure 22-14

Examples of transtibial amputation techniques. ***A,*** *When a long lateral flap is used, the suture line will be on the distal medial aspect of the residual limb.* ***B,*** *When equal anterior and posterior flaps are used, the suture line lies in the frontal plane, side to side across the distal inferior residual limb.* ***C,*** *When equal medial and lateral sagittal flaps are used, the suture line lies in the sagittal plane, front to back across the distal inferior residual limb.* ***D,*** *The most common approach for individuals with dysvascular/neuropathic-related amputation is a long posterior flap, which places the suture line across the anterior surface of the residual limb, distal to the cut end of the tibia. (From Singer JM,* Hershey Board Certification Review Outline Study Guide. *Camp Hill, Pa.: Philadelphia College of Podiatric Medicine, 1993. p. 640.)*

peroneal arteries and veins are clamped. The soleus muscle is then dissected from the medial and lateral heads of the gastrocnemius and removed to "debulk" the posterior flap for optimal wound closure. The blood vessels of the posterior and lateral compartments are clamped, transected, and ligated. The tibial, superficial peroneal, and deep peroneal nerves are transected under traction so that they will retract upward, away from the end of the residual limb, in order to minimize the risk of subsequent neuroma formation. The tourniquet is deflated, any bleeding small vessels are electrocauterized or sutured, and hemostasis is restored. The beveled anterior tibia is smoothed with a rasp. The surgical site is then irrigated with sterile saline and antibiotic solutions in preparation for wound closure.

When the residual limb is short, much of the syndesmoses between tibia and fibula will have been lost. The surgeon may opt to use an osteoplastic procedure using preserved periosteum before closure in an effort to stabilize the ends of the transected bones. This, theoretically, minimizes the likelihood of dislocation of the fibular head during subsequent activity and prosthetic use.[121] For midlength and longer residual limbs, closure begins with suturing of the deep fascia and gastrocnemius tendon in the posterior flap to the fascia of the anterior compartment. A closed suction drain can be positioned in the posterior flap toward the medial leg above the incision to reduce the risk of hematoma formation within the residual limb. The limb is then irrigated again with saline and antibiotics, and staples are used to approximate and close the wound, with the goal of uniform tension across the incision.

A nonadherent dressing is laid along the incision, covered with a fluffed-gauze bulky dressing, and then a conforming gauze bandage is applied evenly in a distal to proximal figure-of-eight. At this point the surgeon may apply a layer of Ace wrap for slight compression of the residual limb, use an Unna bandage to create a semirigid postoperative dressing, use a prefabricated adjustable thermoplastic rigid dressing, or apply a plaster or fiberglass cast (with the knee in extension). The reader is referred to Chapter 23 for further discussion of the indications and limitations of each type of postoperative bandaging.

The drain is typically pulled 24 to 48 hours after surgery. The operative dressing remains in place for 3 to 5 days unless signs of infection suggest earlier dressing change (Figure 22-15). In the first postoperative days the individual with new transtibial amputation is encouraged to keep the knee of the residual limb in full extension; elevation over a pillow leads to hip and knee flexion contracture that will be problematic later in rehabilitation. The individual is referred for rehabilitation services on postoperative day 2 or 3 to begin out-of-bed activity, transfers, and single-limb ambulation with a walker or crutches. Bedside commodes and wheelchairs with removable armrests assist self-care and mobility and reduce the risk of falls.

Staples typically remain in place for 3 weeks; if there are indications of delayed healing, the surgeon may opt to leave

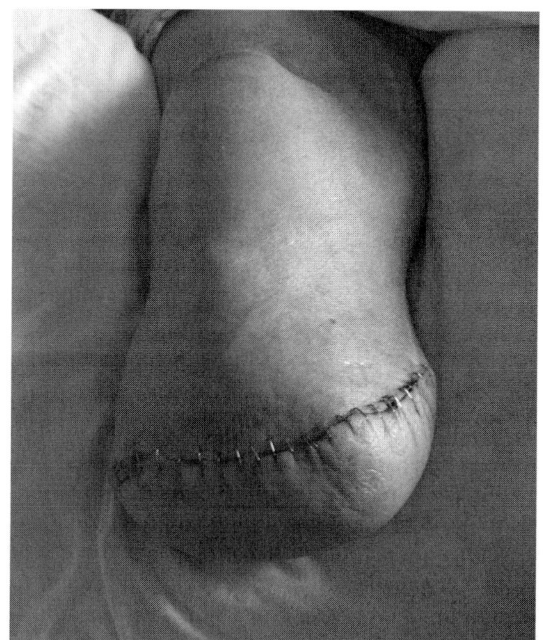
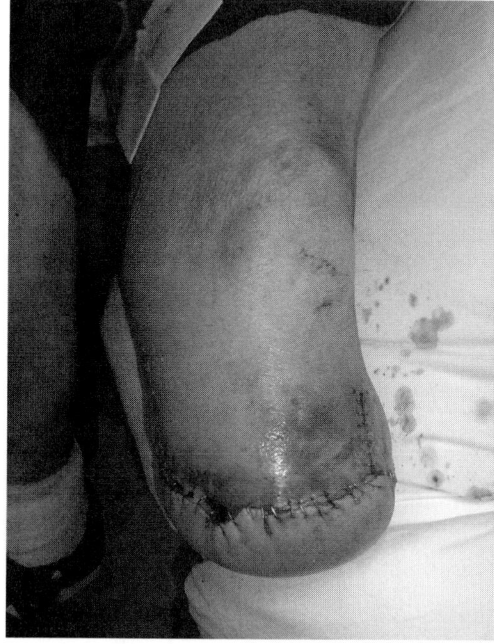

Figure 22-15

A, *A posterior flap transtibial residual limb is healing well but has a slightly bulbous in shape at postoperative day 5.* ***B,*** *A posterior flap transtibial residual limb 3 days postoperatively in a patient with recent failed revascularization. Note the flow of the incision from the previous bypass into the new posterior flap, the serosanguineous drainage medially, and ecchymosis laterally over the tibial tubercle. (Courtesy Algis Maciunas, CPO, FAAOP, Hanger Orthotics and Prosthetics, Wethersfield, Conn.)*

every second or third staple in place longer, reinforcing the incision with Steri-Strips when staples have been removed. Gentle mobilization of soft tissue begins to prevent adherence of the incision scar to underlying fascia and bone. Casting for initial prosthesis occurs only when there has been adequate closure of the surgical wound and the circumference of the distal and proximal portions of the residual limb below the knee is nearly equal. For some individuals this may occur within 3 weeks; for others it may require several months.

KNEE DISARTICULATION AND TRANSCONDYLAR AMPUTATION

In previous centuries, before development of surgical anesthesia and antibiotics, simple knee disarticulation surgery often had a much more favorable outcome than transtibial amputation.[124] Because this surgery does not transect major muscle mass, it can be done quicker and with significantly less blood loss than transtibial or transfemoral amputation. Additionally, simple disarticulation through the knee joint disrupts only the tissue compartment of the joint itself, making postoperative infection in other fascia, muscle, or bone much less likely. The femoral condyles, with their cartilaginous covering, are designed to tolerate weight bearing, and preservation of the entire femur provides mechanical advantage to the prosthetic wearer.[125]

The residual limb heals without much atrophy, requiring less socket replacement or revision early on, allowing fitting with a definitive prosthesis in less time than the typical transtibial or transfemoral residual limb. Additionally, this surgery preserves the growth plate of the distal epiphysis, an important consideration for children with neoplasm or traumatic injury of the proximal tibia. For individuals with severe bilateral vascular disease who are nonambulatory before surgery, the extra length of the femurs provides a larger base of support in sitting, enhancing postural control.[125]

The length of an intact femur, along with the anatomy of the condyles, creates several important challenges to prosthetic fit and function in terms of choice and placement of the prosthetic knee unit, which affects energy cost, as well as efficiency of prosthetic gait. The bony, bulbous residual limb of those who undergo a simple knee disarticulation also creates a challenge regarding donning and doffing the prosthesis (Figure 22-16). Surgical techniques developed by Mazet and Hennessy in the 1960s removed the patella and trimmed the medial and lateral condylar surfaces to address the problems associated with bulbous distal anatomy.[126] In 1977 Burgess recommended removal of 1.5 to 2 cm of distal condyles to permit placement of a newly developed four-bar prosthetic knee unit closer to what had been the anatomical axis of the knee.[127,128] Some surgeons advocate modifying the patella and then fusing it to the intercondylar notch of the femur to create a flat, weight-bearing surface.[129]

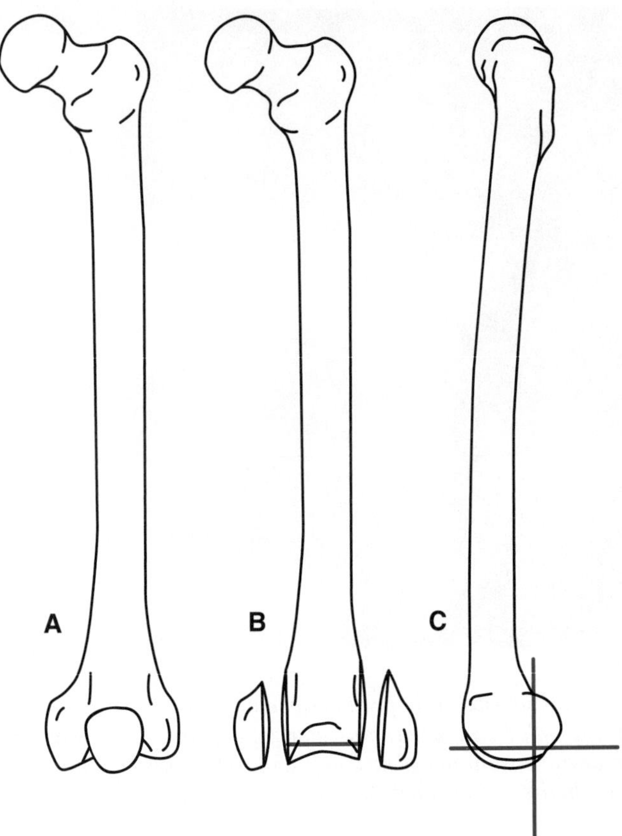

Figure 22-16
A, The residual bony architecture in a simple knee disarticulation, in which no modification of the patella or femur is done. B, Anterior view. C, Lateral view of transcondylar amputation, which shapes the residual femur to resemble a long transfemoral residual limb.

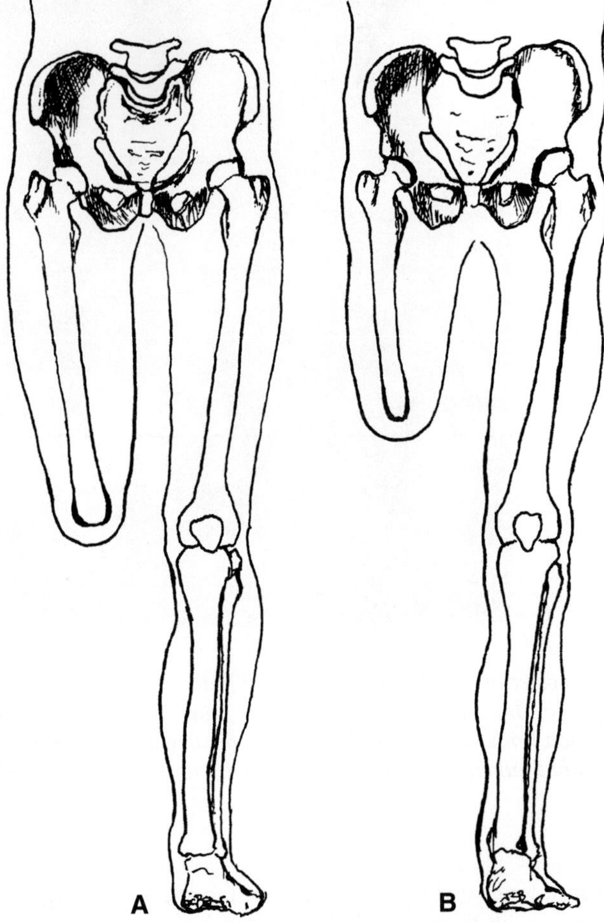

Figure 22-17
Comparison of amputations through the femur. A, Knee disarticulation transects the knee joint, while transcondylar amputation modifies the distal femur and condyles. B, Traditional transfemoral amputation preserves 50% to 66% of femoral length. A long transfemoral residual limb (>66% of femoral length) and knee disarticulation provide a mechanical advantage for prosthetic use but problems with prosthetic cosmesis due to incorporation of a knee unit distal to the socket. A short transfemoral limb (<50% of femoral length) may challenge prosthetic fit and suspension.

Many current transcondylar surgical procedures combine these two approaches to form a residual limb that resembles a long transfemoral limb (Figure 22-17). Typically either equal sagittal flaps or a long posterior flap are used to provide additional "cushion" for weight bearing through the distal residual limb.[125,130] Proponents of simple knee disarticulation, without modification of the distal femur, suggest that the combination of reduced rates of infection, better primary healing, larger surface areas for weight bearing, and advances in prosthetic design and technology lead to better functional outcome and higher rates of prosthetic use.[131,132]

The preparation for knee disarticulation or transcondylar amputation is similar to that of transtibial amputation. The anesthesiologist selects spinal, epidural, or general anesthesia as determined by the health and physiological condition of the person undergoing disarticulation. After application of a tourniquet, the surgeon outlines the incision to guide creation of equal mediolateral flaps (Figure 22-18) approximately half of the anteroposterior diameter of knee in length; some surgeons prefer a long posterior flap as described in the discussion of transtibial surgery. After careful incision of skin and subcutaneous tissue and reflection of the skin flaps, the surgeon transects the patellar tendon at the tibial tubercle, as well as the medial and lateral collateral ligaments just above the menisci. Next, the knee is slightly flexed and the infrapatellar fold is cut. This provides access to the cruciate ligaments, allowing the surgeon to free them from their attachment to the tibia. The posterior joint capsule is carefully cut, with attention to keeping neurovascular structures in the popliteal fossa intact, while exposing the femoral attachment of the gastrocnemius muscle. The popliteal artery and vein and saphenous vein are clamped and ligated,

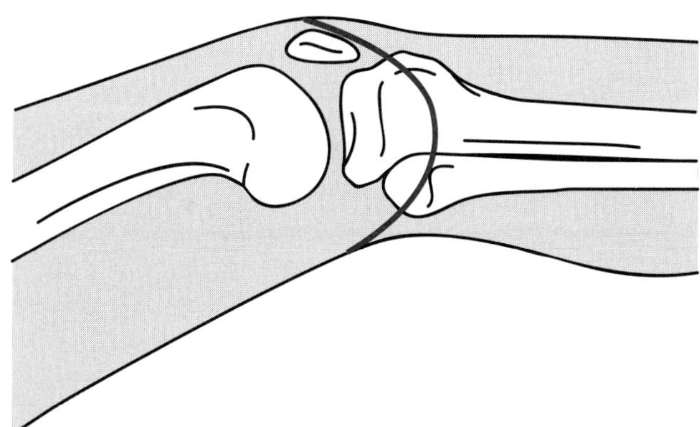

Figure 22-18
A lateral view of the guideline for incision creating equal lateral and medial flaps during knee disarticulation.

and the medial and common peroneal and saphenous nerves are transected under traction and allowed to retract into the residual limb. The surgeon then cuts through the gastrocnemius at the distal edge of the wound, and the lower leg is removed.

For a simple disarticulation the wound is irrigated with saline and antibiotics and prepared for closure at this point. When transcondylar modification is desired, an oscillating saw is used to trim the edges of the condyles before irrigation. The tourniquet is removed, and hemostasis is ensured. In preparation for closure the patellar tendon is sutured to the anterior and posterior ligaments, and the cut edge of the gastrocnemius muscle is sutured to the anterior joint capsule (myoplasty). The hamstring tendons are transected high and allowed to retract. The lateral tendons of the biceps femoris and the iliotibial band are transected low and reconstructed at the time of wound closure to provide muscle stability. The lateral and medial flaps are positioned with approximated edges, and subcutaneous tissues are sutured closed. Finally, the outer layer of skin is closed using staples or external sutures.

A nonadherent gauze is placed over the wound edges, followed by a layer of gauze fluff and a figure-of-eight gauze wrap. The surgeon may choose to apply an Ace wrap, an Unna dressing, a prefabricated adjustable removable rigid dressing, or a plaster or fiberglass cast as the final layer of bandage. The dressing is typically changed at day 5 unless there are indications of infection. Mobility training begins on postoperative day 1, with single-limb ambulation with crutches or walker the next day. A bedside commode and wheelchair allow the individual with new disarticulation who is capable to manage much of his or her own self-care. Some or all of the staples or external sutures are removed at 2 to 3 weeks depending on the condition of the incision. Readiness for a training prosthesis is determined by full healing of the surgical construct, typically between 3 and 8 weeks after surgery.

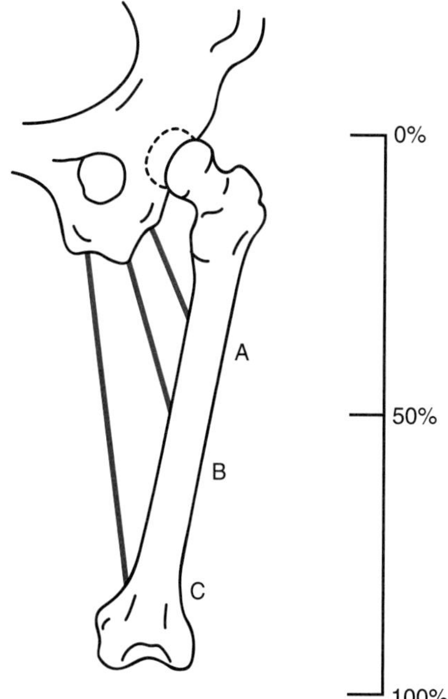

Figure 22-19
*Diagram of point of attachment and line of pull for the **(A)** adductor brevis, **(B)** adductor longus, and **(C)** adductor magnus, as they relate to femoral length. As the length of the residual femur decreases, power and efficiency of adductor muscles groups are more and more compromised.*

TRANSFEMORAL AMPUTATION

Amputation through the femur is chosen when there has been significant trauma to the proximal tibia and knee, when there is a tumor in the proximal tibia or distal femoral condyles that cannot be replaced by allograft or a total joint, and following failed revascularization of the lower leg.[72,133,134] For persons with PAD, the level of choice (if there is adequate circulation for wound healing) is transtibial because functional prosthetic ambulation is most likely when the knee joint has been preserved; some individuals, however, have serious enough circulatory impairment that amputation at transfemoral levels is necessary.[135-137]

Considering not only vascular status, but also muscle attachment and biomechanics of the residual limb in gait, is important when deciding on the precise length of the residual femur. For those needing transfemoral surgeries, function and prosthetic control improves as length of residual femur increases. Preservation or reattachment of the adductor brevis, adductor longus, and especially adductor magnus provides sufficient power for stabilization of the residual limb in adduction in stance so that the abductors can work to keep the pelvis level during prosthetic gait[138] (Figure 22-19). Preservation of femoral length and of muscle mass via myoplasty or myodesis, rather than trisection through muscle belly, results in a stronger residual limb that is more easily fit and has better prosthetic control.[139,140] It also

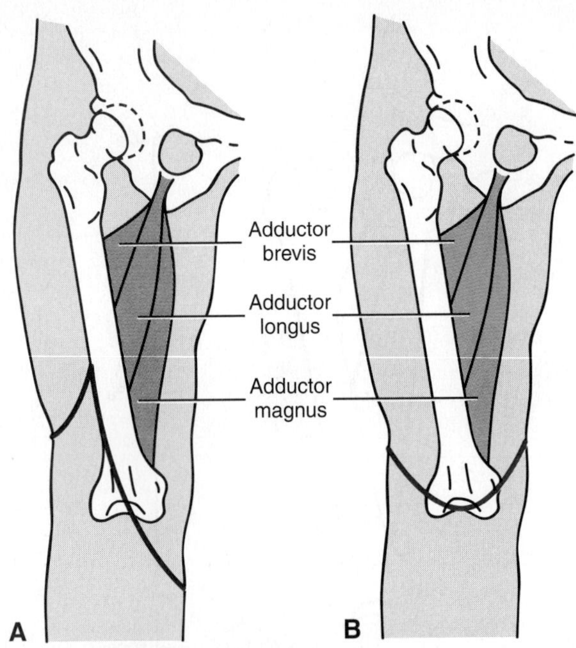

Figure 22-20

*Illustration of incision guidelines for **(A)** a long medial flap and **(B)** equal anterior and posterior flaps for transfemoral amputation surgery. Note that both preserve as much of the adductor magnus as possible for later myoplasty or myodesis when the wound is closed.*

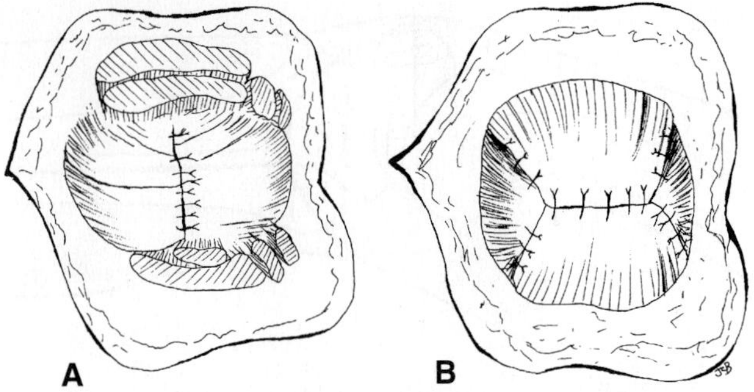

Figure 22-21

*Myodesis of the muscles of the thigh is used to stabilize soft tissue after transfemoral amputation. The initial layer **(A)** attached medial adductor muscles to the vastus lateralis and iliotibial band. The second layer **(B)** connected anterior quadriceps to the posterior hamstrings, covering the first layer. Finally, the two layers are sutured together to stabilize the muscular sling that has been created across the bottom of the residual limb.*

reduces the risk of developing hip abduction and flexion contracture during rehabilitation and over the individual's lifetime. The surgeon must work with the viable thigh tissue to create a residual limb that is balanced in muscular power, provides a long enough lever to allow hip extensors to control prosthetic knee stability in stance, and has as smooth and sensate a skin surface as possible.[135]

In preparation for surgery the patient is placed in a three-quarters supine position, lying on the side of the body opposite the limb to be amputated. The surgeon may or may not choose to use a tourniquet depending on the etiology of amputation. The surgeon may opt to use equal anteroposterior flaps, equal mediolateral flaps, or a long flap from any one limb surface that will be approximated to the opposite limb surface at closure[135,136,141] (Figure 22-20). The skin is opened, followed by subcutaneous tissue, according to the flap pattern chosen. The lower leg may be disarticulated at this point to provide a less cumbersome operative area for subsequent revision. The fascia and muscle of the quadriceps and adductors are transected as far distally as possible, and the femur is scored at the desired level of amputation. The periosteum is elevated and reflected upward and will be used during myoplasty later in the procedure. The femur is cut with an oscillating saw, and the distal bone is retracted (pulled) anteriorly so that the surgeon can access posterior structures. The hamstrings and tensor fascia lata are incised and transected as distally as possible. Major vessels are clamped and then sutured or ligated. The sciatic nerve is sutured or ligated, cut while under traction, and allowed to retract into hamstring muscle tissue. The sharp edges of the residual distal femur may be shaped and smoothed with a rasp or file. The wound is irrigated with sterile saline and antibiotics, the tourniquet is released, and hemostasis is restored. A drain may be placed, at the surgeon's discretion, as residual tissues are positioned for wound closure.

Some surgeons perform a multiple-layer myoplasty to close the surgical wound, suturing medial and lateral soft tissue and muscle groups together as a deep first layer, anterior and posterior soft tissue and muscle groups as a second layer, and then the skin for an outer layer (Figure 22-21). Others prefer myodesis, first pulling the adductor magnus under the distal femur medially to laterally and suturing it to the lateral surface of the femur, and then pulling the quadriceps under the distal femur in an anterior-to-posterior direction over the repositioned adductor, attaching it to the posterior surface of the femur, before closing the skin with staples or removable sutures.[126] An alternative closure places multiple single sutures from the deep posterior subcutaneous tissue, through hamstrings, posterior and anterior periosteum, quadriceps, and finally anterior subcutaneous tissue, and finishing by stapling the skin surface closed.[131] The goal is to create a tapered, cylindrical residual limb with few "dimples" or redundant tissues.

A nonadherent dressing is placed over the suture line, followed by fluffed gauze and a figure-of-eight and spica gauze bandage. A layer of microporous tape may be applied at this joint to keep the wound clean and decrease the risk of contamination by urine or feces. The outer dressing may be by Ace wrap or Unna bandage for a semirigid dressing. The first dressing change occurs 3 to 5 days postoperatively unless there are indications of infection or excessive bleeding

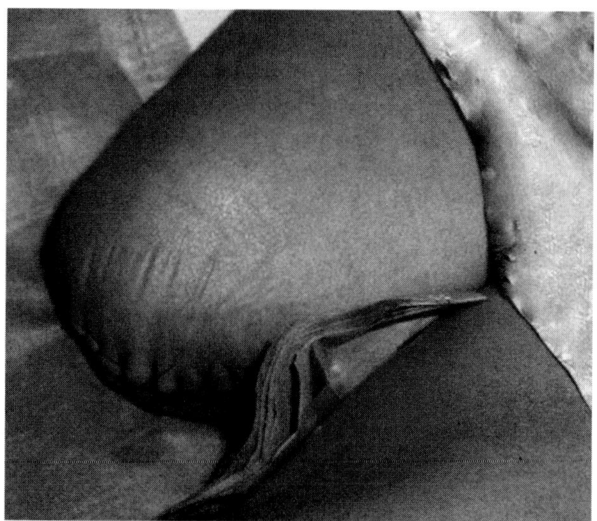

Figure 22-22
Postoperative appearance of a transfemoral residual limb before bandaging. An equal anteroposterior flaps approach has been used, placing the surgical incision in the frontal plane on the underside of the residual limb. (Courtesy Algis Maciunas, CPO, FAAOP, Hanger Prosthetics and Orthotics, Wethersfield, Conn.)

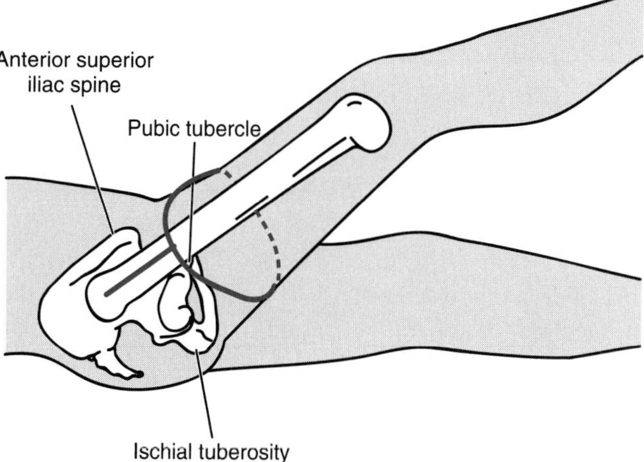

Figure 22-23
An example of the location of incision for a hip disarticulation, creating a posterior flap that will be used when the wound is closed.

(Figure 22-22). If a drain has been placed, it is usually pulled at the first dressing change. Mobility training and early pre-prosthetic positioning exercises (to encourage positioning of the residual limb in hip extension and adduction) are optimally initiated the day after surgery, and single-limb gait training with an appropriate assistive device follows as soon as the individual can tolerate increasing activity. The environment must be set up to minimize the risk of falls; a prefabricated, thermoplastic, adjustable, removable rigid dressing might be used to protect the healing residual limb. Strategies for consistent gentle soft tissue compression are initiated as soon as possible using an Ace wrap, elasticized stockinette, and eventually a commercially available "shrinker." External staples or sutures remain in place for 3 weeks or more, perhaps being removed in successive stages to ensure a solid wound closure. Fitting for initial prosthesis is, as in all other levels of amputation, determined by the condition of the suture line; for some patients this may occur as early as 3 or 4 weeks postoperatively, and for others several months after surgery.

HIP DISARTICULATION AND HEMIPELVECTOMY

Amputation at the level of the hip or pelvis is an extreme surgery that is undertaken to preserve life in the presence of extreme infection or damage of proximal structures: recurrent deep decubitus ulcers in individuals with paralysis, necrotizing wounds with wet gangrene and risk of systemic sepsis, severe crush or shrapnel injury damaging blood vessels in the groin when revascularization is not possible, or invasive tumor of the proximal femur or pelvis when limb-sparing strategies are not possible.[142-147] With these surgeries, significant body mass is removed and there is the likelihood of significant blood loss; careful monitoring of hydration and electrolytes is necessary during surgery and the immediate postoperative period. These are complex surgeries best performed in facilities with an experienced interdisciplinary team available for preoperative, perioperative, and postoperative care.

In the operating room the patient is placed in a three-quarters supine position, with the limb to be amputated uppermost. The limb is prepped and draped for surgery, and a racquet-shaped guideline for incision is traced on the skin, with the goal of creating a large posterior flap of skin, subcutaneous tissue, and gluteal muscle mass for wound closure (Figure 22-23). The incision begins at the medial edge of the anterior superior iliac spine (ASIS), continues along the inguinal ligament to just below the ischial tuberosity and gluteal crease, and then arches upward over the greater trochanter and anterior thigh back to the ASIS.[142] The surgeon must carefully free and then stabilize neurovascular structures in the inguinal region, as well as detach each of the many surface and deeper muscles that cross the hip joint, starting with the anterior and medial groups, then moving laterally and posteriorly.

The gluteals are detached from the greater trochanter but kept in place on the pelvis to be part of the posterior flap. The head of the humerus is forcefully dislocated from the acetabulum. The wound is irrigated with saline and antibiotics, and hemostasis is secured. Pairs of antagonistic muscles may be sutured together in myoplasty or to periosteum of the pelvis in myodesis as wound closure begins. Drains are placed; the posterior flap is positioned against anterior, medial, and lateral edges of the wound; subcutaneous closure is secured by a series of sutures; and skin is closed with staples. The wound is dressed with a layer of nonadherent gauze; then fluff; and then a spica wrap of gauze and elastic bandage, directing soft tissue in a posterior-to-anterior medial direction consistent with the line of the posterior flap. Dressings are changed every 3 or so days, more frequently if there is significant drainage. There is considerable risk of deep venous thrombosis of the intact limb during the immediate postoperative period; low-dose heparin or Coumadin (warfarin) may be used as prophylactics. Limited periods of sitting, mobility, and transfer training, as well as ambulation on the remaining limb using a walker or crutches, begins as soon as the patient is medically stable and able to tolerate increasing levels of activity, optimally within 2 to 3 days after surgery. Special attention must be paid to the sitting posture, with minimal time spent in a posteriorly tilted "sacral sitting" position, to ensure skin integrity. Staples or external sutures remain in place for 2 to 3 weeks postoperatively. Patient and family education must include efforts to carefully protect the surgical site during movement and activities of daily living. An early referral to the prosthetist for fabrication of a custom thermoplastic removable rigid dressing may occur in the week immediately following surgery. Fitting for initial prosthesis, as in amputation at all other levels, is determined by rate and adequacy of healing of the surgical site.

Hemipelvectomy (transpelvic amputation) is a more aggressive and invasive surgery that leaves the individual without a bony case to support abdominal contents on one side of the body. Postoperatively, there is significant risk of developing ileus; many individuals with hemipelvectomy are ill enough to require nasogastric tube and limited feeding in the immediate postoperative period. Mobilization and transfer training may need to be deferred until the individual is well enough and nutritionally supported enough to tolerate increased levels of activity.

SUMMARY

This chapter has presented the strategies used to examine a vascularly compromised or traumatically injured lower extremity and discussed the surgeon's evaluative process when making decisions about limb revascularization, thrombolytic intervention, limb salvage, disarticulation, or amputation. Several factors must be carefully considered: the likelihood of successful healing of the surgical construct; the preservation of the ankle and knee (if possible) to minimize the impact on energy cost of gait and postural control; and the creation of a residual limb with adequate skin surface (pressure tolerance), length (lever arm), and dimension for prosthetic fitting and function. The most common approaches for surgery at each level of amputation were discussed so that rehabilitation professionals could appreciate the manipulation of tissues and postoperative wound healing process. The authors have explored the commonalities and differences in amputations performed because of dysvascular/neuropathic disease, bone infection, lower extremity trauma, neoplasm, or revision in children with congenital limb deficiency. The authors hope that readers have developed an appreciation of the complexity and challenges presented to the surgeon and the rehabilitation team when an individual undergoes amputation.

REFERENCES

1. Aronow W. Management of peripheral arterial disease of the lower extremities in elderly patients. *J Gerontol* 2004;59A(2):172-177.
2. Barnes RW, Cox B. Amputation principles. In *Amputations: An Illustrated Manual.* Philadelphia: Hanely & Belfus, 2000. pp. 1-3.
3. McGuire J. Coping with amputation. *Diabetes Self-Manag* 2001;18(4):96-103.
4. Aulivola B, Hile CN, Hamdan AD, et al. Major lower extremity amputation: outcome of a modern series. *Arch Surg* 2004;139(4):395-399.
5. Lavery LA, van Houtum WH, Armstrong DG, et al. Mortality following lower extremity amputation in minorities with diabetes mellitus. *Diabetes Res Clin Prac* 1997;37(1):41-47.
6. Van Ross ER. After amputation: rehabilitation of the diabetic amputee. *J Am Podiatr Med Assoc* 1997;87(7):332-225.
7. McCollum PT, Raza Z. Vascular disease: limb salvage versus amputation. In Smith DG, Michaels JW, Bowker JH (eds), *Atlas of Amputation and Limb Deficiencies. Surgical Prosthetic and Rehabilitation Principles,* 3rd ed. Rosemont, IL: American Academy of Orthopaedic Surgeons, 2004. pp. 31-45.
8. Misuri A, Lucertini G, Nanni A, et al. Predictive value of transcutaneous oximetry for selection of the amputation level. *Cardiovasc Surg (Torino)* 2000;41(1):83-87.
9. Niinikoski JHA. Clinical hyperbaric oxygen therapy, wound perfusion, and transcutaneous oximetry. *World J Surg* 2004;28(3):307-315.
10. Pinzur MS. The metabolic cost of lower extremity amputation. *Clin Podiatr Med Surg* 1997;14(4):599-602.
11. Murin MC, Espejo-DeGuzman MC, Boninger ML, et al. Predictive factors for successful early prosthetic ambulation among lower limb amputees. *J Rehabil Res Devel* 2001;38(4):379-384.
12. Hosch J, Quiroga C, Bosma J, et al. Outcomes of transmetatarsal amputations in patients with diabetes mellitus. *J Foot Ankle Surg* 1997;36(6):430-444.
13. Gugulakis AG, Lazaris AM, Vasdekis SN, et al. Rehabilitation outcome in patients with lower limb amputations because of arterial occlusive disease: is it worth trying for the lowest possible amputation level? A prospective study. *Int J Rehabil Health* 2000;5(1):65-70.
14. Bowker JH. Transtibial amputation: surgical management. In Smith DG, Michaels JW, Bowker JH (eds), *Atlas of Amputation and Limb Deficiencies. Surgical Prosthetic and Rehabilitation Principles,* 3rd ed. Rosemont, IL: American Academy of Orthopaedic Surgeons, 2004. pp. 481-501.

15. Miroslav J. Rehabilitation following major traumatic amputation of lower limbs—a review. *Crit Rev Phys Med Rehabil* 2003;15(3/4), 235-253.
16. McCollum PT, Raza Z. Vascular disease: limb salvage versus amputation. In Smith DG, Michael JW, Bowker JH (eds), *Atlas of Amputation and Limb Deficiencies: Surgical, Prosthetic, and Rehabilitation Principles,* 3rd ed. Rosemont, IL: American Academy of Orthopaedic Surgeons, 2004. pp. 31-45.
17. Gregg E W, Sorlie P, Paulose-Ram R, et al. Prevalence of lower-extremity disease in the U.S. adult population ≥ 40 years of age with and without diabetes. *Diabetes Care* 2004;27(7):1591-1597.
18. Ward K, Schwartz ML, Thiele R, et al. Lower extremity manifestations of vascular disease. *Clin Podiatr Med Surg* 1998;15(4):629-672.
19. Migliacco-Walle K, Caro JJ, Ishak K, et al. Costs and medical care consequences associated with the diagnosis of peripheral arterial disease. *PharmacoEconomics* 2005;23(5): 733-742.
20. Ebskov LB, Schroeder TV, Holstein PE. Epidemiology of leg amputation: the influence of vascular surgery. *Br J Surg* 1994;81(11):1600-1603.
21. Moreland ME, Kilbourne AM, Engelhardt JB, et al. Diabetes preventive care and non-traumatic lower extremity amputation rates. *J Health Care Qual* 2004;Sep-Oct;26(5):12-17.
22. Bowker MH. Infection: limb salvage versus amputation. In Smith DG, Michael JW, Bowker JH (eds), *Atlas of Amputation and Limb Deficiencies: Surgical, Prosthetic, and Rehabilitation Principles,* 3rd ed. Rosemont, IL: American Academy of Orthopaedic Surgeons, 2004. pp. 47-53.
23. Watkins PJ. Cardiovascular disease, hypertension, and lipids. *BMJ* 2003;326(7394):874-876.
24. Smith DG, Assal M, Reiber GE, et al. Minor environmental trauma and lower extremity amputation in high-risk patients with diabetes: incidence, pivotal events, etiology, and amputation level in a prospectively followed cohort. *Foot Ankle Int* 2003;24(9):690-695.
25. Patout CA Jr, Birke JA, Horswell R, et al. Effectiveness of a comprehensive diabetes lower-extremity amputation prevention program in a predominantly low-income African-American population. *Diabetes Care* 2000;23(9):1339-1342.
26. Carrington AL, Abbott CA, Griffiths J, et al. A foot care program for diabetic unilateral lower-limb amputees. *Diabetes Care* 2001;24(2):216-221.
27. Nelson JP. The vascular history and physical examination. In Robbins J (ed), *Clinics in Podiatric Medicine and Surgery: Peripheral Vascular Disease in the Lower Extremity.* Philadelphia: Saunders, 1992. pp. 1-17.
28. Sieggreen MY, Kline RA. Arterial insufficiency and ulceration: diagnosis and treatment options. *Adv Skin Sound Care* 2004;17(5):242-253.
29. Santilli JD, Rodnick JE. Claudication: diagnosis and treatment. *Am Fam Physician* 1996;53(4):1245-1253.
30. Fontain R, Bubost C (eds). *Les Greffes Vascularies.* Paris: Brodard et Taupin, 1954.
31. Novo S. Classification, epidemiology, risk factors, and natural history of peripheral arterial disease. *Diabetes Obesity Metab* 2002;4(Suppl 2):S1-S6.
32. Dormandy JA, Rutherford RB, Bakal C. Management of peripheral arterial disease: TransAtlantic Inter-Society Consensus Tract. *Int Angiol* 2000;19(Suppl 1)1-310.
33. Rob CG. Clinical evaluation of patients with peripheral vascular disease of the lower extremity. In Jarret F (ed), *Vascular Surgery of the Lower Extremity.* St. Louis: Mosby, 1985. pp. 3-11.
34. Ouriel K. Comparison of surgical and thrombolytic treatment of peripheral arterial disease. *Rev Cardiovasc Med* 2002;3(Suppl 2):S7-S16.
35. Cassady SL. Peripheral arterial disease: a review of epidemiology, clinical presentation, and effectiveness of exercise training. *Cardiopulm Phys Ther J* 2004;15(3):6-12.
36. McCullough JM. Evaluation of patients with open wounds. In McCullough JM, Kloth LC, Feedar JA (eds), *Wound Healing: Alternatives in Management,* 2nd ed. Philadelphia: F.A. Davis, 1995. pp. 111-134.
37. McNeely MJ, Boyko EG, Ahronic JH, et al. The independent contribution of diabetic neuropathy and vasculopathy in foot ulceration. *Diabetes Care* 1995;18(2):216-219.
38. Mueller MJ. Identifying patients with diabetes mellitus who are at risk for lower extremity complications: use of Semmes Weinstein monofilaments. *Phys Ther* 1996;76(1):68-71.
39. Young MJ, Marshal A, Adams JE, et al. Osteopenia, neurological dysfunction, and the development of Charcot neuroarthropathy. *Diabetes Care* 1995;18(1):34-38.
40. Kidawa AS. Vascular examination. *Clin Podiatr Med Surg* 1993;10(2):187-203.
41. Rob CG. Clinical evaluation of patients with peripheral vascular disease of the lower extremity. In Jarrett F (ed), *Vascular Surgery of the Lower Extremity.* St. Louis: Mosby, 1985. pp. 3-11.
42. Baker JD. The vascular laboratory. In Moore WS (ed), *Vascular Surgery: A Comprehensive Review,* 6th ed. Philadelphia: Saunders, 2002. pp. 235-250.
43. Kaufman JA. Vascular imaging with x-ray, magnetic resonance, and computed tomography angiography. In Coffman JD, Eberhardt RT (eds), *Peripheral Arterial Disease Diagnosis and Treatment.* Totowa, NJ: Humana Press, 2002. pp. 75-92.
44. Reid SK, Pagan-Martin HR, Menzoian JO, et al. Contrast-enhanced moving table MR angiography: prospective comparison to catheter arteriography for treatment planning in peripheral arterial occlusive disease. *J Vasc Interv Radiol* 2001;12(1):45-53.
45. Wikström J, Holmberg A, Johansson L, et al. Gadolinium-enhanced magnetic resonance angiography, digital subtraction angiography, and duplex of the iliac arteries compared with intraarterial pressure gradient measurements. *Eur J Vasc Endovasc Surg* 2000;19(5): 516-523.
46. Ouriel K. Current status of thrombolysis for peripheral arterial occlusive disease. *Ann Vasc Surg* 2002;16(6):797-804.
47. Working Party on Thrombolysis in the Management of Limb Ischemia. Thrombolysis in the management of lower limb peripheral arterial occlusion—a consensus document. *J Vasc Surg Interv Radiol* 2003;14(9 pt 2):S337-S349.
48. Giannini D, Balbarini A. Thrombolytic therapy in peripheral arterial disease. *Curr Drug Targets Cardiovasc Haematolog Dis* 2004;4(3):249-258.

49. Kim CK, Schmalfuss CM, Schfield RS, et al. Pharmacological treatment of patients with peripheral arterial disease. *Drugs* 2003;63(7):637-647.
50. Dorffler-Melly, Koopman MM, Prins MH, et al. Antiplatelets and anticoagulant drugs for prevention of restenosis/ reocclusion following peripheral endovascular treatment. *Cochrane Database Syst Rev* 2005(1). Cochrane AN: CD002071.
51. Doggrell SA. Pharmacology and intermittent claudication. *Expert Opin Pharmacother* 2001;2(11):1725-1736.
52. Archdeacon MT, Sanders R. Trauma: limb salvage versus amputation. In Smith DG, Michaels JW, Bowker JH (eds), *Atlas of Amputation and Limb Deficiencies. Surgical Prosthetic and Rehabilitation Principles,* 3rd ed. Rosemont, IL: American Academy of Orthopaedic Surgeons, 2004. pp. 69-75.
53. Dougherty PJ. Wartime amputee care. In Smith DG, Michaels JW, Bowker JH (eds), *Atlas of Amputation and Limb Deficiencies. Surgical Prosthetic and Rehabilitation Principles,* 3rd ed. Rosemont, IL: American Academy of Orthopaedic Surgeons, 2004. pp. 77-97.
54. Sheehy BD, Blansfield JS, Danis DM, et al (eds), *Manual of Clinical Trauma Care: the First Hour,* 3rd ed. St. Louis: Mosby, 1999.
55. Pezzin LE, Dillinhamv RT, MacKenzie EJ. Rehabilitation and the long-term outcomes of persons with trauma-related amputation. *Arch Phys Med Rehabil* 2000;81(3):292-300.
56. Bosse MJ, MacKenzie EF, Kellam JF, et al. An analysis of outcomes of reconstruction or amputation of leg-threatening injuries. *N Engl J Med* 2002;347(24):1924-1931.
57. Dagum AB, Best AK, Schemitsch EH, et al. Salvage after severe lower extremity trauma: are the outcomes worth the means? *Plast Reconstr Surg* 1999;103(4):1212-1220.
58. Gregory RT, Gould RJ, Peclet M, et al. The mangled extremity syndrome: a severity grading system for multisystem injury of the extremity. *J Trauma* 1985;25(12):1147-1150.
59. Howe RH, Poole GV, Hansen KJ, et al. Salvage of lower extremities following combined orthopedic and vascular trauma; a predictive salvage index. *Am Surg* 1987;53(4): 205-208.
60. Helfet DL, Howey T, Sanders R, et al. Limb salvage versus amputation: preliminary results of the Mangled Extremity Severity Score. *Clin Orthop Relat Res* 1990;July(256):80-86.
61. Russell WL, Sailors DM, Shittle TB, et al. Limb salvage versus traumatic amputation: a decision based on a seven-part predictive index. *Ann Surg* 1991;213(5):473-481.
62. McNamara MG, Heckman JD, Corley FG. Severe open fractures of the lower extremity: a retrospective evaluation of the Mangle Extremity Severity Score. *J Orthop Trauma* 1994;8(2):81-87.
63. Durham RM, Mistry BM, Mazuski JE, et al. Outcome and utility of scoring systems in the mangled extremity. *Am J Surg* 1996;172(5):569-573.
64. Caudle RJ, Stern PJ. Severe open fractures of the tibia. *J Bone Joint Surg Am* 1987;69(6):801-807.
65. Gopal S, Giannoudis PV, Murray A, et al. The functional outcome of severe open tibial fractures managed with early fixation and flap coverage. *J Bone Joint Surg Br* 2004;86(8): 861-867.
66. Lange RH, Bach AW, Hansen ST, et al. Open tibial fractures with associated vascular injuries; prognosis for limb salvage. *J Trauma* 1985;25(3):203-208.
67. Persson BM. Amputations for tumors. In Murdoch G, Bennett Wilson A (eds), *Amputation: Surgical Practice and Patient Management.* Oxford: Butterworth-Heinemann, 1996. pp. 195-200.
68. Davis AM. Bone neoplasms. In Lundon K (ed), *Orthopedic Rehabilitation Science: Principles of Clinical Management of Bone.* Woburn, MA: Butterworth-Heinemann, 2000. pp. 143-154.
69. Phillips LL. Managing the pain of bone metastasis in the home environment. *Am J Hosp Palliative Care* 1998;15(1): 32-42.
70. Levesque J, Marx RG, Bell RS, et al. *A Clinical Guide to Primary Bone Tumors.* Baltimore: Williams & Wilkins, 1998.
71. Malawar MM, Link MP, Donalson SS. Sarcomas of bone. In Devita VT, Hellman S, Rosenberg ST (eds), *Cancer Principles and Practice of Oncology,* 6th ed. Philadelphia: Lippincott Raven, 2001. pp. 1891-1936.
72. Mnaymneh W, Temple HT. Tumor: limb salvage versus amputation. In Smith DG, Michaels JW, Bowker JH (eds), *Atlas of Amputation and Limb Deficiencies. Surgical Prosthetic and Rehabilitation Principles,* 3rd ed. Rosemont, IL: American Academy of Orthopaedic Surgeons, 2004. pp. 55-75.
73. Kumta SM, Cheng JC, Li CK, et al. Scope and limitations in limb-sparing surgery in childhood sarcomas. *J Pediatr Orthop* 2002;22(2):244-248.
74. Karakousis CP, Zigratis GC. Radiation therapy for high grade soft tissue sarcomas of the extremities treated with limb preserving surgery. *Eur J Surg Oncol* 2002;28(4):431-436.
75. Bickels J, Wittig JC, Kollender Y, et al. Distal femur resection with endoprosthetic reconstruction: a long term follow-up study. *Clin Orthop Relat Res* 2002;July(400):225-235.
76. Letson GD, D'Amato G, Windham TC, et al. Extendable prostheses for the treatment of malignant bone tumors in growing children. *Curr Opin Orthopaed* 2003;14(6): 413-418.
77. Eggermont AMM, DeWilt JH, Hange TL. Current uses of isolated limb perfusion in the clinic and a model system for new strategies. *Lancet Oncol* 2003;4(7):429-437.
78. van Etten B, van Geel AN, DeWilt JH, et al. Fifty tumor necrosis factor-based isolated limb perfusions for limb salvage in patients older than 75 with limb-threatening soft tissue sarcomas and other extremity tumors. *Ann Surg Oncol* 2003;10(1):32-37.
79. Davidson AW, Hong A, McCarthy SW, et al. En-bloc resection, extracorporeal irradiation, and re-implantation in limb salvage for bony malignancies. *J Bone Joint Surg Br* 2005;87(6):851-857.
80. Refaat Y, Gunnoe J, Hornicek FJ, et al. Comparison of quality of life after amputation or limb salvage. *Clin Orthop Relat Res* 2002;Apr(397):298-305.
81. Nagarajan R, Clohisy DR, Neglia JP, et al. Function and quality of life of survivors of pelvic and lower extremity osteosarcoma and Ewing's sarcoma: the Childhood Cancer Survivor Study. *Br J Cancer* 2004;91(1):1858-1865.
82. Parsons JA, Davis AM. Rehabilitation and quality of life issues in patients with extremity soft-tissue sarcoma. *Curr Treat Options Oncol* 2004;5(6):477-486.
83. Clark MA, Thomas JM. Major amputation for soft-tissue sarcoma. *Br J Surg* 2003;90(1):102-107.

84. Clark MA. Amputation for soft tissue sarcoma. *Lancet Oncology* 2003;4(6):335-342.
85. Ghert MA, Abudu A, Driver N, et al. The indications for and the prognostic significance of amputation as the primary surgical procedure for localized soft tissue sarcoma of the extremity. *Ann Surg Oncol* 2005;12(1):10-17.
86. Stojadinovic A, Jaques DP, Leung HD, et al. Amputation for recurrent soft tissue sarcoma of the extremity: indications and outcomes. *Ann Surg Oncol* 2001;8(6):509-518.
87. Blackley HR, Wunder JS, Davis AM, et al. Treatment of giant cell tumors of long bones with curettage and bone grafting. *J Bone Joint Surg Am* 1999;81(6):811-820.
88. Ferrari S, Bacci G, Pici P, et al. Long term follow-up and post-prelapse survival in patients with non-metastatic osteosarcoma of the extremity treated with neoadjuvant chemotherapy. *Ann Oncol* 1997;8(8):765-771.
89. Musculoskeletal practice patterns H, I, J. In *Guide to Physical Therapist Practice,* 2nd ed. *Phys Ther* 1991;81(1):S251-S303.
90. Kahle AL. Psychological issues in pediatric limb deficiency. In Smith DG, Michaels JW, Bowker JH (eds), *Atlas of Amputation and Limb Deficiencies. Surgical Prosthetic and Rehabilitation Principles,* 3rd ed. Rosemont, IL: American Academy of Orthopaedic Surgeons, 2004, pp. 801–812.
91. Fisk JR, Smith DG. The limb deficient child. In Smith DG, Michaels JW, Bowker JH (eds), *Atlas of Amputation and Limb Deficiencies. Surgical Prosthetic and Rehabilitation Principles,* 3rd ed. Rosemont, IL: American Academy of Orthopaedic Surgeons, 2004. pp. 773-777.
92. Edelstein JE. Developmental kinesiology. In Smith DG, Michaels JW, Bowker JH (eds), *Atlas of Amputation and Limb Deficiencies. Surgical Prosthetic and Rehabilitation Principles,* 3rd ed. Rosemont, IL: American Academy of Orthopaedic Surgeons, 2004. pp. 783-788.
93. Watts H. Surgical modification of residual limbs. In Smith DG, Michaels JW, Bowker JH (eds), *Atlas of Amputation and Limb Deficiencies. Surgical Prosthetic and Rehabilitation Principles,* 3rd ed. Rosemont, IL: American Academy of Orthopaedic Surgeons, 2004. pp. 931-943.
94. Kant P, Koh SH, Neumann V, et al. Treatment of longitudinal deficiency affecting the femur: comparing patient mobility and satisfaction outcomes of Syme amputation against extension prosthesis. *J Pediatr Orthop* 2003;23(2):236-242.
95. Brown KL. Resection, rotationplasty, and femoropelvic arthrodesis in severe congenital femoral deficiency: a report of the surgical technique and three cases. *J Bone Joint Surg* 2001;83A(1):78-85.
96. Hamel J, Winderlmann W, Becker W. A new modification of rotationplasty in a patient with proximal femoral focal deficiency Pappas type II. *J Pediatr Orhtop B* 1999;8(3):200-202.
97. Trode IP, Gillespe R. The classification and treatment of proximal femoral deficiencies. *Prosthet Orthot Int* 1991;15(2):117-126.
98. Glancy GL. Fibular deficiencies. In Smith DG, Michaels JW, Bowker JH (eds), *Atlas of Amputation and Limb Deficiencies. Surgical Prosthetic and Rehabilitation Principles,* 3rd ed. Rosemont, IL: American Academy of Orthopaedic Surgeons, 2004. pp. 889-896.
99. Schmitz ML, Biavendoin BJ, Coulter-O'Berry C. Tibial deficiencies. In Smith DG, Michaels JW, Bowker JH (eds), *Atlas of Amputation and Limb Deficiencies. Surgical Prosthetic and Rehabilitation Principles,* 3rd ed. Rosemont, IL: American Academy of Orthopaedic Surgeons, 2004. pp. 897-904.
100. Stanitski DF, Shahcheraghi H, Nicker DA, et al. Results of tibial lengthening with the Ilizarov technique. *J Pediatr Orthop* 2003;16(2):168-172.
101. Birch JG, Walsh SJ, Small JM, et al. Syme amputation for the treatment of fibular deficiency: an evaluation of long-term physical and psychological functional status. *J Bone Joint Surg Am* 1999;81(11):1511-1518.
102. Simmons ED, Ginsburg GM, Hall JE. Brown's procedure for congenital absence of the tibia revisited. *J Pediatr Orthop* 1996;16(1):85-98.
103. Carranza-Bencano A. Unilateral tibial hemimelia with leg length inequality and varus foot: external fixator treatment. *Foot Ankle Int* 1999;20(6):392-396.
104. Moulik PK, Mtonga R, Gill GV. Amputation and mortality in new-onset diabetic foot ulcers stratified by etiology. *Diabetes Care* 2003;26(2):491-492.
105. McCollum PT, Harrison DK. Amputation level selection. In Murdoch G, Donovan RG (eds), *Amputation Surgery and Lower Limb Prosthetics.* Edinburgh: Blackwell Scientific, 1988. pp. 155-165.
106. Levin AZ. Functional outcome following amputation. *T Geriatr Rehab* 2004;20(4):253-261.
107. Tisi PV, Callam MJ. Type of incision for below knee amputation. 2004, *Cochrane Database Syst Rev (1),* Cochcrane AN: CD003749.
108. Carlson T, Reed JF. A case control study of the risk factors for toe amputation in a diabetic population. *Int J Lower Extremity Wounds* 2003;2(1):19-21.
109. Baumgarten R. Partial foot amputations. In Murdoch G, Donovan RG (eds), *Amputation Surgery and Lower Limb Prosthetics.* Edinburgh: Blackwell Scientific, 1988. pp. 94-103.
110. Barnes RW, Cox B. Toe amputation: phalangectomy and transmetatarsal. In *Amputations: An Illustrated Manual.* Philadelphia: Hanley & Belfus, 2000. pp. 15-26.
111. Bowker JH. Amputations and disarticulations within the foot: surgical management. In Smith DG, Michaels JW, Bowker JH (eds), *Atlas of Amputation and Limb Deficiencies. Surgical Prosthetic and Rehabilitation Principles*, 3rd ed. Rosemont, IL: American Academy of Orthopaedic Surgeons, 2004. pp. 429-448.
112. Barnes RW, Cox B. Transmetatarsal amputation. In *Amputations: An Illustrated Manual.* Philadelphia: Hanley & Belfus, 2000. pp. 37-47.
113. Bowker JH, San Giovanni TP. Amputations and disarticulations. In Myerson MS (ed), *Foot and Ankle Disorders.* Philadelphia: WB Saunders; 2000. pp. 466-503.
114. Condie DN, Bowers R. Amputations and disarticulations within the foot; prosthetic management. In Smith DG, Michaels JW, Bowker JH (eds), *Atlas of Amputation and Limb Deficiencies. Surgical Prosthetic and Rehabilitation Principles,* 3rd ed. Rosemont, IL: American Academy of Orthopaedic Surgeons, 2004. pp. 449-457.
115. Jain AS. The Syme amputation. In Murdoch G, Wilson AB (eds), *Amputation: Surgical Practice and Patient Management.* Oxford: Butterworth-Heinemann, 1996. pp. 79-86.
116. Barnes RW, Cox B. Syme amputation. In *Amputations: An Illustrated Manual.* Philadelphia: Hanley & Belfus, 2000. pp. 49-66.

117. Bowker JH. Ankle disarticulation and variants: surgical management. In Smith DG, Michaels JW, Bowker JH (eds), *Atlas of Amputation and Limb Deficiencies. Surgical Prosthetic and Rehabilitation Principles,* 3rd ed. Rosemont, IL: American Academy of Orthopaedic Surgeons, 2004. pp. 459-471.
118. Dougherty PJ. Transtibial amputees from the Vietnam war: twenty eight year follow-up. *J Bone J Surg Am* 2001;83(3): 383-389.
119. Allcock PA, Jain AS. Revisiting transtibial amputation with the long posterior flap. *Br J Surg* 2001;88(5):683-686.
120. Burgess EM. The below-knee amputation. *Bull Prosthet Res* 1968;Fall(10):19-25.
121. Sanders GT. Below knee. In *Lower Limb Amputations: a Guide to Rehabilitation.* Philadelphia: F.A. Davis, 1986. pp. 163-204.
122. Bowker JH. Transtibial amputation: surgical management. In Smith DG, Michaels JW, Bowker JH (eds), *Atlas of Amputation and Limb Deficiencies. Surgical Prosthetic and Rehabilitation Principles,* 3rd ed. Rosemont, IL: American Academy of Orthopaedic Surgeons, 2004. pp. 481-501.
123. Barnes RW, Cox B. Below-knee amputation. In *Amputations: An Illustrated Manual.* Philadelphia: Hanley & Belfus; 2000. pp. 67-86.
124. Pinzur MS. Knee disarticulation: surgical management. In Smith DG, Michaels JW, Bowker JH (eds), *Atlas of Amputation and Limb Deficiencies. Surgical Prosthetic and Rehabilitation Principles,* 3rd ed. Rosemont, IL: American Academy of Orthopaedic Surgeons, 2004. pp. 517-523.
125. Sanders GT. Knee disarticulation and transcondylar/ supracondylar amputation. In *Lower Limb Amputations: A Guide to Rehabilitation.* Philadelphia: F.A. Davis, 1986. pp. 206-229.
126. Mazet R, Hennessy CA. Knee disarticulation: a new technique and a new knee joint mechanism. *J Bone Joint Surg Am* 1966; 48(1):129-139.
127. Burgess EM. Disarticulation of the knee: a modified technique. *Arch Surg* 1977;112(10):1250-1255.
128. Pinzur MS, Bowker JH. Knee disarticulation. *Clin Orthop Relat Res* 1999;April(361):23-28.
129. Duerksen F, Rogalsky RJ, Cochrane IW. Knee disarticulation with intercondylar patello-femoral arthrodesis, an improved technique. *Clin Orthop* 1990;July(256):50-56.
130. Bowker JH, San Giovanni PT, Pinsur MS. North American experience with knee disarticulation with the use of a posterior myofasciocutaneous flap: healing rate and functional results in 77 patients. *J Bone Joint Surg Am* 2000;82(11):1571-1574.
131. Barnes RW, Cox B. Through-knee amputation (knee disarticulation). In *Amputations: An illustrated manual.* Philadelphia: Hanley & Belfus, 2000. pp. 87-102.
132. Jensen JS. Surgical techniques of knee disarticulation and femoral transcondylar amputation. In Murdock G, Wilson AB (eds), *Amputation: Surgical Practice and Patient Management* Oxford: Butterworth-Heinemann, 1996. pp. 127-134.
133. Van Niekirk LJ, Steward CP, Jain AS. Major lower extremity amputation following failed infrainguinal vascular bypass study, a prospective study on amputation levels and stump complications. *Prosthet Orthot Int* 2001;25(1):29-33.
134. Gottschalk F. Traumatic amputation. In Bucholz RW, Heckman JD (eds), *Rockwood and Green's Fractures in Adults,* 5th ed. Philadelphia: Lippincott Williams & Wilkins, 2001. pp. 391-414.
135. Gottschalk F. Transfemoral amputation, surgical management. In Smith DG, Michaels JW, Bowker JH (eds), *Atlas of Amputation and Limb Deficiencies. Surgical Prosthetic and Rehabilitation Principles,* 3rd ed. Rosemont, IL: American Academy of Orthopaedic Surgeons, 2004. pp. 533-540.
136. Gottschalk FA, Jaegers SM. Transfemoral amputation. In Murdock G, Wilson AB (eds), *Amputation: Surgical Practice and Patient Management.* Oxford: Butterworth-Heinemann, 1996. pp. 111-118.
137. Sanders GT. Above knee amputation. In *Lower Limb Amputations: A Guide to Rehabilitation.* Philadelphia: F.A. Davis, 1986. pp. 230-254.
138. Gottschalk FA, Stills M. The biomechanics of transfemoral amputation. *Prosthet Orthot Int* 1994;18(1):12-17.
139. Jaegers SM, Arendzen JH, deJongh HJ. Changes in hip muscles after above knee amputation. *Clin Orthop* 1995;Oct(319):278-284.
140. Jaegers SM, Arendzen JH, deJongh JH. Prosthetic gait of unilateral transfemoral amputees: a kinematic study. *Arch Phys Med Rehabil* 1995;76(8):736-743.
141. Barnes RW, Cox B. Above-knee amputation. In *Amputations: An Illustrated Manual.* Philadelphia: Hanley & Belfus, 2000. pp. 103-117.
142. Chansky HA. Hip disarticulation and transpelvic amputation: surgical management. In Smith DG, Michaels JW, Bowker JH (eds), *Atlas of Amputation and Limb Deficiencies. Surgical Prosthetic and Rehabilitation Principles,* 3rd ed. Rosemont, IL: American Academy of Orthopaedic Surgeons, 2004. pp. 557-564.
143. Persson BM. Hip disarticulation, transiliac, and sacroiliac amputations. In Murdock G, Wilson AB (eds), *Amputation: Surgical Practice and Patient Management.* Oxford: Butterworth-Heinemann, 1996. pp. 141-148.
144. Unruh T, Fisher DF, Unruh TA. Hip disarticulation: an 11 year experience. *Arch Surg* 1990;125(6):791-793.
145. Merimsky O, Kollender Y, Inbar M, et al. Palliative major amputation and quality of life in cancer patients. *Acta Oncol* 1997;36(2):151-157.
146. Barnes RW, Cox B. Hip disarticulation. In *Amputations, An Illustrated Manual.* Philadelphia: Hanley & Belfus, 2000. pp. 119-143.
147. Carroll KM. Hip disarticulation and transpelvic amputation: prosthetic management. In Smith DG, Michaels JW, Bowker JH (eds), *Atlas of Amputation and Limb Deficiencies. Surgical Prosthetic and Rehabilitation Principles,* 3rd ed. Rosemont, IL: American Academy of Orthopaedic Surgeons, 2004. pp. 565-573.

23

Postoperative and Preprosthetic Care

MICHELLE M. LUSARDI

LEARNING OBJECTIVES

On completion of this chapter, the reader will be able to do the following:

1. Plan a comprehensive examination for an individual with recent lower extremity amputation, selecting appropriate tests and measures and documentation strategies.
2. Use information gathered in the examination, evidence from the clinical research literature, and knowledge of postoperative care to evaluate individuals with recent lower extremity amputation.
3. Formulate an appropriate physical therapy (PT) movement dysfunction diagnosis and prognosis for rehabilitation for individuals with recent lower extremity amputation.
4. Develop appropriate short-term goals and long-term goals and estimate duration, frequency, and intensity of care in the postoperative, preprosthetic care of an individual with recent lower extremity amputation.
5. Develop an appropriate PT plan of care for single limb mobility, residual limb care and wound healing, and preprosthetic rehabilitation.
6. Describe strategies to monitor progress and to adapt and advance the plan of care during the preprosthetic period of rehabilitation.
7. Describe strategies to evaluate outcomes of postoperative, preprosthetic rehabilitation.

PATIENT-CLIENT MANAGEMENT AFTER AMPUTATION

Individuals with New Amputation

In the immediate postoperative period the person with a new amputation is likely to experience acute surgical pain and will be grieving the physical loss of the limb. The immediacy of pain and feelings of loss may make it difficult for him or her to recognize the potential for a positive rehabilitation outcome. Older persons with dysvascular or neuropathic limb loss may have had time to physically and psychologically prepare for an "elective" amputation after a prolonged period of managing a poorly vascularized foot or nonhealing neuropathic ulcer and therefore may be somewhat less distressed about the loss of their limb than younger persons who have suddenly lost a limb in a traumatic accident or other medical emergency. Whatever the circumstances leading to amputation, however, the loss of one's limb requires significant psychological adjustment.[1] Early education and discussion about the process of rehabilitation and the person's ultimate goals are extremely important.

The Interdisciplinary Team

Ideally the physical therapist and prosthetist, as members of the interdisciplinary rehabilitation team, will be involved in discussion with surgeons, patients, and family members about surgical levels, potential for prosthetic use, and optimization of rehabilitation before actual surgery.[2] In the days immediately after amputation, the goals of the members of the interdisciplinary team vary, but all ultimately lead toward the person with a newly amputated limb's independence and return to his or her preferred lifestyle. Surgical and medical members of the team are most concerned about the healing suture line and overall health status, especially for individuals with vascular insufficiency or for those at risk of infection after traumatic amputation.[3] Nursing professionals provide general medical and wound care as the suture line heals. Registered dieticians assess the patient's nutritional needs related to wound healing and exercise demands. Physical and occupational therapists focus on enhancing the patient's early single limb mobility, self-care, assessment of the potential for prosthetic use, control of edema and pain management, optimal shaping of the residual limb for prosthetic wear, and prevention of secondary complications.[4]

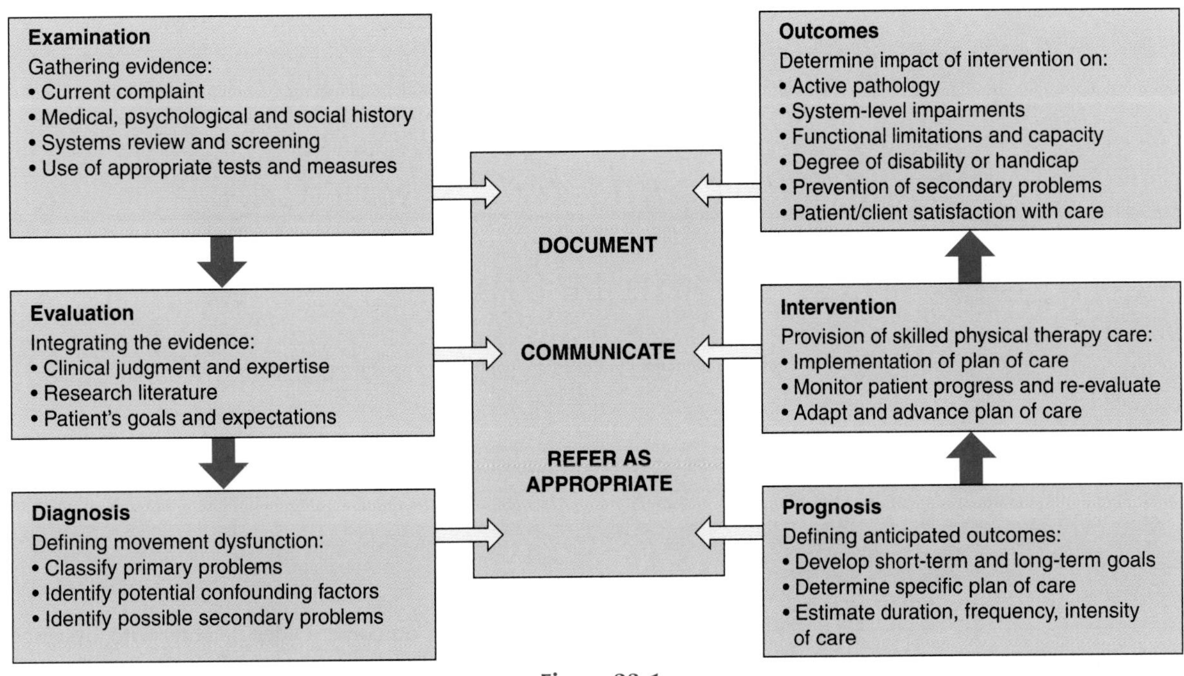

Figure 23-1

The components of a systematic and effective patient-client management process. (Modified from The guide to physical therapist practice. Phys Ther *2001;81[1]:43.)*

The prosthetist may fabricate an immediate or early postoperative prosthesis or semirigid dressing and begins to consider which prosthetic components and suspension systems will ultimately be most appropriate, given the individual's characteristics and functional needs.[5] The person with new amputation and his or her family are often most concerned about pain management and what life will be like without the lost limb.[1] A psychologist, social worker, vocational counselor, or school counselor is involved as needed to help with psychological adjustment and to organize long-term rehabilitation care or community resources in preparation for discharge. A clergyman can also be a valuable resource for the person with new amputation, the family, and the team.

Although the multidisciplinary team can vary in size, depending on patient needs and practice settings, the members at the center are the individual with new amputation and his or her caregivers.[6] Communication among all team members, especially the opportunity for the person and family members to ask questions and voice concerns, is more important in this early postoperative and preprosthetic period than it is during the process of prosthetic prescription and training later in the rehabilitation process. This early period sets the stage for the individual's expectations, and ultimately success, as a person with an amputation.[1]

The unique training, clinical expertise, and individual roles of each team member contribute, in a collaborative process, to the development of a plan for rehabilitation that best meets the needs and optimizes the potential of the individual who has lost a limb.[6] The team must come to agreement on the timing and prioritization of specific rehabilitative interventions to meet the goals defined for each patient. Effective communication and strong relationships among the surgeons, orthopedists, or trauma teams who perform the majority of amputations and the rehabilitation team substantially improve the quality of patient care and assist the rehabilitation process.

This chapter focuses on the roles of rehabilitation professionals who work with persons with new amputation in the days and weeks immediately after surgery. The author explores how surgical pain and phantom sensation are managed, strategies for controlling postoperative edema, and methods to assess a patient's readiness for prosthetic fitting. Interventions that help a person with new amputation gain competence with single limb mobility tasks and exercises that provide the foundation for successful prosthetic use are identified. The strategies for patient management are organized around the model outlined in the American Physical Therapy Association's *Guide to Physical Therapist Practice* (Figure 23-1).[7]

EXAMINATION

Ideally, for those undergoing a "planned" or "elective" amputation, the rehabilitation team will meet with the individual and caregivers before surgery to begin collecting information that will be used to guide intervention and provide information about the rehabilitation process. In some instances input from rehabilitation professionals may be

sought by trauma surgeons to assist patients and families in making informed decisions when faced with amputation after severe injury of the limb. Preoperative interaction may not always be possible, especially when amputation occurs subsequent to failed revascularization, acute and severe limb ischemia, severe infection, or traumatic injury. If preoperative assessment is not possible, referral to rehabilitation should be made as soon after surgery as possible; delaying referrals often leads to contracture formation, further cardiovascular and musculoskeletal deconditioning, delayed prosthetic fitting and training, and a greater risk of dependency.[2] The components of a comprehensive assessment for persons with lower extremity amputation are summarized in Box 23-1.

Whenever the first contact with the individual and family occurs, the rehabilitation team begins by gathering baseline information that will guide planning for and implementing the rehabilitation process. This initial information is gathered in three ways: developing a complete patient-client history, performing a review of physiological systems to identify important comorbidities that will affect the rehabilitation process, and using appropriate tests and measures to identify impairments and functional limitations to be addressed in the rehabilitation plan of care.[7] The volume and complexity of information needed to guide planning for prosthetic rehabilitation means that information gathering is a somewhat continuous process and must be integrated with early mobility training in preparation for the individual's discharge from the acute care setting. Examination in the acute care setting likely focuses on four priorities: initial healing of the surgical site, pain management and volume control of the residual limb, bed mobility and transfers, and readiness for single limb ambulation. Examination later in the preprosthetic period (in an outpatient, home care, or subacute setting) would add more detail to determine potential for prosthetic prescription.

Patient-Client History and Interview

Rehabilitation professionals use several strategies to gather information about an individual's medical history. In the acute care setting the process usually begins with a review of the individual's current medical record or chart, as well as previous medical records (if available). The *chart review* process provides a broad overview of the individual's health, comorbidities, and functional status, as well as details about the surgical procedure. Data that other members of the health care team have generated in their examination and evaluative processes are quite relevant to PT care, not only to avoid redundancy in examination but also in planning what additional information will be necessary to collect during subsequent interviews and discussion with the individual and family caregivers.

The *interview process* provides key information about the individual's priorities and concerns so that they can be appropriately integrated into the plan of care. The physical therapist may also choose to gather supplementary information from the *clinical research literature* at this point to assist in the subsequent development of prognosis and plan or care, especially if the individual's situation is unusual or complex.[8]

Demographic and Sociocultural Information

The information gathered when reviewing history often begins with basic *demographics* such as age, gender, race/ethnicity, primary language, and level of education. These data help us to appropriately target communication during our interaction with an individual with recent amputation. It is also important to build an understanding of the individual's *sociocultural history* including beliefs, expectations and goals, preferred behaviors, and family and caregiver resources, as well as access to and quality of informal and formal support systems.[9,10] Each of these is a potentially important influence on the individual's engagement in the rehabilitation process. Rehabilitation professionals also gather information about the individual's employment status and task demands, roles and responsibilities within the family system, and leisure interests and hobbies, as well as previous and preferred involvement in the community (access, transportation, and key activities). This information is important in developing a prognosis and plan of care; it helps rehabilitation professionals to better define the long-term goals and anticipated outcomes of rehabilitation.

Developmental Status

Another piece of information that informs an appropriate rehabilitation plan of care is the physical, cognitive, perceptual, and emotional *developmental status* of the individual and his or her caregivers, as well as an understanding of the family system as an organization.[11,12] Although the relevance of developmental status is most obvious when the individual being examined is a child, the perspective afforded by understanding of lifespan development is valuable for individuals with recent amputation of any age. Examples of factors that evolve over the lifespan that affect an individual's participation in rehabilitation include postural control, motor abilities, perceptual abilities, willingness to take risks, problem solving, coping styles and strategies, and limb dominance. Observation and interchange during the interview process help the therapist to determine if further clinical examination of developmental status will be necessary.

Living Environment

Rehabilitation professionals gather information about the characteristics of an individual's physical *living environment*.[13] They ask about getting into and out of the house (e.g., how far is it from the car to the house? Are there steps at the entry? What are the distances between the major living areas that the person will have to navigate? How accessible and functional are each of the major living areas in the home

Box 23-1 *Comprehensive Assessment for Patients with Lower Extremity Amputation*

HISTORY (DATA COLLECTED FROM CHART REVIEW AND INTERVIEW)	
Demographics	Age, gender, primary language, race/ethnicity
Social history	Family and caregiver resources, other social support systems
Occupation history	Employment or retirement status, typical work and leisure activities
Developmental status	Physical/motor, perceptual, cognitive, and emotional dimensions
Living environment	Characteristics and accessibility of "home" environment, projected discharge destination
Current condition	Reason for referral, current concerns/needs, previous medical/surgical interventions for current condition
Past medical history	Prior hospitalizations and surgeries; smoking, alcohol, or drug use (past and present)
Family history	Health risk factors for vascular and cardiac disease
Medications	Prescription medication for current and other medical conditions Over-the-counter medications typically used
Functional status	Current and prior abilities and functional limitations [ADLs/IADLs]

SYSTEMS REVIEW (CONCURRENT/COMORBID DISEASE AND IMPAIRMENT RELATED TO PROGNOSIS FOR AND PARTICIPATION IN REHABILITATION)

Cardiopulmonary and cardiovascular systems
Endocrine and metabolic systems
Musculoskeletal system
Neuromuscular system
Gastrointestinal and genitourinary systems

TESTS AND MEASURES (AREAS FOR SPECIFIC ASSESSMENT)	
Pain	Presence of phantom limb sensation or pain Postoperative pain and pain management strategies Muscle soreness related to altered movement patterns Joint pain related to motion or comorbid arthritis, etc.
Anthropomorphic characteristics	Residual limb length (bone length, soft tissue length) Residual limb girth, redundant tissue ("dog ears," adductor roll) Residual limb shape (bulbous, cylindrical, conical) Assessment of type and severity of edema Effectiveness of edema control strategy being used Overall height, weight, body composition
Skin/integument	Assessment of surgical wound healing Assessment/management of adhesions and existing scar tissue Other skin problems (other incisions, grafts, psoriasis, cysts, etc.) Integrity of remaining foot/limb, especially if neuropathic or dysvascular etiology of amputation
Circulation	Palpation/auscultation of lower extremity pulses, residual and intact limbs Skin temperature and presence of trophic changes, residual and intact limbs Skin color and response to elevation or dependent position, residual and intact limbs Claudication time and distance, impact on function
Range of motion/muscle length	Range of motion, soft tissue length, and joint contracture
Joint integrity	Ligamentous integrity or joint instability Structural alignment or joint deformity Integrity or inflammation of synovium, bursae, cartilage
Muscle performance	Current muscle strength of upper extremity, trunk, lower extremity Muscular power for functional activity Muscular endurance for functional activity Potential for improvement
Motor function	Motor control including dexterity, coordination, agility, tone Motor learning including previous use of ambulatory aids, prostheses

Box 23-1 *Comprehensive Assessment for Patients with Lower Extremity Amputation—cont'd*

Upper extremity function	Power and strength of upper extremity and of trunk Ability to use upper extremity in functional activities
Aerobic capacity	Blood pressure, heart rate, respiratory rate (at rest, as well as during and following activity) Perceived exertion, dyspnea, angina, during functional activity Overall level of physical fitness and functional capacity
Attention/cognition/emotion	Level of consciousness, sleep patterns Ability to learn and preferred learning style Cognitive dysfunction screening (delirium, depression, dementia) Motivation, attention/distractibility, learning styles
Sensory integrity	Protective sensation of residual and remaining limb Superficial sensation: light touch, sharp/dull, pressure, temperature Proprioception: kinesthesia, position sense
Mobility	Changing position in bed (rolling, scooting, coming to sitting)
Postural control	Static, anticipatory, reactionary balance, in sitting, standing, during functional activities
Transfers	Ability to transfer to/from bed, toilet, wheelchair, mat, tub/shower
Assistive/adaptive equipment	Assistive devices/adaptive equipment currently being used
Ambulation and locomotion	Ability to use ambulatory aid safely for single limb gait Ability to use wheelchair safely Adaptations/equipment necessary for patient's living environment
Gait and balance	Assessment of postural control in quiet standing, reaching, ability to stop/start, change direction, and alter velocity while walking Reaction to unexpected perturbation, at rest and during activity Observational gait assessment, identification of gait deviations Kinematic gait assessment (e.g., speed, stride length, cadence) Energy cost or efficiency of locomotion/gait, perceived exertion and dyspnea Ability/safety to manage uneven terrain, stairs, ramps, etc.
Posture	Resting posture in sitting, standing, other positions Alteration in posture due to loss of limb segment
Self-care	Ability to perform basic ADLs Ability to perform IADLs Availability of assistance and preparation of caregivers
Community/work reintegration	Analysis of roles/activities/tasks Functional capacity analysis, determination of essential functions Analysis of environment, safety assessment Assessment of need for adaptation
Prosthetic requirements	Potential for functional prosthetic use Readiness for prosthetic fitting/prescription Appropriate prosthetic design, components, suspension

Modified from *Phys Ther* 2001;77(11):1354-1367.
ADLs, Activities of daily living; *IADLs,* instrumental activities of daily living.

for those using ambulatory aids or a wheelchair for mobility? Is it possible to adapt the home if necessary? What adaptive equipment is already available? What type of assistance is likely to be routinely available? What type of equipment is likely to be acceptable for the individual and family?)

Asking about the individual's ability to drive, access public transportation, or plans for alternatives for transport once discharged from the acute care setting is important. This may determine what services will be necessary and where they will be provided. Will the individual be returning to his or her home environment on discharge from acute care? If so, will he or she require home care or is transportation available for follow-up appointments with physicians and for outpatient rehabilitation? Alternatively, will the individual have an interim stay in another health care facility for further rehabilitation? This information will help set rehabilitation priorities and begin the process of discharge planning.

Health, Emotional, and Cognitive Status

During the interview the rehabilitation professional's impression of the individual's general health status that began to develop during chart review becomes broadened. The rehabilitation professional asks questions to discern how the person perceives his or her health and his or her ability to function in self-care, family, or social roles. They assess the individual's understanding of the current situation and prognosis, as well as expectations about the rehabilitation process. They may explore the person's coping style and response to stress, as well as preferred coping skills and strategies.[14] This conversation also provides an indication about the individual's current emotional status, ability to learn, cognitive ability, and memory functions.

Because rehabilitation involves physical effort, it is important to understand the person with recent amputation's usual level of activity and fitness, as well as his or her readiness to be involved in exercise. Is physical activity a regular part of the preamputation lifestyle? Will any additional health habits such as smoking and use of alcohol or other substances affect the individual's ability to do physical work and ability to learn or adapt?

Medical, Surgical, and Family History

Potentially important medical conditions that may influence the postoperative/preprosthetic rehabilitation include diabetes, cardiovascular disease, cerebrovascular disease, obesity, neuropathy, renal disease, congestive heart failure, uncontrolled hypertension, and preexisting neuromuscular or musculoskeletal pathologies or impairments such as stroke or osteoporosis.[15-17] Each of these has a potential impact on wound healing, functional mobility, and exercise tolerance during rehabilitation. Healing and risk of infection are also concerns for those with compromised immune system function, whether from diseases such as human immunodeficiency virus (HIV)/acquired immunodeficiency syndrome (AIDS), those on transplant medications, those involved in chemotherapy or recent stem cell transplant, or those using medical steroids. Wound healing, skin condition, and endurance may be issues for persons who are currently undergoing radiation treatments for cancer.

Review of the individual's past surgical history provides additional information that helps rehabilitation professionals anticipate what the individual's response to physical activity might be like. Has the individual had a cardiac pacemaker or defibrillator implanted? Has there been previous amputation of toes or part of the foot of either the newly amputated or "intact" limb? Are there recent surgical scars to be aware of (e.g., following revascularization before amputation)? Has there been total joint replacement or lower extremity fracture that might affect rehabilitation activities and prosthetic component selection?

The "laundry list" of comorbidities and previous surgeries identified in chart review does not necessarily mean that the individual is in poor health.[18] Many individuals manage chronic illnesses and conditions quite effectively, and although they may have less functional reserve than those without pathology, they have the potential for positive rehabilitation outcomes.

Physical therapists must also be aware of the results of tests and diagnostic procedures that other team members have undertaken as part of their examination and evaluation. These might include preoperative cardiac or peripheral vascular studies, electrocardiogram (ECG), stress tests, pulmonary function tests, radiographs and other scans, urinalysis, and laboratory tests for various components of blood (e.g., hemoglobin, cell counts, cultures). Comparison of the individual's test results to established norms provides an index of overall health status and tolerance of levels of activity.

Because many of the medications used to manage postoperative pain affect thinking and learning, it is important to understand what pain management strategies are in place and when medication is typically administered.[19] Given the likelihood of cardiovascular comorbidity in older adults with vascular disease and diabetes, it is also important to understand what cardiac medications are being administered and how these medications affect response to physical activity and position change.[20] It is not unusual for persons who have been immobile or on bed rest to be at risk of postural hypotension, especially if they are taking medications to manage hypertension. Additionally, given the stress of the surgery and hospital environment, especially if the amputation was performed under general anesthesia, there is the possibility of a temporary postoperative delirium or difficulty with learning and memory.[21] If confusion is observed it is important to clarify typical preoperative cognitive status by speaking with family and caregivers.

Current Condition

Reading the operating room report in the medical record is important to become familiar with the surgical procedure, drain placement, method of closure, and planned postoperative wound and limb-volume strategies being used (Chapter 22 provides an overview of the most common surgical procedures at the transtibial and transfemoral levels). This information, when combined with knowledge of pain management strategies and demographic information, guides early postoperative/preprosthetic care. Physical therapists use this information to identify potential issues with healing, educational needs for the person with new amputation, early positioning of the residual limb, potential issues affecting prosthetic fit, and preparation of the residual limb for wearing a prosthesis. Determining how comorbidities and injuries are being actively managed is also important, as these affect readiness for early mobility, learning, and memory. Impressions of the individual's psychological state, fears, and expectations round out the baseline with which the person will begin early rehabilitation.

Systems Review

In the acute care setting there has likely been a fairly comprehensive review of physiological systems as a component of preoperative work-up or emergency care (in the case of traumatic injury). Rehabilitation professionals find the results of such review in the physician notes and intake forms in the medical record. The therapist may choose to screen or evaluate in more detail if the information in the record is insufficient in depth or detail, especially as it relates to functional status and response to increasing activity and exercise. This includes anatomical and physiological status of the cardiovascular, cardiopulmonary, integumentary, musculoskeletal, and neuromuscular systems, as well as communication, affect, cognition, language, and learning style.[22]

Ongoing screening as rehabilitation progresses will help to identify the onset of secondary problems and postoperative complications that require medical intervention or referral to other members of the team. Deterioration in cognitive status or onset of new confusion over a relatively short period of time is especially important to watch for, as it is often the first indication of dehydration, adverse drug reaction, or infection in older adults.[21]

Test and Measures

In the postoperative, preprosthetic period, physical therapists employ a variety of objective tests and measures to determine the severity of impairment and functional limitation and to establish a baseline that will be used to determine PT movement-related diagnosis, determine prognosis, and assess outcomes of the rehabilitation process.[23] Examples of tests and measures appropriate for the postoperative, preprosthetic period are listed in Table 23-1. Although most strategies are similar to those used in general PT practice, some may need to be adapted to accommodate the condition or length of the residual limb (e.g., the point of application of resistive force during manual muscle testing of knee extension strength after transtibial amputation). Whenever measurement technique is altered, however, the reliability and validity of the data collected may be questionable and the data generated less precise. Therapists often begin with examination at the level of impairment and then move into functional assessment.

Assessing Postoperative Pain and Phantom Sensation

The individual with new amputation is likely to be coping with significant acute postoperative pain and may be distressed by the sense that the limb is still in place (phantom sensation) after amputation. Pain is a subjective sensation; each person defines his or her own level of tolerance. Physical therapists have a number of strategies available to document the nature of pain, location of pain, and the intensity of discomfort that the individual is experiencing. These include descriptors generated by the individual with recent amputation or circled on a pain checklist, body maps, visual analog scales, provocation tests, or specific pain indices or questionnaires for developed for postsurgical patients (Figure 23-2).[24] It is also important to assess how severely that pain interferes with functions, what activities or conditions increase the pain, and what positions or strategies have been helpful in managing the postoperative pain.

Commonly, persons with recent amputation experience a sense that the amputated limb remains in place in the days and weeks after surgery.[25] As many as 70% of persons with new amputation have noticeable phantom limb sensation.[26,27] Most experience a sense of numbness, tingling, or pressure in the missing limb, and some complain of itching toes or mild muscle cramps in the foot or calf.[4] A small percentage of those with new amputation experience significant phantom pain, described as shooting pain, severe cramping, or a distressing burning sensation that may be localized in the amputated foot or present throughout the missing limb. If the individual reports significant phantom sensation or pain, careful inspection of the residual limb helps to rule out other potential sources of pain such as a neuroma or an inflamed or infected surgical wound. Phantom pain is often intermittent, although some individuals report constant discomfort.[28] Onset of phantom pain may or may not be linked to activities such as exercise or dressing change.

Those who experienced significant dysvascular limb pain in the weeks and months before surgery are more likely to experience phantom pain in the immediate postoperative period and for up to 2 years after surgery.[29] Severity or duration of preoperative pain does not appear to be predictive of long-term phantom pain. Phantom limb sensation and pain tend to decrease over time whether the amputation was the result of a dysvascular/neuropathic extremity or a traumatic injury.[25] Although a number of models or theories for phantom limb sensation and phantom pain have been proposed, the neurophysiological mechanism that underlies this phenomenon is not well understood.[30,31]

The likelihood of postoperative phantom limb sensation must be discussed with the individual and family before amputation surgery, as well as in the days immediately after operation. Phantom limb sensation is quite vivid; its realistic qualities can be disturbing and frightening to those with recent amputation. Candid discussion about phantom limb sensation as a normally anticipated occurrence helps to reduce an individual's anxiety and distress should phantom sensation occur. It also alerts him or her to issues of safety in the immediate postoperative period. Individuals with recent amputation are at significant risk of falling when they awaken from sleep and attempt to stand and walk to the bathroom in the middle of the night, thinking in their semi-alert state that both limbs are intact. Ecchymosis or wound dehiscence sustained during a fall can lead to major delays in rehabilitation and prosthetic fitting; some fall-related injuries require surgical revision or closure.

Table 23-1
Examples of Tests and Measures Important in the Postoperative, Preprosthetic Period

Category	*Examples of Test or Measurement Strategy*
Pain	Description of nature or type of pain Visual analog scale for intensity of pain Body chart for location of painful areas Description of factors to increase/decrease discomfort
Anthropometric characteristics	Residual limb length Residual limb circumference Description of edema type and location
Integumentary integrity	Condition of the incision Nature and extent of drainage Condition of "intact" limb Skin color, turgor, temperature
Circulation	Palpation of peripheral pulse Skin temperature
Arousal, attention, cognition	Mini-mental State Examination Depression scales
Sensory integrity	Protective sensation (Semmes-Weinstein filament) Proprioception and kinesthesia Visual acuity, figure-ground, light/dark accommodation Vestibulo-ocular function during position change Hearing impairment (acuity, sensitivity to background noise)
Aerobic capacity, endurance	Heart rate at rest, % maximal attainable in activity Respiratory rate at rest, during activity Ratings of perceived exertion or dyspnea
Mobility	Observation of bed mobility (e.g., rolling) Observation of transitions (e.g., supine–sit) Observation of transfers (various surfaces, heights) Description of level of assistance, cueing required
Balance	Static postural control (various functional positions) Anticipatory postural control in functional activity Reaction to perturbation Specific balance tests (e.g., Berg, Functional Reach)
Gait and locomotion	Use of assistive devices Level of independence, cuing or assistance required Time and distance parameters (velocity, cadence, stride) Pattern and symmetry Perceived exertion and dyspnea
Joint integrity and mobility	Manual examination of ligamentous integrity Documentation of bony deformity
Neuro-motor function	Observation of quality of motor control in activity Observation of efficiency of motor planning Determination of stage of motor learning with new or adapted tasks Muscle tone Reflex integrity
Muscle performance	Strength: manual muscle test, handheld dynamometer Power: isokinetic dynamometer, manual resistance through range at various speeds of contraction Endurance: 10RM or maximum number contractions, time to fatigue
Range of motion/muscle length	Goniometry Functional tests (e.g., Thomas test, straight leg raise)
Self-care and home management	Observation of BADLs and IADLs BADL and IADL rating scales

BADLs, Basic activities of daily living; *IADLs,* instrumental activities of daily living.

McGill Pain Questionnaire

Part 1: Where is Your Pain?

Please mark, on the drawings below, the areas where you feel pain.

Put "E" if the pain is external
Put "I" if the pain is internal
Put "EI" if the pain is both internal and external

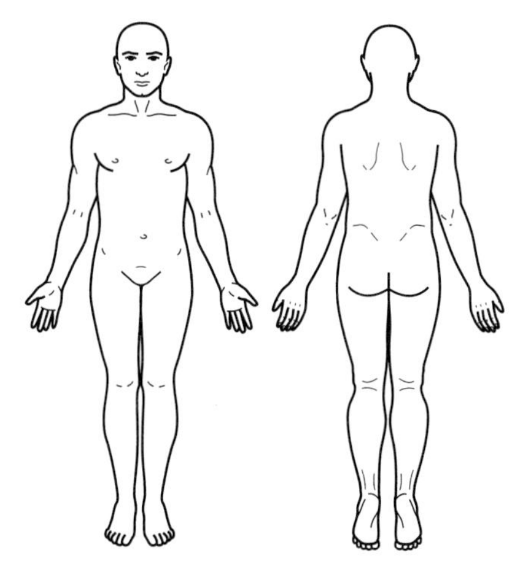

Part 2: What Does Your Pain Feel Like?

Some of the words below describe your PRESENT pain. Circle ONLY those words that best describe your pain right now. Leave out any category that is not suitable. Use only a single word in the appropriate category—the one that applies the best.

1	2	3	4
Flickering Quivering Pulsing Throbbing Beating Pounding	Jumping Flashing Shooting	Pricking Boring Drilling Stabbing Lancinating	Sharp Cutting Lacerating
5	**6**	**7**	**8**
Pinching Pressing Gnawing Cramping Crushing	Tugging Pulling Wrenching	Hot Burning Scalding Searing	Tingling Itchy Smarting
9	**10**	**11**	**12**
Dull Sore Hurting Aching Heavy	Tender Taut Rasping	Tiring Exhausting	Sickening Suffocating
13	**14**	**15**	**16**
Fearful Frightful Terrifying	Punishing Grueling Cruel Vicious Killing	Wretched Blinding	Annoying Troublesome Miserable Intense Unbearable
17	**18**	**19**	**20**
Spreading Radiating Penetrating Piercing	Tight Numb Drawing Squeezing Tearing	Cool Cold Freezing	Nagging Nauseating Agonizing Dreadful Torturing

Part 3: How Does Your Pain Change With Time?

1. Which word or words would you use to describe the *pattern* of your pain?

1	2	3
Continuous	Rhythmic	Brief
Steady	Periodic	Momentary
Constant	Intermittent	Transient

2. What kind of things *relieve* your pain?

3. What kind of things *increase* your pain?

Part 4: How Strong is Your Pain?

People agree that the following five words represent pain of increasing intensity. They are:

1	2	3	4	5
Mild	Discomforting	Distressing	Horrible	Excruciating

To answer each question below, write the number of the most appropriate word in the space beside the question.

1. Which word describes your pain right now? __________
2. Which word describes your pain at its worst? __________
3. Which word describes it when it is least? __________
4. Which word describes the worst toothache you ever had? __________
5. Which word describes the worst headache you ever had? __________
6. Which word describes the worst stomach-ache you ever had? __________

A

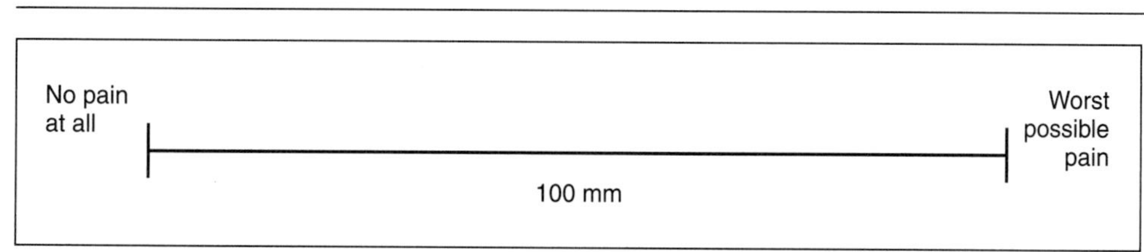

B

Figure 23-2

Examples of tools used to document pain and discomfort. ***A,*** *McGill Pain Questionnaire. Descriptor groups: sensory (1-10), affective (11-15), evaluative (16), and miscellaneous (17-20). (Modified from Melzack R. The McGill pain questionnaire; major properties and scoring methods.* Pain *1975;1(3):280-281.)* ***B,*** *The visual analog scale. (From Bijur PE, Silver W, Gallagher EJ. Reliability of the visual analog scale for measurement of acute pain.* Acad Emerg Med *2001;8(12):1153-1157.)*

Assessing Residual Limb Length and Volume

The length and volume of the residual limb are important determinants of readiness for prosthetic use, as well as socket design and components chosen for the training prosthesis. Initial measurements can be made at the first dressing change. Changes in limb volume are tracked by frequent remeasurement during the preprosthetic period of rehabilitation.

The two components of *residual limb length* are the actual length of the residual tibia or femur and the total length of the limb including soft tissue. Measurements are taken from an easily identified bony landmark to the palpated end of the long bone, the incision line, or the end of soft tissue. In the transtibial limb the starting place for measurement is most often the medial joint line; an alternative is to begin measurement at the tibial tubercle (Figure 23-3, *A*). In the transfemoral limb the starting place for measurement can be the ischial tuberosity or the greater trochanter (Figure 23-3, *B*). Clear notation must be made about the proximal and distal landmarks that are used for the initial measurement to ensure consistency in the subsequent measurement process.

A standard-length transtibial amputation, which preserves 5 to 6 inches of tibia (measured from the tibial plateau), ensures a sufficient lever arm for effective prosthetic control. Transtibial limbs of less than 3 inches may be insufficient in length for prosthetic control and in surface area for skin tolerance of weight-bearing pressures applied by the socket.[32] Persons with long transtibial residual limbs may be unable to flex the knee beyond 90 degrees in sitting when wearing their prosthesis because of distal anterior discomfort or skin irritation where the limb contacts the socket. For those with transfemoral amputation, preservation of as much of the length of the femur as possible enhances control of the prosthetic knee unit; however, the choice of knee units may be limited when the transfemoral limb is long.[33]

Residual limb volume is assessed by serial circumferential girth measurements. For persons with transtibial amputation, circumferential measurement begins at either the medial tibial plateau or the tibial tubercle and is repeated at equally spaced points to the end of the limb (Figure 23-4). For those with transfemoral amputation, measurement begins at either the ischial tuberosity or the greater trochanter and is

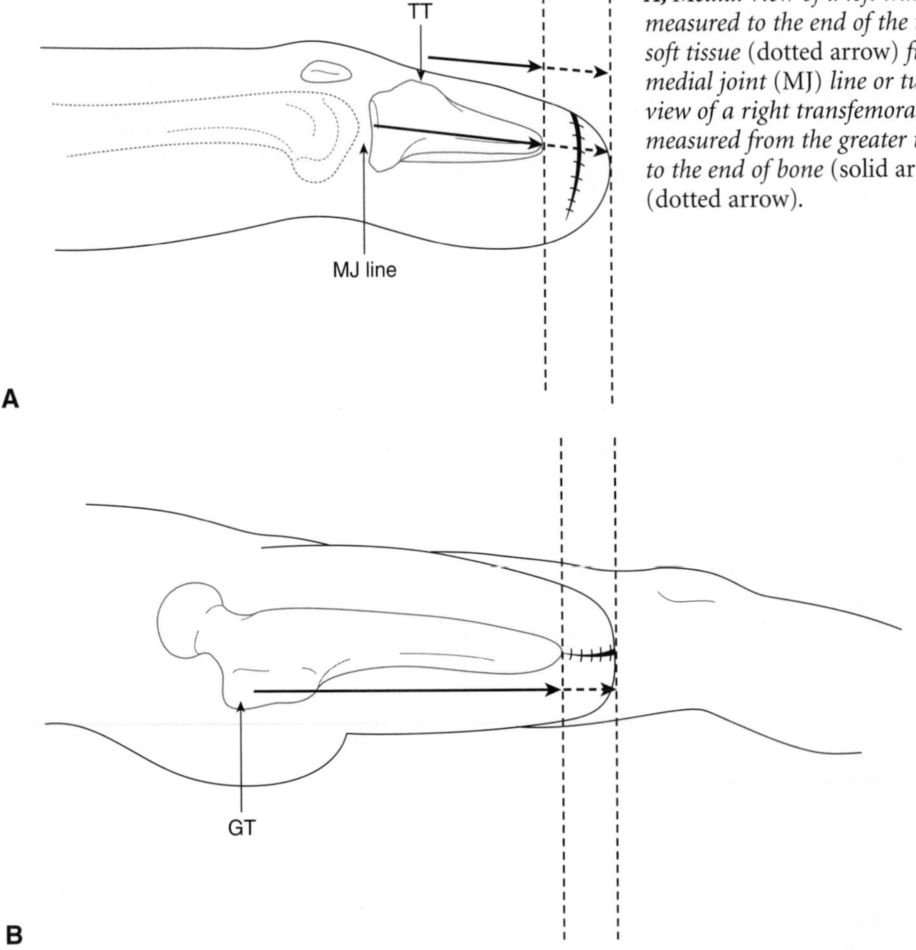

Figure 23-3
A, *Medial view of a left transtibial residual limb. Limb length is measured to the end of the tibia* (solid arrow) *and to the end of soft tissue* (dotted arrow) *from a bony landmark such as the medial joint* (MJ) *line or tubercle of the tibia* (TT). **B,** *Lateral view of a right transfemoral residual limb. Limb length is measured from the greater trochanter* (GT) *or ischial tuberosity to the end of bone* (solid arrow) *and to the end of soft tissue* (dotted arrow).

also repeated at equally spaced points to the end of the residual limb. The interval between measurements should be clearly documented (i.e., every 5 cm or every inch) for consistency and reliability in future measurement.

One of the determinants of readiness for prosthetic fitting is comparison of the proximal and distal circumference of the limb. Often, referral for prosthetic fit is made when the distal limb circumference measurement is equal to or no more than $\frac{1}{4}$ inch greater than proximal limb circumference. Ideally, with effective control of edema and compression, the transtibial residual limb will mature into a tapered cylindrical shape with distal circumference slightly less than proximal circumference. The transfemoral limb typically matures into a more conical shape, with distal circumference significantly less than proximal circumference. A smaller distal circumference is desirable so that shear forces on soft tissue will be minimal when the prosthesis is donned and used.

Assessing Integumentary Integrity and Wound Healing

Assessment of skin condition and the vascular, sensory, and motor status of the patient's limbs (especially the remaining limb) is important. During assessment there is an opportunity to introduce the individual with new amputation and family to strategies that are likely to be used for compression/edema control after surgery. Instructing the individual and family about proper positioning of the residual limb is also important, as well as the need to maintain knee extension and neutral hip alignment to minimize soft tissue tightness and joint contracture.

In most settings the surgeon who performed the amputation assesses the condition of the surgical site at the initial dressing change. This can occur as early as the first postoperative day when soft dressings and elastic wraps have been used or on the third postoperative day if the residual limb has been casted in a rigid dressing.[34] After this initial appraisal the status of the surgical wound is assessed by the nurse or physician at each dressing change. In some settings the physical therapist is charged to inspect the residual limb to monitor the stage of healing of the incision and the limb's shape, length, sensory integrity, and volume; he or she works closely with the surgeon in postoperative wound management and timing of prosthetic replacement.

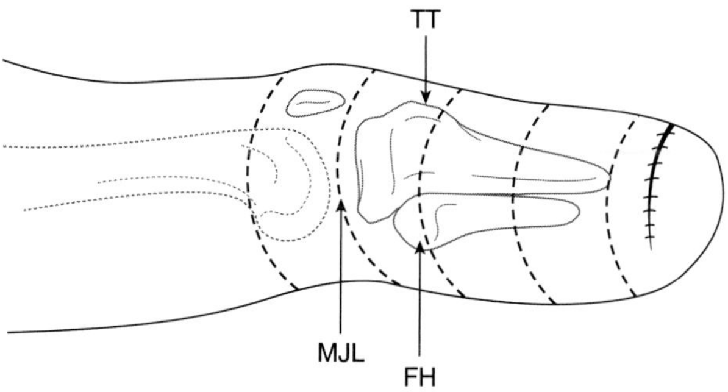

Figure 23-4
Limb volume and shape of a transtibial residual limb is assessed by taking successive circumferential measures (dotted lines) *from a bony landmark such as the medial joint line* (MJL) *to the suture line.* (FH, *Fibular head;* TT, *tibial tubercle).*

With each dressing change, the wound is carefully examined and the quantity and quality of drainage from the wound are documented. Noting a fair amount of serosanguineous drainage absorbed by the dressing is typical as the surgical wound begins to heal. The amount of drainage is expected to decrease over time as healing occurs. Significant amounts of bright red arterial blood or darker venous blood should be reported to the surgeon for further assessment. Thickening, discolored drainage may be a signal of infection of the wound, especially if accompanied by a foul odor.

Wound closure and tissue integrity are monitored closely. In the first several postoperative days, signs of mild to moderate inflammation may be present along the incision line secondary to tissue trauma.[5] The edges of the wound should be closely approximated for effective primary healing; any areas of wound separation (dehiscence), scab or eschar formation, ecchymosis, or other signs of tissue fragility or decreased viability are carefully documented and monitored.

Many persons with traumatic or other nondysvascular amputation have achieved sufficient healing and limb volume control within 2 weeks to use a prefabricated adjustable prosthesis or to be casted for their initial (preparatory, training) prosthesis.[36] Some persons who required amputation secondary to vascular disease may also have healed sufficiently for prosthetic casting as soon as 14 days after the operation (Figure 23-5); for others, sufficient healing may not be achieved for 6 to 8 weeks.[37,38]

When primary healing has been achieved the surgeon can begin to remove sutures or staples from the incision.[37] Initially, every other or every third suture/staple can be left in place to guard against wound dehiscence and be removed over successive days. One or two sutures can be left in place for longer periods if healing has been delayed in one or more areas of the incision. The surgical wound can be reinforced with Steri-Strips when sutures or staples are removed to protect the incision from shearing forces during preprosthetic activity and early prosthetic training. The Steri-Strips can remain on the limb for 2 or more additional weeks after the sutures/staples have been removed. Gait training with a prosthesis can begin, with the approval of the surgeon, when clear evidence of primary healing is found, even if several sutures have been left in place to protect an area along the incision line that has been slow in closing.

Delayed healing of the surgical wound necessarily delays prosthetic use. Older persons with diabetes and vascular insufficiency are particularly at risk for delayed healing.[39] The healing process can also be delayed as a consequence of

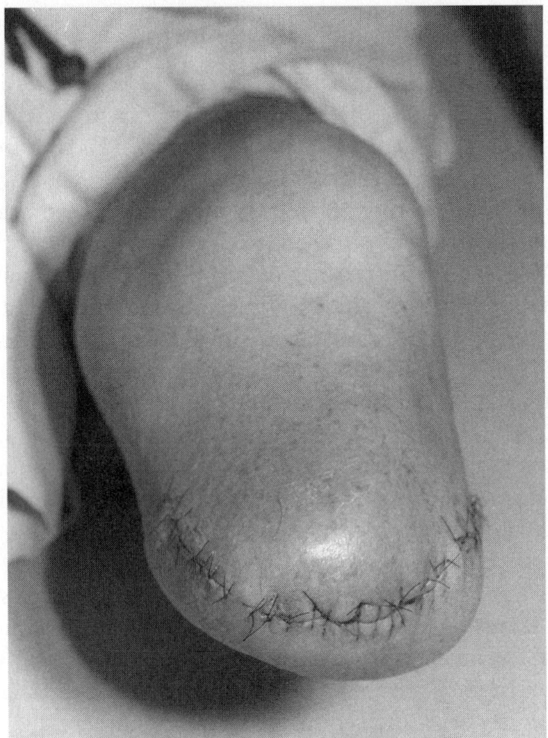

Figure 23-5

A well-healed, transtibial residual limb with a "fish mouth" incision 14 days after amputation. The edges of the wound are approximate, and although several small scabs have formed between sutures, primary healing is well established. Strategies for control of edema and initial limb shaping have been successful as well; this residual limb could be described as cylindrical, with little redundant tissue present.

infection, immunosuppression, or traumatic damage sustained during activity or in a fall in the days or weeks after surgery.[40] Nutritional status is another important determinant of wound healing in the early postoperative and preprosthetic period; individuals with compromised nutritional status are more likely to experience delayed wound healing and are at greater risk of postoperative infection, as well as cardiopulmonary and septic complications.[41]

Assessing Circulation

Because so many amputations are associated with the dyad of vascular insufficiency and polyneuropathy, it is particularly important to examine and monitor vascular status and skin integrity of the remaining (intact) limb, as well as of the residual limb. One criterion for determining the level of amputation is the likelihood of healing of the surgical construct.[3] Surgeons caring for persons with dysvascular limbs typically determine the status of peripheral circulation using both noninvasive and invasive tests before amputation; however, delayed healing or failure of the suture line to close sometimes occurs even with careful preoperative evaluation. In the days and weeks after amputation surgery, members of the team watch for signs of vascular compromise that might threaten adequate closure of the surgical wound.

The remaining limb becomes more vulnerable to skin and soft tissue damage because of increased biomechanical stress associated with single limb mobility. The noninvasive strategies to assess the adequacy of blood flow (described in detail in Chapter 21) include skin temperature and turgor, skin color at rest and after position change, palpation or auscultation of pedal and popliteal pulses, segmental blood pressures, and calculation of an ankle-brachial index. A thorough baseline assessment enables the team to identify and respond to any circulatory problems that might develop as rehabilitation continues.

Assessing Range of Motion and Muscle Length

Having near-normal range of motion (ROM) in the remaining joints of the residual limb is essential for effective prosthetic use.[42] Persons with recent amputation are much at risk for developing soft tissue contracture at the joint proximal to amputation during the preprosthetic period. The risk of hip and knee flexion contracture formation is associated with spending long periods of time sitting in a wheelchair or resting in bed, before and after amputation surgery. Other factors that contribute to the risk of flexion contracture formation include the protective flexion withdrawal pattern associated with lower extremity pain, muscle imbalances that result from loss of distal attachments, and the loss of tonic sensory input generated by weight bearing on the sole of the foot.[30,43] Because limitation in the lower extremity ROM can have a significant impact on the quality and energy efficiency of prosthetic gait, it is essential to assess and monitor ROM. Equally important is implementing strategies to prevent or minimize contracture development as early in the postoperative, preprosthetic period as possible.

For persons with transtibial amputation, definitive measurement of the hip is possible with standard goniometric techniques. With the loss of the malleolus as a distal reference point, accurate measurement of knee extension ROM can be challenging, especially when there is a short residual limb (Figure 23-6). Familiarity with the normal anatomy of the tibia improves the therapist's positioning of the mobile arm of the goniometer and the accuracy of measurement. For individuals with transtibial and transfemoral amputation, the Thomas test may be an effective tool for determining the severity of hip flexion contracture (Figure 23-7). Full hip extension is critical for prosthetic knee stability when walking with a transfemoral prosthesis.[42] The accuracy of standard goniometric measurement of hip adduction and abduction decreases as residual limb length decreases. There is no effective way to assess rotation of the transfemoral residual limb.

Hip flexor tightness is likely to result in increased lumbar lordosis when standing and walking with a prosthesis later in the rehabilitation process. Attempts to achieve an upright

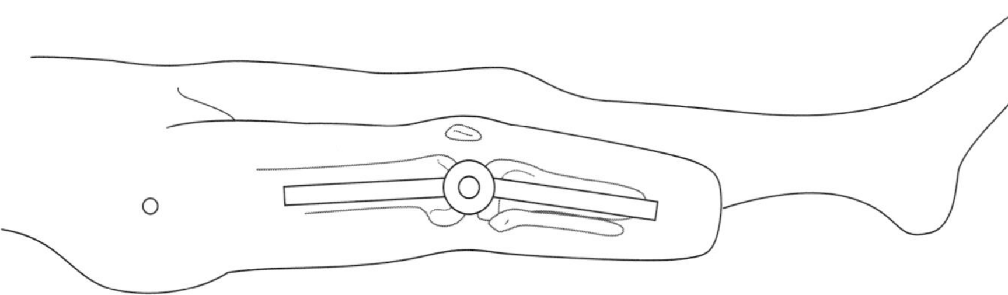

Figure 23-6
Measurement of knee extension for persons with transtibial amputation requires an understanding of the normal anatomy of the tibia to compensate for loss of the distal malleolus as a point of reference for the mobile arm of the goniometer.

posture over the prosthesis in the presence of hip flexion contracture can lead, over time, to excessive mobility of the lumbosacral spine. Individuals with bilateral transtibial amputation, as well as those who wear a transfemoral prosthesis, are much at risk for this problem: Secondary spinal dysfunction and back pain can be more disabling than the original amputation.[44] Attention to the importance of achieving near-normal joint ROM and soft tissue excursion early in the preprosthetic period has a powerful impact on effective prosthetic use over the long run.

When sitting or lying in bed, the natural tendency is for the lower limb to roll outward into a slightly flexed, abducted, and externally rotated position. Excursion of the hip is important to assess; tightness of external rotators may be masked by apparent tightness of hip flexors or abductors. The functional length of two-joint muscles is also important to consider. Adequate hamstring length is essential if the person with recent transtibial amputation is to maintain a fully extended knee when seated. If the knee is held in extension by a rigid dressing or thermoplastic splint, hamstring tightness will pull the pelvis into a marked posterior tilt. Instead of sitting squarely on the ischial tuberosities, the person with hamstring tightness sits in a kyphotic position with weight shifted onto the sacrum. This compromised postural alignment increases the risk of spinal dysfunction and of skin irritation and decubitus ulcer formation. Tightness in the rectus femoris, sartorius, and tensor fascia latae can interfere with advanced mobility skills such as the ability to kneel while transferring to and from the floor.

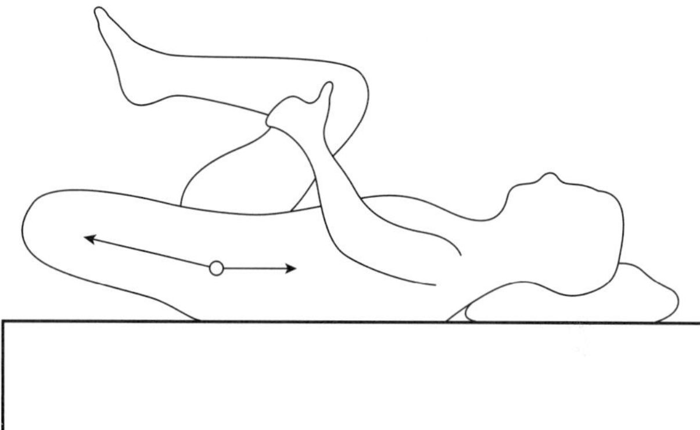

Figure 23-7
The Thomas test can be used to assess the tightness or contracture of hip flexors for patients with transtibial and transfemoral residual limbs. The patient is positioned in supine with both limbs flexed toward the chest and the pelvis in slight posterior tilt. While the opposite limb is supported in place, the residual limb is gently lowered toward the support surface. Tightness or contracture of hip flexors causes the pelvis to move into an anterior tilt before the limb is fully lowered.

Assessing Joint Integrity and Mobility

For individuals with transtibial residual limbs, the alignment and ligamentous integrity of the knee will be an important determinant of socket design, suspension strategy, and eventually the dynamic alignment of the prosthesis. Specific assessment of joint function of the residual limb is often deferred to later in the preprosthetic period when there has been primary healing of the surgical site; however, history of previous ligament injury or tear of the meniscus and concurrent degenerative joint disease or existing bony deformity (e.g., genu recurvatum, genu valgus, genu varum) should be noted during initial assessment.

The special tests used to assess knee function in those with amputation are the same as those used to assess joint integrity in individuals with musculoskeletal dysfunction in intact limbs. They include joint play, medial and lateral gap tests to assess the integrity of the collateral ligaments, anterior and posterior draw test to assess cruciate integrity, and the various tests for meniscus tear.[45,46] The techniques, however, must be adapted to the length of the residual limb; the loss of the foot means that the examiner's distal point of stability is moved upward on the limb, compromising the biomechanical advantage, as well as the accuracy, of the examiner. It may be helpful to first examine the knee of the intact limb using traditional hand placement to get a sense of the individual's baseline, then move the distal hand upward on the intact limb and repeat the examination using hand placement appropriate for the residual limb. Comparison of distal and proximal test results of the intact limb provides a frame of reference for subsequently testing the knee of the residual limb.

Assessing Muscle Performance and Motor Control

Although assessment of strength and muscle function is a key component of preprosthetic and prosthetic rehabilitation, definitive strength assessment beyond active, nonresisted antigravity motion at the joint just proximal to the amputation is usually postponed until there is adequate healing of the surgical site. Strength of key muscle groups at the next most proximal joints can be specifically assessed with standard manual muscle testing or handheld dynamometry techniques.[47] Given time constraints during initial assessment, the therapist may opt to use functional antigravity activities to screen for impairments of strength and power of the remaining limb and trunk, specifically testing strength of particular muscles if functional problems are identified.

For those with transtibial amputation, observation of active knee flexion and extension strength is used to determine if at least fair (full antigravity) strength is present until the physician determines sufficient wound healing has been accomplished. For those with transfemoral amputation, assessment of hip muscle strength beyond active antigravity fair muscle grade must also be postponed pending incisional healing.

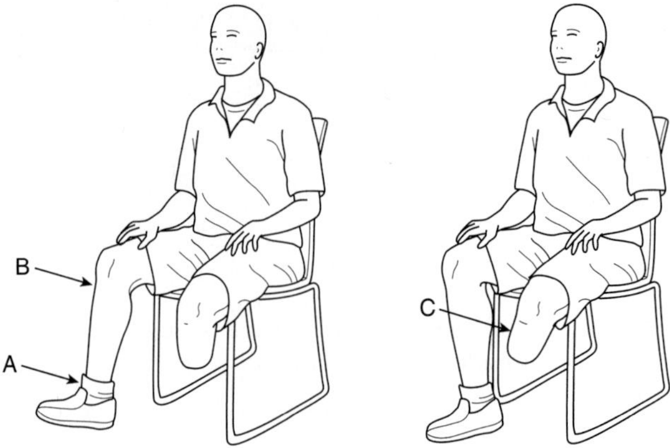

Figure 23-8
Suggested points of force application for to improve accuracy of manual muscle test (MMT) for knee extension strength in a transtibial residual limb. ***A,*** *Standard MMT position on the remaining limb.* ***B,*** *Moving the point of force application proximally on the intact limb provides a frame of reference for subsequent testing* **(C)** *of the residual limb.*

Once the surgeon and rehabilitation team are confident that enough healing has occurred so that the incision cannot be compromised by externally applied resistance, definitive strength testing can be implemented at the joint proximal to amputation. Because of the length of the residual limb, the examiner must apply the resistive force at a more proximal position on the extremity than is defined by the standard manual muscle test technique. With an altered manual contact, the mechanical advantage of the examiner is reduced and the subjective sense of strength grade may be somewhat inflated. This altered point of force application affects the validity of test results. Many therapists attempt to maximize validity by first testing the intact or remaining limb (assuming similarity of strength between the patient's limbs), using standard technique to assign a muscle grade (Figure 23-8, *A*). The intact limb is then retested with a more proximal hand placement, simulating the position for testing of the residual limb (Figure 23-8, *B*). This grade serves as a point of reference when the residual limb is then tested (Figure 23-8, *C*).

Because a healing transtibial suture line is vulnerable to resistive forces applied during strength testing and strengthening exercise, resistance to knee extension should only be applied if and when the suture line can be observed. Resistance must not be applied through a soft dressing or compressive garment during the first several weeks of the preprosthetic program. Unless healing has been delayed, most surgeons consider initiation of conservative resistive exercise a few days after sutures have been removed, perhaps as early as the seventh postoperative day for those with traumatic amputation or 12 or more days for those with dysvascular-neuropathic amputation. Surgeon preference, tissue integrity, and the individual's cardiovascular condition must be factored into strength assessment and strengthening exercise programs.

Function is influenced not only by the maximal force that the individual can generate (as examined in standard manual muscle test), but it also depends on the rate and efficiency at which the individual can generate force (power); the ability of the individual to grade and sustain an effective contraction during activity (endurance); and the ability to control muscle length in concentric (shortening), isometric (holding), and eccentric (lengthening) contractions. Observation of functional activities can identify if there are impairments of these types of muscle function. More specific testing of power can be accomplished using an isokinetic apparatus set at varying speeds or by asking the person to move at varying speeds against manual resistance.

The ability to switch between types of muscle contraction can be accomplished by providing manual resistance while asking the individual to "contract," "hold," and "let go slowly" for key muscle groups. An example of a key functional activity in which this type of control is important is the task of rising from sitting to standing and then returning to a seated position. Many persons can generate adequate force in the intact lower extremity to stand up but have difficulty controlling their descent back to sitting—"plopping" back into their seat. This is especially true for individuals who have been inactive or on prolonged bed rest.

If there is any indication of previous or current neuromuscular dysfunction, examination of tone and motor control is also important. Assessment of muscle tone includes deep tendon reflexes (DTRs), response to passive movement of limbs and trunk (hypotonicity or hypertonicity, rigidity), placement and drop tests, coordination and fine motor tests (e.g., rapid alternating movement; fine, quick tapping or clapping), as well as observation of any abnormal synergy pattern, tremors, or involuntary movement.[48,49] Qualitative assessment of the individual's ability to initiate, sustain, and terminate movement during functional activities will help the therapist identify issues of motor control that may need to be addressed as part of the plan of care.

Assessing Upper Extremity Function

Because most individuals use an ambulatory aid while on a single limb and until they are ready for prosthetic training, it is important to screen for deformity or other musculoskeletal or neuromuscular impairments involving the upper extremity. Many of those with dysvascular- and neuropathic-related lower extremity amputation have age-related degenerative joint disease that might make use of a walker or crutches challenging. Screening for functional strength and muscle endurance of muscles that stabilize the shoulder and elbow identifies individuals who would benefit from a progressive resistive exercise program targeting the upper extremity to enhance their ability to transfer, as well as ambulate.

Polyneuropathy, in a "stocking-glove" distribution, is the most common neuromuscular impairment encountered in those with diabetes who have undergone lower extremity amputation. Diabetic polyneuropathy affects all extremities and not only the sensory system but also the voluntary motor and autonomic systems.[50] For this reason, it is important to at least screen for distal upper extremity sensory loss, weakness of intrinsic muscles of the hand, and autonomic impairment during the preprosthetic period. Compromised upper extremity sensation and functional strength may affect the type of assistive device used for mobility; compression strategy for the residual limb; and, eventually, selection of a suspension strategy for the prosthesis.

Assessing Aerobic Capacity and Endurance

Determining baseline (resting) vital signs (e.g., pulse, blood pressure, respiratory rate, blood oxygen levels via pulse oximetry) is the first step in assessment of aerobic capacity and endurance. Screening for orthostatic (postural) hypotension is important for any individual who has sustained a period of inactivity and bed rest, especially if he or she is older, is on medications that blunt blood pressure response, or has a history of autonomic dysfunction from peripheral or systemic pathology. Change in vital signs during transfers or early mobility training and the time to return to resting baseline values provide information about responsiveness to exercise. Importantly, soon after surgery, anxiety about pain or risk of injury during activities may contribute to a physiological "fight or flight" response, influencing vital signs.[51] A calm and focused demeanor on the part of the therapist, as well as explanation and education about what will happen and the reason for the assessment, can help an individual with recent amputation better manage fears and concerns.

Ratings of perceived exertion and dyspnea are useful assessment strategies in the postoperative/preprosthetic period,[52,53] both to assess how the person with new amputation is tolerating increasing activity and to help the individual target an appropriate level of activity. Upper extremity ergometry may be another useful index of aerobic capacity for those who have recently lost a limb if definitive testing is indicated.[54,55]

Given the similarities in etiology and impact of peripheral vascular, cardiovascular, and cerebrovascular disease, many persons with dysvascular amputation are likely to be at risk for, or have even had, myocardial infarction (MI) or brain attack (stroke).[56] The rehabilitation team must be alert for early signs and symptoms of cardiac compromise as the person with new amputation begins transfer and single limb mobility training. Individuals who have had previous cardiac rehabilitation following MI, angioplasty, or coronary artery bypass may understand the importance of conditioning exercise as part of their preprosthetic program. Assessment of quality of motor control and tone is important if there is history of stroke.

Assessing Attention and Cognition

The tool most commonly used to assess cognitive status in the acute care setting is the Mini-Mental State Examination (MMSE)[57] (Figure 23-9). Typically, scores of 24/30 or less indicate some form of cognitive impairment; however, the MMSE does not identify the etiology or type of cognitive dysfunction.[58] In older adults the most common form of cognitive impairment is a reversible acute brain syndrome (delirium) that is associated with physiological stressors (e.g., clearing from anesthesia, psychotropic effects of narcotic pain medications, stress of hospitalization, dehydration, onset of infection).[59] Cognition and the ability to learn may also be compromised by an acute depression associated with mourning the loss of one's limb.[60] It can be more informative to track how the MMSE score changes over a period of time than to interpret a single value.

Additionally, the therapist may choose to examine more closely the ability to pay attention (distractibility), and communication and language function (both receptive and expressive), as well as level of anxiety and motivation, as each relates to the ability to problem solve and effectively master adaptive motor behaviors.

Assessing Sensory Integrity

Early in the postoperative period, screening of sensory function (vision, hearing, and somatosensation) is aimed at determining if strategies for enhancing communication may be necessary and if the individual has sufficient "data collection" mechanisms in place to monitor the surgical wound condition and health of the remaining foot and limb and to scan the environment in preparation for and during functional activities. Sensory integrity is also a factor influencing selection of prosthetic components and suspension method.

The Mini-Mental State Exam

Patient ______________________ Examiner ______________________ Date __________

Maximum	Score	
		Orientation
5	( )	What is the (year) (season) (date) (day) (month)?
5	( )	Where are we (state) (country) (town) (hospital) (floor)?
		Registration
3	( )	Name 3 objects: 1 second to say each. Then ask the patient all 3 after you have said them. Give 1 point for each correct answer. Then repeat them until he/she learns all 3. Count trials and record. Trials ________
		Attention and Calculation
5	( )	Serial 7's. 1 point for each correct answer. Stop after 5 answers. Alternatively spell "world" backward.
		Recall
3	( )	Ask for the 3 objects repeated above. Give 1 point for each correct answer.
		Language
2	( )	Name a pencil and watch.
1	( )	Repeat the following "No ifs, ands, or buts"
3	( )	Follow a 3-stage command: "Take a paper in your hand, fold it in half, and put it on the floor."
1	( )	Read and obey the following: CLOSE YOUR EYES
1	( )	Write a sentence.
1	( )	Copy the design shown.
	____	Total Score
		ASSESS level of consciousness along a continuum ______________ Alert Drowsy Stupor Coma

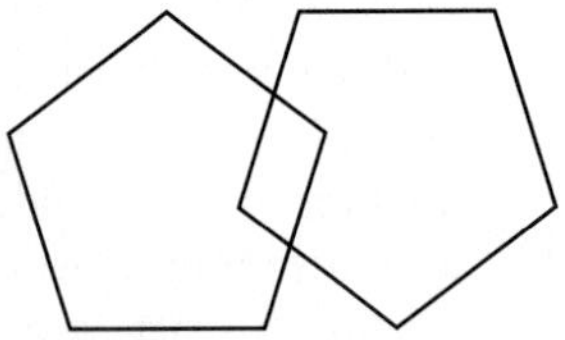

Figure 23-9

The Mini Mental State Examination. (From Folstein MF, Folstein SE, McHugh. "Mini-mental state." A practical method for grading the cognitive state of patients for the clinician. J Psychiatr Res *1975;12(3):189-198.)*

Given the age and common morbidities of those with vascular and neuropathic etiology of amputation, it is quite likely that some degree of visual impairment will be present in this group (Box 23-2).[61] Simple strategies to reduce glare, increase contrast (e.g., handgrips on walkers), and enhance acuity (e.g., large, simple, bold type on written instructions) can be used to help those with common age-related visual changes be more functional during the postoperative/preprosthetic period.[62] If the individual typically wears glasses for daily function, glasses should be worn during examination and subsequent intervention as well.

Similarly, there are cumulative age-related changes in both structure and physiology of the auditory system to be aware of (see Box 23-2) when interacting with older persons with recent amputation, especially for those with concurrent confusion due to postoperative delirium or acquired brain injury after trauma who may have impairment of attention as well. Simple strategies to enhance the ability to listen and hear include dropping the pitch of the speaking voice; speaking more slowly and projecting the voice without shouting; maintaining direct eye contact; interacting in as quiet an environment as possible; and augmenting what is said with directive gestures, simple diagrams, or brief written instruction in large print.[62] Ensuring that hearing aids are in place and functional is especially important during interviews and for patient/family education. Importantly, hearing aids typically amplify all sound; attention to volume and complexity of background noise must always be considered. Many individuals with hearing impairment, however, do not routinely use amplification.

In examining somatosensation the therapist is screening for areas of diminished sensation and areas of hypersensitivity or dysthesias on the surface of the residual limb, as well as on the remaining limb. Age- and pathology-related

Box 23-2 *Age-Related and Pathological Conditions of the Sensory Systems in Later Life*

VISUAL SYSTEM

Age-Related Changes

Diminished visual acuity
Diminished ability to accommodate between near/far visual targets
Delayed dark-light adaptation, especially sudden changes in lighting
Diminished contrast sensitivity and figure-ground discrimination
Diminished color discrimination
Diminished depth perception and visual-spatial sensitivity
Slowed pupillary light responses
Diminished corneal reflex
Diminished ability to converge eyes
Decreased ability to gaze upward/diminished upper visual field
Diminished lateral peripheral field
Increased likelihood of ptosis
Diminished efficiency of vestibular-ocular reflexes

Functional Consequences

Susceptibility to glare
Increasing need for sharp contrast (in text style and color)
Difficulty recognizing and responding to subtle changes in the visual environment
Need for gradual transition from dark-to-light environments
Need to keep directional signs at eye level
Use of bifocals/trifocals to improve visual clarity at near/far distances

Pathologies Affecting the Visual System

Cataract
Age-related maculopathy/macular degeneration
Diabetic retinopathy
Glaucoma
Homonymous hemianopsia consequent to cerebrovascular accident

AUDITORY SYSTEM

Age-Related Changes

Gradual progressive bilateral hearing loss, beginning with high frequencies
Diminished sensitivity to low-volume sounds
Increasing pure tone auditory threshold
Diminished ability to screen background noise
Diminished discernment of speech sounds
Diminished word and sentence recognition
Decreased ability to accommodate to rapid speaking rates
Distortion of sound/sensitivity to shouting and emotional cues

Functional Consequences

Less efficient listening, especially in noisy environment
Compensation by watching facial expression, movement of mouth
Need for adaptation of learning/listening environment:
- Lower tone speech
- Slower rate of speaking
- Higher volume (loudness) without shouting

Use of hearing aids (most effective is conductive hearing loss)

Pathologies Affecting the Auditory System

Buildup of cerumen in the external auditory canal
Traumatic hearing loss from exposure to excessively loud sounds
Acoustic neuroma
Vascular insufficiency in the brainstem auditory system
Cerebrovascular accident affecting auditory cortex function
Ototoxic medications

SOMATOSENSORY SYSTEM

Age-Related Changes

Decrease in number and distribution of receptors for discriminatory touch
Loss of afferent nerve fibers in peripheral nerves
Degeneration of dorsal columns (central sensory discriminatory pathway)
Increased latency for sensory stimulation (diminished conduction velocity)
Increased threshold of stimulation and decreased sensitivity
- Point localization
- Vibration (toe and ankle > UE)
- Two-point discrimination
- Cutaneous pain
- Temperature detection
- Passive movement/joint position sense (LE > UE)

Functional Consequences

Reduced ability to monitor environmental conditions
Less efficient postural responses
Increased risk of tissue damage under low-load, repetitive conditions

Pathologies Affecting Somatosensory Systems

Diabetic neuropathy
Entrapment neuropathy (e.g., carpal tunnel syndrome)
Toxic neuropathy (e.g., chronic alcoholism)
Sensory and perceptual impairment consequent to cerebrovascular accident

LE, Lower extremity; *UE*, upper extremity.

changes in sensation are summarized in Box 23-2. For those with neuropathic-dysvascular disease, it is especially important to ascertain if there is adequate protective sensation (ability to consistently perceive the 5.07 Semmes-Weinstein filament) on weight-bearing surfaces of the intact limb, which will be subject to repeated loading during single limb ambulation.[63] Standard sensory testing protocols for light touch, point and generalized pressure (am I touching you? yes/no), the ability to localize (where am I touching you?), and temperature discrimination (hot/cold) are employed and often documented on a body chart.[64] This information will be used to guide patient-family education about skin inspection and wound care, as well as decisions about appropriate socket-limb interface for prosthetic prescription. Screening for proprioceptive and kinesthetic awareness at intact joints provides information that will be useful when designing interventions for postural control and, eventually, prosthetic gait training.

Sensory testing requires that the individual be able to concentrate and focus in order to respond when a stimulus is presented. The reliability of sensory testing is diminished in individuals with confusion or delirium or if the examiner uses a consistent (predictable) pattern or rhythm during testing.[65] To minimize the likelihood of "lucky guesses" in those with suspected sensory impairment, it may be helpful to test specific sites multiple times, in random order and uneven timing, documenting the number of accurate responses versus number of times stimulated (e.g., 0/3 1/3, 2/3, or 3/3) at each testing site.

Noting how the individual with new amputation perceives the residual limb is also important; is he or she willing to look at it, watch it during dressing changes, touch it, or freely move it? One challenge in the preprosthetic period is to assist the incorporation of this "different" limb in the person's body image and self-perception.[66] Some individuals with dysvascular-neuropathic disease continue to perceive their limb as fragile and needing protection. Those with traumatic amputation may become emotionally distressed when confronted with the real evidence of their loss. These situations may interfere with readiness to wear and use a prosthesis effectively. Awareness of the person's emotional response to his or her altered body guides the therapist in patient education and intervention activities aimed to accomplish adaptation of body image necessary for effective prosthetic use.

Assessing Locomotion and Balance

One of the most functionally important aspects of preoperative assessment is determination of the person with new amputation's *usual* (previous) and *current* (postoperative) ambulatory status. The therapist is interested in the individual's familiarity with the use of assistive devices (e.g., walker, crutches, canes), need for assistance to assume standing and while walking, typical distances walked before surgery, the overall effort (energy cost) of walking, the frequency of walking, any other factors or comorbidities that limit walking, and the type of walking environment that the person is most likely to encounter after discharge from acute care (e.g., level inside, uneven outside, stairs and ramps). Self-reports and direct observation of walking provide this information. Preamputation ambulatory status is a strong predictor of functional postoperative prosthetic use.[67,68]

At this point in rehabilitation the quality and preciseness of the gait pattern are less important than the safety and functionality of walking. Detailed observational gait analysis is typically deferred until training with the prosthesis begins. Quantitative kinematics (e.g., cadence, gait speed, step or stride length) and ratings of perceived exertion can be used to establish a baseline early in the postoperative period, as a benchmark for progression and readiness for discharge. Individuals with new amputation must be able to use a step-to or swing-through gait pattern with the type of walker or crutches that provides adequate stability and energy efficiency with the least activity restriction.[4] In acute care settings, initial examination and training of gait is likely to focus on level, predictable surfaces in a relatively closed environment.

The ability to manage on a variety of surfaces in active and open environments is examined as care progresses; discharge from acute care approaches; and preprosthetic rehabilitation continues at home, in subacute settings, or on an outpatient basis.[4] Familiarity with and effectiveness of propulsion and maneuverability of a wheelchair are likely to be important in the preprosthetic period for both the individual and family caregivers.

Determining the effectiveness of the individual's postural control is also important. This includes *stability* in quiet sitting and standing; *anticipatory* postural adjustments in reaching, transitions from sitting to standing, and during locomotion; and *reactionary* postural adjustments when there is unexpected perturbation or unpredictable environmental conditions (e.g., a wet area on the floor, an area rug that may shift when stepped on). Although testing protocols such as functional reach, Tinetti Performance Oriented Mobility Assessment, and measures of balance confidence are used clinically for persons with recent amputation, the reliability, validity, and norms for safe or impaired performance are not well documented in the research literature.[69-71] Subjective assessment of postural control (poor, fair, good, excellent) is somewhat influenced by the therapist's level of experience and comfort with allowing an individual to move toward his or her limits of stability.[72] Providing an opportunity for the individual to practice moving from sitting to standing and ambulation with an appropriate assistive device allows the therapist to identify potential problems with balance and postural control. This also helps the individual anticipate what mobility will be like while the residual limb heals and while awaiting the prosthesis.

With the loss of some or all of a lower extremity, the body's center of mass (COM) in standing and in sitting shifts slightly upward and toward the remaining limb; the degree of shift increases as residual limb length decreases.[73] These alterations in COM may require adaptation of strategies used before surgery for postural control; most persons with recent amputation can effectively adapt their postural control mechanisms by practicing activities that require them to anticipate or respond to postural demands.

Assessing Posture, Ergonomics, and Body Mechanics

In the assessment of symmetry of alignment in sitting and standing, it is important to differentiate habitual or preferred postures from fixed postures, malalignments, and deformities.[74] This might be accomplished by noting whether a particular postural orientation is maintained during different functional activities, as well as whether the individual with new amputation can change position or alignment when so directed. Quantitative measures to document abnormalities in posture and alignment include comparison with vertical and horizontal using plumb line and grids, goniometry and angle assessment, and passive movement.

Given the typical age group of persons with dysvascular-neuropathic etiology of amputation, there may be kyphosis associated with osteoporosis, especially if there is history of pathological compression fractures of the spine.[75] Assessing the health and function of the lumbar spine in standing and during reaching and lifting activity (including excursion of hamstrings and flexibility of hip flexors and adductors) is important because of the likelihood of developing low back pain with the use of a prosthesis if there is contracture. This is especially true for individuals with a transfemoral or any bilateral amputation level. Considering back health early in the preprosthetic program is a health promotion/wellness activity that is a worthwhile investment in time and effort.

Assessing Self-care and Environmental Barriers

The individual's ability to transfer to and from the toilet, in and out of the shower or bathtub, and in and out of a car, bus, or subway; to manage stairs and escalators; and to get up from the floor (in case of a fall) are examined as the preprosthetic period advances. This is part of the assessment of readiness to return to the home environment. The rehabilitation team must consider the individual's ability to dress, perform self-care and grooming activities, inspect his or her residual and remaining limbs, and function in typical food preparation roles and other instrumental activities of daily living (ADLs).

The team assesses the family caregiver's ability to provide appropriate and effective assistance at home if the individual needs help or guarding during functional activities. Discussion about what work and leisure activities are important for the individual to resume once home will guide selection of appropriate adaptive equipment and adaptive movement strategies necessary to carry out important tasks and roles before receiving the prosthesis. Instruments such as the Functional Independence Measure (FIM) are used in the acute care setting to document the level of assistance that the person with new amputation requires during functional activities.[76] Because of ceiling effects inherent in the scoring system, FIM scores may not be particularly useful as indicators of improvement once an individual has reached relative modified or full independence, especially on the locomotion and mobility subscales.

CASE EXAMPLE 1A

An 89-Year-Old Facing "Elective" Transtibial Amputation for Severe Arterial Occlusive Disease of Her Right Foot

N. H. is a slight but energetic woman who is referred to your interdisciplinary team for preoperative examination and education about the rehabilitation program she will be involved in after her planned transtibial amputation. She stands 5′2″ tall with slight kyphosis and weighs 101 lb. She rises to standing by scooting to the edge of her wheelchair (used for community mobility), then rocking back and forth several times to build momentum. She tells you that she spends her days reading the *New York Times,* writing to grandchildren and the few long-term friends still alive, cooking (with help to assemble ingredients and take things in and out of the oven), and talking to other "shut ins" from her church on the phone. N. H. lives in the home of her youngest son, a 67-year-old who has recently undergone quadruple coronary artery bypass grafting and is recovering from an embolic stroke that left him with mild left hemiparesis. Grandchildren and great-grandchildren visit fairly often. According to her chart, N. H. has hypertension controlled by β-blockers, had a mild MI 15 years ago, has never smoked cigarettes, and enjoys a glass of wine with her evening meal. She had lens implants for cataracts bilaterally but still wears glasses to read. Over the past year, claudication has become an increasing problem, making it difficult for her to walk from her bedroom at one end of the ranch-style home to the kitchen and family room at the other. When presented with the choice of revascularization versus amputation, she decided that, in the long run, she would rather take her chances with amputation surgery with spinal anesthesia than bypass graft with general anesthesia. She expresses concern that she is "very out of shape" because her walking has been so limited by ischemic pain. She has a good friend whose husband used a transtibial prosthesis for many years after losing his foot in a lawn mower accident; this has assured her that a prosthesis will allow her adequate mobility and function once she heals after surgery. She tells you she has come through many difficult times during her long life, and although sad at the prospect of losing her leg, she looks forward to being free of claudication pain and anticipates she will muster the determination necessary to get back on her feet.

Questions to Consider

- What additional data might you want to gather from the medical record to build your understanding of her current condition and medical prognosis?
- What are the most important questions to ask during your interview with N. H. and her son as you begin to formulate her PT diagnosis and plan of care?
- Given her age and general health status, what additional review of physiological systems would be important to carry out before surgery? Why have you chosen these systems? How might they affect her ability to participate in rehabilitation?
- What specific tests and measures, at an impairment level, will be important to do during your physical examination? How long do you think the assessment might take? How might you prioritize if your time with N. H. is limited? How reliable are the strategies that you have chosen? How precise does the information you are collecting at this preoperative visit need to be?
- What functional activities would you choose to assess before her surgery? What tests and measures will you use to document her functional status?
- What information would be important for you to share with N. H. and her son about the first few days after her surgery? Before discharge from acute care? During the preprosthetic period until she is ready to be casted for her initial prosthesis?
- Given the limited information currently available to you, what impression or expectations do you have about her postoperative care? How might this be different if she had a medical diagnosis of type 2 diabetes?

CASE EXAMPLE 2A

A 25-Year-Old with Bilateral Traumatic Transtibial Amputations Sustained in a Construction Accident

P. G. is a construction worker who was pinned between the fenders of two vans when the driver of one van put the vehicle in reverse as P. G. was walking between them. He sustained severely comminuted and open fractures of the mid tibia and fibula and significant damage to soft tissue and neurovascular structures. Tourniquets were placed on his limbs by emergency medical technicians responding to the 911 call. In the emergency department trauma surgeons determined that neither of P. G.'s limbs met criteria for limb salvage. Because the limbs were contaminated by dirt and debris from the job site, the surgeon performed bilateral open transtibial amputations to allow for frequent wound inspection. P. G. was placed on intravenous antibiotics. Three days after the operation, there is no sign of infection in either limb. Revision and closure of his residual limbs is scheduled for tomorrow, using a fishmouth closure, leaving approximately 5 inches of residual tibia in length. Adjustable polypropylene, removable, semirigid dressings are planned for compression and protection of the wound postoperatively.

Review of the medical record indicates that P. G. was in generally good health before his injury, although he has been a pack-per-day smoker since the beginning of high school. He was 6′4″ tall, weighing 210 lb before his injury. His only previous hospitalization was at age 17, for open-reduction, internal fixation of a mid-shaft right femoral fracture sustained in a motorcycle accident. P. G. has been married for slightly more than 1 year, and his wife is seven months' pregnant. They live on the 3rd floor of a three-family home in the ethnic city neighborhood in which they grew up. Extended family members have kept vigil at the hospital since the accident to support P. G. and his wife. When not working, P. G. is an avid motorcycle and quad rider, competing locally in both speed and distance events. He also participates in an intracity adult basketball league.

Pain management has been via a morphine pump; even with this, P. G. reports typical pain levels of 5 to 6 out of 10, increasing in severity during dressing changes. When you come to discuss his postoperative rehabilitation with him, he is in a semireclined position in bed, with both lower limbs abducted and externally rotated at the hip, resting in apparent 20 degrees of knee flexion. He is anxious and quite angry over the situation, stating that he "can't believe this has happened" and "doesn't want to end up in a wheelchair" unable to work. The only experience he has with persons with amputation is an uncle with poorly controlled diabetes who had successive amputations of multiple toes due to vascular insufficiency, subsequently revised to transmetatarsal because of osteomyelitis of a neuropathic wound, and then to transtibial because of delayed healing. P. G.'s uncle's rehabilitation was complicated by a significant stroke a week after transtibial amputation, and although he wears a prosthesis, his mobility limitations keep him homebound.

Questions to Consider

- What additional data might you want to gather from the medical record to build your understanding of P. G.'s current condition and medical prognosis?
- What are the most important questions to ask during your interview with P. G. and his family as you begin to formulate his PT diagnosis and plan of care?
- What additional review of physiological systems would be important to carry out before surgery? Why have you chosen these systems? How might they affect his ability to participate in rehabilitation?
- What specific tests and measures, at an impairment level, will be important to do during your physical examination? How long do you think the assessment

might take? How might you prioritize if your time with P. G. is limited? How reliable are the strategies that you have chosen? How precise does the information you are collecting at this preoperative visit need to be?

- What functional activities would you choose to assess before his surgery? What tests and measures will you use to document his functional status?
- What information would be important for you to share with P. G. and his family about the first few days after the next surgery? Before discharge from acute care? During the preprosthetic period until he is ready to be casted for his initial prostheses?
- Given the limited information currently available to you, what impression or expectations do you have about his postoperative care? How might P. G.'s care be similar to or different from that of his uncle and the older woman in the previous case?

THE PROCESS OF EVALUATION, DIAGNOSIS, AND PROGNOSIS

Understanding an individual's rehabilitation needs emerges as baseline data are collected and integrated with health professionals' clinical expertise and judgment, as well as evidence from the clinical research literature. As part of the evaluative process, the team weighs factors that are likely to influence the rehabilitation program and begins to formulate a plan of care to address the individual's specific needs. The team identifies key problems that will need to be addressed, formulates a PT (rehabilitation) movement dysfunction diagnosis, estimates the level of function that will likely be reached and the time and intensity of intervention necessary to reach it, specifies measurable goals that will be used to judge progression over time, and prioritizes interventions to be carried out as part of the rehabilitation program. Readers are referred to the *Guide to Physical Therapist Practice* patterns for a typical and comprehensive overview of the complete patient-client management process (Box 23-3).[77]

Box 23-3 *Guide to Physical Therapist Practice Patterns Relevant for Individuals with Amputation*

MUSCULOSKELETAL SYSTEM

Impaired motor function, muscle performance, range of motion, gait, locomotion, and balance associated with amputation

NEUROMUSCULAR SYSTEM

Impaired motor function and sensory integrity associated with acute or chronic polyneuropathies

CARDIOVASCULAR/CARDIOPULMONARY SYSTEM

Primary prevention/risk reduction for cardiovascular/pulmonary disorders or

Impaired aerobic capacity/endurance associated with deconditioning

INTEGUMENTARY SYSTEM

Primary prevention/risk reduction for integumentary disorders

Impaired integumentary integrity associated with skin involvement extending into fascia, muscle, or bone and scar formation

Physical Therapy Diagnosis

The PT diagnosis reflects the limitations in function and mobility that the person with recent amputation encounters as a consequence of their particular constellation of impairments and active pathologies. The PT diagnosis differs from the medical diagnosis in that it focuses on the functional consequences of a condition at the level of the system and, more importantly, at the level of the whole person.[7]

The disablement model provides a framework with which to build a PT diagnosis.[78,79] For students and new therapists, it may be helpful to complete an organizational table on the basis of the disablement model that lists all relevant descriptors of active pathology, impairment, functional limitation, and disability on a single page (Table 23-2). The entries in each column in the table can be prioritized, with notations about which issues are likely to improve or change and which will require adaptive equipment or alternative strategies. The statement of PT diagnosis for the particular individual begins with a prioritized list of functional limitations or disabilities to be addressed during the episode of care, followed by the impairments contributing to limitations that are related to or result from the individual's constellation of active pathologies and comorbidities. Formulating the PT diagnosis in this way clearly guides establishment of goals and appropriate interventions.

Plan of Care: Prognosis

Forecasting the potential for prosthetic replacement and rehabilitation can be challenging. Decisions must be informed by several factors:

1. The overall health, cognitive, and preamputation functional status of the individual
2. The level of amputation as it affects prosthetic control and the energy cost of walking
3. The likely contribution of prosthetic use to perform basic and instrumental ADLs, for the individual or for the caregivers who will be assisting and managing daily function
4. The resources (financial and instrumental) available to the individual during the entire rehabilitation process

Table 23-2
Example of a "Disablement Grid," Completed Postoperatively, for Case Example 1A: N. H., an 89-Year-Old with Elective Transtibial Amputation Secondary to Severe Peripheral Arterial Disease

Active Pathologies, Comorbidities, Surgeries, and Medications	*Impairments (problems at the level of the physiological system)*	*Functional Limitations (problems at the level of the individual)*	*Disabilities (problems that the individual has fulfilling social roles)*	*Buffers and Confounding Factors*
Peripheral arterial disease R transtibial amputation • posterior flap (7/15/05) • removable rigid dressing • 2″ square ecchymosis lateral suture line • moderate amount of serosanguineous drainage at mid suture line • postoperative pain (morphine pump) Possible osteoporosis Possible sarcopenia Hypertension (β-blockers) s/p MI (1990) Cataract (lens implants 6/12/02) Recent fall in hospital bathroom (7/17/05) Mild postoperative delirium with sundown syndrome Stress incontinence	Postoperative pain (4/10 VAS) Phantom sensation (cramping) Potential for delayed healing due to injury to surgical site sustained in fall Postoperative edema Limited excursion R knee flexion and hip extension ROM Less than F muscle strength R knee extension, hip abduction, hip extension Diminished functional core and UE muscle strength Limited muscular endurance Limited cardiovascular endurance Limited short-term memory and distractibility (MMSE preop 28/30, postop 18/30) Hypersensitivity to touch and pressure bordering suture line Inadequate protective sensation L forefoot postural control in single limb support (static)	Difficulty with transitions • effortful but functional rolling side to side • minimal assistance to shift upward in bed (difficulty sustaining "bridge" position) • minimal assistance supine to/from sitting with directional cueing • moderate assistance sit to stand, with directional cueing • maximal assistance stand to sit with poor eccentric control UE and LLE Inability to ambulate functionally, moderate assist of 1, hop-to pattern in parallel bars, requires consistent cueing Step length 6 inches, perceived exertion 7/10, distance 10 ft. Diminished exercise and activity tolerance Difficulty with toileting, dressing, and other self-care activities Quickly becomes frustrated and agitated when encounters difficulty with mobility and self-care tasks	Inability to function in typical premorbid roles in interactions with family at home Inability to function in premorbid roles in interactions with members of her communities (church, friends, extended family)	Significant emotional and instrumental support available by a number of family caregivers Knowledge of successful prosthetic use by friend Active and engaged in community (church) Previous use of walker and wheelchair Previous participation in cardiac rehabilitation Lives in 1-story home, with ramp at entry Determined to eventually return to own home LLE claudication may limit activity

Table 23-2—cont'd

Example of a "Disablement Grid," Completed Postoperatively, for Case Example 1: N. H., an 89-Year-Old with Elective Transtibial Amputation Secondary to Severe Peripheral Arterial Disease

Active Pathologies, Comorbidities, Surgeries, and Medications	*Impairments (problems at the level of the physiological system)*	*Functional Limitations (problems at the level of the individual)*	*Disabilities (problems that the individual has fulfilling social roles)*	*Buffers and Confounding Factors*
	and dynamic) Diminished visual acuity and upward gaze; difficulty tracking fast motion	Possible difficulty with carryover of new learning from session to session Difficulty self-monitoring status of residual limb and remaining limb		

Physical Therapy Diagnosis:
N. H. is unable to independently function in mobility and transfers, ambulation, and self-care activities secondary to transient cognitive impairment, pain, impaired muscle strength and motor control, diminished endurance, limited range of motion at key LE joints, impaired postural control and visual impairment related to recent transtibial amputation, postoperative delirium, and various comorbidities.
L, left; *LE*, lower extremity; *LLE*, lower left extremity; *MMSE*, Mini-Mental Status Examination; *R*, right; *UE*, upper extremity; *VAS*, visual analog scale.

Premorbid level of mobility, ADL status, and level of amputation contribute more to an accurate projection of rehabilitation potential and prosthetic use after amputation than any single factor or combination of comorbid health factors.[80] A long list of past or chronic illnesses does not predict poor rehabilitation potential: Many individuals can manage multiple chronic conditions effectively and become highly functional prosthetic users. Most individuals with new amputation can return to their presurgical activities with only slight adaptation of movement and mobility strategies.[17,81] Long-term outcome is more difficult to forecast: The relatively high morbidity and mortality for patients with amputation secondary to vascular disease have been well documented.[82-84] Unless there is clear evidence that ambulation will not be possible and that provision of prosthesis will not improve the patient's mobility (e.g., reducing the amount of assistance that is necessary to transfer), prosthetic replacement should and must be considered.[5]

A key component of prognosis is delineation of the frequency, intensity, and duration of the episode of care. In the acute care setting, hospitalization for an uncomplicated amputation may be 4 to 7 days and PT may occur for 30 to 45 minutes, once or twice daily. For individuals with amputation as a result of trauma affecting multiple systems, the period of hospitalization depends on the severity of damage across all systems, so that duration of care may be longer. In subacute settings, for those on Medicare, the rehabilitation stay may be for a month or more and care is much more intense, with PT typically occurring twice daily with an hour of more of PT and occupational therapy planned each day. Care provided at home and in outpatient settings may be somewhat less intense, occurring three times a week for an hour or more, but is certainly supplemented by an active home program.

Plan of Care: Determining Appropriate Goals

Goals to be achieved during a particular episode of care are influenced by the setting in which care is provided. Although the overall goal of the preprosthetic period is to prepare the individual for prosthetic fitting and training, the specific goals of the acute care setting may be to achieve primary wound closure, initiate an effective strategy for compression, and achieve supervision or minimal assist in transfers and in locomotion using a wheelchair or ambulatory device on level surfaces during the days or week that the person is hospitalized. In subsequent subacute, home care, and outpatient settings, goals expand to include strengthening of core and key muscle groups; ensuring adequate range of motion for prosthetic use; improving cardiovascular fitness; and achieving more advanced ADLs, IADLs, and mobility skills over a longer period of intervention.[85] An effective goal is directly linked to the impairments and functional limitation identified in the PT diagnosis and is stated in measurable terms so that progression can be assessed as postoperative and preprosthetic care continues (Box 23-4).

Box 23-4 *Acute Care Goals for Case Example 1A*

N. H. is an 89-year-old woman with recent transtibial amputation secondary to peripheral arterial disease. By the conclusion of this episode of care (projected 4 to 5 days), N. H. will be able to do the following:

- Actively participate in inspection of her surgical wound during dressing changes and of her remaining limb.
- Describe and recognize signs of inflammation, dehiscence, ecchymosis, and infection along her incision site and of inflammation or developing neuropathic or vascular ulceration of her remaining extremity.
- Direct caregivers in the proper application of her compressive dressing and removal of her rigid dressing.
- Safely perform rolling and bridging activities, without assistance, for effective bed mobility with perceived exertion of no more than 3/10.
- Demonstrate active contraction into full-knee extension in supine and seated positions.
- Demonstrate understanding of proper stretching and flexibility for knee extension and hip extension in multiple functional positions.
- Safely rise and return from sitting to standing position from a standard arm chair or wheelchair with minimal assistance and occasional verbal cues, with perceived exertion of 4/10.
- Ambulate with contact guard and occasional cues, using a hop-to pattern using a standard walker for 25 feet, with a perceived exertion of 4/10.
- Direct caregivers in assisting her with toilet transfers and clothing management during toileting and other self-care activities

CASE EXAMPLE 2B

Determining a Physical Therapy Diagnosis for P. G. following Revision of Bilateral Transtibial Amputations

You have collected the following information in your chart review, interview, and brief initial examination:

- Surgery: Underwent revision and closure of bilateral open amputation 2 days ago (under general anesthesia) with fishmouth closures; 5.25 inch residual tibia on left, 4.75 inch residual tibia on right. Placed in bulky dressing and Ace wrap for compression, then into bilateral adjustable prefabricated semirigid dressings to hold knees in full extension and protect surgical construct. Moderate serosanguineous drainage noted at first dressing change. Wound edges slightly inflamed consistent with operative trauma. No dehiscence noted. Proximal circumference at joint line 10.25 inches bilaterally, distal circumference (4 inches below) of right residual limb 11.25 inches and of left residual limb 11 inches.
- Postoperative health: Elevated temperature postoperatively, with diminished breath sounds in posterior bases of lungs bilaterally. Radiograph suggests early pneumonia. Cough nonproductive.
- Cognition/affect: Signs of agitation and distress in recovery room, being mildly sedated for combination of pain relief and calming. Currently lethargic and somewhat distractible, requiring consistent cueing to stay on task during examination.
- Pain/phantom sensation: Reports postoperative pain at 7/10 level. Complains of shooting pains in phantom RLE and is distressed by "itchy" toes on phantom LLE. Currently IV narcotics q 3 hours for pain management.
- ROM/muscle length: Reports "pulling" behind knees when head of bed elevated into long sitting position. Requests time out of semirigid dressing to allow knee flexion and be more comfortable.
- Muscle performance/motor control: Able to actively extend both knees to −10 degrees from full extension, stops because of "pulling" behind knee.
- Upper extremity function and transfers: Able to "push up" to lift body weight when assisted to bedside chair recliner in contact guard/minimal assist sliding board transfer.
- Aerobic capacity/endurance: Reports transfer effort 6/10 on perceived exertion scale. Reports dyspnea 5/10 immediately following transfer.
- Rolls independently: Able to come to sitting from sidelying with minimal assistance.
- Postural control: Maintained static sitting balance on edge of bed 2 minutes. Able to reach forward 7 inches, sideward > 10 inches bilaterally, reluctant to turn and reach behind due to discomfort. Effective postural responses to mild perturbations forward and backward, moderate perturbations sideways.

Questions to Consider

- List all of the active pathologies and comorbidities that will influence P. G.'s postoperative/preprosthetic care.
- List and prioritize the impairments, across physiological systems and from a psychological perspective, that should be directly addressed or considered in his rehabilitation plan of care.
- List and prioritize the functional limitations that will be addressed during his acute care stay. Suggest additional functional limitations that will be addressed as his rehabilitation progresses at home or at a subacute or rehabilitation facility.
- List and prioritize disabilities that P. G. is likely to be concerned about and that the rehabilitation team will be attempting to minimize over the course of his care.

- Develop a definitive PT diagnosis for P. G. on the basis of the disablement model.
- Develop a rehabilitation prognosis for P. G. and explain or justify your expectations.
- Develop a list of prioritized goals for P. G. for the next 2 weeks in the acute care hospital. Expand these goals as if care would continue after discharge in a rehabilitation center, at home, or on an outpatient basis. What will frequency, duration, and intensity of his rehabilitation sessions be? How will you judge if he is making progress toward achieving these goals?

INTERVENTIONS FOR PERSONS WITH RECENT AMPUTATION

After amputation surgery the focus shifts to preparation for prosthetic use. Strategies for control of edema, pain management, and facilitation of wound healing are implemented. The person with a new amputation and his or her caregivers receive instruction and the opportunity to practice single limb mobility with an appropriate assistive device. Handling of the residual limb during dressing changes and skin inspection, as well as the consistent use of compression devices, helps to desensitize the residual limb, enhancing readiness for prosthetic use. Exercises to strengthen key muscle groups in the residual and remaining limb and to assist effective postural responses are implemented to assist function and prepare for prosthetic gait. Functional training in self-care and transfers begins in the acute care setting and is followed up in home care, subacute, or outpatient settings. The therapist may employ a combination of manual therapy, therapeutic exercise, facilitation techniques, physical agents, and mechanical or electrotherapeutic modalities to help manage pain, assist healing, minimize risk of soft tissue contracture, and enhance mobility. A rigid dressing or temporary socket may be fabricated or adapted to protect the residual limb while it heals.

Postoperative Pain Management

In addition to reducing acute discomfort, effective postoperative pain management is important for several other reasons. Pain is a significant physiological stressor that affects homeostasis, as well as the patient's ability to concentrate and learn.[51,59] In the early postoperative period persons with recent amputation are faced with learning how to care for their new residual limb including monitoring for signs of infection, using strategies to control edema, and appropriate positioning to minimize the risk of contracture formation. They must also learn a variety of new motor skills including exercises to preserve strength and ROM and how to protect their healing suture while moving around with crutches or a walker on their remaining limb. If postoperative discomfort and pain are kept to a minimum, they can better learn and retain these new cognitive and motor skills.

Pain can also be fatiguing and demoralizing; those with significant pain may be reluctant to participate fully in active rehabilitation programs because they fear that movement will only increase their pain. Individuals with significant pain may be erroneously labeled as unmotivated or uncooperative, when their primary goal is to find a way to escape their discomfort. Importantly, although certain types of pain medications (opioid and narcotic analgesics) are effective in providing relief, they may compromise cognitive function or increase the risk of postural hypotension.[86] Therapists must be aware of the actions and side effects of the pain medication being used.

In the days immediately after amputation the goal is to minimize the severity of acute postoperative pain. Because prevention is more effective than reduction of significant pain, those with recent amputations are encouraged to request pain medication before pain becomes severe.[24] Preoperative and intraoperative pain management also affects postoperative pain: In patients undergoing amputation due to vascular insufficiency who receive epidural analgesia before surgery, problematic phantom limb pain after amputation may be less likely to develop.[87] Effective management of postoperative edema is an important element in the control of postoperative pain as well.

Dealing with Phantom Limb Sensation and Phantom Pain

A variety of interventions have been used for individuals with significant phantom limb sensation or pain, although management of phantom pain is often challenging and frustrating for all involved.[88] Nonnarcotic and narcotic pain medications alone are typically ineffective in the presence of phantom pain.[4] Medications that are used to prevent seizure, as well as certain antidepressants prescribed alone or in conjunction with low-dose narcotic agents, may be helpful in some cases. When a clear locus or trigger point is present, some persons receive temporary relief after local injection of a steroid or analgesic. Continuous analgesic infusion to create a nerve sheath or interneural block has been used to control the severity of phantom limb pain in the immediate postoperative period: The success of this intervention varies with pharmacological agents and the rate of their administration.[89-91] Noninvasive alternatives such as relaxation techniques, hypnosis, or therapeutic touch may be effective for certain patients as well.[92]

Physical Therapy Management of Postoperative Pain

The success of early rehabilitation is influenced by the effectiveness of postoperative pain management; for this reason, physical therapists must be aware of medications being used and be involved in assessing the effectiveness of the pain management strategy and its impact on patient learning and function.[93] When epidural anesthesia has been used during

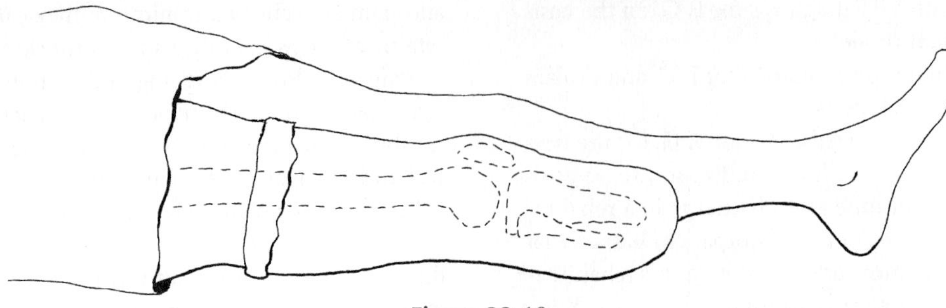

Figure 23-10

A plaster or fiberglass cast, applied immediately after amputation in the operating room, is an effective method of edema control, protection of the residual limb, and prevention of knee flexion contracture.

surgery or in the immediate postoperative period, it is imperative that the patient's cognitive, sensory, and motor function is carefully evaluated before transfer training and single limb mobility activities are begun. In whatever setting PT care is provided, it is important that administration of medications be timed so that pain control is optimal during physical therapy activities. If the patient is experiencing phantom sensation or pain, the physical therapist plays an important role in educating the patient and family about these sensations and often incorporates imagery and relaxation methods into the treatment program.

Transcutaneous electrical nerve stimulation can be an effective adjunct modality for patients with acute surgical pain and may also play a role in the management of troubling phantom sensation or pain in the immediate postoperative period.[94] Some evidence indicates that transcutaneous electrical nerve stimulation may contribute to wound healing after amputation, reducing the need for revision or reamputation, in addition to reducing the severity of postoperative phantom pain.[95] Physical therapists have also used acupressure, ultrasound, application of cold or ice, and a variety of massage techniques to assist pain management, with varying degrees of success.[93,96,97] Careful attention to the healing status of the wound is imperative: Wound closure must not be compromised by any intervention that is aimed at reducing discomfort or pain.

Limb Volume, Shaping, and Postoperative Edema

The management of postoperative edema is important for four reasons: Edema control strategies are important components of pain control, enhance wound healing, protect the incision during functional activity, and assist preparation for prosthetic replacement by shaping and desensitizing the residual limb.[3] A variety of postsurgical dressing and edema control strategies are available. These include soft dressings with or without Ace wrap compression, semirigid dressings, various removable rigid dressings (RRDs) applied over soft dressings, or the application of a rigid cast dressing in the operating room.[9] An immediate or early postoperative prosthesis (IPOP or EPOP) is a rigid dressing with an attachment for a pylon and prosthetic foot.[99] Each option contributes to pain control, wound healing and protection, and preparation for prosthetic use in a significantly different way. The choice of strategy is determined by the etiology and level of amputation, the condition of the skin, the medical and functional status of the patient, access to prosthetic consultation and care, the preference and experience of the surgeon, and established institutional protocol.

Rigid Dressings and Immediate Postoperative Prostheses

Many persons with elective transtibial amputation are placed in a cylindrical plaster or fiberglass cast immediately after amputation while in the operating room (Figure 23-10).[100,101] A simple postoperative cast, used as a rigid dressing, is applied in much the same way as a cast that is used to immobilize a fracture of the proximal tibia or distal femur. If the cast is to be used as an IPOP, a prosthetist often joins the surgical team in the operating room during cast application to incorporate the features of a patellar tendon–bearing socket and an attachment for a pylon into the cast (Figure 23-11).

Several steps are necessary in the application of a rigid postoperative dressing.[102] First, a surgical dressing is applied over the suture line and one or more layers of cotton stockinet or lightly compressive Lycra spandex are pulled over the limb to the upper thigh. Next, a layer of protective padding is applied, with particular attention to protection of the skin over the bony prominences. If the cast will be the socket for an IPOP, several felt or gel pads are positioned on the limb to direct and distribute weight-bearing forces more effectively onto pressure-tolerant areas including the medial tibial flare, the anterior muscle compartment, and the patellar tendon. The residual limb is then supported with the knee extended, and several layers of elastic or nonelastic plaster of Paris or fiberglass casting material are applied. The proximal edges of the cast are finished at the upper thigh (2 to 4 inches below perineum) level. Modifications of the cast (as it is setting) are used to aid suspension or, for an IPOP, to ensure that weight-bearing forces are directed to pressure-tolerant areas. Pressure applied to the outside of the cast just above the femoral condyles captures normal femoral anatomy to

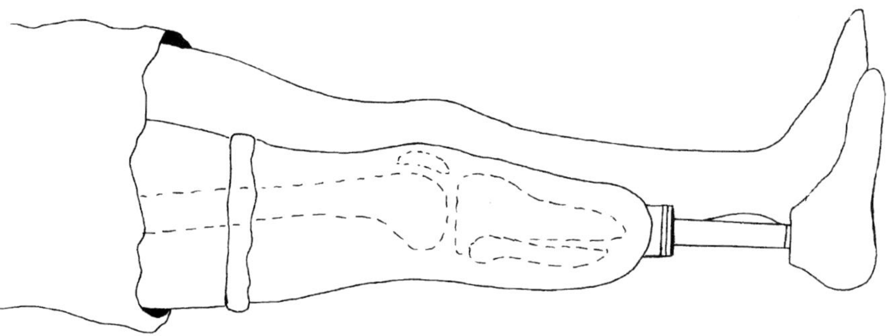

Figure 23-11
Incorporation of a pylon and features of a patellar tendon–bearing socket in an immediate postoperative prosthesis (IPOP) can facilitate early mobility in selected patients.

create supracondylar suspension. For an IPOP the prosthetist incorporates a patellar tendon bar, a broad "shelf" for the medial tibial flare, and a stabilizing popliteal bulge by applying manual pressure to these areas as the cast begins to set. He or she also incorporates a point of attachment and alignment into the distal cast for subsequent attachment of a pylon and prosthetic foot. Finally, the prosthetist or surgeon can incorporate a suspension attachment, which will connect to a waist belt, into the proximal anterior surface of the cast. Recently, bivalved custom and prefabricated removable immediate postoperative prostheses have begun to be used as alternatives to plaster casts (Figure 23-12).[103,104]

A rigid dressing or IPOP is left in place for 2 or more days postoperatively, depending on the patient's condition and the surgeon's preference. When the cast is removed, the status of the wound is carefully inspected. If the wound is healing well, the physician may opt for reapplication of the cast or IPOP for an additional period. If the status of the wound is questionable, an alternative method of edema control that allows more frequent wound inspection and care must be used. Some physicians opt to replace a rigid dressing with a RRD after the first cast is taken off, regardless of wound status.

Rigid dressings are among the most effective strategies for controlling postoperative edema and, as a result, reducing postoperative pain.[105] The rigid cast or semirigid shell protects the vulnerable suture line from unintentional trauma as the patient moves around in bed, transfers to and from bed (or toilet or mat table), is transported by wheelchair, and begins single limb mobility training. Enclosure of the limb in an extended knee position is also effective in preventing problematic knee flexion contracture formation. As a result, those who wear rigid dressings or IPOPs are often ready for prosthetic fitting slightly sooner than those managed by other edema control strategies.[106-108]

Several important disadvantages or drawbacks are associated with rigid dressings and IPOPs, however.[107] Application of a cast precludes visual inspection of the healing incision,

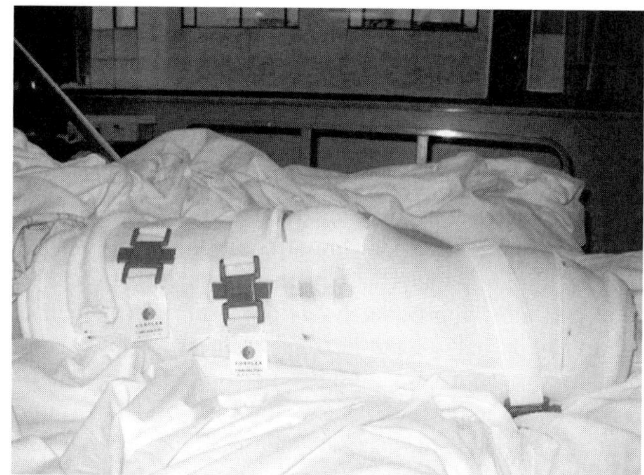

A

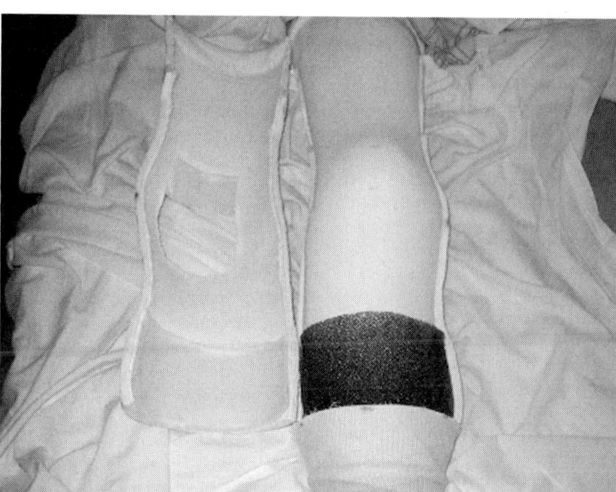

B

Figure 23-12
*Example of a custom, removable, immediate postoperative cast (**A**) bivalved at first dressing change and held closed with Velcro straps. **B**, Interior view of the immediate postoperative prosthesis with gel pads placed to protect the distal anterior tibia and patella. (From Walsh TL. Custom removable immediate postoperative prosthesis.* J Prosthet Orthot *2003;15(4):160.)*

and wound care can only occur when the cast is removed or changed. For this reason a rigid dressing may not be appropriate for those with significant risk of infection, especially if wounds were potentially contaminated during traumatic injury. Wound status can only be monitored indirectly, using body temperature, white blood cell count, size and color of drainage stains on the cast, and patient reports of increasing discomfort and pain as indicators of a developing infection. Application of a rigid cast, especially if it is the base of an IPOP, also requires careful attention to anatomy and alignment, well-developed manual skills, and a clear understanding of prosthetic principles. A poorly applied or inadequately suspended rigid dressing can lead to skin abrasions or pressure-related ulcerations over bony prominences, delaying prosthetic fitting until wound healing occurs. Pistoning or rotation of the rigid dressing on the residual limb can apply distracting forces over the suture line, compromising healing and increasing the risk of ecchymosis or dehiscence.

The early mobility afforded by application of an IPOP may be important for individuals with new amputation who would otherwise be unable to achieve single limb ambulation with a walker or crutches, especially those who are at significant risk of functional decline, physiological deconditioning, or atelectasis and pneumonia secondary to inactivity and immobilization. Importantly, although an IPOP replaces the amputated limb with a pylon and prosthetic foot, it is most appropriately used with limited, protected, toe-touch partial weight bearing.[103] Shearing forces that result from excessive weight shift and repeated loading of the residual limb in an IPOP can compromise or delay wound healing.[109] Because of this risk, an IPOP is inappropriate for frail or confused individuals who are likely to be unreliable about limiting weight bearing. Many proponents of IPOP suggest that gradual controlled application of mechanical stress to healing connective tissues actually assists tissue modeling for better tolerance of the mechanical stresses of prosthetic wear and ambulation.[101,109] Although the early application of mechanical stresses is apparently well tolerated by wounds with adequate blood supply, ischemic wounds tolerate only minimum stress in their healing phase.[109]

Removable Rigid Dressings

RRDs are used in three circumstances.[110,111] For some individuals managed with a rigid dressing applied in the operating room, the next step in postoperative edema control may be fabrication of an RRD. For others the RRD is applied instead of a cylindrical cast in the operating room. The RRD can also be fabricated several days after surgery for those initially managed with soft dressings and elastic bandages. The physical therapist may be responsible for fabrication of the RRD, working in collaboration with the surgeon, surgical nurse, or prosthetist.

The RRD is a "cap" cast worn over a soft or compressive dressing (Figure 23-13). This edema control strategy effectively protects the healing residual limb and helps to limit the development of edema. One of its major advantages, when compared with a cylindrical cast, is the ability to doff (remove) and don (apply) the RRD quickly and easily to monitor wound healing and provide daily wound care.[110,111] Use of an RRD also assists residual limb shaping and shrinkage; patients who wear RRDs are often ready for prosthetic fitting more quickly than those managed with soft

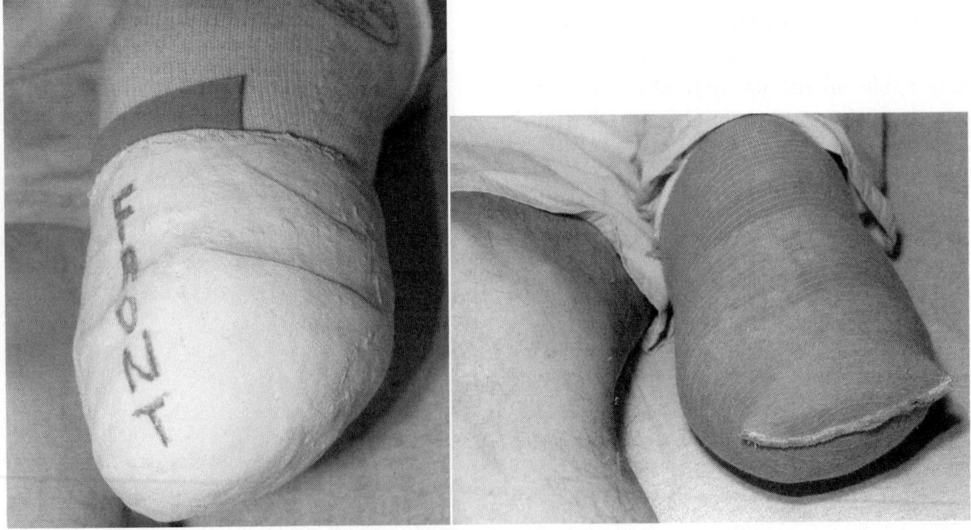

Figure 23-13

A, *This removable rigid dressing has been donned over a nylon sheath and five-ply wool prosthetic sock, with an additional foam pad at the proximal anterior edge for comfort and protection of the skin. Marking the anterior midline of the cast ensures that it will be applied in optimal alignment.* ***B,*** *The removable rigid dressing is held onto the limb by application of an elasticized Tubigrip, sewn closed at one end and pulled up to midthigh level for a sleeve suspension. A Velcro-closing thermoplastic or woven supracondylar strap is applied over the sleeve to ensure suspension.*

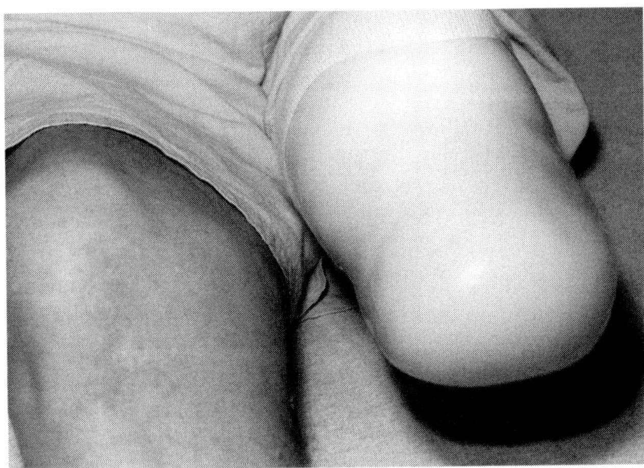

Figure 23-14

A flexible, polyethylene semirigid dressing is fabricated by a prosthetist over a positive model of the patient's residual limb. This ensures an intimate fit for effective control of edema, protection of the healing incision, and optimal "shaping" of a new residual limb.

smaller RRD. Significant change in the shape or configuration of the residual limb also requires fabrication of a new RRD.

Wu and colleagues[110,114] suggest a variety of weight-bearing exercises for patients who are wearing an RRD between the seventh and fourteenth postoperative days, depending on the state of wound healing. These exercises are designed to prepare for eventual standing and walking in a prosthesis. The referral for fabrication of the initial (preparatory or training) prosthesis can occur within 12 to 17 days of surgery if the incision has healed sufficiently. Many individuals continue to use their RRD in conjunction with a shrinker for control of edema and limb protection whenever they are not wearing their prosthesis for as long as 6 months after surgery.

Semirigid Dressings

An alternative to a plaster RRD is a polyethylene semirigid dressing (SRD; Figure 23-14).[115] Like the RRD, the SRD is an effective strategy for control of edema, protection of the healing incision, and shaping of the residual limb. Unlike the RRD, however, the SRD requires the skill of a prosthetist for fabrication. The prosthetist may take a negative mold of the patient's residual limb while in the operating room or when the rigid dressing is removed on the third or fourth postoperative day. A positive model is created using the negative mold and is modified to incorporate reliefs for pressure-intolerant areas of the residual limb. The polyethylene is heated and vacuum molded over the positive model in the same way that a thermoplastic socket would be. The SRD is often ready for delivery in 2 or 3 days after casting. When someone is initially casted for an SRD in the operating room before being placed in a plaster or fiberglass cast, the SRD may be delivered on the day that the rigid plaster dressing is removed.

The polyethylene SRD has several advantages when compared with the plaster of Paris RRD. First, polyethylene is easier to clean; as a result, hygiene of the residual limb may be improved. The SRD is lighter in weight and somewhat more durable than a plaster RRD; it does not melt if exposed to liquids. The flexibility of the material makes it easier to don and doff than the stiff plaster RRD. Because the SRD closely resembles a transtibial socket, greater carryover about proper use of prosthetic socks for optimal fit in the socket of the initial (preparatory, temporary, or training) prosthesis is likely.[116] The major disadvantage of a polyethylene SRD is the cost associated with casting and fabrication. Because most residual limbs become progressively smaller with maturation in the weeks and months after amputation, several successfully smaller SRDs may need to be fabricated as the limb shrinks. In some settings plaster RRDs are used until the initial prosthetic fitting. At that point the prosthetist makes a polyethylene SRD in addition to the socket for the training prosthesis. Some companies now offer a prefabricated adjustable SRD with Velcro closures as an alternative to the custom-molded SRD. Recently, adjustable prefabricated RRDs have become available as alternatives to custom SRDs.

An alternative method for semirigid dressing after amputation is the application of Unna's paste dressing to the residual limb immediately after wound closure in the operating room.[117-119] This dressing was initially developed for the management of venous stasis ulcers. Zinc oxide, glycerin, calamine, and gelatin are impregnated into a roll of gauze to create a pasty dressing that easily adheres to the skin. An Unna dressing typically dries to a semirigid leathery consistency within 24 hours. Although not as rigid and protective as a rigid dressing or RRD, Unna paste dressings are more effective in limiting postoperative edema than are soft dressings and Ace wrapping.[119] An Unna's semirigid dressing can be left on for as long as 5 to 7 days; if more frequent wound inspection is desired, it can be easily removed with bandage scissors. Because the Unna dressing remains in place for an extended period, fewer opportunities are available for limb desensitization and patient education about socket fit compared with those for the RRD and polyethylene SRD.

Pneumatic Compression

Several air-filled options exist for compression in the postoperative and preprosthetic periods. The simplest and least expensive is an air splint, similar to those used to stabilize lower extremity fractures.[122,123] The suture line is covered with smooth gauze pads, and then prosthetic sock, stockinet, or Tubigrip is donned over the residual limb before the air splint is inflated. Although air splints can be easily applied and removed for frequent inspection of the surgical construct, the major drawbacks are that compression is uneven, so shaping of the residual limb is not as effective as other methods, and the splint can be uncomfortably hot if worn for more than 20 to 30 minutes. Air splints also allow early protected weight bearing for physically or medically frail dressings or Ace wraps alone.[112] Because the RRD limits the development of edema, it is an important adjunct in the management of postsurgical pain. The protective cap limits shearing across the incision site as the person recovering from amputation surgery moves around in bed or during therapy; this soft tissue immobilization can assist wound healing.

The RRD is not likely to become displaced or dislodged during activity, a problem that often renders Ace wrap compression ineffective. The ease of donning and doffing means that individuals with new amputation can quickly become responsible for this task component of caring for their residual limb. Because the RRD is removed and reapplied several times a day for wound care, the residual limb quickly becomes desensitized and tolerant of pressure, which assists transition to prosthetic wear. Fabrication and use of an RRD provide the opportunity to educate those new to prosthetic use about the fabrication of a preparatory prosthesis and the use of prosthetic socks to obtain and maintain socket fit.

The RRD is most appropriate for patients whose transtibial incision appears to be in the initial stages of healing. Although the wound may be inflamed secondary to the trauma of surgery, no signs of infection, significant ecchymosis, or large areas of wound dehiscence should be present.[113] Those with substantial drainage from their surgical wound requiring bulky soft dressings and frequent dressing changes are not good candidates for RRD; it is difficult to accommodate distally placed bulky dressings within the RRD shell. Those with fluctuating edema secondary to congestive heart failure or dialysis can be managed with an RRD if it is fabricated when limb volume is high: Layering prosthetic sock ply over the limb before putting on the RRD accommodates for volume loss.[113] The RRD works best if distal residual limb circumference is no more than 0.5 inch larger than its proximal circumference. Compressive dressings may be more appropriate for patients with extremely bulbous residual limbs.

The residual limb is prepared for casting by first placing a protective layer of gauze fluff over the suture line.[113] The limb can be loosely wrapped in plastic wrap to assist removal of the completed RRD after casting. Next, a "sock" made from elasticized cotton stockinet or Tubigrip (Seton Health Care Group TLC, Oldham, England) is applied over the limb, with particular care to avoid shearing across the suture line. Pieces of Webril or a similar filler material are layered around the limb to create reliefs within the RRD for bony prominences (tibial crest, fibular head, distal tibia) and the hamstring tendons. When the distal residual limb has a larger circumference, additional padding is added proximally to ensure that the RRD will be cylindrical and easily donned. A long sock made from regular cotton stockinet is carefully donned over the padding; this will be the inner layer of the finished RRD. The outline of the patella marked on the stockinet guides trimlines as plaster is applied. Typically, two rolls of fast-setting plaster cast material are sufficient for an RRD. The residual limb is supporte knee extension, and successive layers of plaster are sm into place, building a cast with an anterior trimline patella and a slightly lower posterior trimline to allo flexion without tissue impingement.

The cotton stockinet sock is then folded down o cast at the knee, and several additional circumferentia of plaster are used to finish and reinforce the proxima (to ensure that the RRD can subsequently witl repeated donning/doffing). An Ace wrap can be app provide additional compression while the plaster sets. the RRD has hardened sufficiently, the patient is asked the knee slightly and the cast is carefully removed fro residual limb. The extra Webril or padding is pulled the RRD, and the inner surface is inspected for poter problematic rough areas or ridges. Because the RI almost cylindrical, it is helpful to mark the front of th to ensure that it is correctly donned.

Before the completed RRD is applied, one or two pads are placed over the suture line for protection. A thetic sock, Tubigrip, elasticized stockinet sock, or com cially manufactured "shrinker" is carefully donned, minimal shear stress across the suture line. Additional p prosthetic socks are used as needed to ensure a snu within the RRD. A small amount of Webril or other fl padding is placed in the distal anterior RRD to protect distal tibia and suture line; then the RRD is carefully slip onto the residual limb, aligning the markings on the fron the RRD with the patella for optimal fit (see Figure 23- *A*). A small foam filler or cushion can be placed between anterior brim and residual limb to minimize the risk of f tion during activity. The outer Tubigrip or stockinet susp sion sleeve is then rolled over the RRD and onto the thi the supracondylar strap is secured in place, and the sock folded back down over the strap to minimize the risk of l of suspension.

The skin must be inspected within the first 60 to 90 minu of initial fitting with an RRD to assess skin integrity ar identify potential pressure-related problems. If no sk problems develop, routine wound inspection once p nursing shift is usually adequate. The RRD is designed to b worn continuously, even when sleeping, except durin routine wound care or bathing.[110,111] If the individual wit recent amputation is expecting to be out of the RRD fo more than several minutes, another form of compressior such as a shrinker or several layers of Tubigrip must be available to minimize the development of edema. The individual wearing an RRD must be encouraged to report any localized pain or discomfort as signs of potential problems with RRD fit or function. Layers of prosthetic sock are added, over time, as the residual limb "shrinks." Sometimes short distal socks are necessary to provide for distal compression without excessive proximal bulkiness that can prohibit donning. The consistent use of 12- to 15-ply socks to achieve appropriate fit usually indicates the need for fabrication of a

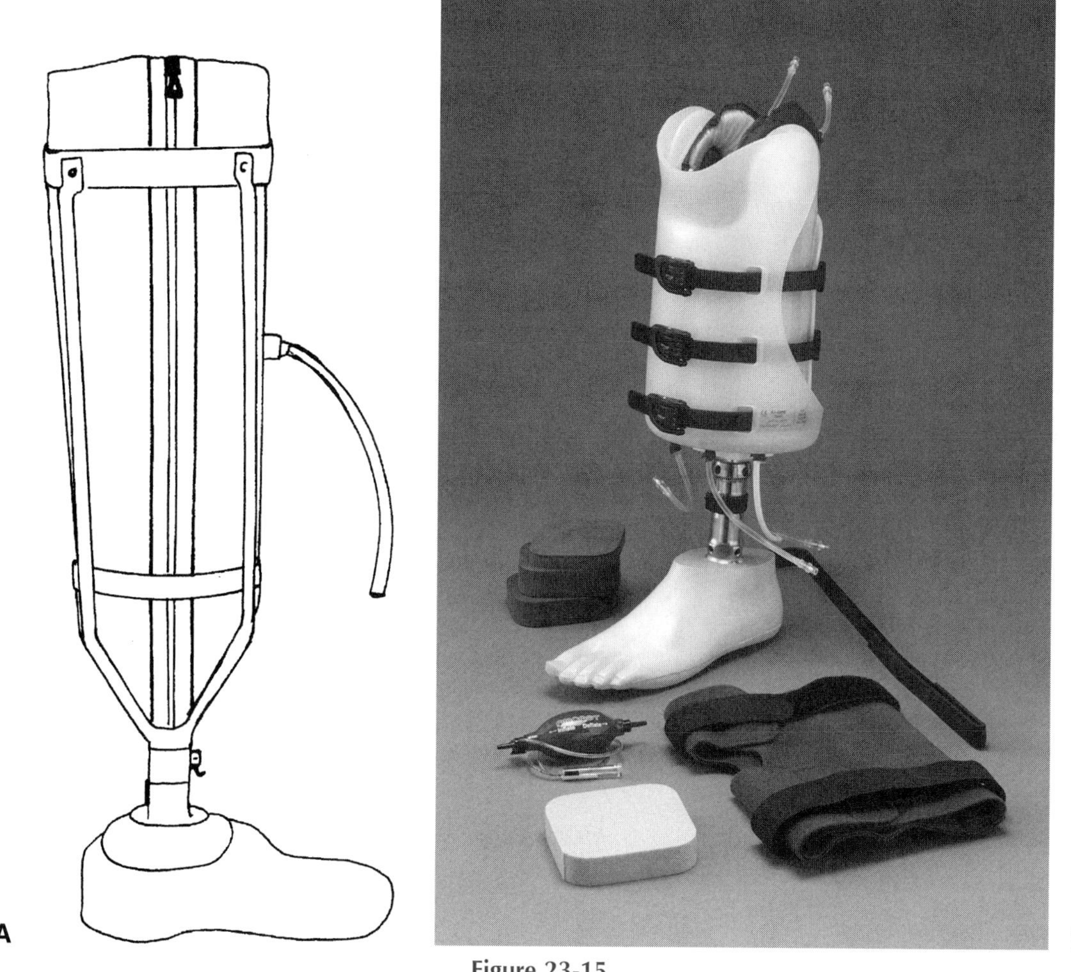

Figure 23-15

A, *An air splint and prosthetic frame may provide limited ambulation for patients who are unable to accomplish single limb gait with an assistive device. The splint is inflated within the frame to 35 to 40 mm Hg, allowing toe touch to partial weight bearing, with minimal risk to the healing incision.* ***B,*** *The Aircast Airlimb, an example of a commercially available, noncustom, pneumatic, immediate postoperative prosthesis. (Courtesy Aircast Inc., Summit, N.J.)*

persons[124-125] (Figure 23-15, *A*). Felt pads are strategically placed over the residual limb's soft dressing, or a shrinker loads pressure-tolerant areas (medial tibial flare and patellar tendon) while protecting pressure-sensitive areas (crest of the tibia and fibular head) after inflation of the air splint. The sleeve is zipped into place around the limb, and the limb is positioned in the frame before inflation. The sleeve is inflated with a hand or foot pump to an air pressure of 35 to 40 mm Hg. This low pressure sustains toe touch to partial weight without compromising capillary blood flow to the healing suture line. The air splint provides limited mobility for patients who would not otherwise be ambulatory and may be a useful means of assessing the potential for prosthetic rehabilitation. Recently a prefabricated pneumatic immediate postoperative prosthesis, with inflatable air bladders within an adjustable closure polyethylene "socket," has become available (Figure 23-15, *B*).[126]

Soft Dressings and Compression

The traditional postoperative edema control and wound management strategy is a soft gauze dressing with compressive Ace bandage wrap. This method continues to be the most frequently used immediate postsurgical option for patients with transfemoral amputation. Although Ace wrapping may be the most viable option when significant wound drainage and a high risk of infection are present, this method of compression is not nearly as effective in limiting postoperative edema as those described previously.[4,120] Soft dressings cannot protect a healing incision from bumps, bruising, or shearing during activity or from fall-related injury. The other practical disadvantage of elastic Ace bandage compression of the residual limb is the need for frequent reapplication: Movement during daily activities quickly loosens the bandages, compromising the effectiveness of the compression. Most rehabilitation professionals

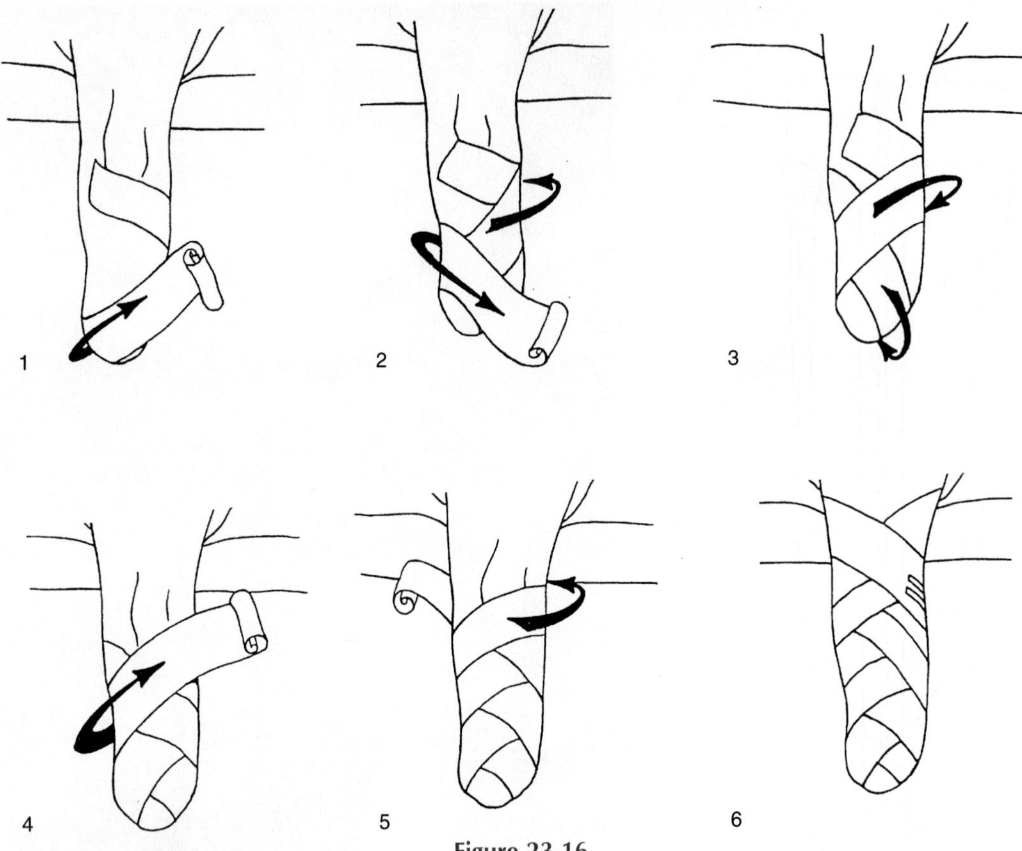

Figure 23-16

The application of an effective Ace wrap to a transtibial residual limb uses successive diagonal figure-of-eight loops between the distal residual limb and thigh to create a distal-to-proximal pressure gradient. This creates a distal-to-proximal, tapering, cylindrical residual limb with minimal excess distal soft tissue. (Modified from Karacollof LA, Hammersley CS, Schneider FJ. Lower Extremity Amputation. *Gaithersburg, MD: Aspen, 1992. pp. 16-17.)*

suggest that Ace bandages should be removed and reapplied every 4 to 6 hours and should never be kept in place for more than 12 hours without rebandaging.[121]

Effective application of an Ace wrap requires practice, manual dexterity, and attention to details if the desired distal-to-proximal pressure gradient is to be achieved[4,97,120] (Figures 23-16 and 23-17). It may be difficult for patients with limited vision, arthritis of the hands and wrist, limited trunk mobility, or compromised postural control to master this technique for independence in control of edema. Nurses, residents, surgeons, therapists, prosthetists, and family members (and anyone else who may be taking down the soft dressing to care for the wound) must be consistent and effective in reapplication of the Ace bandage if maximal control of edema is to be achieved. Ineffectively applied elastic wraps can lead to a bulbous, poorly shaped residual limb, which is likely to delay prosthetic fitting.[112] Tight circumferential wrapping can significantly compromise blood flow, compromising healing of the incision and even leading to skin breakdown.[112]

Several alternatives are available for elastic compression when Ace wrap proves to be cumbersome or problematic. One method that is effective for patients with a bulbous or pressure-sensitive residual limb is application of a elasticized stockinet or Tubigrip sock. Both materials are available with various levels of elasticity; minimal to significant compression can be achieved, depending on the patient's tolerance of pressure. Wu[114] describes a double-layer method in which a long piece of elastic stockinet or Tubigrip is carefully applied over the transtibial residual limb to midthigh level (Figure 23-18). The extra length of elastic stockinet or Tubigrip is then turned or twisted 180 degrees (to minimize pressure over the new incision) and rolled over the residual limb as a second layer of compression. As residual limb volume decreases and the limb becomes more pressure tolerant, stockinet or Tubigrip with progressively narrower diameters is used to increase compressive forces and assist limb shrinkage and maturation. These materials are relatively inexpensive, but they are not as durable as commercially available elastic shrinker socks.

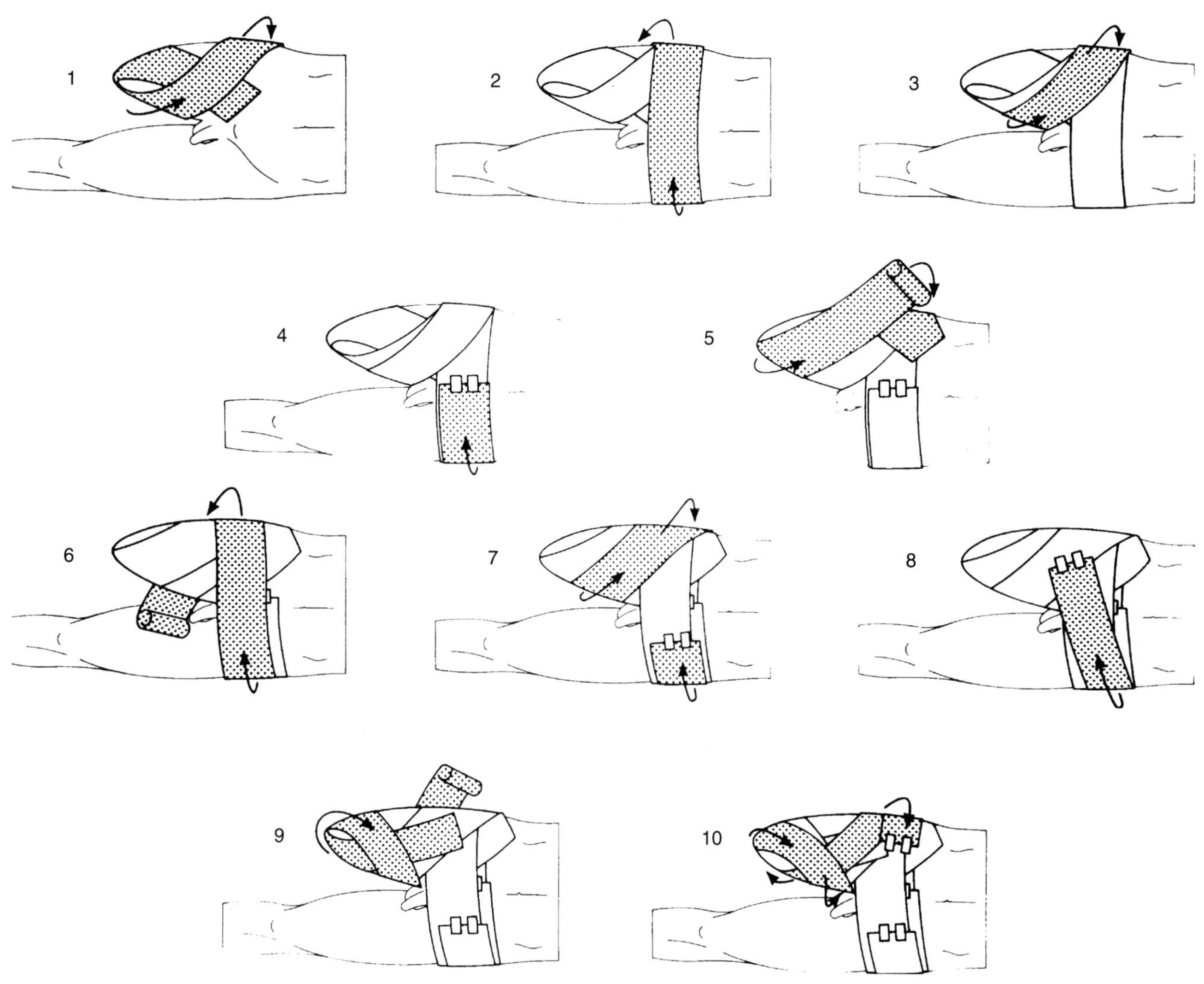

Figure 23-17

The application of an effective Ace wrap to a transfemoral limb also strives to create a distal-to-proximal pressure gradient using a modified figure-of-eight pattern. For patients with transfemoral amputation, the wrap is anchored around the pelvis and applied to pull the hip toward hip extension and adduction. Note the importance of capturing soft tissue high in the groin within the Ace wrap, to reduce the risk of developing an adductor roll of noncompressed soft tissue. (From May BJ. Amputation and Prosthetics: A Case Study Approach. *Philadelphia: F.A. Davis, 1996. p. 84.)*

Commercially Available Pressure Garments

Once the suture line has healed sufficiently, many prosthetists and therapists recommend the use of a commercially manufactured elastic shrinker garment whenever the prosthesis is not being worn (Figure 23-19). Most shrinkers are designed to apply significant compressive force to the residual limb, and it may be difficult for individuals with limited manual dexterity or upper extremity strength to apply them. Patients with recent amputation must be careful to minimize or avoid excessive shear forces over the incision as the shrinker is being applied. Although shrinkers are effective for control of edema and limb volume, it is not possible to create "relief" for bony prominences or pressure-vulnerable areas on the residual limb. As with other soft dressings, commercial shrinkers cannot protect the residual limb from trauma during daily activities or in the event of a fall. It is not unusual for patients to continue to use a shrinker for limb volume control, whenever they are not wearing their prosthesis, for 6 months to a year after amputation.

Although a number of edema control options are available for persons with transtibial amputation, those with transfemoral residual limbs have fewer strategies from which to choose. Commercially manufactured shrinkers are more convenient to don and are more likely to remain in place than the more cumbersome Ace wraps, but those who choose this option must be just as careful to capture all the soft tissue high in the groin within the shrinker to avoid the

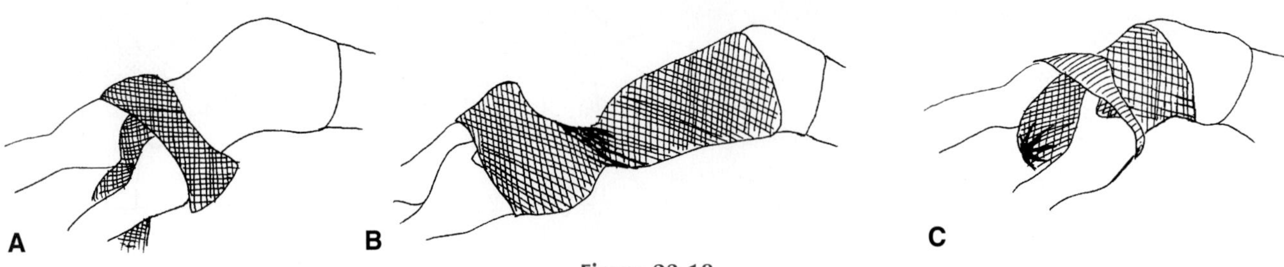

Figure 23-18

*One strategy to control edema and manage limb volume is to use a double layer of an elastic stockinet or Tubigrip to apply compressive forces to the limb. After the initial layer (**A**) has been smoothly applied, the stockinet is twisted closed (**B**) at the end of the limb and the excess is applied (**C**) as a second layer of compression.*

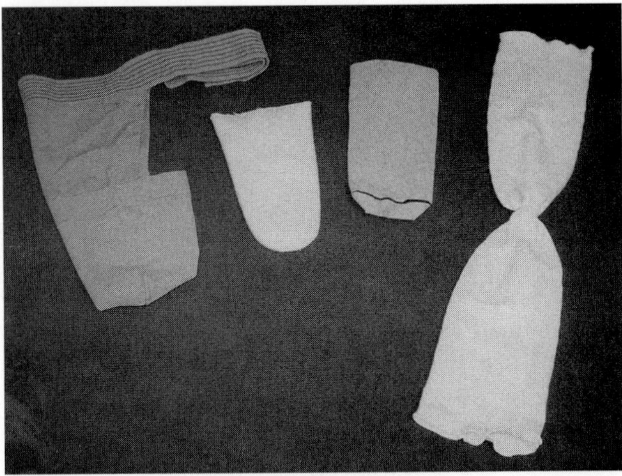

Figure 23-19

Examples of commercially available transfemoral (left) *and transtibial shrinkers used for edema control and shaping of the residual limb.*

development of an adductor roll. Another alternative for those with transfemoral amputation is a custom-fit Jobst pressure garment. Jobst garments can be fabricated either as a half-panty or full pant garment; the full pant garment achieves a more consistent suspension and compression, especially for patients who are obese. A Jobst garment may be the only effective alternative for patients with short transfemoral amputation.

Because shrinkers, Tubigrip, and prosthetic socks worn over a healing residual limb are permeable, they absorb perspiration from the skin of the residual limb, as well as any drainage from the suture line. For this reason they must be laundered daily in warm water and a mild soap. Cotton, wool, or elasticized materials do not tolerate the heat and turbulence of a clothes dryer; most prosthetists recommend that shrinkers and socks be smoothed out on a flat surface to dry. The person wearing the garment must have a sufficient number available in order to apply compression around the clock.

Selecting the Appropriate Compression Strategy

In deciding which edema control and limb-shaping strategy is most appropriate, the rehabilitation team considers the following questions[112,120]:

1. Can the person don/doff the device independently? If not, is a family member available who can assist with this task?
2. Given the individual's physical characteristics and likely level of activity, will the device remain securely in place on the residual limb?
3. Will the device apply enough compression for effective progressive limb shrinkage?
4. Will the device apply enough compression for symmetric shaping of the residual limb?
5. Will the device protect the skin and healing suture line during daily activities, and does use of the device carry any risk of skin irritation or breakdown?
6. Is the device comfortable for the patient to use or wear over the long periods of time that are required for effective control of edema and limb shaping?
7. Is the device relatively cost effective in terms of fabrication, modification, and replacement?

Monitoring tissue tolerance and potential areas of pressure closely in whatever edema control method is chosen is important, especially in the first few days and weeks after amputation. Although rigid dressings, IPOPs, and Unna dressing remain on the limb for extended periods, each other method of edema control and shaping should be removed and reapplied a minimum of three times each day to assure appropriate fit and tissue tolerance in the acute phase of healing. When a rigid cast or IPOP is removed, it must be quickly replaced with an alternative compression device so that limb volume does not increase substantially. Individuals with recent amputation must wear the compression device at all times unless walking in a training prosthesis (even time out of compression during bathing should be as short as possible). Most people find that a compression device is necessary to maintain the desired limb volume for 6 months to a year after surgery. Some persons with mature residual limbs who have fluctuation in volume due to concurrent medical conditions continue to require compression well beyond the first postoperative year.

Many people with amputation experience a transient increase in residual limb volume after a shower or bathing; they often choose to bathe in the evening so that volume change does not interfere with prosthetic use. Those who prefer to bathe in the morning may need to use a compression device immediately after bathing to achieve optimal prosthetic fit and suspension, especially if suction suspension (which requires consistent limb volume) is used. Those who use prosthetic socks may require a few less ply of sock immediately after bathing but need to add a few more ply after a few hours as limb volume decreases.

Skin Care and Scar Management

Importantly, the incision must not adhere to underlying deep tissue or bone as healing progresses. Ideally, enough gliding movement will be present between the skin and the underlying layer of soft tissue after healing that shear forces will be minimal while the prosthesis is donned and used for function. An adherent scar at the distal tibia can be quite problematic: If a point of adherence is present along an incisional scar, the mobility of tissues will be compromised. The resulting traction and shear forces are likely to lead to discomfort, skin irritation, and often recurrent breakdown of soft tissues with prosthetic use. Once primary healing has been established, the person with recent amputation learns to use gentle manual massage to enhance tissue mobility in preparation for prosthetic use. Initially, this is performed above and below, but not across, the incision to minimize the risk of dehiscence.

When the wound is well closed and Steri-Strips are no longer necessary to support and protect the incision, gentle mobilization of the scar itself can begin. Handling of the limb during soft tissue mobilization and massage not only minimizes adhesion formation but also helps the individual to adapt his or her body image to include the postamputation residual limb and prepare for the sensory experience of prosthetic use.

Persons with new amputation may have surgical scars from previous vascular bypass or from harvesting veins for coronary artery bypass surgery. These may require carefully applied soft tissue mobilization or friction massage to free adhesions and restore the mobility of the skin. Those with traumatic amputation may have healing skin grafts or abrasions from road burn, thermal injury, or electrical burn. In such cases wound care and debridement are important components of preprosthetic rehabilitation. For individuals with healing burns or skin graft, the use of an appropriate compression garment or shrinker assists healing and maturation of skin, controls postoperative edema, and shapes the residual limb.

Once the sutures have been removed, normal bathing resumes and a routine for daily skin care is established. Most physicians, prosthetists, and therapists recommend daily cleansing of the residual limb with a mild, nondrying soap. Patting or gently rubbing the limb with a terry cloth towel until it is fully dry also helps to desensitize it in preparation for prosthetic use. A small amount of moisturizer or skin cream can be applied if the skin of the residual limb is dry or flaky. A limb with soft, healthy pliable skin is much more tolerant of prosthetic wear than a limb with tough, dry, easily irritated skin. Persons with new amputation and their caregivers are taught to inspect the skin of the entire residual limb carefully, using a mirror if necessary to visualize difficult-to-see areas. Areas over bony prominences that may be vulnerable to high pressure within the socket are especially important to assess.

Persons with amputation are as likely to have other dermatological conditions such as eczema or psoriasis as the general population. Those with hairy limbs or easily irritated skin may be more at risk of folliculitis and similar inflammatory skin conditions once the prosthesis is worn consistently. Effective early management of skin irritation or other skin problems is important: Serious skin irritation or infection precludes prosthetic use until adequate healing has occurred.

Some persons with new amputation mistakenly assume that something must be used to "toughen" the skin in preparation for prosthetic use. They may opt to rub the skin with alcohol, vinegar, salt water, or even gasoline, erroneously thinking that this will make the skin thicker and more pressure tolerant. In fact, these "treatments" can damage the skin, making it more susceptible to pressure-related problems. Patient and family education about effective cleansing and skin care strategies is essential in the early postoperative/preprosthetic period.[4,120]

Range of Motion and Flexibility

Because of the high risk of knee flexion contracture for those with transtibial amputation and the negative impact of such contracture on future prosthetic use, proper positioning is a key component of preprosthetic rehabilitation. Prolonged dependence of the residual limb held in knee flexion when sitting also leads to development of distal edema, which can delay readiness for prosthetic fitting. Persons with transtibial amputation must maintain the knee in as much extension as possible, whether in bed, sitting in a wheelchair or lounge chair, or during exercise and activity. Although it may be comfortable to place a pillow under the knee when sitting or lying in bed, a more effective strategy is to position a small towel roll under the distal posterior residual limb to encourage knee extension (Figure 23-20). Use of a wheelchair with elevating leg rests helps to keep the residual limb in an extended position, although a "bridge" between the seat and calf support may be necessary for those with short residual limbs. In some settings the therapist fabricates a posterior trough splint from low-temperature thermoplastic

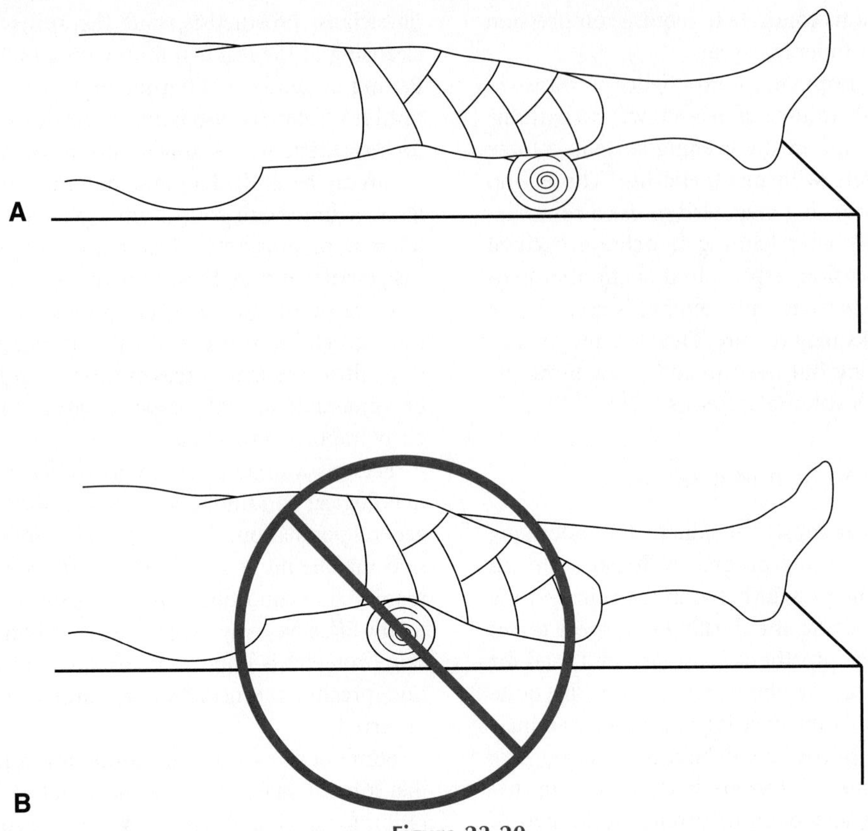

Figure 23-20

The optimal position for individuals with recent transtibial amputation is in full extension. ***A,*** *A small rolled towel, bolster, or pillow placed under the distal posterior residual limb encourages knee extension, while* ***(B)*** *support under the knee makes development of knee flexion contracture more likely.*

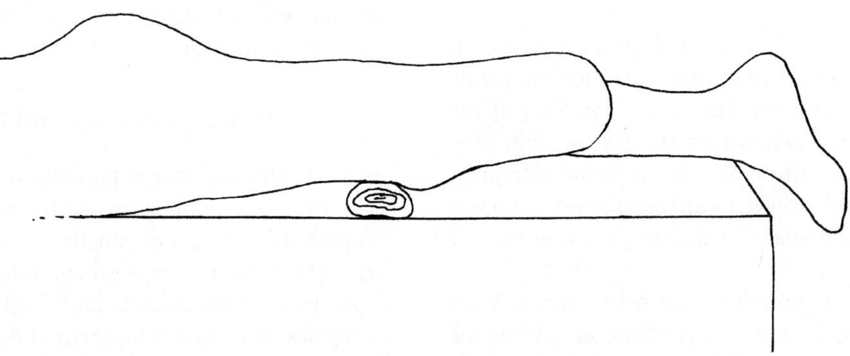

Figure 23-21

Prone positioning for stretching of the posterior soft tissue and prevention of knee flexion contracture. A small towel roll placed just above the patella elevates the residual limb from the surface of the mat or bed. The therapist can use hold-relax or contract-relax techniques, or the patient can actively contract the quadriceps to assist elongation of the hamstrings and posterior soft tissues.

materials; this splint supports the limb in knee extension when the individual with recent amputation is resting in bed or sitting in a wheelchair.

If the person can assume a prone position, the weight of the limb can be used to assist elongation of the hamstring muscles and soft tissue of the posterior knee (Figure 23-21). A small towel roll positioned just above the patella effectively positions the limb for elongation. Modalities such as moist heat or ultrasound, followed by manual physical therapy techniques such as manual passive stretching, proprioceptive neuromuscular facilitation (PNF) hold-relax or contract-relax, or deep effleurage massage, may be effective in reducing existing knee flexion contracture.[127-129] (Readers are referred to *Stretching and Strengthening for Lower Extremity Amputees* by R.S. and A.M. Gailey, Advanced Rehabilitation Therapy Inc, Miami, *www.advancedrehabtherapy.com* for more examples of postoperative flexibility activities.)

Persons with recent amputation are instructed how to perform exercises (done at the bedside while an inpatient or at home while an outpatient) that are designed to elongate muscles and soft tissue to counteract the tendency to development of tightness. Performed independently or with the assistance of a family member or caregiver several times a day, these stretching exercises are important adjuncts to physical therapy sessions during preprosthetic and prosthetic rehabilitation.

Significant hip flexion contracture can render a patient with transfemoral amputation ineffective in controlling a prosthetic knee unit and walking with a prosthesis.[130] Persons with recent transfemoral amputation tend to hold their residual limb diagonally outward when seated, unconsciously and automatically increasing their seated base of support to enhance postural stability. If they spend significant amounts of time in a seated position, development of hip flexor, abductor, and external rotator tightness is almost inevitable. Physical therapy interventions that elongate these soft tissues including manual stretching, active exercise, and functional postural training are used to counteract the tendency for tightness to develop.[127,131,132] Resting in a prone position with a towel roll under the distal anterior residual limb provides prolonged elongation for tight hip flexors. Care must be taken, however, to maintain a neutral pelvis or slight posterior tilt when lying prone. Excessive hip flexor tightness leads to lordosis of the lumbosacral spine.

Muscle Performance

Strengthening programs have two goals: (1) remediation of specific weaknesses detected in the examination and (2) maximization of overall strength and muscular endurance for safe, energy-efficient prosthetic gait. Because functional activities require use of muscles at varying lengths and types of contraction, effective preprosthetic exercise programs include activities that require concentric, holding (isometric), eccentric, and cocontraction in a variety of positions and muscle lengths.[133] In the immediate postoperative period the specific strengthening program is often a combination of isometric and active isotonic exercise within a limited ROM of the joint just proximal to the amputation.[4,85,128,133-135] This strategy minimizes stress or tension across the incision while preserving and improving the strength of key muscle groups.

Incorporation of controlled exhalation during isometric contraction minimizes the risks to cardiac function and fluctuations of blood pressure that are associated with the Valsalva maneuver. For persons with transtibial amputation, exercises to strengthen knee extension that are initiated within the first week of amputation might include "quad sets" in the supine position or "short arc quads" performed in supine or sitting. For those with transfemoral amputation, "glut sets" in the prone or supine position or "short arc" hip extension and abduction in a gravity-eliminated position would be initiated. Gailey[128,136,137] recommends an exercise strategy of slow, steadily controlled, 10-second muscular contraction, followed by 5 to 10 seconds of rest, for 10 repetitions as one that is easily learned and physiologically sound. As wound healing is accomplished, exercises can be progressed to include active exercises through larger arcs of motion, active resistive exercise (using weights or manual resistance), or isokinetic training. Application of manual resistance during functional activities, as in PNF, allows the therapist to provide appropriate resistance as muscle strength varies throughout the active ROM while providing facilitation and augmented sensory feedback to the patient.[138,139] Isokinetic exercise allows the patient to develop muscular strength and control at a variety of movement velocities.[136]

For individuals with transtibial amputation, attachments of the quadriceps and hamstrings are typically intact, and preprosthetic strengthening exercises emphasize control of the knee, as well as hip strength for stability in stance. Those with transfemoral amputation must develop strong hip extension capabilities to control the prosthetic knee unit. They must also have effective hip abduction power if the pelvis is to remain level during stance. It is important to recognize that the distal attachments of the hamstrings, rectus femoris, sartorius, tensor fasciae latae/iliotibial band, adductor longus, and adductor magnus are relocated by myodesis or myoplasty or are lost entirely (for patients with short residual limbs) during transfemoral surgery. The combination of an altered line of pull and loss of muscle mass often creates an imbalance of muscle action around the hip.[132,140] The gluteus maximus, gluteus medius, and iliopsoas, with their intact distal attachments, are more powerful in determining resting hip position than the altered adductor group. If the tensor fasciae latae/iliotibial band and gluteus maximus become secondarily shortened, function of the adductor group is further compromised.

Because of this imbalance, it is important to include activities that strengthen the remaining hip adductors, as well as hip extensors and hip abductors, to prepare the patient for effective postural control in sitting and standing and stance phase stability in prosthetic gait. (Readers are referred to *Stretching and Strengthening for Lower Extremity Amputees* by R.S. and A.M. Gailey, Advanced Rehabilitation Therapy Inc, Miami, *www.advancedrehabtherapy.com*, for more examples of postoperative, preprosthetic strengthening activities.)

General strengthening exercises for the trunk and upper extremities are also essential components of an effective preprosthetic exercise program. Back extensors and abdominal muscles play an important role in postural alignment and postural control. Activities that involve trunk rotation or diagonal movements activate trunk and limb girdle muscles in functional patterns, addressing strength and flexibility for functional activities and enhancing reciprocal arm swing and pelvic control in gait. Upper extremity strengthening, targeting shoulder depressor and elbow extensors, enhances the patient's ability to use an assistive device for single limb ambulation before prosthetic fitting. Many older adults with dysvascular amputation begin rehabilitation with low endurance: Aerobic exercise programs such as upper extremity ergometers help to improve exercise tolerance and endurance and prepare them for the energy demands of single limb and prosthetic ambulation.

Postural Control

Loss of a limb shifts the position of the body's center of mass (COM), moving it slightly upward, backward, and toward the remaining or intact extremity. The magnitude of this shift is determined by the extent of limb loss. The shift may have relatively little impact on postural control and functional ability in patients with Syme or long transtibial amputation. It may, however, have a significant impact on the sitting balance and functional ability of patients with short transfemoral or hip disarticulation amputation. An effective preprosthetic program incorporates activities that challenge patients to improve postural control and equilibrium responses, learning how to control the repositioned COM effectively over an altered base of support. In sitting, this can be accomplished using a variety of reaching tasks including forward reaching, diagonal reaching across and away from the midline, reaching down to a lower surface or objects, reaching up and away from their center, and turning to reach behind them. Anticipatory and reactive postural responses can also be practiced by throwing and catching games that require an automatic weight shift as part of the activity. The difficulty of the task can be advanced by progressively shifting the location of the catch or toss away from the midline of the patient's trunk; alternating locations from side to side or upward or downward; increasing the speed of the activity; increasing the weight of the object or ball that is being used; or performing the activity on a less stable seating surface (e.g., theraball, large bolster, or air-filled balance cushion).

The effectiveness of postural responses is influenced by the flexibility and strength of the trunk and limb girdles, as well as the length and power of the residual limb. The prosthetic replacement of a missing limb increases the functional base of support in sitting; for some individuals the weight of the prosthesis serves as a stabilizing anchor during functional activity. For those with limited flexibility or strength, such a replacement might be essential for effective postural responses and the ability to reach, even if the potential for functional ambulation is small.[140] (Readers are referred to *Balance, Agility and Coordination for Lower Extremity Amputees* by R.S. and A.M. Gailey, Advanced Rehabilitation Therapy Inc, Miami, *www.advancedrehabtherapy.com*, for more activities that can be used to assist postural control.)

Wheelchairs and Seating

Many patients with amputation rely on a wheelchair for mobility during the postoperative, preprosthetic period. Some patients with short transfemoral amputation or bilateral amputation prefer the relative energy efficiency of wheelchair mobility to ambulation with or without a prosthesis. For others, comorbid cardiovascular or cardiopulmonary dysfunction precludes ambulation and the wheelchair becomes their primary mode of locomotion. The shift in COM after amputation has important implications in choice of wheelchairs.

The design of many standard or traditional wheelchairs is based on the anthropomorphic characteristics of an "average" adult male with intact lower extremities. With the loss of a limb, the COM shifts in a posterior and lateral direction; when the patient is seated in a wheelchair, this moves the COM closer to the axis of rotation of the chair's wheels. If the patient with lower extremity amputation turns or reaches backward during a functional activity, the COM shifts even farther toward, or even beyond, the wheel axis, and the chair may tip backward. The provision of simple antitip devices reduces the risk of posterior tipping during functional activities. For those with transfemoral or bilateral amputation, a wheelchair with wheels that can be offset posteriorly is recommended. Patients with recent amputation must also be aware of altered dynamics when they reach forward while sitting in a wheelchair: High downward pressure on the wheelchair foot plate by the intact limb when reaching forward is likely to lead to anterior tipping.

Specific wheelchair assessments and prescription are warranted for all individuals who will be using a wheelchair as their primary means of locomotion and mobility (see Chapter 19). This individual evaluation and prescription process ensures that the wheelchair will provide adequate support of the thighs to increase seating stability and reach, effective seating with an appropriate cushion for pressure distribution, and configuration of components that provides ease of wheelchair locomotion.

Bed Mobility and Transfers

In the acute care setting, physical therapy intervention at the bedside includes instruction about optimal positioning of the residual limb and activities to assist the patient's ability to change position in bed and move to or from a seated position. Early mobility and activity significantly reduce the risk of atelectasis, pneumonia, and further physiological deconditioning.[4] The therapist must, however, be aware of the risk of postural hypotension and of postoperative complications including deep venous thrombosis and pulmonary embolism. Assessment and monitoring of the patient's vital signs (pulse, respiratory rate, blood pressure, pulse oximetry) are recommended as bed mobility and out-of-bed activity begin. Care must also be taken to minimize the risk of trauma to the newly amputated limb during activity, exercise, or transfers.

Many individuals with recent amputation can roll from supine to or from the prone position without great difficulty, although those with transfemoral amputation of the dominant limb may need to develop an adapted movement pattern or sequence. The strategies for transition into sitting are not substantially different from preferred preoperative strategies; however, efficiency of postural responses may be challenged by the alteration in body mass after amputation. Those who have become deconditioned by inactivity in the days and weeks before amputation may find bed rails, a trapeze, bed ladders, or other devices helpful early in rehabilitation. Strategic placement of a bed table or walker near the bedside at night serves as a reminder of the amputation for individuals who are likely to get up during the night to go to the bathroom (without otherwise fully awakening), reducing the risk of falling.

An important goal of postoperative preprosthetic rehabilitation is development of the ability to move between seating surfaces or from sitting to standing as safely and independently as possible. Depending on the individual's preamputation level of activity, this may require some degree of assistance or use of adaptive devices or may be accomplished relatively smoothly and easily. Those who are deconditioned or who have previous neuromuscular-related postural impairment may require a mechanical lifting aid, multiperson lifting, or some level of assistance in the early postoperative period. Others may benefit from a strategically placed transfer board as they develop their ability to perform a pivot transfer on their remaining limb.

Some persons require a walker or crutches for extra stability in single limb stance in the midst of their pivot transfers. Still others quickly master scooting in sitting and pivoting on their remaining limb to become independent in transfers. Persons with single limb amputation initially prefer transferring toward their remaining limb but should be encouraged to master moving in either direction. Individuals with bilateral limb loss or injury that precludes weight bearing on the remaining limb can scoot across a sliding board to a wheelchair or commode that is positioned diagonally from the bed. Those with bilateral transfemoral amputation (and those with bilateral transtibial amputation who have sufficient hamstring excursion) may prefer the surface-to-surface stability that is provided when the entire anterior edge of the wheelchair seat abuts the side of the bed, allowing them to scoot directly forward. Some individuals who require significant assistance to transfer without a prosthesis become nearly independent in pivot transfers when a prosthesis is worn: The sensory feedback that is provided to the residual limb within the socket when there is contact between the prosthetic foot and the floor enhances sitting balance during sliding board or pivot transfers.[141] Persons with transfemoral amputation must learn that, although they can wear a prosthesis when seated, the prosthesis cannot be counted on for stability during transfers. (Readers are referred to *Patient Care Skills,* 5th ed. by S.D. and M.A. Minor, Prentice-Hall, 2005, for suggestions about interventions to enhance bed mobility, transfers, and ambulation with assistive devices.)

Mastery of single limb or non–weight-bearing transfers in the postoperative period is the foundation for functional transfers whenever the person with amputation is not wearing his or her prosthesis. At times in the future, mechanical problems with the prosthesis, skin problems on the residual limb, or a medical problem (e.g., congestive heart failure or renal failure) may affect socket fit, temporarily precluding prosthetic use. Providing opportunities for patients to practice transferring between surfaces at different levels (e.g., wheelchair to stool to floor) in the postoperative preprosthetic period is often helpful, especially if delayed prosthetic fitting is anticipated.

Many individuals with new amputation are discharged from the acute care setting to home before their limb is ready for prosthetic fitting and training. Appropriate adaptive equipment (e.g., tub bench, handheld shower adapter, raised toilet seat, and grab bars) must be identified and correctly installed so that safety in the bathroom is maximized.

Ambulation and Locomotion

Single limb ambulation with an appropriate assistive device provides an opportunity to enhance postural control and to build strength and cardiovascular endurance, in addition to allowing patients with recent amputation to move about in their environment. Many individuals with new amputation can quickly master a two- or three-point swing-through pattern with crutches on level surfaces and are ready to build advanced gait skills on uneven surfaces, inclines, and stairs. Others are fearful of using crutches, preferring the stability provided by a walker to the mobility of crutches. A walker may be appropriate for patients with limited endurance and balance impairment who would otherwise be limited to wheelchair use. Therapists must be aware, however, of the potential long-term limitation in gait patterns imposed by walkers: The halting hop-to gait pattern interrupts forward progression of the COM. Individuals who have adapted to this pattern of motion before receiving a prosthesis may have difficulty developing a smooth step-through pattern or becoming comfortable with a less supportive ambulation aid once they are using their prosthesis. Walkers are also more difficult to use on inclines and are dangerous to use on stairs. Whenever possible, patients are encouraged to use crutches.[4,128,137]

Individuals with limited endurance or poor balance spend much time practicing a hop-to or swing-through gait in the parallel bars before they acquire the confidence and motor skill necessary to move out of the parallel bars with a walker or crutches. Importantly, single limb ambulation with an assistive device is often more energy intensive than walking with a prosthesis.[142,143] Achievement of functional single limb ambulation is *not* a prerequisite for prosthetic fitting. All individuals who can stand and use an assistive device to walk should be encouraged to ambulate as much as possible, even if they are walking for aerobic exercise rather than to accomplish a functional task. For those with single limb amputation, wheelchair use should be reserved for long-distance transportation unless ambulation is not medically advisable. Wheelchairs are appropriate for patients with bilateral amputation; self-propulsion provides some aerobic conditioning, as well as an energy-efficient means of locomotion.[144,145]

Patient and Family Education

Patient and family education begins in the initial interview process and continues throughout the acute hospital stay, as illustrated in the preceding discussions of positioning, residual limb care, and remaining/intact limb care, and enhancing motor performance and functional training.

Patient education about the risk of decubitus ulceration and strategies to reduce this risk are also important components of early postoperative care. Individuals with vascular disease and neuropathy are particularly at risk, with the heel and lateral border of the remaining foot most vulnerable.[146,147] Those with dysvascular limbs may have barely enough circulation to support tissue health in an intact or noninjured foot; once a wound has occurred, circulation may be inadequate for tissue healing. An open wound on the remaining limb would preclude single limb ambulation, increasing the risk of inactivity-related postoperative complications and making prosthetic rehabilitation even more challenging. Pressure-related wounds significantly delay rehabilitation, increase disability, and multiply health care costs for patients with amputation. Vulnerability to pressure increases with sensory impairment; altered mechanical characteristics of injured, calcified, or scarred tissues; poor circulatory status; microclimate of the skin; and (in combination with these factors) advanced age.[148] For those who have limited ability to change position, a pressure-distributing mattress and well-designed, carefully applied heel protectors can reduce the risk of decubitus ulcer formation. A routine of frequent position change, weight shifting, and exercise reduces weight-bearing pressures and enhances circulation to vulnerable tissues.

Before discharge, the rehabilitation team must ascertain how close to functional independence the individual and caregivers are in a variety of self-care activities, in mobility and locomotion, and in performance of preprosthetic exercises (Table 23-3). As the program progresses, the ability of the individual and family in these areas is a key determinant of discharge readiness and placement (home with home care, home with outpatient follow-up, or to a rehabilitation or subacute facility).

Table 23-3
Example of Checklist of Key Patient and Family Knowledge and Skills following Lower Limb Amputation.

Activity:	*Indicator*	
Wound inspection	____	Individual or caregiver is able to independently inspect status of incision and residual limb
	____	Individual or caregiver is able to describe signs of inflammation, infection, dehiscence, bleeding, or ecchymosis requiring contact/visit with health professional
	____	Individual or caregiver is able to effectively inspect and care for intact limb
	____	Supervision or assistance by a health professional is necessary for wound inspection and care of either residual limb or intact limb
Residual limb care	____	Individual or caregiver is able to change wound dressings effectively, maintaining clean environment
	____	Individual or caregiver is able to appropriately cleanse and care for residual limb
	____	Individual or caregiver is able to safely effectively self-mobilize skin around incision site
	____	Individual or caregiver is able to apply appropriate compression strategy (circle: Ace wrap, RRD or SRD, commercial shrinker garment, other)
	____	Individual with transtibial amputation is able to maintain limb in extended knee position
Mobility	____	Individual is able to move around in bed as needed Level of assistance Equipment used
	____	Individual is able to transition from supine to sitting and return Level of assistance Equipment used
	____	Individual is able to transfer from bed or chair to wheelchair and return Level of assistance Equipment used

Table 23-3—cont'd
Example of Checklist of Key Patient and Family Knowledge and Skills following Lower Limb Amputation

Activity:		*Indicator*
	____	Individual is able to transfer sit to single limb standing and return Level of assistance Equipment used
	____	Individual is able to transfer to toilet and return Level of assistance Equipment used
	____	Individual is able to transfer to shower or tub and return Level of assistance Equipment used
Locomotion	____	Individual is able to ambulate on level surfaces using appropriate assistive device Level of assistance Assistive/ambulatory device used Gait Pattern Distance Perceived exertion
	____	Individual is able to ascend/descend stairs using railing and appropriate assistive device Level of assistance Assistive/ambulatory device used Pattern Number of steps Perceived exertion
	____	Individual is able to ambulate on inclines and outdoor surfaces Level of assistance Assistive/ambulatory device used Gait pattern Distance Perceived exertion
	____	Individual/caregiver is able to safely propel wheelchair functional distances Level of assistance Distance Perceived exertion
Self-care activities	____	Individual is able to manage clothing during ADL and dressing activities Level of assistance Positions Adaptive equipment needs Perceived exertion
	____	Individual is able to manage bathing and grooming activities Level of assistance Positions Adaptive Equipment needs Perceived exertion
	____	Individual is able to manage key IADL activities Level of assistance Types of activities Adaptive Equipment needs Perceived exertion
	____	Sufficient and safe transportation is available Type of transportation Level of assistance Equipment used Perceived exertion

Continued

Table 23-3—cont'd
Example of Checklist of Key Patient and Family Knowledge and Skills following Lower Limb Amputation

Activity:	*Indicator*	
Exercise program	____	Individual and caregiver demonstrate mastery of stretching/flexibility component of program Positions/activities Assistance required Equipment used Repetitions and frequency
	____	Individual and caregiver demonstrate mastery of strengthening component of program Positions/activities Assistance required Equipment used Repetitions and frequency
	____	Individual and caregiver demonstrate mastery of aerobic conditioning component of program Positions/activities Assistance required Equipment used Repetitions and frequency
	____	Individual and caregiver demonstrate mastery of balance/coordination components of program Positions/activities Assistance required Equipment used Repetitions and frequency
Follow-up care	____	Plans for return to surgeon for post-op visit are in place
	____	Plans for continued rehabilitation care are in place
	____	Additional services are in place as appropriate Nursing Dietician Counseling Home health Others

CASE EXAMPLE 1B

Interventions for N. H., an 89-Year-Old with "Elective" Transtibial Amputation

N. H. is now 4 days postsurgery, and her delirium is clearing. She is conversing with her typical sense of humor with family and staff. Her casted fiberglass rigid dressing was removed yesterday; the surgical wound is draining moderate amounts of serosanguineous fluid; edges are closely approximate. An area of pressure-related abrasion and inflammation at the anterior distal tibia was noted when the cast was removed; granulation is now evident. N. H. can transfer to a bedside chair with moderate assistance of one person, with noted moderate impairment of postural control. N. H. tolerates being up in a bedside chair for 45 minutes. She rates her postoperative pain as 4/10, except at dressing change, when it increases to 6/10. She laughs but feels concern that she feels mild cramping in the instep of the limb that is no longer there, wanting to stretch her foot and toes into dorsiflexion to relieve her discomfort. She is somewhat reluctant to look at or to touch her residual limb, but does not mind if nurses, physicians, or PT staff handle it during dressing changes or functional activities. She transferred sitting to standing with a walker at bedside with moderate assistance of one person, complaining of dizziness after standing for more than a minute and requesting to return to sitting. She tells you that she is "ready to get going" and wants to return to her own home to use her wheelchair as soon as possible.

Questions to Consider

- Given her postoperative pain and phantom sensation, what physical therapy interventions would be appropriate at this time for N. H.? Why would these be most appropriate from among available options? What are the pros and cons of each, with respect to attention, memory, and ability to learn?

- Given the status of her wound and condition of her residual limb, what strategies for management of edema and limb shaping would you recommend? What are the pros and cons that you considered when deciding among options for compression and residual limb protection? Why do you think the option you selected is the most appropriate? How would this be similar or different if her amputation was at the transfemoral level?
- What strategies for intervention and patient-family education would you implement for skin care and scar management for N. H.? What issues or factors will assist or inhibit her ability to take responsibility for her skin care?
- What specific strategies for intervention and patient-family education aimed at ROM and flexibility do you recommend for N. H.? What impairments or functional limitations are you particularly concerned about for N. H.? What activities will you engage her in? What positions? For what period of time? With what equipment? What would you emphasize if her amputation was at a transfemoral level? What issues or factors will assist or inhibit her ability to take responsibility for exercises aimed at ensuring adequate ROM and flexibility in preparation for prosthetic use?
- What specific strategies for intervention and patient-family education aimed at improving muscle performance do your recommend for N. H.? How do you address strengthening of key muscle groups of extremities and trunk? How do you address power and muscle endurance? How do you address concentric, isometric, and eccentric control and performance? What issues or factors must be considered regarding exercise tolerance, intensity, frequency, and duration during her acute care stay? How will you address her concerns about her low level of aerobic fitness and conditioning?
- What specific strategies for intervention and patient-family education aimed at improving static, dynamic, and reactionary postural control during functional activities do you recommend for N. H.? During which activities is postural control most likely to be problematic? What apparatus, equipment, and activities might you use to assist her postural control?
- What are your concerns about seating and wheelchair mobility for N. H.? Do you think that a standard wheelchair will adequately meet her needs? Do you think she will be able to propel her chair? What tasks does she need to master if the wheelchair will be her primary source of mobility during the preprosthetic period?
- What types of bed mobility and transfer activities are important for N. H. and her family caregivers to master? What specific intervention and patient-family education strategies will you use to help her move toward safe and, hopefully, independent performance of bed mobility and transfer activities? How will you vary environmental conditions and task demands to ensure that she can adapt her strategies and skills?
- What strategies for intervention and patient-family education will you use to get her up and walking? What assistive or ambulatory device do you feel would be most appropriate? Why have you chosen this particular device from among available options? What gait pattern will she use? For what other dimensions or ambulatory skills (in addition to walking forward) will you provide instruction and opportunity for N. H. to practice? How will you address the likelihood that she will experience a fall at some point in her preprosthetic period? What is "functional distance" for ambulation for N. H. and her family?
- Are there any additional interventions that would be appropriate for N. H. at this point in her postoperative, preprosthetic rehabilitation?
- How will you determine her readiness for prosthetic fitting?

CASE EXAMPLE 2C

Interventions for P. G., an Individual with Recent Amputation of Both Lower Extremities following a Construction Accident

Now 3 days postoperation, P. G. is beginning his rehabilitation in preparation for discharge to home until there is adequate healing for prosthetic fitting and prosthetic training. Pain continues to be a serious concern, generally reported as 5 or 6/10 on the visual analog scale. Postoperative agitation has cleared, although P. G.'s wife reports he is more subdued in affect than usual, and she is concerned about possible depression. Low-grade temperature persists, but white cell counts are within normal limits. P. G. can actively flex and extend both knees to within 10 degrees of full ROM, with effort and a "tight pulling sensation" behind the knee, when out of semirigid dressings for dressing changes and wound inspection. Although he reports feeling "weak as a baby" and is quickly fatigued, P. G. can use upper extremity and body strength for contact guard sliding board transfers to and from bed to a bedside chair. Moving between sitting and supine is effortful and fatiguing, but P. G. manages these transitions with occasional standby assistance. He was previously involved in both aerobic and strengthening exercise at the local YMCA, but he is not sure how to use the weights and equipment now that he has lost his limbs. Plans are being made to move temporarily to his parent's home, on the first floor of a three-family house (although there are six steps to reach a front porch and entryway), as it is more accessible than his third-floor walk-up apartment. In the meantime, family and friends are apartment hunting for housing that will be less challenging for P. G. in the months ahead. P. G.'s major goal is to achieve independent mobility with a wheelchair before the birth of his child.

Questions to Consider

- Given his postoperative pain and phantom sensation, what PT interventions would be appropriate at this time for P. G.? Why would these be most appropriate from among available options? What are the pros and cons of each, with respect to attention, memory, and ability to learn?
- Given the status of his wound and condition of his residual limb, what strategies for management of edema and limb shaping would you recommend? What are the pros and cons that you considered when deciding among options for compression and residual limb protection? Why do you think the option you selected is the most appropriate? How would this change if his amputations were at the transfemoral level?
- What strategies for intervention and patient-family education would you implement for skin care and scar management for P. G.? What issues or factors will assist or inhibit his ability to take responsibility for his skin care?
- What specific strategies for intervention and patient-family education aimed at ROM and flexibility do you recommend for P. G.? What impairments or functional limitations are you particularly concerned about for P. G.? What activities will you engage him in? What positions? For what period of time? With what equipment? How would these be similar or different if his amputations were at the transfemoral level? What issues or factors will assist or inhibit his ability to take responsibility for exercises aimed at insuring adequate ROM and flexibility in preparation for prosthetic use?
- What specific strategies for intervention and patient-family education aimed at improving muscle performance do you recommend for P. G.? How do you address strengthening of key muscle groups of extremities and trunk? How do you address power and muscle endurance? How do you address concentric, isometric, and eccentric control and performance? How would this be similar or different if his amputations were at the transfemoral level? What issues or factors must be considered regarding exercise tolerance, intensity, frequency, and duration during his acute care stay? How will you address his concerns about low level of aerobic fitness and conditioning?
- What specific strategies for intervention and patient-family education aimed at improving static, dynamic, and reactionary postural control during functional activities do you recommend for P. G.? During which activities is postural control most likely to be problematic? What apparatus, equipment, and activities might you use to assist his postural control?
- What are your concerns about seating and wheelchair mobility for P. G.? Do you think that a standard wheelchair will adequately meet his needs? Do you think he will be able to propel his chair? What tasks does he need to master if the wheelchair will be his primary source of mobility during the preprosthetic period?
- What additional bed mobility and transfer activities do you think are important for P. G. and his family caregivers to master? What specific intervention and patient-family education strategies will you use to help him move toward safe and, hopefully, independent performance of bed mobility and transfer activities? How will you vary environmental conditions and task demands to ensure that he can adapt his strategies and skills?
- How will you address the likelihood that he will experience a fall at some point in his preprosthetic period?
- Are there any additional interventions that would be appropriate for P. G. at this point in his postoperative, preprosthetic rehabilitation to assist with his coping and adjustment to his limb loss?
- How will you determine his readiness for prosthetic fitting?

SUMMARY

Early rehabilitation in the postoperative preprosthetic period lays the foundation for prosthetic rehabilitation. Initial emphasis is placed on wound healing and control of edema, essential prerequisites for prosthetic use. Early in the process, the individual with new amputation and family caregivers become actively involved in the rehabilitation process and decision making, assuming responsibility for limb compression, skin care, and desensitization. The therapist is alert for postoperative medical complications such as postural hypotension or deep venous thrombosis, as early mobility begins. The therapist implements strategies to prevent secondary impairments and functional limitations such as further deconditioning and contracture formation. Strengthening exercises, targeting the residual limb and overall fitness, begin in the acute or subacute setting and continue as an aggressive home program to prepare the individual for prosthetic training. Persons with new amputation are encouraged to become as independent as possible in transfers, single limb gait, and wheelchair mobility, depending on their medical status and functional capability. As the wound heals and edema subsides, the individual with new amputation, family caregivers, therapist, prosthetist, and physician begin discussion about future prosthetic rehabilitation. The postoperative, preprosthetic period is a time of transition in which many individuals mourn the loss of their limb and question their future yet are challenged and encouraged by the possibilities offered by prosthetic replacement of their limb. If the consensus is that prosthetic fitting is not viable, emphasis shifts to development of wheelchair mobility skills and adaptation of the patient's environment as rehabilitation continues.

REFERENCES

1. Racy JC. Psychological adaptation to amputation. In Smith DG, Michael JW, Bowker JH (eds), *Atlas of Amputation and Limb Deficiencies: Surgical, Prosthetic, and Rehabilitation Principles,* 3rd ed. Rosemont, IL: American Academy of Orthopaedic Surgeons, 2004. pp. 727-738.
2. May BJ. Amputation and prosthetics, then and now. In May BJ (ed), *Amputation and Prosthetics: A Case Study Approach.* Philadelphia: F.A. Davis, 2002. pp. 1-15.
3. Smith DG. General principles of amputation surgery. In Smith DG, Michael JW, Bowker JH (eds), *Atlas of Amputation and Limb Deficiencies: Surgical, Prosthetic, and Rehabilitation Principles,* 3rd ed. Rosemont, IL: American Academy of Orthopaedic Surgeons, 2004. pp. 21-30.
4. May BJ. Post surgical management. In *Amputation and Prosthetics: A Case Study Approach,* 2nd ed. Philadelphia: F.A. Davis, 2002. pp. 74-108.
5. Bowker JH. The art of prosthesis prescription. In Smith DG, Michael JW, Bowker JH (eds), *Atlas of Amputation and Limb Deficiencies: Surgical, Prosthetic, and Rehabilitation Principles,* 3rd ed. Rosemont, IL: American Academy of Orthopaedic Surgeons, 2004. pp. 739-744.
6. Strasser DC, Falconer JA, Martino-Saltzman D. The rehabilitation team: staff perceptions of the hospital environment, the interdisciplinary team environment, and interprofessional relations. *Arch Phys Med Rehabil* 1994; 75(2):177-182.
7. Who are physical therapists, and what do they do? In *The Guide to Physical Therapist Practice,* 2nd ed. Originally published in *Phys Ther* 2001;81(1):39-50.
8. Sackett DL, Strauss SE, Richardson WS, et al. *Evidence-Based Medicine: How to Practice and Teach EBM,* 2nd ed. Philadelphia: Churchill Livingstone, 2000.
9. Spector RE. *Cultural Diversity in Health and Illness,* 6th ed. Saddle River, NJ: Prentice-Hall, 2003.
10. Horgan O, MacLachlan M. Psychosocial adjustment to lower limb amputation: a review. *Disabil Rehabil* 2004;26(14/15):837-850.
11. Kail RV, Cavenaugh JC. *Human Development: A Lifespan View,* 2nd ed. Belmont, Calif.: Wadsworth, 2003.
12. Anderson SA, Sabatelli RN. *Family Interaction: A Multigenerational Developmental Perspective,* 3rd ed. Upper Saddle River, N.J.: Allyn & Bacon, 2002.
13. Taira ED, Carlso JL. *Aging in Place: Designing, Adapting and Enhancing the Home Environment.* Binghamton, N.Y.: Haworth Press, 2000.
14. Miller JF. *Coping with Chronic Illness: Overcoming Powerlessness,* 3rd ed. Philadelphia: F.A. Davis, 1999.
15. Frugoli BA, Guion WK, Joyner BA, et al. Cardiovascular disease risk factors in an amputee population. *J Prosthet Orthot* 2000;12(3):80-87.
16. Stewart CR, Jain AS. Cause of death in lower limb amputees. *Prosthet Orthot Int* 1992;16(2):129-132.
17. Medhat A, Huber PM, Medhat MA. Factors that influence the level of activities in persons with lower extremity amputation. *Rehabil Nurs* 1990;15(1):13-18.
18. Gauthier-Gagnon C, Griese MC, Potvin D. Predisposing factors related to prosthetic use by people with transtibial and transfemoral amputation. *J Prosthet Orthot* 1998;10(4):99-109.
19. Fung DL. Post operative pain. In Gershwin ME, Hamilton ME, Gershwin E (eds), *The Pain Management Handbook: A Concise Guide to Diagnosis and Treatment.* Totowa, NJ: Humana, 1998. pp. 239-260.
20. Powles AC. The effect of drugs on the cardiovascular response to exercise. *Med Sci Sports Exerc* 1981;13(4):252-258.
21. Freter SH, Dunbar MJ, MacLeaod H, et al. Predicting post-operative delirium in elective orthopaedic patients: the Delirium Elderly at Risk (DEAR) Instrument. *Age Ageing* 2005;34(2):169-171.
22. Boissonnault WG, Umphred DA. Differential diagnosis phase 1: medical screening for the therapist. In Umphred DA (ed), *Neurological Rehabilitation*, 4th ed. St. Louis: Mosby; 2001. pp. 31-42.
23. What type of tests and measures do physical therapists use? In *The Guide to Physical Therapist Practice,* 2nd ed. Originally published in *Phys Ther* 2001;81(1):51-103.
24. *Acute Pain Management: Operative or Medical Procedures and Trauma. Clinical Practice Guideline. AHCPR Pub. No. 92-0032.* Rockville, MD: Agency for Health Care Policy and Research, Public Health Service, US Department of Health and Human Services, February 1992.
25. Houghton AD, Nicholls G, Houghton AL, et al. Phantom pain: natural history and association with rehabilitation. *Ann R Coll Surg Engl* 1994;76(1):22-25.
26. Melzack R. Phantom limbs. *Sci Am* 1992;266(4):120-126.
27. Wartan SW, Hamann W, Wedley JR, et al. Phantom pain and sensation among British veteran amputees. *Br J Anaesth* 1997;78(6):652-659.
28. Sherman RA. Limb pain and stump blood circulation. *Orthopaedics* 1984;7(8):1319-1320.
29. Jensen TS, Krebs B, Nielsen J, et al. Immediate and long term phantom limb pain in amputees: incidence, clinical characteristics, and relationships to pre-amputation limb pain. *Pain* 1985;21(3):267-278.
30. Mouratoglou VM. Amputees and phantom limb pain: a literature review. *Physiother Pract* 1986;2(4):177-180.
31. Sherman RA, Ernst JL, Barja RH, et al. Phantom limb pain: a lesson in the necessity for careful clinical research on chronic pain problems. *J Rehabil Res Dev* 1988;25(2): viii-x.
32. Castronuovo JJ, Deane LJ, Deterling RA Jr, et al. Below knee amputation: is the effort to preserve the knee joint justified? *Arch Surg* 1980;115(10):1184-1187.
33. Hagberg K, Branemark R. Consequences of non-vascular trans-femoral amputation: a survey of quality of life, prosthetic use and problems. *Prosthet Orthot Int* 2001;25(3):186-194.

34. Bowker JH. Transtibial amputation: Surgical management. In Smith DG, Michaels JW, Bowker JH (eds), *Atlas of Amputation and Limb Deficiencies: Surgical, Prosthetic, and Rehabilitation Principles,* 3rd ed. Rosemont, IL: American Academy of Orthopaedic Surgeons, 2004. pp. 481-501.
35. Meyers BA. Wound healing. In *Wound Management: Principles and Practice.* Upper Saddle River, NJ: Prentice-Hall, 2004. pp. 9-22.
36. Kapp SL, Fergason JR. Transtibial amputation: prosthetic management. In Smith DG, Michaels JW, Bowker JH (eds), *Atlas of Amputation and Limb Deficiencies: Surgical, Prosthetic, and Rehabilitation Principles,* 3rd ed. Rosemont, IL: American Academy of Orthopaedic Surgeons; 2004. pp. 503-515.
37. Wagner WH, Keagy BA, Kotb MM, et al. Noninvasive determination of healing of major lower extremity amputation: the continued role of clinical judgment. *J Vasc Surg* 1988;8(6):703-710.
38. Barnes RW, Cox B. Below knee amputation. In *Amputations: An illustrated Manual.* Philadelphia: Hanley & Belfus, 2000. pp. 67-86.
39. Frantz RA, Gardner S. Elderly skin care: principles of chronic wound care. *J Gerontol Nurs* 1994;20(9):35-45.
40. Myers BA. Miscellaneous wounds. In *Wound Management: Principles and Practice,* Upper Saddle River, NJ: Prentice-Hall, 2004. pp. 356-368.
41. Pedersen NW, Pedersen D. Nutrition as a prognostic indicator in amputations. *Acta Orthop Scand* 1992;63(6):675-678.
42. Perry J. Amputee gait. In Smith DG, Michaels JW, Bowker JH (eds), *Atlas of Amputation and Limb Deficiencies: Surgical, Prosthetic, and Rehabilitation Principles,* 3rd ed. Rosemont, IL: American Academy of Orthopaedic Surgeons, 2004. pp. 367-384.
43. Gottschalk F. Transfemoral amputation: surgical management. In Smith DG, Michaels JW, Bowker JH (eds), *Atlas of Amputation and Limb Deficiencies: Surgical, Prosthetic, and Rehabilitation Principles,* 3rd ed. Rosemont, IL: American Academy of Orthopaedic Surgeons, 2004. pp. 533-540.
44. Uellendahl JE. Bilateral lower limb prosthesis. In Smith DG, Michaels JW, Bowker JH (eds), *Atlas of Amputation and Limb Deficiencies: Surgical, Prosthetic, and Rehabilitation Principles,* 3rd ed. Rosemont, IL: American Academy of Orthopaedic Surgeons, 2004. pp. 621-632.
45. Hoppenfeld S. Physical examination of the knee. In *Physical Examination of the Spine and Extremities.* Norwalk, CT: Appleton & Lange, 1976. pp. 171-196.
46. Magee DJ. *Knee in Orthopedic Physical Assessment,* 4th ed. Philadelphia: Saunders, 2002.
47. Kendall FP, McCreary EK, Provance PG, et al. *Muscles: Testing and Function,* 5th ed. Philadelphia: Lippincott Williams & Wilkins, 2005.
48. O'Sullivan SB. Assessment of motor function. In O'Sullivan SB, Schmitz TJ (eds), *Physical Rehabilitation: Assessment and Treatment,* 4th ed. Philadelphia: F.A. Davis, 2001. pp. 177-212.
49. Lusardi MM. Tremors, chorea, and other involuntary movements. In Kaufmann TL (ed), *Geriatric Rehabilitation Manual.* New York: Churchill Livingstone, 1999. pp. 155-164.
50. Pauda L, Saponara C, Ghirlanda G, et al. Lower limb nerve impairment in diabetic patients: multiperspective assessment. *Eur J Neurol* 2002;9(1):69-73.
51. Umphred DA. The limbic system: influence over motor control and learning. In Umphred DA (ed), *Neurological Rehabilitation,* 4th ed. St. Louis: Mosby, 2001. pp. 149-177.
52. Borg G, Domserius M, Kaijser L. Psychophysical scaling with applications in physical work and the perception of exertions. *Scand J Work Environ Health* 1990;16(Suppl 1):55-58.
53. Borg GA. Psychosocial bases of perceived exertions, basis of perceived exertion. *Med Sci Sports Exerc* 1982;14(5): 377-387.
54. Davidoff GN, Lampman RM, Westbury L, et al. Exercise testing and training in persons with dysvascular amputation: safety and efficacy of arm ergometry. *Arch Phys Med Rehabil* 1992;73(4):334-338.
55. Finestone HM, Lapman RM, Davidoff GN, et al. Arm ergometry exercise testing in patients with dysvascular amputations. *Arch Phys Med Rehabil* 1991;72(1):15-19.
56. Ness J, Aronow WS, Newkirk E, et al. Prevalence of symptomatic peripheral arterial disease, modifiable risk factors, and appropriate use of drugs in the treatment of peripheral arterial disease in older persons seen in a university general medicine clinic. *J Gerontol A Biol Sci Med Sci* 2005;60(2):255-257.
57. Rabins PV, Folstein MF. The dementia patient: evaluation and care. *Geriatrics* 1983;38(8):99-103.
58. Crum RM, Anthony JC, Bassett SS, et al. Population based norms for the Mini Mental State Examination by age and educational level. *JAMA* 1993;269(18):2386-2391.
59. Jackson-Wyatt O. Brain function, aging, and dementia. In Umphred DA (ed), *Neurological Rehabilitation,* 4th ed. St. Louis: Mosby, 2001. pp. 790-816.
60. Rohling ML, Scogin F. Automatic and effortful memory processing in depressed persons. *J Gerontol* 1993;48(2): P87-P95.
61. Patten C, Craik RL. Sensorimotor changes and adaptation in the older adult. In Guccione AA (ed), *Geriatric Rehabilitation,* 2nd ed. St. Louis: Mosby, 2000. pp. 78-109.
62. Wharton MA. Environmental design: accommodating sensory changes in the elderly. In Guccione AA (ed), *Geriatric Rehabilitation,* 2nd ed. St. Louis: Mosby, 2000. pp. 134-149.
63. Mueller MJ. Identifying patients with diabetes mellitus who are at risk for lower extremity complications. *Phys Ther* 1996;76(1):68-71.
64. Schmitz TJ. Sensory assessment. In Sullivan SB, Schmitz TJ (eds), *Physical Rehabilitation: Assessment and Treatment,* 4th ed. Philadelphia: F.A. Davis, 2001. pp. 133-156.
65. Ross RT. *How to Examine the Nervous System,* 3rd ed. Stamford, CT: Appleton Lange; 1999.
66. Norris J, Spelic SS. Supporting adaptation to body image disruption. *Rehabil Nurs* 2002;27(1):8-12.
67. Moore TJ, Barron J, Hutchinson F, et al. Prosthetic usage following major lower extremity amputation. *Clin Orthop* 1989;Jan(248):227-230.
68. Munin MC, Espejo-DeGuzman MC, Boninger ML, et al. Predictive factors for successful early prosthetic ambulation among lower-limb amputates. *J Rehabil Res Devel* 2001;38(4):379-384.
69. McGuire TL. Performance-based measures following transtibial amputation: a case report. *Topics Geriatr Rehabil* 2004;20(4):262-272.

70. Burger H, Marincek C. Functional testing of elderly subjects after lower limb amputation. *Prosthet Orthot Int* 2001;25(2):102-107.
71. Miller WC, Deathe AB, Speechley M. Psychometric properties of the Activities Specific Balance Confidence Scale among individuals with a lower limb amputation. *Arch Phys Med Rehabil* 2003;84(5):656-661.
72. Allison L, Fuller K. Balance and vestibular disorders. In Umphred DA (ed), *Neurological Rehabilitation,* 4th ed. St. Louis: Mosby, 2001. pp. 616-660.
73. Levangie PK, Norton C. Joint structure and function, 4th ed. Philadelphia, F.A. Davis, 2005.
74. Moncur C. Posture in the older adult. In Guccione AA (ed), *Geriatric Physical Therapy.* St. Louis: Mosby, 2000. pp. 265-279.
75. Woolf AD, Pfleger B. Burden of major musculoskeletal conditions. *Bull World Health Organization* 2003;81(9): 646-656.
76. Leung EC, Rush PJ, Devlin M. Predicting prosthetic rehabilitation outcome in lower limb amputee patients with the Functional Independence Measure. *Arch Phys Med Rehabil* 1996;77(6):605-608.
77. *Guide to physical therapist practice.* Alexandria, VA: American Physical Therapy Association, 2001.
78. Jette AM, Assmann SF. Interrelationships among disablement concepts. *J Gerontol* 1998;53A(5):M395-404.
79. On what concepts is the guide based? Guide to Physical Therapy Practice, *Phys Ther* 2001;83(1):27-36.
80. Muecke L, Shekar S, Dwyer D, et al. Functional screening of lower-limb amputees: a role in predicting rehabilitation outcome? *Arch Phys Med Rehabil* 1992;73(9):851-858.
81. Pinzur MS, Gottschalk F, Smith D, et al. Functional outcome of below knee amputation in peripheral vascular insufficiency: a multi-center study. *Clin Orthop* 1993;Jan(286):247-249.
82. Hubbard WA. Rehabilitation outcomes for elderly lower limb amputees. *Aust J Physiother* 1989; 35(4):219-224.
83. Stewart CP, Jain AS. Cause of death in lower limb amputees. *Prosthet Orthot Int* 1992;16(2):129-132.
84. Ham R, de Trafford J, Van de Ven C. Patterns of recovery for lower limb amputations. *Clin Rehabil* 1994;8(4):320-328.
85. Gailey RS, Clark CR. Physical therapy. In Smith DG, Michaels JW, Bowker JH (eds), *Atlas of Amputation and Limb Deficiencies: Surgical, Prosthetic, and Rehabilitation Principles,* 3rd ed. Rosemont, IL: American Academy of Orthopaedic Surgeons, 2004. pp. 589-619.
86. Ciccone CD. Geriatric pharmacology. In Guccione AA (ed), *Geriatric Rehabilitation,* 3rd ed. St. Louis: Mosby, 2001. pp. 182-208.
87. Bach S, Noreng MF, Tjellden NU. Phantom limb pain in amputees during the first 12 months following limb amputation, after preoperative lumbar epidural blockage. *Pain* 1988;33(3):297-301.
88. Halbert J, Crotty M, Cameron ID. Evidence for the optimal management of acute and chronic phantom pain: a systematic review. *Clin J Pain* 2002;18(2):84-92.
89. Danshaw CB. An anesthetic approach to amputation and pain syndromes. *Phys Med Rehabil Clin North Am* 2000;11(3):553-557.
90. Lambert AW, Dashfield AK, Cosgrove C, et al. Randomized prospective study comparing preoperative epidural and intraoperative perineural analgesia for the prevention of post-operative stump and phantom limb pain following major amputation. *Reg Anesth Pain Med* 2001;26(4):316-321.
91. Elizaga AM, Smith DG, Sharar SR, et al. Continuous regional analgesia by intraneural block; effect on post-operative opioid requirements and phantom pain following amputation. *J Rehabil Res Dev* 1994;31(3):179-187.
92. Leskowitz ED. Phantom limb pain treated with therapeutic touch: a case report. *Arch Phys Med Rehabil* 2000;81(4): 522-524.
93. Kuiken T. Perioperative rehabilitation of the transtibial and transfemoral amputee. *Phys Med Rehabil State Art Rev* 2002; 16(3):521-537.
94. Salim M. Transcutaneous electrical nerve stimulation in phantom limb pain. *Altern Ther Clin Pract* 1997;4(4): 135-137.
95. Long D. Fifteen years of transcutaneous electrical stimulation for pain control. *Stereotact Funct Neurosurg* 1991;56(1):2-19.
96. Mirabella-Susans L. Pain management. In Umphred DA (ed), *Neurological Rehabilitation,* 4th ed. St. Louis: Mosby, 2001. pp. 889–912.
97. Edelstein JE. Preprosthetic management of patients with lower- or upper-limb amputation. *Prosthet Phys Med Rehabil Clin North Am* 1991;2(2):285-297.
98. Golderg T, Goldberd S, Pollack J. Postoperative management of lower extremity amputation. *Phys Med Rehabil Clin North Am* 2000;11(3):559-568.
99. Slayton SA. Early post-operative prosthesis training in a below knee amputee with diabetes mellitus: a case report. *Acute Care Perspect* 2004;13(4):5-9.
100. Choudhury SR, Reiber GE, Pecoraro JA, et al. Postoperative management of transtibial amputation in VA Hospitals. *J Rehabil Res Devel* 2001;38(3):293-298.
101. Harrington IJ, Lexier R, Woods J, et al. A plaster-pylon technique for below knee amputation. *J Bone Joint Surg* 1991;73(1):76-78.
102. Burgess EM. Immediate postsurgical prosthetic fitting; a system of amputee management. *Phys Ther* 1971;51(2): 139-143.
103. Walsh TL. Custom removable immediate postoperative prosthesis. *J Prosthet Orthot* 2003;15(4):158-161.
104. Pinzur MS, Littcoy F, Osterman H, et al. A safe, prefabricated immediate postoperative prosthetic limb system for rehabilitation of below knee amputations. *Orthopedics* 1989;12(10):1343-1345.
105. May BJ. Assessment and treatment for individuals following lower extremity amputation. In O'Sullivan SB, Schmitz TK (eds), *Physical Rehabilitation: Assessment and Treatment,* 4th ed. Philadelphia: F.A. Davis, 2001. pp. 619-644.
106. Woodburn KR, Sockalingham S, Gilmore H, et al. A randomized trial of rigid stump dressing following trans-tibial amputation for peripheral arterial insufficiency. *Prosthet Orthot Int* 2004;28(1):22-27.
107. Smith DG, McFarland LV, Sangeorzan BJ, et al. Postoperative dressing and management strategies for transtibial amputations: a critical review. *J Rehabil Res Dev* 2003; 40(3):213-224.
108. Folsom D, King T, Rubin JR. Lower extremity amputation with immediate postoperative prosthetic placement. *Am J Surg* 1992;164(4):320-322.

109. Mooney V, Harvey IP, McBride E, et al. Comparison of postoperative stump management: plaster vs. soft dressings. *J Bone Joint Surg* 1971;53A(2):241-249.
110. Wu Y, Krick H. Removable rigid dressing for below-knee amputees. *Clin Prosthet Orthop* 1987;23(1):452-456.
111. Wu Y. An innovative removable rigid dressing technique for below knee amputation. *J Bone Joint Surg Am* 1979;61(5): 724-729.
112. Mueller M. Comparison of removable rigid dressings and elastic bandages in preprosthetic management of patients with below-knee amputations. *Phys Ther* 1982;62(10): 1438-1441.
113. Palma T, Owens L, Jennings S. *Removable rigid dressing protocol.* Hartford, CT: Department of Rehabilitation, Hartford Hospital, 1990.
114. Wu Y. Removable rigid dressings for residual limb management. Appendix D. In Karacoloff LA, Hammersley CS, Schneider FJ (eds), *Lower Extremity Amputation: A Guide to Functional Outcomes in Physical Therapy Management. Rehabilitation Institute of Chicago Procedure Manual.* Gaithersburg, MD: Aspen, 1992. pp. 241-248.
115. Swanson VM. Below knee polyethylene semirigid dressing. *J Prosthet Orthot* 1993;5(1):10-15.
116. Post-amputation care options. In *Prosthetic and Orthotic Currents, Newsletter of Newington Prosthetics and Orthotic Systems, Inc.* Newington, CT, Spring 1995.
117. Maclean N, Fick GH. The effect of semirigid dressings on below knee amputations. *Phys Ther* 1994;74(7):668-673.
118. Sterescu LE. Semi-rigid (Unna) dressing for amputation. *Arch Phys Med Rehabil* 1974;55(9):433-434.
119. Wong CK. Unna and elastic post-operative dressings: comparison of their effects on function of adults with amputation and vascular disease. *Arch Phys Med Rehabil* 2000;81(9):1191-1198.
120. Seymour R. Clinical use of dressings and bandages. In Seymour R (ed), *Prosthetics and Orthotics: Lower Limb and Spinal.* Philadelphia: Lippincott Williams & Wilkins, 2002. pp. 123-142.
121. Muilenburg AL, Wilson AB. *A Manual for Below-Knee Amputees,* 4th ed. Alexandria, VA: American Academy of Orthotists and Prosthetists, 1993.
122. Rausch RW, Khalili AA. Air splint in pre-prosthetic rehabilitation of lower extremity amputated limbs: a clinical report. *Phys Ther* 1985;63(6):912-914.
123. Barraclough BH, Coupland GA, Reeve TS. Air splints used as immediate post operative prostheses after long posterior flap below knee amputation. *Med J Aust* 1972;2(14): 764-767.
124. Little JM. The use of air splints as immediate prostheses after below knee amputation for vascular insufficiency. *Med J Aust* 1970;2(19):870-872.
125. Bonner FJ, Green RF. Pneumatic airleg prosthesis: report of 200 cases. *Arch Phys Med Rehabil* 1982;63(8):383-385.
126. Boucher HR, Low C, Schon MD, et al. A biomechanical study of two postoperative prostheses for transtibial amputees: a custom molded and a prefabricated adjustable pneumatic prosthesis. *Foot Ankle Int* 2002;23(5):452-456.
127. Gailey RS, Gailey AM. *Stretching and Strengthening for Lower Extremity Amputees.* Miami: Advanced Rehabilitation Therapy; 1994.
128. Seymour R. Development of an exercise/functional program. In Seymour R (ed), *Prosthetics and Orthotics: Lower Limb and Spinal.* Philadelphia: Lippincott Williams & Wilkins, 2002. pp. 143-174.
129. Karacoloff LA, Mannersley CS, Snchneider FJ (eds). *Lower Extremity Amputation: A Guide to Functional Outcomes in Physical Therapy Management,* 2nd ed. Austin, TX: Pro-Ed, 2005.
130. Berger N, Edelstein JE, Fishman S, et al. *Lower-Limb Prosthetics.* New York: Prosthetics and Orthotics, New York University, Post Graduate Medical School, 1987.
131. Shurr DG, Cook TM. Above knee amputation and prosthetics. In Schurr DG, Cook TM (eds), *Prosthetics and Orthotics.* Norwalk, CT: Appleton & Lange, 1990. pp. 83-116.
132. Jaegers S, Hans Arendzen J, deJongh HJ. Changes in hip muscles after above-knee amputation. *Clin Orthop* 1995;Oct(319):276-284.
133. Gossman M, Sahrmann S, Rose S. Review of length-associated change in muscle. *Phys Ther* 1982;62(12):1799-1808.
134. Kegel B, Burgess EM, Starr TW, et al. Effects of isometric muscle training on residual limb volume, strength, and gait of below knee amputees. *Phys Ther* 1981;61(10):1419-1426.
135. Kisner C, Colby LA. Therapeutic exercise: foundations and techniques, 2nd ed. Philadelphia: Harper & Row, 1993.
136. Davies GJ. *A Compendium of Isokinetics in Clinical Usage and Rehabilitation Techniques,* 2nd ed. LaCrosse, WI: S&S, 1985.
137. Gailey RS, Clark CR. Physical therapy. In Smith DG, Michael JW, Bowker JH (eds), *Atlas of Amputation and Limb Deficiencies: Surgical, Prosthetic, and Rehabilitation Principles,* 3rd ed. Rosemont, IL: American Academy of Orthopaedic Surgeons, 2004. pp. 589-620.
138. Adler SS, Beckers D, Buck M. *PNF in Practice: an Illustrated Guide,* 2nd ed. New York: Springer, 2000.
139. Voss DE, Ionta MK, Myers BJ. *Proprioceptive neuromuscular facilitation patterns and techniques,* 3rd ed. Philadelphia: Lippincott Williams & Wilkins, 1985.
140. Burger H, Valencic V, Marincek C, et al. Properties of musculus gluteus maximus in above-knee amputees. *Clin Biomech* 1996;11(1):35.
141. Kirby RL, Chari VR. Prostheses and the forward reach of sitting lower-limb amputees. *Arch Phys Med Rehabil* 1990;71(2):125-127.
142. Waters RL, Perry J, Antonelli D, et al. Energy cost of walking of amputees: influence of level of amputation. *J Bone Joint Surg* 1976;58(1):42-46.
143. Waters RL, Mulroy SJ. Energy expenditure of walking in individuals with lower limb amputations. In Smith DG, Michael JW, Bowker JH (eds), *Atlas of Amputation and Limb Deficiencies: Surgical, Prosthetic, and Rehabilitation Principles,* 3rd ed. Rosemont, IL: American Academy of Orthopaedic Surgeons, 2004. pp. 395-407.
144. DuBow LL, Witt PL, Kadaba MP, et al. Oxygen consumption of elderly persons with bilateral below knee amputations: ambulation versus wheelchair propulsion. *Arch Phys Med Rehabil* 1983;64(6):255-259.
145. Wu Y, Chen S, Lin M, et al. Energy expenditure of wheeling and walking during prosthetic rehabilitation in a woman with bilateral transfemoral amputations. *Arch Phys Med Rehabil* 2001;82(2):265-269.

146. Czerniecki JM, Harrington RM, Wyss CR. The effects of age and peripheral vascular disease on the circulatory and mechanical response of skin to loading. *Am J Phys Med Rehabil* 1990;69(6):302-306.
147. Mueller MJ, Sinacore DR, Hoogstrate S, et al. Hip and ankle walking strategies: effect of peak plantar pressures and implications for neuropathic ulceration. *Arch Phys Med Rehabil* 1994;75(11):1196-1200.
148. Brem H, Tomic-Canic M, Tarnovskaya A, et al. Healing of elderly patients with diabetic foot ulcers, venous stasis ulcers, and pressure ulcers. *Surg Technol Int* 2003;11:161-167.

24

Prosthetic Feet

JOHN FERGASON

LEARNING OBJECTIVES

On completion of this chapter, the reader will be able to do the following:

1. Define the four primary functional classifications of prosthetic feet.
2. Restate the functional tasks of stance that prosthetic feet are designed to mimic.
3. Summarize the functional analysis of each foot category.
4. Differentiate between the functional levels of activity used to determine eligibility for prosthetic feet.
5. Formulate a prescription recommendation for a prosthetic foot on the basis of an evaluation of the client's needs.

WHAT IS A PROSTHETIC FOOT DESIGNED TO DO?

The prosthetic foot is designed to replace many functions of the anatomical human foot. As the connection between the prosthesis and the ground, it must mimic the biomechanical characteristics of the human foot as much as possible. Understanding the functions of the anatomical foot enables the prosthetic rehabilitation team to recommend the type of prosthetic foot that best meets the functional needs of each individual.

Prosthetic feet can be classified according to the motions they allow or simulate. Only a few basic foot designs were commonly used until the 1990s, when dozens of options became available. For most members of the prosthetic team, knowledge of the characteristics of groups of prosthetic feet is more efficient for decision making than attempting to remember exact characteristics of each commercially available prosthetic foot. Although the physical therapist provides information about the patient's functional needs, the certified prosthetist is the team member most likely to understand the complexities of the many prosthetic feet and to remain current with the rapid advances in prosthetic foot technology.

In the past decade, many new materials for the keel of the foot have been developed to increase the foot's flexibility and responsiveness. The use of carbon composites, with their superior strength–weight ratio, has been successfully applied to the design of high-performance, dynamic-response prosthetic feet. Traditional prosthetic feet were separate components that were bolted to the shank of the prosthesis, but many current designs incorporate the shank, ankle, and foot as one continuous unit. Other articulating ankle components substitute for movement in or about all three planes of anatomical ankle motion. Additionally, cosmetic appearance and durability of the various feet should be considered in formulating the appropriate prosthetic prescription. The primary goal of this chapter is to provide a basic understanding of the classification and function of prosthetic feet.

HISTORICAL PERSPECTIVE

Before commercially produced prosthetic feet became available, prosthetists had to fabricate prosthetic feet of their own design. Commonly, these early prosthetic feet included some form of an ankle axis to allow plantar flexion and dorsiflexion, as well as a toe-break in the area of the metatarsal heads. The body of the foot was often carved from a block of hardwood such as maple. A compressible bumper was positioned in a recessed area of the heel to simulate ankle plantar flexion motion, which is required for the first rocker (heel rocker) of gait. As weight was transferred onto the heel during loading response, compression of the bumper resulted in a controlled lowering of the prosthetic foot toward the floor, substituting for the ankle plantar flexion motion that is required to attain the foot-flat position.

Similarly, a compressible rubber bumper placed in a recessed area anterior to the ankle axis was used to simulate dorsiflexion, which is required to complete the second rocker (ankle rocker) of gait, from loading response into midstance and terminal stance. As the shank of the prosthesis progressed forward, compression of the bumper allowed controlled dorsiflexion of the foot. A third bumper in the anterior of the prosthetic foot was used to simulate dorsiflexion of the metatarsophalangeal (MP) joints, which is required for the third rocker (toe rocker) of gait. As the gait cycle progressed from terminal stance into preswing, compression of the toe bumper facilitated the transition from stance into swing. The plantar surface of the prosthetic foot was often reinforced with flexible belting or felt to provide additional stability and durability. The unidirectional location of the toe-break, which limited motion to a single plane, was the major disadvantage of this early design. Any deviation from this one plane caused an inefficient gait from midstance to heel rise.

The weight, lack of flexibility, and maintenance needs associated with a custom-fabricated foot prompted the development of commercially manufactured prosthetic feet that are more accommodating to the functional concerns, energy costs, and cosmetic preferences of prosthetic users. The basic characteristics of early prosthetic feet provide the biomechanical foundation for many of the feet currently in use. The articulating-ankle single-axis foot uses a similar principle for its axial motion. The early prototypes of the solid-ankle cushioned-heel (SACH) foot developed by Foort and Radcliff[1] in the early 1950s used a slightly different approach to achieve the functional goals of earlier prosthetic feet. This commercially available, simple, lightweight design was a significant improvement and provided acceptable function for most people with amputation. Early SACH feet were generally maintenance free and considerably lighter than the earlier conventional, individually created or manufactured, articulating wooden feet.[2,3]

The SACH foot and the single-axis wooden foot remained the only options for prosthetic users for many years. In the late 1970s, Campbell introduced the stationary-ankle flexible endoskeletal foot (SAFE). This foot maintained the basic characteristics of the SACH foot, adding a component of flexibility that was missing in previous designs. Although heavier than the SACH foot, it allowed for some multiaxial motion that substituted for the accommodation to uneven surfaces, which is possible in the anatomical foot-ankle complex.

Development of articulated multiaxial foot-ankle assemblies followed the institution of the U.S. Artificial Limb Program in 1945. Early versions were relatively unsuccessful, but a number of later designs found commercial success.[4] These basic designs were the primary options until the early 1980s.

The "technology boom" for prosthetic foot design began in the early 1980s, sparked by the development of the Seattle Foot (Seattle Systems, Inc., Poulsbo, Wash.) by the Prosthetic Research Study at the University of Washington.[5] This foot was the first in the class of dynamic-response energy-storing feet that provided an elastic keel for use in higher-level activities, such as running and jumping. Many current designs use the original Seattle Foot principle of elasticity to offer a higher level of performance to prosthetic wearers who are involved in athletics and other active functional and leisure activities.

FUNCTIONAL DESIGN CRITERIA FOR THE PROSTHETIC FOOT

The design of a prosthetic foot offers the same functional characteristics that are seen in the human foot-ankle complex. Ideally, the prosthetic foot duplicates each biomechanical motion with a mechanical substitute. Given the complexity of the human foot-ankle complex, however, this goal may not be completely attainable. During the gait cycle, the human foot performs many functions. It adapts to uneven surfaces and provides shock absorption at heel strike, torque conversion, knee stabilization, transfer of weight-bearing forces, limb lengthening and shortening during forward progression, and a stable weight-bearing base.[6-8]

In the early stance phase, the human foot is flexible to allow accommodation to uneven terrain and to maintain balance. Toward the end of the stance phase, the human foot converts to a rigid lever arm for push-off at preswing. This unique biomechanical progression from a flexible to a rigid position is dependent on the position of the components of the foot, as well as on their motion and structure.[9] An individual with an amputation has no physical connection between the musculature of the residual limb and the prosthetic foot: the prosthetic foot must substitute for the function of the bony anatomy, as well as the loss of muscle action. None of the currently available prosthetic feet are designed to actively dorsiflex during swing phase; most focus on performance in stance. Design variations affect how well the prosthetic foot addresses the functional tasks of stance. These tasks include the following:

1. Shock absorption and controlled plantar flexion in loading response
2. Accommodation to uneven terrain and controlled advancement of the prosthetic shank (shin) during midstance
3. Heel rise and weight transfer during terminal stance
4. Transition through double support and preparation for the swing phase

Initial Contact into Loading Response

The two functional tasks in early stance are shock absorption and transition to foot-flat position. The prosthetic foot is designed to absorb much of the heel's impact as it contacts the ground, in order to minimize forces that are transferred to the residual limb. For people with transtibial amputation, shock absorption must also provide for a normal knee flexion moment and position as the gait cycle progresses to loading response.

In early stance, the ground reaction force vector is posterior to the ankle, creating a plantar flexion moment that drives the foot toward the floor. In the human foot-ankle, eccentric contraction of the foot dorsiflexion or pretibial muscle group allows smooth, controlled plantar flexion of the foot toward the floor during the heel rocker of gait. As the foot progresses to the floor, the tibia begins to advance forward during the ankle rocker of gait and limb progression continues. Proper control of plantar flexion prevents the tibia from advancing either too slowly or too rapidly.

Midstance

In early stance, the anatomical foot and ankle are flexible and capable of accommodating variations in terrain. The ability of the prosthetic foot to simulate the inversion and eversion of the subtalar joint mechanically determines how effectively it substitutes for this function.

The momentum of the swing limb and forward fall of the body weight create a dorsiflexion torque that moves the tibia over the weight-bearing foot from approximately 8 to 10 degrees of plantar flexion at loading response to 5 to 8 degrees of dorsiflexion at end stance. This motion is necessary for the forward progression of the stance leg as the opposite limb moves forward in swing. Eccentric contraction of the gastrocnemius and soleus muscles controls the speed of this progression and helps to maintain stance stability.[6] The prosthetic foot simulates this muscle activity by providing stance phase stability through a rigid, semirigid, or flexible keel within the foot.

Terminal Stance into Preswing

In terminal stance, the anatomical foot-ankle complex locks into position to provide for heel rise as the tibia continues to advance. The body weight is transferred forward onto the forefoot and rolls over the MP joints during the toe rocker of stance. This allows the foot to roll over at the metatarsal heads instead of at the tips of the toes.[6] The design of the prosthetic foot must provide terminal stance phase support, as well as simulate MP dorsiflexion, which is necessary for the toe rocker. Although a true articulation is unnecessary, the design of the foot should allow for an amount of forefoot flexibility to provide for a smooth rollover motion.

During dual limb support, the weight of the body is transferred from the preswing limb to the opposite side. The muscle force of the gastrocnemius-soleus complex is reduced as the ankle begins to plantarflex. The well-designed prosthetic foot provides sufficient support of the amputated side to assist in balance and facilitate smooth transfer of weight to the sound side. This is a primary factor in reducing the force placed on the sound side foot[10] and may be particularly important for the individual with compromised vascular and neurological systems.

Rapid knee flexion during preswing results in relative shortening of the limb to allow adequate clearance as the swing phase begins. A slight spring action of the prosthetic foot at the end of terminal stance simulates this muscle activity.

CATEGORIES OF PROSTHETIC FEET

Prosthetic feet are most often categorized by the combinations of functional tasks they are designed to simulate. Prosthetic feet can generally be grouped into one of four designs:

1. Nonarticulating feet (e.g., SACH feet)
2. Articulating designs (e.g., single-axis and multiaxial feet)
3. Prosthetic feet with elastic keels (e.g., SAFE feet)
4. Dynamic-response or energy-storing designs (e.g., Seattle Foot and the Flex-Foot [Ossur North America, Aliso Viejo, Calif.])

Nonarticulating Designs: Solid-Ankle Cushioned-Heel Feet

The SACH foot has been available in its most basic form since the late 1950s.[2] Today's SACH foot differs little in principle from its early designs. It continues to be commonly prescribed because of its simplicity, low cost, and durability. It has no articulations and relies on the flexibility of its structure for joint motion simulation. The internal keel SACH foot is available with various heel densities and can be obtained in heel heights ranging from 0 to 3½ inches.[7] The SACH foot is composed of a firm keel that is surrounded by dense yet flexible foam to give shape to the foot (Figure 24-1). The keel ends distally at the toe-break area of the foot. Molded toes are available if desired. A heel cushion wedge is placed under the keel in the posterior of the foot. In some designs, rubberized belting is attached to the distal area of the keel and extends to the end of the toes. This belting simulates the toe flexors and assists in giving a slight resistance to MP extension during preswing. This motion aids in

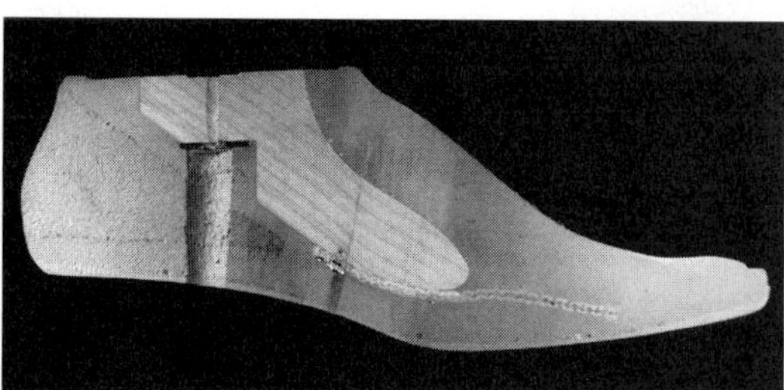

Figure 24-1
Solid-ankle cushioned-heel foot in cross section. The heel cushion, wooden keel, and belting extend toward the toe.

preventing a feeling of dropping off of the toe during this phase of gait.

Functional Analysis of the Solid-Ankle Cushioned-Heel Foot in Stance

At initial contact and into loading response, the cushioned heel of the SACH foot adequately provides for shock absorption as body weight is transferred onto the stance foot. The compression resistance of the heel cushion can vary from soft to firm, depending on body weight. Compression of the heel cushion also simulates the eccentric contraction of the ankle dorsiflexors in controlling plantar flexion into a foot-flat position (Figure 24-2). This compression of the heel cushion allows for a controlled progression into the early stance phase. A soft heel cushion can be chosen for individuals who need to reach a stable foot-flat position quickly, such as those with balance impairment. A firmer heel might be chosen for those who are overweight or involved in relatively higher impact mobility activities.

During the transition to midstance, the SACH foot has no true inversion or eversion to assist in accommodating uneven terrain. The flexible structure of the outer foot may accommodate small deviations in terrain but should not be depended on for this function. Simulation of ankle rocker (as the shank of the prosthesis rolls forward over the foot) is controlled through the keel of the foot. The rigid keel offers resistance to tibial advancement until the weight line is past the toe-break of the foot.

Control of heel rise during toe rocker in terminal stance and progression onto the forefoot in preswing are functions of the length of the keel in the SACH foot. Although some manufacturers make available SACH feet of various keel lengths or densities, most SACH feet have standard keel lengths that correspond to the size of the foot. In late stance, the prosthetic foot is stable and resists rapid heel rise until the weight line passes the toe-break, where the keel ends. As the shank of the prosthesis continues forward, the end of the keel is reached and toe dorsiflexion begins. If the keel is too short, an early heel rise and an unwanted knee flexion moment occur, often perceived by the prosthetic user as a "buckling" of the knee. If the keel is too long, heel rise is delayed and a knee extension moment occurs. This interrupts forward tibial progression and prevents smooth weight transfer to the opposite limb.

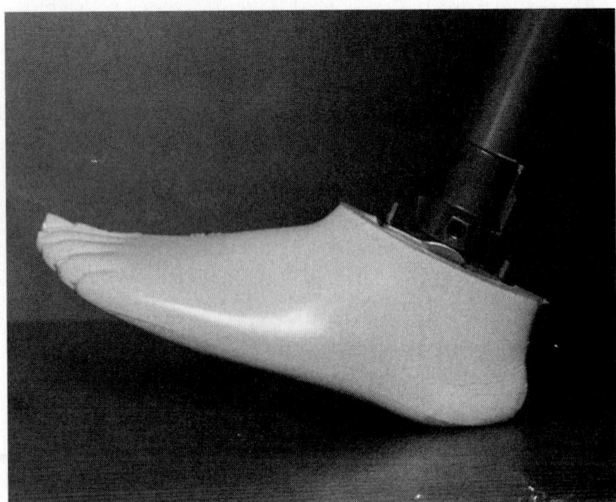

Figure 24-2
Compression of the heel cushion in the solid-ankle cushioned-heel foot during loading response simulates controlled plantar flexion of the ankle toward the foot-flat position. The firmness (durometer) of the heel cushion and weight of the prosthetic user determine how quickly the foot-flat position is attained.

The toe-break on the SACH foot is located at the end of the keel. The toe-break simulates dorsiflexion of the toes and shortens the effective length of the foot. The dorsiflexed toes of the SACH foot offer little weight-bearing support: the alignment of the foot under the socket determines how effectively the keel provides support as weight is transferred to the sound side. As the prosthetic user moves toward the end of preswing and the limb begins to rise, the toe flexibility adds a small elastic motion to help assist in knee flexion. This motion, however, is minimal compared with the elastic keel and dynamic-response categories of prosthetic feet.

Advantages and Indications of the Solid-Ankle Cushioned-Heel Foot

Because it has no moving parts, the SACH foot is durable and requires little maintenance. The wide range of available heel heights may still make it the foot of choice for many new prosthetic wearers. The SACH foot has excellent shock absorption characteristics because of its large heel cushion. Prosthetists often recommend it for use in temporary or preparatory prostheses because of its light weight and low cost. The SACH foot is most appropriate for prosthetic users at the level of household and limited community ambulation.

Disadvantages and Contraindications of the Solid-Ankle Cushioned-Heel Foot

The primary disadvantage of the SACH foot is its inherent lack of flexibility, especially its inability to accommodate to uneven surfaces. Its design and construction target optimal performance during relaxed walking cadence and in a single alignment configuration. It should seldom be recommended for the active community ambulator. The SACH foot is inappropriate for those who are involved in high-level activities and sports or those who must traverse uneven terrain.

Articulating Designs: Single-Axis Feet

Articulating or axial designs include a simulated ankle joint that actually permits motion about a joint axis. The single-axis foot design was the first true articulating, or axial, foot. This foot is a direct descendant of the historic conventional wooden foot. The modern single-axis foot is composed of a keel within a molded rubber foot shell. Most single-axis, articulating prosthetic feet allow up to 15 degrees of plantar flexion and 5 to 7 degrees of dorsiflexion.[1] This is accomplished by foot rotation about a horizontally positioned axis located in the ankle area of the foot. Compression of the rubber bumper located posterior to the axis mimics plantar flexion. Its density determines the speed of foot descent in loading response. For dorsiflexion, most single-axis feet have a rubber bumper located anterior to the axis. When compressed, this anterior bumper resists rapid forward movement of the prosthetic shank. Other designs may instead use a "stop" that limits motion after 5 to 7 degrees of dorsiflexion is reached.

Functional Analysis of the Single-Axis Foot

A single-axis foot provides excellent shock absorption during initial contact and loading response because of the combined compression of the heel and the plantar flexion bumper. At initial contact, the heel begins to compress and cushion shock. As the heel reaches full compression, the force is transferred to the plantar flexion bumper (Figure 24-3). This rubber plantar flexion bumper begins to compress and continues to absorb the shock of loading as the foot descends toward the grounds. Changing the durometer (resistance to compression) of the plantar flexion bumper can control the rate of descent of the foot toward the ground. All manufacturers of single-axis feet supply numerous interchangeable bumpers of varying durometers or firmness. If a firm heel bumper is used, the foot is resistant to plantar flexion and a knee flexion moment results. If a softer heel bumper is used, the knee flexion moment is reduced and the foot quickly reaches a foot-flat position. Considerations for determining bumper firmness revolve around patient weight, activity level, and the need for knee stability.

The articulation in the single-axis foot allows movement in the sagittal plane only. This provides more accommodation to uneven surfaces than does a nonarticulated foot but does not allow articulated movement in the coronal plane when inversion and eversion may be desired. Advancement of the tibial shank of the prosthesis during midstance is controlled by the combination of the dorsiflexion bumper (or dorsiflexion stop) and the solid keel in the foot. Once the full range of dorsiflexion is reached, the keel of the foot acts as a rocker to continue the controlled progression of the tibial shank.

Heel rise in terminal stance is determined by the effect of the dorsiflexion bumper or stop. For the prosthetic foot with a dorsiflexion bumper, the firmness of the bumper determines when the tibia stops advancing. Once the bumper is maximally compressed (stopping tibial advancement), the force is applied to the foot and heel rise is initiated. For the foot with a dorsiflexion stop, force is transferred to the foot and heel rise is initiated once the stop is fully engaged. The length of the keel in the foot also contributes to the control of heel rise. Once the end point of ankle dorsiflexion is reached, the distal portion of the keel acts as a rocker. When the end point of this rocker is reached, toe dorsiflexion begins.

As preswing is approached, the mechanics of the single-axis foot become similar to that of the SACH foot. The toe break of the foot is located where the keel ends. Once the end of the keel is rolled over, the toes begin to dorsiflex. The alignment of the foot under the prosthetic socket and the overall length of the keel determine the support necessary to allow smooth transfer of weight to the sound side. As the end of preswing is reached, the toes offer a slight spring action that encourages knee flexion into the swing phase.

Advantages and Indications of the Single-Axis Foot

The primary advantage of a single-axis foot is its ability to reach a stable foot-flat position quickly in early stance. This may be advantageous for activities that affect knee stability, such as walking down a ramp or other inclines. Although most individuals with amputations at the transtibial level have adequate knee extensor strength for controlled loading response, those who have significant nonremediable strength impairment or a particularly short residual limb may benefit from a single-axis foot. At the transfemoral level of amputation, knee stability during loading response is related to hip extensor strength and length of the residual limb; as a result, knee stability can be more challenging to achieve. A single-axis foot increases knee stability, reducing the knee flexion moment during loading response. An additional advantage is the capability of changing the durometer of the bumpers in the foot to suit the needs and activity level of the prosthetic user.

Contraindications and Disadvantages of the Single-Axis Foot

The major disadvantages of a single-axis foot include its increased weight (compared with the SACH and other nonarticulating feet) and its need for occasional maintenance. The

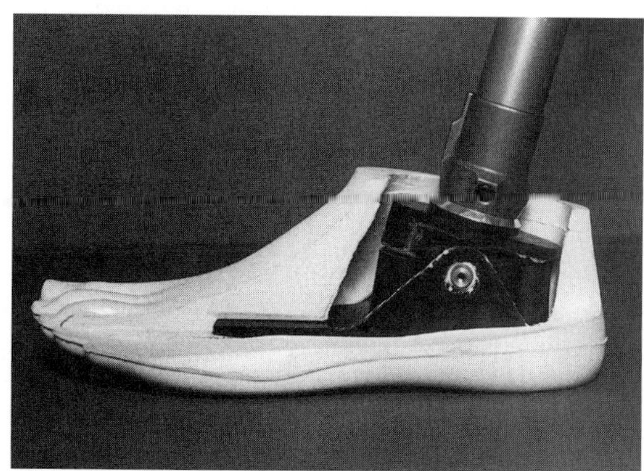

Figure 24-3
Compression of the plantar flexion bumper during initial contact and loading response. The pylon has a posterior leaning angle as the prosthetic foot approaches the foot-flat position.

benefit of extra stability in early stance may be countered by the increased energy cost of a heavier foot for prosthetic users with significant strength impairment or poor aerobic capacity. Because the foot has moving parts, it needs occasional service for the normal wear and tear that can alter the function of the foot and gait pattern of the user.

Articulating Designs: Multiaxis Feet

The multiple-axis (multiaxis) foot operates similarly to the single-axis foot, using various combinations of rubber bumpers. The multiaxis foot offers coronal and transverse plane motion in addition to motion in the sagittal plane. True inversion, eversion, and rotation allow this prosthetic foot to absorb more of the torque forces that would otherwise be transferred to the patient's residual limb. As a result of the large availability of range, stability is found only at the extremes of each plane of motion.

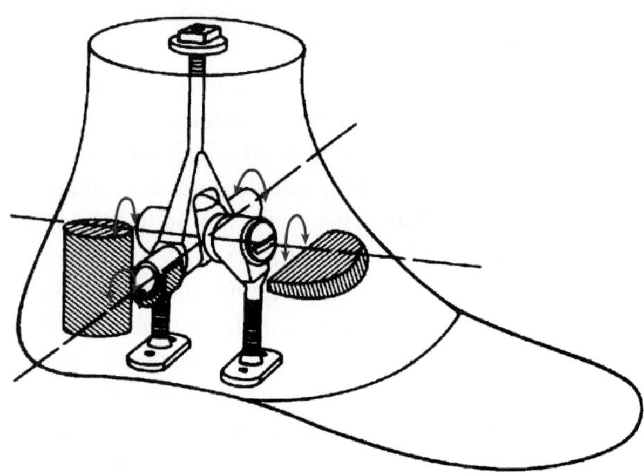

Figure 24-4
Internal mechanisms of a multiaxial foot. This design allows movement in the sagittal, coronal, and transverse planes.

Feet that offer multiaxial motion are available in various styles. The Greissinger foot (Otto Bock Healthcare, Minneapolis) has the longest history of commercial availability, with widespread use in Europe and limited but steady success in the United States.[4] It consists of a wooden keel surrounded by a molded rubber foot. A set of rubber bumpers and mechanical articulations allow inversion and eversion, plantar flexion and dorsiflexion and axial rotation (Figure 24-4). More recent, successful multiple-axis designs allow the same triplanar motion with use of composite structural materials (Figure 24-5).

Functional Analysis of the Multiaxis Foot

As with the single-axis foot, the primary method of shock absorption in early stance occurs from compression of a plantar flexion bumper. Because the ankle components take up space in the heel that is commonly used for a heel cushion in other foot designs, almost all shock absorption occurs by this bumper compression. As weight is applied to the foot, the plantar flexion bumper compresses to provide a controlled progression to midstance. Plantar flexion resistance is adjusted to meet specific user needs by changing the plantar flexion bumper to one with a different stiffness.

During midstance, the true multiaxial features of the foot become engaged. The multiaxial foot accommodates to uneven ground in the sagittal, coronal, and transverse planes (Figure 24-6). Because the multiaxial foot also allows transverse motion, rotational forces are absorbed in the foot-ankle complex rather than being transferred to the socket-limb interface. Tibial advancement is controlled by

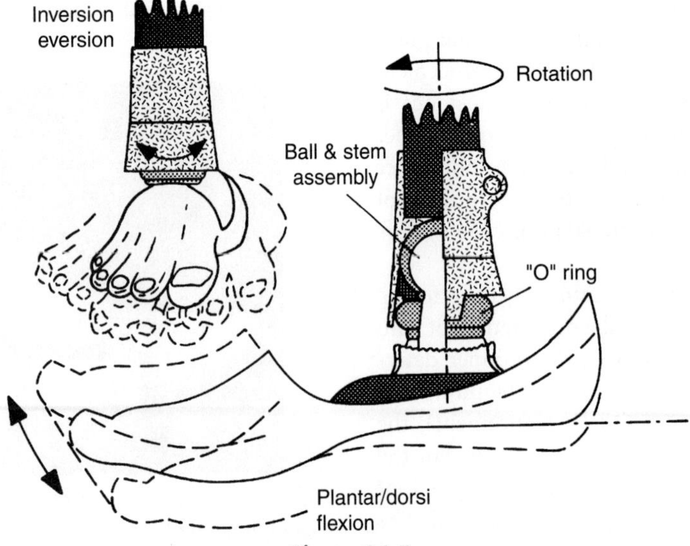

Figure 24-5
The ball and stem assembly and "O" ring of this multiaxial foot design mimic inversion and eversion of the foot and ankle, allowing accommodation when the patient is walking on uneven surfaces. (Courtesy Endolite North America, Centerville, Ohio.)

the stiffness of the rubber components of the ankle. Once full compression of the rubber component is reached, the force is transferred to the foot. The length and stiffness of the keel determines the continued amount of resistance as terminal stance is reached.

Heel rise in terminal stance is controlled first by the effect of the rubber components in the foot that act to control dorsiflexion and then by the length of the prosthetic keel. The foot's resistance to dorsiflexion determines when the tibial advancement is slowed and heel rise is initiated. Once the dorsiflexion limit is reached, tibial advancement is slowed, the force is applied to the foot, and heel rise begins. Multiaxial feet have varying keel lengths specific to their design and manufacturer. As the heel rises, the foot pivots over the edge of the keel and toe dorsiflexion begins. Toe dorsiflexion is controlled by construction of the foot in the toe area (Figure 24-7). Various foot shell designs allow some toe elasticity, and as previously discussed, the prosthetic alignment of the foot under the prosthesis and the overall length of the keel determine how much support is available for smooth transfer of weight to the opposite limb. As preswing is completed, the elasticity in the rubber toes and their inner supporting structure again provides a slight spring action to encourage knee flexion into the swing phase.

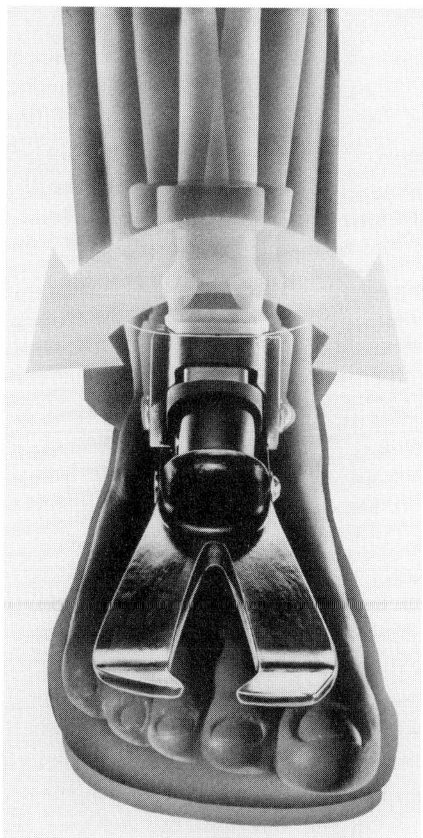

Figure 24-6
Multiaxial feet allow movement in the sagittal and coronal planes, giving the person with amputation additional accommodation for uneven terrain. (Courtesy College Park Industries, Inc., Fraser, Mich.)

Advantages and Indications of Multiaxial Foot Designs

The multiaxial foot has several specific indications for use. The primary advantage is the ability of the foot to accommodate uneven terrain in more than one plane. Although the transverse movement does not mimic normal human motion exactly, it is extremely useful for reducing torque forces on the residual limb during stance. The prosthetic user who anticipates being on uneven terrain would certainly appreciate this feature. Those with mechanical instability of their anatomical knees, poor postural control, or vulnerable residual limbs would also benefit from reduction of torque forces during stance. The density or resistance of the rubber bumpers can be changed for accommodation to the prosthetic user's weight and activity level. For instance, when recommending a foot for an individual with a recent amputation, the clinician would expect to see gait changes as rehabilitation progresses. Most multiaxial designs would allow adjustment in plantar flexion and dorsiflexion resistance by interchanging the durometer of bumpers in the foot. This allows the foot to enhance ambulation ability and negates the need for frequent upgrade or replacement.

Disadvantages and Contraindications of Multiaxial Foot Designs

Because movement is allowed in all three planes, the multiaxial foot provides less static stability than does the nonaxial foot.[11] An individual with specific muscle weakness may not feel stable or supported when using this foot. These factors can be accommodated by use of a bumper of different durometer, determined by individual needs. Multiaxial feet are often heavier than nonarticulating, elastic keel, or dynamic-response prosthetic feet. The moving parts within the foot make regular maintenance a necessity. Bushings and

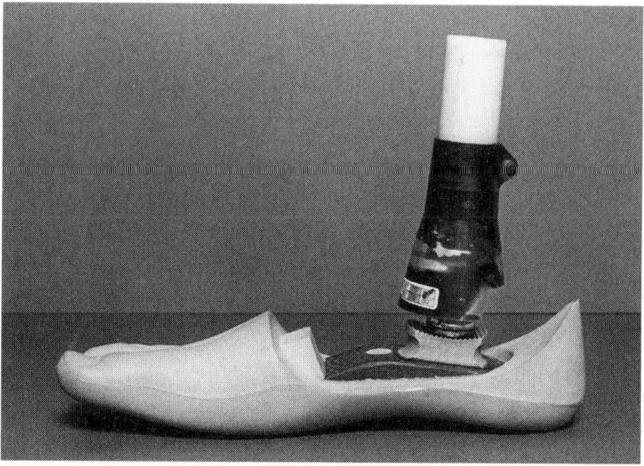

Figure 24-7
The preformed keel with dorsiflexed toes of this multiaxial foot's shell facilitates rollover and initiation of heel rise in terminal stance.

bumpers wear with use; performance of the foot deteriorates as this occurs. If gait deviations develop, replacement of worn components will in many instances restore performance to acceptable levels. Multiaxial feet should not be used if an individual is unwilling to schedule regular maintenance checks or is inaccessible to the prosthetist.

Elastic Keel Feet

The elastic keel foot is designed to mimic the movement characteristics of the human foot without the use of true articulations and moving parts. Such a task requires the design attention to be placed primarily on the keel of the foot and the material of the surrounding foot shell. In the anatomical foot, the plantar fascia (plantar aponeurosis) works in combination with the intrinsic muscles of the foot to transmit force across the longitudinal arch of the foot.[12] A "windlass effect" occurs as the MP joints are dorsiflexed and the plantar fascia is tightened. The collagen fibers of the plantar fascia resist the tensile forces and become progressively stiffer. This tension promotes inversion of the calcaneus and supination of the subtalar joint to establish a rigid lever for push-off.[9] The elastic keel foot is designed to mimic this motion by increasing stiffness of the foot as it moves through midstance, terminal stance, and preswing. Several versions of elastic keel feet are commercially available. The SAFE II foot is used to represent this class of prosthetic feet in the following functional analysis, because this design most closely resembles the motion of the anatomical foot. Other feet in the elastic keel category can be analyzed with the same criteria given the variations in design and manufacturing techniques.

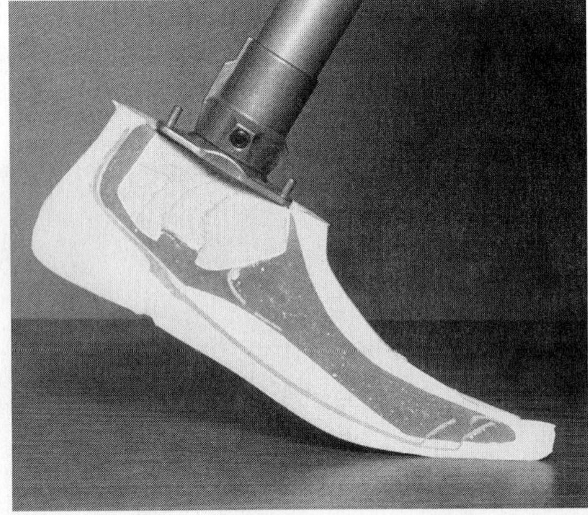

Figure 24-8
Elastic keel class, stationary-ankle-flexible endoskeletal (SAFE II) foot. The plantar bands originate on the posterior surface of the keel and insert into the distal keel. These bands simulate the action of the plantar fascia in the human foot. As the SAFE II foot is loaded in terminal stance, the tension applied to the plantar bands creates the semirigid level necessary for efficient transition from stance into swing.

Functional Analysis of an Elastic Keel Foot

Most elastic keel feet use a cushioned heel similar to that of the SACH foot for shock absorption in initial contact and loading response. Many manufacturers offer the soft-, medium-, and firm-heel durometer to allow for variations in patient weight, activity level, and need for shock absorption. Other feet may not have a separate foam compartment in the heel area, instead using keel flexibility and the foot shell foam to provide shock absorption.

The differences in the design of elastic keel feet become apparent during the transitions from early stance through midstance and into terminal stance. Certain elastic keel feet rely primarily on compression of the heel cushion to control the rate of foot plantar flexion toward foot flat in early stance, using principles similar to those of the SACH foot. Others involve the biomechanical properties of their keel design. The SAFE II has a two-part keel. The most proximal section is a rigid block containing the foot bolt that connects the foot to the prosthesis shank. Inside the foot, this rigid block is connected to the flexible portion of the keel that extends to the distal end of the foot at the toes. Once the cushion heel reaches its limit of compression during loading, the rigid block moves relative to the foot shell and flexible portion of the keel. This movement provides additional cushion to the patient's residual limb.

Inversion and eversion are simulated by the nature of the flexibility in the elastic keel foot. The foot provides moderate accommodation to uneven terrain because of the movement allowed between the keel and its surrounding rubber foot shell. Tibial advancement is controlled by the plantar bands embedded under the keel of the SAFE II foot. These two bands originate at the heel area of the keel. The first band crosses the arch and attaches proximal to the toe break. This band serves to stabilize the arch of the keel and prevent excessive flexibility while standing during midstance. The second band crosses the toe-break and attaches in the distal end of the keel. As the tibia advances, the keel begins to bend and the foot starts to dorsiflex. The plantar bands begin to tighten, controlling the rate that the keel bends. This resistance to rapid bending of the keel acts to control the tibial advancement. Other elastic keel feet achieve the same effect through the use of only a flexible keel within the foot. Most elastic keel feet tend to offer limited rotational ability. Rotation occurs by minimal movement of the flexible keel within the rubber housing of the foot.

Heel rise during terminal stance is controlled by the stiffness of the keel. As the prosthetic tibial shaft advances, the keel continues to flex as the foot dorsiflexes and weight progresses onto the forefoot. The keel in most elastic keel feet extends all the way into the toe area. The flexible keel eliminates the need for a rocker effect and provides a considerably smoother rollover throughout this phase. The SAFE II foot has additional control during dorsiflexion and heel rise as tension is applied to the plantar bands (Figure 24-8). These bands allow for gradual stiffening of the forefoot to create a semirigid lever during this phase, as does the aponeurosis in the anatomical foot. The plantar fascia band crosses the toe-break and offers control and support as the toes dorsiflex. Other elastic keel feet rely on the flexibility of the keel alone without incorporating a mechanical toe break.

The elastic keel of these feet is compressed as the prosthetic tibial shank advances from midstance to terminal stance. As the prosthetic limb is unweighted during preswing and weight is transferred to the opposite limb, the patient has a sense of "energy return" as the prosthetic foot returns to its uncompressed or resting state. The spring action of this elastic response serves to encourage knee flexion of the amputated side and aid initiation of the swing phase.

Advantages and Indications of an Elastic Keel Foot

Elastic keel feet provide a smooth gait pattern because no mechanical rocker motions occur during the subphases of stance. Individuals with a moderate need for accommodation to uneven terrain appreciate the flexibility of elastic keel feet. The benefit of flexibility of an elastic keel is also evident during activities such as stair climbing or descent and incline negotiation. An elastic keel foot is an alternative for the prosthetic user who would benefit from the features of a multiaxial foot but does not want the maintenance or weight characteristics associated with those designs. Although the range of motion and torque absorption are not as extensive as those in multiaxial designs, the characteristics of the elastic keel foot functionally approximate them for many prosthetic users.

Disadvantages and Contraindications of an Elastic Keel Foot

The "spongy" feel of an elastic keel foot may be disliked by prosthetic users who are in need of, or accustomed to, a greater sense of stability during stance. Active or athletic individuals often prefer a foot with a stiffer keel than those that are available in the elastic keel class, preferring instead those of the dynamic-response class.

Dynamic-Response Feet

The dynamic-response, or energy-storing, class of prosthetic feet is most often chosen for high-performance prosthetic users. An early survey of recreational activities of lower limb prosthetic users by Kegal and colleagues[13] in 1980 suggested that the major factor affecting performance during and enjoyment of athletic activities is the inability to run effectively. Enoka and associates,[14] in studying performance characteristics and kinetics of running and jumping while wearing a prosthesis, demonstrated that the ground reaction force may be two to three times greater while running than walking. Most prosthetic feet have been designed to substitute for ankle and foot motion during walking; many are unable to meet the increased performance demands of running and jumping. Recognition of these limitations prompted development of prosthetic feet with energy-storing capabilities to absorb and store forces during loading and release this stored energy during push-off or preswing.

One of the first dynamic-response designs to become commercially available was the Seattle Foot (Figure 24-9). This foot has a one-piece keel of synthetic composite material embedded in a foam foot shape.[15] The keel provides a unique combination of stiffness and flexibility to absorb the forces applied early in the gait cycle. As cadence increases from walking speed toward running speeds, the amount of time spent on the forefoot increases. The increasing amplitude of the dorsiflexion moment is accommodated during the terminal stance by greater distortion in the keel as it compresses, and absorbs more and more energy. As the foot is unloaded in preswing, this stored energy is released quickly, simulating push-off and aiding the forward propulsion of the limb into swing.

Most current designs use similar biomechanical principles but differ in the materials used for the keel. The inherent strength, durability, and light weight of carbon graphite composites have made this the material of choice for many dynamic-response feet. For example, Carbon Copy feet (Ohio Willow Wood, Mt. Sterling, Ohio) use a carbon graphite leaf spring solid keel that is embedded in a foam foot shell (Figure 24-10). Other designs, such as Flex-Foot (Ossur North America) or Springlite (Otto Bock Healthcare, Minneapolis), use a single carbon graphite component

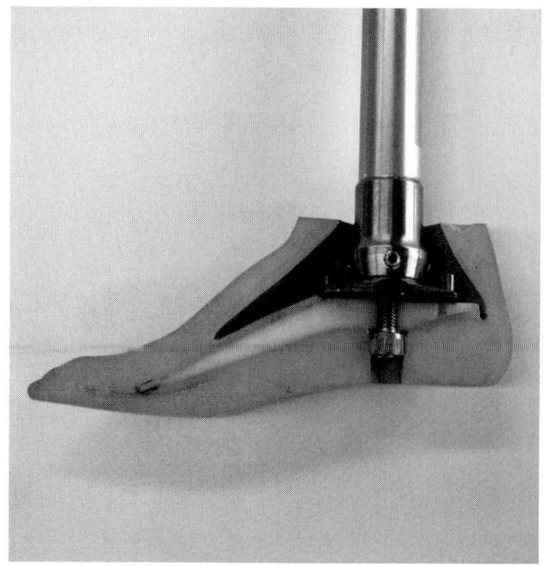

Figure 24-9
Seattle Foot (Seattle Systems, Poulsbo, Wash.) with Delrin (Dupont, Inc., Wilmington, Del.) dynamic-response keel. The combination of stiffness and flexibility of the keel enhances function in early stance. Compression of the keel in late stance is returned as push-off as the swing phase begins.

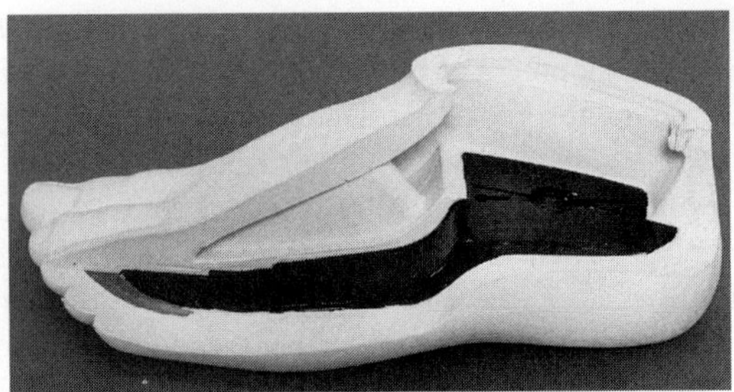

Figure 24-10

Carbon Copy II dynamic-response foot (Ohio Willow Wood, Mt. Sterling, Ohio). The carbon graphite composite keel acts as a leaf spring, storing energy as it is compressed with forward progression of body weight during stance, and returning that energy as push-off when the foot is unloaded and the swing phase begins.

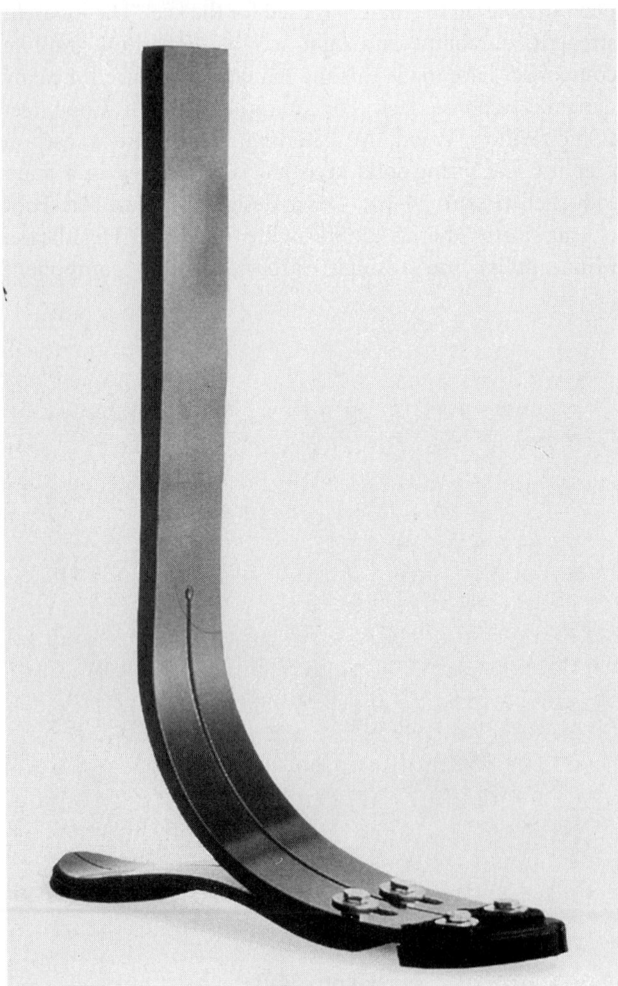

Figure 24-11

Example of a one-piece dynamic-response carbon graphite design incorporating the shank, ankle, and foot. This type of prosthetic foot can be encased in a foam cosmetic cover. (Courtesy Ossur North America, Aliso Viejo, Calif.)

incorporating the shin, ankle, and foot in a combined design (Figure 24-11). These offer the advantage of increased flexibility, because the entire length of the shin and foot deforms under loading conditions. The functional analysis of these two dynamic-response foot designs (foot only and shank/ankle/foot combination) illustrates the similarities and differences among dynamic-response designs.

Functional Analysis of Dynamic-Response Feet

Shock absorption of dynamic-response feet during early stance is comparable to that of the other classes. Many dynamic-response feet have a cushioned heel to absorb shock during compression. Control of plantar flexion is also affected by the stiffness of the heel in the foot. Some of the dynamic-response feet offer various heel foam densities to correspond to the prosthetic user's weight and activity level. The combination systems provide different degrees of heel stiffness with an interchangeable heel plate.

Most dynamic-response feet do not have significant uneven ground accommodation characteristics. Because the keel of dynamic-response feet is designed to be stiffer than that of elastic keel class feet, it is less adaptable to uneven surfaces. The rubber and foam foot shell may absorb a minimal amount of torque forces from stepping on uneven surfaces. Because of the stiff keel, no true inversion/eversion is available in most of these feet. In response to this limitation is a split-toe version that has a longitudinal separation in the forefoot and heel that allows some range of inversion/eversion. The Re-Flex VSP (Ossur North America) foot has a vertical compression shaft designed to absorb axial forces during high-load activities (Figure 24-12).

The most significant functional differences between dynamic-response feet and other classes of prosthetic feet are found in control of tibial advancement. Dynamic-response feet are chosen for individuals with high activity levels. During these activities, control of the rate of prosthetic tibial shaft advancement is crucial. As cadence increases to running, extra stiffness is necessary during midstance into terminal stance. Tibial shaft advancement is controlled by the stiffness of the keel in the foot. As the shaft advances, the keel deflects, absorbs forces generated during deflection, and resists rapid advancement.

Progression of heel rise is also related to stiffness of the keel in the foot. As the shaft continues to advance, the keel continues to deflect, and the foot dorsiflexes as weight progresses onto the forefoot. The keel in most dynamic-response feet extends into the toe or all the way to the distal end of the foot. The stiffness and deformation qualities of the dynamic-response keel eliminate the need for a rocker effect as seen in the SACH foot. Simultaneously, this extended keel provides stability necessary for support during controlled heel rise during high activity use. In a high loading activity such as running, progression onto the forefoot occurs through a smooth arc of dorsiflexion as the keel continues to deform under the increasing load throughout this phase. Keel deformation and dorsiflexion are now at their maximum points.

The stiffness of the keel now has an effect as body weight is completely transferred to the sound side. Support that allows comfortable transfer of weight to the sound side is provided. Because the stiff yet flexible keel has allowed maximal dorsiflexion without sacrificing support to the amputated side, the runner is allowed a longer sound side stride length. As it is unloaded, the keel begins to decompress as it returns to its original shape, creating a spring action that effectively simulates a true push-off. The spring action of this dynamic response also encourages knee flexion of the amputated side and aids in the initiation of a rapid swing phase.

Advantages and Indications of Dynamic-Response Feet

The primary indication for use of the dynamic-response foot is the potential for and desire to engage in high-demand activities. Many prosthetic users report that they can walk with less difficulty and more energy efficiency over a range of grades and speeds.[16] Because the many feet that are available in this class have varying degrees of stiffness, matching prosthetic users to the optimal feet for their preferred activities is critical. Walking velocity and type of activity directly affect the decision as to which dynamic-response foot to choose. Dynamic-response feet are available in a wide range of stiffness, specific to the weight and activity of the user. Manufacturers can custom fabricate a foot to the patient specifications if a standard design is not appropriate.

Dynamic-response feet are indicated when maximum late stance dorsiflexion is desired (e.g., during running), when frequent changes in cadence or velocity are necessary, or when walking on inclines.[17,18]

Disadvantages and Contraindications of Dynamic-Response Feet

The dynamic response foot is designed to deform under the loading conditions associated with high activity. For users whose activities are unable to generate enough loading force, dynamic-response feet often are perceived as being stiff and unaccommodating. Because most dynamic-response feet are manufactured from materials such as carbon graphite composite, cost is often significantly higher.

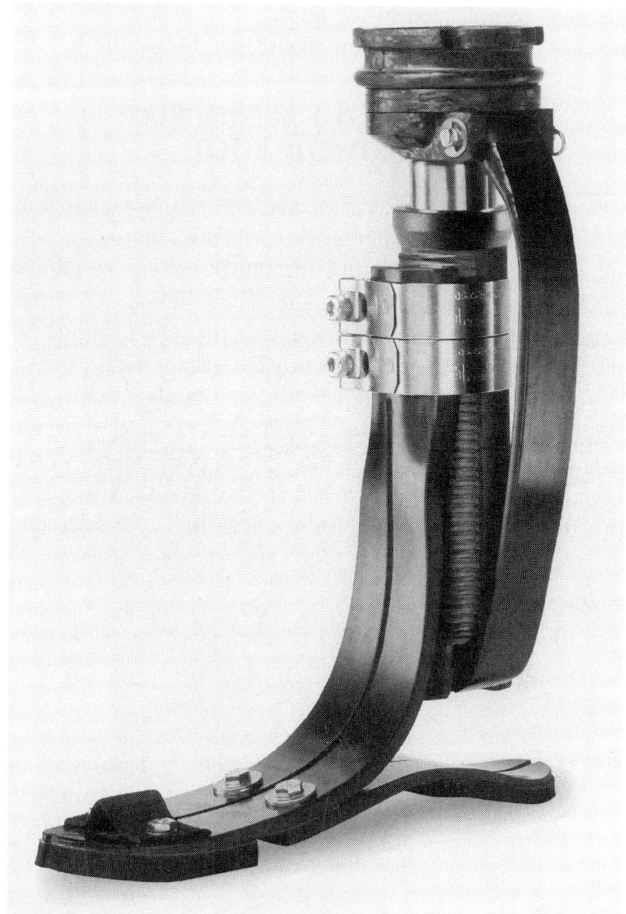

Figure 24-12
The carbon fiber side spring and telescoping tubes of the Re-Flex VSP foot absorb shock and return energy for prosthetic users who are involved in high-load activities. Split-foot and heel sections of this dynamic-response foot articulate to allow limited movement in eversion and inversion. (Courtesy Ossur North America, Aliso Viejo, Calif.)

Prosthetic Feet That Are Combinations of Classes

Most current prosthetic feet belong to one of the four classes described earlier. Several feet, however, may combine characteristics from more than one class. For instance, a dynamic-response keel can be combined with a multiaxis ankle to give increased accommodation to uneven terrain, as well as the spring motion associated with the dynamic-response class (Figure 24-13). In general, the prosthetic foot that combines the characteristics of several classes is likely to

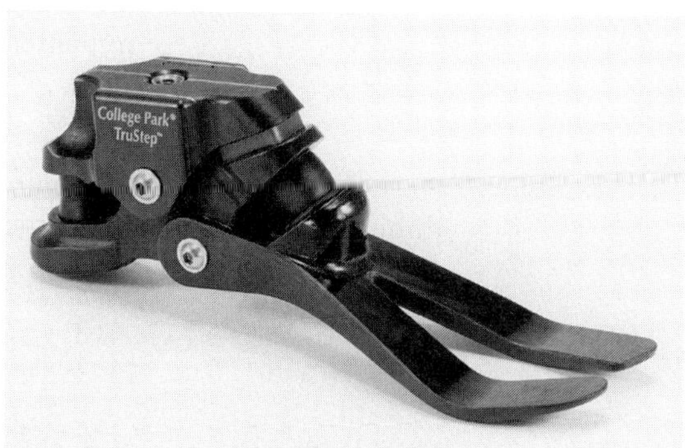

Figure 24-13
A dynamic-response keel combined with a multiaxial ankle offers the benefits of two classes of prosthetic feet. The construction includes plantar flexion and dorsiflexion bumpers and carbon graphite. (Courtesy College Park Industries, Fraser, Mich.)

be more complicated to use and requires additional maintenance. Each foot must be evaluated on its own merit.

CHOOSING THE APPROPRIATE PROSTHETIC FOOT

When a prescription recommendation for a prosthetic foot is formulated, many different characteristics should be considered in conjunction with the functional classes of feet (Table 24-1). In addition to the functional classes, other issues must be considered, first among them heel height and the type of shoes that will be worn. For instance, if a Western boot is to be worn, the foot must accommodate the overall height of the heel. If the heel height is not considered, severe gait deviations can occur and the overall performance of the prosthesis will be compromised (Figure 24-14). A standard prosthetic foot is designed for a ¾-inch heel and is suitable for most standard dress shoes designed for men. If frequent heel height changes are necessary, a foot/ankle that allows the user to adjust for various heights should be considered (Figure 24-15).

Another characteristic to consider is the foot's ability to resist moisture. Some feet are essentially waterproof; others should be kept as dry as possible. Many feet can be made water resistant by the prosthetist; however, the manufacturer should always be consulted (Figure 24-16). The cosmetic appearance of the foot is mainly a matter of preference. Some feet appear more lifelike, whereas others are mechanical in appearance by design. Surface features such as toes, veins, and malleoli can be provided if desired.

The choice of foot initially centers on the prosthetic user's activity level. The optimal prosthetic foot allows the prosthetic user to walk faster and achieve an equal step length of both amputated and intact limbs.[19] Decisions

Table 24-1
Identifying Factors of Foot Classifications

Class	*Characteristic Function*	*General Indications*	*Advantages*	*Disadvantages*
SACH	Absorbs impact of initial contact Provides stable walking surface	Household or limited community ambulation Infrequent cadence changes	Low cost Durable Entry level	Lack of structural flexibility
SINGLE AXIS	Ensures rapid foot-flat Assists knee stability at loading response	Reduced knee flexion moment at loading response	Increases early stance phase stability Provides effective transfemoral knee stability	Increased weight, cost, and maintenance
MULTI-AXIAL	Triplanar motion	Uneven terrain Reduced knee flexion moment at loading response	Reduces shear stress on limb Ensures rapid foot-flat at loading response Adapts to terrain	Increased weight, cost, and maintenance
ELASTIC KEEL	Smooth transition through gait cycle	Community ambulation	Enables smooth gait phase transitions May reduce residual limb skin shear	Limited response in terminal stance
DYNAMIC RESPONSE	Flexible structure compresses Keel deforms to absorb and release energy	Variable cadence High activity Exercise activity	Highly responsive Stores and releases energy	Cost May be difficult to cosmetically finish

SACH, Solid-ankle cushioned-heel.

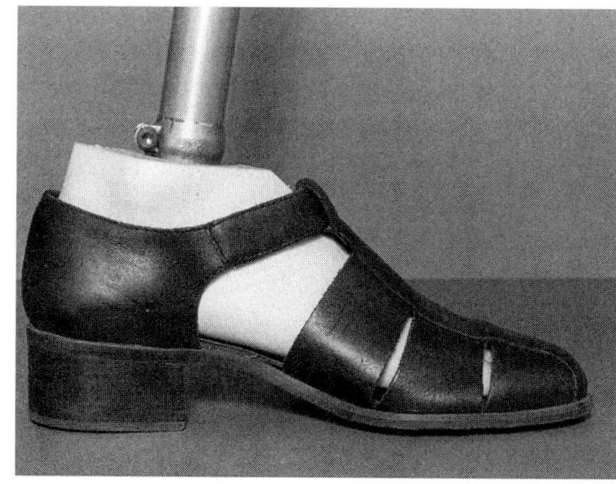

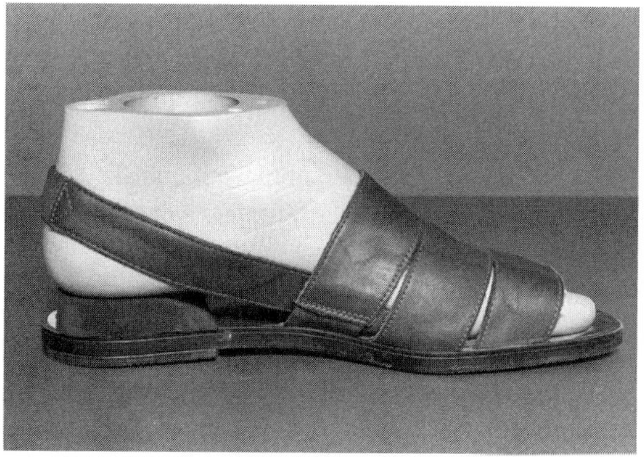

Figure 24-14

A, Prosthetic foot in a shoe with excessive heel height. The top of the foot should be level when in a shoe. Gait deviations occur if the heel rise of the prosthetic foot and the heel height of the shoe are mismatched. ***B,*** *A firm heel wedge positioned under the prosthetic foot in a flat sandal aligns the foot correctly for all phases of the gait cycle.*

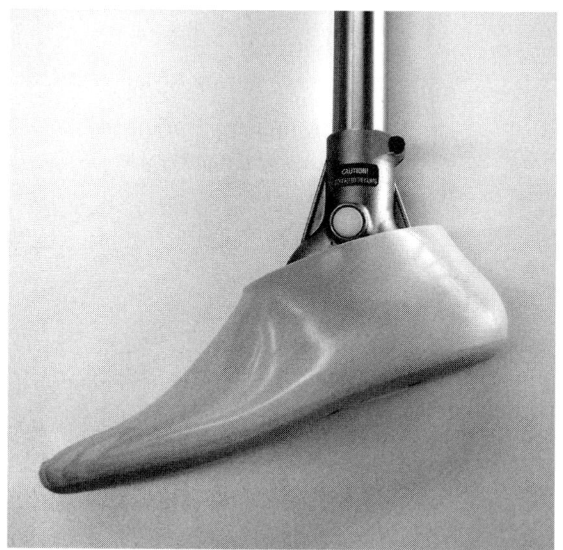

Figure 24-15

This foot may be adjusted by the user to accommodate frequent heel height changes. Shown here is a position to accommodate the maximum heel height.

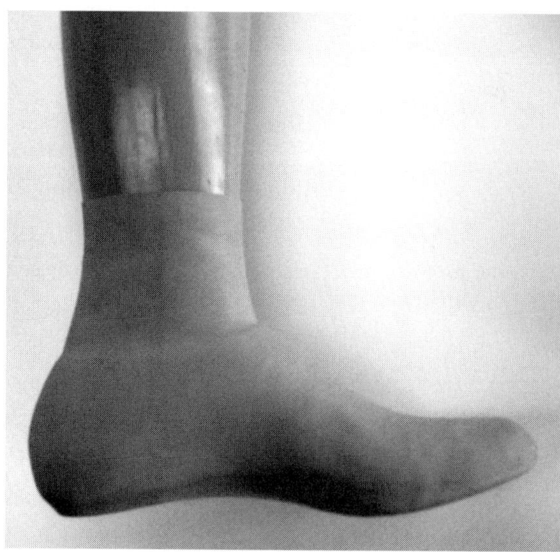

Figure 24-16

This foot has been made water resistant by applying a flexible latex covering. This is recommended if water immersion is anticipated.

about the prosthetic foot must consider accommodating not only a user's current activity level but also the potential to reach a higher level. The Center for Medicare Services has adopted prescription criteria on the basis of ability or potential to reach certain levels (Table 24-2). Vocational and recreational interests must be considered to ensure that the foot coincides with the functional needs of the prosthetic user. Although the most commonly reported reasons for delay back to work after amputation are related to the residual limb condition, the entire prosthetic prescription will have an effect on the type of work task to which the individual can return.[20] These needs should be clearly delineated and then balanced with the cost of the desired component.

The least expensive prosthetic foot is the simple SACH foot. The most expensive foot tends to be the sophisticated dynamic-response foot. Many functional and energy-efficient feet that will optimally meet the needs of the prosthetic user fall on a cost continuum between these two extremes. A study by Schmalz and colleagues[21] in 2002 demonstrated that for the slower self-selected walking speeds, there is little difference in oxygen consumption among several classes of feet. However, energy consumption may increase substantially in some classes as the walking speed increases.[21] In general, the more sophisticated designs have significantly higher cost and more frequent and complicated maintenance requirements. The prosthetic user who

Table 24-2
CMS Functional Level Categories Are Used to Determine Eligibility for Prosthetic Feet

Activity Level Modifier	*Ability Eligible*	*Components*
K0	**Nonambulatory** Cannot ambulate or transfer safely with or without assistance. Prosthesis does not enhance quality of life or mobility.	None
K1	**Limited or unlimited household ambulation** Can use the prosthesis for transfers or ambulation on level surfaces at fixed cadence.	SACH Single axis
K2	**Limited community ambulation** Can traverse low-level environmental barriers such as curbs, stairs, and uneven surfaces.	SACH Flexible (elastic) keel Single axis Multiaxial
K3	**Community ambulation** Can ambulate with variable cadence and traverse most environmental barriers. Has vocational, therapeutic, or exercise activities that demand prosthetics use beyond simple locomotion.	SACH Flexible (elastic) keel Single axis Multiaxial Energy storing (dynamic response)
K4	**Higher Activity** Child, active adult, or athlete who exceeds basic ambulation skills including high impact, stress, or energy levels.	Any foot appropriate for the individual's activity level

CMS, Center for Medicare Services; *SACH,* solid-ankle cushioned-heel.

is wearing a foot that requires regular maintenance must be willing to schedule periodic visits to the prosthetist who designed and provided the prosthesis.

SUMMARY

The choice of foot for any prosthesis should always be a team effort with the prosthetic user as a key participant. The prosthetist is responsibility for educating the prosthetic user about the available options and the characteristics of the feet. The individual with an amputation who has an active role in decision making regarding components is more vested in the use of the prosthesis. The proper choice of foot has a drastic effect on the performance of the prosthesis. An improperly prescribed foot leads to poor functional performance and contributes to discouragement on the part of the user. Because so many feet available today are interchangeable, a foot can be changed or upgraded as the needs of the person with amputation change. A SACH foot may be completely appropriate in the early stages of rehabilitation, but as the prosthetic user who becomes more adept in gait desires to resume higher-level activities, a high performance foot may be indicated. This can be accomplished if the prosthesis is based on a modular system that allows for interchangeability of components.

When developing a prescription recommendation for a prosthesis, special attention should always be given to the choice of foot. The foot is a critical component because it is the base of the entire prosthesis. A properly prescribed and fitted prosthetic foot can help each prosthetic user reach and maintain the desired level of activity and integrate the use of the prosthesis into daily activities.

REFERENCES

1. Sanders GT. Ankle foot mechanisms. In Sanders GT (ed), *Lower Limb Amputations: A Guide to Rehabilitation.* Philadelphia: F.A. Davis, 1986. pp. 143-162.
2. Radcliff CW, Foort J. *The Patellar Tendon Bearing Prosthesis.* Berkeley, CA: Regents of the University of California, 1961. pp. 104-113.
3. Murphy EM. Lower extremity components. In *American Academy of Orthopaedic Surgeons, Orthopedic Appliance Atlas,* vol 2. Ann Arbor, MI: Edwards, 1969.
4. Condie DN. Ankle foot devices. In Murdock G, Donovan RG (eds), *Amputation Surgery and Lower Limb Prosthetics.* Oxford, England: Blackwell Scientific, 1988. pp. 52-60.
5. Burgess EM, Wittenberger DA, Forsgren SM, Lindh D. The Seattle prosthetic foot: a design for active sports. *J Prosthet Orthot* 1983;37(1):25-31.

6. Perry J. *Gait Analysis; Normal and Pathological Function.* New York: McGraw-Hill, 1992. pp. 61-69.
7. Cummings D, Kapp SL, MacClellan B. *Below Knee Prosthetics.* Dallas: University of Texas Prosthetics Orthotics Program, 1987. pp. 4/14-4/20.
8. Shurr DG, Michael JW. *Prosthetics and Orthotics,* 2nd ed. Norwalk, CT: Appleton & Lange, 2002. pp. 69-74.
9. Donatelli R. *The Biomechanics of the Foot and Ankle.* Philadelphia: F.A. Davis, 1990. pp. 9-27.
10. Pitkin MR. Mechanical outcomes of a rolling-joint prosthetic foot and its performance in the dorsiflexion phase of transtibial amputee gait. *J Prosthet Orthot* 1995;7(3):114-123.
11. Kapp S, Cummings D. Prosthetic management. In Bowker JH, Michael JW (eds), *Atlas of Limb Prosthetics.* St. Louis: Mosby-Year Book, 1992. pp. 463-466.
12. Perry J. Anatomy and biomechanics of the hindfoot. *Clin Orthop* 1983;July-Aug(177):9-15.
13. Kegal B, Webster JC, Burgess EM, et al. Recreational activities of lower extremity amputees: a survey. *Arch Phys Med Rehabil* 1980;61(6):258-264.
14. Enoka RM, Miller DI, Burgess EM, et al. Below amputee running gait. *Am J Phys Med* 1982;61(2):66-84.
15. Burgess EM. The Seattle Prosthetic Foot. In Murdock G, Donovan RG (eds), *Amputation Surgery and Lower Limb Prosthetics.* Oxford, England: Blackwell Scientific, 1988. pp. 61-62.
16. MacFarlane PA, Nielsen DH, Shurr DG, et al. Perception of walking difficulty by below-knee amputees using a conventional foot versus the Flex-Foot. *J Prosthet Orthot* 1991;3(3):114-119.
17. Barth DG, Schumacher L, Thomas SS, et al. Gait analysis and energy cost of below-knee amputees wearing six different prosthetic feet. *J Prosthet Orthot* 1992;4(2):63-75.
18. Snyder RD, Powers CM, Fontaine C, et al. The effect of five prosthetic feet on the gait and loading of the sound limb in dysvascular below-knee amputees. *J Rehabil Res Dev* 1995;32(4):309-315.
19. Mizuno N, Aoyama T, Nakajima A, et al. Functional evaluation by gait analysis of various ankle-foot assemblies used by below-knee amputees. *Prosthet Orthot Int* 1992;16:174-182.
20. Bruins M, Geertzen JH, Groothoff JW, Schoppen T. Vocational reintegration after a lower limb amputation: a qualitative study. *Prosthet Orthot Int* 2003;27(1):4-10.
21. Schmalz T, Blumentritt S, Jarasch R. Energy expenditure and biomechanical characteristics of lower limb amputee gait: the influence of prosthetic alignment and different prosthetic components. *Gait Posture* 2002;16(521):255-263.

25

Postsurgical Management of Partial Foot and Syme Amputation

EDMOND AYYAPPA

LEARNING OBJECTIVES

On completion of this chapter, the reader will be able to do the following:

1. Differentiate among the various disarticulation and transaction surgeries used when amputation of the forefoot, midfoot, or rearfoot is necessary.
2. Describe usual gait performance and limitations of individuals with a partial foot and with Syme amputation.
3. Compare the advantages and disadvantages of prosthetic options for individuals with partial foot amputation.
4. Compare the advantages and disadvantages of the various prosthetic designs for persons with Syme amputation, including donning and pressure tolerance.
5. Compare how the various nonarticulating and dynamic response Syme prosthetic feet mimic the three rockers of gait.
6. Describe typical static and dynamic alignment variables or issues affecting gait for patients with a Syme or partial foot prosthesis.
7. Use knowledge of prosthetic options to suggest prosthetic prescriptions and plans of care for patients with partial foot and Syme amputation.

Partial foot and Syme level amputations present advantages and challenges to the patient and the rehabilitation team. Preservation of the ankle and heel (in partial foot amputation) and most of the length of the lower limb (in Syme amputation) has an important advantage of distal weight-bearing capability: the individual with partial foot or Syme level amputation is often able to ambulate without a prosthesis if necessary. The prosthesis, however, provides protection for the vulnerable distal residual limb for patients with vascular compromise and neuropathy.

The length and shape of the residual limb present three challenges for successful fitting and prosthetic training for patients with partial foot or Syme amputation: suspension of the prosthesis on the residual limb, distribution of weight-bearing forces within the prosthesis, and attachment and alignment of the prosthetic foot. This chapter defines the most common partial foot and Syme amputations and reviews the prosthetic management options currently available. Also identified are specific indications and contraindications for the various prosthetic designs.

PARTIAL FOOT AMPUTATIONS

Until the advent of antibiotics, disarticulation through the joints of the foot reduced the risk of sepsis and shock and improved the prognosis for healing compared with amputations that transected bone. The earliest partial foot amputation was recorded in 434 BC by the Greek historian Herodotus,[1] who told of a Persian warrior who escaped death while in the stocks by disarticulating his own foot. He hobbled 30 miles to a nearby town, where he was nursed to health until he could construct a prosthesis for himself. Later he became a soothsayer for the Persian army but ultimately was recaptured by the Spartans and killed.

At present, partial foot amputations include a wide variety of ray resections, digit (phalangeal) amputations, and metatarsal transections (Figure 25-1). Midfoot amputations include surgical ablation at Chopart and Lisfranc levels (Figure 25-2).[2] The Chopart disarticulation involves the talocalcaneonavicular joint and separates the talus and navicular as well as the calcaneus and cuboid.[3] The Lisfranc disarticulation separates the three cuneiform bones and the cuboid bone from the five metatarsal bones of the forefoot.

The three hindfoot amputations are the Pirogoff, Boyd, and Syme. The Pirogoff amputation is a wedging transection of the calcaneus, followed by bony fusion of the calcaneus and distal tibia with all other distal structures removed. In the Boyd amputation, the calcaneus remains largely intact

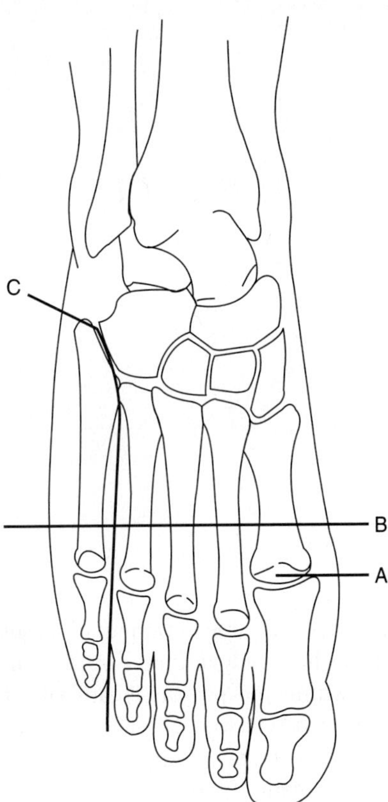

Figure 25-1
Examples of amputations involving the forefoot. A, *This digit (phalangeal) amputation involves disarticulation at the tarsal-metatarsal joint. More distal digit amputations remove either the distal phalanx or the middle and distal phalanges.* B, *In this complete transmetatarsal amputation, transaction occurred just proximal to all five metatarsal heads.* C, *Ray resections involve disarticulation of one or more metatarsals and their phalanges from the tarsal and neighboring metatarsals. Ray resections often require skin graft to achieve adequate tissue closure.*

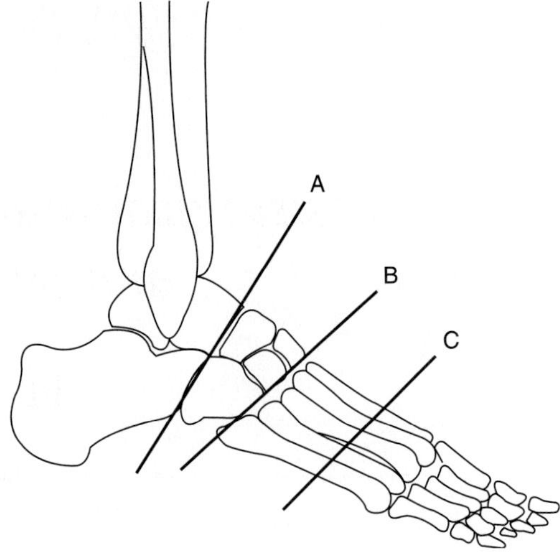

Figure 25-2
In a Chopart amputation (A) *there is disarticulation of the midfoot from the forefoot at the level of the talus and calcaneus. In a Lisfranc's amputation* (B) *there is disarticulation of the forefoot (metatarsals) from the midfoot (tarsals). In a transmetatarsal amputation, there is transaction through the length of one or more metatarsals, usually just proximal to the metatarsal heads.*

rather than being wedged before arthrodesis with the tibia. Today these amputations are infrequently performed on adult patients. Neither provides an easy fit with a prosthesis. The Boyd amputation has received positive clinical reviews when used in the management of congenital limb deficiencies in children in which the amputated limb is shorter than the sound limb.[4,5] In this case, there are usually fewer post-operative complications, such as scarring and heel pad migration, and less susceptibility to the bony overgrowth common in children with congenital limb deficiencies. The Syme amputation is performed more frequently in adults because of the ease of prosthetic management at this level (Figure 25-3). Because of the length of the residual limb in the Pirogoff and Boyd amputations, the attachment of a prosthetic foot lengthens the limb when a prosthesis is worn. A heel lift on the contralateral sound limb is usually necessary to counteract this artificially long prosthetic limb.

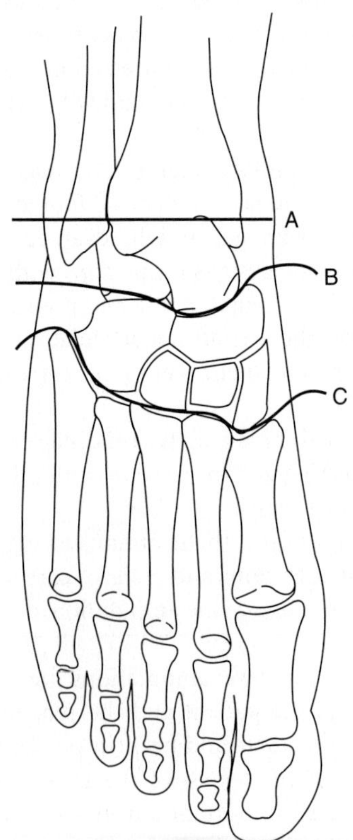

Figure 25-3
A, *The Syme amputation involves removal of the inferior projections of the tibia and fibula and all bone structures distally while preserving the natural weight-bearing fat pad of the heel.* B, *The Chopart amputation preserves the talus and calcaneus.* C, *The Lisfranc amputation has disarticulation of metatarsals from the midfoot.*

Proximal partial foot amputations often result in equinus deformities because of muscular imbalance created by severed dorsiflexors and intact triceps surae.[6-8] Nevertheless, many individuals with a partial foot amputation function extremely well. In one survey, physicians and prosthetists reported that patients with partial foot amputation function better than those with Syme amputation.[9] Although surgeons and prosthetists have long supported Syme amputation in preference to Lisfranc or Chopart amputations, many patients with midfoot amputation achieve high levels of function. For example, Jack Dempsey, a professional football player with a midfoot amputation, set several all-time field goal records wearing a custom-designed kicking boot.[10]

Gait Characteristics after Partial Foot Amputation

A person with a partial foot amputation typically has vascular insufficiency, is usually between the ages of 60 and 70 years, has compromised proprioception and sensation, and has weak lower limb musculature. After Syme or partial foot amputation a patient may be able to ambulate without a prosthesis but has a loss of the anterior lever arm in ambulation and an inefficient, somewhat dysfunctional gait. The primary need immediately after amputation is to protect the remaining tissue, which is vulnerable to vascular or neuropathic disease. The neuropathic walker developed at Rancho Los Amigos Medical Center locks the ankle in a custom-molded, foam-lined, thermoplastic ankle-foot orthosis (AFO) (Figure 25-4). A rocker bottom is contoured to promote a smooth rollover as a substitute for the second and third rockers of gait, and the orthosis provides optimum protection for the insensate residual foot. For patients with adequate protective sensation, the risk of tissue breakdown is less and a custom shoe insert with in-depth or postoperative shoes often provides adequate protection.

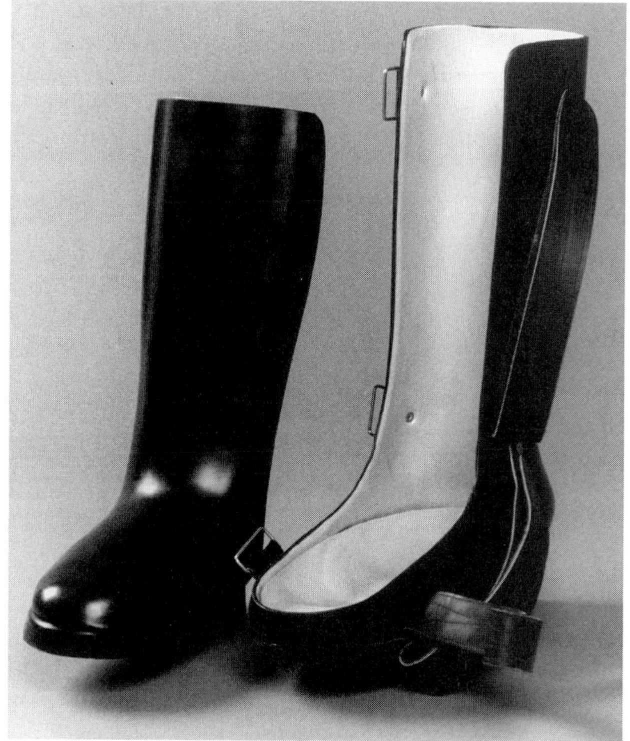

Figure 25-4
The neuropathic walker provides maximum protection for the denervated foot at risk for amputation. The combination of custom-molded multidurometer liner, locked neutral ankle, and rocker bottom permits a rollover with minimal plantar pressure and shear.

A review of gait in partial foot case histories showed variations in single-limb support time directly related to the reduction of the forefoot lever arm of a partial foot and subsequent increase in the force concentration on the distal end during terminal stance, reflected as reduced time in single-limb support on the limb with amputation (Figure 25-5).[11]

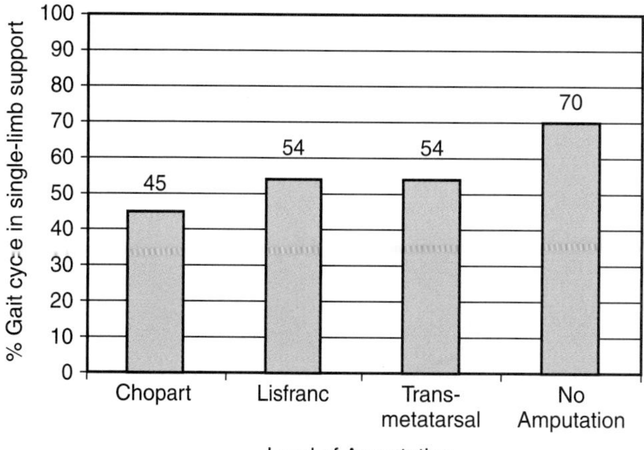

Figure 25-5
Percent of the gait cycle spent in single-limb support for patients with midfoot Chopart or Lisfranc amputations and forefoot transmetatarsal amputation. Healthy older adults with intact feet typically spend between 65% and 75% of their gait cycle in single-limb support.

In a person with a whole foot, a fully intact anterior lever arm preserves elevation of the center of mass at terminal stance. With normal quadriceps strength and eccentric control, slight knee flexion (15 to 20 degrees) provides shock absorption as weight is rapidly transferred onto the limb during loading response (Figure 25-6). Most people with dysvascular partial foot and Syme amputation demonstrate significant weakness of the quadriceps. This functional weakness threatens eccentric control of the usual knee flexion angle that occurs during loading response. To compensate, the patient may keep the knee extended during loading response. This strategy shifts the ground reaction force vector to a position anterior to the knee joint axis, thus reducing the workload of the quadriceps. Although this compensatory strategy enhances early stance phase stability, it sacrifices the shock absorption mechanism at the knee and hip joints, increasing the likelihood of cumulative joint trauma at both joints (see Figure 25-6, *B*). Neuropathic impairment of proprioception and sensation may further complicate

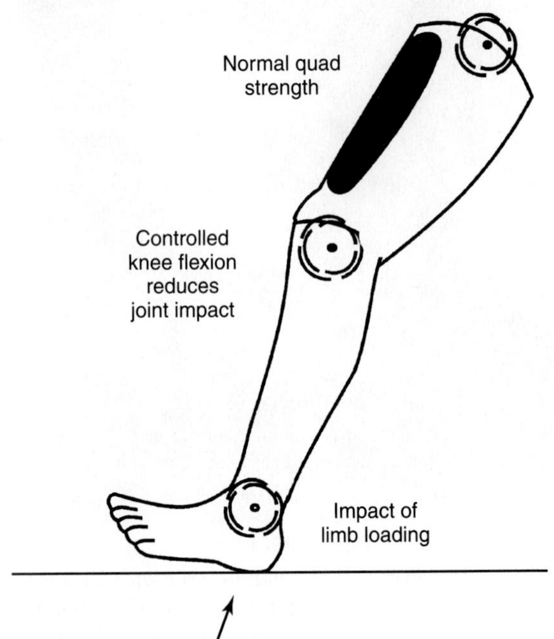

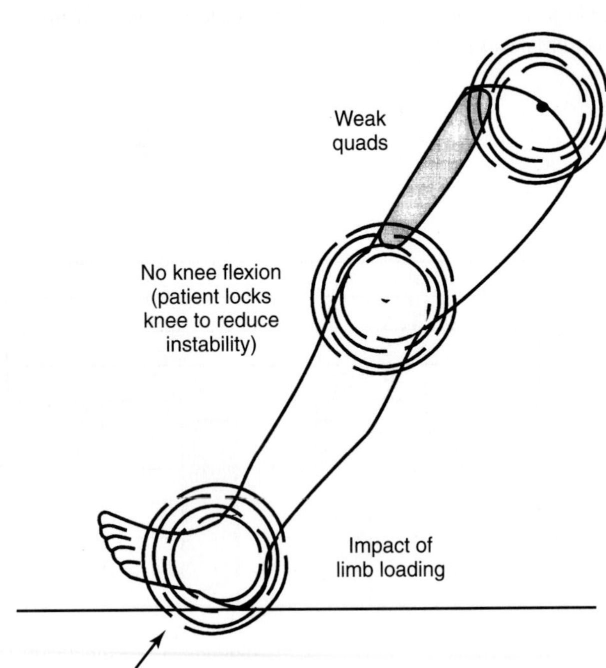

Figure 25-6

A, *During loading in normal gait, knee flexion provides a significant shock absorption mechanism to protect the proximal joints.* ***B,*** *The patient with weakness associated with dysvascular disease avoids knee flexion to increase stability, with a penalty of increased trauma to the proximal joints as a consequence of repeated higher impact loading.*

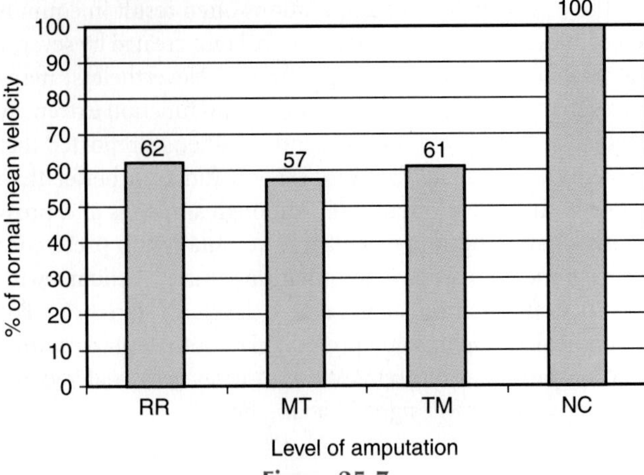

Figure 25-7

Reduced gait velocity in patients with partial foot amputations. On average, patients walked at 62% of gait velocity of control subjects with intact lower limbs. RR, *Ray resection;* MT, *metatarsal amputation of 1 to 4 rays;* TM, *complete transmetatarsal amputation;* NC, *normal control subjects.*

control of the knee in early stance. In addition, compromised forefoot support increases center of gravity displacement. A penalty of higher energy cost results.

A recent study of the gait of persons with partial foot amputation included 18 patients with transmetatarsal amputations, 11 with one or more metatarsal amputations, 15 with ray resections, and 2 with either Lisfranc or Chopart amputations.[11-13] One portion of the analysis focused on the mechanics of the residual limb rockers. Partly because of a delay in the forefoot rocker, patients with all types of partial foot amputations walked with a significantly slower velocity than control subjects with healthy, intact feet (Figure 25-7). Peak ankle dorsiflexion was also significantly delayed for all three partial foot groups compared with those with intact feet. Although the control group with intact lower limbs reached peak ankle dorsiflexion at a point 43% into the gait cycle, patients with partial foot amputation did not reach peak dorsiflexion angle until nearly the halfway point of the gait cycle (Figure 25-8). This delay in reaching peak dorsiflexion subsequently delays forward progression over the shortened stance limb and the transition to double-limb support.

The rise rate of the vertical ground reaction force is the amount of force that occurs in 1% of the gait cycle and can be expressed as Newtons divided by the percent of the gait cycle. After controlling for variation in velocity, the rise rate of the vertical ground reaction force from mid to terminal stance (as the force pattern nears its F2 peak) was significantly lower for all three amputation groups compared with the control group (Figure 25-9). Peak vertical ground reaction forces were significantly higher for the sound limb than the affected limb, likely reflecting an abrupt unloading of the partial foot amputation limb.

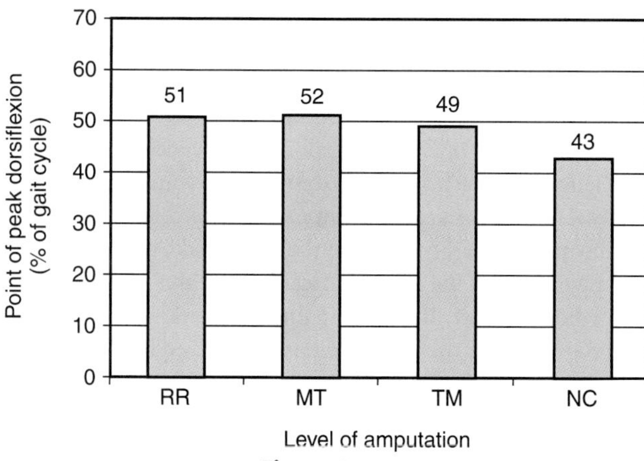

Figure 25-8
For persons with partial foot amputations, maximum dorsiflexion is delayed during stance phase of the gait cycle. Although control subjects with intact feet achieved a maximum dorsiflexion angle at a point 43% into the gait cycle, those with partial foot amputation did not reach the maximum dorsiflexion angle until halfway through the cycle. The consequence of this delay is a slowed forward progression of the body's center of mass and transition to the subsequent period of double-limb support. RR, *Ray resection;* MT, *metatarsal amputation of 1 to 4 rays;* TM, *complete transmetatarsal amputation;* NC, *normal control subjects.*

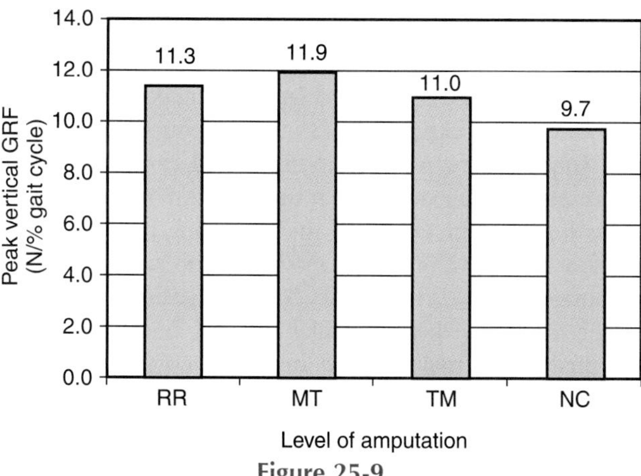

Figure 25-9
Comparison of peak vertical ground reaction force (GRF) *of the intact limbs of patients with partial foot amputations and persons without amputation, expressed as Newton divided by % of gait cycle.* RR, *Ray resection;* MT, *metatarsal amputation of 1 to 4 rays;* TM, *complete transmetatarsal amputation;* NC, *normal control subjects.*

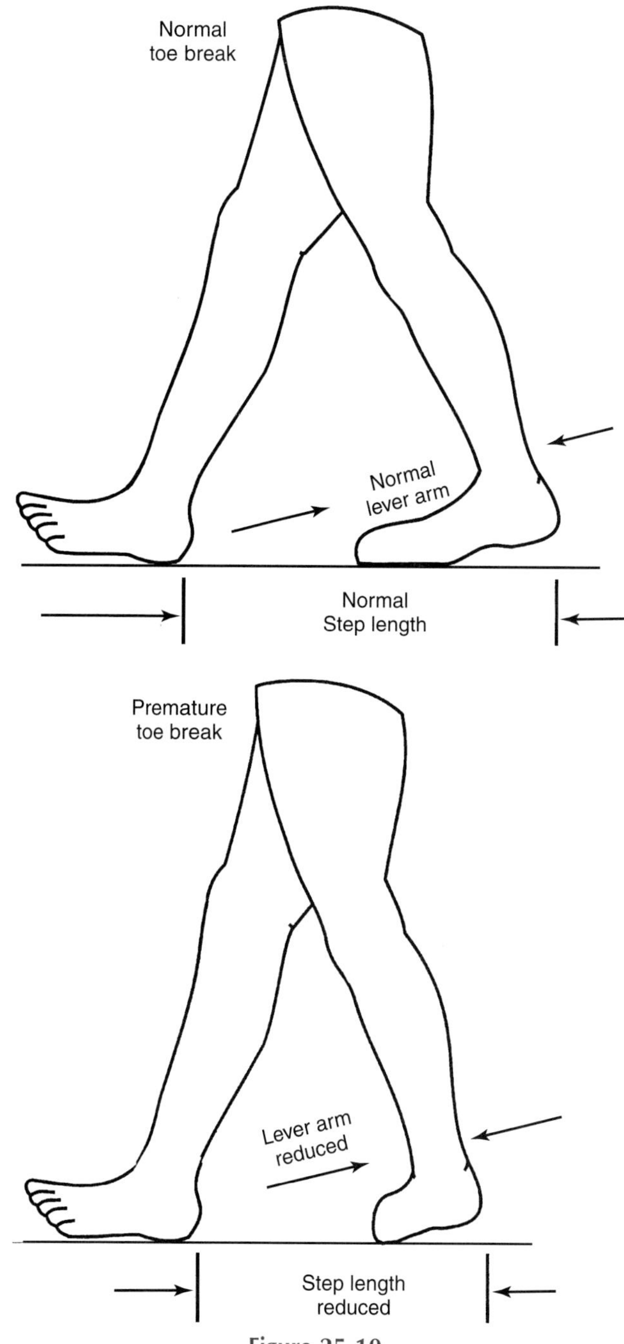

Figure 25-10
A, *The forefoot lever arm contributes to a normal step length.* ***B,*** *Reduction of the forefoot support after partial foot amputation produces a consequent reduction in contralateral step length.*

The forefoot lever arm of the trailing limb typically provides anterior support and results in adequate terminal stance support time (Figure 25-10). This results in appropriate step length of the advancing limb. By contrast, inadequate anterior support of the trailing limb of the partial foot amputee reduces the lever arm, resulting in premature toe break and forefoot collapse. The step length of the advancing limb may be correspondingly reduced (see Figure 25-10, *B*).

An inverse relation exists between surface area and peak pressure when body weight is loaded on the foot during stance. This relation is especially important for individuals with partial foot amputation during terminal stance. As the

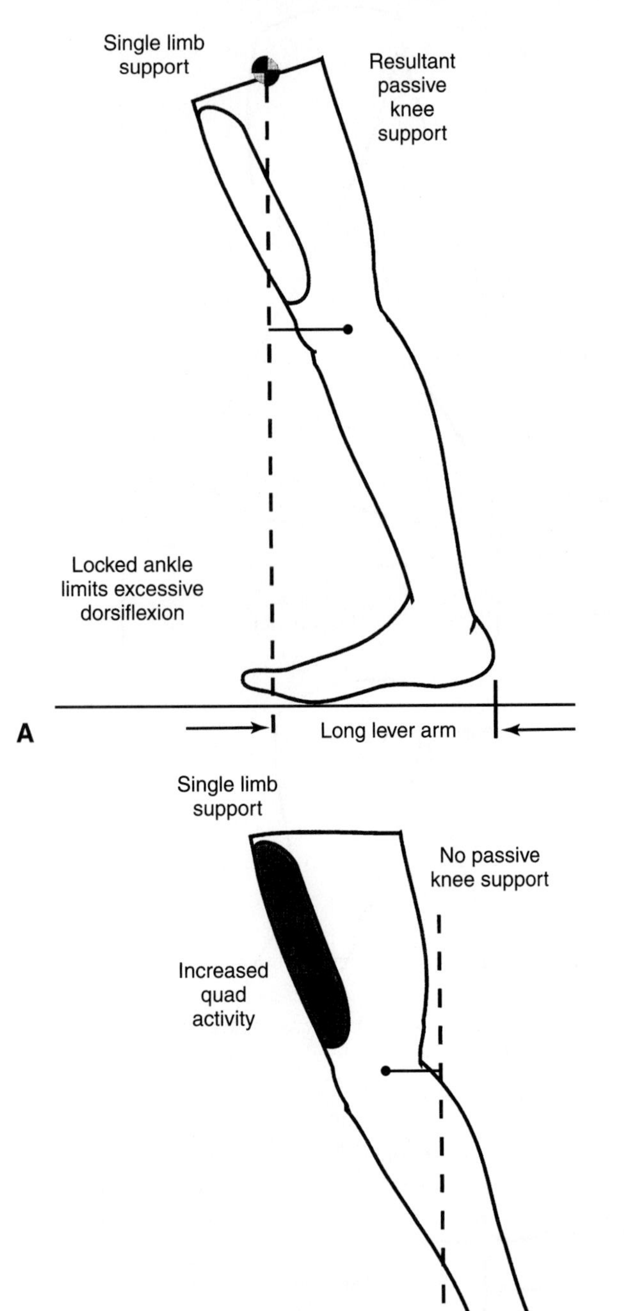

Figure 25-11

A, *Normal energy-efficient passive knee support in late stance relies on a locked or rigid forefoot that limits further dorsiflexion at the ankle and a normal forefoot lever arm to maintain the ground reaction force anterior to the knee during late stance.* ***B,*** *After partial foot amputation, the reduced forefoot lever arm often leads to increased quadriceps activity to compensate for reduced passive knee support and ensure stability in late stance.*

plantar surface area of the supporting forefoot is reduced, the magnitude of the pressure is increased.[11-13] The reduced forefoot lever arm also creates abrupt weight transfer to the contralateral side and can reduce step length, stride length, and velocity. Without prosthetic support, the advancing sound-side step length diminishes. Fear, insecurity, and pain aggravated by increased pressure near the amputation site collectively create an abrupt transfer of weight to the sound side, thus increasing the magnitude of the initial vertical force peak.[14]

In normal gait, the weight line is positioned more and more anterior to the knee joint as the gait cycle moves from midstance into terminal stance and preswing phases (Figure 25-11). As a result, the limb is held in a passive, energy-efficient extended knee position, effectively supporting body weight and increasing stability in late stance. The length of the forefoot lever arm is one of the key determinants of this support. For persons with partial foot amputation, the lever arm of the foot is greatly reduced, leading to a less-effective, premature loss of support at the end of stance phase. This shorter lever places the ground reaction force closer to or behind the knee in late stance (see Figure 25-11, *B*). Because much of the passive stability provided by a normal forefoot lever in late stance is absent, the quadriceps must contract to maintain stance phase stability, contributing to an increased energy cost of walking for persons with partial foot amputation.

Pinzur and colleagues[15] described a functional relation between gait velocity and the level of amputation at the foot. As the amputation level becomes more proximal (as the length of the residual foot decreases), changes in temporal and kinetic gait characteristics include reduced sound-side step length, decreased velocity, increased energy cost, and increased vertical load on the sound side. An inverse relation exists between the length of the remaining portion of the forefoot and the time spent in single-limb support on the amputated side.[14] When the level of amputation is proximal to the metatarsal heads, medial support is lost at loading response. This may require orthotic "posting" to limit resultant valgus deformity. Patients with partial foot amputation frequently have plantar flexion contracture develop from muscle imbalance. Any plantar flexion contracture, in turn, increases pressure at the distal residual limb during terminal stance, causing discomfort, pain, and risk of ulceration.[16] A contracture is even more problematic for individuals with Hansen's disease or diabetic neuropathy because they already have compromised sensation.[17,18] Shoes worn without prosthetic replacement of the missing forefoot quickly become disfigured, collapsing at a displaced toe break, further endangering the vulnerable areas of the residual limb.[19] The areas of the residual foot most vulnerable to tissue damage during walking include the distal end, first and fifth metatarsal heads, navicular, malleoli, and tibial crest. The longitudinal and transverse arches, the heel pad, and the area along the pretibial muscle belly are pressure-tolerant areas for loading in a custom shoe or prosthesis.

Prosthetic Management

During the 1800s, digit amputations were fitted by a wood or cork sandal with a leather ankle lacer.[20,21] Partial foot amputations were sometimes fitted with a socket and keel fashioned from one piece of carefully chosen root wood, the grain of which followed the curve of the ankle. This was referred to as the *natural crook technique*. Another commonly used historical design incorporated steel-reinforced leather sockets.[22]

In recent decades, a wide variety of prosthetic options for individuals with partial foot amputation have emerged. The prescribing physician and patient care team must familiarize themselves with the broad array of options available in prosthetic components and design so that prescription considerations can best accommodate the special needs of each patient. Because of variability in level of amputation, sensitivity or insensitivity of the residual limb, concurrent foot deformity, and patient activity, no single prosthetic prescription can be used for all patients with foot amputation.[23] As the amputation level becomes more proximal and the length of the residual foot decreases, prostheses are more likely to incorporate supramalleolar containment or more superior support. This is especially true as a patient's activity level increases. Commonly used prosthetic approaches include toe fillers placed inside the shoe, a foot orthosis or an arch support, the University of California Biomechanics Laboratory (UCBL) orthosis to control heel position, and a boot or slipper made of flexible urethane resin (Smooth-On, Easton, Pa.). Cosmetic restoration of silicone and several variations of AFOs are also in common use.

The length and degree of flexibility of the prosthetic forefoot affect the anterior lever arm and consequently foot and ankle motion. The biomechanical goal is to allow anterior support in the area of the lost metatarsals as well as a controlled fulcrum of forward motion as the foot-ankle complex pivots over the area of the lost metatarsal heads in the third rocker of late stance. An additional goal is to minimize pressure at the amputated distal end within the socket or shoe.

Toe Fillers and Modified Shoes

If a simple filler is prescribed, an extended steel shank or band of rigid spring steel should also be placed within the sole of the shoe, extending from the calcaneus to the metatarsal heads. The challenge that faces the prosthetist is to match the appropriate degree of forefoot flexibility to the needs of each patient. For an energy-efficient and cosmetic gait, relative plantar rigidity should give way to at least 15 degrees of forefoot flexibility distal to the metatarsal heads. The extended steel shank is helpful in providing a limited degree of buoyancy that substitutes for the lost anterior support of the foot.[24] Stiffening the sole with a spring steel shank increases the lever arm support, but often at the expense of additional pressure on the distal end of the residual limb.[25]

For a patient with a more complex partial foot amputation, a rocker bottom shoe modification distributes force

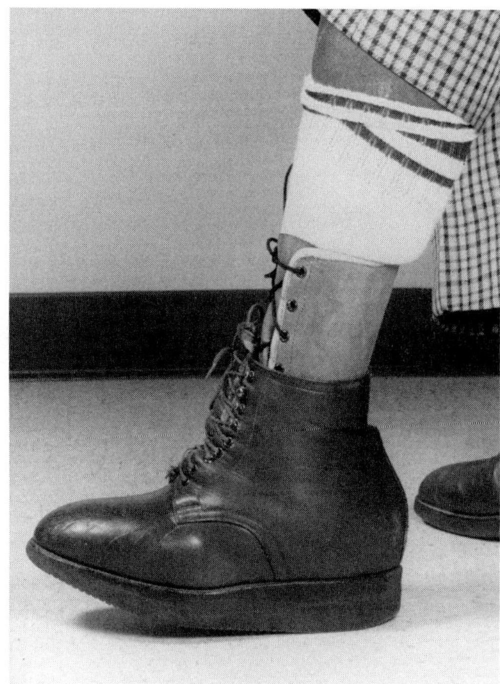

Figure 25-12
A supramalleolar leather lacer, worn inside a high-top extra-depth shoe with toe filler and rocker bottom, is an effective prosthetic choice for this patient with a Chopart amputation.

over a greater area and advances stance more quickly and efficiently. A curved roll or buildup on the plantar surface of the shoe encourages tibial advancement while minimizing weight-bearing pressures on the distal amputated end (Figure 25-12). For optimal function the plantar contour of a rocker bottom should follow a radius originating from the knee joint center but break or roll more abruptly just distal to the metatarsal heads. Although a rocker bottom assists rollover, it also compromises symmetry of gait. It is often prescribed for individuals with chronic pain or in conjunction with a custom-molded accommodative interface for those with a neuropathy-related risk of reamputation. Extra-depth shoes have 6 to 8 mm or more of space inside the shoe on the plantar surface to accommodate an orthotic insert or prosthesis and may be useful for patients with digit or ray amputations.[23]

Custom-molded shoes, when used in conjunction with a filler and shank, improve the comfort level and reduce the risk of ulceration in many dysvascular patients with amputation. They are not as subject to forefoot collapse, provide major protection to the endangered foot, and may last longer than stock shoes.[26]

Custom Shoe Inserts and Toe Fillers

A custom-molded, flexible, plantar shoe insert is one of the options for individuals with amputation of the hallux or first ray. This orthotic approach is typically used in combination with extra-depth shoes. The goal is to provide a flexible

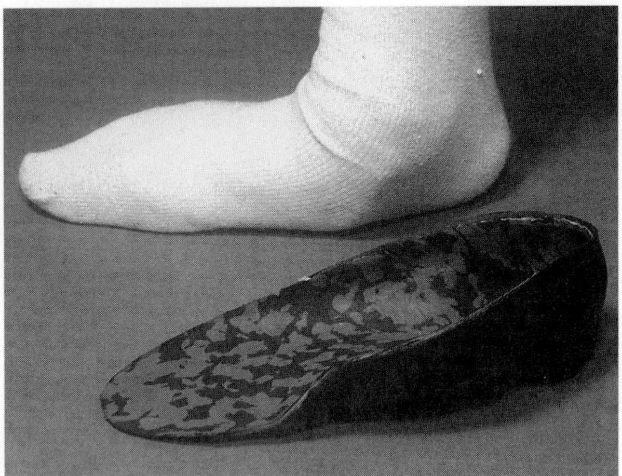

Figure 25-13
The custom-molded University of California Biomechanics Laboratory orthosis attempts to obtain a purchase over the os calcis and is thought to influence alignment of the subtalar joint. This patient has ray resection of the hallux and first metatarsal.

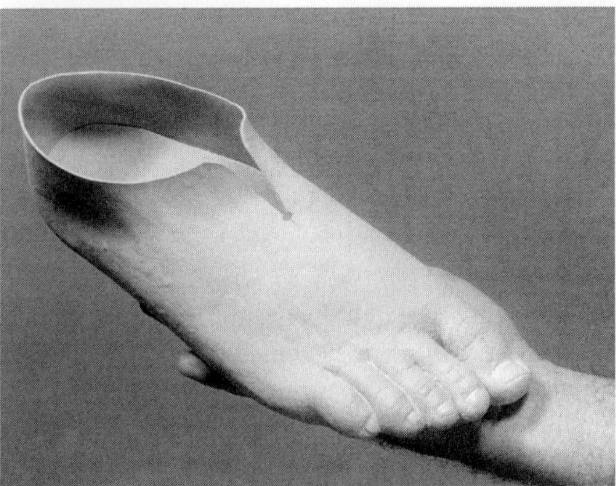

Figure 25-14
The life cast prosthesis provides excellent cosmesis with little or no biomechanical assistance. Without additional reinforcement a silicone slipper-style prosthesis does not provide adequate forefoot support.

anterior extension to compensate for a missing or shortened first ray to improve the third rocker and yet support and protect the amputation site during the simulated metatarsophalangeal hyperextension in late stance and preswing.[27] This provides some relief for metatarsal head pressure, supports the arch, and probably assists in normalizing the ground reaction force pattern during terminal stance and preswing. It may incorporate a toe filler to prevent premature forefoot shoe collapse.[28-30] Toe fillers consist of soft foam material such as room-temperature vulcanized elastomer, which fills the voids in the toe box of the shoe. They provide limited extension of the shoe life and a moderate degree of cosmesis. They also act as spacers, keeping adjoining toes properly positioned and reducing abnormal motion that can otherwise lead to ulceration. The toe filler alone provides limited mechanical advantage. A spring steel shank within the sole of the shoe and extending from mid-calcaneus to the metatarsal heads can further improve gait. An alternative to the spring steel shank is a longitudinal support built into a flexible custom insole. Either support device must end at the metatarsal heads to allow hyperextension of the metatarsophalangeal joints. A foot orthotic with arch support and filler is preferable to the simple filler because it can be used in different shoes and because it provides plantar support to an already compromised weight-bearing surface.[31] Custom insoles can also be made from a sawdust and epoxy resin instead of foams and thermoplastics.

The UCBL, a foot orthosis that encapsulates the calcaneus, was developed at the University of California Biomechanics Laboratory during the 1960s and was comprehensively described in 1969.[32,33] The UCBL is designed to provide better control of subtalar and forefoot position than custom-made shoe inserts, reducing motion and thus friction with a closer fit or purchase over the calcaneus and forefoot (Figure 25-13).[34] The UCBL design can be effectively incorporated into a custom orthosis and filler for persons with partial foot amputation.

Cosmetic Slipper Designs

The slipper, one variation of which has been referred to as the *slipper-type elastomer prosthesis*, is fabricated from semi-flexible urethane elastomer.[35] A similar design in silicone may not provide adequate forefoot support without the addition of an extended steel shank in the patient's shoe. Another similar variation is made from a combination of silicone Silastic (Dow Corning, Midland, Mich.), polyester resin, and prosthetic (polyurethane) foam. These designs provide much of the support and control of the UCBL approach but with added cosmesis. These designs may be appropriate for individuals with transmetatarsal amputations or disarticulations. They are ideal for swimming or water sports because most are water impervious, cosmetic, and capable of providing a flexible whip action, which is useful with swim fins.

Some slipper-type prostheses are cosmetic restorations made of silicone or vinyl and based on a "life cast," or an alginate impression of a human model (Figure 25-14). This prosthesis is made for patients who consider cosmesis paramount. This custom prosthesis is most often produced in special manufacturing centers and frequently requires a considerable amount of time for delivery. It can be ordered with hair, freckles, and in a large variety of skin tones; however, it is most often a less than perfect match when compared with the intact contralateral foot. The patient should always share responsibility in the color swatch selection. The material itself is easily stained and changes color with time when exposed to sunlight. The cosmetic restoration provides little ambulation advantage but does increase shoe life. It may be appropriate for patients with transmetatarsal amputations who place a premium on cosmesis.

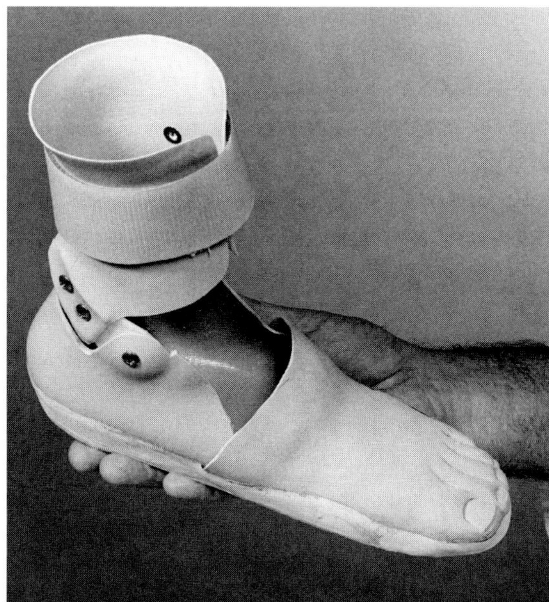

Figure 25-15
A prothetic boot, composed of epoxy-modified acrylic resin combined with supramalleolar containment and free motion, single-axis ankle joints, may be helpful at the transmetatarsal level. Without the circumferential containment above the ankle, patients often report joint pain toward the end of the day.

Prosthetic Boots

The prosthetic boot, with laced or hook-and-loop material ankle cuff closures, has greater proximal encompassment to reduce distal motion and increase control (Figure 25-15). This design is appropriate for individuals with Lisfranc's or transmetatarsal disarticulation or amputation. One variation, the Chicago boot, or Imler partial foot prosthesis, combines a thermoplastic UCBL-type heel cup with a flexible urethane prosthetic forefoot.[36,37] Other designs incorporate urethane with a modified solid-ankle, cushion heel foot; some are fabricated from leather, laminated plastic, or Silastic elastomer (Dow Corning), Plastazote (Bakelite Xylonite Ltd, United Kingdom) combinations, as an insert for a boot, or as an outer boot with inner filler to accommodate bony prominences.[38-41] Such boots often have an anterior or medial tongue and laces or some other means of obtaining a firm purchase above the ankle.[42-45] Some variation of the prosthetic boot may be the general prosthesis of choice for most patients with midfoot amputations.

Ankle-Foot Orthoses

The AFO is another option for persons with partial foot amputation. The polypropylene or copolymer shell supports the plantar aspect of the foot, incorporates the heel, and extends up the posterior leg to the belly of the gastrocnemius (Figure 25-16). A circumferential anterior strap stabilizes the limb in the AFO. As an alternative, metal uprights may be attached to a shoe but have obvious cosmetic drawbacks. The AFO, whether metal or plastic, provides advantages of the arch support/UCBL and boot with maximum containment and a lever arm for support and substitution of the rocker mechanism. It offers enhanced stability and control because of its high proximal trimline. It has been an excellent solution for many patients with partial foot amputation and may be the prosthesis of choice for the active patient with Chopart or Lisfranc amputation. Supramalleolar thermoplastic or laminated versions are fit with Tamarack (Blaine, Minn.) or Gillette (Gillette Children's Specialty Healthcare, St. Paul, Minn.) joints to provide free plantar and dorsiflexion motion. This biomechanical solution is popular for the higher activity level of midfoot amputations.

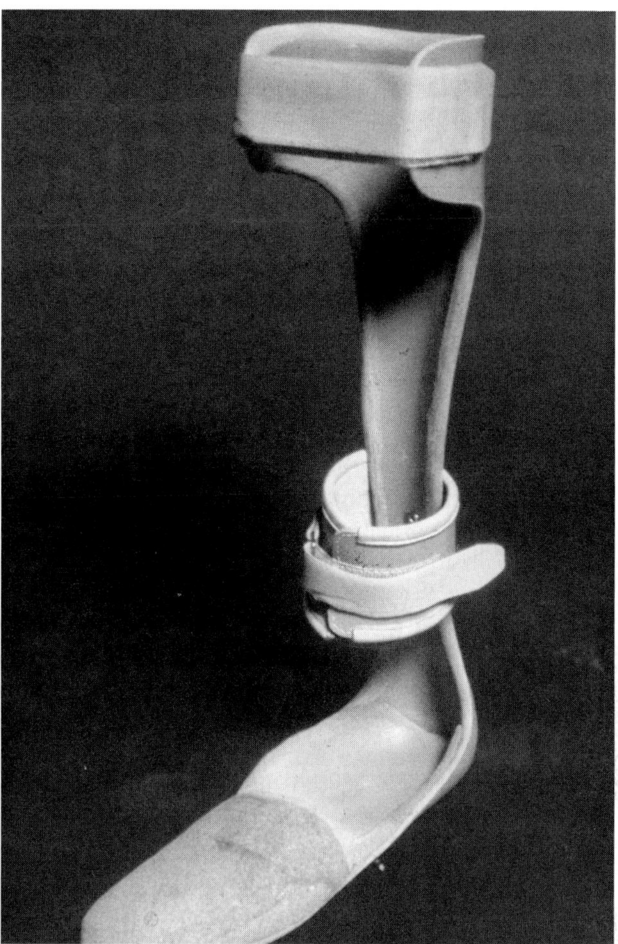

Figure 25-16
A posterior leaf spring AFO with toe filler and anterior strap is successful for many patients with partial foot amputation.

CASE EXAMPLE 1

An Individual with Bilateral Chopart's Amputation

A. E. is a 64-year-old man with a 23-year history of peripheral vascular disease, diabetes, and recurring foot ulcers. He underwent a Chopart amputation of his left lower extremity 7 years ago and has since successfully worn an orthopedic shoe with a toe filler. When needing to walk for long distances, A. E. uses a straight cane on the right to reduce distal anterior discomfort of his residual limb. Twelve months ago a neuropathic ulcer developed on his right plantar forefoot. Despite conservative management with felted foam and a Darco heel wedge shoe (Sammons-Preston, Bolingbrook, Ill.). the ulcer failed to heal and ultimately became infected and developed into osteomyelitis. He underwent Chopart amputation without complication, healed successfully, and now is able to stand unsupported without shoes or orthosis (Figure 25-17). He is able to ambulate in shoes with prosthetic fillers; however, he walks with a remarkably slow velocity and an observable shortened step length.

Questions to Consider

- Given his medical history, what concerns exist about the condition of his residual feet? What areas are most vulnerable to pressure from repetitive loading during walking in Chopart residual limbs?
- Are there muscle imbalances as a result of Chopart amputation that place him at risk for development of contracture? How should joint excursion of his shortened feet be examined? What indicators of muscle performance are important to assess? What measures should be used to assess muscle function and strength? How should any impairments be addressed?
- How will his shortened feet affect his progression through the gait cycle? Will he have compromise of the first rocker from initial contact through loading response? Of the second rocker from loading response through midstance to terminal stance? Of the third rocker in terminal stance into preswing? Why will there be shortened step and stride length of the opposite swing limb?
- What are the major goals for prosthetic intervention for A. E.? What specific recommendations should be made and why? What is his prognosis for functional ambulation? Should an assistive device be recommended for long-term use? Why or why not? How should the efficacy of intervention be assessed?

Recommendations

After reviewing his overall gait performance and discussing his functional needs, the team recommends bilateral rocker bottom walking boots (Figure 25-18). (Walking boots are most often recommended for individuals with single-limb Chopart amputation.) After prosthetic fitting with bilateral rocker boots, temporal parameters significantly improved over orthopedic shoes. Although A. E. had identical cadence with both conditions (shoe and boot), his step length dramatically increased and single-limb support time decreased when wearing the rocker boots. The overall result is a significantly higher gait velocity. Although he initially used a straight cane on the left for balance and to reduce anterior distal pressures of his newly amputated limb, A. E. is now able to ambulate functional distances without assistive devices. He uses his cane only when in crowds to "buy himself more space" and reduce the likelihood he will be bumped or jostled by others.

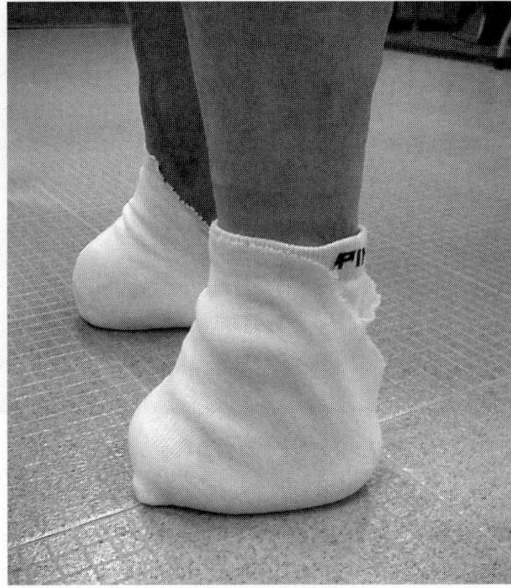

Figure 25-17
An individual with bilateral Chopart amputation is able to stand steadily. Because of the short forefoot lever, however, the "sway envelope" for dynamic postural control is likely narrowed. Plantar flexion contracture, if present, would compromise stability and increase pressure at the distal plantar surface of the residual limb. In this illustration, the patient is wearing several layers of socks before putting on his prostheses.

SYME AMPUTATION

In 1867 E.D. Hudson, the surgeon general of the United States, described Syme amputation with a litany of superlatives: "No amputation of the inferior extremity can ever compare in value with that of the ankle joint originated by Mr. Syme. Twelve years of experience with that variety of operation have afforded me assurance that it is a concept which is complete in itself and not capable of being improved in its general character."[46]

The Syme, or tibiotarsal, amputation is a disarticulation of the talocrural joint. The forefoot is completely removed, but the fat pad of the heel is preserved and anchored to the distal tibia. This allows distal end bearing and some degree of ambulation without a prosthesis (Figure 25-19; see also Figure 25-3).[47] It gained popularity during the late 1800s primarily because the likelihood of survival with this technique was substantially greater than with other surgical choices, given the reduced degree of sepsis and shock that occurred when bone was not severed.[48]

Two possible problems exist in amputations at the Syme level: migration of the distal heel pad (which may be surgi-

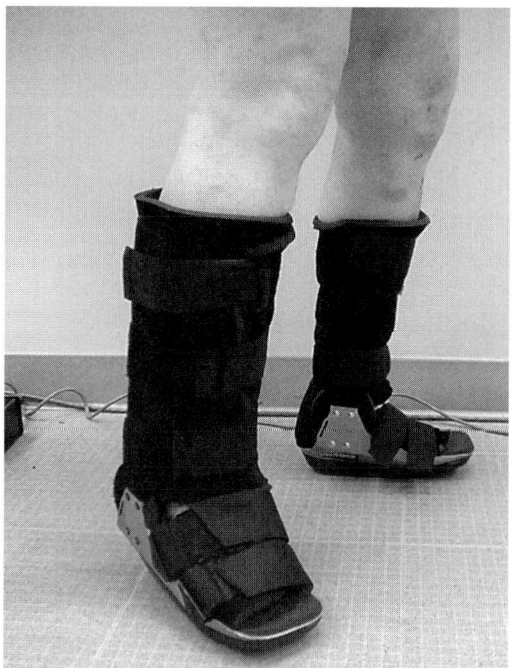

Figure 25-18
This individual with bilateral Chopart amputation has been fit with bilateral rocker bottom walkers. The rocker bottom mimics second and third rockers of the gait cycle, whereas the extension of the anterior lever provides additional dynamic stability in gait. These combine to increase stride and step length for improved functional mobility and a more energy-efficient gait.

cally avoidable) and poor cosmetic result (which can sometimes be partially addressed by removal of the malleoli). For a positive outcome, the vascular supply must be adequate to ensure healing. The resurgence of popularity of Syme amputation today is from an increased awareness of its energy efficiency in gait compared with transtibial levels as well as improved vascular evaluation techniques and medical procedures that increase the likelihood of more distal primary wound healing.[49,50] In addition, the dramatic weight-bearing potential of a well-performed Syme surgery (with or without a prosthesis) has always been considered.[51] Pressure-sensitive areas of a Syme residual limb include the tibial crest, lateral tibial flair, fibula head, and the bony prominence around the distal expansion.[52,53] Pressure-tolerant areas include the midpatella tendon, medial tibial flair, and anterior tibialis.

Postoperative Care: Walking Casts

To avoid medial migration of the heel pad in the postoperative period, gait training and other therapy that involve weight bearing should be encouraged only after delivery of the prosthesis. The prosthesis is designed to hold the ankle and bulbous distal residual in an appropriate relation. A fully mature residual limb is less likely to displace. Early prosthetic fitting may involve a definitive prosthesis or a temporary walking cast with a patten bottom (Figure 25-20). The temporary walking cast may be especially preferred if the patient has edema, is obese, or has other medical conditions in which significant volume loss is anticipated. The initial walking cast should be applied as soon as the sutures have been removed, usually within 2 weeks of surgery. The successful application of a Syme walking cast requires a more thorough knowledge base in prosthetics than might be readily appreciated. Application of a walking cast should be done by a clinician with a solid prosthetic background.

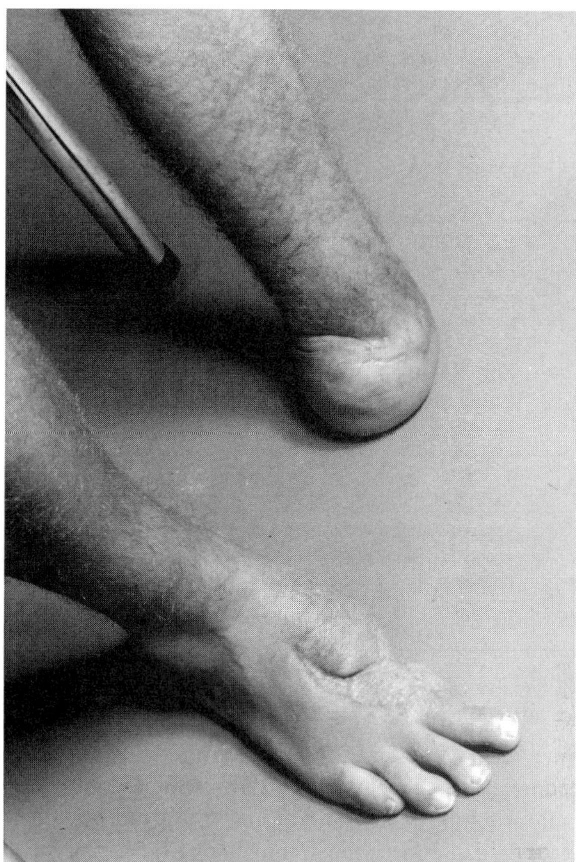

Figure 25-19
This individual has had a Syme level amputation of the left lower extremity and a first ray (hallux) resection in the right lower extremity. Early weight-bearing before prosthetic fitting can aggravate migration of the heel pad after Syme amputation, even though migration is primarily a function of surgical technique.

Prosthetic Management

The prosthesis for a Syme amputation must be strong enough at the ankle section to withstand the forces of tension and compression that are produced by the long tibial lever arm throughout the gait cycle and at the same time provide an acceptable degree of cosmesis over the bulbous expansion at the ankle. All prosthetic designs strive to

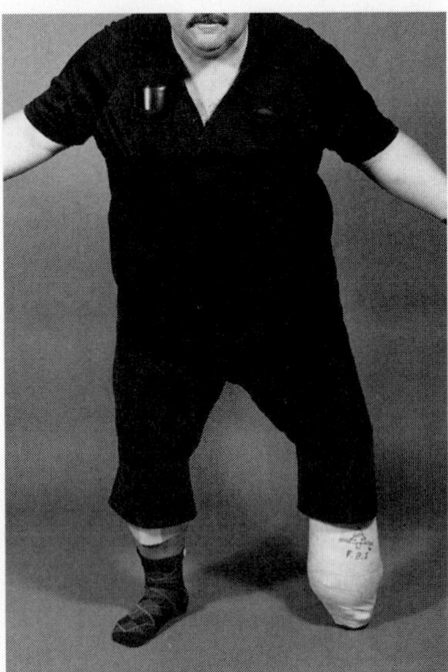

Figure 25-20
The patten bottom in a walking cast is used when the clinic team anticipates gross volume changes in a patient with Syme amputation.

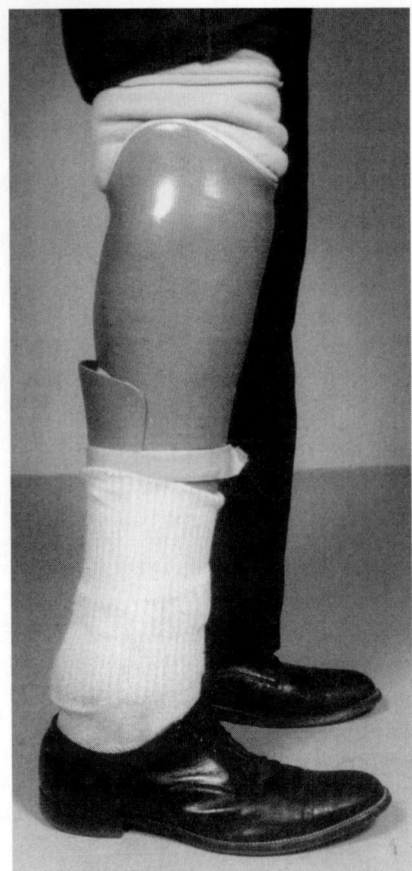

Figure 25-21
The Canadian Syme prosthesis has a posterior opening access panel that diminishes its strength at the ankle. It may be inappropriate for heavy-duty wearers.

encompass the tibial section above the distal expansion firmly and still permit donning and doffing. Although prostheses designed for Syme amputations may be appropriate for Pirogoff's and Boyd's amputations, use of such prostheses requires that a lift be placed on the contralateral shoe to achieve bilateral limb length symmetry.

Before World War II, most patients with Syme amputations were fit with anterior lacing wooden sockets or leather sockets supported by a superstructure of heavy medial and lateral steel sidebars.[53,54] The prostheses most frequently fabricated today include the Canadian, medial opening, sleeve suspension, and flexible wall (bladder) designs.

Canadian Syme Prostheses

The *Canadian Syme prosthesis* design was introduced during the 1950s as the first major improvement over the traditional steel-reinforced leather (Figure 25-21).[55-58] When viewing the ankle in the coronal plane, no obvious buildups, windows, or hardware is present to increase the ankle diameter. The Canadian Syme prosthesis has a removable posterior panel to facilitate donning and doffing. This donning window extends from the apex of the distal expansion, moving proximal as far as necessary to provide clearance for the bulbous end.[59] Breakage may be higher than with other Syme prostheses because the ankle area, which undergoes the most compression and tension during ambulation, is weakened by the window cutout around the ankle in the posterior region. Modern carbon fiber and acrylic lamination materials and techniques have aided in meeting this challenge.[60,61] The Canadian prosthesis is a relatively cosmetic approach, but more recent options have limited its use.

Medial Opening Syme Prostheses

The *medial opening Syme prosthesis,* also known as the *Veterans Administration Prosthetic Center Syme,* followed the introduction of the Canadian Syme. Developed at the New York City Veterans Administration Medical Center in 1959,[62] it has a removable donning door that extends proximally from the distal expansion to a level approximately two thirds of the height of the tibial section on the medial side (Figure 25-22).[63] Like the Canadian design, the medial opening prosthesis is relatively cosmetic at the ankle and compares favorably with the Canadian design. The medial placement of the donning panel provides much more opportunity for anteroposterior strengthening of the prosthesis. All other factors being equal, this design is stronger than the Canadian design and is the approach of choice for many patients with Syme amputation.

Sleeve Suspension Syme Prostheses

The *sleeve suspension Syme prosthesis* is sometimes referred to as the *stovepipe Syme* because of the cylindrical appearance of its removable liner (Figure 25-23). It is constructed with an inner flexible insert or sleeve that has filler material in the

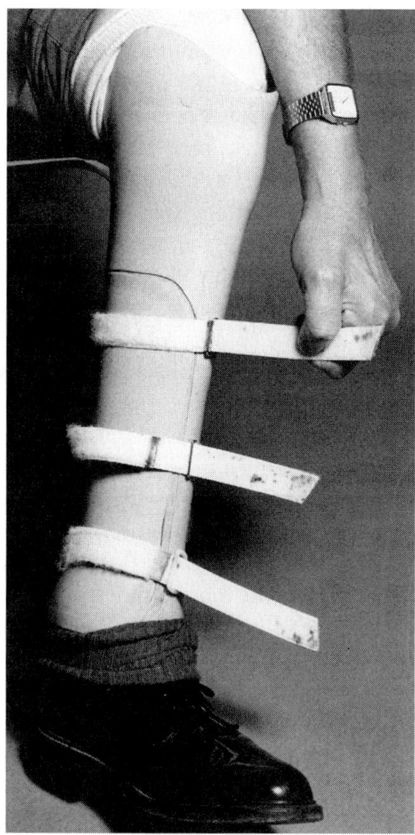

Figure 25-22
The Veterans Administration Prosthetic Center Syme prosthesis has a medial opening window and has long been a popular approach to fitting the Syme amputation.

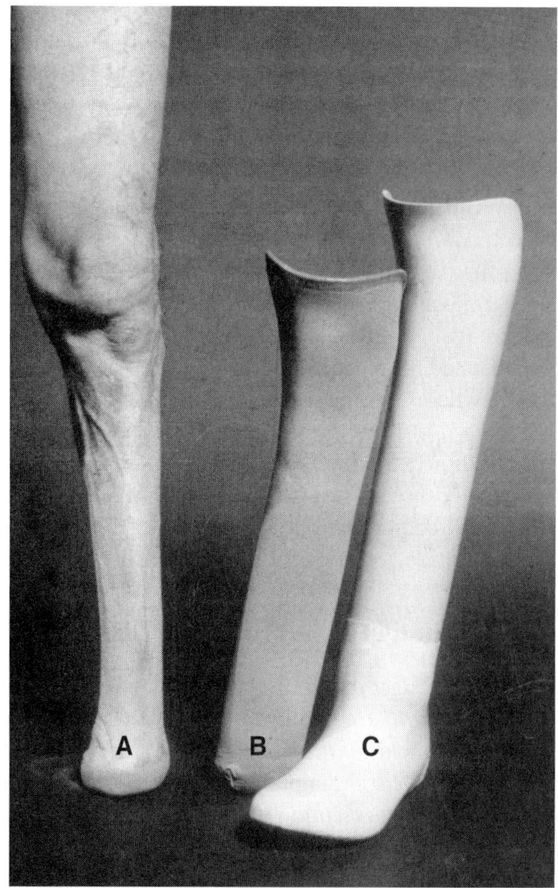

Figure 25-23
*A mature Syme residual limb (**A**). The sleeve suspension Syme's prosthesis has a full-length liner (**B**) that slips into the prosthetic socket (**C**). This design accommodates adjustments well. It offers excellent strength at the cost of cosmesis and is an excellent option for the obese or heavy-duty wearer.*

areas just proximal to the distal expansion.[64,65] Before slipping into the outer shell or socket, the wearer first pulls on the flexible liner.[66] The outside sleeve then telescopes within the outer prosthetic shell. In another version the leather and foam inner sleeve does not cover the entire residual limb but wraps around the leg and fills up the void areas above the expansion.[67] The sleeve suspension prosthesis is bulky and not very cosmetic, but its strength is significantly better because no window is present to create a structural weakness. It is often chosen for the obese or very heavy-duty wearer or for the patient with recurring prosthetic breakage with other designs. It is more adjustable and forgiving than the other Syme designs and is often chosen when major fitting problems are anticipated.

Expandable Wall Prostheses

The *flexible, expandable wall*, and *bladder Syme prostheses*, of which several varieties are available, vary more by materials used than by mechanism of action. All are based on the concept of an inner socket wall just proximal to the distal expansion that is elastic or expandable enough to allow entry of the limb into the prosthesis and still provide a level of total contact around the ankle once donned.[68,69] This design normally requires a double prosthetic wall. The original bladder Syme prosthesis described by Marx[70] in 1969 obtained expansion by using flexible polyester resin in the neck area. The more recent Rancho Syme prosthesis uses a flexible inner socket, supported by a frame or superstructure of laminated thermosetting plastic. The use of flexible thermosetting plastics and silicone elastomer for expandable wall sockets has gradually eclipsed the use of Surlyn (DuPont, Wilmington, Del.) and other thermoplastics as a material of choice for the inner liner. Expandable wall Syme prostheses are slightly bulkier and less cosmetic at the ankle than their Canadian or medial opening counterparts because they require a flexible inner socket and a rigid exterior superstructure. The fabrication process is more involved, and fitting adjustments to the flexible inner socket can be difficult. Creating either a silicone elastomer or a Surlyn inner socket flexible enough for comfortable donning and doffing may significantly limit its durability. A Syme residual limb presents greater pressure distribution challenges to a prosthetist than do other types of lower limb prosthetics.

A test socket is especially recommended for all Syme's prostheses. Because the act of donning and doffing with this system is relatively simple, it may be the prosthesis of choice for patients with upper limb dysfunction or cognitive impairment.

Tucker-Winnipeg Syme Prostheses

The *Tucker-Winnipeg Syme prosthesis,* rarely seen in the United States, ignores the traditional requirement of comprehensive total contact by introducing lateral and medial donning slots.[71] The design is well suited for children. It is contraindicated for patients with severe vascular disease and for others who are prone to window edema. A loss of total contact can also affect proprioception and control of the prosthesis. In general, the method permits a prosthesis that is relatively cosmetic, easy to don, and not prone to the noises that are sometimes created by rubbing at the window covers of the medial opening and Canadian Syme's prostheses.

Prosthetic Feet for Syme Prostheses

One of the challenges in selecting prosthetic components for patients with Syme amputation is fitting a prosthetic foot and ankle bolt within the very limited space under the residual limb while still maintaining equal leg lengths and a level pelvis. The rare exception to this is when bilateral ankle disarticulation has occurred; Syme's bilaterality fits many more choices of foot designs. When there is unilateral Syme amputation, great care must be given to the minimal amount of space available between the distal end and shoe so that a heel lift on the contralateral side would not be necessary.

Determining the Prosthetic Clearance Value

In determining whether a particular Syme foot can accommodate a patient, the available space between the distal end of the residual limb and the floor is measured with the pelvis level, and the anatomical clearance value is derived. Most Syme feet are attached to the socket by a foot bolt screwed upward from below the prosthetic heel into a Syme nut, a threaded disk that is laminated into the socket. The nut, shaped to approximately match the contours of the distal residual limb, is approximately $^5/_8$ inches tall, and this height must be considered when constructing the prosthesis. In addition, the typical Syme's foot has a liner with distal end thickness which is $^1/_8$- to $^1/_4$-inch thick. To determine the applicability of a particular foot for a patient the space between the bottom of the heel of the foot and the top of the foot is added to height of the Syme nut and the liner and end pad thickness. This measurement is the prosthetic clearance value.

Nonarticulating Syme Feet

Many prosthetic feet used for transtibial amputation have been adapted for Syme amputation. The first was the *solid-ankle, cushion heel* (SACH) foot, patented in 1863 by Marks and further developed at the University of California Berkeley after World War II. It was introduced as a component of the Canadian Syme prosthesis in the 1950s. The Syme SACH is distributed in the United States primarily by Kingsley (Costa Mesa, Calif.). It is available in a regular men's shoe heel height and a running shoe heel height.

The SACH-type Syme foot was the historical foot of choice for patients with Syme amputation in previous decades and remains a highly durable, cost-effective foot design today.The SACH foot design simulates plantar flexion as the patient rolls over a compressible heel, but because of a rigid wooden (typically maple) keel, it is neither flexible nor elastic in late stance.

The *stationary-ankle flexible endoskeletal* Syme foot has the advantage of providing a modest inversion and eversion component of motion, through elasticity of the forefoot, and is useful for uneven terrain ambulation. Not including the thickness of the Syme's nut, the SAFE II (Campbell-Childs, White City, Ore.) the Syme foot requires $1^3/_8$ inches of space between the distal end and the floor or shoe with pelvis leveled.

Dynamic Response Syme Feet

In the last decade a variety of dynamic response foot designs have emerged for more active Syme walkers. The Impulse Syme foot (Ohio Willow Wood, Mt. Sterling, Ohio) which has a Kevlar (DuPont, Wilmington, Del.) keel with carbon deflection toe-spring plates, carries a weight limit of up to 250 lb (113 kg). The toe spring is a carbon-epoxy composite. A unique manufacturing technique allows carbon fibers to be optimally oriented and avoid wrinkling, buckling, and deformation. The most interesting part of the foot is alignment adjustability. Ohio Willow Wood also has a Carbon Copy II Syme's foot available in two heel heights and with all the toe resistances and sizes of the standard (non-Syme) Carbon Copy II. The Carbon Copy II is available with a medium heel density for patient weights up to 250 lb (113 kg).

The Steplite Foot (Kingsley) provides a compressible heel design with the buoyancy of a carbon keel. It is quite durable and applicable to almost every patient with Syme amputation because it requires only $1^5/_8$ inches of prosthetic clearance value. That accounts for 1 inch for the foot itself and $^5/_8$ inches for the nut and socket thickness. The low-profile version accommodates a typical man's heel height. The Strider is made for a man's running shoe, and the Flattie is a narrow foot for female which accommodates a flat heel. The Steplite provides a buoyant elastic forefoot but, like many Syme feet, is limited in its heel compression.

Ossur (Aliso Viejo, Calif.) offers a low-profile carbon Syme version for a very active prosthetic wearer weighing up to 285 lb. The same foot can be worn by a low-activity amputee weighing up to 365 lb. The Ossur Low Profile requires 2 inches of clearance from the floor to the distal end of the socket and is designed with a flexible double-spring keel. It uses a fenestrated heel, which allows greater compression, thus reducing shock. The upper spring bumper is coated with Teflon (DuPont), which reduces squeaks, a characteristic not uncommon to feet with more than one keel in the forefoot. Another Syme foot that may be used for patients up to 500 lb is the Vari-Flex (Ossur), which requires only 1¾ inches of space under the socket and is attached with epoxy filler and lamination. Another dynamic elastic foot choice for the active individual is the Seattle Light Foot (Seattle Orthopedic Group, Seattle, Wash.).

Almost all prosthetic feet for Syme prostheses have ankles that are essentially locked. This characteristics results in increased work for the quadriceps for controlled knee flexion during loading response. Incorporation of several degrees of adjustable articulated plantar flexion (at the risk of increasing the weight of the prosthesis) might improve function for certain patients.

Alignment Issues

With most prosthetic feet, the small area between the distal residual limb and floor limits the prosthetist's ability to refine the special relation between the socket and foot in the dynamic alignment phase. Adjustable alignment devices, similar to those available for transtibial prostheses, have historically not compact enough to fit in the available space between the prosthetic foot and the end of the socket. Two component options have been introduced with the goal of addressing this limitation.

A novel functional alignment device for the Impulse Syme, available from Ohio Willow Wood, permits some degree of dynamic alignment by enabling the prosthetist to adjust the angular positions of the foot during the fitting process. This Impulse Syme socket adapter kit (Figure 25-24) allows angular adjustments during the dynamic phase of 4 to 8 degrees, depending on the direction. In addition, ⅛-inch carbon spacers allow for length additions up to ⅜ inch. The kit is used with a 1-inch Syme "dished" nut contoured to interface with the distal end of the limb.

The SL Profile and the Lo Rider Syme feet (Otto Bock, Minneapolis, Minn.) provide angular adjustability by a pyramid. Unfortunately, the height of the pyramid may preclude the use of these feet for many patients with Syme amputation. The newest and very promising addition is the 1C20 ProSyme's (Otto Bock), which can be fitted on most patients and is a moderately dynamic urethane carbon fiber foot for Syme amputees up to 275 lb (Figure 25-25). It has a wide range of alignment adjustability as well as heel height changes.

Placing the Syme prosthesis in slight dorsiflexion relative to the shin mimics normal gait patterns, encourages a smooth cosmetic and energy-efficient rollover during stance phase, and optimizes the weight-bearing potential of the socket contours. For individuals with quadriceps weakness, the dorsiflexion angle can be reduced to minimize excessive demands on the quadriceps. The telltale clinical sign of excessive demand is trembling of the knee during midstance. Although early alignment recommendations placed optimal initial dorsiflexion up to 12 to 15 degrees, current practice is to set the foot at a smaller angle of approximately 5 degrees.[72] The long Syme residual limb does not easily accommodate itself, cosmetically or functionally, to more than 5 degrees of dorsiflexion.

Alignment can be significantly compromised when knee flexion contracture is present. To prevent breakage and premature wear from the anterior lever arm, the degree of anterior (linear) displacement of the socket over the foot is generally reduced from that of a transtibial prosthesis.

A Syme socket is positioned in an angle of adduction that matches the anatomical adduction angle of the tibia. The adduction of the socket should be positioned to create as

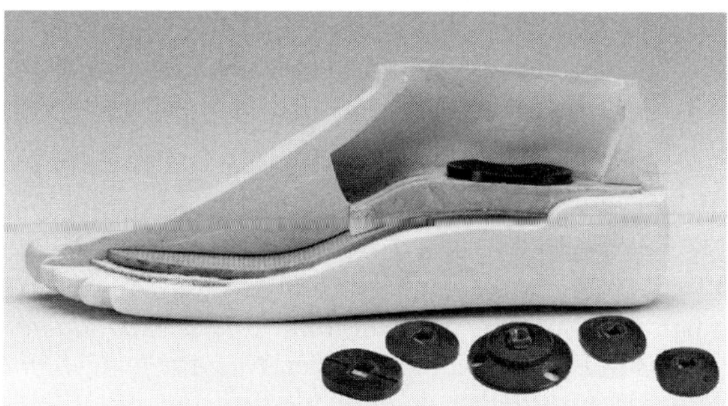

Figure 25-24
The Impulse Foot is a dynamic response foot system for Syme prostheses. This foot is particularly useful when prosthetic clearance value is limited. The adaptable design allows the prosthetist to fine tune during the dynamic alignment process to achieve a gait pattern that is energy efficient and cosmetic. (Courtesy Ohio Willow Wood, Inc., Mt. Sterling, Ohio.)

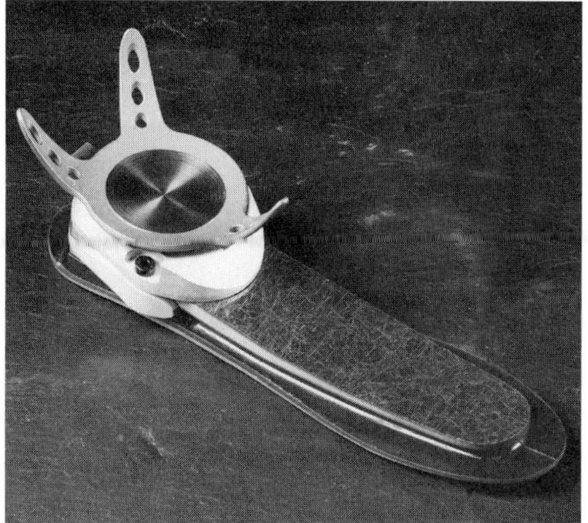

Figure 25-25
The 1C20 ProSyme, similar to the Impulse, is unique in its alignment adjustability. Angular and linear alignment as well as heel height adjustments make it an exceptional choice. (Courtesy Otto Bock, Minneapolis, Minn.)

smooth a transition as possible at the ankle and knee so that the prosthetic foot rolls over with the sole flat on the floor. The optimal spatial relation in the coronal plane is one that creates a slight varus moment. Socket adduction angle, foot eversion angle, and linear displacement affect the external varus moment at the knee during midstance. For an efficient and cosmetic gait, the knee must displace approximately 12 mm laterally at midstance. Insufficient displacement implicates malalignment, most often at an inadequate eversion angle. Excessive displacement may be the result of malalignment or lateral collateral ligament laxity at the knee. The most successful strategy to address chronic weight-bearing ulceration at the knee that has not responded to a silicone liner, or to address major laxity of the collateral ligaments, is the addition of orthotic components (external knee joints and a thigh lacer) to provide extra support and protection.

CASE EXAMPLE 2

A Patient with Bilateral Dysvascular Syme Amputation

H. P. is a 56-year-old man with an 18-year history of insulin-controlled diabetes. Eight years ago, a left hallux ray resection failed to heal and became infected, necessitating a left Syme amputation. After healing, he became proficient with a Syme prosthesis, ambulating functional distances without assistive devices. One year ago a large neuropathic wound developed under the second through fourth metatarsal heads of his right foot. The wound failed to heal despite several trials of total contact casting. H. P. and his vascular surgeon agreed that a Syme amputation on the right would improve his functional status and allow him to return to work as a junior high school teacher and baseball coach. Amputation occurred 7 months ago, and both residual limbs are well healed. He has Rancho-style expandable wall Syme prostheses with SACH feet (Figure 25-26). He has been on an exercise program and is walking 2 miles per day. He ambulates at a relatively high speed (120 steps/min) and can walk long distances (more than 1 mile) at that velocity. He has poor socket fit wearing 10-ply socks. Stress cracks can be seen on the foot. The team agrees that a change in prosthetic design and components would improve his function and satisfaction.

Questions to Consider

- Given his medical history, what concerns exist about the condition of his residual feet? What areas are most vulnerable to pressures from repetitive loading during walking in Syme residual limbs?
- What types of muscle performance at his knee and hip are important to assess? What measures should be used to assess muscle function and strength? How will any impairments be addressed?
- How does Syme's amputation affect progression through the gait cycle? How might a prosthesis substitute for compromise of the first rocker from initial contact through loading response? Of the second rocker from loading response through midstance to terminal stance? Of the third rocker in terminal stance into preswing? How might Syme amputation affect step and stride length of the opposite swing limb?
- What are the major goals for prosthetic intervention for H. P.? What specific recommendations should be made for socket design, suspension, and prosthetic feet? What options should be chosen from among those available? What is his prognosis for functional ambulation? Is an assistive device recommended for long-term use? Why or why not? How should the efficacy of intervention be assessed?

Recommendations

The clinical team determines he is a candidate for a dynamic response foot and a design consistent with an active lifestyle. His is provided with a Medial Opening

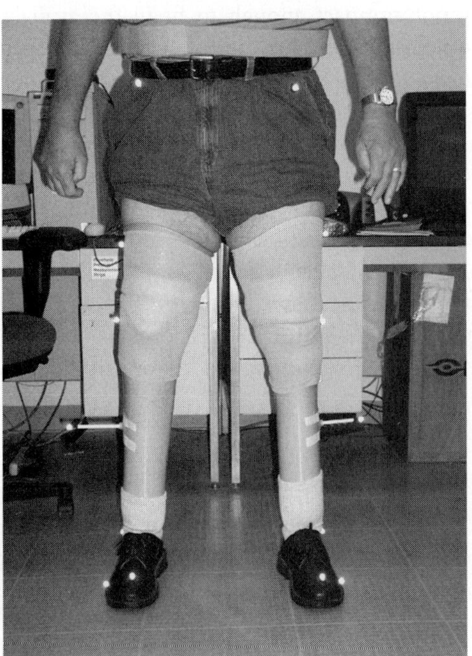

Figure 25-26

This patient is wearing bilateral Rancho-style expandable wall Syme prostheses with SACH feet. Note the wide diameter at the ankle, necessary to accommodate the bulbous distal residual limb during donning. His prostheses incorporate a patellar tendon–bearing design at the knee, and he wears neoprene suspension sleeves as auxiliary suspension. Note also the widened base of support that he has adopted to enhance stability in quiet standing. Reflective markers have been placed at the pelvis, greater trochanter, lateral lower thigh, lateral prosthesis, lateral malleolus, and the shoe in preparation for comprehensive gait analysis.

Syme prosthesis (Medicare code L5050), test socket (L5618), acrylic socket (L5629), expandable wall (Rancho style) (L5630), extended PTB style brim (L5632), total contact (L5637), suspension sleeve (L5675), ultralight construction (L5940), Freedom Innovation FS-2000 Low Profile Foot (L5981) and alignable system (L5910), and six prosthetic socks for each limb (Figure 25-27). After delivery of the limbs, H. P. reports immediate improvement of long-distance walking.

SUMMARY

This chapter has explored the options for prosthetic management for patients with partial foot and Syme amputations. Because of the variability in surgical procedures, condition of the residual limb, and altered biomechanics of the residual limb in gait, no single best option exists for prosthetic design. Instead, the characteristics of each patient (weight, skin condition, desired activity level, and length of residual limb) must be carefully considered in prosthetic prescription. The goal is to find the best match of the person's status and needs from the growing array of prosthetic design options for the partial foot and Syme amputations. This places an increasing demand on the knowledge base of medical professionals. More than ever the physician, physical therapist, and prosthetist are challenged to function as a cohesive team, drawing on each others' strengths to achieve the best possible outcome for each patient.

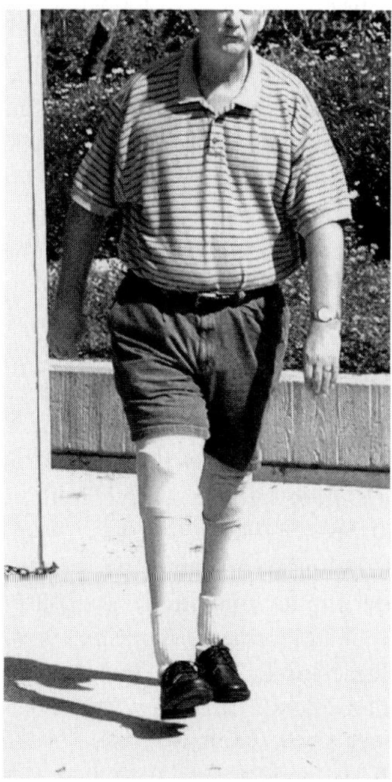

Figure 25-27
The same individual as in Figure 25-26 after receiving his new prostheses with dynamic response feet. Distance between heels has been reduced in both standing and walking, stride length has increased substantially, and he reports greater comfort and ease in walking long distances required for his job and leisure activities.

ACKNOWLEDGMENTS

The author thanks James Tomoush for graph preparation and artwork; Dana Craig, BS; and the staff of the National Veterans Administration Prosthetics Gait Lab for data collection of case studies.

REFERENCES

1. Herodotus. Library IX, 37, *Loeb Classical Edition*, vol 4. London: Heinemann, 1924. pp. 202-205.
2. Bowker JH. Partial foot and Syme amputations—an overview. *Clin Prosthet Orthot* 1988;12(1):10-13.
3. Bahler A. The biomechanics of the foot. *Clin Prosthet Orthot* 1986;10(1):8-14.
4. Frankovitch KF, Farrell WJ. Syme and Boyd amputations in children. *Int Clin Info Bull* 1984;19(3):61.
5. Oglesby DG, Tablada C. The Child Amputee: Lower Limb Deficiencies: Prosthetic and Orthotic Management. In *American Academy of Orthopaedic Surgeons, Atlas of Limb Prosthetics* (2nd ed). St. Louis: Mosby, 1992. pp. 83.
6. Burgess EM. Prevention and correction of fixed equinus deformity in mid-foot amputations. *Bull Prosthet Res* 1966; 10(5):45-47.
7. Pritham CH. Partial foot amputation—a case study. *Newsletter Prosthet Orthot Clin* 1977;1(3):5-7.
8. Wagner FW. Partial Foot Amputations. In *American Academy of Orthopaedic Surgeons, Atlas of Limb Prosthetics*. St. Louis: Mosby, 1981. pp. 315-325.
9. Wilson AB. Partial foot amputation results of the questionnaire survey. *Newsletter Prosthet Orthot Clin* 1977;1(4):1-3.
10. Kay HW. Limb deficits no bar to record performance. *Int Clin Info Bull* 1970;10(3):17.
11. Dorostkar M. Ayyappa E. & Perry J: Gait Mechanics of the Partial Foot Amputee, Rehabilitation Research & Development Final Report, Project #A861-RA -2000, July 11, 1999.
12. Dorostkar M. Ayyappa E. & Perry J: Gait Mechanics of the Partial Foot Amputee, Project #A861-RA - RR&D Progress Reports, Vol 35, pp 17-18. July 1998.
13. Dorostkar M. Ayyappa E. & Perry J: Gait Mechanics of the Partial Foot Amputee, Project #A861-RA - RR&D Progress Reports, Vol 36, July 1999.
14. Ayyappa E, Moinzadeh H, Friedman J. Gait characteristics of the partial foot amputee. Proceedings of the 21st Annual Meeting and Scientific Symposium of the American Academy of Orthotists and Prosthetists, New Orleans, March 21-25, 1995.
15. Pinzur MS, Gold J, Schwartz D, Gross N. Energy demands for walking in dysvascular amputees as related to the level of amputation. *Orthopedics* 1992;15(9):1033-1037.
16. New York University Post Graduate Medical School. *Lower Limb Prosthetics*. New York: New York University, 1979; 233-234.

17. Enna CD, Brand PW, Reed JK, Welch D. The orthotic care of the denervated foot in Hansen's disease. *Orthot Prosthet* 1976;30(1):33-39.
18. Menon PBM. A new type of protective footwear for anesthetic feet. *ISPO Bull* 1976;18:4.
19. Veterans Administration Prosthetics Center. Semiannual report of the VA Prosthetics Center. *Bull Prosthet Res* 1965;10(3):142-146.
20. Marks AA. *Manual of Artificial Limbs*. New York: AA Marks, 1931;27-36.
21. Marks GE. A *Treatise on Artificial Limbs with Rubber Hands and Feet*. New York: AA Marks, 1888. pp. 40-47.
22. American Academy of Orthopaedic Surgeons. *Orthopedic Appliance Atlas. Vol 2: Artificial Limbs*. Ann Arbor, MI: J.W. Edwards, 1960;212-281.
23. Cestaro JM. Comments on partial foot amputations. *Newsletter Prosthet Orthot Clin* 1977;1(3):7.
24. Levy SE. Total contact restoration prosthesis for partial foot amputations. *Orthot Prosthet* 1961;15(1):34-44.
25. Lunsford T. Partial foot amputations: Prosthetic and orthotic management. In *American Academy of Orthopaedic Surgeons, Atlas of Limb Prosthetics*. St. Louis: Mosby, 1981. pp. 320-325.
26. Staros A, Peizer E. Veterans Administration Prosthetic Center research report. *Bull Prosthet Res* 1969;10(12): 340-342. pp. 155.
27. Zamosky I. Shoes and their modifications. In Light S, Kampuetz H. (eds), *Orthotics Etcetera* (2nd ed). Baltimore: Williams & Wilkins, 1980. pp. 368-431.
28. Potter JW, Stockwell JE. Custom foamed toe filler for amputation of the forefoot. *Orthot Prosthet* 1974;28(3):57-60.
29. Young RD. Functional positioning toe restoration. *Orthot Prosthet* 1985;39(3):57-59.
30. Young RD. Special Chopart prosthesis with custom molded foot. *Orthot Prosthet* 1984;38(1):79-85.
31. Platts RGS, Knight S, Jakins I. Shoe inserts for small deformed feet. *Prosthet Orthot Int* 1982;6(2):108-110.
32. Henderson WH, Campbell JW. UC-BL shoe insert, casting and fabrication. *Bull Prosthet Res* 1969;10(11):215-235.
33. Inman VT. UC-BL dual axis ankle control system and UC-BL shoe insert; biomechanical considerations. *Bull Prosthet Res* 1969;10(11):130-145.
34. Quigley MJ. The present use of the UCBL foot orthosis. *Orthot Prosthet* 1974;28(4):59-63.
35. Stills M. Partial foot prosthesis/orthosis. *Clin Prosthet Orthot* 1988;12(1):14-18.
36. Imler CD. Imler partial foot prosthesis IPFP—the Chicago boot. *Orthot Prosthet* 1985;39(3):53-56.
37. Imler CD. Imler partial foot prosthesis IPFP "Chicago boot." *Clin Prosthet Orthot* 1988;12(1):24-28.
38. Wilson MT. Clinical application of TRV elastomer. *Orthot Prosthet* 1979;33(4):23-29.
39. Fillauer K. A prosthesis for foot amputation near the tarsal-metatarsal junction. *Orthot Prosthet* 1976;30(3):9-12.
40. Pullen JJ. A low profile pediatric partial foot. *Prosthet Orthot Int* 1987;11(3):137-138.
41. Rubin G, Danisi M. A functional partial-foot prosthesis. *ISPO Bull* 1972;3(7):6.
42. Collins JN. A partial foot prosthesis for the transmetatarsal level. *Clin Prosthet Orthot* 1988;12(1):19-23.
43. Rubin G, Danisi M. Functional partial-foot prosthesis. *Bull Prosthet Res* 1971;10(16):149-152.
44. Staros A, Goralnik B. Lower limb prosthetic systems. In *American Academy of Orthopaedic Surgeons, Atlas of Limb Prosthetics*. St. Louis: Mosby, 1981. pp. 293-295.
45. LaTorre R. The total contact partial foot prosthesis. *Clin Prosthet Orthot* 1987-1988;12(1):29-32.
46. Hudson ED. *Mechanical Surgery; Artificial Limbs, Apparatus for Resections, by U.S. Soldiers*. New York: Commission of the Surgeon-General, 1867 (Library of Congress Call No. RD 756.H86).
47. Jansen K. Amputation—principles and methods. *Bull Prosthet Res* 1965;10(4):19-20.
48. Harris RI. *The History and Development of the Syme's Amputation: Selected Articles from Artificial Limbs*. Huntington, NY: Krieger, 1970. pp. 233-272.
49. Burgess EM, Romano RL, Zettl JH. *The Management of Lower-Extremity Amputations*. Washington, DC: U.S. Government Printing Office, 1969. pp. 74-84.
50. Wagner FW. The Syme amputation: surgical procedures. In *American Academy of Orthopaedic Surgeons, Atlas of Limb Prosthetics*. St. Louis: Mosby, 1981. pp. 326-334.
51. Quigley M. The Rancho Syme prosthesis with the Regnell foot. *Clin Prosthet Orthot* 1988;12(1):33-40.
52. Hanger HB. *The Syme and Chopart Prostheses*. Chicago: Northwestern University Prosthetic-Orthotic Center, 1965.
53. Wilson AB. Prostheses for Syme amputation. *Artif Limbs* 1961;61(1):52-75.
54. Leimkuehler J. Syme's prosthesis—a brief review and a new fabrication technique. *Orthot Prosthet* 1980;34(4):3-12.
55. Foort J. The Canadian type Syme prosthesis. *Abstracts Artif Limbs* 1954;4(2):75-76.
56. Murphy EF. Lower extremity components. In *American Academy of Orthopaedic Surgeons, Orthopedic Appliance Atlas*, vol 2. Ann Arbor, MI: J.W. Edwards, 1960. pp. 212-217.
57. Voner R. The Syme amputation: prosthetic management. In *American Academy of Orthopaedic Surgeons, Atlas of Limb Prosthetics*. St. Louis: Mosby, 1981. pp. 334-340.
58. Boccius CS. The plastic Syme prosthesis in Canada. *Artif Limbs* 1961;6(1):86-89.
59. Department of Veterans Affairs. *Syme Amputation and Prosthesis*. Toronto: Department of Veterans Affairs, Prosthetic Services Centre, 1954.
60. Dankmeyer CH, Doshi R, Alban CR. Adding strength to the Syme prosthesis. *Orthot Prosthet* 1974;28(3):3-7.
61. Radcliffe CW. *The Biomechanics of the Syme Prosthesis: Selected Articles from Artificial Limbs*. Huntington, NY: Krieger, 1970. pp. 273-282.
62. Schwartz RE, Bohne WO, Kramer HE. Prosthetic management of below knee amputation with flexion contracture in the child. *J Assoc Child Prosthet Orthot Clin* 1986;21(1):8-10.
63. Iuliucci L, Degaetano R. *V.A.P.C. Technique for Fabricating a Plastic Syme Prosthesis with Medial Opening*. New York: New York University Medical School, 1969.
64. Byers JL. Fabrication of Cordo, Plastizote, or Pelite removable liner for closed Syme sockets. *Bull Prosthet Res* 1972;10(18):182-188.
65. Warner R, Daniel R, Lesswing A. Another new prosthetic approach for the Syme's amputation. *Int Clin Info Bull* 1972;12(1):7-10.
66. Byers JL. The closed Syme socket with removable liner. *ISPO Bull* 1973;7:4-5.

67. McFarlen JM. The Syme prosthesis. *Orthot Prosthet* 1966;20(3):23-27.
68. Eckhardt AL, Enneberg H. The use of a Silastic liner in the Syme's prosthesis. *Int Clin Info Bull* 1970;9(6):1-4.
69. Meyer LC, Bailey HL, Friddle D. An improved prosthesis for fitting the ankle-disarticulation amputee. *Int Clin Info Bull* 1970;9(6):11-15.
70. Marx HW. An innovation in Syme prosthetics. *Orthot Prosthet* 1969;23(3):131-141.
71. Lyttle D. Tucker-Syme prosthetic fitting in young people. *Int Clin Info Bull* 1984;19(3):62.
72. Hanger of England. *Prosthesis for Below-Knee Amputation—Roelite Instruction Manual.* Bath, England: Trowbridges, 1982. p. 20.

26

Transtibial Prostheses

GARY M. BERKE

LEARNING OBJECTIVES

On completion of this chapter, the reader will be able to do the following:

1. Describe the principles underlying current transtibial socket design.
2. Discuss the pros and cons of the various options for prosthetic suspension.
3. Identify key weight-tolerant and pressure-intolerant surfaces of a typical transtibial residual limb.
4. Identify key determinants of appropriate transtibial prosthetic alignment.
5. Recognize and differentiate the various factors that may lead to transtibial prosthetic gait deviations.
6. Suggest appropriate strategies to address transtibial gait deviations.

Amputation at the transtibial level occurs at least twice as often as amputation at other levels.[1] Because approximately 90% of all amputations involve the lower extremity, the majority of patients with amputation who are seen by health care professionals have amputation at the transtibial level. Today, many people with transtibial amputations actively participate in professional or amateur sports and leisure activities.[2] These achievements are enhanced by modern techniques and theory, coupled with prostheses that are properly and carefully fit by qualified prosthetists and gait training and exercise guided by skilled physical therapists.[2-4]

Historically, amputations have been perceived by surgeons as a last resort, perhaps because they view amputations as an admission of failure. Until recently, surgical technique often resulted in residual limbs that were difficult to fit comfortably with prostheses,[5] which in turn limited the rehabilitation potential of persons with lower limb amputation.[6] Research and education about the relation between surgical technique and prosthetic options has led to improved surgical and rehabilitation outcomes.[5]

A prosthesis is a complex device that must be custom fit to each patient. To achieve optimal fit and alignment, a sequence of several fittings and careful follow-up are necessary to maintain the prosthesis and make occasional repairs and adjustments as warranted by the patient's activity level and lifestyle. For this reason, patients should work with prosthetists who can be seen regularly so that simple but necessary adjustments can be made to ensure long-term comfort and function.

In the last 10 years, the concepts and materials used in fabricating transtibial prostheses have dramatically changed, allowing patients to become much more active and use their prostheses for longer periods of time.[2,7] For effective rehabilitation outcomes for patients with new amputations, physical and occupational therapists must be well versed in the mechanical and biomechanical principles of transtibial prostheses.

This chapter describes the various types of transtibial prostheses, discusses the performance characteristics and constraints of the materials and methods currently available for rehabilitation interventions, and identifies the biomechanical principles and alignment issues for energy-efficient and natural prosthetic gait.

DETERMINING POTENTIAL FOR PROSTHETIC REHABILITATION

One of the most important roles of the interdisciplinary rehabilitation team is to determine a patient's potential for limited or functional ambulation with a prosthesis. Although a true team approach may be difficult in some situations, the importance of interdisciplinary communication cannot be overstated. Positive outcomes appear to be related to the ability of the core team members to communicate. The core team may include the patient and patient's family, the prosthetist, the surgeon, the physiatrist, the physical and occupational therapists, and the social worker or case manager.

Another powerful indicator of outcome is the patient's presurgical level of function. If the patient was able to stand and walk before amputation surgery, even if assistance or an ambulatory aid was necessary, it is likely that, at minimum, limited ambulation with a prosthesis will be possible.[8] This criteria does not mean that someone who was nonambulatory before surgery should not be evaluated for potential prosthetic use. Having a prosthesis may allow family caregivers to safely assist frail, older patients who have an amputation to perform transfers (to or from the bed, wheelchair, toilet, or car) that would otherwise be too difficult or unsafe. The evaluation of all patients with transtibial amputations as candidates for prostheses is important because many factors, such as aerobic conditioning, comorbid medical conditions, cognitive status, and motivation and drive, interact to determine the success or failure of prosthetic rehabilitation.

Consider the case of an 85-year-old man with degenerative joint disease of the hip and bilateral transtibial amputations whose ability to ambulate has been restricted in the 6 months before amputation because of nonhealing neuropathic ulcers. Although he may not reach independent ambulation, a prosthesis may enable him to transfer independently from a wheelchair to or from a toilet. This functional ability may allow the patient to remain at home with occasional assistance with shopping and cleaning, rather than residing in a long-term care facility.

Medicare has taken the first step in acknowledging various levels of prosthetic use by creating functional level codes (Table 26-1).[9] These codes help guide the prosthetist in choosing components on the basis of the goals and activity level of the patient. This evaluation process ensures that all patients, regardless of age or functional status, are candidates for a prosthesis appropriate for their needs.

TABLE 26-1
Medicare Guidelines: Functional Classification for Patients with a Prosthesis

Code	*Description*
K0	The patient does not have the ability or potential to ambulate or transfer safely with or without assistance, and a prosthesis does not enhance quality of life or mobility.
K1	The patient has the ability or potential to use a prosthesis for transfers or ambulation on level surfaces at a fixed cadence. With a prosthesis, the patient achieves limited or unlimited household ambulation status.
K2	The patient has the ability or potential for ambulation, including the ability to traverse low-level environmental barriers such as curbs, stairs, or uneven surfaces. With a prosthesis, the patient is considered a limited community ambulator.
K3	The patient has the ability or potential for ambulation with variable cadence. He or she is likely to achieve community ambulation, with the ability to traverse most environmental barriers, and may have vocational, therapeutic, or exercise activity that demands prosthetic use beyond simple locomotion.
K4	The patient has the ability or potential for prosthetic ambulation that exceeds basic ambulatory skills, exhibiting high impact, stress, or energy levels during activity. This category includes most children, active adults, or athletes with amputation.

From DMERC Medicare Advisory Bulletin. Columbia, SC: DMERC, 1994. pp. 95-145.

COMPONENTS OF A TRANSTIBIAL PROSTHESIS

A transtibial prosthesis has four key components: the socket and its interface, the suspension mechanism, the shank (or pylon), and the prosthetic foot. The various types of prosthetic feet and their functional characteristics are discussed in Chapter 24. This chapter focuses on the socket, suspension, and alignment issues.

Transtibial Socket Design: A Historical Perspective

The socket is the portion of the prosthesis that makes contact with and disperses pressure around the patient's residual limb. It is designed to contain and support the residual limb during weight bearing and transmit forces from the limb to control the placement of the foot.[10] The patellar tendon-bearing (PTB) prosthesis, first developed in the 1950s, has been the most commonly prescribed and fabricated transtibial socket.[11] In early versions of the PTB design, the socket was open ended and typically fabricated from carved wood or aluminum. The weight-bearing surfaces of the limb were limited to the patellar tendon and the popliteal space. Pressure in these areas would suspend the residual limb inside the socket and enable the prosthetic wearer to ambulate with a relatively normal gait. Early PTB designs had problems, however. In some cases, the end of the residual limb was unable to tolerate pressures caused by the movement of the bone within the soft tissue envelope. A lack of distal contact often led to an edematous distal residual limb, making the prosthesis difficult to don, uncomfortable, and sometimes impossible to use.

The concept of total contact or total surface bearing has emerged to address the limitations of early PTB socket designs.[11,12] In theory, the total surface-bearing design distributes loading pressures over the entire surface of the residual limb, including some over the distal end. Distribution of pressure over a larger surface area reduces loading at any one location, making the prosthesis more comfortable to use. Total surface contact also reduces the likelihood of the development of distal edema during prosthetic use. It is important to note that most modern socket designs incorporate characteristics of both total surface-bearing design and the original PTB socket design.[13] For ease of nomenclature, all references in this section to PTB (unless otherwise noted) refer to the modern total surface bearing/PTB socket, not the historical model.

Recent development in materials used for liners has led to the exploration of hydrostatic fit within a socket that has not been modified with the traditional relief areas and pressure-directing areas that are built into a PTB socket.[11] Although there is little evidence to support any socket design theory, there is a clinical evolution toward minimizing local forces as much as possible.[14,15]

Pressure-Tolerant Areas of the Transtibial Residual Limb

The PTB/total surface bearing design distributes the primary loading pressures of weight bearing over several surfaces of the transtibial residual limb (Figure 26-1).[11] These areas include the patellar tendon, the posterior popliteal tissues, the fibular shaft, the anterior-medial tibial shaft and soft tissue of the neighboring anterior compartment, the medial tibial (metaphyseal) flare, and the medial and lateral femoral condyles. Pressure-intolerant areas, most notably the fibular head and the distal anterior tibia, are protected by relief areas incorporated into the socket.

The PTB design positions the residual limb appropriately within the socket with an *anterior patellar bar* that loads the patellar tendon above its insertion on the tibial tubercle and a *posterior popliteal bulge* designed to stabilize the limb on the patellar bar (Figure 26-2). Force applied to the pressure-tolerant soft tissue of the posterior compartment pushes the limb forward onto the PTB surface (the patellar bar). This action helps suspend the limb within the prosthesis, minimizing excessive distal weight bearing as the limb is loaded during the stance phase of gait. Although the amount of pressure applied on the patellar tendon is reduced with a total surface-bearing socket, a PTB bar still maintains the role of rotation control and helps the patient evaluate the fit, aiding in the determination of the appropriate sock ply.

Pressure along the *lateral fibular shaft* (distal to the peroneal nerve) helps control the distal segment of the residual limb during the stance phase of gait, stabilizing the prosthesis against the varus thrust that normally occurs at the knee at midstance. This distribution of weight-bearing pressures along the shaft of the fibula reduces forces on the pressure-intolerant distal fibula and fibular head. Patients who have had a fibulectomy because of disease or trauma often have a difficult time maintaining medial-lateral stability between the residual limb and the socket and often require additional medial-lateral support from their socket.

Pressures applied on either side of midline, along the *medial tibial shaft* and the *anterolateral muscular compartment,*

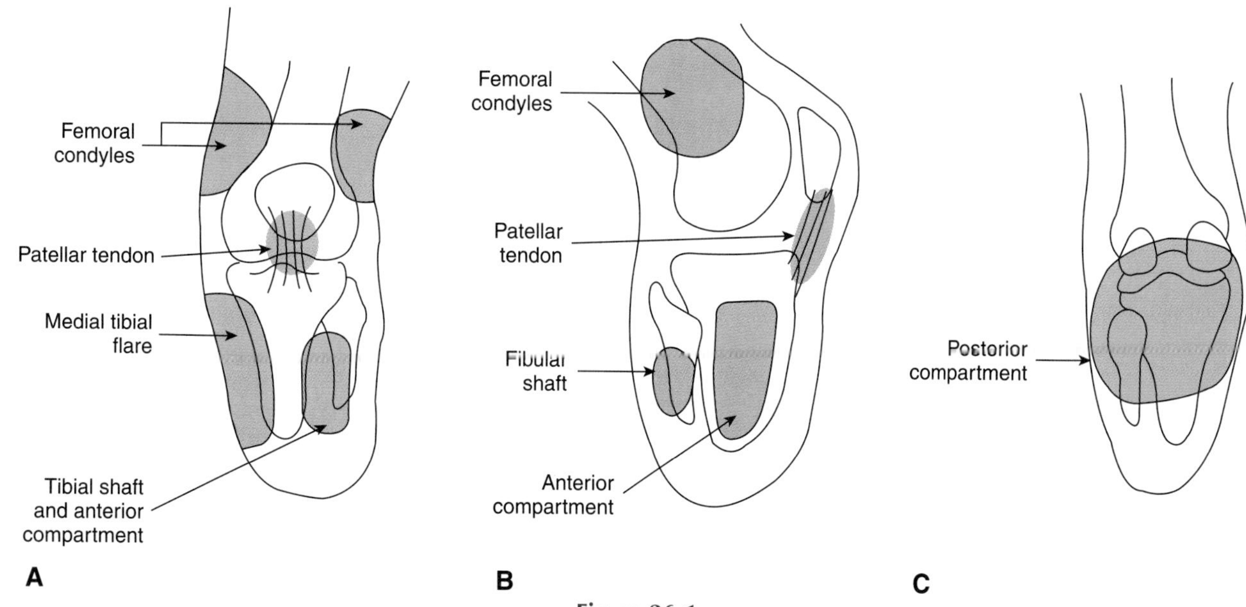

Figure 26-1

Pressure-tolerant areas of the transtibial residual limb. ***A,*** *On the anterior surface, pressure-tolerant surfaces include the patellar tendon, the medial tibial flare, both sides of the tibial shaft, and the medial and lateral femoral condyles.* ***B,*** *On the lateral view, pressure-tolerant areas include the patellar tendon, anterolateral compartment, and the shaft of the fibula.* ***C,*** *On the posterior surface, most structures within the popliteal fossa are pressure tolerant.*

are also used to control the tibia during the stance phase of gait; this enhances vertical support of the limb in the prosthesis as well.[15] The PTB design also incorporates a slight relief area for the crest of the tibia and vulnerable anterior distal end of the tibia.

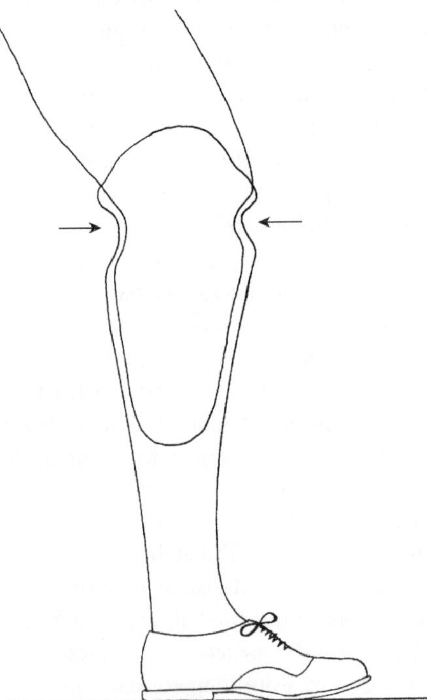

Figure 26-2
The patellar tendon bar and posterior popliteal bulge of a PTB socket apply anteroposterior forces to suspend and stabilize the residual limb within the socket.

The *medial tibial (metaphyseal) flare* is one of the most weight-tolerant areas of the residual limb. The PTB socket is carefully contoured so that the medial tibial flare rests against a carefully contoured supporting surface within the socket to aid in vertical support of the limb in the prosthesis during stance, keeping the distal end from banging on the bottom of the socket.

Pressures along the *medial and lateral femoral condyles* are used to provide mediolateral stability during the stance phase of gait. The prosthesis is carefully contoured to accept the forces in this area because excessive pressure over either condyle may cause discomfort.

Pressure-Intolerant Areas of the Transtibial Residual Limb

In the evaluation of prosthetic fit, understanding where weight-bearing pressures must be minimized along the residual limb is probably more important than understanding where they are most effectively applied. Excessive pressure over intolerable areas increases the risk of compensatory gait deviation as the patient attempts to minimize discomfort. Excessive pressure over vulnerable areas also increases the risk of skin irritation or breakdown; waiting for irritated skin or wear-induced open wounds to heal can significantly delay rehabilitation and gait training. The areas most vulnerable to excessive pressures include the fibular head and peroneal nerve, the anterior distal tibia (the cut end of the bone), the hamstring tendons, the tibial crest, the anterior tibial tubercle, the distal fibula, the patella, and the adductor tubercle (Figure 26-3).

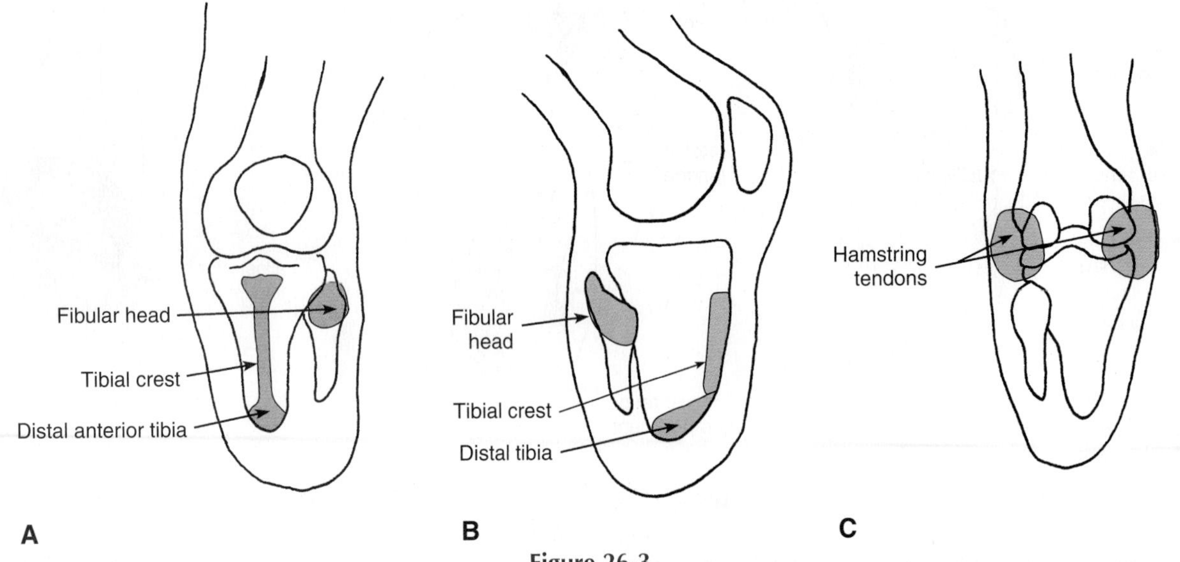

Figure 26-3
Pressure-intolerant areas of the residual limb. ***A,*** *From an anterior view, areas that are pressure intolerant include the head of the fibula, crest of the tibia, and distal anterior tibia.* ***B,*** *Laterally, the fibular head must be relieved of pressure.* ***C,*** *On the posterior surface, tendons of the hamstring muscles need to be protected.*

Transtibial Socket Interfaces

A variety of options are available as an interface between the transtibial socket and the skin of the residual limb.[11] Each material and design has specific advantages and disadvantages that must be carefully considered in the process of prosthetic prescription and fitting. The most commonly used variations are the hard socket (worn with prosthetic socks); the soft liner, roll-on liners, and other cushioning interfaces; and the flexible socket supported by a rigid frame.

Hard Socket

For some patients, the prosthetist might recommend a hard socket, which is a rigid plastic interface worn with prosthetic socks but no additional liner. Often a soft, closed-cell foam pad is placed in the distal end to make the socket more comfortable during weight bearing. This design has several important advantages. First, if an intimate fit is achieved, shearing and friction between the socket and residual limb are minimized, enhancing function. Second, overall cosmesis is enhanced because no liners add bulk around the residual limb, making the prosthesis less obvious when worn under clothing. Third, a hard socket is easy to keep clean and bacteria-free. Finally, the socket is quite durable, with no compressible components to pack down or change shape over time.

Several constraints or disadvantages should also be considered. The intimate fit necessary for an effective hard socket requires careful skill and exactness on the part of the prosthetist in manufacture, modification, and fitting of the prosthesis. A hard socket is difficult to adjust or modify as the residual limb changes shape or matures. The hard socket alone, without an additional liner, may not be appropriate for patients with fragile skin or significant bony prominences or for new amputees because their limbs are continuously changing and the hard socket may be difficult to adjust appropriately.

Prosthetic Socks

The most common interface used between a socket and the residual limb is a prosthetic sock. Prosthetic socks accomplish three goals: (1) they help cushion the forces applied to the residual limb during ambulation, (2) they help accommodate changes in the volume of the residual limb, and (3) they wick moisture that might accumulate during wear away from the skin.

For most prosthetic users, residual limb volume varies during any given day as a result of normal activity. Minor though these changes may be, they have the potential to compromise the fit of the prosthesis and increase the risk of skin irritation and discomfort. The addition or subtraction of sock layers (ply) accommodates changes in the limb and helps maintain the fit. Prosthetic wearers may need to add several additional ply of sock in the middle of the day after a morning of moving about in their prosthesis to maintain optimal fit and function. Discerning when and how many ply of sock to add or remove is a skill developed during prosthetic training and rehabilitation.

Prosthetic socks are available in several materials and multiple thicknesses. They are sized to best fit the circumference and length of the patient's residual limb. The prosthetist usually provides several sets of socks of various weights (ply) and materials (wool, cotton, or blended material) with each prosthesis. During prosthetic training, the new prosthetic user learns to layer socks of various ply to achieve the most comfortable and functional fit in the socket. Once the layers of sock reach 10-ply or more, however, the fit of the socket is so compromised that a new socket may be necessary.

Socks must be donned and smoothed carefully so that no wrinkles occur in any of the layers. A wrinkle increases pressure inside the prosthesis, which can lead to discomfort, skin irritation, and ultimately ulceration. Many prosthetists design a new hard socket to fit with a single three-ply wool sock. This baseline provides adequate cushioning while preserving intimacy of fit. As the limb shrinks or swells, socks are added or taken off, one ply at a time, until a comfortable fit is achieved.

For new prosthetic wearers, the distal residual limb may shrink more rapidly than the proximal limb around the knee. In this case, a sock is trimmed to fit only halfway up the residual limb; current sock manufacturing prevents unraveling of cut edges. This shortening improves prosthetic fit distally without compromising proximal fit.

Many patients with amputation wear a nylon sheath (similar to a stocking) between the residual limb and their prosthetic socks. The sheath wicks perspiration away from the skin toward the socks, resulting in a dryer, more comfortable feeling inside the socket.[16] The sheath also helps decrease the sheer forces between the socket and the residual limb. Daily cleaning and changing of socks are essential because the bacteria levels in a closed prosthetic environment are often quite high. In warmer climates, socks may need to be changed several times a day.

Soft Liner

For patients with fragile skin or significant bony prominences and for prosthetic users with high levels of activity, a soft liner may provide additional protection and comfort during gait and other activities. A soft liner is often fabricated in conjunction with the rigid outer shell for an exact fit. The materials for a soft liner are chosen on the basis of their elastic properties and frictional characteristics.[17]

Most commonly, the patient first puts on a sheath and the appropriate ply of sock and then dons the liner. Once all are in place, the residual limb and liner are fit into the socket. This external liner often eases the application of a snugly fit prosthesis. Sock ply is added or removed between limb and liner as needed to ensure comfortable prosthetic fit.

A soft liner provides additional protection and padding for the residual limb and can be easily adjusted or modified.

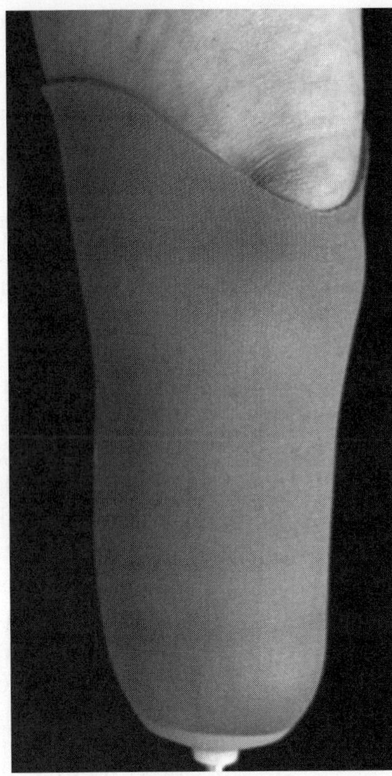

Figure 26-4
Roll-on liners are currently available in a variety of thicknesses and styles. Some provide only protection of the limb within the prosthesis whereas others incorporate socket suspension as well.

Some liner materials, however, absorb perspiration and may be difficult to clean. Liner materials also compress with repeated loading and use; eventually the quality of prosthetic fit may be compromised. Liners also add an additional layer, increasing the bulk of the prosthesis, which may be problematic for prosthetic users who are concerned about cosmesis. In some cases, especially for very active prosthetic users, the liner presents an opportunity for shearing and friction between the socket and residual limb, increasing risk of skin irritation and breakdown. Regardless of these potential disadvantages, liners continue to be used by the prosthetic community with excellent results; the benefits of added limb protection usually outweigh the detriments or disadvantages.

Roll-on Liners and Other Interfaces

Advances in prosthetics have made a third option available as an interface for transtibial sockets. These new liners are designed to absorb some of the shearing forces that normally occur between the limb and prosthesis during gait.[11] These elastomeric liners are usually made of silicon or similar materials (Figure 26-4). These liners differ from traditional soft liners in that they must be worn directly against the skin to minimize shearing. Prosthetic socks are still used to accommodate limb volume changes; however, they are donned over the liner rather than between the liner and the skin.

Such liners such have several important advantages compared with prosthetic socks or other soft liners.[15] First, they appear to be effective in dispersing forces during gait, including shear forces that can irritate or ulcerate the skin, making the prosthesis more comfortable to use. Often these liners also provide a mechanism for suspension of the prosthesis. These types of liners may be helpful for patients with fragile skin or recurrent discomfort or breakdown over bony prominences. Some of these liners can accommodate minor changes in residual limb volume without the need for prosthetic socks; moderate to major changes can be addressed by the addition of prosthetic socks over the liner.

As with any skin/socket interface, liners have disadvantages that must be considered. Occasionally, prosthetic wearers may not tolerate the skin/material interface, leading to skin reaction and blistering. First-time users of these liners should carefully and frequently monitor their skin condition. Some wearers will also have minor skin reaction and blistering just at the proximal edge of the liner. This reaction is often caused by the change in tension of the skin at the liner interface. Manual release of this tension or a small amount of non–water-soluble lubricant under the top edge of the liner or even a slightly larger liner may be necessary to resolve this problem.

These roll-on liners require significant dexterity and upper extremity strength to don; they may be difficult to put on if a patient has arthritis, sensory loss, or other impairments of the upper extremities. Some patients complain about the increased time and attention required to don the liner properly. All these liners require greater care in cleaning to reduce odor and bacteria. For some patients, this type of liner can cause skin problems such as contact dermatitis, bacterial infections, or follicular irritation.

Flexible Socket in a Rigid Frame

In a variation of a transtibial prosthesis, a prosthetist can use thin thermoplastic material to create a flexible socket, which is supported within a rigid external frame fabricated from either a thicker thermoplastic material or composite material hardened with polymer resin in a thermosetting process (Figure 26-5). The flexible socket is, essentially, the same PTB design previously described, worn with a sheath or prosthetic sock and providing total contact with the residual limb. Its flexibility, however, allows it to change shape slightly as underlying muscle contracts or as the knee joint moves further into flexion range of motion. Theoretically, the flexibility of the thinner and softer socket will improve comfort and better disseminate body heat during wear; however, little current evidence is available to support these claims.

The external rigid frame is designed to direct forces to the pressure-tolerant areas of the residual limb, particularly the medial tibial flare, the anterolateral muscular compartment, the fibular shaft, and the patellar tendon. Cutaways may be present in the frame (not the liner) over pressure-intolerant areas such as the tibial crest and distal tibia and the head of the fibula.

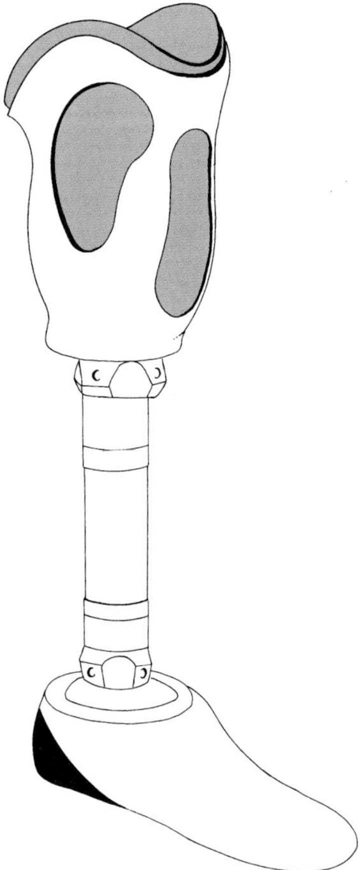

Figure 26-5
Example of a flexible socket in a rigid frame (anterolateral view). A thin thermoplastic socket is supported by a rigid external frame that transmits weight-bearing forces from pressure-tolerant areas of the residual limb to the pylon and prosthetic foot while open space around the fibular head and anterior tibia minimizes forces on these pressure-intolerant areas.

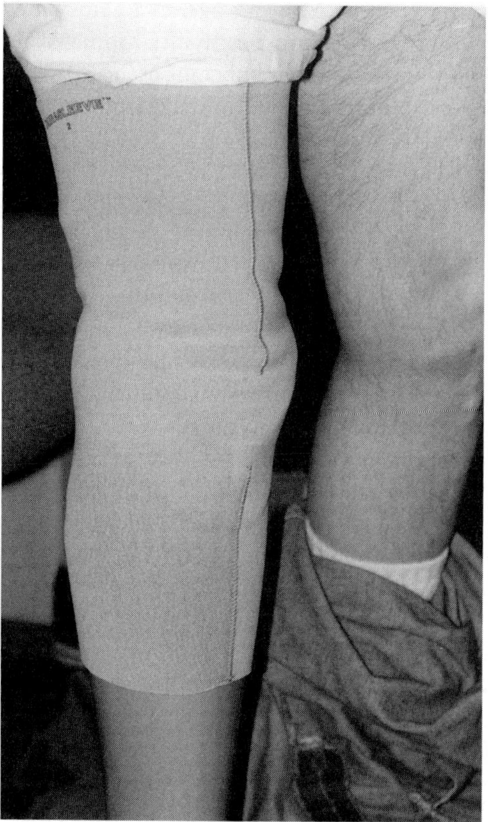

Figure 26-6
Neoprene suspension sleeve placed around the shank of the prosthesis and rolled upward against the skin of the thigh to hold the prosthesis in place. Note the seam at the anterior midline and the slight bump where the underlying prosthetic socks have been trimmed to ensure contact with the skin several inches from the top of the sleeve.

Suspension Systems

Safe and effective prosthetic use requires that the prosthesis be suspended comfortably and consistently on the limb during patient activity.[18] All suspension mechanisms must accomplish two goals: holding the prosthesis firmly to the limb during gait and allowing the patient to sit comfortably. A good suspension reduces the risk of skin irritation or breakdown by minimizing movement (pistoning and torque) between the socket and the limb. In the prosthetic prescription process, the choice of suspension is influenced by the patient's current and future activities, goals and physical abilities, and the climate in which the patient lives.

Sleeve Suspension

One commonly prescribed suspension system is a sleeve made of neoprene, urethane, silicone, or latex (Figure 26-6), which is positioned around the shank of the prosthesis and is rolled (or pulled) upward over the thigh once the prosthesis has been donned. Although the outer surface of the sleeve has a smooth covering, the inner surface tends to "grab" the surface of the skin. Sleeves are manufactured in various lengths and diameters to ensure a snug fit against the patient's thigh. To be effective, the sleeve must be in direct contact with several inches of skin above the top of the prosthetic socks (occasionally, the tops of the socks need to be trimmed). Suspension sleeves use friction and negative pressure (a result of the air-tight fit) to hold the prosthesis to the residual limb. Circumferential constriction is minimal, so suspension sleeves are appropriate even for patients with vascular insufficiency.

Suspension sleeves have a number of advantages over other suspension strategies. Many patients find these relatively thin sleeves to be more cosmetic than other suspension mechanisms. Because suspension sleeves are fit to be air tight, they are often the suspension of choice for patients who prefer to wear the prosthesis while showering or swimming because water does not enter the socket. Although some upper extremity strength and dexterity are required to pull the tight sleeve up into place, many prosthetic wearers find them easy to use. Suspension sleeves allow unrestricted knee motion during most activities. Some very active wearers dislike the posterior bunching of the material during kneeling or other activities that require maximal knee flexion.

One of the major disadvantages of suspension sleeves is their limited durability. They are susceptible to tearing or stretching from repeated donning and doffing and should be replaced fairly frequently. Even a small hole can reduces the sleeve's ability to suspend the prosthesis.[19] Suspension sleeves create a closed environment, retaining heat inside the socket and sleeve, which is especially problematic if the patient lives in a hot or humid environment. Constant friction against the skin can cause skin irritation or hygiene or sweating problems, especially in wearers with significant body hair. Although the sleeve is similar in appearance to an elastic knee orthosis, it does not directly stabilize the knee. For patients with upper extremity arthritis, weakness, or sensory loss, suspension sleeves may be difficult to don or doff.

Supracondylar Suspension

Supracondylar suspension captures the femoral condyles as they taper into the shaft of the femur to hold the prosthesis on the residual limb (Figure 26-7). To do this, the medial and lateral walls of the socket rise proximally around the femoral condyles. Because the walls are designed to taper rapidly to a narrow mediolateral dimension above the condyles, the prosthesis literally hangs from the condyles. This type of suspension is often abbreviated as PTB-SC (PTB-supracondylar) or PTS suspension (patellar tendon-supracondylar). The high walls of the PTB-SC prosthesis also provide mediolateral stability to the knee joint itself, a major advantage for patients with collateral ligament damage or insufficiency. For those who have no residual fibula, the PTS socket helps stabilize medial-lateral pressure during stance phase. This suspension is ineffective, however, for obese or muscular patients for whom clear definition of the femoral condyles is not available.

Most prosthetic users, even those with visual impairment or upper extremity dysfunction, find supracondylar suspension fairly easy to don and doff. The extra medial and lateral support provided by PTB-SC prostheses is important for those with moderate mediolateral instability of the knee and for those with short residual limbs that require additional control of the prosthesis. As long as the condyles are accessible, PTB-SC suspension is so effective that no additional means of suspension are necessary. Some wearers, however, choose to use a secondary suspension in conjunction with the PTB-SC.

One disadvantage of this type of suspension is that the proximal walls of the socket are significantly taller than those of a standard socket. As a result, some wearers may be concerned about the cosmesis of the PTB-SC or PTS suspension. The proximal walls are quite obvious through clothing when the knee is flexed during sitting. Although this suspension incorporates mediolateral support for the knee, it does not provide additional stability in the anteroposterior direction and should not be used to address anterior or posterior cruciate ligament instability. Fabrication of the PTB-SC prosthesis is also more time consuming and somewhat more difficult than other forms of suspension.

In a supracondylar-suprapatellar prosthesis (PTB-SCSP), a high anterior wall is added to the supracondylar design, encapsulating the patella (see Figure 26-7, *C*). This high anterior wall increases the stiffness and stability of the mediolateral walls and facilitates suspension with the addition of a quadriceps bar over the proximal patella. Because this bar maintains the patient's knee in slight flexion during the

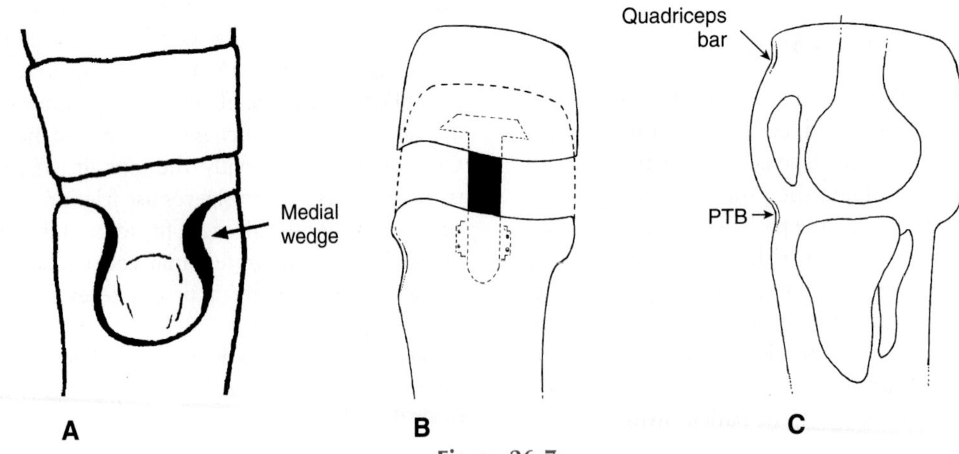

Figure 26-7

Variations of supracondylar suspension. ***A,*** *The medial and lateral walls of this hard socket extend upward to encompass the femoral condyles. Note the medial wedge incorporated in the soft liner to enhance suspension.* ***B,*** *Some PTB-supracondylar prostheses have a removable medial brim that opens to facilitate donning and closes once the limb is in the socket to achieve suspension.* ***C,*** *A lateral view of a supracondylar-suprapatellar socket also encompasses the patella within a raised anterior wall. Note the patellar tendon bar and relief for the patella.*

stance phase, PTB-SCSP suspension may be appropriate for wearers who have a very short residual limb and for those who tend to hyperextend their knee in the stance phase of gait. A soft liner is often used with PTB-SCSP sockets to facilitate donning and doffing. This suspension is, however, even less cosmetic than the PTB-SC in sitting because of the high anterior wall and patellar relief. Wearers of PTB-SCSP prosthesis often are uncomfortable when kneeling. Placement of the patellar relief and quadriceps bar requires skill and extra time and attention during fabrication. Finally, the PTB-SCSP may not be appropriate for those who are obese or highly muscular if the condyles cannot be sufficiently "captured" to ensure consistent suspension.

Cuff Suspension

Another method of suspension that captures the femoral condyles is cuff strap suspension (Figure 26-8).[20] In this method, a leather or webbing strap in the shape of a broad "X" is attached to the medial and lateral walls of the prosthesis, slightly posterior to midline. The X of the strap is positioned directly above the patella, then wraps around the limb posteriorly above the femoral condyles and is secured with hook-and-loop material, a D-ring, or a buckle closure. The cuff suspends the prosthesis by being snug over the top of the patella, not by circumferential tightness around the residual limb. The quality of suspension is controlled by the cuff's point of attachment on the prosthesis. The attachment points should be posterior to the center of the socket so that the line of pull falls posteriorly at the proximal portion of the patella. This attachment point is also critical for the patient to sit comfortably. If the cuff is not suspending well, wearers may be tempted to tighten the posterior strap inappropriately. A tight circumferential pressure actually compromises circulation and does nothing to enhance the efficiency of prosthetic suspension.

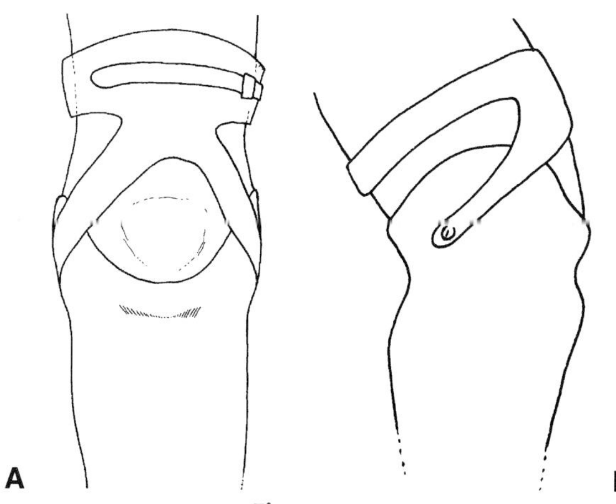

Figure 26-8
*Anterior (**A**) and medial (**B**) views of cuff strap suspension. Note the center of the cuff positioned above the patella (**A**) and the points of attachment slightly posterior to midline (**B**), which are necessary for efficient suspension.*

Cuff strap suspension is easy to don and doff and is readily adjustable. A cuff strap is an efficient suspension system for most patients with a mid-length residual transtibial limb. The points of attachment can be varied slightly to help control unwanted knee hyperextension. Some wearers find the cuff restrictive when knee flexion is needed for kneeling or sitting. In some cases, inaccurate placement of the points of attachment can lead to rotation of the socket on the limb during gait. In some individuals, especially those who are heavy, impingement of soft tissue may be present between the strap and posterior brim of the socket. In obese or very muscular wearers, achieving adequate purchase above the patella and around the femoral condyles may be difficult. Unlike the PTB-SC suspension, a cuff strap does not provide any mediolateral or anteroposterior stability to an unstable knee joint. If the cuff is made of leather, it may become misshapen over time and need to be replaced (fortunately a cuff strap is fairly inexpensive and relatively simple to replace).

Waist Belt and Anterior Strap

A historic method of prosthetic suspension uses a waist belt and anterior strap to suspend the prosthesis from the pelvis (Figure 26-9). The waist belt, usually made of webbing or leather, can be worn outside clothing during early prosthetic training when frequent skin inspection is warranted, but it is generally worn under the clothes during regular use. An elastic strap extends from the belt toward the prosthesis.

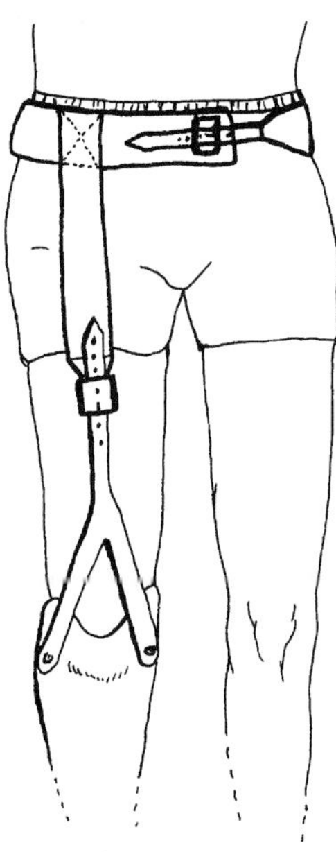

Figure 26-9
A waist belt with an anterior elastic strap can be hooked or buckled to a cuff or can directly attach to the prosthesis, as shown. In either method, the elastic elongates to allow flexion for sitting and for late stance and early swing of gait and then recoils to assist forward progression of the prosthesis during swing.

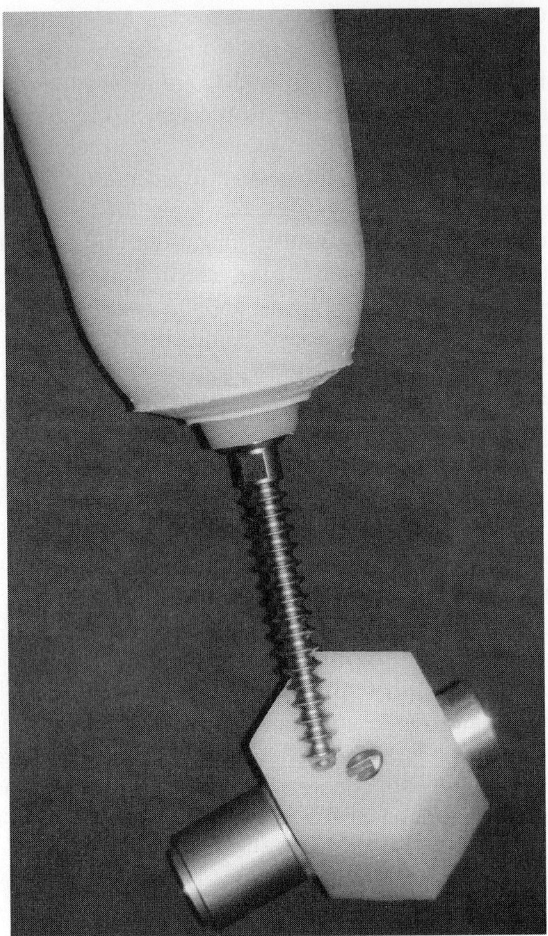

Figure 26-10
Silicone suspension sleeve with its distal pin and the locking mechanism to be embedded in the base of the prosthetic socket. Once the sleeve is in place, the wearer steps down into the prosthesis until the pin lock has engaged. When doffing the prosthesis, the wearer pushes a button that is recessed into the wall of the socket to disengage the lock and release the pin.

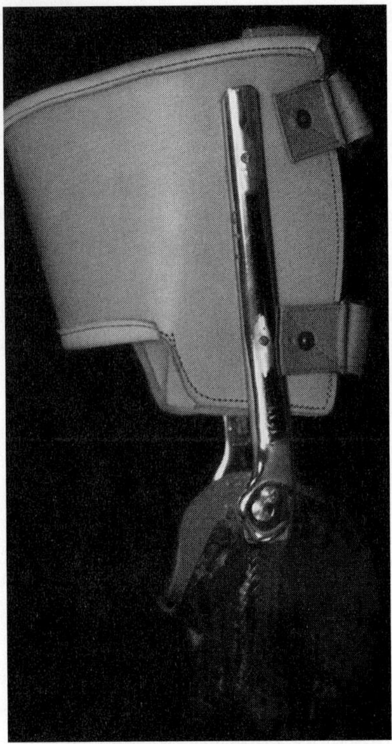

Figure 26-11
Example of a transtibial prosthesis with thigh cuff and side joints. Prosthetic knee joints are incorporated at the medial and lateral walls of the prosthesis. Weight-bearing forces are distributed around the thigh through a snugly fit leather or thermoplastic corset.

This strap can hook or buckle to a cuff strap or can fork to anterior-medial and anterior-lateral points of attachment directly on the prosthesis. This anterior strap incorporates an elastic material for two reasons: (1) to accommodate the extra length needed for knee flexion from terminal stance to initial swing and when the wearer is sitting and (2) to provide some assistance with knee extension as the elastic recoils from initial swing to initial contact during gait. Although the waist belt has been quite effective for suspension, it is bulky and at times difficult to manage under clothing and is now used much less frequently as a primary means of suspension. It may still be used as the first strategy for suspension in patients who are fit with a prosthesis immediately after surgery or for individuals who are frail or deconditioned who would benefit from the assistance provided by elastic recoil for limb advancement in swing.[17] Waist straps are also used when other forms of suspension are contraindicated or have proved unsuccessful. Athletes with amputation often opt to use a waist belt as auxiliary suspension in case their preferred suspension fails during demanding activity or competition.

Although the waist belt and elastic strap provide excellent suspension and are easy to don and doff, the elastic anterior strap can become overstretched with time and must be occasionally replaced. The various straps and buckles may be difficult to manage for patients with visual impairment, sensory loss, or limited upper extremity dexterity. The waist belt may be difficult to keep clean. The waist belt and strap cannot provide any external stability for those with ligamentous instability or weakness of the muscles around the knee.

Roll-on "Suction" Suspension with Pin Lock

Prosthetists have experimented with various types of suction suspension for transtibial prostheses for a number of years, but until recently most attempts at suction suspension had limited success. Unlike the transfemoral residual limb with its abundant and compliant soft tissue, the irregular topography of the transtibial residual limb presents a challenge for achieving the consistent air lock needed for suction. Widespread use of suction suspension became possible only with the development of silicone materials. In 1986, Ossur Kristinsson presented the first roll-on silicone sleeve that would suspend a prosthesis.[21] Today, several manufacturers market prefabricated roll-on suction suspension mechanisms (Figure 26-10). A silicone suspension mechanism has two components. The first is a pliable sleeve, usually made of a silicone polymer or thermoplastic elastomer, which is 1 to 9 mm thick and has a short peg or pin incorporated at the distal end. This pin inserts into a locking mechanism embedded at the base of the prosthetic socket. Once the pin is locked in place, the friction between the sleeve and skin suspends the prosthesis. A sock or sheath (with a hole cut in the bottom for the pin) is worn over the sleeve to ease donning into the socket. Additional layers of sock can be added to adjust for volume change during daily wear.

Many prosthetic wearers enjoy the increased sense of limb position awareness afforded by roll-on suspension.[22] Roll-on sleeves may attenuate sheer forces and are excellent alternatives for prosthetic wearers with fragile or sensitive skin. Suction suspension sleeves vary in price but tend to be more expensive than some of the other forms of suspension. This is sometimes problematic if sleeves are damaged or torn during frequent donning and doffing. Cleanliness is sometimes a problem; sleeves must be consistently cleaned and maintained to minimize odor and bacterial buildup. Skin problems are frequently noted.[23] The locking mechanism can also add weight to the finished prosthesis.

Contraindications for this type of suspensions are deep scarring, skin adhesions, and patient tolerance. Often the distally directed tension on the distal aspect of the residual limb is not tolerated well. Finally, many roll-on suspension systems may require more frequent maintenance and repair, which increase the overall cost of caring for the device.

Thigh Cuff or Lacer with Side Joints

A transtibial prosthesis may be difficult to use for a variety of reasons. If the patient has significant pain, scar tissue, knee instability, a very short residual limb, or an unsuitable limb for fitting, alternative techniques for fitting and suspension must be investigated. One such alternative is the thigh corset (also called thigh cuff or lacer) with side joints (Figure 26-11). Although traditional versions use a leather thigh corset closed by laces, a long thermoplastic thigh cuff with hook-and-loop material closures is more often used. Compression of soft tissue in the thigh by the snugly closed thigh cuff during weight bearing distributes the pressure proximally, reducing forces on the residual limb. The side joints control knee instability in the mediolateral plane. They also direct the varus and valgus forces generated during walking away from the knee center onto the thigh. If anteroposterior instability of the knee is present, a posterior "check strap" can be attached between the posterior distal thigh cuff and the posterior brim of the socket to limit excessive knee extension while the prosthesis is worn. The posterior check strap also reduces noise and limits wear of the prosthetic joint surfaces. Drop locks may be attached to the uprights to further enhance stability if necessary.

Although the thigh cuff and side joint provide significant external stability for a biomechanically unstable knee, aid in suspension of the prosthesis, and absorb vertical loading, many patients find the combination to be very bulky and reject its use. The thigh cuff, if fabricated from leather, may be difficult to keep clean. Although it is designed to be worn under clothing, cosmesis and adjustability may be problematic. For persons with limited flexibility or upper extremity dysfunction, the thigh cuff may be difficult to don. For many users who require the stability and force distribution afforded by a thigh cuff, additional suspension in the form of a waist belt is often necessary, adding to the difficulty of donning and the bulkiness under clothing.[24]

Additional Design and Suspension Variations

Patients who cannot tolerate the thigh lacer or whose residual limb is extremely short (less than 2 inches from knee center to distal tibia) have a limited number of alternatives. The prosthetist may suggest a gluteal-bearing prosthesis or bent-knee prosthesis. Both designs are quite difficult to fit and are cumbersome to use. Although preservation of the knee joint is associated with reduced energy cost during walking, some patients with very short, extensively scarred, or painful residual limbs may opt for surgical revision to knee disarticulation or transfemoral amputation so that prosthetic fit can be more effective, comfortable, and cosmetic.

CASE EXAMPLE 1A

A Patient with Recent Dysvascular-Neuropathic Transtibial Amputation

N. M. is a 6-foot, 2-inch 77-year-old man weighing 155 lb who underwent transtibial amputation of his right lower extremity approximately 24 days ago. Currently living with his 73-year-old wife in a senior housing complex, N. M. has been ambulating within the apartment with a standard walker in a hop-to gait pattern. He uses a wheelchair for long distances within the community. His medical history includes adult-onset (type 2) diabetes mellitus currently controlled by oral hypoglycemic medication and diet. He has a history of peripheral vascular disease of the lower extremities with associated neuropathy. The ankle-brachial index of his left limb is 0.8. He also has a history of three-vessel coronary artery bypass grafting approximately 1 year ago after myocardial infarction. His amputation was the result of infection of a chronic neuropathic ulcer at the fist metatarsal head. Before amputation, he and his wife walked daily for approximately 1 mile and were active volunteers at the local hospital. His favorite leisure activity is fly fishing.

Examination of his lower extremities reveals a mid-length (approximately 7 inches from knee center to distal end) transtibial amputation of his right lower extremity. A majority of N. M.'s incision has healed well; however, a 0.2-cm area at the center of his incision continues to drain a small amount of serosanguinous fluid and is reinforced by several elastic skin closures. He has been using an elastic "shrinker" on his limb for volume control. Range of motion at the knee and hip on the amputated side is within normal limits, and he has been working with the physical therapist on continued gait, strength, and range of motion exercises. His knee stability is excellent, and strength of both lower extremities is 4+ at all levels except for his left ankle, which is swollen and has decreased strength and range of motion. Examination of his left foot demonstrates decreased Semmes-Weinstein sensation (5.17) up to the knee. His skin is mottled but intact. Further examination of his right residual limb demonstrates that the circumference of his distal residual limb (measured 6 inches below the medial joint line) is 0.5 inches larger than proximal circumference (measured 2 inches below the medial joint line). He is meeting with the prosthetic team to determine an appropriate prosthetic prescription for his first temporary prosthesis.

Questions to Consider

- What tests and measures should be used in the examination? What is the current evidence of reliability and validity of such measures?
- What information about joint integrity and strength will be important in the formulation of a prosthetic prescription? What strategies should be used to examine joint integrity and strength? What is the current evidence of reliability and validity of such measures?
- Given the information provided, how should N. M.'s potential to use a transtibial prosthesis be assessed? Which of Medicare's functional classification levels would he likely be assigned? Why?
- Given his age, body type, and potential activity level, what are the pros and cons of each type of transtibial socket interface (hard socket with prosthetic socks, soft liner, roll-on liner, or flexible socket in a rigid frame) for this patient? Which one should be recommended? Why?
- What are the pros and cons of each option for suspension (sleeve, supracondylar, cuff strap, roll-on sleeve with pin lock, waist belt, or thigh cuff with side joints) for this patient? Which should be recommended? Why?

Recommendations

The prosthetic clinic team decides that N. M. is ready to be measured for his first prosthesis. They recommend a preparatory endoskeletal system for ease of adjustment of alignment and interchangeability of prosthetic components. They also choose a total contact socket with a Pelite (Bakelite Xylonite Limited) liner and suspension sleeve because a slight wound is present and the residual limb will be drastically changing once he begins wearing a prosthesis. This type of socket is easily adjusted. The suspension sleeve is easy to don, extremely reliable, and easily replaced if it becomes torn. Given his premorbid level of activity, age, and desire to regain mobility, they also recommend a SAFE foot (Campbell-Childs, White City, Ore.) because it has been demonstrated to be the most stable foot at early and late stance phase. The prosthetist informs N. M. and his wife that initial fitting will take place the following week once the prosthesis has been designed and fabricated.

CASE EXAMPLE 2A

A Patient with Traumatic Amputation and Concurrent Compound Fracture of the Intact Limb

S. P. is a 17-year-old high school senior and avid soccer player who sustained a traumatic amputation of his left lower extremity 1 year ago. He was hit by a car while skateboarding on the street near his home, sustaining an open comminuted fracture of his left tibia and fibula, tear of the left medial collateral ligament, strain of his anterior cruciate ligament, and a displaced fracture of his distal right tibia and fibula. In the emergency department, he was determined not to be a candidate for limb salvage, so he underwent a short transtibial amputation on the left (4 inches of tibia remain, measured on radiograph) and open reduction, internal fixation of his right tibial and fibular fractures.

Postoperatively significant ecchymosis, inflammation, and localized infection of the lateral suture line of his residual limb developed, which required revision and closure with split thickness skin grafting. Limb volume was managed by soft dressing and compressive wrap until the surgical wound and graft site were stable. Twelve weeks after his initial injury he was fit with a temporary prosthesis. His mobility was limited by his contralateral limb injuries. He is being seen in the prosthetic clinic for development of prosthetic prescription and evaluation of his temporary prosthesis. He is doing well with his temporary device but is limited in his activities by the prosthesis type and continuing discomfort at his right ankle. Hardware removal is planned for the right leg. He is anxious to "get a new leg" and wants to be able to skateboard and play soccer in the future.

Questions to Consider

- What tests and measurements should be used in the examination at this time? What is the current evidence of reliability and validity of such measures?
- What information about joint integrity and strength are important in the formulation of a prosthetic pre-

scription? What strategies should be used to examine joint integrity and strength? What is the current evidence of reliability and validity of such measures?

- Given the information provided about his preinjury functional status, how should S. P.'s potential to use a transtibial prosthesis be assessed? Which of Medicare's functional classification levels would he likely be assigned? Why?
- Given his age, potential activity level, and the condition of his residual limb, what are the pros and cons of each type of transtibial socket interface (hard socket with prosthetic socks, soft liner, roll-on liner, and flexible socket in a rigid frame) for this patient? Which one should be recommended? Why?
- What are the pros and cons of each option for suspension (sleeve, supracondylar, cuff strap, roll-on sleeve with pin lock, waist belt, or thigh cuff with orthotic joints) for this patient? Which should be recommended? Why?

Recommendations

The prosthetic team is somewhat concerned about tissue tolerance of pressure within the socket, especially around the graft, which has broken down a few times over the past year. These skin breakdown periods were most likely caused by reduction of volume of the limb and lack of protective sensation over the grafted area. These skin issues were early in the process and S. P. now understands the importance of volume and sock use. Regardless, concern about shear forces within the socket during dynamic activity, given S. P.'s skin graft and short residual limb, are a concern for the team. They are also concerned about medial-lateral stability at his knee. Anticipating that he has the capacity to progress quickly in his mobility and activity level, the team recommends a patellar tendon-bearing–supracondylar transtibial system to be used in conjunction with a 6-mm silicone liner with pin and lock. There is some concern over skin reaction to the liner and this will be watched for, but the benefits of the thicker elastomeric liner outweigh the other concerns at this early stage. Because of S. P.'s athleticism, the team also chooses a dynamic response foot. S. P. is casted for a negative mold of his limb, and the prosthetist informs the patient, his family, and the team that fittings will occur over the next few weeks.

PROSTHETIC PROGRESSION: FROM TEMPORARY TO DEFINITIVE PROSTHESIS

Often the first prosthesis received by a patient with a new amputation is called a *temporary* or *preparatory* prosthesis. The goal of the preparatory prosthesis is allow the patient to begin ambulation and prosthetic rehabilitation, reduce and stabilize the volume of the residual limb, and prepare the patient for definitive prosthesis use. The temporary prosthesis is most often an endoskeletal system consisting of a socket, suspension system, pylon, and prosthetic foot with no cosmetic cover or finishing. This strategy permits the prosthetist to interchange components as necessary and helps minimize production costs when many adjustments and adaptations to the socket and prosthetic alignment are anticipated. The size and shape of the residual limb usually change significantly when the new patient is ambulating on his or her first prosthesis. During this period the residual limb may shrink so much that the patient must wear 10 or more ply of sock to compensate for the loss of limb volume; prosthetic fit is therefore significantly compromised. For many preparatory prosthetic users, a smaller preparatory socket needs to be fabricated within the first 3 to 6 months of prosthetic use. Because the limb continues to shrink up to 1 year after amputation, the prosthetist often must fabricate a series of progressively smaller preparatory sockets until limb size and volume stabilize.

The definitive prosthesis is fit when the size of the patient's limb has stabilized, typically indicated when the patient consistently uses the same number of socks with the prosthesis over several weeks or months or when girth measurements remain the same over a similar period. Unfortunately, not much can be done to speed the process of limb maturation. Preparatory devices are required for at least 6 months; some new wearers may remain in their temporary prostheses for 1 year or more if further significant volume changes are anticipated.[25] Once the residual limb has matured, the definitive prosthesis is fabricated and fit. Most definitive prostheses should fit comfortably and maintain their structural integrity for 3 to 5 years for normal levels of activity.

The definitive prosthesis can be fabricated as either an endoskeletal (having a central pylon with a foam cosmetic cover) or exoskeletal (having a hard outer shell between the socket and prosthetic foot) system. Definitive prostheses are usually cosmetically enhanced to match the contours and skin color of the remaining limb as closely as possible before final delivery to the patient. In deciding whether to use an endoskeletal or exoskeletal system, the prosthetist and patient must weigh the various advantages and disadvantages of each to determine which system will best meet the patient's individual needs.

Endoskeletal Finishing

In an endoskeletal system, body weight is supported by a central rigid pylon (Figure 26-12),[26] and cosmesis is achieved by a soft, contoured foam cover with a nylon stocking, rubberized paint, or latex "skin" as a finishing external layer. The pylon (endoskeleton) may be the same steel alloy, titanium, or aluminum tube used in the temporary prosthesis or may be a lighter-weight non-adjustable material. The choice of pylon is influenced by the patient's weight, level of endurance, and types of activities anticipated; the material

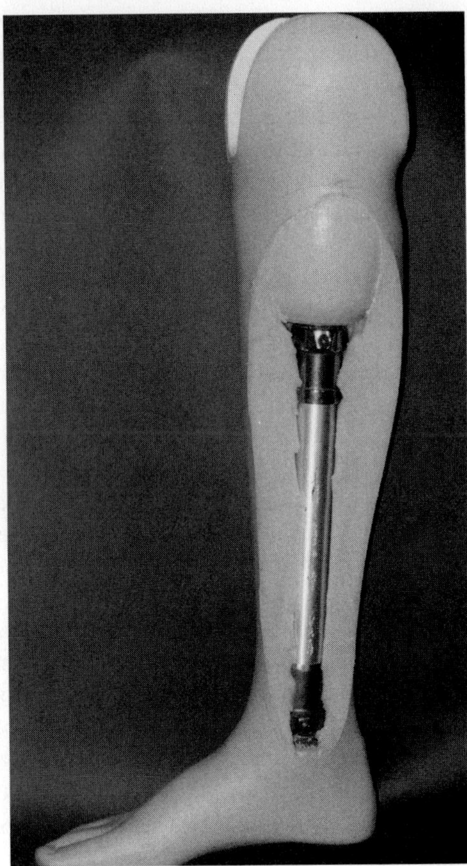

Figure 26-12
Cutaway view of an endoskeletal transtibial prosthetic system. Note the hard socket and upright pylon and the foam filler covered by a rubberized "skin." Alignment couplings between the socket and pylon, and between the pylon and prosthetic foot, are used to fine tune alignment for an efficient and comfortable gait.

must be strong enough to support the patient's body weight and sustain repeated loading during activities. A prosthetist might recommend a shock-absorbing pylon for very active wearers who engage in activities that involve high levels of loading to the socket and limb or who ambulate consistently at a high rate of speed.[27,28] The outer cover of a finished endoskeletal prosthesis (whether nylon, rubberized paint, or latex) is matched as closely as possible to the patient's skin color to maximize prosthetic cosmesis.

Prosthetic wearers often find that their endoskeletal systems are soft to the touch, much like real skin, and thus are cosmetically appealing. The use of a rubber or latex "skin" over the soft cover increases the durability and water resistance of the prosthesis. The major advantage of an endoskeletal system is its adjustability. Components, such as prosthetic feet, can be interchanged, and realignment of the prosthesis can occur as necessary.

A disadvantage of the endoskeletal system is that the soft foam cover and its protective finish are susceptible to damage during activity and are much less durable than an exoskeletal system. The colored cosmetic hose tends to run or tear and may be somewhat expensive to replace. The soft foam cover itself is not water resistant unless it has a rubberized or latex outer layer. Given the need for a protective finish over the foam cover and the risk of damage or staining, endoskeletal systems may be somewhat more expensive in the long run than the more durable exoskeletal system.

Exoskeletal Finishing

The outer walls of an exoskeletal prosthesis provide support to body weight during stance in the same way that the pylon does in an endoskeletal prosthesis. The socket is in a fixed position within a skin-colored hard shell, which continues over the entire shank of the prosthesis. The strength of the prosthesis is provided by the hard outer shell. The area below the socket within the shell can be hollow or filled with lightweight foam material. The outer shell (exoskeleton) can be fabricated from multiple layers of materials impregnated with thermosetting plastic resins or from a variety of other plastic materials.

The major advantage of exoskeletal systems is their durability, a feature important for prosthetic wearers who are involved in heavy physical activity or athletics. For skilled prosthetists, exoskeletal finishing may be less expensive and require less fabrication time than endoskeletal systems. The hard outer shell ensures that the prosthesis is waterproof. Some patients find exoskeletal prostheses to be less cosmetically acceptable and somewhat heavier to wear than endoskeletal systems. The major disadvantages of an exoskeletal system, however, are its fixed alignment and difficulty in adjusting the socket once it has been finished and delivered.

Prosthetic Feet and Footwear

Prosthetic feet are designed to work when the patient is wearing both shoes. The height of the heel space of the prosthetic foot should correspond with the height of the heel of the shoe. A prosthetic foot is well matched with a shoe when the top surface of the foot (at the attachment to the pylon) is parallel to the surface on which the prosthesis is sitting. If the foot is tilting backward, lifts should be added to the heel on the inside of the shoe to make the top of the foot level. If the foot is tilting forward, the heel height of the shoe is too high, and the patient needs different shoes for the prosthesis to work properly. The foot should fit snugly into the shoe to prevent movement but not so tightly that the foot cannot compress properly to achieve normal gait. The prosthetic foot alignment in the shoe affects the entire prosthesis and should be examined carefully before the patient dons the prosthesis.

EVALUATION OF PROSTHETIC FIT

The ability to evaluate the fit of the transtibial prosthesis requires attention to detail, training, and cumulative practical experience. Because so many patients with transtibial amputation have sensory impairment of their residual limbs, they are prime candidates for abrasions, skin ulceration, and infection. Socket fit should be assessed objectively, and teaching patients to inspect their skin for marks that indicate appropriate force distribution within the socket and for signs of irritation in pressure-sensitive areas is important.

Initial Evaluation

The first component of assessment of socket fit is visual inspection of the residual limb as the prosthesis is donned and after the patient has stood and walked in the prosthesis for a short period. Ideally, the residual limb should slide smoothly in and out of a snugly fit prosthesis or liner, and the patellar bar (if present) should make contact with the skin at the mid-patellar tendon. Although a total contact fit is desired for most patients, for some a small amount of space may be present at the liner's anterior distal end. If the newly delivered prosthesis is comfortably donned and the patient is able to stand, then he or she should shift weight onto the residual limb and then walk a short distance (perhaps in the parallel bars if external support is required). After this brief walk, the prosthesis, any liner, and socks are removed, and the skin is visually inspected once again. The prosthetist and therapists should look for areas of reactive hyperemia (areas of redness where pressure has been applied by the prosthesis) and the markings from the socks or sheaths over pressure-tolerant areas (the medial tibial flare, the patellar tendon, and the lateral shaft of tibia and fibula) as well as the absence of such redness and markings over pressure-intolerant areas (especially the distal anterior tibia and the fibular head). Areas of significant redness over a sensitive or nontolerant area indicate a potential problem with prosthetic fit, and the prosthesis should not be worn until an appropriate adjustment can be made. For most patients, reactive hyperemia should blanch on palpation and should dissipate back to normal skin color within a few minutes of this brief ambulation. If redness persists or any areas of irritation or abrasion are present, the prosthesis should not be worn until the contours of the socket can be appropriately adjusted and the skin is sufficiently healed.

Finding the source of discomfort within a prosthetic socket is sometimes a challenging task. Discomfort may be the result of excessive pressure or inadequate contact and too little pressure. Discoloration may be caused by too much pressure in one spot or too much pressure proximal to the discolored area. Several tricks are used by a prosthetist or therapist to help determine the causes of discomfort noted on initial evaluation: the visual evaluation, the powder test, the ball of clay test, and the lipstick test.

Visual Evaluation

The most immediate assessment of fit occurs when the prosthetist and therapist make a quick visual inspection of the limb immediately after the removal of the prosthesis. Areas that are blanched but quickly turn deep red often indicate areas of excessive pressure. The shape or contour of the blanched area and the patterns of reactive hyperemia (redness) help the practitioner identify potential problems based on a knowledge of total surface bearing (total contact) and the areas of support designated by socket design. In many instances, problems are the result of changes in limb circumference or shape and can be successfully corrected by altering the number of socks within the socket. If a change in sock ply fails to solve the problem, the prosthetist must use other strategies to identify the source of pain, skin irritation, or excessive pressure.

Powder Test

The powder test works best in cases in which the discomfort is caused by a loss of total contact between the residual limb and the socket, often at the bottom of the socket. A small amount of powder (baby powder or cornstarch) is sprinkled on the sides and bottom of the socket, especially in areas where firm contact between the socket and residual limb is desired. The prosthesis is then donned with care so that the powder within the socket is not disturbed or rubbed away. The patient stands, walks a short distance, and sits. The prosthesis is carefully removed, and the socks and interior of the socket are inspected. In a well-fitting prosthesis, a minimal amount of powder remains at the bottom of the socket because most of the powder will transfer to outermost prosthetic sock. Powder at the bottom or on the sides of the socket indicates loss of total contact fit. The number of sock ply can be adjusted, and the test is repeated. If the powder pattern does not change and the patient is not more comfortable, it may be time to consult the prosthetist about socket fit.

Ball of Clay Test

The ball of clay test helps identify if the residual limb is seated appropriately within the socket, is descending too far down into the socket (e.g., bottoming out), or is not going deep enough into the socket. A small, penny-sized ball of soft clay is placed in the bottom of the socket before the patient dons the prosthesis. The patient then stands, shifts weight onto the prosthesis, walks a short distance, and sits to remove the prosthesis. This test is not valid when the patient is using an elastomeric lining with a locking pin system.

In a well-fitting prosthesis, the clay is compressed into a flat disk approximately 1/8 to 1/4 inch thick, indicating that proper pressure is being applied around the distal end. If the ball is smashed against the bottom of the socket and is very thin, too much pressure is being borne on the distal end of the limb. If this is the case, the addition of another ply or two of sock will usually help position the residual limb correctly within the socket, and discomfort will be reduced. If the clay ball is hardly deformed, the limb is not descending far enough into the socket for proper support. Fit often improves and discomfort is eliminated by removing several ply of sock to reposition the limb correctly within the socket. For patients whose distal residual limb is hypersensitive or very pressure intolerant, the prosthesis may be designed with a moderate amount of space at the distal end to enhance comfort. For these patients, and patients with roll-on liners, the ball of clay test does not give an appropriate analysis of fit.

Lipstick Test

The lipstick test is used when prosthetic wearers have localized pain. When a patient points to a sensitive area, which is also tender on palpation, the lipstick test is used to determine if the sensitive area is touching the prosthesis. This test is effective in determining if the pain is referred from another location on the limb. This test also helps the therapist or prosthetist to determine if the limb is correctly positioned within the socket.

A small amount of lipstick is applied to the outer surface of snugly applied prosthetic socks over the pressure-sensitive area. The patient then dons the prosthesis, stands, shifts his or her weight, and walks a short distance. After the patient sits again, the prosthesis is carefully removed and the inside of the socket is inspected. The lipstick transfers from the sock to the socket where contact has occurred. If the mark is below the relief for a bony prominence in the prosthesis, the limb is probably positioned too deeply within the socket and an additional layer of sock may be necessary. Conversely, if the mark is above a relief area for a bony prominence, the limb is not far enough into the socket to fit properly and a layer or more of sock may need to be removed. The lipstick test can be repeated until comfort is achieved or other problems occur. If changing sock layers does not solve the problem, the prosthetist who designed the prosthesis should be contacted.

If, after walking, no lipstick remains on the liner or interior socket and the patient is still experiencing pain, the discomfort may be referred from another location on the residual limb. To determine if this is the case, other areas of the residual limb are palpated with moderate pressure. If pain can be reproduced by pressing on a different area of the residual limb (e.g., the peroneal nerve or posterior compartment) it is referred from this other location away from the actual sensation pain. The possibility of neuroma must also be considered if local discomfort or pain persists when these tests (especially the lipstick test) indicate proper positioning and fit of the prosthesis. Further surgery may be required if discomfort from a neuroma cannot be relieved by adjustment within the prosthesis.

Troubleshooting

In many instances problems with prosthetic fit can be solved in a systematic troubleshooting process that considers the location and pattern of pain, the potential prosthetic fit, and patient-related factors that may explain the symptoms. Common problems encountered in new transtibial prosthetic wearers, their most likely causes, and possible solutions are summarized in Table 26-2. Prosthetic problems can often be resolved by the therapist or the patient by simply altering the prosthetic socks. If problems persist, however, contact the prosthetist who designed and fabricated the prosthesis for more extensive evaluation and adjustment of prosthetic fit is appropriate. The most common causes of new discomfort in a prosthesis that was previously comfortable are often related to changes in the volume of the residual limb (possibly from discontinuing use of a prosthetic shrinker when not wearing the prosthesis), shoes with different heel heights or widths, and changes in activity level.

Table 26-2
Guidelines for Troubleshooting Transtibial Prosthetic Problems

Description	*Possible Cause*	*Other Indicators*	*Possible Solutions*
Inferior patella pain	Knee pathology (patellar-femoral syndrome)	Discomfort duplicated on examination of knee without prosthesis	Refer to physician
	Limb descends too far into socket	Fibular head pressure or redness Pressure or discoloration of anterior distal tibia or distal residual limb Inability to flex knee fully Positive ball of clay test	Add additional sock ply
Anterior tibial tubercle and/or proximal anterior tibial shaft pain	Limb not fitting far enough into socket	Distal discoloration Distal end pain Pain at fibular head Significant pistoning Difficulty controlling prosthesis	Remove sock ply
	Inadequate relief of tibial tubercle	No other problems noted Positive lipstick test	Refer to prosthetist for socket adjustment

Continued

Table 26-2
Guidelines for Troubleshooting Transtibial Prosthetic Problems—cont'd

Description	*Possible Cause*	*Other Indicators*	*Possible Solutions*
Tibial crest pain	Long heel lever	Rapid descent of foot at IC Anterior distal tibial pain	Check heel height and tightness of shoe Instruct patient to fully load the limb in early stance Refer to prosthetist for alignment adjustment
	Inadequate relief of tibial crest	No other problems may be noted Positive lipstick test	Refer to prosthetist for socket adjustment
Fibular head pain	Limb descends too far into socket	Anterior distal tibia pain Pain at distal pole of patella Feeling of "looseness" within socket Inability to flex the knee fully Positive lipstick test	Add additional sock ply
	Limb not far enough into socket	Distal discoloration Distal end pain Lack of control of prosthesis Anterior tibial tubercle pain Increased mediolateral movement of residual limb within socket Positive lipstick or powder test	Remove sock ply
	Prosthesis rotates on residual limb	Foot pointing into toe-out or toe-in General discomfort	Re-don prosthesis with patella centered above patellar tendon bar Add or subtract ply of socks
Anterior distal tibia pain	Limb descends too far into socket	Pain on distal pole of patella Feeling of looseness within socket Pistoning during gait cycle Inability to flex knee fully Positive ball of clay test	Add additional sock ply
	Excessively long heel lever	Rapid forward motion at IC	Refer to prosthetist for adjustment of alignment
	Shoes with higher heels	Anterior tilt of foot at MSt	Change to more appropriate heel
	Shoes too tight for prosthetic foot	Inadequate heel compression at IC/LR	Change to larger shoe to smaller foot
Inadequate relief of anterior distal tibia	No other problems noted	Refer to prosthetist for adjustment of socket	
	Pain referred from elsewhere	Positive lipstick test Pain or redness over another area reproduces discomfort at distal tibia	Address source of problem Refer to prosthetist for socket or alignment adjustment
	Limb not far enough into socket	Distal discoloration Distal end pain Pistoning within socket Increased mediolateral movement within socket Anterior tibial tubercle pain Positive powder, lipstick, or ball of clay tests	Remove sock ply

Continued

Table 26-2
Guidelines for Troubleshooting Transtibial Prosthetic Problems—cont'd

Description	*Possible Cause*	*Other Indicators*	*Possible Solutions*
	Bone or skin adhesion at distal tibia	Discomfort within skin traction Decreased skin mobility over tibia	Intervention to reduce adhesion Refer to physician Refer to prosthetist for socket adjustment
Posterior calf pain	Distal socket tightness	Blanching proximal to distal end, turning deep red with observation	Reduce sock ply
	Excessive proximal posterior pressure	Pistoning of limb in socket Popliteal abscess Distal end pain Cramping in limb	Loosen cuff or clothing on thigh Reduce sock ply Refer to prosthetist for further evaluation
	Circulatory disorders	Cool limb Aching residual or contralateral limb (especially after activity) Lack of color in residual limb Patient reports night pain in leg or limb	Refer to physician for evaluation
Vertical movement of limb inside prosthesis (pistoning)	Poor suspension	Old or worn suspension system	Replace or repair suspension system
	Too few socks	Pain at distal patella Loose feeling in prosthesis Inability or flex knee fully Pain on anterior distal tibia or crest	Add additional sock ply
	Too many socks	Distal discoloration Loose feeling in prosthesis Lack of control of prosthesis Anterior tibial tubercle pain	Remove sock ply
Distal looseness with proximal tightness of limb inside prosthesis ("bell clapping")	Normal limb shrinkage with prosthetic use	Distal anterior discomfort Lack of control of prosthesis Patient reports "looseness" Inability to add sock ply comfortably	Cut half-length sock to add ply to distal residual limb only Refer to prosthetist

IC = initial contact; MSt = midstance; LR = loading response.

CASE EXAMPLE 1B

A Patient with Recent Dysvascular-Neuropathic Transtibial Amputation

Today N. M. receives his first prosthesis. He and his wife are impatient to "get going" with his prosthesis and they hope to go on a cruise planned 1 month from now.

Visual inspection of N. M.'s residual limb before he dons his new prosthesis reveals a nearly closed and mobile suture line with no significant areas of tenderness. The wound is covered with a very thin skin layer and is no longer draining. He and his wife have been consistent with a home program that includes desensitization, handling of his residual limb, stretching, and strengthening of his residual limb as well as his trunk and upper limbs. He continues to use a "shrinker" nearly 24 hours each day. The prosthetist teaches and assists N. M. in the proper donning of the liner and socket, emphasizing that the socks are donned first and then the liner. The prosthetist stresses that the liner must be applied to the limb before placing the limb into the socket. Accommodations have been made to the liner to allow it to slide easily into the socket despite the difference in circumference of his limb at the proximal and distal ends. A sheath is worn over the liner so that it will slide more easily into the socket. After the socket is donned correctly, the prosthetist evaluates fit and assesses if there are appropriate tensions. The suspension sleeve is also applied.

Next, N. M. stands in the parallel bars with his feet shoulder width apart and is instructed to shift his weight onto his prosthesis so that each leg bears equal weight. The appropriate length of the device is then evaluated and adjusted before any ambulation. He reports that the prosthesis feels "tight" around his limb but no areas of noticeable high pressure are present. He then sits and removes the prosthesis and sleeve so that the prosthetist can inspect his limb and adjust the height. Evaluation shows no areas of excessive pressure or inappropriate pressures. N. M. is instructed to re-don his prosthesis and is then asked to ambulate the length of the bars. After this short walk, which occurs with minimal assistance, his prosthesis is once again removed for inspection of limb condition. This time an area of marked redness is present at the distal edge of the patella, fibular head, and distal anterior tibia.

Questions to Consider

- How is weight bearing optimally distributed within a patellar tendon-bearing socket? What areas of the transtibial residual limb are the most pressure tolerant? Where in the patellar-tendon bearing socket will there be areas of relief for non–pressure-tolerant areas? Where would reactive hyperemia areas be seen if a correct fit has been accomplished?
- Why is the prosthetic team so conservative about N. M.'s initial time in the socket, especially when he is so anxious to "get going"?
- What do the markings on his residual limb suggest when the prosthesis is removed after his walk down and back in the parallel bars? How would current fit of his prosthesis be described? What recommendations should be made about improving fit of the prosthesis? Does the socket need any revision at this point? Why or why not?

Recommendations and Interventions

The prosthetist determines that the limb is descending too far down into the socket. A single-ply sock is added to the residual limb and the prosthesis is re-donned. The height of the device is reevaluated because the addition of socks can affect the functional length of the device. N. M. ambulates the length of the bars again and his limb is reevaluated. After a few trials, the prosthetist decides that, at least for the moment, two 1-ply socks provide the most appropriate fit. Because N. M. is able to achieve fairly equal (if a bit cautious) reciprocal strides, with upper extremity support for balance, in the parallel bars, he is encouraged to walk approximately 50 feet down the hallway with a rolling walker for support as necessary. After this trial, no areas of pronounced redness are present. After a short rest, N. M. takes a final walk down the hallway for 100 feet. Once again the marks from the socket on his limb appear appropriate. Greatly encouraged, N. M. and his wife make an appointment to begin outpatient gait and functional training with the therapist the next day.

CASE EXAMPLE 2B

A Patient with Traumatic Amputation and Concurrent Compound Fracture of the Intact Limb

S. P. and his parents arrive at prosthetic clinic for initial fitting of his new left transtibial prosthesis. He is not required to wear his fracture brace on his right lower extremity; however, he continues to report ankle pain and decreased mobility. The prosthetist explains the donning procedure, placing the liner against the skin and the socks over the liner. The removable medial brim supracondylar system is applied after the socket is donned. S. P. then stands in the parallel bars, shifting weight cautiously onto his new prosthesis. He reports that the socket feels very tight and points to areas of noticeable pressure at the anterior tibial tubercle, fibular head, and lateral surfaces of the femoral condyles.

On removal of the prosthesis, several areas of reactive hyperemia are present well below the patellar tendon and on the proximal surface of the fibular head as well as on the femoral condyles. A small area (1 cm diameter) of serous drainage is present on the liner, corresponding to the top edge of the skin graft at the lateral suture line, although no apparent dehiscence or continued drainage is noted. The team decides to have S. P. re-don the prosthesis with a nylon sheath over the liner, stand and shift weight, and then walk the length of the parallel bars. He reports that the prosthesis, although still snug, is more comfortable. He sits down, removes the prosthesis, and the team inspects his skin once again. This time reactive hyperemia occurs in the expected areas.

Questions to Consider

- How is weight bearing optimally distributed within a patellar tendon-bearing–supracondylar socket? What areas of the transtibial residual limb are the most pressure tolerant? Where in the patellar tendon-bearing–supracondylar socket will there be areas of relief for non-pressure-tolerant areas? Where would reactive hyperemia be seen if a correct fit has been accomplished? How does residual limb length affect pressure tolerance and reactive hyperemia?

- What do the markings on S. P.'s residual limb suggest when the prosthesis is removed after his initial period of standing? Why did the prosthetist make a switch from 1-ply sock to a nylon sheath? What do the markings after S. P.'s walk down the parallel bars suggest? How would the current fit of his prosthesis be described? What recommendations should be made about improving fit of the prosthesis? Does the socket need any revision at this point? Why or why not?

Recommendations and Interventions

S. P. begins ambulating in the parallel bars and soon afterwards independently with a straight cane in his left hand. After walking approximately 75 feet, S. P. now reports distal anterior tibial discomfort. On doffing the prosthesis, marked reactive hyperemia is present over the distal anterior tibia as well as the bottom edge of the patella. The team concludes that because of this short ambulation, fluid has been forced from the limb, thereby reducing his limb volume. He is now descending too far into the socket, requiring a return to the single-ply sock. Once again, the inappropriate hyperemia resolves within the expected timeframe.

PROSTHETIC ALIGNMENT

Prosthetic alignment is defined as the relationship between the socket and the prosthetic foot. Proper alignment is influenced by the patient's natural gait pattern, the functional characteristics of the prosthetic foot, the condition and pressure tolerance of the residual limb, and the functional goals of the patient. Alignment has an impact on comfort and energy expenditure during gait. Three steps are necessary to achieve optimal alignment: bench alignment in the prosthetic laboratory, static alignment while the patient is standing in the prosthesis, and dynamic alignment based on gait analysis. Each step in this process further refines alignment, tailoring the socket-foot relation to the individual patient.

Confusion is often present when using standard anatomical terminology in relation to a prosthesis. For example, the term *flexion refers to flexion of the knee or flexion of the socket, which are essentially the same. The* confusion occurs because a pseudoarthrosis is present at the distal end of the socket that allows the foot position to change relative to the socket. In an anatomical model, when a person flexes the knee in standing (assuming a stable thigh segment), the foot becomes relatively more posterior to midline. In a prosthesis, flexion of the socket may or may not change the position of the foot relative to the midline because the socket (hence the knee) can be flexed and the foot put back in the original position (Figure 26-13). This independence of socket and foot posi-

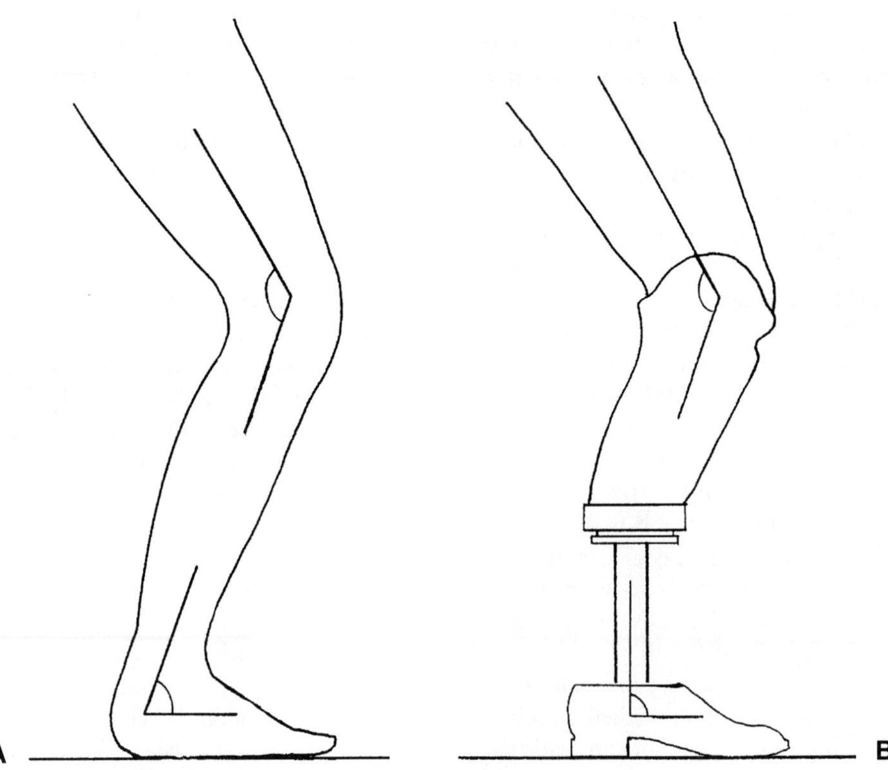

Figure 26-13

A, *In an intact limb, knee flexion is linked to ankle position and dorsiflexion.* ***B,*** *In a prosthesis, socket position can be changed without altering the balanced position of the prosthetic foot.*

tion allows the prosthetist to compensate for fixed deformity or minor contracture without significant compromise of the quality of prosthetic gait. Currently, no specific terminology exists to adequately describe this phenomenon.

Static Evaluation

The first step in the alignment process is static evaluation. The patient dons the prosthesis and stands while the practitioner systematically evaluates fit, comfort, and force distribution in quiet standing (Box 26-1). The patient should attempt to stand with the feet approximately shoulder width apart. First, the ability to bear weight equally on both legs without discomfort is assessed. Patients with recently healed amputations who are receiving their first prostheses may need encouragement to shift weight toward the prosthetic side until body weight is equally shared by the prosthesis and the intact limb. Next, relative length equality of prosthetic and intact leg length is determined. Palpation of the patient's anterior superior iliac spines, posterior superior iliac spines, and iliac crests is used to determine whether the pelvis is level. If the pelvis is not level, adjustment of the length of the prosthetic pylon is indicated. Although some patients may not be concerned with slight leg length discrepancy, over time asymmetry in gait may contribute to the development of secondary back pain. Before the length of the prosthesis is adjusted, however, double checking the position of the limb within the socket is wise. Inappropriate sock ply can mimic a leg-length discrepancy.

Attention is then turned to the contact between the foot and the floor. Ideally, the foot should be flat on the floor. If obvious differences in weight bearing between the heel and forefoot, or between medial and lateral borders of the foot, are noted, the position of the socket established during bench alignment probably needs adjustment or refinement.

The top surface of the prosthetic foot is designed to be parallel to the ground. If this surface is inclined, heel height of the shoe may be incorrect. In an endoskeletal prosthesis that has a pylon between the foot and the socket, the verticality of the pylon is not an appropriate indicator of alignment. A pylon does not have to be perpendicular to the floor in a well-aligned prosthesis. The top of the foot, rather than the position of the pylon, is the most important reference in assessing alignment. Additionally, the prosthetic foot may not be flat on the floor if a knee flexion contracture has developed or if an existing knee flexion contracture has not been well accommodated by initial alignment of the prosthesis. Mild knee flexion contractures sometimes reduce with use of the prosthesis over time.

Finally, forces applied to the lower extremity above the socket are assessed. A sense by the patient that the knee is forced into flexion or extension may indicate incorrect alignment or incorrect heel height of the shoe.

Pressure on the residual limb is greatly affected by the inclination of the supporting surfaces in the socket.[5] When the socket is placed in a relatively flexed position (Figure 26-14), the area of the socket providing vertical support for the residual limb is increased when compared with a socket that is mostly vertical.

If the patient does not exhibit any of the previously mentioned problems, he or she is ready to walk and participate in the dynamic alignment process. If the prosthesis does not pass static alignment, however, ambulation in a normal fashion is nearly impossible. Much of the guesswork and time spent in gait analysis can be saved by performing a thorough static alignment evaluation before the patient walks with the prosthesis.

Box 26-1 *Checklist for the Evaluation of Static Alignment*

- Is weight bearing equal between the prosthesis and the intact limb?
- Is the patient experiencing any pain or discomfort?
- Are the anterior superior iliac spines, posterior superior iliac spines, and iliac crests level?
- Is the foot flat on the floor?
- Is the top of the foot parallel to the ground in the anteroposterior and mediolateral planes?
- Is the knee being forced into flexion or extension?

Transmission of Forces during Prosthetic Gait

When a patient walks in the prosthesis, the forces generated by weight bearing must be absorbed by the residual limb.

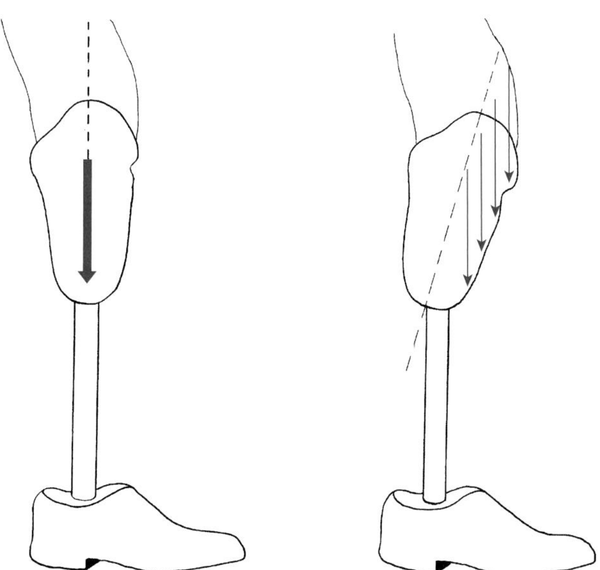

Figure 26-14
Setting the socket in slight flexion rather than in the vertical or upright position increases comfort and function by distributing weight-bearing forces along the entire anterior surface of the residual limb.

The amplitude and effect of these forces on the residual limb depend on several interconnected factors: the loading characteristics of the liner and socket materials, the intimacy and quality of prosthetic fit, the health and characteristics of the skin and soft tissue of the residual limb, and the effectiveness of the alignment between the foot and socket.[28]

No matter how well the socket fits the residual limb, there will be a torque about the residual limb generated by the prosthetic foot position with respect to the center of the socket. Considering the residual limb and the socket as two separate entities is often helpful. When force is directed on one, it must be resisted by the other. The residual limb/prosthetic interface can be thought of as a pseudarthrosis with a center of motion at the center of the residual limb.[29] The residual limb is, essentially, a stationary object. If the foot is offset from the center of the socket, the socket tends to rotate around the residual limb during weight bearing. Because the residual limb is a stationary object, it will resist this rotation with an equal but opposite force (Figure 26-15).

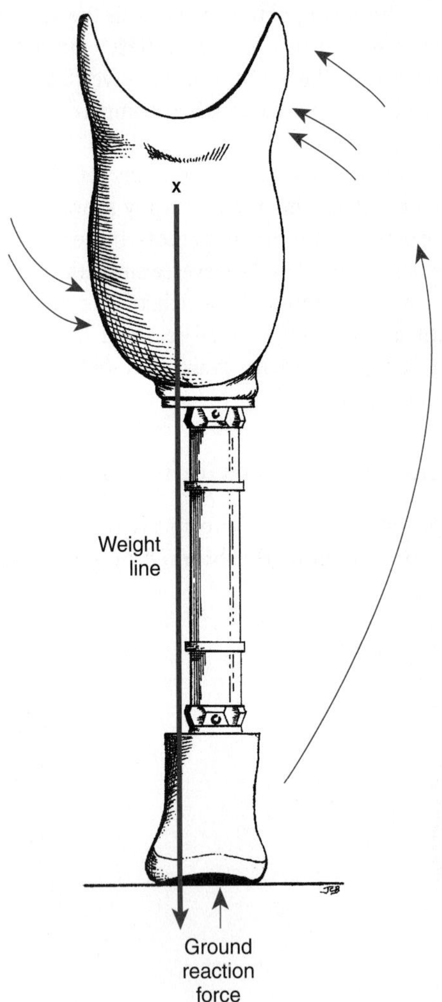

Figure 26-15

Understanding rotation of the socket on the residual limb. If the residual limb is thought of as a stationary object, the weight-bearing forces transmitted upward from the center of the foot during gait and applied at the socket-limb interface can be better understood. For example, when the foot is medially inset, the resulting force acts to rotate the socket on the residual limb in the frontal plane. This rotational force creates pressure at the proximal medial limb (at the medial tibial flare) and distal lateral limb (along the lateral shaft of the tibia).

As an example, consider a prosthesis used after transtibial amputation of the right lower extremity. If the prosthetic foot is slightly inset with respect to the socket, the resulting force causes rotation (if viewed from the front) in a counterclockwise direction, which in turn exerts pressures at the bottom left (distal lateral) and top (proximal medial) surfaces of the residual limb. The proximal medial surface makes contact with the medial tibial flare; the distal lateral surface makes contact with the shaft of the fibula and anterior compartment musculature. Both these areas are pressure tolerant; a slightly inset prosthetic foot appropriately loads the limb for weight bearing.

If the foot is instead positioned slightly laterally (outset) with respect to the center of the socket, the direction of the rotational force reverses, with pressures exerted at the top left (proximal lateral) and bottom right (distal medial) surfaces of the residual limb, and the most pressure-tolerant areas of the limb cannot be efficiently loaded for weight bearing. Position of the foot relative to the limb is one of the major determinants of amplitude and location of pressure that the patient feels inside the prosthesis.

DYNAMIC GAIT ANALYSIS

Observational gait analysis is used to evaluate whether the alignment of the prosthesis allows the patient to achieve the most energy-efficient and highest quality pattern of walking.[30,31] In the dynamic alignment process, the gait characteristics of a person with amputation are compared with the norms of able-bodied individuals of the same age and activity level.[31-33] The symmetry of distance and time parameters (e.g., stride length, single limb support time) of the intact and prosthetic limb are also assessed.[28] The goal of the dynamic alignment process is to achieve a gait that is as close to normal as possible. Gait deviations can be attributed to malalignment of the prosthesis or to the physical limitations (e.g., joint contracture, weakness, skeletal deformities) of the patient.[34] Determining whether a gait deviation is specifically caused by the prosthesis or if a physiological/anatomical problem is at the root of the problem can be difficult. This challenge reinforces the importance of a team approach to care and open communication among the team members. Care always seems to improve if the team member who identifies a possible gait deviation thoroughly assesses whether the deviation is something that can be addressed by his or her special skills and knowledge. If the problem falls outside that team member's scope of practice, then the other members should be consulted.

Prosthetic causes of gait problems are numerous and are often easily repaired by adjusting alignment. Patient-perceived quality of life may not be directly related to the ability to perform physical tasks, highlighting the concept that gait analysis and rehabilitation protocols are truly individual.[36] Prosthetic gait should be energy efficient and comfortable; it does not have to be perfect. Mild visual deviations may in some cases be preferable in terms of wearer comfort and function.

For effective gait analysis, the patient must be viewed from the anterior, posterior, and lateral perspectives because certain gait deviations are best observed in each of these planes. Once a prosthetic problem has been identified by the prosthetist or therapist, the prosthetist adjusts the alignment of the prosthesis. The prosthetist, rather than the therapist, is responsible (and liable) for making the necessary changes in prosthetic alignment. Systematic gait assessment requires evaluation of function in each of the subphases of gait. One strategy is to systematically assess early stance (transitions from initial contact until midstance), late stance (transitions from midstance through preswing), and swing (initial swing to the subsequent loading response). If gait deviations are observed, the therapist or prosthetist must first determine the possible prosthetic or nonprosthetic (wearer-related) causes of the deviation before deciding on the best strategy to correct the problem.[24]

Initial Contact, Loading Response, and Midstance

Initial contact is when the heel makes first contact with the ground surface. As the limb is loaded, controlled flexion of the knee should occur for shock absorption, along with a controlled "lowering" of the prosthetic foot to the floor.[36] The transition to single-limb support during midstance should, optimally, be smooth and stable. The functional goals of early prosthetic stance are effective weight acceptance and smooth forward progression of weight bearing from the rearfoot toward the midfoot. This allows the contralateral limb to have an effective early swing phase.

Alignment in the Frontal and Transverse Planes

The optimal position for the prosthetic foot in the frontal plane is directly under or slightly medial to the center of the proximal socket. This foot position imparts a rotation that applies pressure over the medial condyle of the tibia (medial tibial flare, a very tolerant area) and the distal lateral shaft of the fibula and tibia (see Figure 26-15). This rotational force also creates a slight varus thrust to the knee joint at midstance, which is necessary for comfort.

If the foot is in an *excessive outset position* (placed too far laterally) with respect to the center of the socket, the prosthesis rotates on the limb in the opposite direction, and the patient experiences increasing pressure on the proximal lateral and distal medial portions of the residual limb. This lateral foot placement may exert enough pressure on the fibular head and peroneal nerve to cause noticeable discomfort in the prosthesis. When the prosthetic foot is positioned too far laterally, an abnormal *valgus thrust* of the knee will also be present at midstance.

The quality and comfort of gait can also be significantly compromised when the prosthetic foot is in an *excessive inset position* (too far medially) with respect to the center of the residual limb. The rotation forces lead to excessive proximal-medial pressures and distal-lateral pressures as well as a marked *varus thrust* at the knee at midstance.

The position of the foot relative to the socket must be changed if excessive varus thrust or a valgus thrust is present as neither is well tolerated by the patient for any length of time. The contours of the lateral wall of the socket must protect the distal fibula and should direct pressures to the tolerant fibular shaft.

Abnormal *transverse rotation* of the foot is usually observed at initial contact. Typically, the foot rotates externally (laterally), pivoting around the point of floor contact at the heel to compensate for difficulty in moving into a foot-flat position. This rotation occurs for a variety of reasons. First, the shoe on the prosthetic foot might be too tight or the heel of the shoe too rigid (e.g., cowboy boots). If the problem persists with different shoes, prosthetic causes must be suspected. A socket that is too loose on the residual limb may also rotate as the foot makes contact with the ground. The addition of more ply of prosthetic sock to improve the fit of the limb in the socket may address this problem. A patient who is very deconditioned or weak may not have adequate strength or endurance of hip and knee musculature to control the prosthesis effectively. A strengthening program that targets improved concentric and eccentric control is necessary in this instance.

Early in gait training, a new prosthetic user might be reluctant to bear weight fully on the prosthesis, limiting compression of the heel cushion and leading to rotation of the prosthetic foot at loading response. Similarly, discomfort within the socket can lead to cautious initial contact and inadequate heel cushion compression and result in rotation of the prosthetic foot. If none of these precipitating problems is occurring, the most likely prosthetic problem is a heel cushion that is too stiff. The solution is to replace the prosthetic foot with one that has a heel cushion more appropriate for the patient's weight and activity level.

Occasionally, the patient will report the sensation of "sinking down" into the socket during this phase of gait. This sensation is often accompanied by distal end, patella, or fibular head discomfort. In a majority of cases when the patient had previously been ambulating comfortably, the cause is a reduction of the size of the residual limb relative to the socket, which may be easily corrected by increasing the ply of sock used.

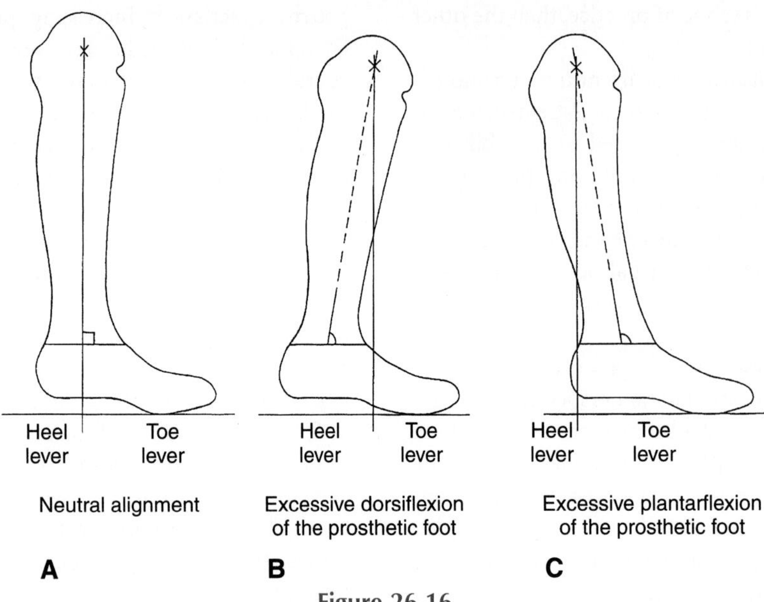

Figure 26-16

***A,** Toe lever is the distance between the center of the socket and the distal end of the prosthetic foot; heel lever is the distance between the center of the socket and the back of the heel. Both levers are influenced by alignment and stiffness of the prosthetic foot as well as relative position of the socket over the foot. **B,** The toe lever is relatively shortened and the heel lever is lengthened when the foot is dorsiflexed, the socket is flexed, or the foot is positioned slightly posterior to the socket center. **C,** The toe lever is relatively lengthened and the heel lever is shortened when the foot is plantar flexed, the socket is extended, or the foot is positioned slightly anterior to the socket center.*

Alignment in the Sagittal Plane

The relation between the socket and foot becomes more complicated when evaluating gait in the sagittal plane. The prosthetist must balance heel and toe levers to provide a smooth and natural gait pattern and to ensure socket comfort (Figure 26-16). The *heel lever* is the distance between the back of the heel of the prosthetic foot and the point on the foot that intersects a perpendicular line from the proximal center of the socket. The *toe lever* is the distance between the end of the toe and the same perpendicular line from the center of the socket. The heel and toe levers are influenced by three factors: the angle of attachment of the prosthetic foot (relative dorsiflexion or plantar flexion), the sagittal position of the socket over the foot, and the flexion or extension of the socket.

For a true understanding of gait the weight line and the center of pressure must be defined. For this discussion the *weight line* is defined as a line that drops from the center of the proximal aspect of the socket through the foot, perpendicular to the top of the foot (the same line that defines the heel and toe levers). The *center of pressure* is the point at which the foot makes contact with the floor at any moment in time. The *ground reaction force* is the resultant force between the weight line and the center of pressure, which is directed from the floor through the prosthesis. The relation between the center of pressure and the weight line changes as stance phase progresses.

In most nonarticulating prosthetic feet, no actual plantar flexion or dorsiflexion is possible. Instead, the heel or posterior portion of the foot must compress with weight bearing to simulate an articulation and provide a natural gait pattern. As weight is transferred onto the prosthesis in loading response, the heel compresses and the center of pressure moves forward on the foot toward the weight line. This decreases the torque about the socket and allows a smooth transition to the midstance portion of the cycle.

As the patient wearing a prosthesis begins stance phase (initial contact), the center of pressure is posterior to the weight line, causing a forward moment of the socket (Figure 26-17). The larger the difference between the weight line and the center of pressure (i.e., a long heel lever), the more quickly the prosthesis wants to rotate forward. This rotational force increases pressure on the residual limb at the proximal posterior and anterior distal segments as the patient attempts to control the rapid forward movement of the socket.

As the patient moves forward and begins the midstance portion of the cycle, the center of pressure moves directly under the center of the prosthesis. Little difference is present between the position of the weight line and center of pressure in the sagittal plane; hence, little torque is being applied to the limb. When patients report discomfort during midstance, the most likely problem is improper vertical support within the prosthesis.

Three prerequisites must be met for an effective prosthetic loading response.[37] First, the patient's knee must be able to flex an additional 15 to 20 degrees for shock absorption as weight is transferred onto the prosthesis in preparation for single-limb support. Second, approximately a $^3/_8$-inch

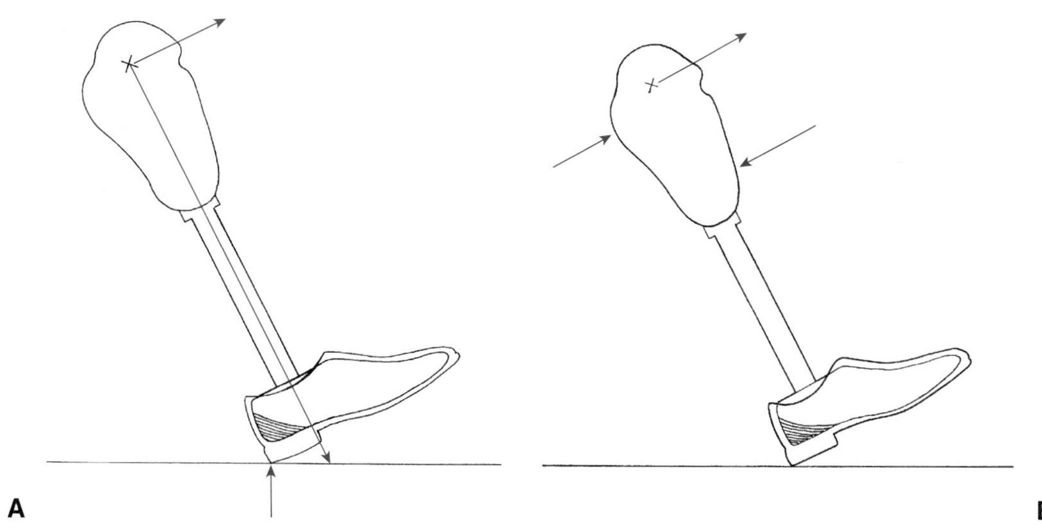

Figure 26-17

***A,** Because the center of pressure is well behind the weight line at initial contact, the resultant force causes a rapid forward movement of the socket. **B,** This creates pressure at the anterior distal and posterior proximal aspects of the residual limb as the user attempts to slow forward progression of the socket.*

compression of the heel cushion or posterior prosthetic foot should be present to simulate the plantar flexion required for an effective first (heel) rocker of gait. Finally, the position of the residual limb in the socket should be consistent as body weight is loaded onto the prosthesis, with minimal movement deeper into the prosthesis. The therapist and prosthetist also evaluate if equal stride length occurs and if the prosthetic foot makes contact with the ground in the line of forward progression without rotation in the transverse plane.

Gait Deviations: Initial Contact Through Midstance

The most typically observed gait deviations in the first half of stance phase include lack of knee flexion in loading response, excessive knee flexion throughout early stance, unequal stride lengths of the prosthetic and intact limb, and poorly controlled or rapid knee flexion as midstance begins. A number of possible prosthetic fit or alignment issues should be considered, as well as wearer-related factors that may contribute to each of these problems.

Knee Remains Fully Extended

One potential cause of excessive knee extension at initial contact and into loading response may be that the suspension system is inadequate, failing to hold the anatomical knee in the desired position of slight flexion. Ensuring appropriate suspension often corrects the problem, which is especially true if cuff suspension is used. In this instance, moving the point of attachment to a slightly more posterior position on the socket better maintains the desired knee flexion. If suspension is not the problem, the focus shifts to a heel lever that may be too short, forcing the knee into extension at initial contact.

Some new patients, nervous about knee instability during stance, might purposefully extend the knee more than is desirable to minimize the perceived risk of buckling. Gait training, rather than prosthetic adjustment, is an appropriate strategy for this wearer-related problem.

Knee Is Flexed More Than 10 Degrees

If initial contact is made with excessive knee flexion, stability in single-limb support stance may be threatened. If this gait deviation is observed, two contributing factors must be considered. First, the suspension system may be poor or incorrectly holding the knee in too much flexion, which is often the case if cuff suspension is adjusted too tightly or if the points of strap attachment are too far posterior on the socket. Adjustment of suspension often solves this problem.

Another factor to consider is a possible knee flexion contracture. Although a prosthetist can make prosthetic accommodations for slight contractures, significant limitations in knee range of motion compromise the quality of gait. Physical therapy interventions to reduce knee flexion contracture may be effective over time in improving knee function during early stance. The best strategy, however, is prevention of contracture formation in an aggressive preprosthetic exercise and positioning program. Patients with knee flexion contractures in excess of 40 degrees will find ambulation with a prosthesis nearly impossible.

Unequal Stride Length

Three contributors to unequal stride length are possible. The first, once again, is adequacy of the suspension mechanism. If suspension limits available knee extension in late swing phase, the prosthetic stride is shorter and stride length will be limited. If inadequate suspension raises the patient's concern about keeping the prosthesis on, prosthetic stride can be shortened as a compensatory strategy that shortens swing time, so the foot can make contact with the ground quickly. Either of these problems is corrected by adjusting the suspension system.

The other two factors are patient related. If the patient has pain or dysfunction of the sound limb, or pain with pressure on the prosthesis, stance time on the prosthesis may be reduced, thus limiting time in swing (and overall stride length) on the contralateral side. Careful evaluation of the painful limb to identify the limiting factor, followed by appropriate intervention, often helps improve the symmetry of stride length. Finally, new prosthetic users may be reluctant to trust that prostheses will support them during stance and will display unequal stride length until they can gain confidence and skill from focused gait training.

Rapid or Poorly Controlled Knee Flexion

Patients who are deconditioned or have weak quadriceps may have difficulty controlling the eccentric contraction of the quadriceps needed for an effective loading response. Exercises that alternate between concentric and eccentric contraction of the quadriceps muscles within the functional range of motion necessary for loading response, and intensive gait training, are the most appropriate physical therapy interventions to address this gait deviation.

In abrupt or forceful knee flexion in the transition to midstance, the socket is propelled forward too quickly as the prosthetic foot moves into the foot-flat position. This action can occur because of a problem with alignment or a problem with footwear. Several footwear issues should be considered before changes in alignment are made. A shoe with a heel too high for the prosthetic foot, a heel that is excessively stiff, or a shoe that is too narrow or tightly closed on the prosthetic foot will cause abrupt or forceful knee flexion in loading response. If the shoe is appropriate, then evaluation of the alignment must occur. Quick forward propulsion of the knee is often the result of an excessively long heel lever. The solution is to shorten the heel lever by sliding the foot slightly forward (anteriorly) with respect to the socket, repositioning the foot in a slightly more plantar-flexed direction, or decreasing the amount of socket flexion. A heel cushion that is too stiff and does not compress quickly enough to lower the forefoot to the floor also propels the prosthesis forward and causes abrupt knee flexion. Changing to a prosthetic foot with a less dense heel cushion might be the solution in this case.

Midstance to Terminal Stance

Stability of the knee and smooth forward progression over the prosthetic foot during late stance are important determinants of an effective stride length and preparation for initial contact of the contralateral, swinging limb. An effective stride and efficient weight transfer contribute to energy efficiency of gait.

Alignment in the Frontal and Transverse Planes

In assessing quality and efficiency of late stance, the prosthetist and therapist look for four key components in the frontal plane: a level prosthetic foot (top of the foot) as the other limb passes in midswing, a varus moment that causes a slight (approximately $\frac{1}{2}$ inch) lateral displacement of the knee, an upright trunk with minimal lateral trunk bending, and an equal reciprocal arm swing. Screening for gait deviations in midstance requires a lateral and a posterior viewpoint.

Alignment in the Sagittal Plane

As midstance is completed and the body continues forward over the anterior aspect of the prosthetic foot, the center of pressure moves anterior to the weight line. The foot begins to resist forward movement of the socket. The center of pressure moves rapidly toward the end of the foot, farther from the weight line (Figure 26-18). The resultant force attempts to maintain the flat foot position while the body continues to move forward. This action rotates the socket on the residual limb, pushing the proximal tibia posteriorly and extending the knee. The greatest pressures on the limb are found on the anterior proximal and posterior distal portions of the residual limb (Figure 26-19). Typically, the prosthetic wearer is more aware of excessive pressure around the patellar tendon because the soft tissue of the posterior distal residual limb is usually able to tolerate significant pressure.

Gait Deviations: Midstance to Terminal Stance

In assessing quality and efficiency of gait in the second half of stance phase, the most frequently observed deviations observed include a prosthetic foot that leans medially or laterally, insufficient varus moment at the knee, and lateral trunk bending.

Prosthetic Foot Leans Medially

If at midstance the top surface of the prosthetic foot is not level but leans medially, the prosthetist or therapist must consider five possible contributing factors. This deviation occurs when the socket is set in excessive adduction or the prosthetic foot is set in a pronated position; gait improves if the components are shifted slightly in the opposite direction toward abduction or toward supination. This deviation can also be caused by a foot that is more outset (lateral to the midline) than necessary and can be corrected by sliding the foot slightly toward the midline. Additionally, uneven shoe wear can mimic a medial leaning foot, so evaluation of the shoe is warranted. This deviation may also be observed in new prosthetic wearers who are reluctant to shift their weight fully onto the prosthesis. Gait training activities or an

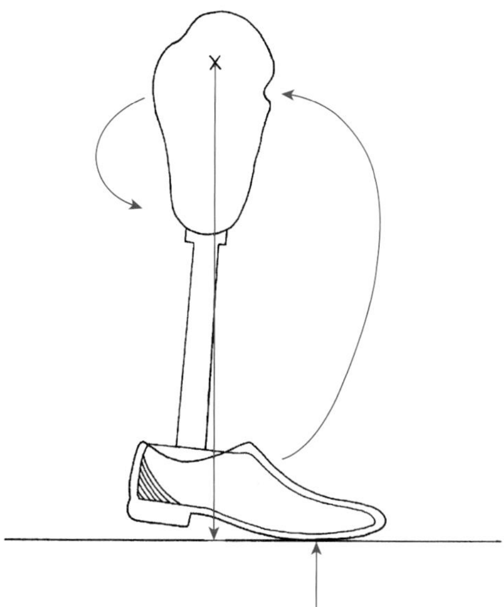

Figure 26-18
As the patient moves into terminal stance, the center of pressure moves anterior to the weight line. The resultant rotational forces lead to an extension moment at the knee. If the toe lever is excessive, the patient has to work harder to counteract this backward force and continue with forward progression. The patient often reports a sense of walking uphill if the toe lever is too long.

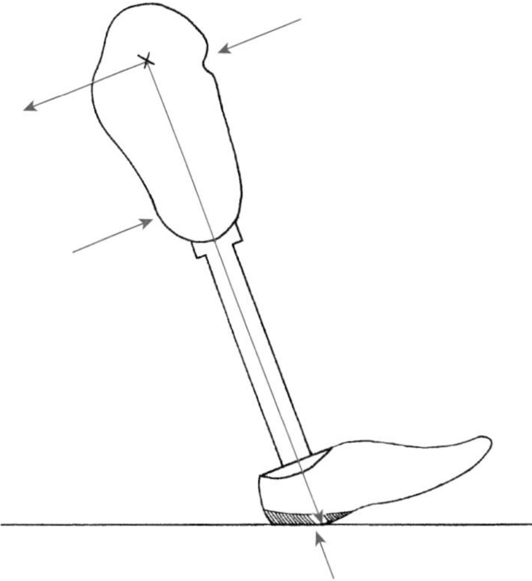

Figure 26-19
If the heel of the prosthetic foot is too soft for the patient's weight or activity level, the center of pressure and weight line almost coincide. Without the resultant forward rotation of the socket, the prosthesis fails to move forward, the patient feels high pressure at the proximal anterior and distal posterior socket, and an extension force is imparted to the knee.

appropriate assistive device helps patients learn to trust their prosthetic limbs. When patients report discomfort or pain, however, the fit of the socket must be reevaluated.

Prosthetic Foot Leans Laterally

The possible causes for a laterally leaning foot are the counterparts of those that cause it to lean medially. The foot may be positioned in too much supination, the foot may be further inset than is appropriate, or the socket may be set in less initial adduction than the patient needs. If so, movement of the foot or socket slightly in the opposite direction improves the quality and efficiency of gait. Uneven wear of the sole or heel of the shoes can shift the prosthetic foot laterally. Finally, an unaccommodated, narrow-based gait can mimic lateral foot lean. Gait training activities are often effective in changing step width to a more functional 3- to 4-inch heel separation.

Abnormal Varus or Valgus Moment at the Knee

If, at midstance, the desired varus moment is not occurring, the prosthetic foot is likely positioned too laterally (outset) relative to the socket. At the opposite extreme, if the varus moment is excessive, the foot is likely too far inset (medial to weight line). Occasionally, an excessive varus moment can be traced to a socket that is too wide in the mediolateral dimension, allowing the socket to shift on the residual limb. In this case, the prosthetist must adjust the width of the socket to improve function at midstance.

Lateral Trunk Bending

Excessive trunk bending during midstance increases energy expenditure during ambulation and disrupts smooth forward progression. This deviation can occur if the prosthesis is too short or too long compared with the contralateral limb, the patient is attempting to reduce discomfort within the socket, the prosthetic foot is positioned too far laterally (outset) with respect to the socket, or weakness of the abductor muscles of the hip is present. The fit of the prosthesis should be carefully reevaluated before adjustments to length are made because too many or too few prosthetic socks can incorrectly position the limb within the socket, resulting in an apparent, artificial leg length problem.

Terminal Stance to Preswing

For an efficient and cosmetic gait, heel off during terminal stance should occur smoothly and effortlessly just before (or simultaneously with) initial contact of the opposite limb. Ideally, a step width of between 2 and 4 inches is present between the medial borders of the feet. The knee should begin to flex as soon as the heel rises in preparation for toe-off. Because the prosthesis is unweighted, the foot should remain within the plane of forward progression with little or no transverse plane rotation of the heel. If these conditions are met, the transfer of body weight from the prosthetic limb to the opposite limb is accomplished smoothly. The socket must also remain adequately suspended on the residual limb as the swing phase is initiated.

Gait Deviations: Terminal Stance to Preswing

A variety of gait deviations can occur at the end of stance phase, including early heel rise, delayed heel rise, abnormal step width, rotation of the heel, and excessive motion between the residual limb and socket.

Premature Heel Rise and a Sense of Dropping Off

Most prosthetic feet are designed so that heel rise occurs in terminal stance subphase. An early heel rise occurs when the toe lever is too short and inadequate support is provided in late stance. If the heel rises during midstance, the foot is probably malpositioned with respect to the socket; it may be set in slightly too much dorsiflexion or set slightly more posterior to the socket than necessary. Alternatively, the socket may be set in excessive flexion. Early heel rise also occurs when the patient is wearing shoes with heels that are higher than appropriate for the prosthetic foot or if a knee or hip flexion contracture is present that has not been adequately addressed by prosthetic alignment. If contracture is a problem, moving the socket into more flexion combined with plantar flexion of the prosthetic foot may enable the prosthetist to establish the desired toe lever. Weakness of muscles around the knee that compromises stability in late stance may also contribute to this pathologic condition.

When the toe lever is too short, patients sometimes also report a sudden sense of "dropping off" or "falling into a hole" as their weight moves forward over the toes of the prosthetic foot. As a result, swing of the opposite limb is shortened for an earlier than normal weight acceptance as lack of foot support hastens entrance into the double-support phase of gait.

Delayed Heel Rise or a Sense of Walking Uphill

During early gait training, some patients report a sense of walking uphill or a strong knee extension moment accompanied by a delay in heel rise as they approach the end of the stance phase. This occurs when the toe lever of the prosthetic foot is functionally too long, preventing the normal rollover of the anterior of the prosthetic foot and the initiation of knee flexion in preparation for foot clearance in swing phase. The most common prosthetic causes of this gait deviation are a foot positioned too far forward (anterior) with respect to the socket or in too much initial plantar flexion, or a socket that is not adequately preflexed. Rollover and forward progression can also be compromised by a prosthetic foot with a keel that is too firm or stiff given the patient's weight or level of activity or by a shoe that is too stiff. Changing prosthetic feet to a more forgiving keel or changing to more flexible footwear may help solve the problem.

Abnormal Step Width

If less than 2 inches are present between the medial borders of the feet, the prosthetic foot may be positioned too far inset (medially) with respect to the socket. Moving the foot laterally (outset) or increasing initial adduction of the socket may help normalize stride width. If the patient habitually ambulates with a narrow base, gait training activities may be necessary to alter this motor behavior.

Step widths that are wider than 4 inches are associated with increased mediolateral displacement during forward progression of gait and a higher energy cost of prosthetic gait. Wide step widths may be related to a problem with alignment (a prosthetic foot that is too far lateral or outset with respect to the socket) or to a fear of instability and reluctance to shift weight completely onto the prosthesis. Gait training that reinforces the need for a narrower base of support or an appropriate assistive device may be helpful for patients who are concerned with instability.

Medial or Lateral Rotation of the Heel

Occasionally, the heel appears to rotate as weight progresses forward over the toes of the prosthetic foot. The prosthetic cause of this deviation is a prosthetic foot that has been set in slightly too much pronation or supination. More commonly, the patient-related cause of this deviation is shortening of hip flexor musculature that prevents the femur from rotating with the pelvis in the transition between stance and swing phase. If this is the case, physical therapy interventions designed to lengthen hip flexor muscles improve the quality of prosthetic gait. This deviation may also be the consequence of inappropriate cuff strap attachment on the socket; adjusting the point of attachment may improve quality of gait.

Excessive Motion between the Residual Limb and Socket

In preswing, as the prosthesis is unweighted in preparation for initiation of swing, the patient may feel the socket drop away (piston) from the residual limb. Two factors should be considered when this occurs: the adequacy of the suspension and the number of sock ply that the patient is wearing. Too few ply of sock and too many ply of sock can cause pistoning between the residual limb and socket.

Swing Phase

Prosthetic gait has two primary goals during swing phase. First, the prosthetic foot should swing forward within the line of progression, without transverse rotations (whips or excessive toe-out or toe-in). Second, toe clearance must be ample as the prosthesis progresses from initial swing into midswing and is finally positioned for the next cycle of gait as terminal swing concludes.

Gait Deviations in Swing Phase

Gait deviations during swing phase are evaluated from the lateral and the posterior perspectives. Prosthetists and therapists watch for abnormal medial or lateral "whips" and inadequate or excessive toe clearance.

Medial or Lateral Whips

A whip occurs when the prosthetic foot rotates in the transverse plane after toe-off. It may move in a medial arc (toward the stance limb) or a lateral arc (away from the stance limb) during swing. The patient's knee, however, moves forward within the line of progression. The differentiation of whips from abducted or adducted gait, in which the entire limb moves in an arc (usually a compensatory deviation when inadequate knee flexion adds relative length to the limb, challenging swing phase clearance), is important. If the patient is using a cuff suspension system, inappropriately placed tabs may lead to a whip during stance phase. If the prosthetic foot is aligned (rotated) with slightly too much toe-out or toe-in, it can change the path of forward progression from a straight line into a whip. Adjustment of foot position or suspension usually solves the problem.

"Catching" the Toes during Midswing

Problems with toe clearance during midswing can compromise safe ambulation and challenge the patient's sense of mastery and safety while walking. "Catching" the toes of the prosthetic foot as the shank of the prosthesis advances forward in midswing is the result of a prosthesis that is either actually or (most commonly) functionally too long. Patients, and sometimes therapists, are quick to assume that the prosthesis is actually too long. No change in length of the prosthesis should be made unless all other potential causes of swing clearance problems have been ruled out and careful reassessment of prosthetic limb length clearly indicates the need to trim length. Prosthetically, the three factors most likely to mimic excessive prosthetic leg length include inadequacy of the suspension mechanism and sock ply, prosthetic foot position (a foot set in excessive plantar flexion also adds relative length to the prosthesis), and limitation in the ability to flex the knee in initial swing and midswing. Only after these factors have been found to be appropriate or normal should the prosthetist consider shortening the pylon of the prosthesis.

CASE EXAMPLE 1C

A Patient with Recent Dysvascular-Neuropathic Right Transtibial Amputation

N. M. is now at clinic for a follow-up appointment with the team. During the last 3 weeks, N. M. has had four outpatient visits for gait training and two follow-up visits to the prosthetist. He wears one five-ply and two single-ply socks to maintain the appropriate fit of his prosthesis. He wears the prosthesis full time, without difficulty, and is able to self-monitor the fit of his prosthesis. He is ambulating independently with a straight cane (on the left) on level indoor surfaces but uses his walker outside or in crowded environments. His stride length and cadence have improved, and he is much less hesitant with this prosthesis than at the initial fitting. He does report that he's come to "trust" his prosthesis more as time goes on. He finds he has a few areas of consistent "discomfort." He notes some increased pressure at the medial tibial condyle and distal lateral residual limb and he feels as if he is walking up a ramp. There seems to be excessive knee extension at terminal stance. He wears a new pair of athletic shoes.

Observational gait analysis during today's session reveals an appropriate initial contact of the prosthetic heel, with smooth transition to foot flat during loading response and midstance. A strong varus moment is apparent at the knee during midstance and a delayed heel rise in the transition from midstance to terminal stance. Terminal swing is effective in preparing for the next phase of the gait cycle.

On evaluation of his limb, the team notes well-circumscribed areas of prolonged reactive hyperemia at the medial tibial condyle and along the shaft of the fibula (without impingement on the fibular head) as well as the patellar tendon. All other skin markings are within normal limits.

Questions to Consider

- What is the procedure for static alignment of the patient in the prosthesis before ambulation?
- What potential patient-related and prosthetic alignment problems do patient self-report and observational gait analysis suggest may be occurring? Why has it taken several sessions of gait training for these problems to emerge? How will the team discern the contributing factors to the observed gait deviations?
- What recommendations might the team make to improve the quality, comfort, and energy efficiency of his walking?

Recommendations and Interventions

The team concludes that two different gait problems are occurring. Excessive point pressure at the medial tibial condyle and excessive varus moment at midstance suggest that the prosthetic foot may be slightly too inset (medial) with respect to the prosthetic socket. This deviation has become more apparent as N. M. has become more confident and aggressive in his use of the prosthesis. The prosthetist makes a slight adjustment in alignment to solve the problem. N. M. reports that socket pressure is more tolerable, and the team notes a reduction in the varus moment at midstance.

The sensation of walking uphill, difficulty moving forward over the prosthetic toes in late stance, and extension moment at terminal stance lead the team to investigate the causes of a long toe lever. Before altering alignment or reducing the length of the pylon, the team looks for patient-related factors to explain the observed changes in gait pattern, especially noting the recent change in footwear. On inspection, heel height of the new shoes is inadequate for the prosthetic foot. A lift is added inside the heel of the shoes, adjusting the shoe to the foot. This allows use of the new athletic shoes and decreases the functional toe lever to a natural level. The team concludes that N. M. should return to the clinic in 6 months for follow-up with his first prosthesis and determination of readiness for his definitive prosthesis. The team also believes he should continue therapy and visits with the prosthetist on a regular basis for adjustment. He was encouraged to take extra socks and his walker on the cruise, as well as his wheelchair just in case.

CASE EXAMPLE 2C

A Patient with Traumatic Left Transtibial Amputation and Concurrent Compound Fracture of the Intact Limb

S. P. has progressed quickly with his prosthesis in the last 2 weeks, and the addition of the silicone sleeve suspension has improved comfort and protected the skin as intended. He walks with a straight cane on the left (as his activity level has increased, he has more discomfort in stance on the fractured right lower extremity than he does on his left prosthetic extremity). He has returned to school and wears his prosthesis during the school day, removing it to rest his residual limb when he gets home in the afternoon. He typically has to apply one or two one-ply socks as the day progresses to maintain appropriate fit. He is ambulating independently on all surfaces and is impatient to use a step-over-step strategy on stairs. His stride length is now within normal limits for his height, and his gait speed is approaching that of his peers. He reports that, as his speed and stride length have increased, his knee "buckles," and he is concerned that he will not be able to resume running.

Observational gait analysis reveals appropriate foot positioning at initial contact; however, a somewhat rapid and uncontrolled foot descent to foot flat occurs at loading response. Although appropriate varus moment is apparent as he enters midstance, premature heel rise and knee instability in the transition to terminal stance occurs, necessitating shortening of swing time (and therefore stride length) of his right limb. During prosthetic swing, the prosthetic foot moves forward in a straight line. Reactive hyperemia is within expected parameters after walking more than 200 feet. The suture line and graft site appears to tolerate pressure and the liner well.

Questions to Consider

- What is the procedure for static alignment of the patient in the prosthesis before ambulation?
- What potential patient-related and prosthetic alignment problems do patient self-report and observational gait analysis suggests may be occurring? Why has it taken several sessions of gait training for these problems to emerge? How will the team discern the contributing factors to the observed gait deviations?
- What recommendations might the team make to improve the quality, comfort, and energy efficiency of his walking?

Recommendations and Interventions

On the basis of the observed gait deviations in stance phase that have occurred as S. P. has gained skill and confidence with his prosthesis, the team concludes that the toe lever length is now functionally less than optimal for this active young man. Because footwear has not changed and S. P. has been managing sock ply appropriately, the combination of rapid foot-flat and a sense of drop-off at late stance lead the team to reevaluate the degree of dorsiflexion and the anteroposterior alignment of the foot with respect to the socket. The straight forward progression of the foot in swing suggests alignment in supination and pronation (rotation) is appropriate.

The prosthetist adjusts alignment by plantar flexing the foot to increase toe lever length as well as a slight socket flexion, retuning the socket to the appropriate flexed position and still increasing the toe lever. S. P. re-dons his prosthesis and then walks down and back in the corridor, varying his gait speed to get a feel for new alignment. After several minor adjustments, his stride lengths are once again symmetrical, and he and the team are satisfied that optimal alignment is achieved. He will see his orthopedic surgeon in 2 weeks for preoperative evaluation of his right leg and makes an appointment to return for reassessment after that appointment. He is anxious to try to walk without assistive devices and to learn to run once again.

SUMMARY

Most patients with transtibial amputation are candidates for prostheses if their functional status and quality of life will be enhanced, whether or not functional community ambulation will be possible. Guidelines have been established to help the prosthetist and therapist determine the appropriate prosthetic components for the patient's anticipated level of function. The PTB/total surface bearing socket design is effective for most transtibial prostheses. The decision regarding whether to fabricate a hard socket worn with socks or some type of liner as an interface or a flexible socket in a rigid frame is made on the basis of the patient's weight, skin condition, bony topography, and anticipated level of activity. The pros and cons of each type of interface must be carefully considered in the prescription process. The ideal suspension system holds the prosthesis securely on the residual limb, minimizing movement of the prosthesis on the residual limb in the transitions between the stance and swing phase and also allows the patient to sit comfortably. Effective upper extremity use in donning the prosthesis and securing suspension is an important determinant in choosing among the various suspension systems currently available. Although the ability to adjust alignment of an endoskeletal temporary prosthesis is advantageous early in rehabilitation when frequent alignment adjustments are anticipated, patients who are very active may benefit from a more durable exoskeletal definitive prosthesis.

In the process of alignment, the prosthetist establishes an initial spatial relation between the socket and prosthetic foot based on biomechanical principles that direct forces toward pressure-tolerant areas and enhance a smooth forward progression during gait. Alignment is first refined statically while the patient is standing. If no problems have been identified, dynamic observational gait analysis is used to fine tune alignment until the most energy-efficient and natural-appearing gait pattern is accomplished. Although some problems identified during this dynamic alignment process require adjustment of socket or prosthetic foot position, many can be traced to inadequate suspension, inappropriate sock ply, shoe condition and heel height, or patient-related factors (such as apprehension about shifting weight fully onto the prosthesis). When assessing the effectiveness of a transtibial prosthesis, therapists who are skilled in prosthetic rehabilitation recognize the interplay of many factors: the characteristics of prosthetic components, adequacy of suspension, fit of the socket, alignment of prosthetic components, importance of footwear, and the patient's musculoskeletal and neuromuscular characteristics. Close collaboration among the prosthetist, therapist, and patient ensures optimal prosthetic outcome.

REFERENCES

1. Bowker JH, Goldberg B, Poonekar PD. Transtibial amputation. In Bowker JH, Michael JW (eds), *Atlas of Limb Prosthetics: Surgical, Prosthetic, and Rehabilitation Principles.* St. Louis: Mosby, 1992. pp. 429-452.
2. Carroll K. Adaptive prosthetics for the lower extremity. *Foot Ankle Clin* 2001;6(2):371-386.
3. Sadeghi H, Alllard P, Duhaime M. Muscle power compensatory mechanisms in below knee amputee gait. *Am J Phys Med Rehabil* 2001;80(1):25-32.
4. Gutfleisch O. Peg leg and bionic limbs: the development of lower extremity prosthetics. *Interdiscip Sci Rev* 2003;28(2):139-148.
5. Pinzur MS, Reddy N, Charuk G, et al. Control of the residual limb in transtibial amputation. *Foot Ankle Int* 1996;17(6): 538-540.
6. Brodsky JW. Amputations of the foot and ankle. In Mann RA, Coughlin MJ (eds), *Surgery of the Foot and Ankle,* 6th ed, vol 2. St. Louis: Mosby, 1993. pp. 959-990.
7. Gailey R. Energy expenditure of trans-tibial amputees during ambulation at self-selected pace. *Prosthet Orthot Int* 1994;18(2):84-91.
8. Penington G, Warmington S, Hull S, et al. Rehabilitation of lower limb amputations and some implications for surgical management. *Aust NZ J Surg* 1992;62(10):774-779.
9. *DMERC Medicare Advisory Bulletin.* Columbia, SC: DMERC, 1994. pp. 95-145.
10. Kapp S. *Below Knee Prosthetics Course Manual.* Dallas: University of Texas Southwestern Medical Center, 1988.
11. Fergusen J, Smith DG. Socket considerations for the patient with transtibial amputation. *Clin Orthop Rel Res* 1999;1(641):76-84.
12. Staats TB, Lundt J. The UCLA total surface bearing suction below knee prosthesis. *Clin Prosthet Orthot* 1987;11:118-130.
13. Engsberg JR, Sprouse SW, Uhrich LM, et al. Preliminary investigation comparing rectified and unrectified sockets for transtibial amputees. *J Prosthet Orthot* 2003;15(4): 119-124.
14. Kapp SL, Fergason JR. Transtibial amputation: Prosthetic management. In Smith DG, Michael JW, Bowker JH (eds). *Atlas of Amputation and Limb Deficiencies; Surgical, Prosthetic, and Rehabilitation Principles*, 3rd ed. Rosemont, IL: American Academy of Orthopaedic Surgeons, 2004. pp. 503-515.
15. Sanders JE, Lam D, Bralle A, et al. Interface presses and sheer stresses at thirteen socket sites on two persons with transtibial amputation. *J Rehab Res Dev* 1997;67:196-199.
16. Thompson D. *Therapeutic Exercise Course Manual.* Oklahoma City: University of Oklahoma Health Sciences Center, 1995.
17. Saunders JE, Greve JM, Mitchell SB, et al. Material properties of commonly used interface materials and their static coefficients of friction with skin and socks. *J Rehabil Res Dev* 1998;35:161-163.
18. Kapp S. Suspension systems for prostheses. *Clin Orthop Rel Res* 1999;1(361):55-63.
19. Chino N, Pearson JR, Cockrell JL, et al. Negative pressure during swing phase in below-knee prostheses with rubber sleeve suspension. *Arch Phys Med Rehabil* 1975;56(1):22-26.
20. Berger N, Fishman S. Lower-limb prosthetics. In Berger N, Fishman S (eds), *Transtibial Prostheses and Components.* New York: New York University, 1998. pp. 47-67.
21. Fillauer CE, Pritham CH, Fillauer KD. Evolution and development of the silicone suction socket. *JPO J Pract Orthod* 1989;1(2):61-72.
22. McCurdie I, Hanspal R, Nieveen R. Iceross—a consensus review: a questionnaire survey of the use of Iceross in the United Kingdom. *Prosthet Orthot Int* 1997;21:124-128.
23. Lake C, Supan TJ. The incidence of dermatological problems in the silicone suspension sleeve user. *J Prosthet Orthot* 1997;9(3):97-104.
24. Kapp SK, Cummings D. Transtibial amputation: prosthetic management. In Bowker JH, Michael JW (eds), *Atlas of Limb Prosthetics: Surgical, Prosthetic and Rehabilitation Principles,* 2nd ed. St. Louis: Mosby–Year Book, 1992. pp. 453-478.
25. Official findings of the Consensus Conference on Post-Operative Management of the Lower Extremity Amputee. *J Prosthet Orthot Suppl 2005;*16(3);S1-S27.

26. Gard SA, Konz RJ. The effect of a shock-absorbing pylon on the gait of persons with unilateral transtibial amputation. *J Rehabil Res Dev* 2003;40(2):109-124.
27. Hsu MJ, Neilsen DH, Yack HJ, et al. Physiological measurements of walking and running in people with transtibial amputations with 3 different prostheses. *J Orthop Sports Phys Ther* 1999;29(9):526-533.
28. Winter DA, Sienko SE. Biomechanics of below-knee amputee gait. *J Biomech* 1988;21(5):361-367.
29. 1996 study guide. *Arch Phys Med Rehabil* 1996;77(suppl):3-5.
30. Waters RL. Energy expenditure of amputee gait. In Bowker JH, Michael JW (eds), *Atlas of Limb Prosthetics: Surgical, Prosthetic, and Rehabilitation Principles.* St. Louis: Mosby–Year Book, 1992. pp. 381-387.
31. Bateni H, Olney SJ. Kinematic and kinetic variations of below knee amputee gait. *J Prosthet Orthot* 2002;14(1):2-10.
32. Berger N. Analysis of amputee gait. In Bowker JH, Michael JW (eds), *Atlas of Limb Prosthetics: Surgical, Prosthetic, and Rehabilitation Principles.* St. Louis: Mosby–Year Book, 1992. pp. 371-379.
33. Tibarewalla DN, Ganguli S. Pattern recognition in tachographic gait records of normal and lower extremity handicapped human subjects. *J Biomed Eng* 1982;4:233-240.
34. Saunders GT. Static and dynamic analysis. In *Lower Limb Amputations: A Guide to Rehabilitation.* Philadelphia: F.A. Davis, 1986. pp. 415-475.
35. Trantowski-Farrell R, Pinzur MS. A preliminary comparison of function and outcome in patients with diabetic dysvascular disease. *J Prosthet Orthot* 2003;15(4):127-132.
36. Perry, J, Boyd LA, Rao SS. Prosthetic weight acceptance mechanics in transtibial amputees wearing the Single Axis, Seattle Lite, and Flex Foot. *IEEE Trans Rehabil Eng* 1997;5(4):283-289.

27

Rehabilitation of Persons with Recent Transtibial Amputation

JULIE D. RIES AND VICTOR G. VAUGHAN

LEARNING OBJECTIVES

Upon completion of this chapter, the reader will be able to do the following:

1. Organize and justify each component of a comprehensive physical therapy examination for the individual with transtibial amputation.
2. Use and synthesize data collected during the examination to establish diagnosis and prognosis for rehabilitation.
3. Create a well-defined and focused treatment plan that addresses the needs of the individual with transtibial amputation.
4. Identify, justify, and prioritize rehabilitation issues about which individuals with transtibial amputation must be educated.
5. Anticipate functional outcomes of an individual with transtibial amputation, on the basis of data collected and available evidence.

Persons who have undergone transtibial amputation may approach rehabilitation with a sense of expectancy, excitement, and apprehension. They may be relieved that they have healed and curious about the prosthesis they are about to receive. They may be anxious to commence their prosthetic rehabilitation and may have realistic or unrealistic expectations. To facilitate optimal rehabilitation outcome, the physical therapist must consider the patient's goals, physical abilities, and mobility needs. As prosthetic skills are mastered, interventions progress from basic gait and mobility skills to more complex, higher-level bipedal activities. With many individuals, vocational, leisure, and sporting activities can be addressed to facilitate the return to a productive and enjoyable lifestyle.

This chapter focuses primarily on strategies for initial and intermediate-level rehabilitation, with a short discussion on more advanced prosthetic training. Anticipated functional outcomes for the transtibial prosthetic user are also addressed. Evidence-based practice requires the integration of best research evidence, clinical expertise, and patient values.[2] The goal of this chapter is to provide a foundation for using evidence-based practice in the management of the individual with transtibial amputation.

COMPONENTS OF THE PHYSICAL THERAPY EXAMINATION

Effective physical therapy management for individuals with amputation begins with a thorough and comprehensive initial examination. In the examination, the physical therapist must obtain a patient history, conduct a systems review, and administer tests and measures to obtain baseline data. This information allows the therapist to establish a diagnostic classification that provides the basis for accurately identifying the appropriate treatment interventions that will lead to optimum outcomes. The examination may occur immediately following amputation, at the time of the prosthetic fitting, or after the individual has already obtained a prosthesis, depending upon the practice setting.

Patient History

The patient history is the collection of health-related data from the past and present. It helps to establish what brought the person to seek physical therapy services and to highlight the individual's desires and expectations. The person's perspective on the illness or injury that caused the amputation and on the resulting functional limitations and possible disability has a powerful influence on the rehabilitation process.[3,4]

A number of important areas must be explored while taking the patient history (Table 27-1). Although all areas provide important information, several are integral to

Table 27-1
*Important Patient History Component of Physical Therapy Examination**

Component	*Issues to Consider*
Social history	Cultural beliefs and behaviors Family and caregiver resources Social interactions, activities, and support systems
Employment/work/leisure	Current and prior work Community and leisure activities
Living environment	Assistive devices and adaptive equipment Living environment Projected discharge destination
General health status	General health perception Physical and psychological functions Role and social functions
Social health habits	Health risks (e.g., smoking, alcohol or drug abuse) Level of physical fitness
Family history	Family health risks
Medical/surgical history	Prior hospitalizations, surgeries, and preexisting medical and other health-related conditions
Chief complaint/current condition	Concerns that led patient or caregiver to seek physical therapy services Current therapeutic interventions Mechanism of injury/disease including date of onset and course of events Patient/caregiver/family expectations and goals Patient/family/caregiver's perceptions of the person's emotional response to the current situation Any previous occurrences of this problem and therapeutic interventions
Functional status and activity level	Current and prior functional status in self-care, home management activities, and ADLs Current and previous functional status in work and community/leisure activities
Medications	Medications for current conditions or other conditions
Other clinical tests	Laboratory and diagnostic tests Review of available records Review of other clinical findings

ADLs, Activities of daily living.
*Format and terminology consistent with *Guide to Physical Therapist Practice.*[1]

establishing the diagnosis and the treatment plan. The person's general health status is critical to understanding overall health perception, physical functions, psychological functions, and role and social functions. Discussion of the current condition or chief complaint gives the therapist a sense of the individual's concerns, previous interventions, mechanism of injury or disease, and course of events. The therapist should also attempt to understand the goals and aspirations of a person with a transtibial amputation. If the individual's initial goals appear to be too ambitious or not ambitious enough, the therapist can address these issues with education and interaction with peers as possible interventions.

The interview process provides valuable insights about the person's communication ability, emotional status, cognitive abilities, preferred coping strategies, insight into the rehabilitation process, and usual learning style, as well as the availability of emotional and instrumental support systems (assistance with activities of daily living [ADLs]). Information about the person's preamputation level of activity and mobility is helpful in establishing a realistic prognosis. Specific and probing interview questions are often helpful in obtaining clear and accurate information. Although many individuals are accurate historians, others may have an incomplete understanding or imprecise memory of what has happened. Information should be confirmed by interviewing family members and reviewing the medical record. The physician should be contacted with any outstanding questions.

The interview also yields important information that can be used to guide treatment interventions and begin the process of education about amputation, treatment, and prosthetic training. Many individuals with transtibial amputation do not understand clearly what to expect during rehabilitation or how their disease processes might progress. Amputation is not selective to patients of a specific age group, cultural background, educational experience, or socioeconomic level. Each individual benefits by being well educated about his or her condition and treatment. For many people, the events that brought them to rehabilitation may be a blur of disjointed experiences and medical jargon or a laundry list of conditions that seem unrelated or independent. The physical therapist can help individuals to place their history and experience in a meaningful context, which, in turn, assists them in forming realistic expectations and may decrease the likelihood of second amputations.

Systems Review

The systems review provides a gross and limited review of the anatomical and physiological status of the person's cardiopulmonary system, musculoskeletal system, integumentary system, and neuromuscular system. Cognitive screening is also an important part of the systems review. This gross screening process aids in focusing and prioritizing the tests and measures portion of the examination. For instance, a gross screen of range of motion (ROM) and strength of all uninvolved extremities may reveal findings to be within normal limits, eliminating the need for further assessment.

Tests and Measures

The third component of the examination is the use of appropriate tests and measures to gather objective data about the individual's various impairments and functional limitations. Combining this data with the history and systems review, the physical therapist can establish a working diagnostic hypothesis. The physical therapist chooses from among an array of possible tests and measures those that will best confirm or deny the developing diagnostic hypothesis. The information gathered in the interview, systems review, and examination allows the therapist to establish a suitable plan of care and develop the most appropriate interventions.[1] Some assessments, such as strength testing or joint play motions, might require modification of technique because loss of limb length necessarily changes where the therapist can hold or resist the limb. Table 27-2 provides categories of tests and measures that might be appropriate for the patient with transtibial amputation and some detail of how the therapist might assess each area.

Table 27-2
*Tests and Measures Used in the Physical Therapy Examination**

Component	*Issues to Examine*
Aerobic capacity	During functional activities During standardized exercise testing Signs and symptoms of cardiovascular system in response to increased oxygen demand during increased activity Signs and symptoms of pulmonary system in response to increased oxygen demand during increased activity
Anthropometric characteristics	Body composition Body dimensions Edema
Arousal, attention, cognition	Motivation
Assistive/adaptive devices	Equipment or devices used during functional activities Components, alignment, fit, and ability to care for devices or equipment Effectiveness of devices or equipment in correcting impairments, limitations, or disabilities Safety during use of equipment or devices
Circulation	Cardiovascular signs Physiological responses to position changes
Cranial/peripheral nerve integrity	Motor distribution and integrity Sensory distribution and integrity

Continued

Table 27-2

Tests and Measures Used in the Physical Therapy Examination—Cont'd*

Component	*Issues to Examine*
Environmental barriers	Physical space and environment
Ergonomics/body mechanics	Coordination and dexterity during functional activities Functional and physical performance during work tasks Safety in work environment Specific work conditions/activities Tools, equipment, and workstation design used during job activities Body mechanics during home and work activities
Gait and balance	Static and dynamic balance with or without the use of assistive devices or prosthetics Balance during functional activities with or without the use of assistive devices or prosthetics Gait during functional activities with or without the use of assistive devices or prosthetics Safety during gait and balance activities
Integumentary integrity	Activities and positioning that produce or relieve trauma to the skin Equipment, devices, or prosthesis that may produce trauma to the skin Current skin characteristics and conditions Activities or positioning that may aggravate the wound or scar Presence of signs of infection Wound/scar characteristics
Joint integrity and mobility	Joint play including accessory movements
Motor function	Dexterity, coordination, and agility Hand function
Muscle performance	Strength, power, and endurance Strength, power, and endurance during functional activities Muscle tension
Orthotic, protective, and supportive devices	Components, alignment and fit of devices Use during functional activities Effectiveness of devices in correcting limitations and disabilities Safety during use of devices
Pain	Location and description of pain Intensity ratings of pain
Posture	Postural alignment and positioning, static and dynamic Alignment of specific body parts
Prosthetic requirements	Components, alignment, fit, and ability to care for prosthesis Use of prosthesis during functional activities Effectiveness of prosthesis at correcting limitations, impairments, and disabilities Residual limb edema, strength, ROM, and skin integrity Safety during use of prosthesis
ROM	Functional ROM Active and passive joint movement Muscle length and flexibility, soft tissue extensibility

Table 27-2

*Tests and Measures Used in the Physical Therapy Examination**—*Cont'd*

Component	*Issues to Examine*
Self-care and home management	Ability to access home Ability to perform self-care and home management activities Safety in home and self-care management
Sensory integrity	Superficial sensation Deep sensation Combined/cortical sensation
Work/community/leisure integration	Ability to return to work, community, and leisure activities Ability to access work site, community, and leisure activities Safety in work, community, and leisure activities

ROM, Range of motion.
*Format and terminology consistent with *Guide to Physical Therapist Practice.*[1]

EVALUATION PROCESS

The evaluation process requires the physical therapist to interpret and integrate the information obtained from the history, systems review, and the tests and measures to identify the primary areas of limitations or impairments. The physical therapist uses professional judgment to predict or make a prognosis as to the likely functional outcome and time required for effective prosthetic rehabilitation. The evaluation must include a summary of the individual's major problems and the presumed underlying cause or causes. Problems are prioritized, with those having the most significant functional implications receiving top priority. This is done on an individualized basis, as the same problem may affect different patients in different ways. An individual with poor sensation of the residual limb who is cognitively intact may be easily educated about compensating for the sensory deficit with visual inspection of the residual limb, effectively reducing the risk of compromise of skin integrity. Another individual with the same sensory deficit who also has cognitive impairment may require a more extensive educational intervention focused on residual limb care. This individual has a much higher risk of skin problems and is likely to require a caregiver's assistance to monitor skin integrity.

Therapists must also be skilled in determining the functional implications of specific problems. For instance, a slight knee flexion contracture can be accommodated for in transtibial socket alignment, whereas a significant knee flexion contracture prohibits prosthetic fitting with a conventional prosthesis. Prosthetic prescription and physical therapy intervention may be quite different for two individuals who both present with knee flexion contractures.

CASE EXAMPLE 1A

Examination and Evaluation of a Patient with Traumatic Transtibial Amputation

P. L., 24, suffered a severe mangle and crush injury to his left foot in a motorcycle accident 4 weeks ago. The foot was determined to be unsalvageable, and P. L. underwent a left transtibial amputation. P. L. is a college graduate with a job in informational technology. He lives with his girlfriend in a two-bedroom, one-story, walk-up apartment. His past medical and surgical history is unremarkable, and his level of physical fitness is excellent. Before the injury, he enjoyed softball, bicycling, and riding his motorcycle. His girlfriend is supportive and involved.

P. L. was hospitalized for 6 days and then discharged with outpatient follow-up by his surgeon's office. He ambulates independently and safely in his home environment and in the community, using a two-point, swing-through, single-limb gait pattern with axillary crutches. P. L. is independent in all single-limb functional mobility activities and ADLs. He is eager to receive a prosthesis and states that his goal is to return to two-legged activities. P. L.'s preprosthetic physical therapy home exercise program includes stretching and strengthening activities for the hip and knee of the residual limb, desensitization techniques, gentle scar management, and balance activities. Currently he presents with good strength and range of motion of the residual limb and excellent soft tissue mobility around the incision site. P. L. has a well-healed and cylindrically shaped residual limb with intact sensory status with the exception of decreased sensitivity to light touch around the fish-mouth incision scar.

Questions to Consider

Given the information collected in the patient history and systems review, as well as examination findings, consider the following:

- Is there any additional information (other tests and measures) that should be gathered for an evaluation of this patient?
- What is the most likely prognosis for this patient? What expectations might there be for the rehabilitation process? What are the immediate short-term goals? Long-term goals?
- How long might rehabilitation intervention take to achieve these goals? In what setting will rehabilitation take place? What are some suggestions in terms of frequency of care? Intensity of care?
- What factors (intraindividual and environmental) might influence P. L.'s progression and the ultimate outcome of his rehabilitation? How should these factors be monitored over time?

ESTABLISHING A PHYSICAL THERAPY DIAGNOSIS

Establishment of the diagnosis for a person with transtibial amputation is relatively straightforward. The diagnosis is determined by a collection of signs and symptoms that delineate the primary dysfunction of the individual. The physical therapist then directs interventions toward resolving that dysfunction. According to the *Guide to Physical Therapist Practice, Part 2,* the preferred practice pattern for a person with an amputation is impaired motor function, muscle performance, ROM, gait, locomotion, and balance associated with amputation.[1] For the majority of people with transtibial amputations, this will be the pattern of choice.

FORMULATING A PROGNOSIS

The physical therapist uses patient history information and specific test findings, as well as a knowledge base of outcome measures for individuals with transtibial amputation, to predict each person's rehabilitation potential and probable functional outcome. On the basis of the individual's prognosis, measurable short- and long-term goals are defined to guide planning for intervention. These goals are also used to inform assessment of outcomes as rehabilitation progresses. An important component of the prognosis is delineation of the likely time frame for achievement of the optimal final outcome. A young, active, healthy person with traumatic transtibial amputation who has few postoperative complications is likely to progress through rehabilitation more quickly, achieving a relatively high level of function in a short time. In contrast, a medically frail and deconditioned patient who has had an amputation as a result of vascular compromise or nonhealing neuropathic ulcer will likely have a longer rehabilitation time, with a less satisfactory final functional outcome. Advanced age and multiple comorbidities can add significantly to the rehabilitation time and negatively affect the ultimate functional outcome.[5, 6] These differences will be reflected in the plan of care, as well as the specific goals set and the anticipated rate at which goals will be met.

The physical therapy plan of care includes information about the frequency, duration, location, and specific physical therapy interventions to be used. The plan of care is directly related to the goals delineated by the evaluation and prognostic process. The prioritized problem list provides a foundation for determination of functional short- and long-term goals that, in turn, direct rehabilitation activities. If independent donning and doffing of a prosthesis are primary short-term goals, the associated treatment plan must include education strategies, opportunities to practice this skill, and remediation or adaptation of any movement components that, if missing, would compromise the individual's ability to perform this necessary task (e.g., the person may need to improve grip strength or intrinsic hand strength to manipulate prosthetic suspension). The plan includes information about equipment to be ordered, referrals to be made, and the ultimate physical therapy discharge plan.

CASE EXAMPLE 2A

Examination and Evaluation of a Patient with Neuropathic/Dysvascular Bilateral Transtibial Amputation

V. R. is an 80-year-old man with a 4-year history of type 2 diabetes. He had coronary artery bypass graft surgery for three blocked vessels 10 years ago. His medical history also includes a transient ischemic attack and hypertension, which is controlled with medication (beta-blocker). He reports that, over the past 3 years, he had a series of slowly healing "sores" on the bottom of his right foot. Despite 2 months of conservative management with felted foam, a Darco shoe, and limited weight bearing, the most recent sore under the first metatarsal head would not heal. Upon probing the neuropathic wound to bone and finding evidence of osteomyelitis, the vascular surgeon recommended right standard-length transtibial amputation.

V. R. was discharged 1 week following surgery to a subacute rehabilitation center. He participated in preprosthetic training for 4 weeks, and was discharged to home with home health physical therapy (PT) and nursing. Two weeks of home care PT focused on single-limb mobility and therapeutic exercises that did not include his involved limb. V. R. had a delayed fitting of his prosthesis because of slow healing of his surgical wound. Now, 5 months after his amputation, he has been referred for outpatient rehabilitation and prosthetic training.

On examination, V. R. presents as a relatively healthy man with a well-healed surgical amputation site. He is alert and attentive but is a poor historian with notable memory recall difficulties. Therefore his daughter provides medical history. She reports that V. R. spends most of his time sitting in his chair or in a wheelchair. He received his initial prosthesis 2 weeks ago but has been reluctant to use it.

On examination, range of motion (ROM) of the involved knee is found to be 5 to 125 degrees, whereas the ROM of his intact limb is within normal limits. V. R. demonstrates 5/5 strength in his right hip, 4/5 strength in his knee extensors and flexors, and 3+/5 in his abdominals. In standing, wearing the prosthesis, he leans forward slightly with flexed hips and a slightly flexed right knee. His pelvis is level and leg length appears equal. V. R. can transfer his wheelchair to a plinth low mat table independently. He ambulates independently with partial weight bearing on his prosthesis using a walker with a step to gait. His sitting balance is within normal limits. His ability to maintain single limb stance on the left limb is fair and on the right limb, poor.

On examination the skin of V. R.'s residual limb is intact, with a mobile surgical scar and no edema. He has two small, dried blood blisters on his anterior distal residual limb. He currently has an open neuropathic ulcer under his left first metatarsal head. On examination of sensation, he has intact sensibility to light touch in his entire left lower extremity, right residual limb, and both hands. He reports no problems with his vision and no pain of any kind. His residual limb is warm to touch with normal color, whereas his left foot and ankle are slightly cold to touch and dusky in appearance.

His initial prosthesis was a rigid patellar tendon-bearing socket, with a roll-on silicone sleeve and a pin locking mechanism for suspension, and a solid-ankle cushioned-heel foot. He currently wears three-ply wool and one-ply cotton socks over his suspension sleeve for a comfortable fit.

V. R. lives with his wife (who has rheumatoid arthritis) and a developmentally disabled daughter, both of whom have limited mobility and other functional limitations. Another daughter and son live nearby; these adult children act as caregivers and are responsible for housework, maintenance, shopping, and transport to medical appointments.

Questions to Consider

Given the information collected in the patient history and systems review, as well as examination findings, consider the following:

- Is any additional information (other tests and measures) necessary to complete the evaluation of this patient?
- What is the most likely prognosis for this patient? What are the expectations for the rehabilitation process? What are the immediate short-term goals? Long-term goals?
- How long will rehabilitation intervention take to achieve these goals? In what setting will rehabilitation take place? What are some suggestions in terms of frequency of care? Intensity of care?
- What factors (intraindividual and environmental) might influence V. R.'s progression and the ultimate outcome of his rehabilitation? How will these factors be monitored over time?

INTERVENTIONS FOR PERSONS WITH TRANSTIBIAL AMPUTATION

Various skills and physical and functional characteristics create the foundation for successful prosthetic use. These key areas include functional ROM of the hip and knee, functional strength of muscles at the hip and knee, adequacy of motor control and balance, aerobic capacity and endurance, effective edema control and maturation of the residual limb, integrity of the skin and soft tissue, and sensory integrity of the residual limb. These areas must be addressed early in the rehabilitation process. Inability to achieve a certain status or level of performance in one area does not prohibit a good prosthetic outcome; however, difficulties in multiple areas affect prosthetic candidacy and use. Each area should be evaluated carefully, and appropriate interventions should be undertaken to achieve at least minimal requirements for functional prosthetic use, if not optimal level of performance.

Ensuring Necessary Range of Motion

Early and aggressive achievement of functional ROM of the lower extremity, especially of the knee and hip, is of paramount importance.[7] The development of contractures or tightness of hip flexors, abductors, and external rotators and knee flexors of the residual limb can significantly affect functional ambulation and mobility. This flexed posture of the residual limb is consistent with the flexor withdrawal pattern associated with lower extremity pain. The flexion withdrawal posture is reinforced if the residual limb is elevated on pillows when the person is in bed. These factors place individuals with recent amputation at significant risk of contracture formation.

Maintaining or increasing available ROM at the hip and knee of the residual limb continues to be a primary treatment goal as the patient moves from preprosthetic into prosthetic rehabilitation. The prevention of loss of ROM is much easier than efforts to regain lost motion.[8] Prone positioning is an excellent strategy to combat contracture formation of the hip flexors and should be prescribed (60 minutes daily) for all patients who can tolerate prone lying. Low-load stretching of long duration is safe and can yield significant elastic and plastic changes in soft tissues.[8] Active and passive stretching in the side-lying position may be used for those

Table 27-3
Prosthetic Consequences of Limitations in ROM

ROM Limitation	*Potential Functional Limitation*	*Implication*
↓'d hip extension	Inability to achieve upright posture in stance Compensatory knee flexion causes instability in gait	Chronic low back pain due to compensatory anterior pelvic tilt Decreased stride length of contralateral limb in gait
↓'d hip adduction	Abducted stance in gait	Abductor lurch on ipsilateral side in gait
↓'d internal rotation	Toe-out stance and gait	Knee joint pain or pathology due to lack of anterior/posterior orientation of knee joint
↓'d knee extension	Limb functionally shorter, with associated gait deviations	Decreased midstance stability in gait Requires prosthetic alignment adjustments to compensate
↓'d knee flexion	Inability to place foot flat on the floor when sitting	Inability to bear weight through prosthesis during sit-to-stand transfers Difficulty managing steps and curbs

ROM, Range of motion.

unable to lie prone. A knee extension splint or board (extending from between wheelchair seat cushion and wheelchair seat) can be an effective technique early in the process to prevent knee flexion contractures from developing. An individual with a recent amputation should be encouraged to use the knee extension splint as long as tolerable throughout the day, supplemented with frequent active "quad set" exercises. The person must also be taught to regularly check the integrity of skin of the residual limb while using the splint or board, to minimize the risk of pressure-related skin damage that would delay use of a prosthesis.

Although achieving knee flexion ROM is sometimes overlooked in early rehabilitation, full knee flexion ROM is required for efficient step-over-step stair ambulation and for rising from a seated position. Assessment of ROM of the intact limb is also important, as loss of ROM of either limb affects the quality and energy efficiency of gait.[9] The importance of functional ROM is also emphasized in patient education and home exercise routines. Potential prosthetic problems associated with loss of functional ROM are summarized in Table 27-3. Use of a wide variety of active and passive ROM therapeutic exercise techniques is appropriate as early as possible. All exercises that were started during the preprosthetic phase are generally appropriate to continue as prescribed or to be intensified as tolerated during the prosthetic training phase. Once full-functional ROM is achieved, the person must be educated to maintain this level.

Strength and Motor Control

Early in the prosthetic training process, baseline strength must be evaluated in several ways. Standard manual muscle test (MMT) protocols provide a starting point against which gains can be measured. Assessing knee strength of the residual limb becomes somewhat more subjective, as the standard lever arm for providing resistance has been altered by the amputation. Isokinetic machinery or handheld dynamometers may be used to evaluate muscle strength, although the validity and reliability of these tests has not been well established for this population.[10-12] Functional strength of the hip and knee during closed chain activities and eccentric control is equally important, as these activities more closely reflect muscle activity during normal gait. Stability of the hip and pelvis, especially in stance on the prosthetic side, is a key ingredient in achieving forward progression over the prosthesis during gait.[13] Although preamputation weakness of proximal muscles is often subtle with little to no observable abnormality in preamputation gait patterns, these impairments of strength and muscle endurance may significantly affect prosthetic gait. Periods of disuse following amputation typically produce further weakness in much of the involved limb's musculature. Without adequate proximal muscle strength and with the loss of distal musculature because of the amputation, problems with gait are likely.

Attention to strengthening of the hip abductors, adductors, extensors, quadriceps, and hamstrings is paramount in helping the person achieve optimal ambulation abilities. This is best addressed in the early phases of rehabilitation but should continue throughout the process. Strengthening of the abdominal and paraspinal muscles is equally important as these muscles assist with trunk stabilization during gait. Positioning of the individual in a gravity-dependent or gravity-neutral position depends upon existing strength

Table 27-4
Examples of Therapeutic Exercises for Strengthening Used in Early Prosthetic Training

Muscle Group	*Exercises*
Hip extensors	Bridging with residual limb over ball, bolster, or padded stool Prone leg lifts with weights Manual resistance in prone or side lying, or even sitting (early in range) Standing (parallel bars) hip extension with pulley weights or elastic bands
Hip abductors	Side-lying bridges with small ball or padded stool under knee of residual limb Hip abduction in side lying with weights or manual resistance Standing hip abduction with pulleys or elastic bands
Hip flexors	Supine SLR with manual resistance or weights Standing hip flexion with pulleys or elastic bands
Hip ER/IR	Seated hip ER and IR with manual resistance or elastic bands
Knee extensors	Seated knee extension, closed or open chain with manual resistance or weights
Knee flexors	Seated knee flexion with manual resistance or elastic bands Prone knee flexion with manual resistance or weights

ER, External rotation; *IR,* internal rotation; *SLR,* straight leg raise.

levels. Closed-chain (e.g., residual limb on bolster or gymnastic ball, or individual in kneeling position if tolerated) and open-chain exercise techniques and both concentric and eccentric muscle contractions are appropriate and effective. Progressive resistance protocols are often used to improve strength and muscle endurance. Resistance may be applied manually or with equipment, such as cuff weights, resistive elastic bands, or pulley weights. Resistance is generally not applied at or near the suture line until the surgical wound is soundly healed. As an individual's strength improves, exercises become more functionally oriented and more intense. Closed-chain exercises can take on greater emphasis during the latter stages of rehabilitation as the intervention focus may be exclusively on upright functional activities. Table 27-4 highlights some exercises that may be helpful in reducing strength deficits in an individual with transtibial amputation.

The strength and motor control requirements for ambulation with a transtibial prosthesis are similar but not identical to those of normal gait. Both the involved and intact lower extremities display increased muscle activity during their respective stance phases. Specifically, activity of the ipsilateral hip and knee extensors is increased and prolonged during stance as compared with persons without amputation.[14,15] The intact limb is subject to increased ground reaction forces, presumably a result of the absence of the normal foot and ankle mechanism of the involved side.[16,17] Hip abductors and extensors and knee extensors of the intact limb must respond to these increased forces. They demonstrate an increase in power generation and muscle activity.[18] Clearly, physical therapy interventions must address the strength not only of the residual limb but of the uninvolved limb and trunk as well.

Balance and Postural Control

Effective postural control during functional tasks has two fundamental components: (1) controlling the body's position in space for purposes of stability (maintaining center of mass over base of support), and (2) orientation of the trunk and limbs in space (appropriate relationship between body segments and between body and environment).[19] The normal postural control mechanism relies on visual, vestibular, and somatosensory input. Visual and vestibular information adds awareness of position in space with respect to objects in the environment and to gravity, and somatosensation provides information about the position of the foot and ankle and the pressures through the lower extremity joints. With loss of the distal limb to amputation, somatosensation and proprioception can no longer provide direct information about the limb's interaction with support surfaces.

Discussion of standing balance activities should be prefaced by mention of the difficulty some individuals have in adjusting to changes in sitting balance following transtibial amputation. Before receiving a prosthesis, lack of a second foot on the floor alters the base of support while sitting. Most individuals adjust fairly quickly in achieving static sitting stability, but the inability to shift weight onto that foot can challenge dynamic sitting balance, especially with reaching tasks requiring movement anterior and ipsilateral to the amputated side. For this reason, seated reaching ability is evaluated during the initial examination and is addressed in treatment as necessary. Once an individual is training with a prosthesis, practicing dynamic sitting balance activities usually progresses quickly.

In the preprosthetic phase, standing balance assessment and training might include single-limb standing in the parallel bars or at a support surface with less and less reliance on upper extremity support. The individual who can tolerate a kneeling position with the residual limb or even gentle pressure to the knee or distal end may stand with the intact limb on the floor and the residual limb resting on an elevated surface (e.g., low mat, gymnastic ball, foam block) that allows some weight bearing and balance support. Preprosthetic gait training with an appropriate assistive device is another useful approach to upright balance training.

Because sensory and proprioceptive input from the distal segment is absent after amputation, a new prosthetic user must learn to compensate for this lack of important postural information. The person may learn to deduce the position of the prosthetic foot and contact with the support surface by the angle of the knee and pressures felt within the prosthetic socket. Early in gait training, the person may make an exaggerated effort to dig the heel into the floor at initial contact and loading response. The purpose is to use the resulting pressure at the posterior residual limb as an indicator of contact with the floor with the knee in extension. The individual may learn to interpret this sensory experience as the secure position for proceeding with loading response and progressing into midstance.

In addition to the loss of direct sensory knowledge of contact with the floor, the loss of muscles at the ankle often compromises postural responses. Nashner[20] describes three stereotypical motor responses— ankle, hip, and stepping strategies—used to ensure that the center of mass stays within the base of support in response to unexpected anteroposterior perturbations. These postural strategies are also evident during functional activities such as ambulation.[19] The ankle strategy movement pattern, evident in normal postural sway, requires intact ROM and strength of muscles at the ankle. After amputation, this strategy is no longer available to the involved limb. Therefore the person may not be able to resolve the balance perturbation with intact limb response only and instead may need to rely on a hip strategy (movement of the trunk over the base of support) or a stepping strategy (moving the base of support under the center of mass) when a postural response is necessary.

Individuals with transtibial amputations must be able to respond to environmental demands during ambulation and other functional tasks in anticipatory (feed-forward) and reactive (feedback) modes. Therapists can design activities to assess and encourage postural control in various tasks and environments.[21] For example, successfully catching and throwing a ball requires the person to anticipate postural demands (in an effort to throw) and react to postural disruptions (in an effort to catch). Reaching activities in standing helps individuals develop skill and confidence in their anticipatory postural responses and, should the reach distance be excessive, their reactive postural responses as well. Balance confidence among people with lower limb amputations is closely related to performance in mobility skills, making it a relevant clinical concern.[22,23] Individuals with higher functional demands will require more advanced training. Therapists must consider the person's ultimate likely functional requirements and design various balance tasks to help the individual achieve those levels.

Cardiovascular Endurance

A thorough assessment of a patient's cardiovascular status followed by appropriate cardiovascular endurance training is an integral part of preprosthetic management. The energy requirements for an individual who is using a prosthesis for ambulation are higher than those of an individual who ambulates on two intact lower limbs.[24,25] The oxygen uptake for patients with unilateral transtibial amputation is correlated to residual limb length and may be 10% to 40% higher than that of individuals without amputation.[26] Physical conditioning is an essential component of rehabilitation for patients with lower extremity amputation, especially those with cardiopulmonary or vascular compromise. Improving metabolic efficiency (aerobic capacity) has a direct impact on the potential for functional ambulation even for the frailest and most deconditioned patients.[27] Endurance activities during the preprosthetic rehabilitation phase (such as wheelchair propulsion, single limb ambulation with an appropriate assistive device, and upper extremity ergometry) help improve cardiovascular status before the patient is a functional prosthetic user. Patients often continue these activities as they enter into the prosthetic phase of treatment. As the condition of the patient's residual limb and wearing tolerance permit, ambulation with the prosthesis can be used as an additional cardiovascular endurance activity. The 2-minute walk test with a prosthesis may be a useful tool to document changes in functional exercise capacity for an individual with transtibial amputation.[28]

For patients whose endurance may be a limiting factor for prosthetic ambulation, the physical therapy plan of care must include a cardiovascular exercise component as a priority. Patients who are taught to monitor their own pulse, respiratory rate, and perceived rate of exertion can participate more fully in prosthetic rehabilitation and prosthetic training. To develop an effective cardiovascular conditioning program, the therapist uses knowledge of the person's past medical history and cardiovascular pathophysiology, adapting the program to provide an appropriate challenge without surpassing the patient's physiological capabilities. The therapist must recognize the influence of cardiopulmonary pathology, such as unstable angina or advanced chronic obstructive pulmonary disease, on the patient's ability to improve endurance and adjust goals and intervention strategies as appropriate. For patients with few cardiovascular restrictions, more advanced cardiovascular exercises can be used as rehabilitation progresses. Brisk walking or use of exercise equipment (e.g., treadmill, stationary bicycle, stair climber, elliptical machine, or cross-country skier) are excellent endurance training activities for the appropriate person. A transtibial amputation does not prevent most patients from participating in health and wellness exercise programs during and following their rehabilitation.

Edema Control of Residual Limb

Initiation of weight-bearing activities in the prosthetic socket significantly decreases limb edema and accelerates maturation of the residual limb as a result of total contact within the socket and the pumping of muscle contractions during weight-bearing activities and movement.[29,30] This shrinking of the residual limb in early prosthetic training is accommodated for with the addition of layers of appropriate-ply thickness of cotton or wool socks to maintain a snug residual limb-prosthesis interface. Given fluctuations in residual limb size during early training and the need for an intimate fit in the prosthetic socket, new prosthetic users must carry extra socks with them whenever they will be out more than 2 to 3 hours.

Individuals in the early phases of prosthetic rehabilitation must continue to use a commercial "shrinker" pressure garment when not wearing the prosthesis to reduce the likelihood of insidious edema when the prosthesis is not worn. Patients with fluid volume fluctuations (e.g., those with kidney dysfunction or congestive heart failure) should use such shrinkers indefinitely. For patients whose residual limbs ultimately reach a stable size and shape, shrinkers may not be necessary once they use their prostheses functionally on a daily basis. The decision to discontinue the use of a shrinker permanently is based on two factors: (1) consistency in the number of sock ply worn during the day, and (2) the ability to don the prosthesis without decreasing the usual number of sock ply after a night's sleep without the shrinker.

Soft Tissue Mobility of Residual Limb

Soft tissue and bony adhesions that limit tissue mobility around the incision scar and the surrounding area may affect prosthetic tolerance, comfort, and use. The surgical procedure of a transtibial amputation can include muscle-to-muscle (myoplasty), muscle-to-fascia (myofascial), or muscle-to-bone (myodesis) surgical fixations to stabilize the remaining muscle.[31] Scarring or adhesions can occur among any or all of these tissues. The normal stresses and shearing forces of cyclic weight bearing and non–weight bearing during gait require that soft tissue throughout the residual limb be mobile. If the soft tissue is unable to move independently of the scar tissue or skeletal structures, the stress can lead to tissue breakdown and discomfort. Soft tissue mobilization techniques early in the rehabilitation process can help establish appropriate tissue mobility in the residual limb. Once the surgical incision is closed securely, deep friction massage (DFM) can be an effective tool in maintaining tissue mobility and in managing scar tissue that is restrictively adhered. Patients can be instructed in the use of this modality with specific guidelines for proper technique. Improper DFM technique is ineffective in managing scar tissue and potentially harmful for patients with fragile skin and soft tissue. Appropriate DFM targets movements between skin, subcutaneous soft tissue and fascia, and muscle layers. Inappropriate friction generated between the fingers and skin results in skin irritation, blistering, or breakdown and can delay prosthetic use until adequate healing occurs.

Sensory Status of Residual Limb

Residual limb and sound limb sensitivity is formally assessed during the initial physical therapy examination. Standard sensation testing guidelines (i.e., peripheral nerve distribution, or distal to proximal assessment) are used to assess all sensory modalities (sharp/dull, light touch, deep pressure, warm/cold, proprioception, vibration). Several commonly occurring postamputation sensory phenomena can have serious implications for functional outcome in patients with amputation. These include hyposensitivity, hypersensitivity, phantom sensations, and phantom limb pain.

Hyposensitivity

Hyposensitivity is most often encountered among patients with a history of diabetes, neuropathy, traumatic nerve damage, or vascular disease. In a small study, Kosasih and Silver-Thorn[32] found that superficial pain was often impaired in patients with transtibial amputations. Although deep pressure was not impaired, light touch and vibration sensations were minimally impaired.[32]

Patients with amputations who have impaired sensation are at high risk for skin breakdown because they may not recognize discomfort associated with skin irritation resulting from repetitive stresses and pressures. Inclusion of patient education about the preventive need for visual inspection, as well as practice time to perform visual inspection of the residual limb for signs and symptoms of soft tissue lesions, significantly reduces the risk of skin breakdown. Adaptive equipment, such as mirrors, or the assistance of caregivers may be necessary for patients with concurrent limitations in flexibility or visual impairment, or both.

Hypersensitivity

Early in rehabilitation, a generalized hypersensitivity of the residual limb is commonly encountered. This hypersensitivity is thought to be a consequence of nerve damage from amputation surgery itself.[33] Hypersensitivity can be effectively managed by bombarding the residual limb with tactile stimuli, using various textures and pressures. Strategies for reducing hypersensitivity include gently tapping with the fingers, massaging with lotion, touching with a soft fabric (e.g., flannel, towel), rolling a small ball over the residual limb, and implementing a specific wearing schedule for shrinker socks and rigid dressings. Intensity of intervention is based on the patient's tolerance to the sensory stimulation. The techniques can be progressed in intensity, type of modality used, and duration of stimulus (e.g., touching the limb with a rougher fabric and increasing wearing time for the shrinker socks). Patients with amputations are strongly encouraged to use these techniques independently as part of their home program. Over time these techniques should help reduce the hypersensitivity, with the ultimate goal of tolerance to normal sensory input without discomfort.

Localized hypersensitivity is often an indication that a troublesome neuroma has developed at the distal end of a surgically severed peripheral nerve. A neuroma is suspected when localized tapping sends a shock sensation up the patient's leg. If conservative clinical treatment is unsuccessful in reducing the hypersensitivity and pain caused by a neuroma, injection of a local anesthetic directly into the region or surgical removal may be necessary.

Phantom Limb Sensations

Phantom limb sensations are quite common after amputation.[34-38] Many patients report experiencing feelings of tingling or numbness in the toes or foot of the limb that has been amputated. Although the sensation can include the entire missing extremity, it is most often perceived as toe, foot, or ankle sensation. This predominantly distal presentation of phantom sensation is presumably a result of the large area of somatosensory cortex dedicated to the distal portion of the extremity.[4] Phantom limb sensations are considered to be the brain's erroneous interpretation of sensory nerve impulses traveling along the pathway of the nerves that formerly provided sensory feedback from the amputated limb.[4,34] Phantom limb sensation is a relatively harmless condition that has important functional implications for the patient. This sensation may be functionally useful in providing a semblance of proprioceptive feedback from the prosthesis. It may, however, also present a potential danger: Many patients with phantom limb experience nighttime falls when, half asleep, they attempt to stand and walk to the bathroom, expecting their phantom foot to make contact with the floor.

Phantom Limb Pain

Phantom limb pain is a special type of phantom sensation that can affect the rehabilitation of patients with amputations. Although most patients report phantom sensation, phantom pain is less common. When phantom pain occurs, it is most often described as a cramping, squeezing, or burning sensation in the part of the limb that has been amputated. The spectrum of complaints may vary from occasional mild pain to continuous severe pain. The absence of observable abnormalities of the residual limb is common. Although the etiology of phantom pain is not well understood, it has been theorized to be a product of the central nervous system (central origin theory), spinal cord–mediated mechanisms, or psychological factors.[33] The association between the etiology of amputation (vascular vs. traumatic) and the incidence of phantom pain is unclear.[31,37,38] Whatever the etiology, phantom limb pain is challenging to manage and disabling if the pain is severe. Strategies to address phantom limb pain include desensitization techniques, heat modalities, firm pressure applied to the residual limb, use of analgesics, and consistent use of a prosthesis.[36]

Care of Sound Limb

Ongoing assessment of the intact lower extremity is the responsibility of the therapist and of the patient with amputation. Patients with diabetes, peripheral neuropathy, or peripheral vascular disease who have lost one leg as a result of the disease process have a significant chance of losing the other leg, given the symmetrical distribution of these disease processes. Up to 20% of individuals with diabetes will undergo contralateral amputation within 1 year of the initial amputation surgery, and 5 years after initial amputation 28% to 51% of patients with diabetes will experience a second leg amputation.[39] To minimize the risk of loss of the remaining limb, close monitoring of limb condition (especially for subtle or insidious trophic, sensory, or motor changes) and optimal foot care is essential. Ongoing, systematic, and frequent assessment of pulses, edema, temperature, and skin is suggested. Education about the importance of a daily routine of cleansing, drying, and closely inspecting the foot (including the plantar surface and between the toes) is crucial. Podiatric care of nails, corns, and plantar callus, appropriately fitting footwear or accommodative foot orthoses, and avoidance of barefoot walking are three additional imperatives for the longevity of the remaining foot. If patients cannot perform daily foot inspection independently because of disease, age-related visual impairment, or decreased agility, they must be able to direct a caregiver in inspecting the foot. Even if patients are physically incapable of performing certain tasks for their own health and safety, they are ultimately responsible for their own care. Developing or improving on a patient's skill at directing assistance is a useful and realistic physical therapy treatment goal.

INITIAL PROSTHETIC TRAINING

A general knowledge of the timeline of the prosthetic rehabilitation process is helpful in projecting goals and educating patients about expected outcomes. Prosthetic fitting with an initial prosthesis (also called a temporary or training prosthesis) occurs when the surgical incision is healed and girth measurements at the distal residual limb are equal to or less than proximal girth measurements. This can occur as early as 10 to 14 days postoperatively to as long as 8 to 12 weeks or more after surgery. As a new residual limb matures and shrinks in size, the person will add additional ply (layers) of prosthetic sock to ensure adequate fit in the prosthesis. Typically, when the intimacy of fit within the socket is compromised by 15 or more ply of sock, a new prosthetic socket is indicated. How quickly the initial socket must be replaced varies depending on the pattern of shrinkage of the residual limb. For some, the first replacement socket may be necessary in 2 to 3 months, whereas others may use their initial socket for 6 months or more. The socket may be replaced several additional times as the residual limb continues to shrink in the first postoperative year. A definitive prosthesis is prescribed when the residual limb size is stable for an 8- to 12-week period, as indicated by girth measurements and by a consistent number of sock ply for optimal prosthetic fit. Although some patients are ready for their definitive prosthesis within 6 months after surgery, others do not achieve stable residual limb size for 12 to 18 months or longer. With each new socket, close monitoring of the residual limb throughout the adjustment period is necessary.

Several important components of rehabilitation involving prevention of skin breakdown and safe use of equipment can be effectively addressed in group classes or through printed materials. These components include care of the sound limb, donning and doffing the prosthesis, establishing a prosthetic wearing schedule, management and prevention of skin breakdown, positioning with the prosthesis, and care of equipment.

Prosthetic Prescription

The members of the interdisciplinary team involved in the care and rehabilitation of patients with amputation include the orthopedic or vascular surgeon, a physiatrist, a prosthetist, a physical therapist, an occupational therapist, a social worker, a rehabilitation nurse, and a vocational rehabilitation counselor. Many hospitals and rehabilitation centers have established prosthetic clinics that bring together the appropriate professionals to address the needs and problems of prosthetic users. Determining prosthetic candidacy is the first major clinical decision to be made. Although the research literature has identified predictors of outcome of prosthetic use, the team considers the individual's needs, motivation, and functional capacity in deciding prosthetic candidacy.[40-43] Factors most often considered in determining whether to fit with a prosthesis include the following:

1. *The patient's medical history.* Disabling medical conditions may prohibit successful prosthetic use. Advanced cardiac or pulmonary disease that significantly impairs functional status before amputation affects a person's prosthetic candidacy. A history of cerebrovascular accident with residual hemiplegia of the side opposite the amputation may limit functional prosthetic use. If a prosthesis would make transfers and mobility more efficient or safer for caregivers, a prosthesis may be appropriate even if independent ambulation is not anticipated.
2. *The patient's premorbid and present level of function.* A patient who required substantial assistance for functional mobility before amputation may have limited prosthetic training goals. Patients who are independent with functional activities, ADLs, and ambulation with an assistive device after amputation tend to do well with a prosthesis. If, before receiving a prosthesis, a patient can dress himself or herself, transfer independently from a bed to a chair, and safely stand and walk using an assistive device, the potential for functional prosthetic use is excellent.
3. *The patient's body build and type.* Patients with morbid obesity or fixed deformities (e.g., extreme kyphotic posture) that interfered with mobility before an amputation may present a significant challenge in prosthetic training activities.
4. *ROM.* Significant hip and knee flexion contractures are best addressed before prosthetic fitting if the patient is to achieve efficiency and functional independence with a prosthesis.
5. *Availability of support at home.* Patients who are likely to require assistance must depend on family members, significant others, or formal caregivers to help with one or more prosthetic tasks. The potential to be a limited household ambulator with a prosthesis may be important in reducing the burden of care for caregivers and may allow a patient to remain at home with a caregiver as opposed to living in an institutional setting.

If the patient is considered to be a reasonable prosthetic candidate, these same considerations and others are used in determining a specific prosthetic prescription. Table 27-5 presents suggestions for prosthetic prescription for patients with special needs.

Physical therapists must have a basic understanding of prosthetic components and design to be able to contribute to the prescription process. Because therapists spend much time working with people in one-on-one circumstances, they often have a better perspective about an individual's goals or needs than do other members of the team. Therapists may gain insight or information that is important in the decision-making process. If therapists are familiar with prosthetic components, they may begin to form an opinion about the best prosthetic prescription for a patient during the early rehabilitation phase. Therapists should use the prosthetist and professional literature to stay current with evolving technology in prosthetics. They must be critical consumers of the literature in order to make decisions that are in the best interest of the patients when prescribing prosthetic features. An understanding of the different characteristics of various prosthetic feet will help therapists to identify the type of foot that is most suitable and economical to meet a specific patient's functional needs.[44-48]

Therapists must also be familiar with the special needs of certain clinical populations so that they can assist in the

Table 27-5
Considerations in Transtibial Prosthetic Prescription

Category of Consideration	*Specific Consideration*	*Potential Prescription Implications*
Medical history	Hemodialysis	Socket with removable insert allows for change in residual limb size with fluctuating fluid status
	Ipsilateral hemiplegia	High socket trimlines (supracondylar, suprapatellar suspension) or thigh corset suspension to provide increased knee stability
	Upper extremity involvement	Adaptation of suspension device for ease of donning/doffing
Patient goals	High activity, interest in sports	Energy-storing prosthetic foot Use of suction suspension
	Rigorous outdoor work	Exoskeletal prosthesis for durability
Body build and type	Obesity	Supracondylar cuff to achieve purchase on thigh, with auxiliary fork strap
	Cachexia	Soft socket insert to protect bony prominences
	Short residual limb	High socket trimlines (supracondylar, suprapatellar suspension) or thigh corset suspension
Range of motion	Severe knee flexion contracture	Modification of socket alignment for a bent knee prosthesis

optimal prosthetic prescription to meet the individual patient's needs. Patients with diabetes who are at great risk for additional skin breakdown and poor healing may benefit from a socket with a soft insert or from a silicone sleeve designed to reduce friction during prosthetic use. Frail or deconditioned patients may reach higher levels of function if lightweight components are chosen and stability in prosthetic prescription is emphasized. Active children need durable components, but replacement costs must also be considered, as components must be replaced frequently to accommodate growth. Athletes with amputation desire durable, lightweight, high-technology components for a competitive edge in their sport performance.

Decisions to change socket design or suspension for long-term prosthetic users must be carefully considered. Some patients who have worn a particular type of prosthesis for a long time may have difficulty acclimating to a new type of device. If a patient has no complaints about a prosthesis other than "it's worn out," the prosthetist may prescribe the similar components for a replacement prosthesis. If a patient expresses interest in new goals or activities, however, prosthetic prescription changes may be warranted. A patient who has been using a solid-ankle cushioned-heel foot on an existing prosthesis but wants to increase activity (such as trying race walking or jogging) may benefit from the prescription of an energy-storing foot.

CASE EXAMPLE 1B

Initial Prosthetic Fitting and Early Prosthetic Training for a Patient with Traumatic Transtibial Amputation

The rehabilitation team determines that P. L. is an excellent prosthetic candidate with the need for a device that will allow him to return to his active lifestyle. The prosthetist, physical therapist, and surgeon agree to include an energy-storing foot on his initial prosthesis. Suspension will be accomplished by a roll-on silicone suspension sleeve with a pin locking mechanism, with prosthetic socks worn on top of the sleeve to accommodate for the anticipated rapid shrinkage of the residual limb once P. L. begins to wear the prosthesis.

The prosthesis is delivered 5 weeks after P. L.'s amputation. He quickly masters the process of prosthetic donning, initially using one three-ply cotton sock over his suspension sleeve. During initial gait training, the team notes that P. L. tends to stand up without weight on the prosthetic foot; this may be because he has become so adept at single limb ambulation over the past several weeks. To help him become more comfortable bearing weight through his prosthesis, the team asks P. L. to focus on and practice weight shifting during transfer activities and in static standing.

P. L. takes an initial walk down and back in the parallel bars without any cues or instructions. This allows the team to assess P. L.'s natural instincts during initial prosthetic use and anticipate major issues during prosthetic training. If P. L. continues to be hesitant about loading his prosthesis, early training could focus on weight bearing and weight shifting activities. As soon as P. L. begins to accept full weight during prosthetic stance, training begins to target dynamic balance and postural control issues.

During his early gait attempts in the parallel bars, P. L. progresses from bilateral to unilateral upper extremity support. Because the team notices a tendency toward left knee hyperextension during the single-limb support phase, the prosthetist adjusts alignment to slightly increase the anterior tilt of the prosthetic socket. A skin check of the residual limb after the first 10 minutes in the prosthesis reveals a generalized reactive hyperemia that resolves within 5 minutes.

Because P. L. shows an excellent ability to take weight through the prosthesis, early prosthetic training is geared toward minimizing the need for upper extremity support, challenging balance and mobility skills, increasing tolerance to prosthetic wearing, and prosthetic gait training. P. L. and the team periodically monitor skin condition during every rehabilitation session.

Questions to Consider

- What resources and limitations does this patient bring to his rehabilitation process? What will be his major challenge as prosthetic training begins?
- What key things must this patient understand about the care of his residual limb and remaining limb? What kind of support or services might he need as he takes on this responsibility for himself?
- Should additional issues or goals be addressed in this early rehabilitation period? What are they, and why are they important?
- What is a reasonable progression of the activities in this patient's initial prosthetic rehabilitation program?
- What factors may influence the pace and progression of his rehabilitation and his ability to participate in it?

Preparatory Prosthesis

A patient with a transtibial amputation is fitted for a temporary or training prosthesis as soon as the surgical incision is stable, usually from 2 to 6 weeks after surgery. The initial socket is most often fabricated from high-temperature thermoplastic but can be made of plaster of Paris, fiberglass, laminate, or other materials. The socket is connected to the prosthetic foot using an alignment system at either end of a metal or plastic pylon (pipe). Endoskeletal modular prostheses are preferred to exoskeletal prostheses because modification of alignment can be expected early in the rehabilitation process. Some patients are fitted with a permanent pylon and prosthetic foot at this early stage and progress through a series of sockets until their residual limb reaches its mature contours. Most often, a foam and stocking cosmetic prosthetic cover is not provided until the final socket fitting. Because of significant changes in residual limb size and shape, patients may progress through two or three sockets before being fitted for the definitive socket or prosthesis. The three primary benefits of early fitting with a temporary or training prosthesis include (1) early bipedal ambulation with limited weight bearing through the residual limb, (2) improved edema control of the residual limb, and (3) faster shrinking (maturation) of the residual limb.[6]

Donning and Doffing the Prosthesis

Using Prosthetic Socks

In early prosthetic rehabilitation, prosthetic socks are used to modify the fit between the socket and the shrinking residual limb. Proper use of prosthetic socks enhances residual limb weight bearing in pressure-tolerant areas, decreases the likelihood of skin breakdown in pressure-intolerant areas, and increases patient comfort during ambulation. Wool or cotton prosthetic socks are available in three different ply (thicknesses): 1 (thinnest), 3, and 5 (thickest). Many patients with amputations who use a rigid or flexible socket first apply a thin nylon sheath directly over the skin (under the socks) to minimize friction forces and wick moisture away from the skin. Cotton or wool socks of various ply are then applied before the limb is placed in the socket. If a nylon sheath is not used, socks are applied smoothly directly onto the residual limb.

When silicone suction suspension or a friction reducing liner that requires skin contact is used, socks are applied after the sleeve or liner has been donned. For liners with a pin locking mechanism, a small hole is cut in the bottom of the socks to allow for engagement of the pin into its receptacle. Socks of various thicknesses are combined to create a snug and comfortable fit. Patients are encouraged to don the fewest number of socks to achieve the same amount of thickness (i.e., one 3-ply sock is preferable to three 1-ply socks). Prosthetic socks can also be used creatively to solve problems with socket fit. If, for example, the patient's distal residual limb girth has decreased more quickly than proximal girth, creating a pendulum effect within the socket during ambulation, one of the prosthetic socks can be cut to cover just the lower half of the residual limb. When layered between two full-sized socks, the shorter sock helps to fill the extra space within the socket, ensuring total contact between the limb and socket.

Fluctuations in limb volume associated with edema in the first weeks and months after amputation often mean that the appropriate number of sock ply varies from daily and perhaps within a given day. Because of this variability in limb size, choosing the correct number of prosthetic socks may be challenging for those new to prosthetic use. Limb size can change rapidly. Even a few minutes in a dependent position without a shrinker or Ace wrap in place can substantially increase residual limb size. For this reason, patients should wear their compression device until the moment they are ready to don the prosthesis. Therapists and prosthetists work with the patient to assist the development of problem-solving skills and strategies to determine the appropriate number of socks to don.

Good prosthetic socket fit is extremely important to patients with amputations.[49] New prosthetic users must understand the principles of prosthetic fit and weight bearing. The optimal prosthetic fit is snug, like that of a custom-fit glove on the hand. Total contact between the residual limb and socket is important; significant skin problems can occur when total contact is not achieved. Patients must understand where weight-bearing pressures are best tolerated on the limb and where pressure sensitivity is likely to occur. Although they might initially expect to bear weight through the distal end of the limb, they must understand that most sockets are designed to be total contact and to distribute weight-bearing forces across several areas, including the patellar tendon, anteromedial and anterolateral surfaces of the residual limb, medial tibial flare, and distal posterior aspect of the residual limb.

A number of indicators are used to assess the adequacy of sock ply during prosthetic ambulation. If too few socks are donned, the residual limb descends too far down within the socket. The patient may complain of pistoning during ambulation: The prosthesis slips downward when unweighted during the swing phase and is pushed upward on the residual limb during weight bearing in stance. If pistoning is suspected, a pen or marker is used to mark the prosthetic sock at the anterior or posterior trimline of the socket. If the line becomes more visible when the individual lifts the limb (using a hip-hiking motion), slippage may be occurring and additional sock layers are indicated. When the prosthesis and socks are taken off for inspection of the skin, reactive hyperemia (redness) is seen at the proximal patellar tendon and at the inferior border of the patella, as well as at the distal anterior residual limb. Redness may also be present on the fibular head, which contacted the socket below its intended relief area. These are signs that thickness of the sock is inadequate and additional sock layers should be added.

A different set of signs indicates that too many ply of sock have been donned. The patient may feel that the prosthetic limb is difficult to don, fits too tightly, and is just slightly longer during forward progression at midstance and during foot clearance in swing. When the skin is inspected after ambulation, reactive hyperemia is visible at the distal patellar tendon and the tibial tubercle. Redness may also be present at the head of the fibula, which contacted the socket above its intended relief within the socket. These are indications that one or more ply of socks should be removed to enhance socket fit.

Most patients become adept at judging the adequacy of sock ply when given the opportunity to practice and problem solve early in their rehabilitation. For the functional prosthetic user, donning and doffing the prosthesis becomes as second nature as donning and doffing one's pants or shoes. The initial instruction period in this skill, however, requires attention to detail. Patients should be encouraged to establish a careful routine of donning the appropriate number of prosthetic socks, one layer at a time. The socks should be smoothed free of wrinkles, with any seams facing down and out so as to minimize pressure on the surgical scar. Patients then don the soft insert (if applicable) and palpate to assure that the patellar tendon indentation on the insert aligns appropriately with the patellar tendon. The hard socket of the prosthesis is then applied by gradually increasing weight bearing (from the sitting or standing position) to push the residual limb gently into the socket and checking that the alignment of the socket in the horizontal plane is correct. If great force is required to achieve purchase into the socket, the patient should be instructed to stop and start over. Figure 27-1 illustrates an effective strategy for donning the transtibial prosthesis.

Checking Adequacy of Suspension

Once the patient is comfortably in the socket, adjustment of the suspension device is necessary. Suspension options for transtibial prostheses include neoprene sleeve, supracondylar strap with or without waist belt and auxiliary fork strap, supracondylar socket design, supracondylar or suprapatellar socket design, thigh corset with joint uprights, and suction socket with pin in ring suspension. To complete the donning process, the person stands and bears weight through the socket to ensure proper positioning of the residual limb while adjusting the suspension system.

When donning a prosthesis that uses a roll-on silicone suspension sleeve, the sleeve is rolled on first. Care must be taken that the pin is centered on the inferior surface of the distal residual limb. The appropriate number of socks is applied over the silicon sleeve by sliding the pin through the hole in each sock. The hard socket is donned as the patient aligns the pin with the socket receptacle and pushes into the socket; the pin should click into place. Once the residual limb is seated in the hard socket, the patient stands and bears weight through the prosthesis; the pin should further depress into the ring mechanism three to six clicks. If 10 or more clicks are audible upon initial weight bearing, more ply of sock may be required.

Prevention and Management of Skin Breakdown

Because prolonged wound healing and development of new skin irritation can delay prosthetic training, the prevention and management of skin breakdown on the residual limb are important goals. Open areas frequently preclude weight-bearing and gait-training activities. Pressure, friction, or shearing forces are the primary etiologies of skin breakdown related to prosthetic wear. If, during weight bearing, external pressure exceeds capillary refill pressure (25 to 32 mm Hg)

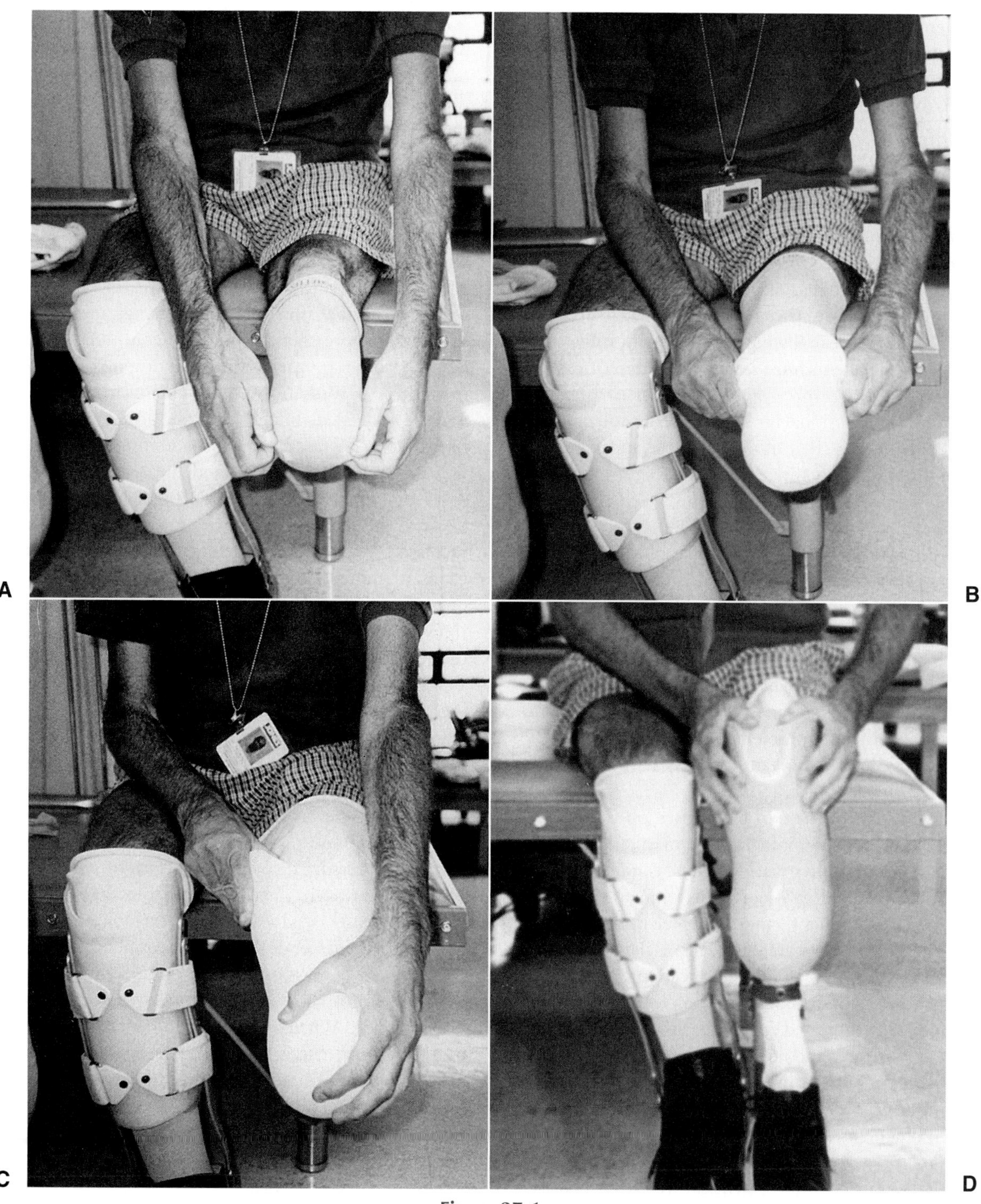

Figure 27-1

This patient with a recent transtibial amputation demonstrates the correct sequence for donning his prosthesis. ***A,*** *First, he applies a nylon sheath, adjusting its fit to prevent formation of wrinkles or folds as additional layers of sock are added. Wrinkles result in uneven distribution of pressure and can increase the likelihood of residual limb discomfort and skin breakdown.* ***B,*** *Once the sheath is positioned, prosthetic socks are added, one at a time, and carefully adjusted for smooth fit until the desired number of ply is reached. The least possible number of socks is used to create a snug, comfortable prosthetic fit.* ***C,*** *This patient's prosthetic design includes a soft Pelite insert. The anterior trimline of the liner is cup shaped to accommodate the patella and is used to guide the position of the liner on the limb during donning. Patients are cautioned against using a twisting motion when applying the insert/liner, to avoid causing wrinkles in the underlying sheath or socks.* ***D,*** *The final step is to insert the residual limb with properly positioned socks and liner into the prosthesis. This patient dons the prosthesis in a sitting position, gradually increasing weight bearing to achieve the desired total contact fit. Note that a patellar tendon–bearing orthosis is used to support and protect his remaining limb, which is vulnerable as a result of Charcot's arthropathy.*

for an extended time, the delivery of oxygen and nutrients and the removal of waste products from active tissues are interrupted. If relief of pressure is provided, this local ischemia is followed by a reactive vasodilation or hyperemia. This is the mechanism that produces the redness over weight-bearing areas, such as the patellar tendon and medial tibial flare and shaft, that is observed in new prosthetic users. A blanchable area of redness over weight-bearing areas, which returns to normal skin coloration within 10 minutes, is to be expected in early prosthetic training and indicates normal reactive hyperemia.[50] If redness persists or does not blanch on firm palpation, tissue damage has likely occurred and the risk of skin breakdown increases significantly.

Therapists and patients must recognize the different implications of redness over pressure-tolerant versus pressure-sensitive areas of the residual limb. If a pressure-tolerant area shows evidence of excessive pressure, socket fit and alignment may be appropriate, but the amount of weight bearing or duration of wearing time may need to be decreased. If pressure-sensitive areas are showing signs of too much pressure, it is more likely that socket fit or alignment needs to be adjusted. When excessive redness is observed, successful problem solving dictates changing a single variable at a time and assessing the impact of this one change on the prosthetic problem. If multiple changes are made at the same time (e.g., wearing time, alignment, and socket fit are all altered), it is unclear which change actually solved the problem, if indeed the problem is solved. If the problem is not solved, there is no way of knowing if the interventions may have been more successful independent of one another.

An individual's risk for skin breakdown on the residual limb is determined by physiological and mechanical factors. The vascular, sensory, and musculoskeletal conditions of the residual limb are the physiological determinants, whereas socket fit, socket alignment, amount of weight bearing, and duration of weight bearing are the mechanical determinants. Each risk factor may have clinical implications. A conservative prosthetic wearing schedule and frequent residual limb inspection may be indicated for those with skin breakdown caused by any of the physiological risk factors. If poor scar and soft tissue mobility of the residual limb leads to tissue breakdown, DFM over the involved area (after healing) or application of a nylon sheath under prosthetic socks may be appropriate interventions.

Improper socket fit or alignment can result in increased weight bearing to pressure-sensitive areas of the residual limb and may result in skin breakdown. If improper fit or alignment is suspected, the first step in problem solving is a thorough reevaluation of donning technique and the number of socks used. Prosthetic fit is then reassessed to determine if total contact between the residual limb and socket has been achieved. If all of these areas are sufficient, potential problems with prosthetic alignment are investigated. Increasing duration of prosthetic wearing too quickly in a well-aligned and appropriately fit prosthesis can also result in skin breakdown to pressure-tolerant areas of the residual limb. An individual who has been ambulating with partial weight bearing using axillary crutches without any problems with skin integrity may, when progressed to full-time unilateral crutch use, present with skin breakdown over the patellar tendon, a pressure-tolerant area, as a result of increased weight bearing.

The presence of skin breakdown is not a direct contraindication to further use of the prosthetic device. The first priority should be to identify the cause of breakdown and eliminate it by making the appropriate changes. Close observation and ongoing assessment and treatment of any lesions with appropriate nonadherent dressings inside the socket should allow prosthetic training to continue. Certainly, if a lesion becomes progressively worse despite clinical management during prosthetic training, a hiatus from prosthetic use may be indicated. In the example presented previously, a return to bilateral crutch use and diminished prosthetic wearing time may be indicated until the lesion is healed. After healing, ambulation time might be divided between bilateral and unilateral crutch use, to build tolerance for increased weight bearing before full-time unilateral crutch use is attempted once more. If the area does not show signs of healing or becomes worse, with increasing lesion size or signs of inflammation or infection, discontinuation of prosthetic use altogether may be necessary for healing to occur.

As a patient begins to ambulate over different terrains, the magnitude and direction of weight-bearing pressures within the socket may change as well, presenting additional mechanical risk factors for skin breakdown. Descending stairs in a step-to-step pattern protects the residual limb by leading with the prosthetic leg; when advancing to a step-over-step technique, the residual limb experiences a different pattern of pressure distribution. Depth of stairs also has an impact on pressure distribution within the socket: As step height increases, so does the total excursion through ROM necessary to descend the stairs. Ambulation on uneven terrain, such as grass or gravel, produces different pressures within the prosthetic socket than walking on a predictable, level surface. When evaluating potential causes of skin breakdown, the characteristics of the environments and the task demands of the activities must be considered. Changing technique by adapting the movement strategy or the environment or adding an assistive device can provide just enough protection for the residual limb to prevent skin irritation and breakdown.

If localized increased pressure is determined to be causing tissue breakdown, pressure relief is the goal, and socket modification by the prosthetist may be necessary. Certain methods of pressure relief are inappropriate and should be avoided. The use of "donut" padding around an area of breakdown or potential breakdown is counterproductive for three reasons. A donut pad will (1) increase pressure to the area surrounding the lesion when the limb is placed in the socket, (2) increase the ischemic effect of weight bearing, and (3) potentially lead to edema or extrusion of the vulnerable tissue through the "hole" of the donut. Any adhesive materials that are in contact with skin should be used with extreme caution. A nylon sheath can be used to hold a dressing in place under the prosthetic socks. Finally, the abrasive quality of certain dressings, including standard gauze, must be avoided inside the socket. Nonadherent dressings or non-stick pads tend to be less textured and less abrasive to an area of skin breakdown. Many new products that are thin and self-adherent, but not noxious to the skin, are available to effectively provide another "tissue" layer to an area that is threatening breakdown or in the process of healing.

Dressings should be used sparingly inside a prosthetic socket, as the socket fit is designed to be snug, and any padded dressing increases pressure over the affected area, which is counterproductive to the goal of wound healing. The therapist must reevaluate the prosthetic fit if a dressing is used within the socket, recognizing that the application of even a thin dressing may require the removal of one ply layer of socks.

Wearing Schedule

Once the evaluation of socket fit and alignment has been completed and any adjustments have been made, it is time to begin prosthetic training. Constant reassessment of socket fit and alignment is necessary during the entire training phase because of changes in residual limb shape and size. The duration of time for initial prosthetic wearing is usually conservative, especially for patients with a history of skin integrity problems. Often, the first prosthetic weight-bearing activities are closely supervised, lasting no longer than 5 to 10 minutes in between skin inspections. Once patients are tolerating 30 to 60 minutes in the prosthesis without problems, total time in the prosthesis is gradually increased, often in increments of 15 to 30 minutes, as skin condition permits. Patients with no history of skin integrity problems (i.e., after traumatic amputation or revision of congenital limb anomaly) often progress quickly with wearing activities, whereas those with sensory impairment or peripheral vascular disease must be progressed much more cautiously.

Inspection of the residual limb after the first few minutes of weight bearing should reveal redness of the skin in predictable pressure-bearing regions: the patellar tendon, medial tibial flare, anterolateral distal tibial shaft, and posterior aspect of the residual limb. Because the socket is intended to have total contact with the residual limb, the entire limb may develop a mild reactive hyperemia that is apparent when the socket is first removed. Increases in wearing time require continued, frequent skin inspection. The patient must understand the importance of gradual progression of wearing time. If a patient is allowed to initiate prosthetic wearing unsupervised or does not take the wearing schedule seriously, the potential for skin breakdown is greatly increased.

Ideally, though not always possible, the prosthetist and physical therapist are present for the delivery of the prosthesis to the patient with amputation so that both may be involved in the final fitting and alignment checkout. After delivery of the prosthesis, the physical therapist and patient with amputation may determine that it is safest to use the prosthesis only when supervised by the therapist during the first week or more of therapy. Once the patient is cleared to use the prosthesis at home, a written wearing schedule is used to guide the patient and prevent misunderstandings about the time permitted for prosthetic use (Figure 27-2).

PROSTHESIS WEARING SCHEDULE

Patient Name: ______________________________

Your wearing schedule for your prosthesis is ____________ on and __________ off.

Check your skin every time you take your prosthesis off. You are looking for areas of redness that do not go away within 10 minutes, areas of blistering or abrasions, or pain in your residual limb.

If you have any of these problems, or any questions, call your therapist at the number below and do not wear your prosthesis again until the problem is addressed with your therapist.

If you do not have any of the problems above, in two (2) days you can increase the "on time" to __________ and maintain the off time as above.

Next scheduled appointment: ______________________________

Therapist name & phone number: ______________________________

Figure 27-2
Example of a wearing schedule used to guide the patient's use of the new prosthesis at home, early in rehabilitation.

Positioning

Patients often need instruction about positioning of the lower extremity in the prosthesis when seated. The trimlines of the socket are designed for optimal pressure distribution during weight-bearing activities. The high posterior wall of the socket is necessary to provide counter pressure to the patellar tendon–bearing surface in stance but can provide undue pressure to the hamstring tendons in sitting. The patellar tendon bar in the prosthesis is designed to take weight in standing but can provide pressure to the anterior aspect of the tibial tuberosity if the prosthesis slips down when the patient is seated. When seated, the patient's prosthetic foot should rest flat on the floor or foot plate of the wheelchair so that the residual limb remains in total contact with the socket, thus avoiding the risk of undue pressure and decreasing the chance of gapping between the prosthesis and the residual limb that may allow edema to collect.

CASE EXAMPLE 2B

Initial Rehabilitation for a Patient with Dysvascular/Neuropathic Amputation

Evaluation of V. R. reveals that his impairments include loss of range of motion (ROM), decreased strength, poor balance, gait abnormalities, and fragile skin. Functional limitations include loss of community mobility, diminished function in activities of daily living, and limited understanding of the care and wear of his prosthetic limb. The prosthetic team agrees on a diagnosis of impaired motor function, muscle performance, ROM, gait, locomotion and balance associated with amputation. They anticipate that, with 3 months of outpatient rehabilitation care, V. R. will be able to use his prosthesis well enough to return to community ambulation on a limited basis, ambulate with an assistive device independently, and participate in all household activities of daily living as necessary.

The physical therapy plan of care focuses on improving functional ROM, general strengthening, balance training, gait training, improving cardiovascular endurance, and education of V. R. and his family on the wear and care of his prosthesis, residual limb, and remaining/intact limb.

Prosthetic training begins with simple weight-bearing and weight-shifting activities in the parallel bars. The skin condition and integrity of his residual limb and remaining foot are monitored carefully, and his "in prosthesis" time is increased as tolerated. V. R.'s daughter assists him with skin inspection. As soon as he gains confidence walking in the parallel bars, he advances to gait training with a step-through pattern using a rolling walker. As his tolerance of prosthetic wear increases, his therapist begins to work with him on a reciprocal gait pattern using two straight canes.

His residual limb continues to "shrink" as his activity level increases. V. R.'s cognitive difficulties make it difficult for him to understand when he should add sock ply when donning his prosthesis. His son and daughter take on the responsibility to monitor limb condition and sock use several times each day. The team anticipates that, once his limb volume stabilizes, V. R. will be able to effectively don the established number of ply of socks. The team emphasizes the need for V. R. to continue using his compression garment (shrinker) at night while sleeping.

V. R. can now wear his prosthesis for 6 to 7 hours each day and ambulate independently with his walker in the house and outside to his social club. He requires the supervision of a family member when walking indoors with his two straight canes. His hip strength has improved to 4+/5 in his hip abductors and extensors. He is now only -3 degrees from full knee extension. His limb volume is stabilized; he wears his prosthesis comfortably with five-ply socks. Although V. R. has attempted to ambulate with a single straight cane, his postural control is insufficient for safety at this time.

Questions to Consider

- What resources and limitations does this patient bring to his rehabilitation process? What will his major challenge be as prosthetic training begins?
- What key things must this patient and his caregivers understand about care of his residual limb and remaining limb? What kind of support or services might he need as he and his family take on this responsibility?
- Are there additional issues or goals that need to be addressed in this early rehabilitation period? What are they, and why are they important?
- How can you determine how quickly to advance or progress the activities in this patient's initial prosthetic rehabilitation program? What factors may affect his ability to participate, tolerate, and improve in his rehabilitation process?

Care of Prosthetic Equipment

Patients with amputations also require explicit instructions about the proper care and maintenance of their prosthetic equipment. The prosthetic socket and liner should be wiped daily with a damp cloth. Prosthetic socks should be washed daily and laid flat to dry (wool socks shrink in a clothes dryer). When not being worn, the prosthesis should be stored in a flat position to minimize the risk of damage should it fall over (hard sockets are particularly vulnerable to traumatic cracks). Patients also benefit from tips for ease of daily activities, such as dressing the prosthesis with sock, pant leg, and shoe before donning.

PROSTHETIC FIT AND ALIGNMENT

As new prosthetic users become comfortable and confident with their prosthetic limb, changes in socket fit and alignment may be necessary to achieve the most energy-efficient and cosmetic gait. Ideally, the prosthetist, the patient with amputation, and therapist work as an interdisciplinary team to solve problems with socket fit and alignment as they arise. The physical therapist should have a thorough foundational knowledge of optimal socket fit and alignment in order to recognize and troubleshoot problems and be ready to refer the patient to the prosthetist should alignment need adjustment.

Prosthetic Socket

An intimate fit between the residual limb and the socket is necessary for successful prosthetic training. The total contact socket is designed to distribute the load of weight bearing over the residual limb to assist in venous blood return from the limb and provide some sensory feedback to the prosthetic user through the residual limb. Although the socket is prepared over a positive model of the patient's limb, either through casting or computerized technology, it is not uncommon for the socket to be modified in the early days of prosthetic training. Frequent and careful inspection of the residual limb and verbal feedback from the patient help to assess socket fit and patient tolerance to prosthetic wear.

Alignment

Prosthetic alignment is evaluated in quiet standing (statically) and during gait activities (dynamically). Static alignment refers to assessment of the relationships among the socket, pylon, prosthetic foot, and floor; the length of the prosthesis; and the overall fit of the socket on the residual limb. Dynamic alignment includes those concepts, as well as prosthetic considerations as they relate to suspension, symmetry of gait, and energy requirements of gait.[51] Because static alignment assessment is the first standing activity in which a patient engages, it is prudent to carry this out in the parallel bars or with substantial support if parallel bars are not readily available. Information gleaned from alignment assessment can reveal clues about pressure distribution on the tissues of the residual limb inside the socket. Problems with alignment affect not only pressures within the socket but also the biomechanics of gait and the translation of forces from the prosthetic foot up the kinetic chain. Static and dynamic alignment are evaluated from an anterior, posterior, and lateral (prosthetic side) view. For a thorough review of transtibial prosthetic alignment, see Chapter 26, Transtibial Prosthetic Options. Table 27-6 provides a basic rationale for standard transtibial static prosthetic alignment.

PROSTHETIC GAIT TRAINING

The ability to move within and over one's base of support with efficient timing and sequencing of muscle activity and appropriate postural control is the key determinant of functional ambulation across the wide variety of environments

Table 27-6
Transtibial Static Prosthetic Alignment and Rationale

Alignment	*Rationale for Alignment*
POSTERIOR VIEW	
Prosthetic height (symmetric leg length)	Prevents gait deviations associated with leg-length discrepancy Prevents orthopedic deformity associated with leg-length discrepancy
Plumb line: midsocket to $\frac{1}{2}$ inch lateral to midheel	Creates slight varus moment during stance, as in normal gait Directs compressive forces to pressure-tolerant areas at medial proximal (medial tibial flare, medial femoral condyle) and lateral distal (fibular shaft) residual limb and minimizes compressive forces on nontolerant areas at lateral proximal (fibular head) and medial distal residual limb
LATERAL VIEW	
Socket in 5-10 degrees of flexion (anterior tilt) with top of prosthetic foot parallel to the floor	Distributes compressive forces to anterior aspect residual limb and loads patellar bar Limits vertical displacement of center of gravity at midstance to decrease energy cost of gait
Plumb line: midsocket to anterior edge of heel	Allows for controlled knee flexion in loading response and late stance, as in normal gait Prevents abnormal hyperextension of the knee in midstance Allows for knee flexion from mid to terminal stance

encountered in daily life. Many transtibial prosthetic users have the potential to ambulate with a near-normal symmetrical gait pattern that is free of significant gait deviations and independent of assistive devices.[52] To do this, however, the patient must meet various challenges, including (1) building tolerance to prosthetic wear and weight bearing through the residual limb, (2) controlling dynamic weight shifting through the prosthesis in all planes of movement, and (3) reintegrating postural control and balance with respect to the lack of ankle joint sensory and proprioceptive input, muscle control, and ROM.

A patient's fears and concerns influence his or her determination and motivation. These are powerful determinants of the ability to ambulate and perform other important functional activities.[22,53] A patient with an amputation who is capable of safe and functional ambulation in the community may choose not to venture outside the home because of lack of physical confidence or fear of being identified as disabled or different. In contrast, a patient whose clinical picture is less promising for functional prosthetic use but who is determined to return to a busy and productive life "on two feet" may well do so.

Initial Training

For the new transtibial prosthetic user, initiation of gait training typically starts with ambulation on level surfaces with few environmental demands. Gait training often begins in the parallel bars, as a protected environment, because they provide a stable and secure setting with minimal environmental challenges. Countertop or table support, raised mats, plinths or chairs, and even assistive devices can all be appropriate alternatives if parallel bars are unavailable. The therapist should limit cues for the patient who is excited about this new activity and simply allow walking in the protected environment of the parallel bars. This helps the therapist to identify potential gait deviations early in training before maladaptive habits become problematic. On the basis of this preliminary gait assessment, individual problem areas can be addressed with pre–gait exercise activities and gait training.

Early therapeutic activities will progress from initially supporting and later challenging the patient's postural stability. Progressing from weight bearing and gait activities with significant bilateral upper extremity support to those with minimal or no support is a common early goal in the rehabilitation process. A typical progression of early prosthetic training activities might include the following:

1. Static weight bearing with decreasing dependency on upper extremity support (i.e., progressing from bilateral open-handed upper extremity support, to contralateral open-handed upper extremity support, to ipsilateral open-handed upper extremity support, to static standing activities without support).
2. Simple dynamic weight-shifting activities consisting of loading and unloading body weight through the prosthesis in multiple directions (anterior/posterior, medial/lateral, and diagonal patterns) as is required in gait and functional activities. These tasks are progressed by decreasing upper extremity support and varying foot positions (parallel stance, step-stance, tandem stance).
3. Reaching activities that require the person to reach to various heights and directions within a functional context. These activities are progressed by increasingly challenging reaching limits in all directions, varying foot position and decreasing upper extremity support.
4. Repeated stepping activities (i.e., break gait cycle into component parts) in all directions and marching in place with decreasing upper extremity support.
5. Stepping with the uninvolved limb onto an elevated surface (low step stool or small ball), forcing increased weight bearing through the prosthetic limb with progressively decreasing upper extremity support.
6. Gait training to minimize gait deviations inside or progressing out of the parallel bars. Early in training, individuals often benefit from cues to "dig in" the heel of the prosthetic foot during forward stepping activities to improve awareness of the location of the prosthetic foot on the floor.
7. Sit-to-stand and stand-to-sit activities, encouraging partial weight bearing through the prosthesis. These activities can progress and vary from high surfaces with arm rests to lower surfaces without arm rests.

Figure 27-3 depicts some of these early prosthetic training activities. Although use of specific weight-bearing activities outside of functional tasks may be contrary to fundamental motor learning principles of encouraging action-directed performance versus motor performance, activities that encourage weight bearing can be successfully practiced and then integrated into functional gait and mobility skills. Repetitive loading of the prosthesis is an appropriate task without continuing with the translation of weight over the foot as in the intact gait cycle. Once patients become accustomed to accepting the weight as in initial contact through loading response of the stance phase of gait, they may progress to practicing more full weight-bearing activities in preparation for the single-limb support phase of gait and finally integrate the activity into the full gait cycle. Regardless of the focus of the intervention (weight bearing, balance, postural control, or coordination and sequencing), the activity can and should be integrated into the gait cycle or the functional task within the same treatment session. Interventions are most effective if they are performed within the context of functional tasks.[54]

Progressing prosthetic training requires increasing challenges to postural control and balance. Dynamic activities without upper extremity support and activities that require both feed-forward and feedback balance strategies (e.g., playing catch) can be used to prepare the prosthetic user for more open, unpredictable environments.[21] Figure 27-4 depicts some of these activities. Coordination and sequencing of an

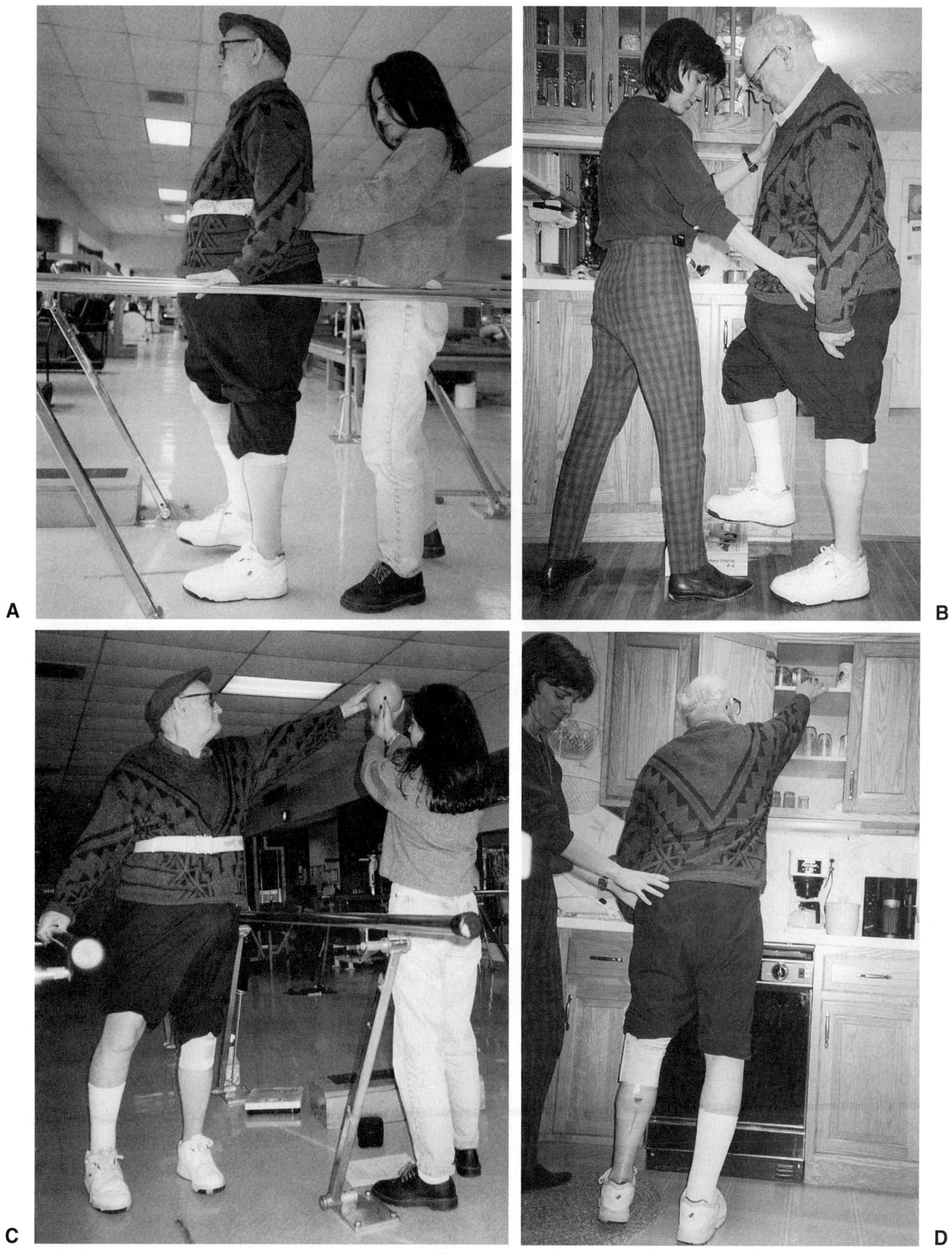

Figure 27-3

Weight-bearing, weight-shifting, and balance activities in early prosthetic training. ***A,*** *A new prosthetic user practices loading weight onto the prosthesis by repeatedly practicing single steps (forward and backward) with the intact limb. Note full weight bearing through the prosthesis, demonstrating good prosthetic alignment and erect trunk and head posture, with a gentle open-handed grip on the parallel bars.* ***B,*** *Stepping up onto a phone book or low stool can increase weight bearing through the prosthesis.* ***C,*** *Reaching activities, using all planes of movement, encourage weight shifting onto and off of the prosthesis and can challenge balance and postural control. Early on, the opposite hand grip on the parallel bar compensates for decreased balance and postural control. This activity can be progressed by decreasing, and ultimately eliminating, upper extremity support.* ***D,*** *Reaching activities in a functional context should be integrated early in the rehabilitation process.*

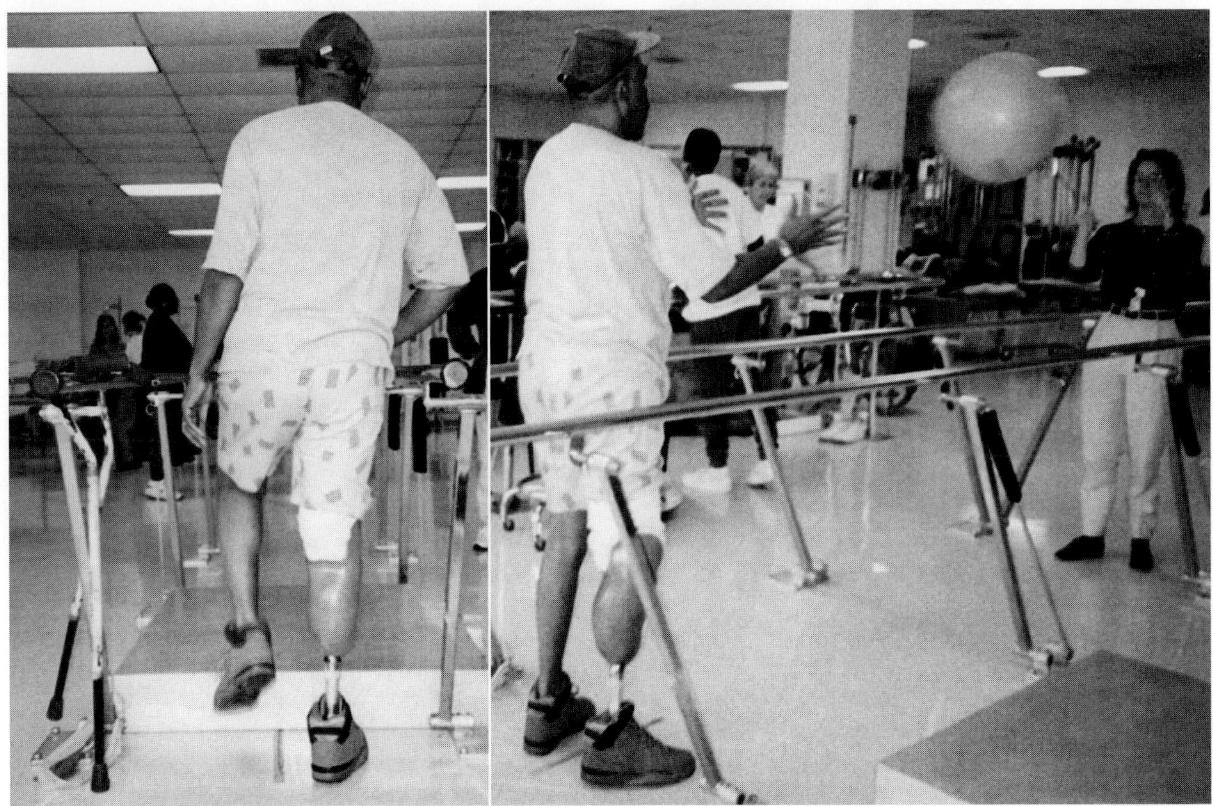

Figure 27-4

Progression of weight-shifting and balance activities in prosthetic training. ***A,*** *Stepping activities become more challenging without the use of the upper extremities for balance or support.* ***B,*** *Throwing and catching activities encompass balance (feed-forward and feedback), coordination, postural control, and weight bearing through the prosthesis.*

appropriate assistive device and activities to promote timing and fluidity of gait (e.g., use of a metronome to facilitate equal stance duration right and left), as well as to encourage appropriate weight bearing (e.g., use of audio biofeedback for weight bearing), are other areas that can be included in this phase of prosthetic training. During all activities with the new prosthetic user, the therapist must remember to check the skin frequently for signs of pressure intolerance and skin irritation.

Patients who are having difficulty accepting weight onto the prosthesis during the gait cycle may be reluctant to shift body weight over the prosthetic limb, rely heavily on weight bearing through the upper extremity in the parallel bars, and express great concern about putting all of their weight through the prosthesis. They may be tempted to use the prosthesis as an "assistive device" for ambulation rather than a true replacement limb. Both the therapist and new prosthetic wearer should recognize that improved prosthetic weight bearing allows for decreased mechanical stresses on the sound limb, which is often vascularly compromised. Other strategies that might help patients improve their ability and confidence in weight shifting in preparation for independent walking include verbal cueing to progress the pelvis toward the parallel bars on the prosthetic side over a stable foot and tactile cueing of the therapist's hand placed on the anterolateral aspect of the involved hip to facilitate anterior progression. If a patient is having difficulty loading the limb, stepping onto a bathroom scale may provide useful objective feedback regarding weight bearing through the prosthesis. The use of mental imagery of successful mastery of the activity may also be an appropriate adjunct to physical therapy.

Assistive Devices

Assistive devices can provide help with balance only (e.g., single-point cane or quad cane) or with weight bearing and balance (e.g., walker, axillary crutches, or Lofstrand crutches). The goal is to provide only the amount of support necessary to protect the healing residual limb and to reduce the risk of falling without hampering the patient's willingness or ability to load the prosthesis. It may be prudent to spend time on prosthetic weight-bearing and weight-shifting activities in the parallel bars or at a stable surface to allow the patient to progress directly to an assistive device that aids in balance only. Patients with transtibial amputations are encouraged to use an open hand versus a closed grip on the parallel bars to minimize the stability gained from pulling on the bars. Optimally, the prosthetic limb can tolerate 100% weight bearing so that upper extremity weight bearing through an assistive device is unnecessary. Patients who demonstrate good weight bearing, strength, and balance may progress directly from the parallel bars to use of a single-point cane or no assistive device. Use of a quad cane is not recommended, as it is frequently misused as a weight-bearing device and its wide base can create a fall hazard. For patients who cannot achieve early full weight bearing through the prosthesis and require a weight-bearing assistive device, the devices of choice are axillary or Lofstrand crutches. Crutches allow patients to progress to a two-point gait using a step-through gait pattern, which closely approximates a normal sequence and pattern of gait. Patients begin with bilateral support and progress to unilateral support with crutches as prosthetic weight bearing improves.

Standard walkers impede development of an efficient reciprocal gait pattern because they limit forward progression to a "step-to" rather than "step-through" movement strategy, limiting gait to a step-to pattern. This interrupts fluid movement, hampers smooth forward progression of the center of gravity over the base of support, and precludes an effective terminal stance and preswing. Walkers are used only when endurance or postural control are significantly compromised. A wheeled walker can minimize interruptions to the gait cycle if it is advanced between each step or if the patient is bearing weight only slightly through the walker (i.e., pushing the walker like a grocery cart).

Although some patients with physical or medical frailty become functional household ambulators only with the aid of a walker, many individuals with transtibial amputation reach functional independence without any assistive device or choose to use just a straight cane for "balance assist" when walking on unpredictable surfaces or in crowded environments.

CASE EXAMPLE 1C

Functional Training for a Patient with Traumatic Transtibial Amputation

Over the next few weeks, P. L. progresses through a series of therapeutic activities of increasing difficulty. The goal is to prepare him for higher-level motor tasks necessary for independent community and athletic function with a prosthesis.

Initial dynamic reaching and stepping activities in the parallel bars with decreasing upper extremity support progress to similar activities outside the parallel bars. Initially, reaching activities are performed in unsupported standing, with feet positioned for a fairly wide base of support. As P. L.'s confidence increases, the team asks him to try feet-together and tandem standing positions. Eventually he can reach with his intact extremity positioned on a series of stools of increasing height, on a rocker board, and finally with his intact extremity on a small Theraball.

As P. L.'s postural control improves, the therapist increases the demand for dynamic postural response by adding random (unexpected) perturbations during standing and reaching activities. Although these activities first occur in the parallel bars with upper extremity support, P. L. progresses quickly to similar activities in unsupported standing on level surfaces. Given his interest in softball, he particularly enjoys playing catch as an activity to facilitate his anticipatory and reactionary balance.

As P. L. masters ambulation on level surfaces using a straight cane, he begins to practice walking on various terrains (carpet, grass, gravel, ramps, stairs, sidewalks) and in various environments (crowded corridors, multiple obstacles, in wet and windy conditions). Until shown a videotape of his walking pattern, P. L. consistently spends more time in stance on his intact lower extremity than his prosthetic limb. After watching the video, he corrects this common gait deviation, eliminating it almost completely.

Once he can wear his prosthesis for 2 to 3 hours, P. L. begins advanced gait activities that involve curbs, steps, ramps, and getting on and off elevators (which requires precisely timed movement), in preparation for using his prosthesis in the community. Although he practices ascent and descent activities with step-over-step gait patterns in the clinic, he is initially reluctant to try this in the community, stating that he feels safer using conservative techniques to reduce the risk of falling. P. L. chooses to continue using his cane as he begins wearing his prosthesis full time in the community, although his gait training activities in the clinic are performed without any assistive device.

Next, P. L. practices sidestepping, tandem walking, cross stepping, and kicking activities as higher-level gait skills. He practices moving to and from the floor, squatting, avoiding stationary and moving obstacles while walking, and picking up objects from the floor. Although these activities begin in the parallel bars to ensure safety, P. L. is motivated to practice them in the open space of the rehabilitation gym, as well in "realistic" environments such as his bedroom and living room. P. L. is excited to work on his softball fielding skills, practicing fielding ground balls to his left and right, back-peddling to catch fly balls, and throwing on the move. He initially attempts these activities in the indoor gym environment before moving to the outdoor field environment.

P. L. is encouraged and highly motivated as his program begins to focus on agility and power activities. Although his initial attempts at rapid running in place with a low center of gravity are frustrating, he consistently gains skill and endurance. As his discharge from rehabilitation nears, he begins to explore how to jump and land effectively. In his initial trials of running, he uses a hop-and-step pattern, but his goal is to master a "true" running pattern without a period of double-limb support. He is eager to carry these activities from the gym to a "real" outside environment.

Questions to Consider

- What are the functional goals for each of these gait training, balance, and agility and power activities?
- How can the right time to progress this patient to activities of increasing difficulty or challenge be determined?
- How can it be determined whether this patient is progressing at the rate predicted in the prognosis? What can be done if improvement is slower or faster than anticipated?
- Could any other activities or exercises have been used to better facilitate this patient's mastery of functional activities? Why are these activities or alternative approaches suggested?
- How often, and how formally, should the patient's progress be "reassessed" during this acute stage of prosthetic rehabilitation?

Gait Analysis

An understanding of the biomechanics of normal gait is crucial for physical therapists because it provides the standard by which prosthetic gait is measured. The main objective of static and dynamic prosthetic alignment and physical therapy intervention is to optimize the energy efficiency and cosmesis of gait. The ultimate goal is a gait that is safe, energy efficient, and symmetrical. When deviations from the norm are observed, the therapist and prosthetist seek to discover the underlying cause or causes of the problem.

Any one of the commonly observed prosthetic gait deviations has many different potential contributors. Gait deviations may be a product of intrinsic factors (pertaining to the individual using the prosthesis) or extrinsic factors (pertaining to the prosthesis and the environment). The observed deviation may be a primary gait problem, caused directly by an intrinsic or extrinsic factor, or a compensatory strategy, a result of the individual's attempt to avoid a primary deviation. If a new prosthetic user is observed to ambulate with a forward-leaning trunk throughout the stance phase of gait, the therapist must determine if this is a primary or compensatory problem. It may be a primary gait deviation resulting from a hip flexion contracture that limits the individual's ability to achieve upright posture. It may also be a compensatory strategy of the patient who is fearful of knee instability during prosthetic stance; a forward-leaning trunk results in the drop of the individual's line of gravity anterior to the knee joint, improving stability at the knee by creating an extensor moment at the joint.

During initial gait training, prosthetic alignment issues may not be immediately evident. Hesitancy to fully load the prosthesis and upper extremity weight bearing through the parallel bars or assistive device will affect the resulting gait pattern. As the individual becomes more willing to bear weight through the residual limb, a "truer" gait pattern emerges and the function of the prosthesis becomes more critical. The therapist, along with the prosthetist, must be attentive to the potential emerging need to correct prosthetic alignment as the individual improves in prosthetic weight bearing and as impairments improve (i.e., changes in strength, ROM, or balance might warrant prosthetic alignment changes).

When problem solving, the clinician must think about why certain gait deviations might occur and whether they are primary or compensatory. Answering these questions allows the therapist to focus treatment on the most salient issues. Physical therapists who work in prosthetic rehabilitation become skilled at recognizing common prosthetic gait deviations and their possible causes. Table 27-7 describes some of the more common transtibial prosthetic gait deviations and their most likely potential causes.

An example of the problem-solving thought process follows. A patient shows knee instability during loading response and throughout midstance, as evidenced by lack of knee extension or excessive knee flexion. The therapist must use deductive reasoning to identify the true sources of the problem. If the instability occurs on level surfaces, environmental causes of the problem can be ruled out. If evaluation of the static alignment of the prosthesis reveals appropriate alignment of the foot and pylon, the socket's being set in excessive knee flexion could contribute to the problem. Thorough evaluation of the problem requires assessment of potential intrinsic causes as well. If examination reveals full, strong, active ROM at the knee and no complaints of pain, the therapist must look to the joints proximal to the problem. Assessment of the hip may reveal a hip flexion contracture that leads the patient to maintain knee flexion as a compensatory strategy to maintain upright posture. If these two distinct potential causes of the problem are found, the therapist can then prioritize and address each cause. Extrinsic causes can be modified immediately: Improvement of quality of gait and elimination of deviations after realignment (typically the responsibility of the prosthetist) suggest alignment as the factor underlying the gait deviation. If a socket alignment adjustment does not have a significant impact, magnifies the observed gait problem, or leads to a new gait deviation, the underlying cause is likely to be intrinsic issues needing physical therapy intervention. In this example, restoration of hip extension ROM through a program of stretching the hip flexors would be appropriate.

Table 27-7
Common Gait Deviations in Transtibial Prosthetic Gait

Phase of Gait	*Problem*	*Category**	*Possible Cause*
Initial contact to midstance	Excessive knee flexion	Intrinsic	Knee flexion contracture Hip flexion contracture Hip extensor muscle strength or timing problem, or both Knee extensor muscle strength or timing problem, or both Anterior distal residual limb pain
		Prosthetic (extrinsic)	Excessive dorsiflexion of the prosthetic foot Excessive socket flexion (anterior tilt) Socket positioned anterior to prosthetic foot Excessive heel cushion stiffness (SACH foot) Prosthesis too long
		Environmental (extrinsic)	Walking down inclines
	Absent knee flexion or knee hyperextension	Intrinsic	Cruciate ligament insufficiency Quadriceps weakness Anterior or posterior distal residual limb pain Excessive soft tissue in popliteal area
		Prosthetic (extrinsic)	Excessive plantar flexion of prosthetic foot Excessive socket extension (posterior tilt) Excessively soft heel cushion (SACH foot) Inadequate cuff suspension Socket positioned posterior to prosthetic foot Prosthesis too short
		Environmental (extrinsic)	Ascending inclines/walking uphill
Midstance	Valgus moment at knee	Intrinsic	Collateral ligament insufficiency Medial distal residual limb pain
		Prosthetic (extrinsic)	Excessive outset of prosthetic foot Inadequate socket fit or suspension
		Environmental (extrinsic)	Walking on uneven surfaces
	Varus moment at knee	Intrinsic	Collateral ligament insufficiency Lateral/distal residual limb pain Weakness of hip abductor muscles
		Prosthetic (extrinsic)	Excessive inset of prosthetic foot Inadequate socket fit or suspension
		Environmental (extrinsic)	Walking on uneven surfaces
	Insufficient weight bearing	Intrinsic	Residual limb pain or hypersensitivity Excessive upper extremity weight bearing on assistive device Instability of the knee joint Decreased muscle strength of residual limb Fear of falling/lack of confidence in prosthesis
		Prosthetic (extrinsic)	Prosthesis is too long Poor socket fit
		Environmental (extrinsic)	Walking uphill Walking on rugged terrain
Midstance to preswing	Early knee flexion (quick drop-off)	Intrinsic	Hip or knee flexion contracture, or both Weakness of hip extensor muscles Anterior/distal residual limb pain

Continued

Table 27-7
Common Gait Deviations in Transtibial Prosthetic Gait—cont'd

Phase of Gait	*Problem*	*Category**	*Possible Cause*
		Prosthetic (extrinsic)	Excessive dorsiflexion of prosthetic foot
			Socket positioned anterior to prosthetic foot
			Inadequate socket fit or suspension, or both
		Environmental (extrinsic)	Walking down inclines or hills
	Delayed knee flexion (walking uphill effect)	Intrinsic	Posterior/distal residual limb pain
			Patient locks knee in extension as compensation for instability or weakness
		Prosthetic (extrinsic)	Excessive plantar flexion of prosthetic foot
			Socket positioned posterior to prosthetic foot
			Excessively long keel of prosthetic foot
		Environmental (extrinsic)	Walking up inclines/uphill
Swing	Inadequate clearance of foot†	Intrinsic	Decreased hip or knee flexion ROM
			Decreased hip or knee flexion strength or motor control
		Prosthetic (extrinsic)	Prosthesis too long
			Excessive plantar flexion of prosthetic foot
		Environmental (extrinsic)	Walking on uneven surfaces

SACH, Solid-ankle cushioned-heel; *ROM,* range of motion.
*Intrinsic problems are due to patient-related factors. Extrinsic problems are associated with prosthetic issues (alignment or fit) or environmental issues (best understood by analyzing the specific conditions or activity in which they are observed).
†Compensations for inadequate swing phase clearance include a lateral lean of the trunk toward the remaining limb, circumduction of the prosthesis and residual limb, or a high-steppage gait.

Gait Training on Level and Alternate Surfaces

To adapt to and meet environmental demands, the patient with a transtibial prosthesis must be able to adjust his or her step length and cadence while ambulating in response to environmental conditions or circumstances. The physical therapy program might begin with practice opportunities until the patient achieves a normal cadence. It might then progress to activities that demand an increased or decreased cadence and transitional gait movements, such as sidestepping, turning, and walking backward. These skills can initially be practiced in the clinic with minimal environmental demands. The patient can then progress to situations in which the environment presents a challenge, such as crossing a street in a timely manner, getting on and off an elevator or escalator, walking through a crowded corridor in a busy store, or walking to a seat in the middle of an aisle in an auditorium or theater. Successful community ambulation also requires management of many different ground surfaces, including steps, curbs, ramps, and varied terrain (Figure 27-5). In providing therapeutic practice opportunities for a patient who is new to prosthetic use, the therapist considers the following important extrinsic variables:

1. Level of assistance required for safe performance
2. The specific demands of the environment, such as the depth and height of steps and curbs or a ramp's degree of slope
3. The need for an assistive device or railing
4. The optimal technique for performing the task safely
5. The ability to superimpose an additional activity while walking or moving in the environment

An initial goal might be to decrease the level of assistance on these alternative surfaces, which can be accomplished by simplifying one or more of the other variables of the task, such as decreasing the depth of the step or curb, allowing the use of a sturdy rail versus a crutch or cane, and allowing the sound limb to "lead" or dominate the task. Once a skill is consistently demonstrated, the task demands are increased. Early skills in stair climbing are generally developed in a step-to gait pattern with the sound limb leading in ascent and the prosthetic limb leading in descent. Advanced gait-training activities may instead require the patient to use the prosthetic limb first while ascending and the sound limb first while descending; these skills are necessary if the patient is to master a step-over-step pattern for stair ascent and descent.

The ultimate goal is to provide a repertoire of strategies for the patient to choose from to respond to environmental demands (e.g., when crossing the street, the patient can ascend the curb with the prosthetic foot without disrupting gait cadence). The unpredictable surface of uneven terrain encountered in walking across a lawn can challenge postural responses significantly if no assistive device is used.

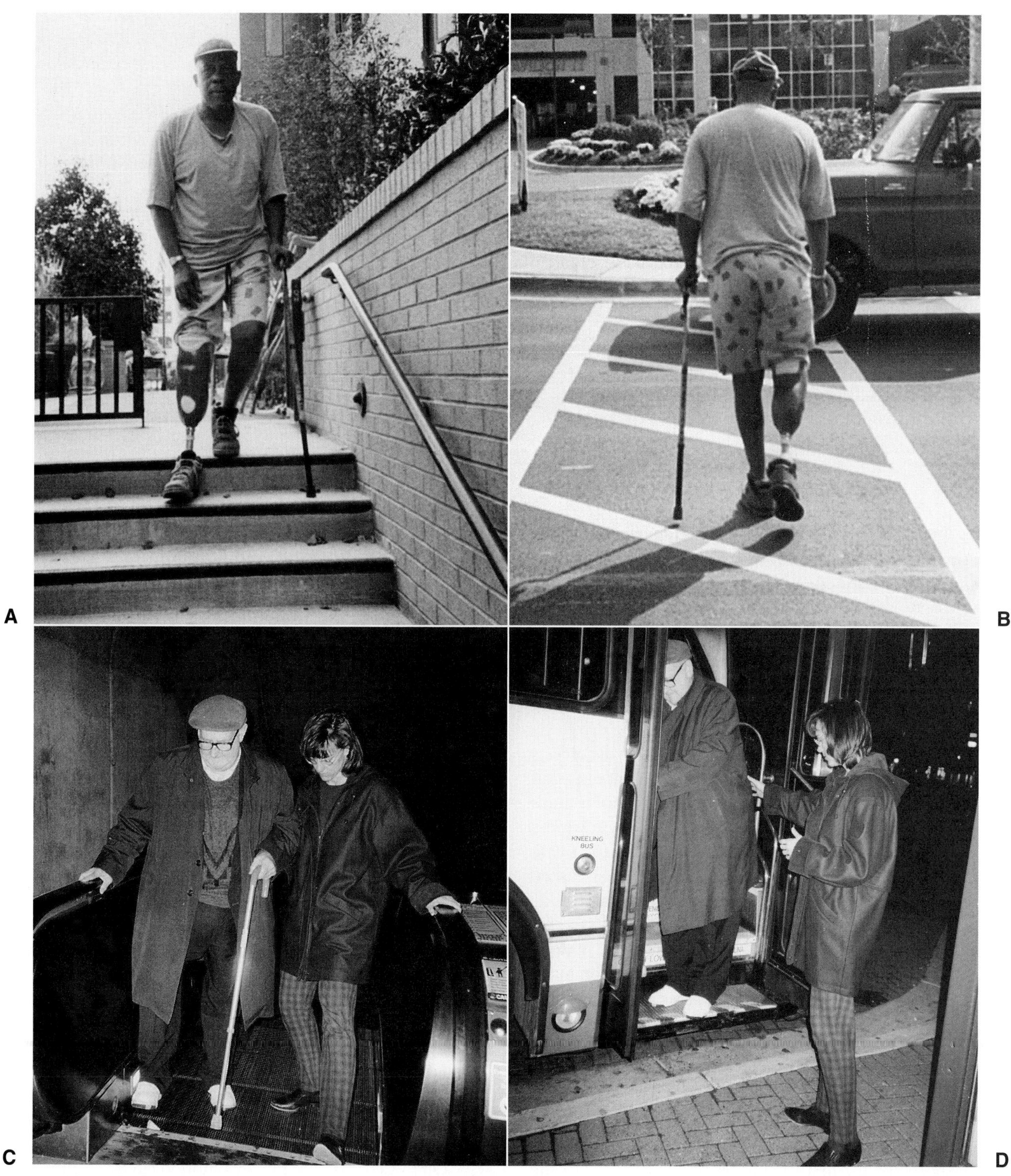

Figure 27-5

In addition to walking on level surfaces, functional community ambulation requires that the patient be able to adapt movement strategies to meet various environmental demands. ***A,*** *When descending stairs, three factors contribute to the level of difficulty: the number and depth of steps, the type of upper extremity support (rail, assistive device, or none), and the movement pattern (step-to-step vs. step-over-step).* ***B,*** *Crossing a street requires the patient to adjust cadence in response to a dynamic and unpredictable environment.* ***C,*** *Managing an escalator requires a quick adaptation from a stable to a dynamic surface when getting on and from a dynamic to stable surface when getting off.* ***D,*** *Training for the use of transportation might include practice in getting in and out of the front and back seats of a car or ascending and descending steps of a bus if using public transportation.*

Box 27-1 *Advanced Exercises and Activities for Individuals with Transtibial Amputation*

Range of motion	Independent stretching of hamstrings, quadriceps, hip flexors, hip internal rotators, and external rotators
Strengthening	Resistance training of hip musculature, quads and hamstrings, closed-chain exercises—step ups, leg press, wall or ball squats, involved limb stance with opposite limb resistance exercises, multiple plane stepping exercises, involved limb lunges; advance to using handheld weights to increase resistances
Balance and coordination	Involved single-limb stance, rocker or BAPS board standing, stool stepping with uninvolved limb stepping to stool, beam walking, involved single-limb stance and UE resistive or dynamic activities such as ball catching
Speed and agility	Figure-of-eight walking, progressing to running, shuttle walk to run, sprinting, obstacle course
Cardiovascular activities	Swimming, running, cycling, treadmill walking, stair/stepper climbing

From Gailey R. *One Step Ahead: An Integrated Approach to Lower Extremity Prosthetics and Amputee Rehabilitation Workbook.* Miami: Advanced Rehabilitation Therapy, 1994.
BAPS, Biomechanical ankle platform system.

Sidestepping is a skill needed in environments such as theaters and can be practiced when the theater is empty or when people are seated. A supervised community outing is an excellent strategy for addressing and achieving high-level ambulation goals.

Superimposing functional activities on gait during therapeutic treatment prepares patients for the daily "real world" challenges that they are sure to encounter. The variety of functional tasks practiced by the patient may be driven by specific patient goals. Safe ambulation while carrying objects of varying weights and sizes is an important functional skill and an appropriate physical therapy activity. The patient's specific goal may be to carry a full laundry basket down the hall or a cup of hot coffee from the kitchen to the living room. As patients become functional prosthetic users, household tasks and leisure or work activities may guide their therapeutic needs.

High-level activities, such as running and athletic endeavors, are appropriate and attainable goals for many transtibial prosthetic users. Some patients with transtibial amputation may wish to resume certain sports or leisure activities that they participated in before their amputation. With current advances in prosthetic components, patients can enjoy a multitude of athletic and recreational activities. Patients with amputation are returning to basketball, running, rock climbing, and cycling, and some are taking up these sports for the first time as prosthetic users! With the technological advances in prosthetics and the growth and exposure of the Paralympics, high-level athletics are no longer limited to a small elite group of prosthetic users. Box 27-1 describes some more advanced rehabilitation activities that can help individuals prepare to take part in their chosen activity.

CASE EXAMPLE 2C

Return to Community Ambulation for a Patient with Neuropathic/Dysvascular Bilateral Transtibial Amputation

Six months after discharge from his outpatient prosthetic rehabilitation program, V. R. undergoes transtibial amputation of his left lower extremity due to a nonhealing and infected neuropathic ulcer of his left first metatarsal head. He is once again treated in a rehabilitation facility followed by home care physical therapy. His postoperative course is uneventful, although wound healing is slow. He receives his prosthesis approximately 6 weeks after surgery and begins outpatient physical therapy 1 week later. V. R. reports that he has worn his prosthesis for much of the day but is not walking much.

On examination, V. R. is found to be in relatively good health, given his comorbidities. Although alert and attentive, his difficulties with memory and recall continue (his son provides an accurate medical history). V. R., his wife, and daughter with developmental disability have recently moved into an "in-law" apartment at his son's home. Since discharge from the hospital, he has spent most of his time watching television and sitting but states that he hopes to return to visiting his social club, if rehabilitation progresses well.

On the left, his knee range of motion (ROM) is limited from 5 to 110 degrees. His left hip ROM is within normal limits in flexion, abduction, and rotation but lacks the final 10 degrees for functional hip extension. On manual muscle testing (MMT) V. R. demonstrates 4/5 strength in hip flexion. hip abduction and adduction, and 3+/5 in hip extension. MMT at the left knee is 4+/5 in extension and 4/5 in flexion. The suture line of his new residual limb is well healed and mobile and of equal circumference at distal and proximal points.

In quiet standing, wearing both prostheses and using a walker, V. R. stands with slightly flexed hips and knees. He cannot stand unsupported. His sitting balance is functional, although reaching distance is reduced in all directions. V. R. responds with 90% accuracy on light touch sensory testing in both residual limbs.

At present V. R. ambulates with standby supervision using a walker and step-to gait pattern for 25 feet. Once set up, V. R. is independent with his activities of daily living, including bathing/showering, dressing, and donning/doffing his prostheses.

The team anticipates that, over the next 6 to 8 weeks, V. R. will be able to use his prosthesis well enough to return to limited community ambulation with his walker.

The plan for this episode of care is much like the one that guided his previous rehabilitation, including therapeutic exercises for ROM of his left hip and left knee, strengthening of his hip and knee musculature, volume control and residual limb care, and balance and gait training. Balance training will likely be more of a challenge in this episode of care, as the loss of ankle strategies in both limbs markedly increases the impairment of balance. The team anticipates that progression through the rehabilitation process will be enhanced by the family's existing understanding of the care and wear of the prosthesis.

The team agrees that limited community mobility requires nearly normal ROM, and 4 to 4+/5 strength at all lower extremity joints. V. R. desires to improve his balance so that he can stand unsupported in his prosthesis for self care and cooking activities. He also wants to be able to walk independently with two canes.

Questions to Consider

- Are there any concerns about this patient's potential for regaining functional, independent ambulation and adequate postural control for ADLs and leisure activities?
- Do the team's prognosis and plan of care make sense? Why or why not?
- What factors make rehabilitation for an older adult with bilateral ambulation challenging?
- How can the right "time" to have this patient progress to activities of increasing difficulty or challenge be determined? How can it be determined whether the patient is progressing at the rate predicted when making the prognosis?
- Given the outcomes of V. R.'s previous rehabilitation and his stated goals, what are the most important goals and activities at present? What activities or exercises might be used to better facilitate this patient's mastery of the key functional activities that have been prioritized?
- How often, and how formally, should the progress during this acute stage of prosthetic rehabilitation be reassessed?

Functional Activities

Prosthetic training is not just a matter of teaching a patient to ambulate—it includes various other functional activities, such as transfer training from various surfaces, kneeling, management of falls, and rising from the floor. Specific functional tasks should also be designed to address the individual patient's goals as they relate to ADLs, job-related activities, or recreational activities. Because occupational therapists have excellent knowledge of adaptive devices and skill in environmental adaptation, working with these team members may prove helpful.

Many patients with amputations have a strong desire or need to return to work. The successful return to employment of such patients has been studied. Schoppen and colleagues[56] found three predictors of success in returning people to work: age at the time of amputation, education level, and wearing comfort of the prosthesis. In their study, 79% of people with lower limb amputations successfully returned to work, but 23% did not regain the ability to work. A change in job was often necessary, especially if the physical demands of the job were high. Older patients with amputations with a lower education level and poor wearing comfort of their prosthesis were at risk for failing to return to work. These patients may need special attention during the rehabilitation process to assist with achieving their goal of returning to work.[56]

Functional tasks that simulate job activities are appropriate to incorporate into the program as the person's abilities allow. With higher-level functional activities, the art of designing activities that are task oriented and that help to develop the patient's problem-solving skills is the goal. Challenging patients' problem-solving skills and assisting them in the development of creative solutions when they are faced with new challenges is a rewarding and important component of prosthetic rehabilitation.

CASE EXAMPLE 1D

Assessing Outcomes of Initial Rehabilitation for a Patient with Traumatic Transtibial Amputation

Within 6 weeks of receiving his prosthesis (not quite 12 weeks after injury), P. L. is ambulating independently in the community without an assistive device, undeterred by environmental obstacles such as stairs, rugged terrain, or escalators. He has returned to work full time without having to request accommodations to his work environment or his job duties. He has just returned to practice softball with his team. Overall he is pleased with his current mobility but wants to return to his other athletic and outdoor interests as soon as he can.

Questions to Consider

- What outcome measures might be appropriate for use with this patient? Are there any other therapeutic goals that might be appropriate at this time?
- What follow-up is recommended for this patient? How frequently will he need to see his prosthetist, surgeon, and physical therapist? What guidelines can be given to determine when it is appropriate to return for follow-up?
- What is this patient's potential for further improvement in walking and for mastering other leisure or athletic activities that might be important or interesting for him? Are there other professionals or support groups that could be beneficial to him?

Outcome Assessment

Recognizing the impact of physical therapy intervention is an important component of the patient management model in physical therapy.[1] Outcome measures may focus on health-related quality of life measures[57] or on components of a disablement or enablement model. An important consideration in measuring outcomes as they relate to components of a model is to establish relationships between changes in different levels of the model.[58] For instance, within the Nagi model are changes in impairment level also reflected as changes in functional limitations or disabilities, or both? Impairment-level changes that may be measured in the patient with transtibial amputation might include increases in ROM, strength, or balance. Functional limitation–level changes might include improvements in ADL abilities, improved ability to transfer (less assistance or improvement in varied surfaces), or better ambulation (less assistance, change in assistive device or increased distance or velocity). Disability-level changes might include improved satisfaction with the ability to carry out specific life roles in the family or with respect to social, work, and leisure activities. Within the context of the International Classification of Functioning, Disability and Health model, introduced by the World Health Organization, it is important to understand how changes in body structure and function may relate to changes in activity and participation. Physical therapists are responsible for assessing and documenting the effectiveness of their interventions. They must always bear in mind that the overriding point of a rehabilitation plan is to return patients with amputations to the highest functional level attainable with the best possible outcomes.

CASE EXAMPLE 2D

Assessment of Outcomes for a Patient with Bilateral Dysvascular/Neuropathic Amputation

V. R. has done well with the gait and balance activities that took priority in the rehabilitation following his second transtibial amputation. With the assistance of his family, he has implemented a home exercise program to address his hip and knee flexion contractures. With occasional reminders from family, he has been consistent in using compression devices (shrinkers) for both residual limbs when he is not wearing his prosthesis. His family reports moderate success with the portion of his home program targeting muscle strength of his hips and knees.

As he approaches discharge after 8 weeks of outpatient rehabilitation, V. R. is once again independent in ambulation with his walker for distances greater than 150 feet. He can also ambulate in the parallel bars walking with one hand hold, perform "step ups" onto a low stool with each limb to facilitate weight bearing and balance, safely perform lunges on either limb, maintain unilateral stance for 10 to 15 seconds, and navigate a "mini obstacle course" designed to promote clearance on swing phase. Although V. R. can walk short distances with close supervision in the rehabilitation gym using bilateral straight canes, judgment, adequacy of postural responses, and overall safety continue to be issues. V. R. and his family agree that he will only use the canes at home when close supervision and assistance is available.

Questions to Consider

- In what ways might the prognosis, goals, and plan of care be similar or different for this patient with a second transtibial amputation, especially considering his concurrent cognitive decline? How could it be assessed how well each initial and long-term goal has been met?
- What is the recommended follow-up for this patient and his family? How frequently will he need to see his prosthetist, surgeon, and physical therapist? What guidelines could be given to him and his family to determine when it would appropriate to return for follow-up?
- What is this patient's potential for further improvement in walking and other leisure or athletic activities that might be important or interesting for him? Are there other professionals or support groups that could be beneficial to him?

SUMMARY

Prosthetic rehabilitation of patients with transtibial amputation is both challenging and rewarding. Early in the rehabilitation process, concern for the integrity of the suture line and skin is a major determinant of progression of time in the prosthesis and the types of activities that are appropriate. As a patient's residual limb matures, emphasis is placed on the quality of ambulation and on developing adaptive motor skills that enable the patient to function safely during various activities under many different environmental conditions. The diversity of patients with transtibial amputation requires that the therapist carefully consider individual circumstances to guide prosthetic prescription and progression of the rehabilitation program. Effective patient education strategies and opportunities for practicing various skills in various settings are essential for mastery of mobility skills and optimal outcomes for rehabilitation.

REFERENCES

1. American Physical Therapy Association. Guide to physical therapist practice. *Phys Ther* 2001;81(1):S31-S124.
2. Sackett DL, Straus SE, Richardson WS, et al. *Evidence-Based Medicine: How to Practice and Teach EBM.* Philadelphia: Churchill Livingstone, 2000. p. 1.
3. Kemp BJ. Motivation, rehabilitation and aging: a conceptual model. *Top Geriatr Rehabil* 1988;3(3):41-51.
4. Friedmann LW. The Physiological Rehabilitation of the Amputee. Springfield, IL: Thomas, 1978. pp. 109-140.
5. Frykberg RG, Arora S, Pomposelli FB, LoGerfo F. Functional outcome in the elderly following lower extremity amputation. *J Foot Ankle Surg* 1998;37(3):181-185.
6. Cutson TM, Bongiorni DR. Rehabilitation of the older lower limb amputee: a brief review. *J Am Geriatr Soc* 1996;44(6):1388-1393.
7. Munin MC, Espejo-DeGuzman MC, Boninger ML, et al. Predictive factors for successful early prosthetic ambulation among lower-limb amputees. *J Rehabil Res Dev* 2001;38(4):379-384.
8. Kisner C, Colby LA. *Therapeutic Exercise Foundations and Techniques.* Philadelphia: F.A. Davis, 2002.
9. Rose J, Ralston HJ, Gamble JG. *Energetics of Walking in Human Walking,* 2nd ed. Baltimore: Williams & Wilkins, 1994. pp. 45-72.
10. Moirenfeld I, Ayalon M, Ben-Sira D, Isakov E. Isokinetic strength and endurance of the knee extensors and flexors in trans-tibial amputees. *Prosthet Orthot Int* 2000;24(3):221-225.
11. Pedrinelli A, Saito M, Coelho RF, Fontes RB. Comparative study of the flexor and extensor muscles of the knee through isokinetic evaluation in normal subjects and patients subjected to trans-tibial amputation. *Prosthet Orthot Int* 2002;25(3):195-205.
12. Isakov E, Burger H, Gregori M, Marin C. Isokinetic and isometric strength of the thigh muscles in below-knee amputees. *Clin Biomech (Bristol, Avon)* 1996;11(4):232-235.
13. Nadollek H, Brauer S, Isles R. Outcomes after trans-tibial amputation: the relationship between quiet stance ability, strength of hip abductor muscles and gait. *Physiother Res Int* 2002;7(4):203-214.
14. Winter DA, Sienko SE. Biomechanics of below-knee amputee gait. *Biomechanics* 1988;21(5):361-367.
15. Powers CM, Boyd LA, Fontaine CA, Perry J. The influence of lower-extremity muscle force on gait characteristics in individuals with below-knee amputations secondary to vascular disease. *Phys Ther* 1996;76(4):369-377.
16. Snyder RD, Powers CM, Fontaine C, Perry J. The effect of five prosthetic feet on the gait and loading of the sound limb in dysvascular below-knee amputees. *J Rehabil Res Dev* 1995;32(4):309-315.
17. Powers CM, Torburn L, Perry J, Ayyappa E. Influence of prosthetic foot design on sound limb loading in adults with unilateral below-knee amputations. *Arch Phys Med Rehabil* 1994;75(7):825-829.
18. Nolan L, Lees A. The functional demands on the intact limb during walking for active trans-femoral and trans-tibial amputees. *Prosth Orthot Int* 2000;24(2):117-125.
19. Shumway-Cook A, Woollacott MH. *Normal Postural Control in Motor Control: Theory and Practical Applications,* 2nd ed. Baltimore: Lippincott Williams & Wilkins, 2001. pp. 163-191.
20. Nashner LM. *Sensory, Neuromuscular, and Biomechanical Contributions to Human Balance: Proceedings of the APTA Forum.* Alexandria, VA: APTA, 1990. pp. 5-12.
21. Gentile AM. Skill acquisition: action, movement, and neuromotor processes. In Carr J, Shepherd R (eds), *Movement Science: Foundations for Physical Therapy in Rehabilitation,* 2nd ed. Gaithersburg, MD: Aspen, 2000. pp. 111-187.
22. Miller WC, Deathe B, Speechley M, Koval J. The influence of falling, fear of falling, and balance confidence on prosthetic mobility and social activity among individuals with a lower extremity amputation. *Arch Phys Med Rehabil* 2001;82(9):1238-1244.
23. Miller WC, Speechley M, Deathe AB. Balance confidence among people with lower-limb amputations. *Phys Ther* 2002;82(9):856-865.
24. Gailey RS, Wenger MA, Raya M, et al. Energy expenditure of trans-tibial amputees during ambulation at self-selected pace. *Prosthet Orthot Int* 1994;18(2):84-91.
25. Hebert LM, Engsberg JR, Tedford KG, Grimston SK. A comparison of oxygen consumption during walking between children with and without below-knee amputations. *Phys Ther* 1994;74(10):943-950.
26. Gonzalez EG, Corcoran PJ, Reyes RL. Energy expenditure in below knee amputees: correlation with stump length. *Arch Phys Med Rehabil* 1974;55(3):111-118.
27. Ward KH, Meyers MC. Exercise performance of lower-extremity amputees. *Sports Med* 1995;20(4):207-214.
28. Brooks D, Hunter JP, Parsons J, et al. Reliability of the two-minute walk test in individuals with transtibial amputation. *Arch Phys Med Rehabil* 2002;83(11):1562-1565.
29. Cutson TM, Bongiorni D, Michael JW, Kochersberger G. Early management of elderly dysvascular below-knee amputees. *J Prosthet Orthot* 1994;6(3):62-66.
30. Redhead RG. The early rehabilitation of lower-limb amputees using pneumatic walking aid. *Prosthet Orthot Int* 1983;7(2):88-90.
31. Smith DG. General principles of amputation surgery. In Smith DG, Michael JW, Bowker JH (eds). Atlas of

Amputations and Limb Deficiencies, 3rd ed. Rosemont, IL: American Academy of Orthopedic Surgeons; 2004. pp.21-30.
32. Kosasih JB, Silver-Thorn MB. Sensory changes in adults with unilateral transtibial amputation. *J Rehabil Res Dev* 1998;35(1):85-90.
33. Kempczinski RF. *The Ischemic Leg.* Chicago: Year Book, 1985. pp. 553-568.
34. Melzak R. Phantom limbs. *Sci Am* 1992;226(4):120-126.
35. Carlen PL, Wall PD, Nadvorna H, Steinbach T. Phantom limbs and related phenomena in recent traumatic amputations. *Neurology* 1978;28(3):211-217.
36. Jensen TS, Krebs B, Neilsen J. Immediate and long-term limb pain in amputees: incidence, clinical characteristics and relationship to pre-ambulation limb pain. *Pain* 1985;21(3):267-278.
37. Houghton AD, Nicholls G, Houghton AL, et al. Phantom pain: natural history and association with rehabilitation. *Ann R Coll Surg Engl* 1994;76(1):22-25.
38. Weiss SA, Lindell B. Phantom limb pain and etiology of amputation in unilateral lower extremity amputees. *J Pain Symptom Manage* 1996;11(1):3-17.
39. Reiber GE, Boyko EJ, Smith DG. Lower extremity foot ulcers and amputation in diabetes. In Harris MI, Cowie CC, Stern MP, et al (eds), *Diabetes in America,* 2nd ed. Washington, DC: National Institutes of Health, 1995. pp. 409-428.
40. Campbell WB, St. Johnston JA, Kernick VF, Rutter EA. Lower limb amputation: striking the balance. *Ann R Coll Surg Engl* 1994;76(3):205-209.
41. Campbell WB, Ridler BM. Predicting the use of prostheses by vascular amputees. *Eur J Vasc Endovasc Surg* 1996;12(3): 342-345.
42. Lundsgaard C. Evaluation of patients with below knee amputation with respect to postoperative prosthesis fitting. *Ugeskr Laeger* 1994;156(49):7360-7364.
43. McWhinnie DL, Gordon AC, Collin J, et al. Rehabilitation outcome 5 years after 100 lower-limb amputations. *Br J Surg* 1994;81(11):1596-1599.
44. Casillas JM, Dulieu V, Cohen M, et al. Bioenergetic comparison of a new energy-storing foot and SACH foot in traumatic below-knee vascular amputations. *Arch Phys Med Rehabil* 1995;76(1):39-44.
45. Postema K, Hermens HJ, de Vries J, et al. Energy storage and release of prosthetic feet. Part 1: Biomechanical analysis related to user benefits. *Prosthet Orthot Int* 1997;21(1):17-27.
46. Postema K, Hermens HJ, de Vries J, et al. Energy storage and release of prosthetic feet. Part 2: Subjective ratings of 2 energy storing and 2 conventional feet, user choice of foot and deciding factor. *Prosthet Orthot Int* 1997;21(1):28-34.
47. Torburn L, Schweiger GP, Perry J, Powers CM. Below-knee amputee gait in stair ambulation: a comparison of stride characteristics using five different prosthetic feet. *Clin Orthop* 1994;June(303):185-192.
48. Torburn L, Powers CM, Guiterrez R, Perry J. Energy expenditure during ambulation in dysvascular and traumatic below-knee amputees: a comparison of five prosthetic feet. *J Rehabil Res Dev* 1995;32(2):111-119.
49. Legro MW, Reiber G, del Aguila M, et al. Issues of importance reported by persons with lower limb amputations and prostheses. *J Rehabil Res Dev* 1999;36(3):155-163.
50. Bullock BL, Rosendahl PP. *Pathophysiology, Adaptations and Alterations in Function.* Boston: Scott Foresman, 1988. pp. 698-700.
51. New York University Medical Center. *Lower Limb Prosthetics.* New York: New York University Medical Center, Prosthetics and Orthotics Division, 1983. pp. 134-138.
52. Radcliffe CW. Prosthetics. In Rose J, Gamble J (eds), *Human Walking,* 2nd ed. Baltimore: Williams & Wilkins, 1994. pp. 165-199.
53. Bandura A. *Social Foundations of Thought and Action: A Social Cognitive Theory.* Englewood Cliffs, NJ: Prentice-Hall, 1986.
54. Shumway-Cook A, Woollacott MH. Motor control: issues and theories. In *Motor Control: Theory and Practical Applications,* 2nd ed. Baltimore: Lippincott Williams & Wilkins, 2001. pp. 1-25.
55. Gailey R. *One Step Ahead: An Integrated Approach to Lower Extremity Prosthetics and Amputee Rehabilitation Workbook.* Miami: Advanced Rehabilitation Therapy, 1994.
56. Schoppen T, Boonstra A, Groothoff JW, et al. Factors related to successful job reintegration of people with a lower limb amputation. *Arch Phys Med Rehabil* 2001;82(10):1425-1431.
57. Jette AM. Using health-related quality of life measures in physical therapy outcomes research. *Phys Ther* 1993; 73(8):44-52.
58. Jette AM. Outcomes research: shifting the dominant research paradigm in physical therapy. *Phys Ther* 1995;75(11):39-44.

28

Transfemoral Prostheses

RICHARD PSONAK

LEARNING OBJECTIVES

On completion of this chapter, the reader will be able to do the following:

1. Describe the indications for, functional characteristics of, advantages, and trade-offs or limitations of the most commonly used transfemoral components and suspension strategies.
2. Compare and contrast the design, fit, and function of two common transfemoral socket designs: ischial containment socket and quadrilateral socket.
3. Describe the interaction of alignment stability, mechanical stability, and muscular stability on the control and function of the prosthetic knee in standing, during gait, and on uneven surfaces.
4. Describe the key influences on static and dynamic alignment in transfemoral prosthetic fit and function.
5. Identify the nine items that will cause variations in transfemoral socket fit and function.
6. Recognize the intraindividual and extraindividual causes of the most common transfemoral gait deviations, and suggest appropriate corrective action.

ADVANCES IN TECHNOLOGY

Advances in technology, materials, and prosthetic components have had a greater impact on the quality of life of individuals with transfemoral amputation than on any other level of amputation. As little as 10 years ago, ambulation in transfemoral prostheses was labored and often painful. Only the most physically fit individuals attempted to run with their prostheses. Now, socket designs better approximate anatomy of the lower limb, materials are friendlier to the residual limb, and dynamic prosthetic feet and knee components offer improved, energy-efficient function. The result has been a significant improvement in quality of gait, allowing more people with transfemoral amputation to walk comfortably and naturally with their prostheses. In addition, athletes with amputations can run in a natural "step-over-step" pattern with a higher degree of stability and comfort than previously possible.

This chapter presents information about current socket design and materials, the major types of prosthetic knee components, and the suspension systems available for individuals with transfemoral amputation. It also provides the reader with a strategy to assess fit and dynamic function and explains the major user- and prosthesis-related reasons for commonly observed gait deviations.

PROSTHETIC MANAGEMENT AFTER KNEE DISARTICULATION OR TRANSFEMORAL AMPUTATION

An amputation proximal to the anatomical knee joint is referred to as a *transfemoral* (above knee) amputation. An amputation through the center of the anatomical knee joint is known as a *knee disarticulation* (Figure 28-1). Individuals with knee disarticulation present with prosthetic challenges and functional advantages when compared with those with transfemoral amputation. The disarticulation residual limb tends to be long and distally bulbous, a result of the preservation of the femur and its condyles. Prosthetically, this creates a challenge in donning the prosthesis and cosmetically fitting a knee component. The bulbous distal end does, however, facilitate prosthetic suspension. The normal adduction angle of the lower extremity is more likely to be preserved, and the long lever arm of the femur facilitates control of the prosthetic knee. Also, as the proximal component of a weight-bearing joint, the distal femur tolerates end-bearing pressures within the socket.

In contrast, the transfemoral residual limb varies in length, depending on how much of the femur has been retained. The shape of the residual limb is likely to be a

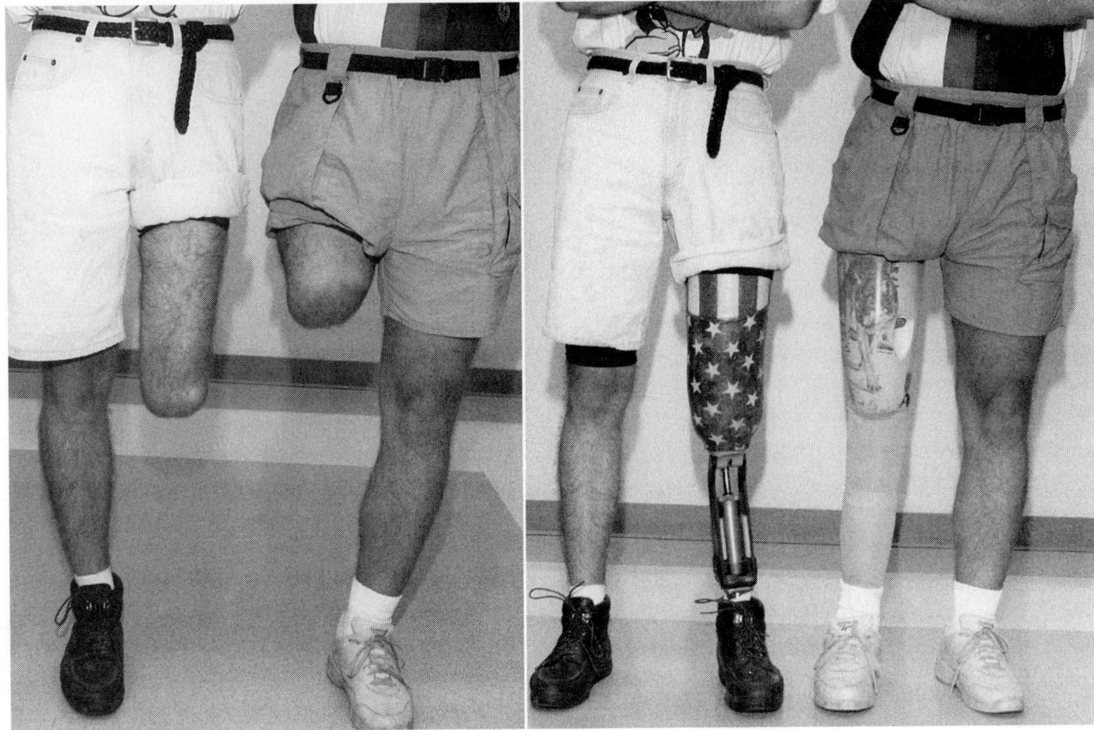

Figure 28-1
The similarities and differences in prosthetic fit and function between amputations at transfemoral and knee disarticulation levels are determined, to a large degree, by the length of femur that is preserved. ***A,*** *The knee disarticulation residual limb is long and bulbous, whereas the transfemoral residual limb is a tapered cylinder.* ***B,*** *In a knee articulation prosthesis, the center of the prosthetic knee is generally lower than that of the intact limb, whereas the knee center of most transfemoral prostheses matches that of the intact limb.*

tapered cylinder so that donning is less difficult. Suspension can be challenging, however, as a result of this cylindrical shape of the residual limb. The fleshiness of the transfemoral residual limb presents an opportunity for suction suspension. As the length of the residual limb decreases, socket suspension and control of the prosthetic knee (anatomical stability in stance) become more problematic.

The successful prosthetic management of transfemoral amputation and knee disarticulation involves providing a prosthesis that is comfortable in containing the residual limb, stable during the stance phase of gait, smooth in transition to the swing phase of gait, and acceptable in appearance.[1] In choosing components for an individual's transfemoral or knee disarticulation prosthesis, the prosthetic team must consider the interrelationships among the component's weight, function, cosmesis, comfort, and cost. Often, the most functional or technologically sophisticated components are also the heaviest, most expensive, most likely to need maintenance, and least cosmetic. Because of the great variation in physical characteristics and preferred activities of many individuals with high-level amputation, no single material, component, or transfemoral design is appropriate for all persons with amputation. The preferences and needs of each individual must be considered carefully, in the context of weight, function, cosmesis, comfort, and cost, for the optimal prosthetic outcome.

ENERGY EXPENDITURE

An individual with a transfemoral amputation faces significant energy expenditure when ambulating with a prosthesis (Box 28-1). The energy cost of gait increases significantly as the length of the residual limb decreases.[2-5] Fisher and Gullickson[6] report the energy cost of walking for healthy individuals (mean gait speed, 83 m/min) as 0.063 kcal/min/kg (oxygen consumption/physical effort) and 0.000764 kcal/m/kg body weight (oxygen cost/energy required to ambulate). Individuals with transtibial amputation walk 36% more slowly, expending 2% more kilocalories per minute and 41% more

Box 28-1 *Prosthetic Features That Affect Energy Expenditure*

- Weight of the prosthesis
- Quality of the socket fit
- Accuracy of alignment of the prosthesis
- Functional characteristics of the prosthetic components

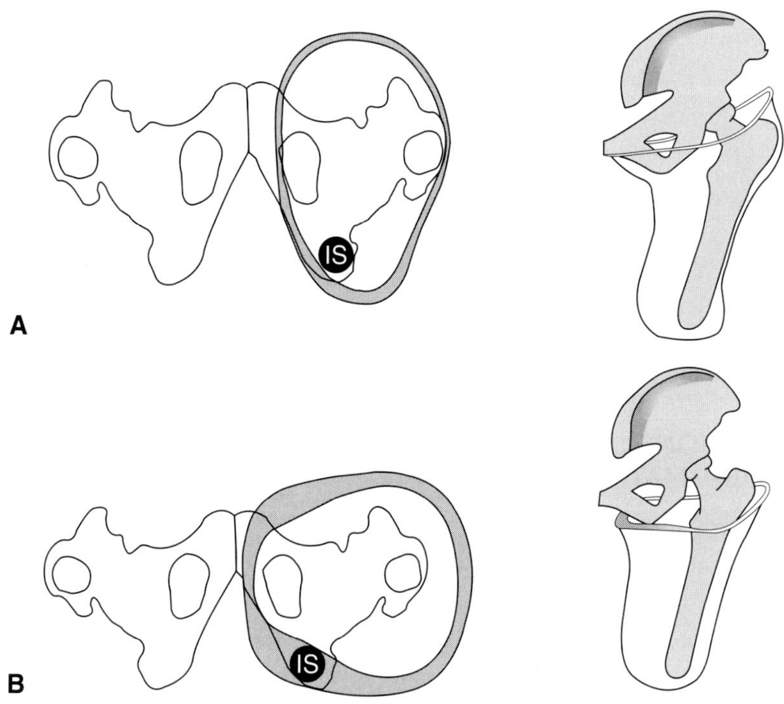

Figure 28-2

Comparison of the design of the quadrilateral (quad) socket ***(A)*** *and the ischial-ramal containment (IRC) socket from a posterior and transverse perspective* ***(B)****. The quad socket has a narrow anteroposterior dimension, and the IRC socket has a narrow mediolateral dimension. In the IRC socket, the ischium* (IS) *sits inside the socket; in the quad socket, the ischium sits on the socket brim (seat).*

kilocalories per meter to cover a similar distance. For individuals with transfemoral amputation, gait speed is 43% slower, whereas energy cost is reflected as 5% less kilocalories per minute and 89% more kilocalories per meter. In other words, the individual ambulating on a transfemoral prosthesis walks more slowly to avoid an increase in energy consumption per minute and is dramatically less efficient in terms of energy expended over distance (per meter). This increase in energy cost is manifested as a higher rate of oxygen consumption, elevated heart rate, and notable reduction in comfortable (self-selected) walking speed.[2,5]

Because of this high energy cost, many older individuals with amputations related to vascular disease may be limited in their ability to become functional community ambulators, instead of walking slowly with the assistance of a walker or cane.[5] Individuals with bilateral transfemoral amputation rarely become community ambulators with prostheses, instead choosing a wheelchair for long-distance mobility.

CONTEMPORARY TRANSFEMORAL SOCKET DESIGN

A significant evolution in the design of the transfemoral socket has occurred over the past several decades. Before the 1950s, prosthetists typically carved a "plug fit" socket from a block of wood, which, depending on the skill of the craftsman, was often uncomfortable and cumbersome while walking and sitting. The traditional quadrilateral (quad) socket, developed at the University of California at Berkeley in the 1950s, offered a notable improvement in fit and function and remained the socket design of choice until the mid-1980s. The quad socket, as its name implies, has four distinct walls fashioned to contain the thigh musculature and to allow the muscles to function at maximum potential (Figure 28-2, *A*).[1,7,8] A flat posterior shelf, the ischial seat, is the primary weight-bearing surface for the ischium and gluteal muscles. The anterior wall contours create a posterior-directed force at the anatomical Scarpa's triangle, which is intended to stabilize the ischium on its prosthetic seat. As a result, the socket is narrower in its anterior-posterior dimension than its medial-lateral direction.

The most recent design development, which has been evolving since the 1980s, is the ischial-ramal containment (IRC) socket[9] (Figure 28-2, *B*). The IRC socket is designed to stabilize the socket on the residual limb and control socket rotation by containing the ischial tuberosity and the pubic ramus within the contours of the socket. This socket also attempts to better maintain normal femoral adduction by distributing pressure through the socket along the shaft of the femur.[10,11] When comparing the IRC socket with the quad socket, the most obvious difference is the narrow medial-lateral dimension that is highly contoured to match the unique shape of the individual user's residual limb.[12] According to Long,[10] an additional advantage of the IRC design is that the wider anteroposterior dimension enhances muscle function by providing more room to accommodate contraction than possible in the crowded anteroposterior dimension of the quad socket. Currently, most prosthetists recommend the IRC socket, unless the individual with amputation is a prior quad socket wearer who has been satisfied with the comfort of the quad socket design. Radcliffe[7] suggests that, regardless of socket design, the primary goals of the transfemoral prosthesis are to achieve comfort in weight bearing, to provide a narrow base of support in standing and walking, and to accomplish as close to normal swing phase function as possible.

SOCKET OPTIONS: RIGID AND FLEXIBLE MATERIALS

Most transfemoral sockets are fabricated from various thermoplastic or thermosetting resin materials. A rigid socket consists of a resin-laminated or thermoformed plastic socket that is intended to have an intimate, total contact fit over the entire surface of the residual limb. Prosthetic socks are often worn as a soft interface between the socket and the residual limb. The rigid socket is durable, easy to clean, and often less bulky and less expensive to produce than flexible sockets. In contrast, it is more difficult to adjust the fit of a rigid socket, especially for individuals with "bony" or sensitive residual limbs.

The flexible socket is vacuum formed using any number of flexible thermoplastic materials.[13,14] It is encased in a rigid frame, which provides support during weight bearing and helps to maintain socket shape. The flexible socket accommodates to change in muscle shape during contraction and can be easily modified after initial fabrication to provide relief for bony prominences. Flexible sockets may also be more comfortable to wear, especially in sitting, because there are no hard edges at the brim to impinge on the groin. Flexible sockets are especially useful if suction suspension is desired. They are, however, somewhat less durable, more bulky to wear (requiring a socket and a frame), and more expensive to produce than rigid sockets.

PROSTHETIC SYSTEMS

A transfemoral prosthesis can be fabricated as either an exoskeletal or endoskeletal system. The weight-bearing strength and cosmetic shape of an exoskeletal prosthesis are provided by a laminated shell that incorporates the socket, shin component, and ankle block (Figure 28-3, *A*). This system is durable and requires little maintenance but cannot be easily realigned or adjusted. In the endoskeletal system, weight-bearing strength comes from an internal pylon that connects the socket to the prosthetic knee unit and then to the prosthetic foot (Figure 28-3, *B*). The cosmetic shape of the prosthesis is provided by a soft foam cover, carved to mirror the remaining limb, which is fit over the socket, knee unit, and pylon. This foam shell is, in turn, covered by several cosmetic stockings or a silicone "skin" to achieve the desired skin color. The endoskeletal system has two distinct advantages: The prosthetist is quickly able to adjust prosthetic alignment, and he or she can easily interchange or replace modular components. This is particularly helpful as new prosthetic users become more competent in controlling their knee unit or when advancing mobility leads to different functional needs (e.g., involvement in athletic activities). The durability of the foam and cosmetic coverings may be an issue for some prosthetic users, especially when work or leisure activities are physically demanding.

PROSTHETIC KNEE UNITS

The function of the human knee joint is difficult to replicate. Henschke Mauch, who developed hydraulic guidance systems for rockets during World War II, turned his considerable knowledge and creativity to designing a hydraulic prosthetic knee for veterans with amputations after the war.[15] He commented that it was far easier to design a large rocket with a guidance system capable of maneuvering hundreds of miles than to duplicate the human knee. The anatomical knee is a modified hinge-type synovial joint. The offset axis of the knee allows rotation in addition to flexion and extension, practically making it three joints rolled into one.[16] Because most prosthetic knees function in a single plane of motion, the action of the anatomical knee is difficult to fully replicate. As a result, it is more difficult for the individual who is using a transfemoral prosthesis to walk as efficiently and cosmetically as someone using a transtibial prosthesis.

Prosthetic knee mechanisms have two primary functions. First, to simulate normal gait, the prosthetic knee must smoothly flex and extend through the swing phase of gait. The speed or rate of shin advancement during swing is determined by the mechanical properties (friction or resistance) of the prosthetic knee unit. Second, the prosthetic knee must remain stable as body weight rolls forward over the prosthetic foot during the stance phase of gait. The major categories of commonly used prosthetic knee units vary with respect to how, and to what degree, they accomplish these two tasks. Various knee units are available in endoskeletal and exoskeletal versions. The recent advancements in microprocessor technology are changing and will continue to improve the functional characteristics of prosthetic knee units.

Single-Axis Knee Units

The single-axis knee (Figure 28-4, *A*) simulates a simple hinge and allows the prosthetic shin to swing freely in flexion and extension. Stance-phase knee stability is achieved by a combination of positioning of the knee unit with respect to the weight line (alignment) and muscular control (activity of hip extensors). This knee is lightweight, durable, and low

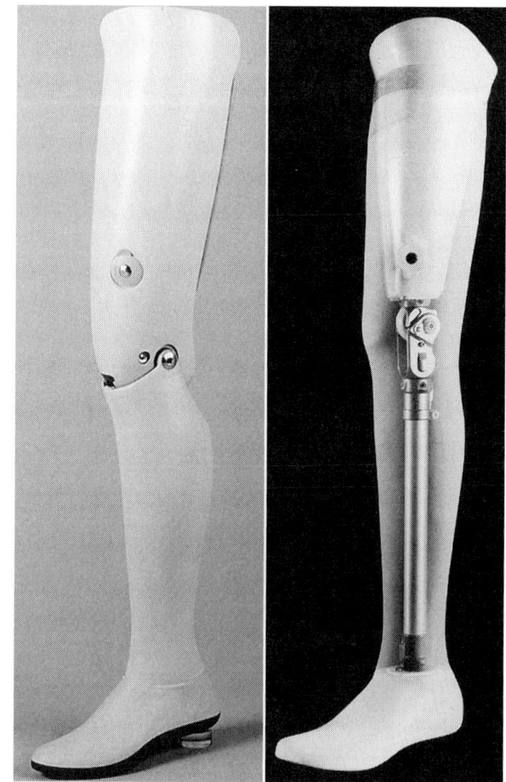

Figure 28-3
*Comparison of the rugged exoskeletal **(A)** and the modular endoskeletal **(B)** transfemoral prosthetic systems. (Reprinted from Otto Bock Health Care, Minneapolis.)*

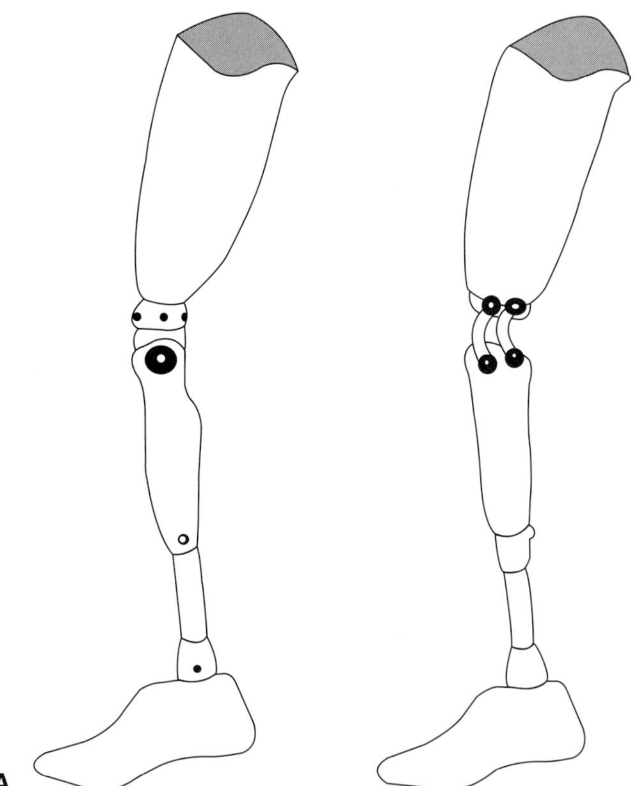

Figure 28-4
*Comparison of a single-axis knee **(A)** and a polycentric knee **(B)**. The single-axis knee has a solitary point of rotation, whereas the polycentric knee uses a four-bar linkage that provides a changing instantaneous center of rotation.*

maintenance, but because of its unrestricted movement, it has no inherent mechanical stability. For this reason, it is not appropriate for individuals with relatively short residual limbs who lack the mechanical advantage of a long femoral lever for muscular control of the knee unit or for those whose stability is compromised for other reasons. Although the rate of advancement of the shin during swing phase (determined by the resistance setting of the knee) can be individualized, cadence responsiveness is minimal once the resistance has been set. The shin of the prosthesis will swing forward at the same rate, regardless of gait speed. As a result, an audible terminal impact often occurs as the knee reaches full extension. To run with a single-axis knee, the individual must use a skipping pattern on the intact stance limb while waiting for the prosthesis to complete the swing phase and begin the initial heel contact. The single-axis knee is primarily for patients with long residual limbs who are able to voluntarily stabilize the knee through active hip extension against the posterior wall of the prosthesis.

Polycentric Knee Units

The instantaneous center of rotation of a polycentric knee unit changes through the range of motion (ROM) because of the linkage provided by its "four-bar" design (Figure 28-4, *B*).[17] In addition to simulating the anatomical axis of motion more closely, the mechanical characteristics of this type of knee unit enhance stance phase stability in gait. As the knee unit flexes during swing phase, the polycentric axis of motion leads to relative "shortening" of the distal prosthesis (shin and foot components), which enhances toe clearance throughout swing phase.[18] It is especially helpful for individuals with long residual limbs or knee disarticulation because the changing center of rotation allows the shin to tuck under the thigh when sitting, resulting in a more natural and cosmetic appearance of thigh and shin lengths. The polycentric knee unit's inherent stance phase stability also makes it an option for individuals who have short residual limbs or significant weakness of hip extensors. The major disadvantage of the polycentric knee, with its multiple mechanical joints, is its durability.

Weight-Activated Stance Control Knee Units

The stance control knee has a braking mechanism that is activated when weight is applied through the knee during the stance phase of gait (Figure 28-5). The intent of the braking mechanism is to prevent (or at least retard) unwanted

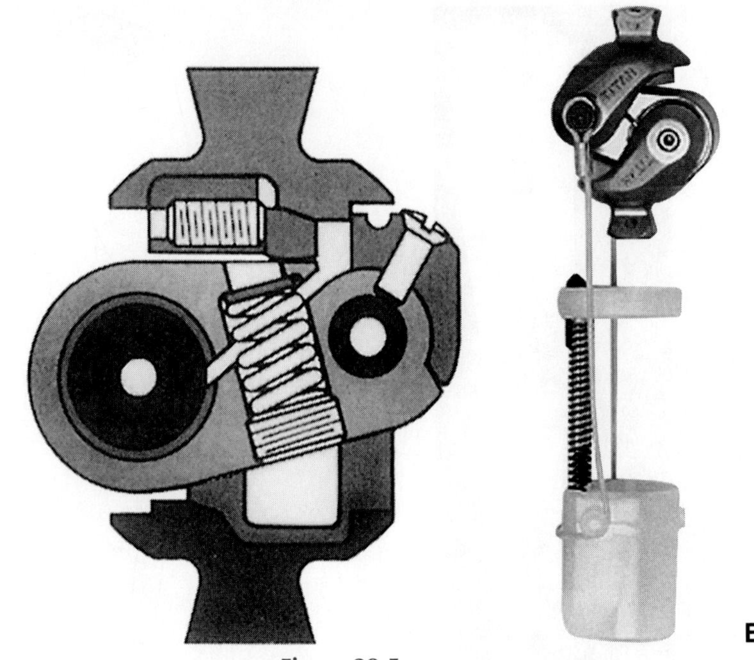

Figure 28-5

*A "cut-away" diagram (**A**) and photo (**B**) of a stance control knee unit for a transfemoral prosthesis. As body weight is shifted on the prosthesis in early stance, compression of the spring causes the cylindrical brake bushing to engage and resist the knee flexion moment associated with loading response. This braking mechanism provides stability even if the knee is slightly flexed during weight shift. When the knee is unloaded in late stance/preswing, decompression of the spring leads to "unlocking" of the brake, allowing free knee flexion for limb clearance during swing phase. (**A,** From Shurr DG, Michael JW.* Prosthetics and Orthotics, *2nd ed. 2002, Prentice Hall. p. 111. **B,** Courtesy Otto Bock Orthopedic Industry, Inc, Minneapolis, Minn.)*

knee flexion during stance. The sensitivity of the braking mechanism can be adjusted to match the individual's level of activity and ability to control the knee voluntarily. If initial contact is made when the knee is not completely extended, as when walking on uneven ground, the braking mechanism provides additional mechanical stability to keep the knee from rapidly buckling. During swing phase, the weight-activated stance control knee unit functions like a single-axis knee and has similar disadvantages. Advancement of the prosthetic shin occurs at the same rate regardless of changes in gait speed; minimal cadence responsiveness is present. This type of knee unit is most often prescribed for individuals who have recently undergone amputation and who have short residual limbs or nonremediable weakness of hip extensors and would otherwise have difficulty in actively stabilizing their prosthetic knees.

Manual Locking Knee Units

For patients who must rely on mechanical stability in stance, the knee of choice is often a manual locking knee. This unit is basically a single-axis knee with the addition of a locking pin mechanism (Figure 28-6). The pin automatically locks with a distinctive click when the knee is fully extended. Individuals who use a manual locking knee unit walk with their prosthetic knees locked in extension. Although a locked knee provides maximum mechanical stability in stance, it also significantly compromises mobility and toe clearance in swing. The prosthesis is often fit to be slightly shorter than the sound side limb to facilitate toe clearance during swing of the prosthesis. The prosthetic wearer can manually unlock the knee by manipulating a pulley or lever system attached to the outside of the socket. This unit is often used in the initial training prosthesis for patients when balance, endurance, or cooperation may be problematic.

Hydraulic Knee Units

Hydraulic knee units are cadence responsive; the forward progression of the prosthetic shin changes as gait speed changes. This is because the flow of hydraulic fluid through narrow channels within the prosthetic knee unit provides a frictional resistance, which increases with the speed of compression (Figure 28-7). This variable resistance permits a swing phase that more closely simulates normal gait. As gait speed increases, the shin of the prosthesis also extends more rapidly. Little swing-phase delay is experienced in knee extension as compared with strictly single-axis or polycentric knee units. This variable cadence characteristic has been helpful for both young, active individuals and older adults with mobility impairment.[19] This enhanced function, however, is associated with increased weight, higher maintenance needs,

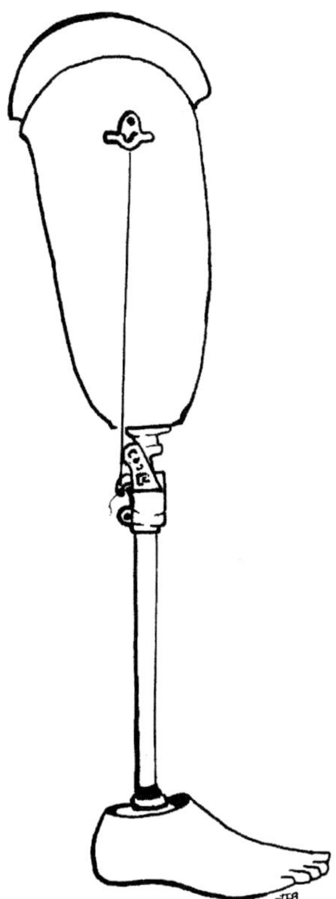

Figure 28-6
A manual locking knee provides maximum stability when the knee is in the locked position. The knee can be unlocked manually by manipulating a lever and cable system connected to the knee.

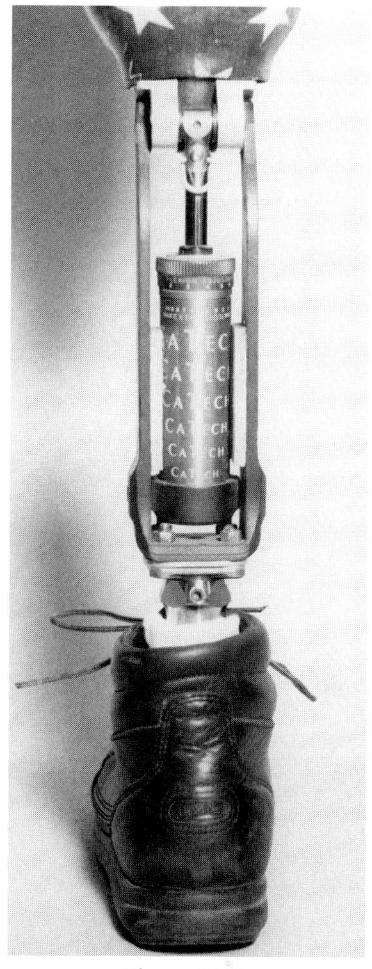

Figure 28-7
Example of a swing and stance, hydraulic, fluid-controlled knee unit. This type of hydraulic unit is fit inside the knee frame of an endoskeletal prosthesis or the shin section of an exoskeletal knee.

and higher cost. Additionally, with colder temperatures the knee may initially be slow to respond to changes in cadence until the hydraulic fluid warms up from typical daily use.

Some manufacturers offer a variation of hydraulic knee units that allow both variable cadence in swing and mechanical stability in stance (swing and stance [SNS] control).[15] Stance control occurs as a result of hydraulic resistance to knee flexion during weight bearing or by a braking mechanism that is activated by weight bearing through the prosthesis. This feature allows the individual to ambulate with greater confidence over uneven surfaces and also permits the use of a more natural step-over-step pattern when negotiating hills and going down stairs.

Pneumatic Knee Units

Pneumatic knee units offer the prosthetic user a varied cadence capability, using air pressure dynamics in much the same way that fluid is used in the hydraulic knee. Because air is compressible, the channels within the knee can be adjusted to affect the rate of swing. Pneumatic knees usually weigh less and are less expensive than their hydraulic counterparts; however, they provide less precise cadence control and require just as much maintenance. This is because hydraulic fluid is denser and has a higher coefficient of viscosity than air.[17]

Microprocessor Technology

The initial theory of microprocessor knee control was developed in Japan in the early 1980s. Charles A. Blatchford & Sons, Ltd, the developer of the Endolite carbon composite prosthetic system, collaborated with a Japanese electronics company to produce the first commercial application of microprocessor control in a transfemoral prosthesis. The microprocessor swing phase control knee is known as the *Intelligent Prosthesis Plus* (IP+).

Currently the most popular computerized system is the Otto Bock C-LEG (Computer-Leg). It is the world's first completely computer-controlled artificial limb. This prosthesis is powered by a rechargeable lithium ion battery with

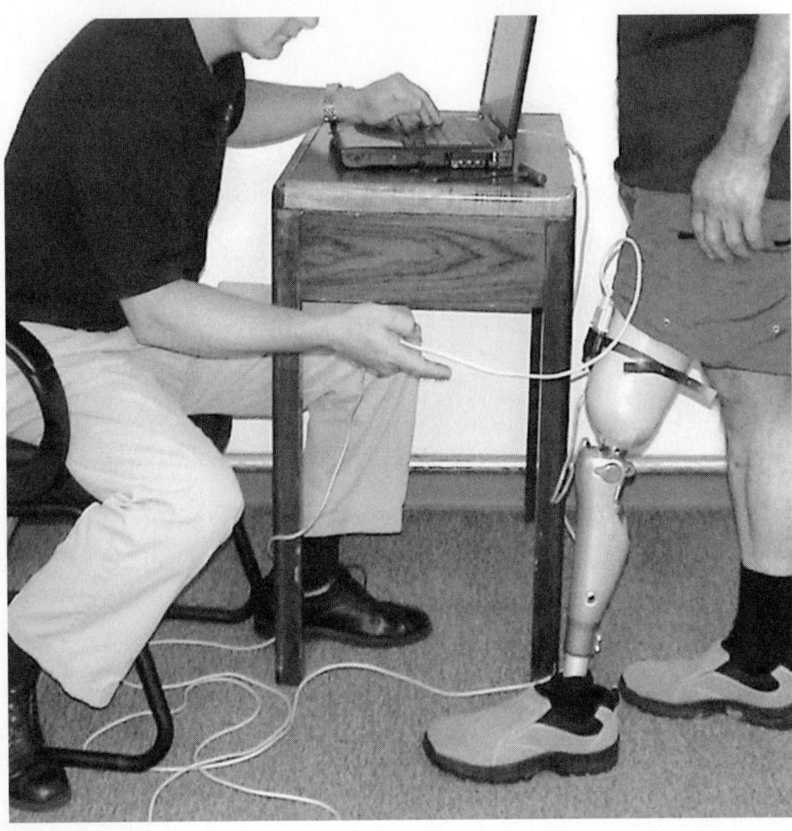

Figure 28-8

Customized stance and swing phase adjustments are made to the microprocessor knee using a personal computer.

25 to 30 hours of functional capacity. The C-LEG incorporates an on-board microprocessor, hydraulics, pneumatics, and servo-motors. A microprocessor controls the single-axis knee with hydraulic stance and swing phase control, as well as the automatic servo-adjustment of the hydraulic resistance valves. The knee position sensor and force sensor in the shin gather data at a frequency rate of approximately 50 times per second.[20] The microprocessor control of the C-LEG is based on kinematic and kinetic gait analysis and biomechanical studies. Electronic sensors in the C-LEG collect real-time data, which are then sent to the hydraulic damper to control stance and swing phase movements. At initial contact with the ground, the user may notice the added hydraulic stance stability, which prevents any unintentional bending of the knee that sometimes occurs when walking on uneven terrain. The microprocessor enables the patient with transfemoral amputation to move in a natural way, which makes it easier to walk downhill or down stairs.

Customized adjustments are made to the C-LEG using a personal computer (Figure 28-8). Unique software algorithms determine the phase of gait, then immediately adjust the knee functions to compensate during both the stance and swing phases of gait. The current disadvantage of microprocessor technology in prosthetics is the significant expense of such devices. The cost of an entire prosthesis that incorporates a computerized knee can be two to three times that of a prosthesis that features a hydraulic knee. The C-LEG comes with a three-year warranty from the manufacturer (Otto Bock Health Care, Minneapolis), including refurbishments and upgrades. As the use of such technology becomes more frequent in prosthetics, the cost of microprocessor-based knee units is expected to decrease.

Additional Components

For individuals who require assistance to initiate knee extension in early swing phase, an extension aid can be incorporated into the prosthesis. An extension aid is usually an internal spring or an elastic strap that recoils from an elongated position to accelerate the prosthetic shin into extension during swing. Extension aids may also be useful to control excessive heel rise in early swing phase.

Torque absorbers (axial rotation devices) are designed to simulate the rotation during stance, which would normally occur in an intact anatomical limb. In the absence of the ankle and knee joint, significant shearing forces can occur at the socket–residual limb interface as the prosthetic user pivots on the prosthesis. Torque absorbers are effective in reducing shearing and may be especially useful for individuals with fragile, sensitive skin or adherent scars. They are also often indicated for those involved with sports or work that requires them to negotiate uneven ground. Although

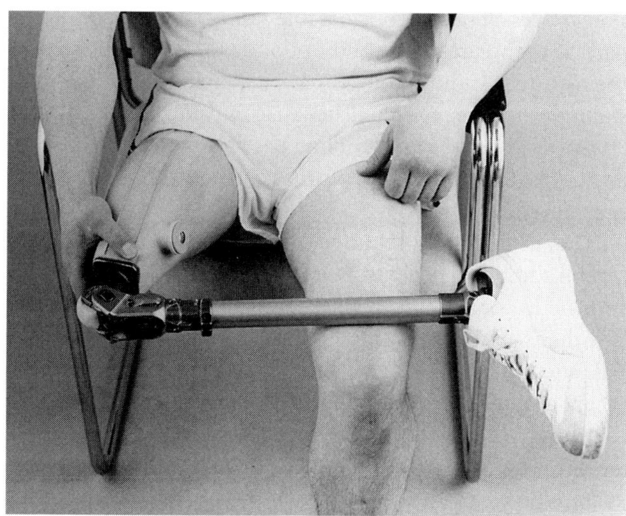

Figure 28-9
A transverse rotational unit is generally installed between the socket and the prosthetic knee. When the unit is unlocked, the individual can sit with legs crossed (e.g., to change shoes without having to remove the prosthesis). (Reprinted from Otto Bock Health Care, Minneapolis.)

these units reduce shear to the residual limb and increase comfort during functional activities, they also add weight to the prosthesis and are susceptible to mechanical failure.

Transverse rotational units have been developed to allow prosthetic wearers to passively rotate the shin section of their prosthesis passively (Figure 28-9).[21] An external button is pushed to unlock the limb, allowing a full 360 degrees of rotation. The unit automatically locks once the knee is moved back into its natural position. This type of device allows the prosthetic wearer to sit in a crossed-legged position, change shoes without having to remove the prosthesis, and enter and exit automobiles with greater ease.

CASE EXAMPLE 1

A Young Man with Multiple Trauma as a Result of a Motor Vehicle Accident

C. J. is a 23-year-old man who lost control of his motorcycle on an icy roadway 10 days ago, sustaining moderate head injury, traumatic amputation of the left lower extremity, and comminuted fracture of the right femur. On admission, he was taken to the operating room for debridement and closure of his amputated limb, and open-reduction/internal fixation of his fractured femur. Initially responsive to pain and voice, C. J. now fluctuates between level 4 (confused and agitated) and 6 (confused and appropriate) on the Rancho Los Amigos Cognitive Scale. C. J. is extremely agitated and combative while in bed but calms somewhat when seated in a bedside chair. He repeatedly requests to be allowed to get up to walk but cannot comprehend the need to limit weight bearing on the fractured side and doesn't seem to understand that he has lost his left limb. The rehabilitation team wonders if his cognitive function will stabilize and advance if he can be upright. After much discussion and debate, the team decides that C. J.'s residual limb is healed sufficiently for early fitting with an ischial-ramal containment socket suspended by a total elastic suspension belt, with a locking knee and solid-ankle cushioned-heel (SACH) foot. The team is hopeful that careful early mobilization into upright posture will reduce his combativeness without compromising his healing residual limb.

When elevated on a tilt table (with a 3-inch lift under the prosthetic side to maintain the non–weight-bearing status of the fractured extremity), C. J.'s cognitive function and behavior improve rapidly. Within several days, he can step off the tilt table and begin to ambulate, non–weight bearing on the right, using a walker for short distances with moderate assistance of one therapist. Over the next three weeks, he becomes independent with crutches and continues to use the locking knee until his fracture site heals enough to safely tolerate full weight bearing safely. The team anticipates that his prosthetic prescription will be significantly modified as he recovers from his head injury and is better able to learn to use and control a more advanced knee unit, prosthetic foot, and methods of suspension.

Questions to Consider:

- Why do you think that an ischial containment socket was selected for C. J.'s initial prosthesis? What are the advantages and disadvantages when compared with a traditional quadrilateral socket?
- Considering his current cognition and nonweight-bearing status, what are the advantages and disadvantages of the locking knee unit that the team recommends? Why do you think that they selected this option from among the other types of knee units that are available?
- Why do you think that the team recommended a SACH foot for C. J.'s initial prosthesis? What are the benefits and tradeoffs of SACH, articulating, or dynamic response feet for individuals with head injury in C. J.'s situation? (See Chapter 24 for detailed information about prosthetic feet.)
- Would an extension aide, torque absorber, or transverse rotational unit be appropriate at this point for C. J.? Why or why not?
- What are the implications for safety, energy cost, and cosmesis of gait when using a locked knee and a SACH foot?
- As C. J. regains cognitive function and the fracture of his right femur heals, what options might the rehabilitation team consider for his next prosthesis, in terms of socket design, suspension, knee unit, and prosthetic foot?

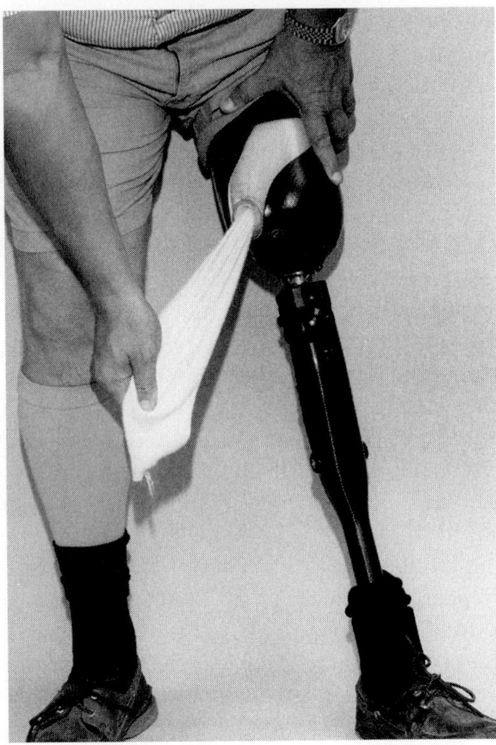

Figure 28-10
Patient donning a suction socket using a pull sock. The air expulsion valve has been removed so that the sock can be pulled completely out of the socket.

TRANSFEMORAL SUSPENSION SYSTEMS

Keeping the prosthesis on in its optimal functional position is more challenging for individuals with transfemoral amputation than with transtibial amputation. The transfemoral residual limb is fleshy and cylindrical, lacking the bony prominences that aid in suspending the transtibial prosthesis. The weight of the transfemoral prosthesis with the addition of its knee unit creates an additional challenge for adequate suspension. Five options for suspension are currently being used. Depending on the nature of the prosthetic wearer's normal activities, a single system or a combination of several systems may be chosen.

Traditional Pull-In Suction Suspension

Traditional pull-in suction suspension uses negative air pressure, skin-to-socket contact, and muscle tension to hold the socket onto the limb (Figure 28-10).[22] A suction prosthesis can be donned in several ways. One option uses donning sock (of cotton stockinette or similar material), donning sleeve (of parachute nylon or similar material), or elastic bandage to pull the residual limb down into the socket. Once the limb is well seated in the socket, the sock, sleeve or elastic wrap is pulled through the valve housing at the distal socket, and the air expulsion valve is then screwed back into place. This process requires considerable agility and balance on the part of the wearer. A second option is to add a lubricant to the skin (e.g., liquid powder) to facilitate the residual limb sliding into the socket. The air-expulsion valve is then "burped," by pushing or pulling the valve button, to release any trapped air. The liquid powder dries quickly, and suction is achieved.

The intimate fit required for suction suspension has several additional benefits: The wearer often reports enhanced prosthetic control and a better proprioceptive sense of the prosthesis during walking. Because an intimate fit is essential, suction suspension is inappropriate for patients with recent amputation who will continue to lose limb volume or for those with a history of fluctuating edema or unstable weight. The high shearing forces associated with donning a suction socket also may preclude its use for patients with fragile or sensitive skin, painful trigger points, or significant scarring or adhesions.

Roll-on Suspension Liners

Growing in popularity as a suspension system is the use of roll-on liners. These liners have become available as an alternative to the standard suction suspension system. Roll-on liners are manufactured from various materials, including silicone, urethane, and elastomer. They are produced by several manufacturers in a variety of sizes, thicknesses, and tapers.[23] Worn against the skin, roll-on liners are donned by first being turned inside-out, then rolled directly over the residual limb. The roll-on suspension liner creates a negative atmospheric pressure and somewhat adhesive bond to the skin. The liner can be used for suspension in three different ways: in a shuttle lock system, as part of a lanyard system, or as a cushion liner used with an air expulsion valve.

Shuttle Lock Systems

This liner is commonly called a locking liner. It is similar to the cushion liner except for a distal stabilizing matrix incorporated into the liner to prevent elongation. This liner also an external distal cap, the center of which a serrated pin screws into and sticks out approximately $1\frac{1}{2}$ inches. The pin engages into the shuttle lock, inside the bottom of the socket, when the individual stands and pushes his or her limb down into the socket. To remove the prosthesis, the individual depresses a release button on the medial aspect of the socket that disengages the serrated pin (Figure 28-11, *A*).

Lanyard System

This system uses the locking liner, but instead of a pin screwed into the liner's distal cap, a lanyard (cord) is attached to the cap and routed through the distal socket and used to pull the residual limb into the socket. The lanyard is then attached to the external lateral aspect of the socket via a locking hook or using Velcro (Figure 28-11, *B*).

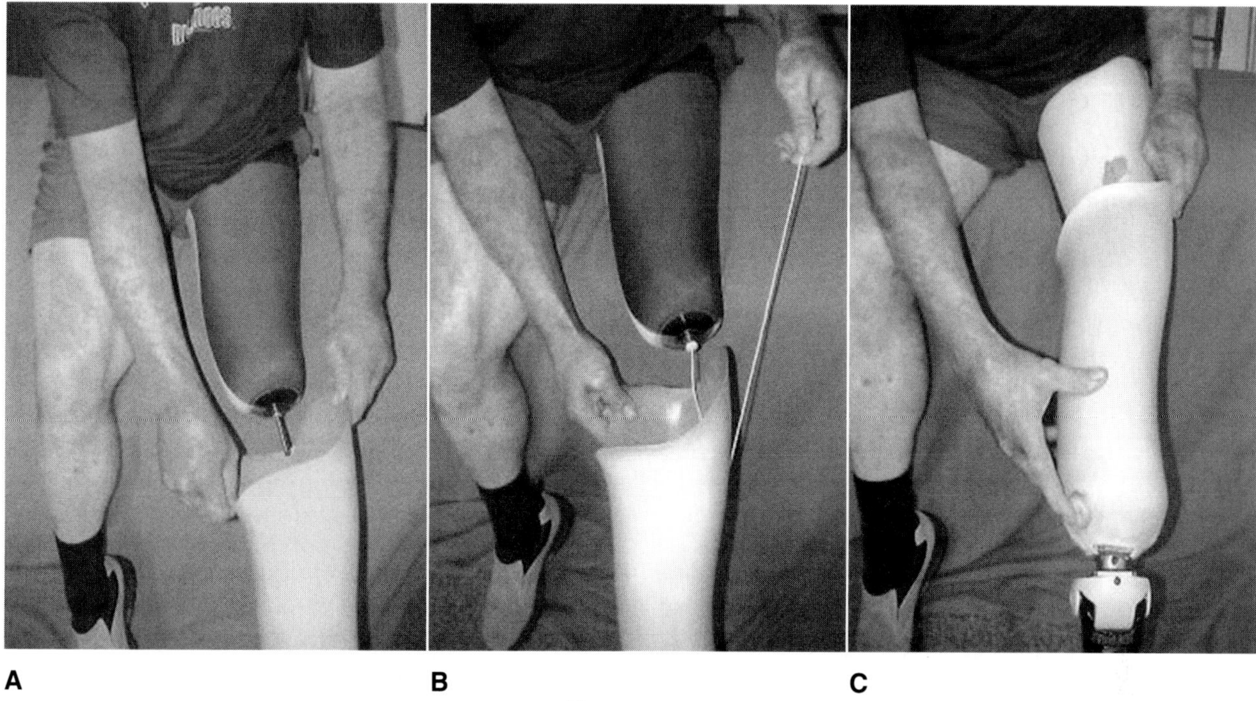

Figure 28-11

Roll-on liners are an alternative to traditional suspension. The liner can be used for suspension in three different ways. ***A,*** *A shuttle lock system uses a pin that engages into the shuttle lock in the bottom of the socket.* ***B,*** *The lanyard system incorporates a cord into the liner that is routed through the distal socket and used to pull the residual limb into the socket.* ***C,*** *An air expulsion valve system is similar to the traditional skin suction socket method. Once the liner is donned, the residual limb is pushed into the socket, creating a negative pressure environment by expelling air through the expulsion valve.*

Cushion Liner with Air Expulsion Valve

This type of liner is generally referred to as a cushion liner. After the liner is donned on the residual limb, it is pushed into the socket, creating a negative pressure environment by expelling air through the expulsion valve (Figure 28-11, *C*). This process is similar to the traditional skin suction socket method mentioned previously.

The major advantage of any type of roll-on suspension is a significant reduction in the amount of friction and shear on the residual limb.[24] The donning procedure is simple and can be accomplished while seated. This suspension system has been useful for individuals with short residual limbs and those who have experienced discomfort using the traditional pull-in suction method. The disadvantages of this system include its expense and durability. Roll-on liners become worn or torn and must be replaced two to three times a year depending on the wearer's activity level. Some wearers have experienced rashes or other types of skin irritation as a result of these types of liners. Wearers who choose this type of suspension must clean the liners daily to prevent the buildup of perspiration and bacteria.[25,26]

Silesian Belt Suspension

A Silesian belt is usually made from leather or lightweight webbing (Figure 28-12). It is attached to the lateral aspect of the socket, encircles the pelvis, and then runs through a loop or buckle on the anterior of the socket. The Silesian belt is most often used as an auxiliary (backup) for traditional suction suspension systems. The problem with choosing the Silesian belt as the sole means of suspension lies with its inability to control residual limb rotation within the socket. For individuals with long residual limbs who are not expected to be vigorous ambulators, the Silesian belt may provide adequate suspension.

Total Elastic Suspension Belt

The total elastic suspension (TES) belt is typically made of an elastic neoprene material. The distal sleeve of the TES belt fits snugly around the proximal half of the thigh section of the transfemoral prosthesis. The neoprene belt encircles the waist and attaches in front with Velcro (Figure 28-13). The TES belt is easy to don, comfortable to wear, and maintains

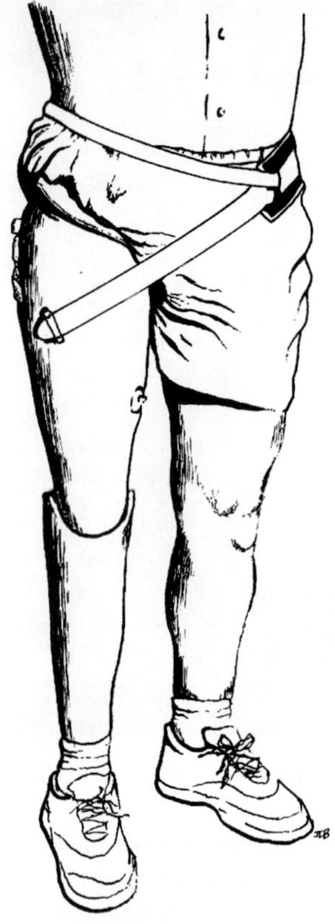

Figure 28-12
Example of Silesian belt suspension. Although the belt suspends the prosthesis to the pelvis, it cannot fully counteract rotary forces between limb and socket during vigorous walking.

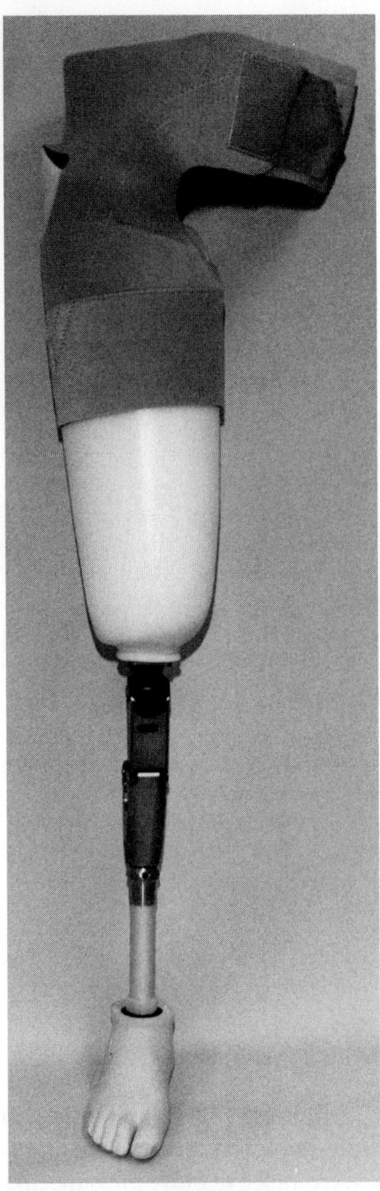

Figure 28-13
The total elastic suspension belt is a simple and comfortable suspension system that is often used as an auxiliary suspension.

good suspension with minimal pistoning between the limb and socket. It is an excellent auxiliary suspension system. This system is generally not recommended as a sole source of suspension for prosthetic users who are active ambulators, because like the Silesian belt, the TES belt cannot control residual limb rotation adequately within the socket. The major disadvantages of the TES system include its limited durability, especially for active ambulators, and its tendency to retain heat. It is often chosen for individuals with recent amputation whose residual limb has not yet matured to a stable size, for older patients who are unable to use the pull-in suction or roll-on liners due to upper extremity weakness or pain, and for those with easily irritated skin or adhesions who are unable to tolerate suction. It may also be used as a backup or secondary suspension system for individuals who use suction suspension when playing sports or engaging in high-activity leisure activities.

Pelvic Belt and Hip Joint

For some patients, a pelvic belt and hip joint are used as a means of suspension (Figure 28-14). Generally, the pelvic belt is made of leather and attached to the prosthesis by means of a metal hip joint. Recently, lighter-weight plastic materials have been used as an alternative to the metal joint. Whatever the material, the joint center should be positioned just superior and anterior to the anatomical greater trochanter. This system not only suspends the prosthesis but also helps to control rotation and increase medial-lateral stability of the residual limb within the socket. Traditionally, this has been the suspension of choice for those with short residual limbs. The major drawbacks of this type of suspension are its bulkiness under clothing, added weight, and tendency to be uncomfortable when sitting.

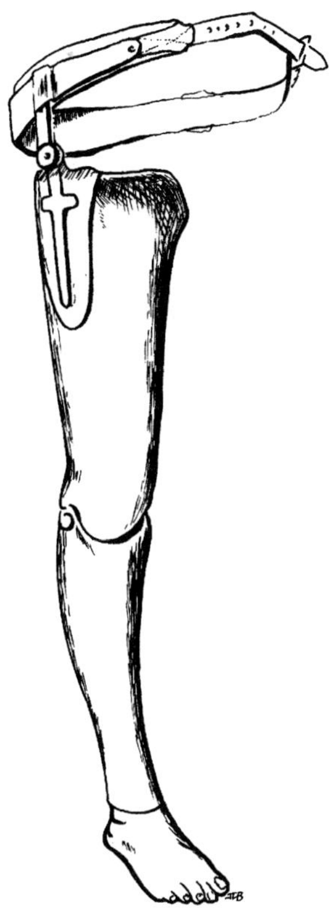

Figure 28-14

A pelvic belt with hip joint not only suspends the prosthesis but also helps to control rotation and increases medial lateral stability of the residual limb within the socket.

CASE EXAMPLE 2

A Grandmother Who Wants to Dance at Her Granddaughter's Wedding

T. F. is a 68-year-old grandmother wants to attend her granddaughter's wedding, so she comes into her prosthetist's office asking for assistance with her 6-year-old transfemoral prosthesis. T. F. underwent elective amputation 6 years ago when she developed osteomyelitis and nonunion of a communuted fracture of her left femur after being hit by a car. Although she was initially deconditioned, her rehabilitation was quite successful, and she returned to her home to live independently after a 2-month stay in a subacute rehabilitation setting. Previously, she smoked ½ pack of cigarettes per day, but she has not smoked since her injury.

T. F.'s residual limb is relatively short: 4½ inches as measured from the perineum to the distal end of her residual limb. She currently wears an endoskeletal prosthesis with rigid socket and prosthetic socks, a polycentric knee, and single-axis foot and ambulates functional distances by using a straight cane. For suspension she uses a pelvic band with a leather belt and hip joint, which is typical for those with her level of amputation. She complains that her prosthesis pistons on her residuum, is heavy and noisy, and pinches her when she sits. Her major goal is that she be able to "blend into the ceremony" such that her prosthesis will not be a distraction. She is also hoping to dance with her son and her new grandson-in-law at the wedding reception.

Her prosthetists consult with her physician and suggest the fabrication of a new flexible ischial-ramal containment socket in a rigid frame, with retainment of the foot and knee that she has been wearing. For suspension, the prosthetist recommends using a roll-on sleeve with a shuttle locking device. This suspension system will eliminate the metal pelvic band with leather belt and hip joint as well as improve suspension and decrease pistoning by means of the locking pin and high coefficient of friction of the urethane sleeve. The new socket and suspension system give T. F. better control of her prosthesis, allowing her to participate in all of the wedding activities without her cane.

Questions to Consider:

- Why was a pelvic band with leather belt and hip joint used for suspension in T. F.'s initial prosthesis? What are the pros and cons of this suspension system? Considering that roll on suspension was not commonly used at the time of her initial fitting six years ago, why did the team not recommend a total elastic suspension belt, Silesian Belt, or Suction Suspension?
- Why do you think the team decided to replace T. F.'s rigid socket with a flexible socket in a rigid frame? What are the advantages and disadvantages of each type of socket?
- Why do you think the team decided to retain the polycentric knee unit when they replaced her socket and suspension system? Are there other knee units that might have been appropriate for someone of her age and activity level? Why or why not?
- Why do you think the team decided to retain the single axis prosthetic foot when they replaced her socket and suspension system? Would you have considered a different prosthetic foot? Why or why not?

CHOOSING A PROSTHETIC FOOT

Individuals with transfemoral amputation and knee disarticulation can use any of the prosthetic feet and ankle options that are available (see Chapter 24, Prosthetic Feet). For someone with transfemoral amputation, one of the important considerations in choosing a prosthetic foot is its impact on stability of the prosthetic knee in stance. A foot that can reach foot flat quickly (e.g., single-axis or multiaxial foot) is preferable because it enhances stance phase stability.[17] Reaching foot flat quickly is especially important for individuals who have a short residual limb or weak hip extensors.

For active individuals, dynamic response feet (e.g., Flex-Foot [Flex-Foot, Inc., Aliso Viejo, Calif.]; Seattle Foot [Seattle Orthopedic Group, Inc., Seattle]) and those with flexible keels (e.g., SAFE II foot [Campbell Childs, Inc., White City, Ore.]) may have advantages. The energy-storing capabilities of these prosthetic feet at push-off promote rapid advancement of the shin section during swing phase. This enhances the ability of the individual who is using a transfemoral prosthesis to walk at faster speeds. Most of these feet are much lighter in weight than the articulating feet. Distal weight is one of the most important determinants of energy consumption for individuals using a transfemoral prosthesis.

GAIT CHARACTERISTICS IN TRANSFEMORAL PROSTHETICS

Normal ambulation is a result of dynamic symmetric relationships of the head, spine, and upper and lower extremities. With a transfemoral amputation, an individual's gait pattern wearing a prosthesis becomes significantly asymmetric, regardless of the functional characteristics of the prosthetic components.[27] The more asymmetric the pattern and uneven the cadence, the greater the energy cost of walking. Asymmetry also increases the demand for postural adaptation and balance reactions. For patients with impairment of musculoskeletal and neuromuscular systems, which are common among those with diabetes or advanced age, the incidence of instability and falls increases significantly.

In normal gait, the muscles of the hip, knee, and ankle work in three ways. First, muscle contraction provides stability during stance by resisting the effects of gravity. Second, during push-off and early swing phase, they act to provide propulsion and accelerate the limb. Third, they also act to decelerate forward progression, especially in late swing in preparation for subsequent initial contact. The loss of ankle and knee musculature as a result of transfemoral amputation compromises energy efficiency and quality of gait.

Knee Stability

The most important goal in transfemoral prosthetics is to obtain optimum knee stability throughout the stance phase. A prosthetic knee that is unstable or difficult to control during stance is a great danger and could lead to a serious fall. Alternately, a knee that is difficult to flex can cause problems with swing phase clearance, increasing the relative length of the limb and the likelihood of tripping and falling.

Three variables influence knee stability during stance:

1. The individual's ability to voluntarily control the knee using muscular power
2. The alignment of the knee unit with respect to the weight line (trochanter-knee-ankle [TKA] line)
3. The inherent mechanical stability of the knee unit

The relationship can be best understood by visualizing the TKA line,[28] representing body weight in stance (drawn from the greater trochanter to the ankle of the prosthetic foot), and considering the position of the knee with respect to the line (Figure 28-15). The most appropriate position of the socket, knee, and ankle components is the one that allows the individual to best use his or her muscle control with the minimum amount of alignment stability and still consistently stabilize the knee. If the prosthetic knee is positioned slightly behind the TKA line, so that the weight line passes anterior to the knee axis, the resulting extensor moment provides alignment stability during stance so that little muscular power is required. However, this alignment also increases the muscular effort and energy required to initiate knee flexion for the swing phase of gait. If the knee is positioned at or slightly in front of the TKA line, so that the weight line passes behind the knee, the resulting flexion moment decreases stance phase stability, making muscular power much more important. It also enhances the ability to flex the knee to initiate swing phase.

An individual's ability to voluntarily control the prosthetic knee is determined by the strength and endurance of muscles around the hip and by the overall length of the residual limb. If stance stability is provided primarily by voluntary control, hip extensors must be forcefully activated at heel strike to create an extensor moment at the knee. For an individual with a knee disarticulation or long residual limb, the long bony lever is a distinct advantage: An inverse relationship between length of residual limb and amount of muscular force necessary to control the prosthetic knee exists. With a long limb, less muscular power is necessary to control prosthetic knee extension or to initiate flexion in the early swing phase, and the prosthetic knee can be placed at or in front of the TKA line. For an individual with a short residual limb, much more muscular power is necessary to achieve the same level of control. For this reason, stance phase stability is provided by using a knee unit with high mechanical stability or by aligning the knee unit posterior to the TKA line. Voluntary control is also compromised for patients with hip flexion contracture, weakness of hip extensors, or physical frailty.

Prosthetists attempt to enhance muscular control by placing the transfemoral socket in a slight amount of flexion (in relation to the hip). Slight elongation of the hip extensors enhance their contractile ability just enough to develop an effective force (against the posterior wall of the socket) to keep the prosthetic knee extended (see Figure 28-15).[1,17] This also reduces the individual's tendency to substitute for the weakness of hip extensor muscles with excessive pelvic lordosis. The amount of initial socket flexion is determined by the initial available ROM at the hip joint. In preparation for initial alignment, the prosthetist sets the socket in 5 degrees of flexion, in addition to the number of degrees of flexion contracture that may be present.

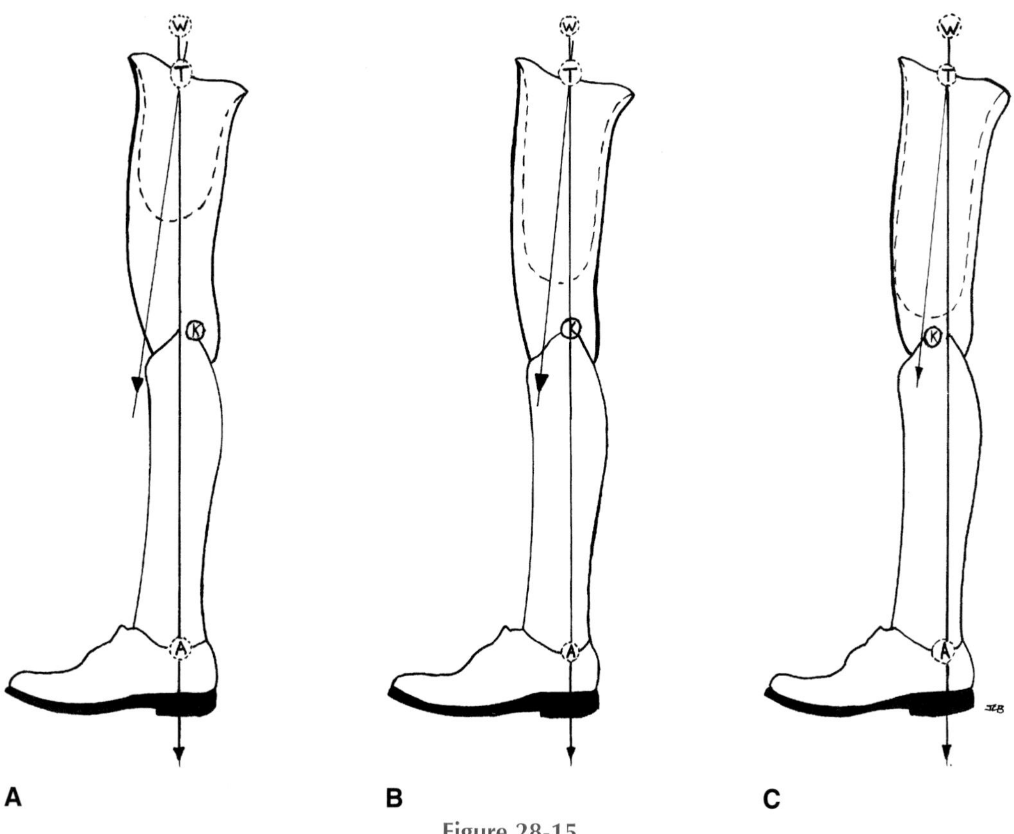

Figure 28-15

The imaginary trochanter-knee-ankle (TKA) line is a useful way to understand the components of stance phase stability at the knee. ***A,*** *Alignment stability is at its maximum when the weight line (W) passes anteriorly to the knee axis. This is often important for prosthetic wearers with short residual limbs or weak muscles or when initial socket flexion is increased more than the typical 5 degrees of preflexion.* ***B,*** *Alignment stability is minimal when the weight line passes through the center of the knee axis, making additional muscular or mechanical stability necessary. Many prosthetic wearers with midlength residual limbs and good muscular power benefit from the enhanced initiation of swing that this alignment provides.* ***C,*** *No inherent alignment stability is present when the weight line passes behind the knee axis; all of the stance phase stability must be provided by the mechanical characteristics of the knee unit or by muscular activity, or both. Prosthetic wearers with long residual limbs can best manage this alignment.*

The stability or, conversely, the mobility of the knee is further influenced by the mechanical properties of the prosthetic knee itself. The degree of inherent stability of the knee varies greatly among the different designs of commercially available prosthetic knees. A manually locking knee offers ultimate mechanical stability; therefore placement with respect to the weight line and muscular power is of lesser importance. At the other end of the continuum, a freely moving single-axis knee offers virtually no mechanical stability; stance phase stability must come from voluntary control, alignment, or a combination of the two. The mechanical stability provided by hydraulic swing and stance, pneumatic, and weight-activated stance control knee units fall between these extremes. Especially important is consideration of the contribution of mechanical stability for individuals with short residual limbs and weak hip muscles and those who routinely negotiate uneven or rough terrain.

Pelvic Stability

Because of transfemoral amputation, the direct anatomical connection between the femur and the ground surface is lost and closed-chain, medial-lateral stability of the pelvis is significantly compromised.[29-31] The femur, without its distal attachment at the knee, is susceptible to marked lateral displacement within the socket during weight bearing in the stance phase. This lateral shift makes it impossible to maintain a horizontal pelvis, even for individuals with strong hip abductor muscles, and results in an apparent Trendelenburg's sign and compensatory gait deviations. Pelvic stability is especially problematic for those with short residual limbs and those who have developed flexion, abduction, and external rotation contracture. The design of a quadrilateral socket primarily applies stabilizing forces in the anteroposterior plane so that there is little to keep the femur from drifting laterally within the socket. As a consequence, the pelvis

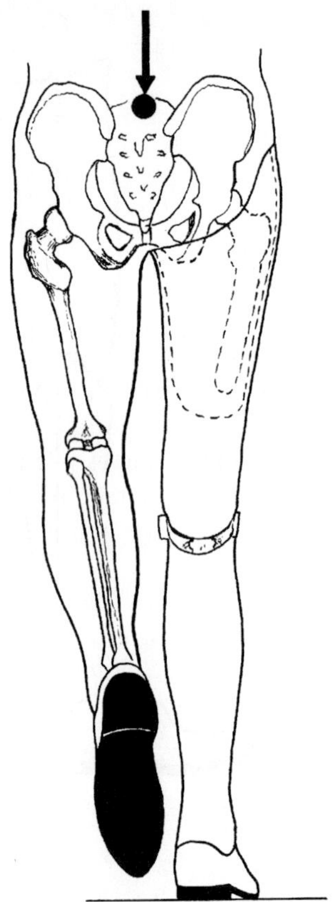

Figure 28-16
Lateral stabilization of the pelvis is maintained by positioning the femur as close as possible to its preamputation adduction angle (usually a mirror image of the intact limb). The resultant narrow base of support also significantly reduces the energy cost of transfemoral prosthetic gait.

drops when the intact limb is in swing phase. To compensate, the prosthetic wearer often leans or lurches laterally toward the prosthetic side. This strategy improves swing clearance but also results in a wide-based, energy-taxing gait. Because the femur is held in an abnormally abducted position, circumduction of the prosthesis during swing is likely to occur. In contrast, the design of the IRC socket attempts to hold the femur in its normal adducted position during stance with an upward and medially directed force along the length of the lateral femur. This strategy enhances the prosthetic wearer's ability to maintain a level pelvis and improves the quality of functional gait (Figure 28-16).

EVALUATION OF SOCKET FIT AND STATIC ALIGNMENT

Despite all the technological advances in prosthetic knee units, prosthetic feet, and materials, the single most important influence on functional outcome in prosthetics is the quality of socket fit. The socket is the interface between the wearer and the prosthesis. It must comfortably contain soft tissue when the patient is standing or sitting, furnish adequate relief for bony prominences, distribute stabilizing pressure to the femur and pelvis, and provide an adequate weight-bearing surface for the ischial gluteal region.

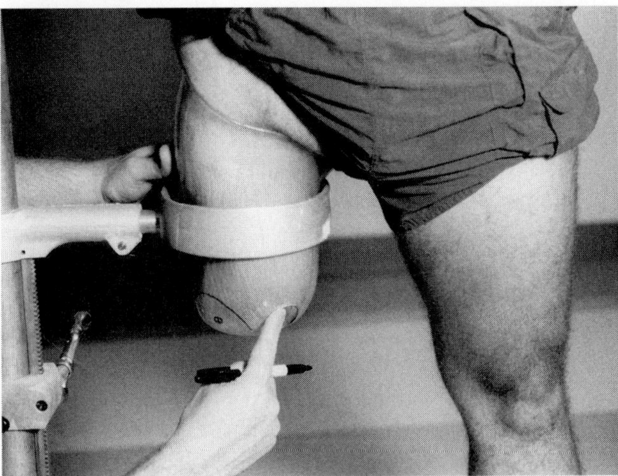

Figure 28-17
Clear diagnostic sockets are used to visually evaluate the prosthetic socket design. Inspection of the skin at the site of the suction valve provides information about adequacy of residual limb containment within the socket.

Transparent diagnostic sockets (test sockets) are routinely used to assess socket fit.[32] These thermoplastic sockets are molded over the modified positive model of the residual limb as an interim step in socket fabrication. They are often donned without a sock or over a thin nylon sheath so that contact with tissues and bony prominences can be clearly viewed (Figure 28-17). Areas of excessive or inadequate pressure can be detected according to the degree of skin blanching. To make necessary reliefs or to enhance total contact, corrections to the diagnostic socket are made by reheating the socket with a hot air gun or torch. The socket may be tried on and then modified several times before optimal fit and comfort are achieved. Once proper fit has been established, the diagnostic socket is filled with plaster or digitized to create a new, accurate positive model for fabrication of the definitive socket.

Donning Procedure

The first step in evaluation of socket fit is to ensure that the socket has been donned properly. If the socket is not positioned correctly on the residual limb because of being rotated or partially put on, its fit cannot be accurately assessed. Optimally, the socket fits easily but snugly over the residual limb. If too many plies of prosthetic sock are worn, donning is difficult and the person will feel as if the residual limb is not fully down in the socket. If too few plies of sock are worn, the limb falls more deeply into the socket and the person will feel medial socket pressure at the pubic ramus as well as a high degree of distal end pressure.

When suction suspension is used, the socket is slightly more difficult to don because of the relatively tight total contact fit that is required to maintain suction. Whether elastic wrap, pull sock, or liquid powder is used, the donning procedure must be consistent each time the prosthesis is donned. Before the air-escape valve is screwed into place, total contact between skin and socket is evaluated. The skin should protrude slightly into the valve housing; however, tissue should not be taut, bulging, painful, or discolored.

The size of the residual limb of individuals with recent amputation can vary if adequate pressure management has not been achieved. Inconsistent use of elastic shrinkers or elastic wrapping can lead to increased limb circumference. Even small increases in limb size can compromise the ability to don a prosthetic socket correctly and can significantly alter the quality of functional gait. The importance of the consistent use of a shrinker or elastic wrap whenever the prosthesis is not being worn cannot be overemphasized.

Total Contact Fit

Most prosthetic sockets are designed so that total contact is present between the skin of the residual limb and the socket. Total contact fit distributes socket pressure over the entire surface of the residual limb. Relief areas are used to reduce pressure over bony prominences, bone spurs, a neuroma, or other pressure-intolerant areas, but total contact is maintained. Total contact also promotes venous return from the tissues of the residual limb and helps to reduce edema. Wherever contact is inadequate, the residual limb is likely to become edematous. Over time, secondary skin problems are likely to develop as well.

Once the socket has been donned, it may be difficult to determine if total contact has been achieved or to locate precise areas of discomfort or excessive pressure. Placing a small amount of clay or powder or a thin film of lipstick inside the socket before donning can assist with assessment of fit. The person dons the socket as usual and then walks (or, if too uncomfortable, stands) for several minutes. When the prosthesis is removed, relatively even traces of the substance should be found on the socks (or skin) of the residual limb. Alternatively, lipstick can be applied to the sock (or skin for suction suspension users) over the area of discomfort before the prosthesis is put on. After donning as usual and wearing for several minutes, the prosthesis is removed and the inside of the socket is inspected. Traces of lipstick identify the area of the socket that requires modification for pressure relief.

Sitting and Kneeling

Most people spend more time sitting than they do standing or walking. How the prosthesis feels when an individual using a prosthesis is seated is important. The sitting surface of the socket should be contoured so that the soft tissue of the upper posterior thigh is not impinged between the socket and the seat.[12] To be comfortable in sitting and in kneeling, individuals with transfemoral amputation must be able to reach at least 90 degrees of hip flexion. If the anterior wall of the socket is excessively high, the brim impinges on the abdomen and the anterior-superior iliac spine (ASIS). For those who are using pelvic belt and hip joint suspension, care should be taken to avoid painful pinching of flesh between the socket and belt.

Another important consideration that relates to standing and sitting is the suspension of the socket. When a person wearing a transfemoral prosthesis sits down or stands up, gaps may occur between the posterior-lateral corner of the socket brim and the proximal residual limb.[12]

This lack of total contact causes a loss of the negative pressure environment that is required for maintaining proper suspension. One way to help prevent this problem is for the individual to take control of the prosthesis and not allow the muscles of the residual limb to go slack within the socket. The individual should expand the muscles of the residual limb, by an isometric contraction of the thigh, whenever going through the motions of sitting down or standing up.[33]

Evaluating Socket Fit and Brim Contours: The Quadrilateral Socket

For the quad socket, the brim shape is rectangular, with a narrow anteroposterior dimension (see Figure 28-2, *B*). The primary weight-bearing surface, the ischial seat, is located on the medial posterior brim. The seat should be widest at the posterior medial corner to adequately support the ischium and gluteal muscles. It should lie parallel to the ground. The overall height of the prosthesis is measured as the distance from this posteromedial corner to the ground with the knee in full extension. A channel for the adductor longus tendon is located at the anteromedial corner of the socket. The anterior brim is higher than the ischial seat as it moves toward the lateral wall. The contours of the anterior wall, at Scarpa's (femoral) triangle, provide a posteriorly directed force to maintain the ischium on its seat.

The medial wall is a flattened surface that represents the line of forward progression. The height of the medial brim is usually the same as that of the ischial seat, fitting well into the groin. It should not, however, create undue pressure on the perineum or pubic ramus. For a person in whom an adductor roll has developed, the medial brim should be flared to accommodate the extra tissue but not lowered. Excessive lowering of the medial wall can exacerbate the problem. The primary function of the lateral wall is to maintain a "normal" femoral adduction angle. This is often difficult to achieve in the quad socket because of the wide mediolateral dimension of the design. Pressure is applied to the limb by flattening the socket along the femoral shaft. A relief area is usually necessary to accommodate pressure sensitivity of the distal lateral femur. The lateral wall completely encases the greater trochanter and fits snugly around the gluteal muscles as the socket wraps toward the posterior wall.[7-9]

Evaluating Socket Fit and Brim Contours: The Ischial-Ramal Containment Socket

A proximal cross section of an IRC socket is more anatomically contoured in shape rather than rectangular, with a narrow mediolateral dimension (see Figure 28-2, *A*). This design more closely resembles the natural shape of the thigh. The brim of this socket captures more of the adductor muscle complex than the quad socket does. The ischial tuberosity and the pubic ramus are contained in a fossa well within the socket. This creates a bony lock that provides mediolateral stability and reduces the likelihood of socket rotation on the residual limb. The contour of the posterior socket captures gluteal muscles. No ischial seat is present because weight bearing occurs predominantly on the soft tissues of the gluteal region and medial aspect of the ischium.[10,11] Because stability is provided in the mediolateral plane, a buildup into Scarpa's triangle on the anterior wall is not as severe.

The medial wall of the IRC socket incorporates an adductor complex channel designed to contain all medial tissues. This minimizes problems with adductor roll pinching. The lateral socket wall is contoured in adduction, with additional pressure against the posterior shaft of the femur for added stability. A pocket hollow or fossa is incorporated into the lateral wall posterior to the greater trochanter for a snug fit against the lateral gluteal muscles.

Static Evaluation in Standing

When an individual receives a new transfemoral prosthesis, the prosthetist and physical therapist first evaluate fit in a secure standing position. Typically, this evaluation is performed with the patient standing within a set of parallel bars to provide upper extremity support and stability. In addition to evaluating socket fit, the static examination focuses on a level pelvis (to check the height of the prosthesis), knee stability, and the width of the base of support.

Height of the Prosthesis

Patients are encouraged to shift weight mediolaterally until they are comfortable with a symmetric standing position with relatively equal weight bearing on the prosthesis and intact limb. The prosthetist or therapist applies a firm downward force through the iliac crests to ensure equal distribution of body weight and then visually evaluates the position

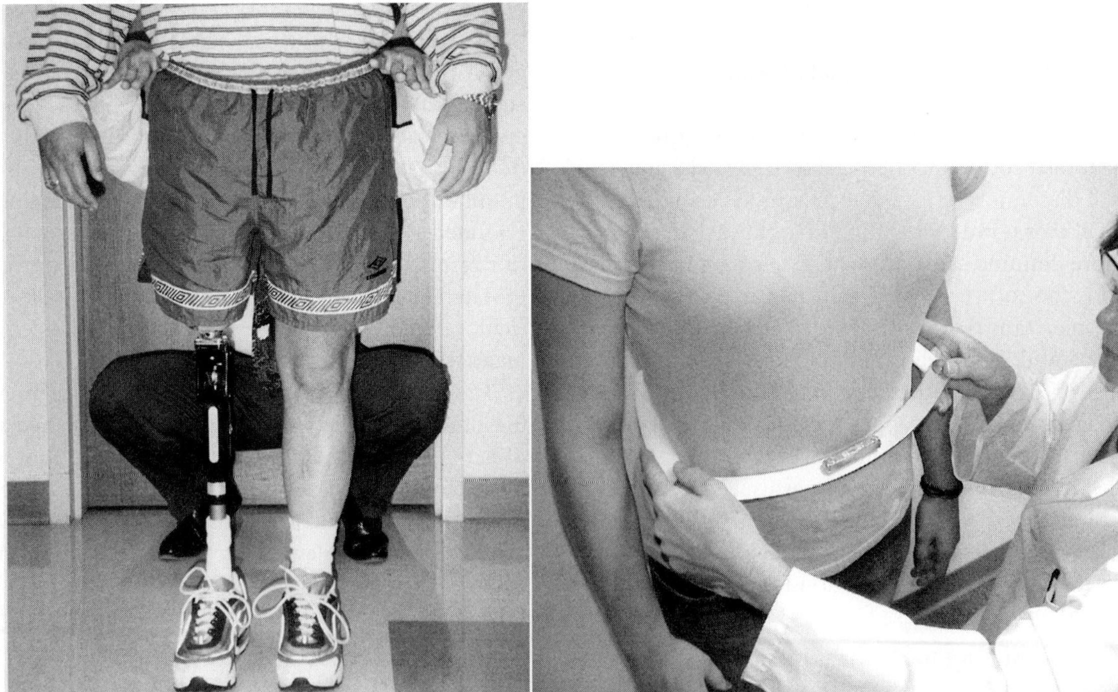

Figure 28-18

The overall height of the prosthesis should approximate that of the sound limb. ***A,*** *One method of checking for adequate prosthetic height is to assess whether the pelvis is level, by comparing the planes of the examiner's hands as they rest on the patient's iliac crests.* ***B,*** *A hip leveling guide is a device that uses a bubble level to determine if the pelvis is level. If the hips are level, the bubble is centered. If the pelvis is not level, the bubble moves off center in the direction of the longer limb.*

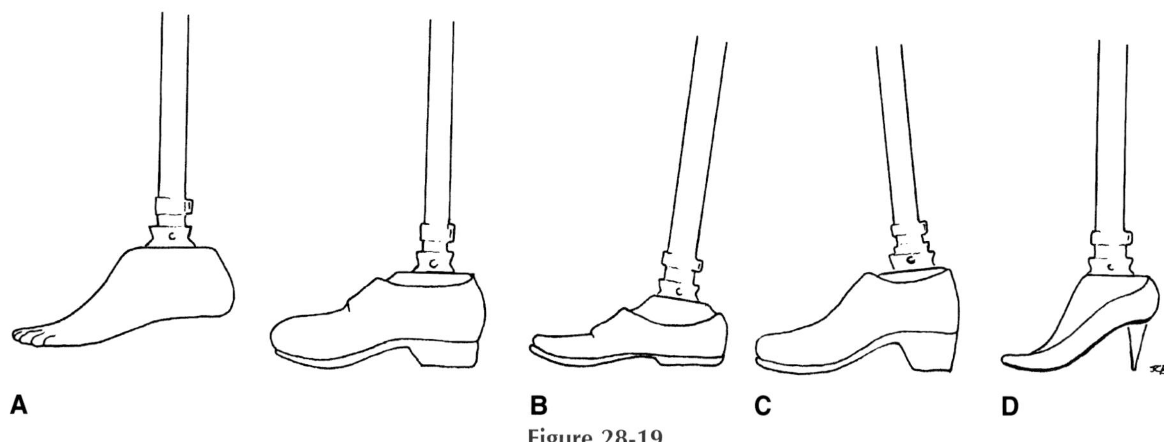

Figure 28-19

Shoes with differing heel heights affect kneel stability for individuals who are using a transfemoral prosthesis. ***A,*** *Most prosthetic feet are designed for a standard* $^3/_4$*-inch heel.* ***B,*** *Decreasing heel height creates an extension moment at the knee, leading to an excessively stable knee.* ***C,*** *Increasing heel height creates a flexion moment, leading to instability of the prosthetic knee.* ***D,*** *Special prosthetic feet are made especially for shoes with high heels.*

of the pelvis. Ideally the examiner's hands over the iliac crests will be in the same plane, and the pelvis will be level (Figure 28-18, *A*). Another way to evaluate this is by using a hip-leveling guide. This device, which has a bubble level at its center, is placed over the individual's iliac crests. If the hips are level, the bubble will be centered. If the pelvis is not level, the bubble will move off center in the direction of the longer limb (Figure 28-18, *B*).

The prosthesis may be up to $^1/_4$ inch shorter than the intact side to enhance toe clearance in swing phase. Leg-length discrepancy of more than $^1/_4$ inch leads to back pain, gait deviation, and higher energy cost in gait. The examiner can place one or more shims or boards (cut in various increments of thickness) under the "short" limb to determine the extent of the discrepancy if the prosthesis appears to be too short or too long.

Evaluation of Knee Stability

The examiner must recognize if the prosthetic wearer has a sense of security or fears that the knee will buckle under full weight bearing. It must be determined if he or she can easily extend the knee and maintain it in a stable position. Stability of the knee can be altered significantly if shoes other than those for which the prosthesis has been aligned are worn (Figure 28-19). Shoes with lower heels create an extension moment at the knee; the resulting stability is often excessive and can interfere with the knee flexion that is necessary in late stance and early swing phase. Shoes with higher heels create a flexion moment at the knee, reducing stance stability and increasing the likelihood of buckling or drop-off at mid-stance. Accommodating for higher heels is difficult unless the individual uses a prosthetic foot designed specifically for high heels.

CASE EXAMPLE 3

Why Should Changing Shoes Be an Issue?

P. O. is 21-year-old man who is learning the hard way about the effects of improperly changing heel heights. Having lost his leg just above the knee as the result of a motor vehicle accident two weeks ago, he is fitted with a transfemoral prosthesis a flexible socket in a rigid frame, total elastic suspension system, weight-activated stance-control knee unit, and dynamic-response Seattle foot while in the hospital. His knee unit is positioned at the trochanter-knee-ankle (TKA) line because of the long lever and muscular control afforded by his residual limb.

After only a few days of inpatient therapy and education concerning his prosthesis, P. O. is able to ambulate by using a straight cane in a fairly symmetrical step-through pattern. He often attempts to ambulate without aids, but whenever he does, his physical therapist stops him immediately and cautions him against varying from the therapy program until his residual limb is sufficiently healed and tolerant of full weight bearing on the prosthesis. At this point, he is able to tolerate up to 3 hours at a time in his prosthesis and is anxious to begin full-time "all-day" wear.

Despite his need to complete a therapy program, P. O. discharges himself from the hospital against his physician's recommendations. Before discharge, he is instructed on the care of his prosthesis, the accommodation of limb volume fluctuation, the way to properly negotiate inclines and stairs, and the impact of changing heel heights. He is also cautioned to gradually increase his "in prosthesis" time to minimize risk of skin breakdown or dehiscence of his healing suture line. P. O. ignores the booklets and instructions he receives. He wants to "get back to life," and 2 days after discharge he wears his favorite pair of high-heeled cowboy boots to go out partying with his friends. While negotiating the first step out of his house, his prosthetic knee buckles and he falls down the next two steps, fracturing the femur of his residual limb and cracking the frame of his socket. He is readmitted to the hospital for open-reduction internal fixation and eventually learns to ambulate with a swing-through pattern, using bilateral axillary crutches. He is discharged from the hospital after 1 week but is not able to return to prosthetic use for the next three months. He returns to physical therapy on an out patient basis to begin the process of prosthetic training once again. This time, he is more cautious and attentive to the instruction and advice of his rehabilitation team. His story now serves as a warning about "what not to when you go home" to everyone who attends the prosthetic clinic that assisted him.

Questions to Consider

- Describe the functional relationships among (1) mechanical stability of P.O's weight-activated stance control knee, (2) its alignment and position with respect to the TKA line, and (3) the length of his residual limb. How might the alignment of his knee unit be adjusted as his limb heals and is better able to tolerate forces generated during normal walking?
- What are the advantages of moving the axis of rotation of the knee unit forward with respect to the TKA line? Under what conditions would the prosthetist move the axis of rotation of the knee until it is behind the TKA line? What would you recommend for P. O. as he begins his outpatient rehabilitation after his fractured femur heals?
- Why would the rehabilitation team be concerned about the time P. O. spends in his prosthesis only 2 weeks after the amputation? What would be an appropriate wearing schedule for someone like P. O. who has been had an early prosthetic fitting? In what ways might the team's recommendation about in-prosthesis time be different as P. O. begins his second period of rehabilitation?
- Why did P. O.'s weight-activated stance control knee become unstable when he changed into his cowboy boots? What forces were acting at the knee at the time that it buckled? Is there anything he could have done to counteract the instability associated with higher heels?
- What would have happened if he had instead put on a pair of sandals with no heels at all? What types of functional problems might he have encountered during gait? How might he minimize the effect of changing to shoes with lower heels and preserve his functional abilities?
- What is the message does P. O.'s situation send to individuals new to prosthetic use?

Base of Support

The ideal distance between heels during comfortable stance is relatively narrow, approximating the normal base of individuals without amputation (2 to 3 inches). The prosthetic foot and shoe should lie flat on the ground with relatively equal weight bearing on medial and lateral borders. This can be assessed by slipping a piece of paper under both sides of the forefoot and rearfoot—the distances should be fairly equal. The individual must also be able to shift weight comfortably between the intact and prosthetic limbs. The adequacy of the suspension system is evaluated by asking the patient to lift the prosthetic foot off of the ground using a hip-hiking motion. Minimal pistoning of the residual limb should occur within the socket.

DYNAMIC EVALUATION

Once appropriate socket fit has been ascertained, a process of dynamic evaluation is used to customize alignment and make adjustments to components to optimize prosthetic function. The goal is to achieve a gait pattern that is safe, comfortable, cosmetic, and energy efficient. The individual's ambulatory history, strength, endurance, usual activity level and preferred activities, concurrent medical conditions or health issues, previous experience in wearing prostheses, and current goals are as important to consider as the prescribed prosthetic components. The dynamic evaluation may occur in the prosthetist's office, physical therapy gym, or prosthetic clinic settings. It begins with a walk down the length of the parallel bars. Having an assistant or aid guard or assist new prosthetic users as they walk is helpful so that the examiner can focus on gait characteristics. For a complete understanding of the dynamic interaction of patient and prosthesis, gait must be observed from lateral/sagittal and anterior/posterior perspectives.

Lateral/Sagittal View

Four key areas evaluated from the lateral perspective are (1) knee stability throughout stance, (2) transition from initial contact to foot-flat position, (3) symmetry of step length and step duration, and (4) quality of knee flexion during late stance and swing phase.

Stability of the knee is the major determinant of safety in ambulation. The new prosthetic wearer must learn to extend the hip at initial contact (heel strike) to stabilize the prosthetic knee adequately. Optimally, the knee will extend smoothly, with little hesitation.

Initial contact (heel strike) is the most unstable point in prosthetic gait. Stability in stance increases significantly when a foot-flat position is reached. The transition from initial contact to foot-flat position should occur relatively quickly and smoothly, with the goal of reaching a position that promotes knee stability without obvious "foot slap." Quality of prosthetic gait and commonly occurring gait deviations are discussed later.

Optimally, the prosthetic and intact limb's step lengths are equal in distance, symmetric in pattern, and even in cadence. The individual should have little hesitation in initiation of swing on the prosthesis or intact limb. Asymmetry in step characteristics impedes the momentum necessary for energy-efficient forward progression, increasing the work of walking significantly.

Step length and swing phase function are influenced by knee flexion during late stance phase. As the patient moves from midstance into initial swing, a controlled and gradual knee flexion must occur to provide adequate toe clearance during the swing phase of gait. Knee flexion that occurs too early compromises stance stability, whereas excessive knee flexion during swing causes rapid heel rise.

Anterior/Frontal View

When viewing gait from an anterior or posterior perspective, the examiner is most interested in adequacy of suspension, width of the base of support, control of the pelvis during prosthetic stance, and quality and pattern of the prosthetic swing.

Suspension can be effective only if it is donned properly and fit adequately to the individual. The examiner wants to determine if the prosthesis remains in optimal orientation on the limb through all phases of the gait cycle. Pistoning or rotation of the prosthesis should be minimal on the residual limb at any point in the gait cycle, but especially during unweighted swing. Because pistoning results in a relative lengthening of the prosthetic limb, patients must use a compensatory strategy to achieve toe clearance. One of the most common gait deviations observed when suspension is incorrectly applied or inadequate is circumduction of the prosthetic limb during swing.

Optimally, a normal narrow base of support and swing path is present with a 2- to 3-inch separation between feet as they alternate between stance and swing. A wide base increases energy expenditure and results in a less cosmetic gait pattern.

The pelvis should remain relatively horizontal during the prosthetic stance phase with a maximum drop of 5 degrees on the intact swing side for optimal cosmetic and energy-efficient gait.[1,7] For those with short residual limbs or weakness of hip abductors, a level pelvis is a challenge to maintain. In these instances, the pelvis drops noticeably on the intact limb during swing. A compensatory pattern, such as lateral trunk bending, can be used to assure adequate toe clearance of the intact swing limb. The frontal plane alignment of socket, knee, and foot plays a significant role in stabilizing the pelvis and trunk. This relationship is established by the prosthetist during diagnostic fitting and alignment sessions before delivery of the finished prosthesis.

The line of progression of the prosthetic foot and knee during swing phase is also assessed. Ideally the foot and knee move forward in the same plane. If the prosthesis has been donned improperly, evidence of a medial or lateral whip may be seen with the foot circumscribing with an inward or outward arc during swing phase.

Variations in Quality of Gait

The pattern and quality of gait with a transfemoral prosthesis can vary a great deal between treatment sessions, especially for those who are new to their prosthesis or have recently had a change in prosthetic components. Most often, these variations in performance can be traced to intraindividual factors, rather than to malalignment or dysfunction of the prosthesis itself. If unrecognized, some of these quite controllable factors can significantly impede progress in gait training and functional mobility. The most common problems encountered include inadequate volume control and edema management, continued shrinkage of the residual limb as it matures, inappropriate number of sock ply, inappropriate heel heights, skin irritation from overuse of a new prosthesis, improper donning, inadequate suspension, worn or loose components, and "patient innovation." Effective patient education and communication between the prosthetic clinical team and the patient can solve many of these problems.[33]

Edema and Limb Volume

For a new prosthetic user who is having difficulty with prosthetic fit and donning, one of the first questions asked should concern compliance in wearing compression garments. An increase in limb circumference after only 15 to 30 minutes without wearing a shrinker or compressive elastic wrap is common. The importance of routine use of a compressive garment whenever the prosthesis is not being worn (including overnight while sleeping) cannot be overstated, especially for those within 6 months of amputation. Even in an experienced prosthetic wearer, limb volume can vary over the course of the day. Adding or subtracting one or more ply of prosthetic socks at some point during the day is not unusual. For those who need the snug fit of suction suspension, edema is a serious problem that can prevent donning the prosthesis and achieving suction. In this case, the compression garment or elastic wrap should be applied for 15 to 20 minutes before donning the prosthesis again.

Maturation and Shrinkage of the Residual Limb

New prosthetic users often experience rapid reduction of limb volume as their time in the prosthesis increases over the first few weeks and months after delivery of the prosthesis. Although this limb maturation may require several socket adjustments until limb size stabilizes, it is a natural and important process that should be supported by the use of compression whenever the prosthesis is not worn. The loss of limb volume is usually accommodated by the need to increase the number of ply of prosthetic socks being worn to a 10- to 15-ply maximum. When more than 15 plies of sock are worn, intimacy of fit is compromised and a new socket should be fabricated. Traditionally, the use of suction suspension is not recommended until limb volume has stabilized. For those using suction suspension who experience further reduction in limb size (e.g., due to weight loss, increased activity, time in the socket), the prosthetist can add padding to the socket to restore the intimate skin-socket fit that is necessary to restore suction.

Inappropriate Number of Sock Ply

Because of the normal mild fluctuation in limb volume, the number of prosthetic sock ply that are required for appropriate fit also can vary from day to day and within the same day. New and experienced prosthetic users often carry several 1-ply cotton socks with them during the day so that they are prepared should adjustment become necessary. Individuals who are wearing too many ply of sock lose total contact with the distal portion of the socket, complain of tightness at the proximal socket, and feel as if the prosthesis is excessively long (this may be manifested as difficulty with toe clearance in swing). Those who have too few ply of sock experience increasing distal end pressure or discomfort in the perineum because they are seated too far down in the socket. New prosthetic users should keep a record of the number of socks and overall ply (thickness) they wear, as well as the frequency with which they adjust ply during the day. This helps them to better understand the dynamic nature of limb volume size and enhance proper care of the residual limb.

CASE EXAMPLE 4

Problem Solving When the Prosthesis Suddenly Doesn't Fit

A physical therapist calls a prosthetist colleague one morning to warn him that T. M., a businessman who recently sustained a transfemoral amputation as the result of diabetes, has called complaining about his preparatory prosthesis. T. M. had been comfortably fit with an ischial-ramal containment socket 9 weeks earlier without difficulty. However, he now reports that his socket is too small and he is not getting all the way down into his prosthesis. He is fearful that the tightness he is experiencing will cause skin breakdown, a frightening prospect for a person with diabetes. T. M. is wearing a transfemoral prosthesis with a stance control knee and dynamic response foot, and he is using a total elastic suspension belt with partial suction suspension.

The prosthetist and physical therapist set up an appointment with the patient for reevaluation in the physical therapy office the next morning. Their goal is to determine why T. M., who has been wearing his prosthesis in excess of 10 hours a day for 9 weeks, is just now complaining about the fit. When T. M. enters the clinic, he is obviously experiencing discomfort and is not shifting his weight equally over the prosthesis during the stance phase of gait. He has chosen to return to using bilateral axillary crutches in an effort to reduce his discomfort. The prosthetist and physical therapist ask T. M. to take his prosthesis off so that they can visually check whether any skin damage has occurred. They find only minimum proximal redness and tenderness over the hip adductors. The prosthetist inspects the prosthesis as the therapist examines her office notes from the man's last visit.

While watching the patient put on his socket, the physical therapist recognizes the source of the problem. During T. M's previous visit she had documented that he was wearing a three-ply sock over a 3-mm roll-on liner. Today he is donning five- and three-ply socks over his roll-on liner. When asked why he has increased sock ply, T.M. reports that since he had progressed from a liner-only fit to wearing an additional three ply in 3 weeks, he thought that by 9 weeks he should be wearing about eight to nine ply of sock. The prosthetist and therapist clarify with him the indicators of need to increase sock ply. The patient returns to using a three-ply sock over the liner and returns to the comfort he experienced before the arbitrary addition of socks. He is relieved to be able to ambulate once again without his crutches.

Questions to Consider

- What is the typical strategy for managing volume control and limb shrinkage in the first months following amputation? Is there a typical rate of maturation of limb volume that can be predicted? Why or why not? When might a new user expect that his or her limb will reach a stable size or volume?
- What are the indicators that additional sock ply is necessary in the first months of prosthetic wear? What must a new prosthetic wearer understand to adjust sock ply appropriately? How can the therapist or prosthetist help a new prosthetic wearer master the art of changing sock ply to adjust prosthetic fit?
- How would T. M.s complaints about fitting be different if he were wearing too few prosthetic socks?
- How many sock ply must a new user be wearing before it is time for the prosthetist to fabricate a new socket? What other indicators might there be that it is time for a change in socket or suspension?
- How might improper socket fit (whether too many or too few socks are worn) affect the prosthetic wearer's stability in stance and mobility during swing phase of gait?

Changing Footwear: Improper Heel Heights

All prosthetic feet are designed to be worn with shoes of a particular heel height (see Figure 28-19). They are available in various heel heights, ranging from a heel rise of 0 mm for sandals and flats to a 45-mm heel rise for women's high heels. Matching the heel rise of the prosthetic foot to the shoes that are most often worn by the patient is essential. A heel wedge placed inside the shoe can be used to accommodate for the occasional use of shoes with slightly lower heels. Change to a shoe with significantly lower heels results in excessive knee stability in stance. Conversely, a change to shoes with much higher heels compromises alignment stability of the knee and places much greater demand on the patient for muscular control of knee position during stance.

Impact of Overuse

Whether learning to use a training prosthesis for the first time since amputation or being fit with a new definitive prosthesis, most prosthetic users benefit from a gradual break-in period. This strategy allows the skin, soft tissue, and musculature to grow accustomed to the forces acting on the residual limb. Failure to adhere to such a plan can lead to muscle soreness, skin irritation, and, in some cases, skin breakdown. New users should be advised to increase the length of time in their prosthesis gradually, carefully inspecting their skin each time the prosthesis is removed and wearing an appropriate compression garment when not in the prosthesis.

Improper Donning

When a prosthesis is not properly oriented on the residual limb as a result of improper donning technique or incomplete donning, it cannot operate efficiently. The wearer may experience discomfort within the socket or may exhibit various gait deviations. Emphasis on developing a careful systematic method of donning is essential when working with new prosthetic wearers. Attention to details when donning the prosthesis can minimize the frustration, inconvenience, and discomfort of having to reapply the prosthesis multiple times until the desired position is achieved.

Inadequate Suspension

Inadequately tightened or badly worn suspension straps, belts, or Velcro closures should be suspected when the wearer experiences pistoning of the residual limb within the socket. The prosthesis drops down slightly when it is unweighted during swing, resulting in a relatively longer swing limb and challenging toe clearance. Additionally, the prosthesis may rotate on the residual limb, leading to various compensatory gait deviations. New prosthetic users should be encouraged to assess the adequacy of suspension carefully and systematically each time they don the prosthesis. All prosthetic users must periodically inspect belts, straps, or Velcro closures for signs of fraying, stretching, or significant wear and tear.

Worn or Loosened Components

As for any mechanical device that is subjected to daily use, the prosthesis should be periodically inspected for signs of excessive wear or loosening of the components. Periodic maintenance check-ups with the prosthetist should be scheduled, especially if the prosthetic wearer is involved in physically demanding leisure or work activities. In some circumstances, the prosthesis may be misused or abused, increasing the likelihood of damage to prosthetic components. Fixing a small problem in the making is much less expensive than having to replace major components or fabricate a new prosthesis because of complete mechanical failure.

Patient Innovation

Prosthetic users who do not fully understand the intricate alignment and design specifics of their prostheses may attempt to modify them. If a patient who has been progressing well in gait training and compliant with compression strategies suddenly has difficulty with socket fit, patient innovation should be suspected. It may be that padding has been added or removed from inside the socket. If knee stability has suddenly changed without any change in footwear, the wearer may have attempted to fine-tune alignment or knee unit function. Individuals who have questions about alignment (including most physical therapists) should not make random small alignment adjustments, but instead rely on the knowledge, equipment, and skilled experience of the prosthetist if adjustment is necessary.

QUALITY OF TRANSFEMORAL PROSTHETIC GAIT

The goal of a well-designed and accurately fit transfemoral prosthesis is an energy-efficient gait in as natural a pattern as possible. Quality of gait is inconsistent early in the gait-training phase but improves as the individual becomes more experienced with the prosthesis during therapy. If gait problems persist, especially if the risk of instability and falls or skin irritation is present, the source of the problem should be identified, and an attempt made to correct it. A number of classic transfemoral prosthetic gait problems may be the result of prosthetic malalignment. Before changing alignment or adjusting mechanical settings of the prosthetic knee or foot, it is wise to rule out patient-related factors (e.g., hip flexion contracture, weakness, habit) as potential contributors.

Problems in Early Stance Phase

At initial contact, the prosthetic knee should be fully extended to position the prosthetic foot appropriately for smooth loading as body weight is transferred onto the prosthesis. As loading occurs, the prosthetic foot rolls smoothly into a foot-flat position. Problems with either of these functions increase the risk of instability and shorten the swing time and step length of the contralateral limb.

Knee Instability: Initial Contact to Midstance

If the prosthetic knee is unable to maintain the necessary extension as the heel strikes the ground and the prosthesis

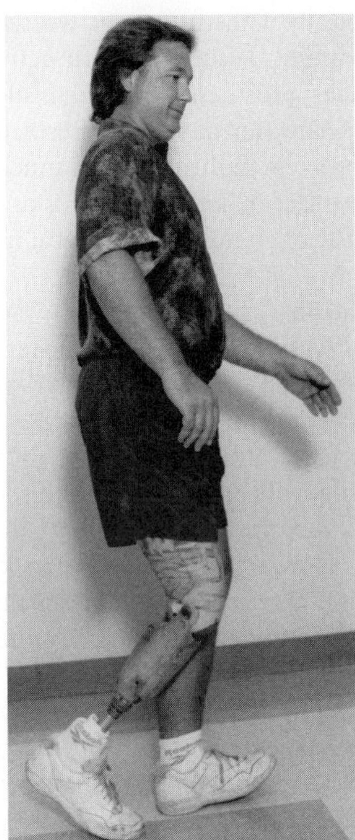

Figure 28-20

An unstable prosthetic knee during stance phase often results in a quick, short step taken by the sound limb. The problem may be due to patient factors (e.g., hip extensor weakness, hip flexion contracture) or inappropriate alignment of the prosthetic knee, anterior to the trochanter-knee-ankle line. If the knee is unstable, the opposite swing phase (stride length) is necessarily shortened to regain postural stability.

is loaded, several possible prosthetic and patient-related factors should be considered (Figure 28-20). The most common patient-related problems that lead to knee instability at initial contact include significant hip flexion contracture or weakness of hip extensor muscles, which compromise the patient's ability to stabilize the prosthetic knee by using active hip extension. If strength and ROM are adequate, four different prosthetic factors might lead to knee instability:

1. The knee axis may be aligned too far anterior to the TKA line, promoting a flexion moment.
2. The socket may not have been set in the optimal preflexed position, which places the hip extensor muscles at a biomechanical advantage for stabilizing the knee.
3. The prosthetic foot may have been aligned in excessive dorsiflexion.
4. The plantar flexion bumper or SACH heel may be too stiff.

Foot Slap

The speed that the prosthetic foot descends to the floor is determined by the durometer of the heel cushion or stiffness of the plantar flexion bumper and by how quickly or forcefully the individual loads the heel of the foot. If the prosthetic foot functions with an apparent foot slap, two factors should be considered. The heel cushion or plantar flexion bumper may be too soft for the user's weight and activity level. Alternatively, those prosthetic wearers who are fearful of instability in the early stance phase may be forcefully driving their heels into the ground to ensure complete knee extension. For those using a locking knee component, the ability to reach a foot-flat position quickly is essential for a smooth transition throughout the stance phase of gait. For most other knee units, the goal is to strike a balance between cosmesis and function.

External Rotation of the Prosthetic Foot

One of the gait deviations observed in the frontal plane is an external rotation of the prosthetic foot at initial contact and loading response as weight is transferred onto the prosthesis. This creates a rotary torque that is transmitted up the length of the prosthesis to the residual limb/socket interface and can lead to skin irritation and discomfort. The most common prosthetic cause of this deviation is an excessively firm heel cushion or plantar flexion bumper. Inappropriate toe-out alignment of the prosthetic foot must first be ruled out. When girth of the residual limb is decreasing (for individuals in whom the whole limb is shrinking as it matures or in anyone who has recently lost weight), fit within the socket may be too loose so that the effect of even a small rotary torque is manifested. Three user-related factors must also be considered. First, if there is weakness of hip muscles, the wearer may be unable to maintain the limb in optimal alignment as transition to stance phase takes place. Second, a wearer who is fearful of knee instability in early stance may be extending the prosthetic knee too vigorously at heel strike to ensure full knee extension has been reached. Third, the shoe may be too tight for the prosthetic foot.

Problems in Midstance to Late Stance Phase

In early stance phase, the primary goal is to ensure sufficient stability of the knee while body weight is loaded onto the prosthesis. In midstance to late stance phase, two additional but equally important goals must be met: (1) smooth forward progression of the body over the prosthetic foot and (2) efficient preparation for the upcoming swing phase.

Pelvic Rise

Excessive pelvic elevation during the transition through midstance and terminal stance is often a compensatory strategy to achieve a smooth progression from foot-flat position to heel off. The prosthetic wearer may make the classic statement: "I feel as though I am walking up a hill." The individual must exert an extra effort, substituting a rise of the pelvis to roll over the toe-break area of the foot. This is most often a consequence of inappropriate alignment of the prosthetic foot, which may be excessively plantarflexed. Alternatively, the foot may be positioned too far anteriorly with respect to the knee and socket. Both conditions create a relative increase in foot length, moving the fulcrum of the third rocker of gait (toe rocker) farther forward.

Drop-Off at Midstance

When relative shortening of the foot is present, the third rocker is reached prematurely and stability of late stance is compromised, just as relative lengthening of the prosthetic foot leads to delayed forward progression and difficulty in reaching the third rocker of gait. Prosthetic wearers may sense knee instability and report that they feel like they are stepping into a hole. A dropping off or lowering of the pelvis often occurs because rollover occurs too early in the transition between midstance and terminal stance, rather than during terminal stance to preswing. The stride of the swing limb must be shortened to compensate for lack of stability in late stance. Most often, this deviation is a consequence of inappropriate prosthetic alignment. The prosthetic foot may be positioned in too much dorsiflexion. If an articulating/axial foot is used, the dorsiflexion bumper may be worn out or excessively soft. The durometer of heel cushion on a SACH foot may be inappropriately soft for the patient's weight or activity level. Finally, the transfemoral socket may be positioned too far anteriorly so that the weight line falls toward the front of the foot at midstance. All of these conditions functionally decrease the length of the prosthetic foot, lead to premature rollover, and instability in later stance.

Lateral Trunk Bending

One of the most common gait deviations observed in the frontal plane is lateral trunk bending toward the prosthetic side during midstance and late stance (Figure 28-21). If the lateral prosthetic wall is not contoured to stabilize the femur in a natural position of adduction, drift of the femur into an abducted position causes a drop of the pelvis on the swinging side. An exaggerated lateral lean toward the stance (prosthetic) side ensures adequate toe clearance. Lateral trunk bending is used to avoid discomfort or excessive pressure in the perineum. This may be a result of a medial wall that is excessively high or rigid when fleshy tissue of an adductor roll is being pinched between the socket and the pubic ramus, or when too few prosthetic socks are worn and the residual limb is positioned too deeply in the prosthesis. Other possible explanations include a socket that is aligned in excessive initial abduction or a prosthetic foot excessively outset from the midline position. In both instances, the base of support is functionally wider than normal, and the only effective way to shift weight onto the prosthetic side is by leaning laterally. Finally, it is difficult to provide lateral stabilization within the socket and align prosthetic components in the ideal narrow base of support for individuals with short residual limbs.

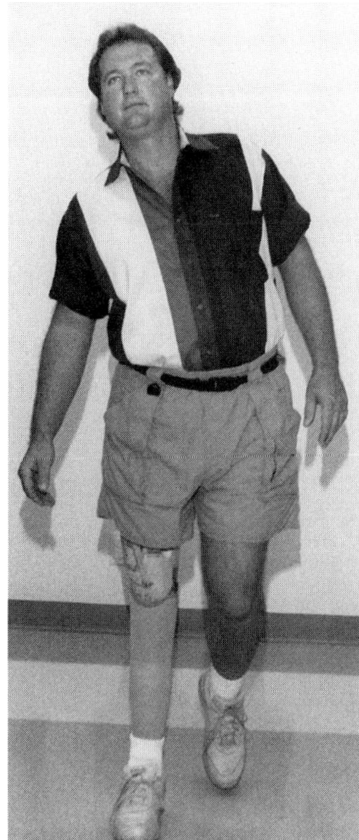

Figure 28-21
Lateral trunk bending during prosthetic stance helps to clear the swinging limb. This gait deviation is observed in the frontal plane.

Problems in Swing Phase

The functional goal of swing phase is advancement of the unweighted limb. The prosthetic wearer has two tasks: (1) to initiate swing with enough hip flexion momentum to achieve the prosthetic knee flexion that is necessary for toe clearance and (2) to position the knee in extension in preparation for initial contact.

Excessive Lumbar Lordosis

Some prosthetic users move into excessive lumbar lordosis in late stance and into the early swing phase. This may be the result of an alignment problem: The transfemoral socket may not have been positioned in an appropriate amount of initial flexion, especially for patients with hip flexion contracture. Patients with weakness of hip flexors or abdominal muscles may compensate by using exaggerated lumbar motion to initiate hip flexion necessary for a functional swing. Finally, lumbar lordosis may be a functional compensation for an ineffective femoral lever in those with short residual limbs.

Excessive Knee Flexion and Heel Rise

Excessive knee flexion/heel rise, a problem that occurs in initial swing phase, can be observed in the sagittal plane of

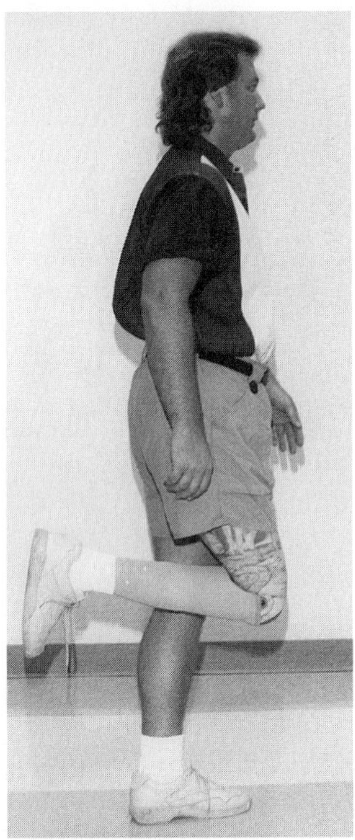

Figure 28-22
Excessive knee flexion/heel rise in early swing delays the extension of the knee, which is necessary to prepare for the next initial contact.

motion (Figure 28-22). When the knee of the prosthesis flexes as swing phase begins, the prosthetic knee continues in flexion with the foot rising quickly away from the floor. If this heel rise is excessive, it delays extension of the prosthetic knee as the swing phase progresses. Prosthetic causes of this gait deviation include inadequate flexion resistance settings in the knee unit, or inadequate adjustment of the knee extension aid. Adjustment of friction or flexion resistance of the knee unit or replacement of worn extension aids generally solves the problem.

Medial and Lateral Whips

Optimally, forward progression of the prosthetic knee and foot occurs in the same line of progression, perpendicular to the floor. A whip occurs when forward progression of the distal parts of the prosthesis follows an oblique path. Whips differ from circumducted gait because the thigh advances in the expected, straight, forward line of progression, whereas the shin and foot travel in an arcing pattern. Whips are most easily observed while evaluating gait in the frontal plane. In a lateral whip (Figure 28-23, *A*), the prosthetic knee seems to rotate internally and the foot traces an arc of motion that moves away from the midline. The possible causes of a lateral whip are the exact opposite of those for a medial whip: The knee unit may be prepositioned in too much internal rotation, or the socket may have been positioned in a slightly internally rotated position during donning.

In a medial whip (Figure 28-23, *B*), the prosthetic knee appears to rotate externally so that the prosthetic foot moves in an arc of motion that carries the foot toward midline during swing. For some patients, the heels of the swing and stance limbs narrowly miss contact at midstance and midswing. Although this occurs when the prosthetic knee is aligned in too much external rotation, it also can be the result of several user-related factors. Medial whips occur when the prosthesis is donned incorrectly in too much external rotation or when the Silesian belt is worn too tightly and pulls the socket into external rotation. Medial whips may also be the consequence of poor purchase between skin and socket for individuals who are using suction suspension, especially those with "flabby" thigh tissue.

Terminal Impact

Excessive terminal impact is a gait deviation observed in the sagittal plane during terminal swing. The shin of the prosthesis moves forward so quickly that the fully extended position is reached early, often with an audible or visible impact against the prosthetic knee. Prosthetic factors that contribute to this deviation include insufficient resistance to extension of the knee unit, an excessively strong extension aid, or worn extension bumper. Prosthetic wearers who are fearful of knee instability in early stance may choose to flex the hip forcefully in initial swing to build momentum for knee extension, then forcefully extend the hip in terminal swing to snap the knee into full extension in preparation for initial contact.

Vaulting

If the prosthetic wearer must rise up on the toes during stance on the nonamputated limb to provide adequate clearance for the prosthesis through midswing (Figure 28-24), several possible prosthetic factors should be evaluated. First, the adequacy and correct application of suspension should be assessed. Second, if suspension is appropriate, adjustment of swing resistance in the prosthetic knee should be considered. Too much resistance to knee flexion and a foot set in excessive plantar flexion may relatively lengthen the prosthesis and compromise toe clearance in swing. Finally, if suspension and knee unit friction are appropriate, the overall height of the prosthesis should be double-checked to determine if the prosthesis is really too long.

Circumduction during Swing

Optimally, forward progression of the prosthesis during swing occurs in a straight line with enough knee flexion for adequate toe clearance (Figure 28-25). If the prosthetic knee is maintained in extension instead, one compensatory strategy would be to swing the limb in a wide lateral arc. In this strategy, the peak distance from midline occurs during

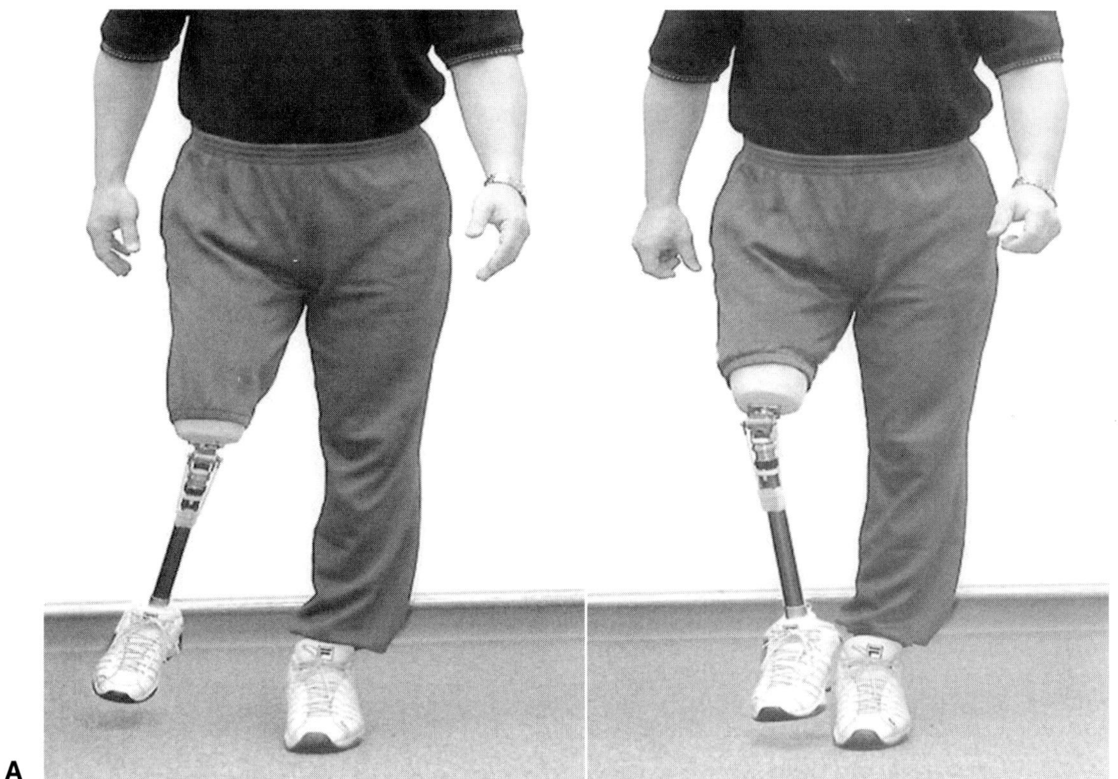

Figure 28-23

***A,** In a lateral whip, the shin and foot describe a lateral arc, appearing to be in excessive internal rotation. **B,** In a medial whip, the thigh moves forward as expected, whereas the shin and foot progress in a medial arc, appearing to be in excessive external rotation. Most whips are the consequence of improper donning or suspension.*

midswing, but the limb moves back toward midline during terminal swing, in preparation for a normal heel strike at initial contact. This deviation, most easily observed from a position in front or behind the patient (frontal plane), is an attempt to compensate for a prosthesis that is functionally or actually too long. Circumstances that can lead to this compensation are similar to the vaulting deviation and include (1) adequate suspension, in which the prosthesis pistons downward due to the force of gravity when unweighted during swing and (2) a prosthetic knee unit that is locked in extension or set with an excessive friction setting, preventing the knee flexion necessary during swing phase. The pattern is also adopted by prosthetic wearers who are nervous about catching their toe during swing or who are reluctant to use knee flexion because of anticipated instability in the subsequent early stance period. Circumduction can also be the result of a foot set in excessive plantar flexion, which makes the prosthesis functionally longer.

Other Issues

Ideally a reasonably narrow base with minimal sway is present, as well as symmetry and evenness in stride length, cadence, and arm swing so that the gait pattern appears to be as natural as possible when the transfemoral prosthesis is used. Excessive side-to-side sway and asymmetry in place of fluid reciprocal movements increase the work and energy cost of walking and are obviously different from a normal gait pattern.

Abducted Gait Pattern

In an abducted gait pattern, the prosthesis is held away from the midline throughout the gait cycle. Functionally, this is most notable in the stance phase of gait. In initial contact, the prosthetic foot lands several inches lateral to the normal or ideal foot position, resulting in a wide base of support and requiring excessive side-to-side sway to accomplish weight transfer from one limb to the other. This deviation has a number of possible causes. The overall length of the prosthesis may need to be reduced. The socket may be aligned in a position of too much initial abduction. Uncomfortable or painful pressure may occur in the groin area (as in lateral leaning). An abducted gait pattern may be a compensatory strategy when pelvic instability is a result of inadequate lateral wall stabilization of the femur or weakness of hip abductors. The prosthetic wearer may be attempting to minimize lateral-distal femoral pain within the socket. Finally, for those who are fearful of falling, an abducted gait pattern may be a habitual movement strategy to minimize feelings of insecurity.

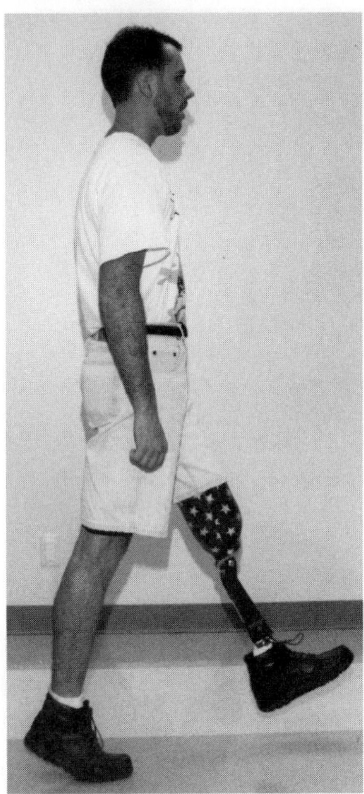

Figure 28-24
Vaulting is a compensatory strategy for a prosthesis that is functionally too long. It may be due to inadequate suspension, excessive friction of the knee unit, an excessively plantarflexed foot, or, sometimes, to excessive length of the prosthesis.

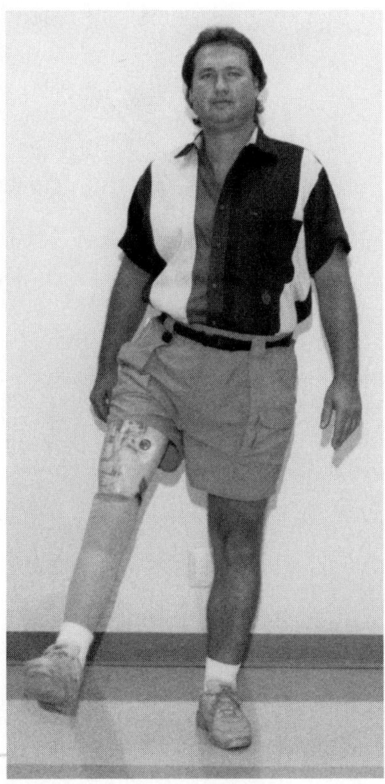

Figure 28-25
In a circumduction gait pattern, the prosthesis swings in a wide lateral arc to facilitate toe clearance in swing. Prosthetic causes of circumduction include inadequate suspension, a locked knee unit, or excessive friction in the knee unit.

Uneven Step Length and Swing Time

Early in prosthetic training, new prosthetic wearers may be cautious and reluctant to use the prosthesis to its full capacity. The goal of equal step length and swing time must be emphasized. Patients gain confidence by practicing single-limb support on the prosthetic side and performing gait training exercises that provide appropriate visual, kinesthetic, and auditory feedback (e.g., equally spaced target marks on the floor, use of mirrors or videotape). Several possible patient-related issues or prosthetic problems, or both, should be considered if gait pattern asymmetry persists. First, the fit of the socket and condition of the skin should be examined carefully. Anyone would be reluctant to spend time in weight bearing if tissue is being pinched or irritated within the socket, if relief for bony prominences is inadequate, or if an inflamed or open area or unrecognized neuroma is present. Second, hip flexion contracture on the prosthetic side may limit excursion in hip extension in late stance, compromising forward progression of the opposite swing limb. If fit, skin condition, and ROM are adequate, the mechanical and alignment stability of the knee unit should be reevaluated. A wearer who senses that the knee cannot provide adequate support in stance will compensate by shortening stance time to minimize sense of security. Finally, individuals with impaired postural responses (poor balance) who are fearful of falling may decrease the time spent in single-limb support by reducing step length.

Uneven Arm Swing

Many individuals with amputations demonstrate diminished or absent reciprocal arm swing when walking with their prostheses. They may hold their arms on the prosthetic side stiffly and relatively still throughout the gait cycle. This is especially common in a new prosthetic user who has not yet developed confidence in the stability of the prosthesis, as well as someone with a painful residual limb. This behavior is also observed in some proficient prosthetic users. The mechanism that underlies this alteration in motor behavior is not clearly understood, but it may be related to loss of sensation from the distal contact between the foot and the ground.

SUMMARY

Advances in technology and improved prosthetic components have greatly benefited individuals with transfemoral amputation. This chapter has explained that the successful functional outcome for individuals needing prosthetic care requires more than advanced technology. A prosthetic team in which the prosthetist and physical therapist are key contributors is necessary. A thorough understanding of the interrelationship between the prosthesis' weight, function, cosmesis, comfort, and cost is also required. Attention to socket design, knee biomechanics, and prosthetic alignment is important in providing optimal patient care. The prosthetic clinical team's goal is not merely to present an individual with a prosthetic product but to provide ongoing comprehensive care that focuses on the individual's needs, physical condition, and personal goals. In this way, patients who require a transfemoral prosthesis have an opportunity to reach their full functional potential.

REFERENCES

1. Radcliffe CW. Functional considerations in the fitting of above-knee prostheses. In *Artificial Limbs.* New York: Krieger, 1970. pp. 35-60.
2. Huang CT, Jackson JR, Moore, et al. Amputation: energy cost of ambulation. *Arch Phys Med Rehabil* 1979;60(1):18-24.
3. Waters RL. Energy expenditure. In Perry J (ed), *Gait Analysis: Normal and Pathological Function.* Thorofare, NJ: Slack, 1992. pp. 443-487.
4. Waters RL. Energy cost of walking amputees: the influence of level of amputation. *J Bone Joint Surg* 1976;58A:42-46.
5. Waters R, Yakura J. Energy expenditure of normal and abnormal ambulation. In Smidt GL (ed), *Clinics in Physical Therapy: Gait in Rehabilitation.* New York: Churchill Livingstone, 1990. pp. 65-93.
6. Fisher SV, Gullickson G. Energy cost of ambulation in health and disability: a literature review. *Arch Phys Med Rehabil* 1978;59(3):124-132.
7. Radcliffe CW. Prosthetics. In Rose J, Gamble JG (eds), *Human Walking.* Baltimore: Williams & Wilkins, 1981. pp. 165-199.
8. Schuch CM. Report from the international workshop on above-knee fitting and alignment techniques. *Clin Prosthet Orthot* 1988;12:81-98.
9. Pritham CH. Workshop on teaching materials for above-knee socket variants. *J Prosthet Orthot* 1988;1(1):51-67.
10. Long IA. Normal shape-normal alignment (NSNA) above knee prosthesis. *Clin Prosthet Orthot* 1985;9:9-14.
11. Sabolich J. Contoured adducted trochanteric-controlled alignment method (CAT-CAM): introduction and basic principles. *Clin Prosthet Orthot* 1985;9:15-26.
12. Carroll K. Getting down to basics: improving life with an above-knee prosthesis. *In Motion* 2001;11(5):14-15.
13. Jendrezejczk DJ. Flexible socket systems. *Clin Prosthet Orthot* 1985;9:27-30.
14. Kristinsson O. Flexible above-knee socket made from low density polyethylene suspended by a weight transmitting frame. *Orthot Prosthet* 1983;37:25-27.
15. Mauch Laboratories. *Manual for the Henschke-Mauch Hydraulic Swing-N-Stance Control System.* Dayton, OH: Mauch Laboratories, 1976.
16. Moore KL. *Clinical Oriented Anatomy.* Baltimore: Williams & Wilkins, 1980. p. 553.
17. Mooney V, Quigley MJ. Above knee amputations: prosthetic management. In Bowker JH (ed), *Atlas of Limb Prosthetics.* St Louis: Mosby-Year Book, 1981. pp. 381-401.
18. Gard SA, Childress DS, Uellendahl JE. The influence of four-bar linkage knees on prosthetic swing-phase floor clearance. *J Prosthet Orthot* 1996;8(2):34-40.
19. Schuch CM. Prosthetic management. In Bowker JH, Michael JW (eds), *Atlas of Prosthetics: Surgical, Prosthetic, and Rehabilitation Principles,* 2nd ed. St Louis: Mosby, 1992. pp. 528-529.
20. Otto Bock Orthopedic Industry, Inc. *Manual for the 3c100 Otto Bock C-LEG.* Duderstadt, Germany, 1998.
21. Otto Bock Orthopedic Industry, Inc. *Prosthetic Compendium: Lower Extremity Prostheses.* Duderstadt, Germany, 1994.
22. Dietzen CJ, Harshburger J, Pidikiti RD. Suction sock suspension for above-knee prostheses. *J Prosthet Orthot* 1991;3(2):90-93.
23. Ohio Williow Wood Company. Advanced alpha solutions. Presented at the Summit Seminars, Mt. Sterling, OH, 2002.
24. Covey SJ, Muonio J, Street GM. Flow constraint and loading rate effects on prosthetic liner material and human tissue mechanical response. *J Prosthet Orthot* 2000;12(1):15-32.
25. Lake C, Supan TJ. The incidence of dermatological problems in the silicone suspension sleeve user. *J Prosthet Orthot* 1997;9(3):97-106.
26. Haberman LJ, Bedotto RA, Colodney EJ. Silicone-only suspension (SOS) for the above knee amputee. *J Prosthet Orthot* 1992;4(2):76-85.
27. Padula PA, Friedman LW. Amputee gait. In Friedman LW (ed), *Physical Medicine and Rehabilitation Clinics of North America.* Philadelphia: Saunders, 1991. pp. 423-432.
28. Radcliff CW. Biomechanics of above-knee prostheses. In *Prosthetic and Orthotic Practice.* London: Edward Arnold, 1970. pp. 191-198.
29. Saunders JB, Inman M, Eberhart HD. The major determinants in normal and pathological gait. *J Bone Joint Surg* 1953;35A:543-558.
30. Perry J. *Gait Analysis: Normal and Pathological Function.* Thorofare, NJ: Charles B Slack, 1992.
31. Gard SA, Childress, DS. The effect of pelvic list on the vertical displacement of the trunk during normal walking. *Gait Posture* 1997;5:233-238.
32. Quigley M. The role of test socket procedures in today's prosthetic practices. *Clin Prosthet Orthot* 1985;9(3):11-12.
33. Kahle JT, Highsmith JM. Isometric training helps prevent socket replacement. *In Motion* 2003;13(3):66-67.
34. Nielsen CC, Psonak RP, Kalter TL. Factors affecting the use of prosthetic services. *J Prosthet Orthot* 1989;1(4):242-249.

29

Rehabilitation for Persons with Transfemoral Amputation

DAVID M. THOMPSON

LEARNING OBJECTIVES

On completion of this chapter, the reader will be able to do the following:

1. Develop an intervention plan to help those with transfemoral amputations appropriately don and adjust suspension of their prostheses.
2. Determine appropriate strategies to help new prosthetic users develop skills necessary for safe and efficient ambulation with transfemoral prostheses.
3. Describe the key determinants of effective transfemoral gait in each subphase of the gait cycle.
4. Select appropriate strengthening, stretching, and functional exercises to improve muscle performance, postural control, and quality of gait for those using transfemoral prostheses.
5. Develop a plan to facilitate motor learning of functional activities (moving between standing and kneeling, standing and the floor, standing and sitting) for those using transfemoral prostheses.
6. Develop a plan to assist motor learning for safely managing stairs, curbs, inclines, and uneven terrain and for retrieving objects from the floor for those using transfemoral prostheses.
7. Describe strategies that individuals wearing transfemoral prostheses use to safely and effectively increase their gait speed or run.
8. Describe key indicators of readiness for a new socket or transition to a definitive prosthesis.

PREDICTORS OF REHABILITATION OUTCOMES

Rehabilitation specialists sometimes assume that a person's ability to use a prosthesis and be functional after amputation is determined by the level of amputation: Those with transfemoral amputations, for instance, might be more dependent or use their prostheses less frequently than those with transtibial amputations. Although there is evidence to support this claim, the level of amputation alone is not the only predictor of outcome to consider; etiology of amputation and overall health status also play significant roles. Because of the chronic nature of dysvascular and neuropathic disease and the likelihood of comorbidity, rehabilitation outcomes in this group are different than in those with traumatic, congenital, or cancer-related amputation.[1]

Moore and colleagues[2] reviewed records for 157 patients with lower limb amputation in a North Carolina hospital, most of whom came to amputation because of dysvascular or neuropathic disease. Of the 129 who received prostheses, 88 (68.2%) could walk with them, while 41 (31.8%) could not. Functional use of a prosthesis also varied with the level of amputation: 66% of those with unilateral transtibial amputation, 46% of those with unilateral transfemoral amputation, and only 19% of those with bilateral amputation used their prostheses for walking. DeLuccia and associates[3] found that 48% of those with transtibial amputation and 22% of those with transfemoral amputation used prostheses to walk 5 years after their initial prescription. They suggest these data reflect the impact of continued disease and comorbidities. In a study of outcomes of a British rehabilitation program following 281 persons with amputation, Davies and Datta[4] report that, 1 year after completion of rehabilitation, 26% of those whose transfemoral amputations related to vascular disease, including diabetes, could ambulate in the community whereas 48% were household ambulators.

A growing number of studies, however, suggest that pre-amputation functional status is a better predictor of rehabilitation outcome than level amputation alone. Pinzur and colleagues[5] followed 95 adults with peripheral vascular insufficiency receiving 3 years of care in the Veterans Administration health system. They used a seven-level functional grading system to rate patients' ambulation before amputation and found that 84% eventually walked within one functional level of their preamputation status. They found that those with higher preamputation functional ambulation levels were more likely to use prostheses and less likely to require ambulatory assistive devices than those with limited ambulation before their surgery, regardless of level of amputation. A study by Penington and colleagues[6] of 200 persons with amputation in Australia had similar outcomes; the authors concluded that "any person previously walking [should] be considered for a trial of prosthetic walking." On balance, the most recent evidence from the rehabilitation research literature cautiously shares this view.

Older people whose amputations relate to diabetes or vascular problems contend with various problems. Cutson and Bongiorni[7] point out that the 2-year postamputation survival rate among older Americans with amputation (40% to 50%) and incidence of loss of the contralateral limb (15% to 20% in the first 2 years) has not markedly improved in more than 40 years. Prosthetists and therapists should concentrate on improving patients' mobility and independence in the months and years following surgery.

DONNING THE TRANSFEMORAL PROSTHESIS

Patients with new transfemoral amputations must understand that their new prostheses cannot help them stand or transfer. Patients must gain skills in standing and balancing on the remaining extremity so that they can safely and independently apply the prostheses to their residual limbs. Most patients learn to don their prostheses using a systematic process that begins with dressing the prosthesis, donning socks, and prepositioning the prosthesis while sitting. Finally, the patient stands to don the prosthesis and secure suspension.

Managing Clothing

Many training (temporary) transfemoral prostheses are suspended on patients by using a system of straps, bands, or belts.[8] A neoprene belt, called "total elastic suspension" (TES), or various Silesian belts are the most commonly used suspension strategies. Given the likelihood of frequent adjustments of suspension during early prosthetic training, many patients choose to wear loose-fitting shorts that can fit easily over their prostheses for early gait training sessions. Many elect to don their prostheses, especially the suspension straps, over these clothes. This strategy is successful only if clothing does not interfere with inserting of the residual limb into the prosthetic socket.

Patients with amputations should be encouraged to incorporate their prostheses into their daily lives as soon as possible by wearing them under clothing. This will permit use of the prosthesis for longer periods of time throughout the day. A patient wearing a prosthesis under clothing need not, for example, remove it to use the bathroom, unlike the patient who chooses to wear the prosthesis and its suspension over a pair of shorts.

Because the transfemoral prosthesis is somewhat large and cumbersome, most persons with amputations "dress the prosthesis first" (socks, pants, shoes), don the prosthesis, then dress the remaining limb. While sitting, holding the prosthesis and the clothing in their laps, the patient can insert the prosthesis into the appropriate pant leg. Some persons with amputations prepare their prostheses before retiring for bed in the evening and joke that they are "already half-dressed" when they arise the next morning.

Applying Prosthetic Socks

Most patients in the initial stages of prosthetic rehabilitation wear prosthetic socks inside their training prostheses in order to accommodate anticipated changes in the residual limb's volume. Additionally, socks absorb perspiration and decrease friction between the socket and the residual limb, making the prosthesis more comfortable to wear and protecting the residual limb.

After "dressing" the prosthesis and placing the prosthetic foot on the floor, the patient can insert the nonamputated limb into the remaining pant leg and apply the appropriate number of socks on the residual limb. Prosthetic socks are made from wool or cotton and are available in various thicknesses (ply), widths, and lengths. New prosthetic users are provided with a quantity of one-, three-, and five-ply socks.

Prosthetic socks are donned in much the same way that socks are put on a sound foot, by rolling or pulling the prosthetic sock onto the residual limb (Figure 29-1, *A*). New prosthetic users learn that socks should be relatively "wrinkle free" and fit snugly on the residual limb; however, the shape of the residual limb may preclude a perfect fit. Because prosthetic sockets contact but do not concentrate pressure on the residual limb's distal end, a small wrinkle in the sock should not pose a threat to the skin. A larger wrinkle or bunching can, however, create high-pressure areas within the socket, making ambulation uncomfortable and potentially damaging skin. The therapist may cut off some length from a sock's proximal end if it is too long for a patient's residual limb. Woolen prosthetic socks are woven so that they do not unravel when they are cut in this way. Once the socks are in place, the prosthetic knee joint is flexed so that the prosthesis can be donned from an initial sitting or supported standing position.

Those whose residual limbs are somewhat conical in shape, with a much larger proximal than distal circumference, may find that their socks migrate distally when they don their prostheses. The socks may even descend into the socket, where they bunch, wrinkle, and interfere with the prostheses' fit. To prevent this, a person with an amputation can place a single-ply sock in the prosthetic socket so that it overlaps the entire proximal brim. When the patient inserts

the leg into the prosthesis, this outer sock forms a "sling" that remains anchored to the socket brim and prevents additional socks from sliding into the socket. The prosthetist or therapist can apply strips of Velcro to the brim's outer wall, onto which prosthetic wearers can overlap the outermost sock improve anchoring.

Some individuals with transfemoral amputation continue to wear at least a thin sock even after they receive the definitive prosthesis, depending on the type of suspension they ultimately choose. Suspension systems that require skin contact, either with the socket's inner wall or with a gel liner, are worn without socks.

Positioning the Prosthesis

With the socks, prosthesis, and clothing in place, persons with transfemoral amputations must rise from sitting into standing and position the prosthesis under them before they can fasten its suspension device (see Figure 29-1, *B*). Most new prosthetic wearers use assistive devices, typically a walker, to provide support while they stand on the intact limb and don the prosthesis; a wearer with impaired balance may need help from a family member.

New prosthetic wearers, their family members, and their rehabilitation team must recognize that most prosthetic knee units are designed to support body weight when in an extended position. This means that, although the prosthesis can be positioned on the limb while still sitting in a chair, it cannot support body weight during the transition from sitting to standing. Individuals with transfemoral amputation must rely on the nonamputated limb for strength and balance to stand. Only after a stable, erect standing posture is achieved can the prosthesis be positioned, fully donned, and effectively support body weight.

Current transfemoral sockets are designed to fit as intimately as possible on the residual limb. Contouring for muscle compartments and bony architecture means that the socket will fit comfortably only when donned with the correct orientation on the residual limb. A key factor in learning and reproducing this comfortable and efficient positioning is the angle at which the socket is rotated on the residual limb. New prosthetic wearers learn to monitor the angle at which the prosthetic foot rests beneath them as an indicator of proper donning position.

The prosthetic foot is usually aligned in a slightly "out-toe" or externally rotated position with regard to the socket and knee joint axis. New prosthetic wearers must take care not to don the prosthesis in an internally rotated position, as this is the most common cause of discomfort during standing and walking. Donning the socket in internal rotation causes the socket's relatively high anterior-lateral wall to move medially, where it can contact the patient's sensitive groin area.

Donning the socket in the appropriate orientation also ensures that the ischium rests in its proper place. Most

A

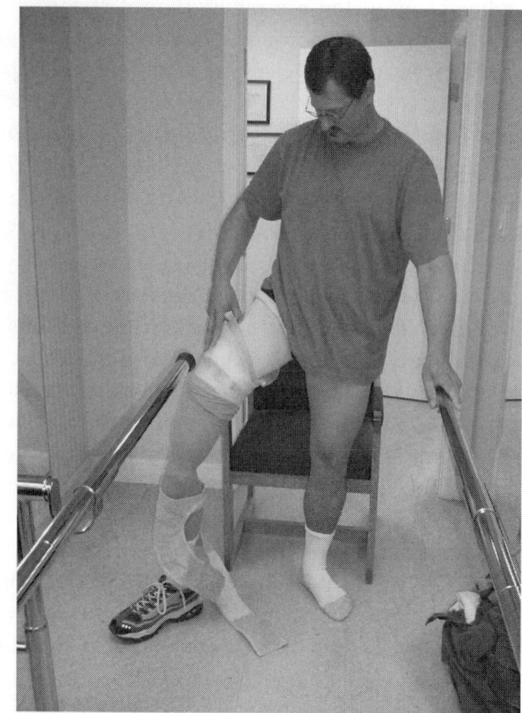

B

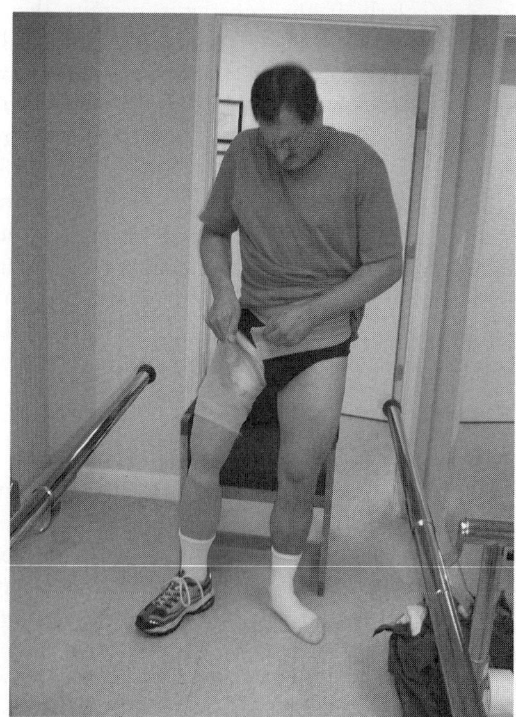

Figure 29-1

A, *To don the prosthesis properly, prosthetic socks are applied to the residual limb and the prosthesis is prepositioned so that the residual limb can more easily enter the socket.* ***B,*** *The individual balances on the intact limb, seats the residual limb within the socket, stands upright, and then adjusts suspension.*

ischial containment sockets nest this important weight-bearing bony contour on a carefully shaped region on the socket's posterior-medial border. New prosthetic wearers can learn to discern whether they have seated the ischium properly within the socket's surface. By firmly palpating the ischial tuberosity before donning, therapists can help new prosthetic wearers become more aware of the location of this important landmark so that they can better detect for themselves its location within the socket.

The ischial tuberosity can be most easily palpated when the individual with amputation bends forward from the hips while standing. This tilts the pelvis anteriorly and lifts the tuberosity from its resting place against the socket wall. Once the therapist has identified the tuberosity, the individual can return to an erect posture; the therapist should feel the ischium squeeze the palpating finger against the socket. If the ischium does not rest on the surface intended for it, adding or removing prosthetic socks from the residual limb should help it attain the proper position.

New prosthetic wearers must learn to judge the appropriate number and combination of socks to wear inside the initial prosthesis. The prosthetic socket is usually initially fit to accommodate a single three-ply wool sock. Individuals with recent amputations may lose residual limb volume rapidly, particularly if the prosthesis permits them to increase their accustomed level of activity. Residual limb volume may also decrease rapidly once new wearers become more comfortable with forcefully using the muscles of the residual limb. A new prosthetic wearer learns that the groin discomfort may indicate the need to apply an additional prosthetic sock. As a residual limb matures and its overall volume shrinks, it will "sink" too far down into the socket, causing uncomfortable pressure at the groin and perhaps at the distal anterior surface of the limb. The application of another ply or more of sock makes up for the lost volume and more optimally positions the limb within the socket.

Adjusting the Suspension

Sometimes the solution to a problem with fit or comfort lies with the suspension strategy rather than the number of socks being worn. The purpose of the suspension system is to hold the prosthesis on the residual limb so that it stays in place throughout the gait cycle. "Pistoning" can result from either inadequate sock ply or poorly applied suspension. The residual limb descends too far down into the socket as weight is transferred onto the prosthesis in early stance and subsequently feels as if it is coming out of the socket as body weight moves off the prosthesis at the beginning of swing. Another problem often related to inadequate suspension is a sense that the prosthesis is rotating or twisting on the residual limb during gait. The need to control socket rotation on the residual limb's soft tissue mass makes it more difficult to suspend a transfemoral socket than a transtibial prosthesis.

Because prosthetists cannot fit new and rapidly changing residual limbs with prostheses that employ suction suspension, they frequently suspend temporary prostheses with straps, belts, or elastic bands. A typical system is the Silesian belt or TES that encircles the wearer's waist and closes with Velcro.

A skill that persons new to prosthetic use must master is how much to tighten suspensions enough to prevent pistoning but not so much to cause rotation of the socket on the residual limb. They must resist the temptation to overtighten the suspension, in the mistaken belief that tight suspension will provide more stability. Overtightening occurs unwittingly when new wearers overlook key details while donning the prosthesis. Both the Silesian belt and the TES are tightened by pulling on a strap or belt located over the lower abdomen. The new user must learn to shift weight onto the prosthesis before the belt is pulled toward the body's opposite side to tighten suspension. If there is inadequate weight shift, pulling on the belt will cause the prosthesis to rotate internally on the residual limb.

Overtightening the suspension in this way causes two problems. Donning the prosthesis in an internally rotated position can produce socket pressure and discomfort in the groin during the stance phase of gait. Although an overly tight suspension belt may not immediately internally rotate the socket, this rotation becomes apparent after even a few steps are taken. The toe of the prosthetic foot will begin to point more medially during both stance and swing phase, and groin pressure soon increases to uncomfortable levels. New prosthetic wearers must temper their natural desire for a tight and firm prosthetic fit with the knowledge that they can easily overdo it. They must learn instead to tighten the suspension only to the point where the prosthesis does not piston on the residual limb.

Anytime pistoning or socket rotation occurs, the first remedy should be an examination and adjustment of prosthetic suspension. If the problem is due to inadequate suspension or overtightening, adding prosthetic socks to "fill in the gaps" will worsen the situation. Even if there seems to be a temporary improvement in fit, the inappropriate addition of prosthetic socks increases the residual limb's overall circumference so that it cannot descend properly into the socket. This sacrifices the intimate fit between the socket's medial and posterior brims and the ischium and pubis. Without appropriate contact at these bony contours, rotation between the residual limb and socket occurs; this makes the prosthesis more difficult to control and compromises stability during the gait cycle. If the pistoning remains after suspension has been adjusted appropriately, then applying an additional layer of sock usually corrects the problem.

Most problems associated with socket rotation are solved when the residual limb attains a stable volume and the prosthetist can safely proceed to fitting the definitive prosthesis. The definitive socket can fit so intimately with the residual limb itself or with a silicone gel liner that is rolled onto the

residual limb that the excellent advantages of suction suspension are available. When suction suspension is impossible or inappropriate, a pin incorporated into the distal end of a roll-on liner can lock mechanically into a receptacle in the socket.[8]

GAIT TRAINING

Learning to effectively use a prosthesis begins with ensuring that the prosthesis is correctly positioned (aligned) on the residual limb, that there is a controlled ability to shift weight onto and off of the prosthesis, that dynamic postural control is sufficient on various walking surfaces, and that there is sufficient endurance for functional walking.

Assessing Alignment

During the static and dynamic alignment process, the prosthetist ensures that the prosthesis' initial alignment is appropriate for the patient. The physical therapist reevaluates this alignment to verify that the new user has properly donned the prosthesis. Additionally, the therapist may need to help the new prosthetic user recognize and sort out any difficulties associated with changing residual limb size or increasing comfort and security in using the new prosthesis.

With the patient wearing the prosthesis and standing, perhaps in parallel bars or using a walker, the therapist begins by checking the pelvis's frontal orientation; the anterior superior iliac spine and iliac crests of the pelvis should be level. If the pelvis is not level or is rotated forward or backward on one side, the therapist should first help the patient shift weight to achieve weight bearing across the prosthetic and intact limbs.

Many new prosthetic users find it difficult or frightening to bear weight on the prosthesis through the residual limb. Ironically, those who have been active during their preprosthetic rehabilitation, ambulating without the prosthesis by using a walker or crutches, may find this especially difficult. These individuals stabilized themselves on an assistive device by placing the nonamputated foot directly under the center of gravity. In doing so, they may have acquired a postural imbalance in which their hip joint positions are asymmetrical; the nonamputated hip joint may be adducted while the residual hip joint is abducted (Figure 29-2).

Traditional "Pregait" Skills

Traditional approaches to gait training patients with recent transfemoral amputations include activities and exercises designed to equalize weight bearing on either leg while patients

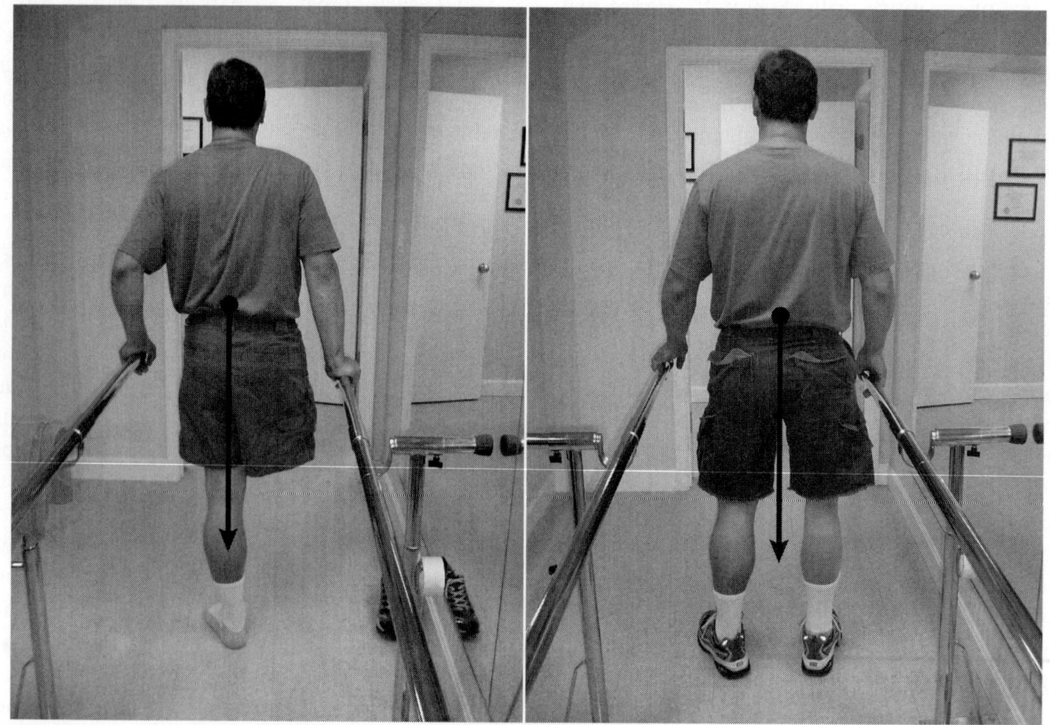

Figure 29-2

A, *In the weeks after surgery and before the delivery of the prosthesis, individuals with amputations shift their center of mass directly over the intact limb during ambulation with an assistive device.* ***B,*** *After a long period of walking on a single limb, some individuals may have difficulty distributing their weight equally between the prosthesis and intact limb and be reluctant to shift total body weight onto the prosthesis.*

are standing.[9-11] These exercises are part of a sequential approach that emphasizes the perfection of pregait skills, such as weight shifting, alternate knee bending, and repetitive stance and swing drills that simulate components of the total movement pattern of walking. Although these exercises help the new prosthetic wearer to gain confidence in the stability of the prosthesis, mastery of isolated skills is no longer considered a prerequisite to walking with the prosthesis.

Motor Learning Approach to Gait Training

Many traditional gait training drills and exercises are valuable in isolated instances in which individuals must remedy specific deficits. However, therapists have several reasons to choose a more direct and functional approach. First, researchers who have studied motor learning suggest that practicing specific gait training exercises does not ensure transfer or integration of these isolated skills into the functional task of walking. Winstein and colleagues,[12] for example, discovered that patients recovering from cerebrovascular accidents bore their body weight more symmetrically on either leg by adhering to a standing balance training regimen that involved augmented feedback. This skill did not carry over into functional ambulation. Patients also did not increase the single-limb stance duration, the amount of time they spent on the paretic limb when they walked.

Other experts in the field of motor learning process question the use of repetitive drills. Schmidt[13] argues that blocked or highly repetitive practice and drill do not effectively facilitate learning, and, in his words, "should almost never be used." Instead, he recommends a more random or varied type of practice that emphasizes solving motor problems in functional tasks. Schmidt[13] believes that random practice, even practice in which one makes mistakes, generates motor learning more effectively than the repetition of accurate performance.

Motor learning researchers also caution therapists against assuming that all motor tasks can be effectively divided into a series of learnable subtasks. Walking, in fact, may be a movement pattern in which timing and energy transfers are so critical that persons cannot perform it in discrete parts but must learn it as a whole.

Finally, society's demands that rehabilitation professionals guide their clients to improve rapidly will lead therapists to avoid relying on "pregait" training unless they can articulate a specific need for it. Therapists need not despair about the health care system's demands that patients accomplish more and that they accomplish it with less therapist-client contact. A growing body of research validates the effectiveness of a rehabilitation approach that requires less direct intervention on the therapist's part and more vigilance on the patient's part. This research suggests, for example, that persons learn and retain motor tasks better when they learn them in situations where feedback is limited, delayed, or intermittent. Subjects in many controlled studies actually learn tasks *less* well when their feedback is complete, instantaneous, or ongoing.[14]

To master ambulation, new prosthetic wearers must discover ways to improve function even as they rely less on their therapists for feedback and guidance. Assuming that feedback necessarily promotes motor learning and that the more extensive and rich the feedback, the better the performance of skill to be mastered might be is erroneous. Feedback actually has negative effects if it promotes dependency, i.e., if patients rely on it and cannot recall and perform tasks in its absence.[13]

Therapists who are sensitive to tightening constraints on the time that they can devote to patient education and treatment must focus on empowering patients so that they learn quickly to "be the boss" and to "tell the prosthesis what to do." This emphasis also redirects patients' energies appropriately during their prosthetic rehabilitation and training. Persons with amputations must resist the assumption that prosthetic technology alone can make them function independently; instead, they must be active and forceful as they learn to walk with a prosthesis.

Walking with an Assistive Device

Many older persons with transfemoral amputations have various medical problems that can complicate their functional recovery. Often they must rely initially on an assistive device, such as parallel bars or a walker, for ambulation. Younger patients with traumatic amputation are even more likely to quickly develop the skills that are necessary for ambulation without an assistive device. For young and older patients, rehabilitation must focus not just on the gait patterns practiced in parallel bars in the clinic but must quickly progress to "real" conditions that they are likely to encounter in their homes and community.

Although standard walkers enhance patients' feelings of security as they learn to negotiate their new transfemoral prostheses, the "step-to" pattern of walker use halts normal forward progression at what would otherwise be midstance position. In this modified gait pattern, the sequence of gait has three components: advancement of the walker, a short step with the intact limb, and another short step to advance the prosthesis. This sequence necessarily entails a "chopping up" of the gait cycle, a sacrifice of fluidity and reciprocal motion, and an increase in the energy cost of walking.

Using a walker safely places an additional restriction on the gait pattern; patients must maintain their center of gravity within the base of support, even when the walker enlarges the dimensions of that base. They must always position the walker and place their feet so that the toes of at least one extremity remain within an imaginary rectangle formed by the walker's four legs. This "rule of thumb" guarantees safety whether the patient walks forward, backward, sideways, or turns while using the walker. For the sake of safety, therapists may advise new users with significantly impaired

balance to keep *both* toes within this rectangular area, even though doing so restricts step length.

Similarly, when the walker is advanced to provide room for the next step with the nonamputated limb, the walker's rear legs cannot be farther forward than the toe of that limb. A modest increase in the height of the walker, such that the handles are slightly above the customary position at the greater trochanter of the femur, may help increase step length; the patient may be able to move the walker farther ahead of his or her front foot without having to incline the trunk forward. The elevated hand rests also support a more normal shoulder girdle posture and provide a kinesthetic cue for erect posture while walking.

CASE EXAMPLE 1A

An Older Person with Dysvascular Transfemoral Amputation

T. C. is a slightly overweight 78-year-old woman with a 10-year history of type 2 diabetes. She underwent a standard left transfemoral amputation 4 weeks ago due to infection and failure of a femoral-popliteal bypass graft. Her medical history includes a complete transmetatarsal amputation of the right forefoot 3 years ago; macular degeneration; hypertension; coronary artery bypass surgery (CABG × 4) to address function-limiting angina 2 years ago; osteoarthritis of wrists and hands, shoulders, and neck; and documented osteoporosis of the thoracic and lumbar spine. Current medications include twice-daily insulin injection, daily antihypertensive medication (calcium channel blocker) and medication for elevated cholesterol and triglycerides (antilipemic), nonsteroidal antiinflammatory drugs as needed for arthritic pain, calcium supplements, and a daily antiosteoporotic (selective estrogen receptor modulator) medication. Her current mini-mental status examination score is 27/30. Before her surgery, T. C. lived with a college-aged granddaughter on the second floor of a three-family home that she owns. Her goal is to return to her lifelong neighborhood and to her activities at a local inner-city senior center and neighborhood housing advocacy, antiviolence, and anti-crime group.

T. C. has been in an active preprosthetic program including flexibility and strengthening of both lower extremities, as well as core stabilization activities, and endurance training at a subacute rehabilitation center near her neighborhood for the past 3 weeks. Friends and neighbors visit daily, serving as her "cheerleading squad" during therapy. Her surgical wound is well healed, but her residual limb is somewhat "fleshy," especially proximally and medially near the groin. She currently ambulates with a regular walker for 125 feet, requiring verbal cuing and contact guarding when transitioning from sitting to standing and returning to sitting. She will soon receive her initial prosthesis, with an ischial-ramal containment (IRC) socket, total elastic suspension belt, weight-activated stance control knee, and solid-ankle cushioned-heel foot. Although she is excited and eager to begin gait training, she is fearful of falling and expresses concern about the risk of hip fracture should she fall (given her osteoporosis).

Questions to Consider

Given the information collected in the patient history and systems review, as well as examination findings, consider the following:

- Is additional information (other tests and measures) necessary to complete the evaluation of this patient?
- What is the most likely prognosis for this patient? What are the expectations for the rehabilitation process? What are the immediate short-term goals? Long-term goals?
- How long should rehabilitation intervention take to achieve these goals? In what settings will rehabilitation occur? What are some suggestions in terms of the frequency of care? Intensity of care?
- What intraindividual and environmental factors might influence T. C.'s progression and the ultimate outcome of her rehabilitation? How can these factors be monitored over time?
- What does this patient bring to her rehabilitation process in terms of resources and limitations? What will her major challenges be at the beginning of prosthetic training?
- What key things must this patient and her caregivers understand about the components of her prosthesis, the donning/doffing process, the functional use of her prosthesis in rising from standing and walking, and early ambulation? How might the principles of motor learning be incorporated into training activities to help her develop this understanding?
- Do additional issues or goals need to be addressed in this early rehabilitation period? What are they, and why are they important?
- How can it be determined how quickly to advance or progress the activities in this patient's initial prosthetic rehabilitation program? What factors may affect her ability to participate, tolerate, and improve in her rehabilitation process?

Mastering Reciprocal Gait

Gait training in the parallel bars or with standard or Lofstrand crutches (and eventually with a straight cane) allows a more effective forward progression, as well as incorporation of the reciprocal motion of efficient gait. The opportunity to practice a step-through, reciprocal gait pattern in a safe and controlled environment is important, especially for those who might be anxious about transitioning from a walker to a less restrictive assistive device.

A therapist may influence a new prosthesis user's walking patterns most effectively by concentrating on those aspects over which the individual has the greatest control: movements in the lower trunk and pelvis. Beginning with the earliest and most classic research, students of human walking have emphasized the critical contributions of pelvic movement patterns to gait efficiency. Saunders and colleagues[15] argue that pelvic movements in the frontal and transverse planes are "determinants of normal gait"; the quality of the gait pattern depends on the normality of pelvic movement. Proper pelvic movement saves energy and ensures proper prosthetic function. Many common gait deficits are remediable if the pelvis moves as closely as possible in the pattern of reciprocal pelvic rotation described in studies of normal gait.

Regaining Pelvic Rotation in Prosthetic Swing Phase

To walk comfortably with the new prosthesis and to avoid gait deficits, new prosthetic users must regain their normal rhythm of pelvic rotation. Pelvic rotation occurs in the transverse plane, the plane parallel to the walking surface. As the user swings the prosthesis forward, the pelvis must rotate forward on that side around the intact stance limb, the way the pelvis moves in a typical gait pattern. Many new prosthetic users use a different and less effective movement strategy; they elevate the pelvis on the prosthetic side and advance the prosthesis primarily by flexing the hip joint within the socket. Some choose an even more inefficient strategy, rotating the pelvis backward, using posterior tilt of the pelvis to afford a more advantageous length to the hip flexors. Unfortunately, the lack of forward pelvic movement robs the prosthetic socket of the velocity necessary to produce prosthetic knee flexion. When either of these less effective strategies is employed, the prosthesis advances slowly, with little of the knee flexion necessary for swing limb clearance, and with unnatural substitutions of pelvic and trunk movement.

For effective swing phase, a combination of hip flexion and forward pelvic rotation is used to advance the prosthesis. To help a new user discover this strategy, the therapist can facilitate pelvic rotation with manual cues. This component of gait is one of the few that can be effectively trained with part-task training designed to perfect the patient's ability to rotate the pelvis forward during swing phase. To practice this pattern of pelvic motion, the person with amputation stands in the parallel bars with the body's weight borne primarily on the nonamputated limb. The person then selects a target on the floor—someone can actually mark the target with tape—and swings the prosthesis forward quickly, planting the prosthetic heel on the target (Figure 29-3). Next, the person extends the residual hip to move the prosthesis *behind* the nonamputated limb and then repeats the entire process. Initially, both hands may lightly contact the parallel bars; complexity of the task is advanced to a single upper limb support and then to a hands-free activity. Motor learning is most effective if a form of random practice is incorporated into the activity (e.g., alternating among targets that require quick steps of different distances and that direct the prosthesis at different angles medially and laterally).

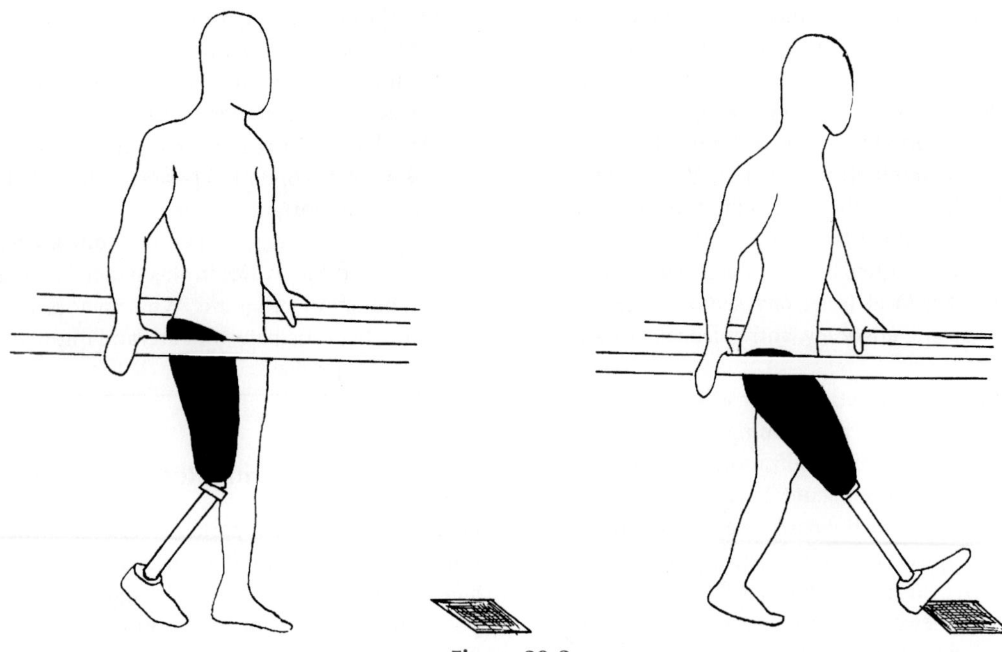

Figure 29-3

Repeated and rapid stepping with the prosthesis toward an anterior target provides an opportunity to practice swing limb advancement of the prosthesis. The step is initiated by forceful hip flexion, leading to flexion of the prosthetic knee. A long stride can only be accomplished with forward rotation of the pelvis.

Although this skill is most easily performed in the parallel bars, patients can also practice at home as their muscle strength and balance improve, using the kitchen counter, a table, or the back of a sofa for support. The drill has two advantages. First, it encourages forceful use of muscles and aggressive control of prosthetic motion, which are especially important for older patients in mastering postural control and balance reactions. Second, this exercise provides patients with a simple but important performance cue—rapidly bringing the prosthesis's distal end to a target on the floor—that automatically produces the pelvic motion necessary to advance the prosthesis efficiently. Even though the focus is on the environment and prosthesis's distal end, the pelvis will move forward during prosthetic swing so that its trajectory is flat and parallel to the floor.

Learning to Use Hip Extension at Loading Response

In the typical gait pattern, ground reaction forces produce knee flexion and hip flexion when the swinging limb finally contacts the walking surface and begins to share the body's weight with the trailing limb.[16] A patient with amputation can generate extension moments to control the hip at this stage of the gait cycle but cannot directly extend the prosthetic knee and must therefore rely on other techniques. Prosthetic alignment causes the ground reaction force to move anteriorly to the prosthetic knee joint during a large portion of the stance phase. An individual with an amputation can extend the prosthetic knee joint when the prosthesis's distal end is fixed on the ground by extending the residual hip joint within the socket.

The need for hip extensor strength is one reason why patients with amputations should continue their preprosthetic exercise programs for at least 3 months after receiving their initial prostheses. Activities that challenge the hip abductors with the resistance of elastic tubing or with the weight of the limb itself, as in the traditional side-lying hip abduction exercise, do not require the muscles to produce a great deal of force. Moreover, the exercises may not be sufficiently specific to the function of walking; they may not cause activation of the hip abductors at the joint angles and muscle lengths in which they are typically active during this portion of the gait cycle. However, a version of the traditional "bridging" exercise satisfies these criteria (Figure 29-4).[17] The individual assumes a supine position, with a firm but slightly forgiving object (e.g., towel roll, blanket, cushioned stool, phone book) under the residual thigh. By pressing the posterior thigh forcefully into the pad, persons with amputations can strengthen their hip extensors at a length and in a range of motion similar to that during loading response. They also learn how to control the pelvis and lumbar spine in a closed kinetic chain using the muscles of the residual limb.

The exercise can be modified to strengthen other muscle groups of both the intact and residual limb. For instance, it can be performed with the nonamputated limb, with the focus on using muscles that produce internal rotation at the nonamputated hip joint to permit the pelvis on the amputated side to move backward eccentrically, and then to move forward through concentric contraction. In doing so, individuals are practicing control of a motion that is identical in direction and muscle control (though different in terms of postural requirements) to the forward pelvic rotation necessary during swing phase.

The patient and family must understand that the prosthesis is designed to distribute the pressures encountered in erect weight-bearing and walking; wearing the prosthesis during strengthening exercises that involve other postures or activities can create areas of high pressure that might damage skin and soft tissue. The prosthesis should always be removed before this type of exercise.

The forward pelvic motion that is necessary during prosthetic swing should persist during loading response. Loading response is an important transition period during which both feet share the body's weight and muscle activity is widespread

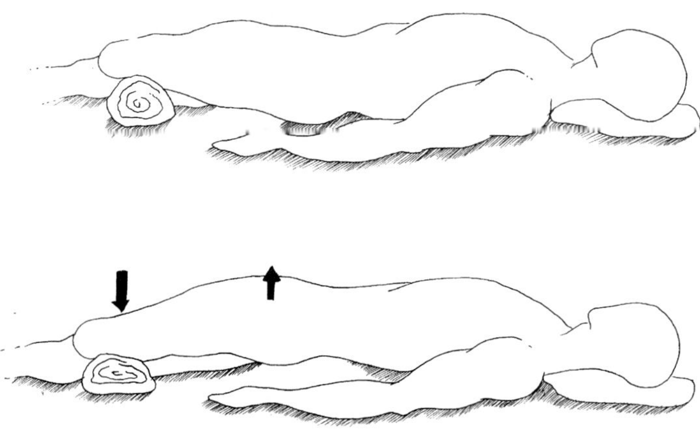

Figure 29-4

Bridging against a rolled towel or low padded stool strengthens the muscles of the residual limb in functional positions that are necessary for stability in early stance phase.

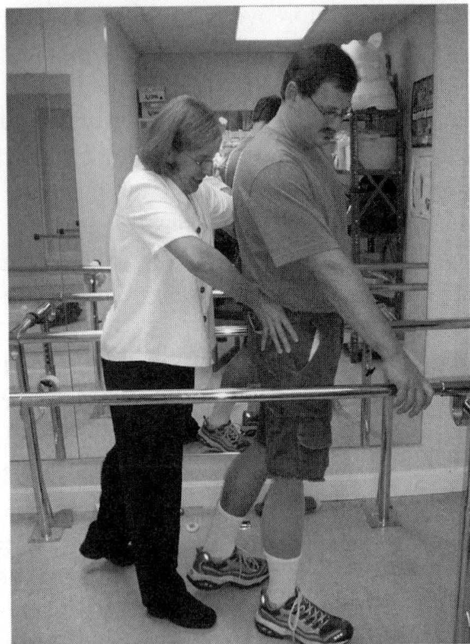

A

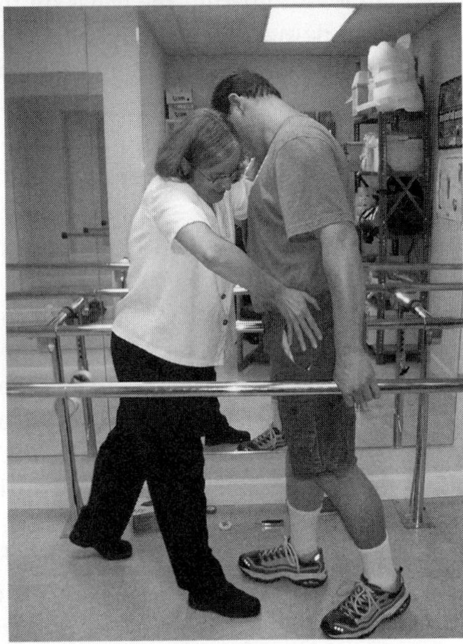

B

Figure 29-5

Facilitation of forward pelvic motion for efficient prosthetic gait. ***A,*** *The therapist can use Neurodevelopmental Treatment–like techniques to cue pelvic position from behind.* ***B,*** *The therapist can also use proprioceptive neuromuscular facilitation manual contacts and appropriate resistance, asking the patient to move the pelvis upward and forward as he or she steps with either limb.*

throughout the trunk and lower extremities. During loading response, as body weight is transferred to the prosthesis, the pelvis's opposite side rotates forward. This rotation, however, is a relative one; no part of the pelvis, including the side on which the limb is amputated, should ever move backward in an absolute sense.

Unfortunately, early in gait training, clients who worry about providing a hip extension force sufficient to stabilize the prosthetic knee may overcompensate, augmenting hip extension with backward pelvic movement. They may appear to sit back somewhat on the socket's posterior brim. Although this pelvic substitution certainly improves the prosthetic knee joint's stability during this critical weight acceptance phase, it diminishes the precious forward inertia necessary for progression into midstance and terminal stance. The energy cost of walking with a prosthesis is high enough without needlessly sacrificing energy by slowing down at every loading response as a result of halting or slowing the forward progress at the pelvis.

Therapists can manually facilitate the pelvic motion that new prosthesis users must perfect. By using augmented extrinsic feedback, such as tapping or brushing techniques of the neurodevelopmental treatment approach or the manual contact and appropriate resistance of proprioceptive neuromuscular facilitation, therapists can help patients with amputations learn to use their pelvises more efficiently and attend to deviations from normal pelvic motion. These techniques reinforce the proper movement pattern in which both sides of the pelvis continue to move forward during loading response, even if the sound side moves ahead of the prosthetic side.

Pelvic movements can be effectively cued from behind the patient. Spreading the fingers wide so that the thumb points upward and the fourth and fingers downward, therapists can place these digits on the muscle masses of the paraspinal muscles and the gluteus medius, respectively (Figure 29-5, *A*). This hand placement is best achieved if therapists hold their elbows close to their sides and extend their wrists. By maintaining contact with the pelvis at those regions on the superior, posterior, and lateral ilium that form the border of the gluteus medius's attachment, therapists may monitor pelvic movement in the transverse plane. Through palpation of the gluteus medius, they may also learn whether the muscles' activity is timely, acting during loading response and midstance. Therapists have excellent leverage to cue and enforce pelvic movement from this position. They should direct pressure from their fingers downward into the gluteus medius and with a slight anterior and medial component. Therapists should apply the pressure at those times during the gait cycle, loading response and midstance, when the hip abductors are active. Additionally, they can use this hand placement to push forward gently on one side of the pelvis when the limb swings forward on that side. Therapists may then maintain that forward pressure to prevent individuals with amputations from "sitting back" or letting the pelvis drift backward during the loading response period. A therapist can perform this facilitation even while using a gait belt to guard a patient early in the rehabilitation process.

Alternatively, repeated stepping with the sound limb "up and over" the stance prosthetic limb, with a downward, posteriorly directed manual contact and appropriate resistance applied at the iliac crest from in front, can be used to provide part-to-whole practice of the forward progression of the pelvis throughout stance phase (see Figure 29-5, *B*). If augmented feedback is provided by either of these facilitation techniques, therapists must be careful to use only that amount of stimulation necessary to achieve the desired response and to decrease the amount of facilitation with successive trials as the desired motor behavior becomes more consistent.

An understanding of pelvic movement and its effect on gait quality helps explain another common gait deviation, in which there is an external rotation of the prosthetic foot during loading response. Therapists often attribute this deviation to overactivity of the gluteus maximus; this hip extensor also externally rotates the hip joint and may do so when a patient new to prosthetic use exaggerates hip extension to stabilize the prosthetic knee. Failure to permit the pelvis to move forward also contributes to this rotational deviation, especially if the failure of forward inertia retards the shift of body weight onto the prosthetic foot. In this case, the foot is not stable on the floor and will move when rotational forces are placed on it from above, either through pelvic or hip joint movement.

Developing an Effective Midstance

Persons with transfemoral amputations frequently lean over their prostheses during midstance, increasing lateral sway and compromising forward progression and energy efficiency of gait. This common deviation stems from an imbalance of abduction and adduction moments at both the residual hip joint and the interface between the residual limb and the prosthetic socket. Stabilization of the femur in the frontal plane inside the prosthetic socket presents prosthetists with one of their greatest challenges.

Therapists should regard a lateral trunk lean as an indication that a person with an amputation is having difficulty controlling adduction, either in the residual hip joint or where the residual limb meets the prosthetic socket. One cause of this compensatory gait deviation is functional weakness or impaired motor control of hip abductor muscles, in particular the gluteus medius and the residual tensor fascia lata. The lateral lean is a compensatory strategy when these muscles are unable to keep the pelvis level as the intact limb swings forward during prosthetic stance. Other common contributors to this deviation include inadequate stabilization of a strong residual limb by the lateral socket wall and discomfort from high-pressure areas within the socket. A lateral trunk lean reorients the residual limb within the socket to avoid pressure either on its medial (proximal) brim or on its lateral distal regions. The prosthetist may need to modify the socket if there is undue pressure in these areas. Lastly, a lateral lean may be used to escape medial brim pressure if a residual limb has shrunk or reduced in volume so that it descends too far into the socket. If limb volume has decreased, additional ply of sock must be added to assure optimal fit and position of the residual limb in the socket. Individuals with short residual limbs may have a consistent lateral lean, even if there is significant strength and motor control, as the short lever arm makes it challenging to control the prosthesis in the frontal plane.

If lateral lean cannot be explained by prosthetic-related discomfort, fit, or alignment issues, the focus of intervention is on developing motor control of hip abductor force. To improve or eliminate lateral trunk lean, an individual using a prosthesis must develop strong hip abductors and then activate them forcefully inside the socket.

The links among strengthening exercises, muscle strength and performance, and the quality of prosthetic gait must be well understood by persons with amputations, their family support system, and the rehabilitation professions with whom they interact. Hip abductor strengthening is a traditional component of rehabilitation programs for those with transfemoral amputations. A modification of the "bridging" exercise, such that it is performed in sidelying, for hip abductor strengthening offers various advantages (Figure 29-6). After removing the prosthesis, the person with an amputation lies on the side of the amputation with the amputated limb resting on a firm supporting surface. The sound limb is flexed comfortably at the hip and knee, perhaps resting on a stool. A rolled towel or blanket is placed under the distal lateral residual limb to elongate hip abductors slightly. Forceful but steady contraction of hip abductors by pressing the residual thigh into the support surface will lift the pelvis from the surface in a lateral "bridge." The pelvis is then lowered slowly, in a controlled eccentric contraction. This exercise is challenging; those with recently healed limbs may be able to perform only three or four repetitions. Initially, some individuals cannot develop enough force to elevate the pelvis from the supporting surface; the goal should be to relieve the hip of at least some portion of body weight.

The exercise's difficulty is outweighed by its specificity in strengthening the important gluteus medius in the very range of motion (ROM) where it must be activated it during midstance. For best results, the exercise should be performed without substitution of other muscles in an effort to clear the pelvis. As muscle fatigue develops, inadvertent repositioning of the pelvis by rolling slightly away from midline position allows other muscle groups to "help" the hip abductors with this difficult exercise. By rolling slightly forward, a degree of hip flexion is introduced into the amputated limb's position. This allows muscles with a flexion-abduction angle of pull, such as the residual tensor fascia lata and other hip flexors, to substitute for the gluteus medius. Conversely, when there is a slight backward repositioning, hip extensor muscles can substitute for the gluteus medius. Each substitution defeats the purpose of the exercise. Therapists must help individuals with amputations recognize these common signs of fatigue and caution them to rest or perform recuperative exercises when substitutions appear. Consistent performance of the exercise will, over time, effectively strengthen hip abductor muscles and improve motor control, even if the pelvis is raised minimally off the support surface.

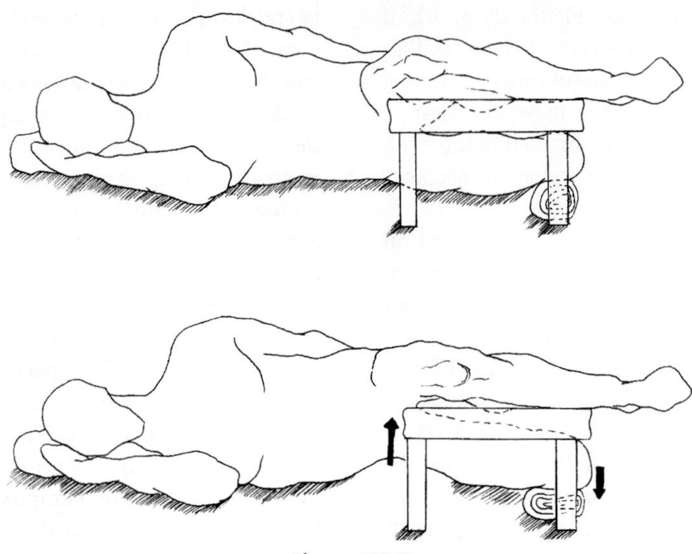

Figure 29-6
When the residual limb is positioned in hip extension, bridging performed in sidelying strengthens hip abductors in a functional range of motion that approximates midstance.

In addition to practicing effective exercise programs, persons with transfemoral amputations can also learn to monitor their pelvic position as they walk throughout the day. Even those who have defeated the tendency to lean their trunks laterally to offset inadequate hip abductor musculature may demonstrate subtle compensations in their pelvic movement patterns. For instance, they may shift the pelvis slightly toward the prosthetic side at midstance even as they maintain a level orientation between the iliac crests. This pelvic movement helps to avoid leaning the trunk laterally and serves a similar purpose; it produces hip adduction during midstance and elongates the hip abductors so that they may develop additional force. Unfortunately, this lateral pelvic shift also permits the center of gravity to migrate farther than it otherwise would toward the midstance side. This practice expends energy unnecessarily over the course of many walking steps.

To combat this compensation and help patients learn appropriate pelvic control throughout the gait cycle, therapists may manually cue pelvic motion using the technique discussed earlier in connection with gait improvement during loading response. They may stand behind the patient with their hands in readiness on the pelvis's posterior and lateral aspects. Spreading their fingers, they can contact the gluteus medius on either side with the fourth and fifth fingers of either hand. These points of control or contact permit therapists to monitor pelvic movement not just in the transverse plane, where they can discern whether the proper rotation is occurring, but also in the frontal plane.

If the pelvis drifts laterally, permitting the hip joint to adduct on that side, therapists have excellent leverage to limit that motion and cue the amputee to activate muscles to prevent it. Once again, the therapist applies pressure to lateral pelvis in a downward, medial, and anterior direction. This facilitation amounts to enforcement of proper pelvic position. The therapist constrains or limits the degrees of freedom within which the pelvis may move and gradually permit the individual to control the pelvis in more dimensions over a larger percentage of the gait cycle.

The use of a straight cane in the contralateral hand can assist with the challenge of keeping the pelvis level during midstance (Figure 29-7). The biomechanical goal is to produce an upward force on the side of the pelvis opposite the prosthesis. Specifically, the prosthetic wearer must create a *reaction* to the force that the cane places on the ground, an upward force that acts through the arm and trunk to elevate the pelvis on the nonprosthetic side. To accomplish, persons with amputations must have strength in their extremities and trunk sufficient to transmit force through the cane into the ground. Further, they must direct a large force straight down, along the cane's shaft, into the ground.

In explaining this concept, therapists must encourage those using a transfemoral prosthesis to push down forcefully into the cane handle, without leaning their upper trunk toward the cane. The goal should be to push the body's center of gravity away from the cane and toward the prosthesis, which appropriately bears the weight during midstance. A straight cane accomplishes this task more readily than a quad cane or one with another type of base. Many persons with amputations would prefer to use quad canes because they "stay put" when not being used (e.g., when opening a door or reaching for an object). They also permit a margin

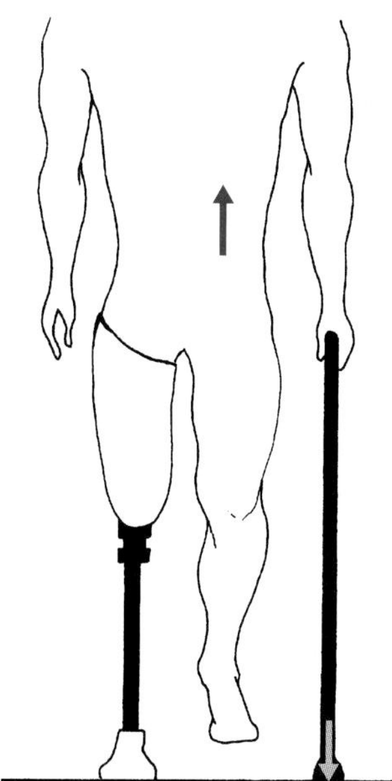

Figure 29-7
A direct downward force applied through a straight cane can assist those who have difficulty maintaining a level pelvis during stance on the prosthesis.

of error while walking; all that is required to remain stable is a force through the cane handle toward a point within the cane's quadrilateral base of support. The problem this creates, in terms of appropriate motor control at midstance, is that the force need not be applied straight downward. A force that is not vertical cannot efficiently support the pelvis at midstance. Because the energy cost of walking with a transfemoral prosthesis is already so high, patients cannot afford to apply upper extremity muscle force in any but the most efficient direction. A straight cane structures the walking task so that it must be used effectively and efficiently.

A "part to whole" exercise in standing that can also be used to assist a new prosthesis wearer to control the pelvis at midstance (and reduce the tendency to laterally lean) is initially performed in the parallel bars (Figure 29-8). The individual concentrates on keeping the trunk erect and the pelvis level and progressing forward while stepping upward onto a stool with the sound limb and then placing it back on the floor. The individual is encouraged to push downward on the parallel bars through an open hand and control the motion by moving slowly. In addition to improving timing and quality of motor control of the residual hip in midstance, this activity also helps to strengthen hip extensors and abductors at lengths necessary for effective gait. The difficulty level of the exercise is progressed by increasing the height of the stool and using a single hand on the parallel bars, and eventually no upper extremity support.

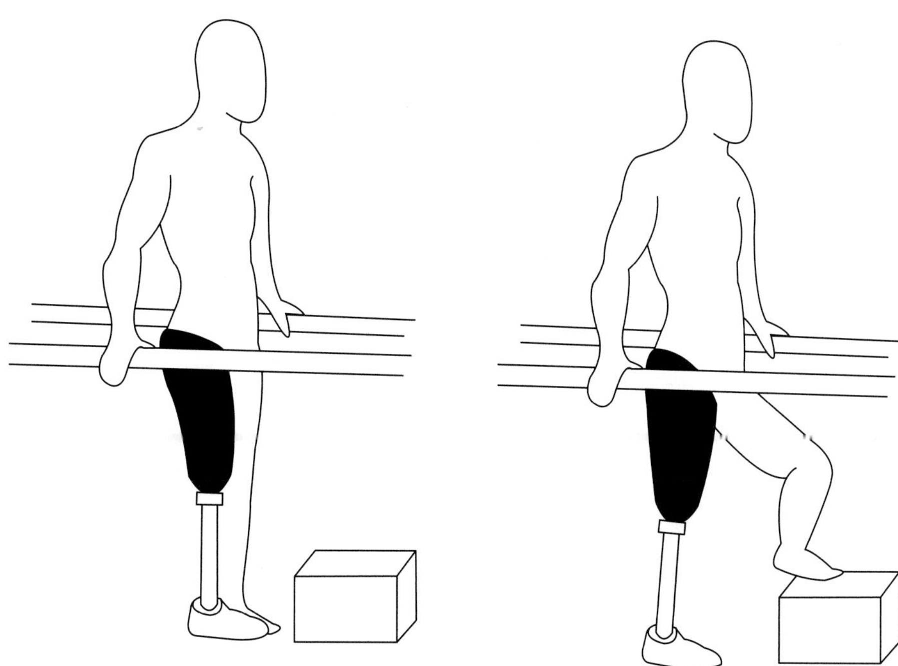

Figure 29-8
In order to step up onto a stool with the intact limb, the individual must shift weight onto the prosthesis to unload the intact limb, stabilize the pelvis with contraction of the gluteus maximus, and allow both sides of the pelvis to move forward as the intact limb is placed on the stool.

CASE EXAMPLE 2

An Individual with Traumatic Transfemoral Amputation and Upper Extremity Injury

B. R., 27, is a previously healthy, 6-foot, 2-inch tall man who recently worked as a relief worker for a nongovernmental agency in the Middle East. His convoy was ambushed by a roadside bomb 8 weeks ago, and he sustained severe blast-related trauma of his right knee and lower leg, a comminuted fracture of the right forearm and wrist, and pneumothorax from a left rib fracture. He was airlifted to a military trauma center for initial care, including amputation at the transfemoral level and open reduction internal fixation of his upper extremity fractures. He was moved to a military hospital in Germany, where infection necessitated revision of his residual limb to a short transfemoral level 7 days after initial injury. He returned to the United States for a short stay in a rehabilitation center near his parents' home. He has been attending an outpatient center for preprosthetic care and early prosthetic rehabilitation twice a week for the past 3 weeks. He reports feeling "deconditioned" and "disillusioned," tiring easily and struggling to believe he will ever return to running and biking, which he enjoyed before his injury.

B. R. received his initial transfemoral prosthesis 1 week ago—an ischial-ramal containment flexible socket in a rigid frame worn with prosthetic socks, total elastic suspension belt, a Total Knee, and hybrid single-axis articulating-dynamic response foot. He now wears his prosthesis comfortably for 3 hours at a time. He requires assistance with donning and adjusting suspension because of his forearm cast. Although he initially used a four-point reciprocal gait pattern with a platform crutch on the right and standard axillary crutch on the left, this has evolved into a slow two-point pattern.

During observational gait examination, the prosthetic rehabilitation team notes the following problems: B. R.'s step length and swing time are larger for the right than for the left limb; left initial contact occurs prematurely at the end of right midstance position, delayed forward progression of the right pelvis from initial contact to midstance, and delayed weight shift onto the prosthesis from loading response to midstance. With the premature termination of right stance (and limitation of forward progression over the prosthetic toe), B. R. has significant difficulty unlocking the prosthetic knee to initiate swing and uses a vaulting pattern to clear his prosthetic foot during midswing. B. R. expresses frustration about his slow gait speed and reliance on crutches, doubting that he will ever "walk normally" again.

Questions to Consider

- What is the "ideal" effective and energy-efficient walking pattern for individuals with transfemoral amputation?
- What are the determinants of an effective prosthetic initial contact and loading response? What characteristics of the individual (e.g., strength, motor control, ROM, fear of falling) influence the quality of early prosthetic stance? What characteristics of the prosthesis influence the quality of early prosthetic stance?
- Considering the length of B. R.'s residual limb, what phases of gait are expected to be most biomechanically challenging for him? Why would these particular subphases be difficult?
- How could B. R.'s early prosthetic stance phase be described? Why is he having difficulty? What type of "part to whole" practice or holistic gait activities could be used to help him develop the most effective early stance period, using a motor learning model?
- How could B. R.'s transition from prosthetic loading response through midstance be described? And his readiness for the terminal stance phase of gait? Why is he having difficulty? How does his shortened prosthetic stance affect the swing phase of the opposite limb? What type of "part to whole" and holistic gait activities could be used help him master an effective single-limb support period of prosthetic stance, using principles of motor learning?
- How could B. R.'s transition from stance to swing phase be described? Why is he having difficulty with this phase of gait? What type of "part to whole" and holistic gait activities could be used to help him master an effective transition from prosthetic stance to swing phase, using principles of motor learning?
- Does B. R. have the potential for functional ambulation without an assistive device? Why or why not? How can the "time" to progress him to a less supportive device or to no supportive device be determined? What type of practice opportunities and augmented feedback can be used to help him move toward unsupported ambulation? How can he progress to more challenging walking environments? How can it be determined whether his progress is occurring at the rate predicted when the prognosis was made?
- How often, and how formally, should his progress be "reassessed" during this stage of prosthetic rehabilitation? What measures can be used to document B. R.'s progress?

Prosthetic Terminal Stance and Stride Length of the Opposite Limb

In the typical gait pattern, muscle activity becomes eccentric in the hip flexors and ankle plantar flexors as the body's mass moves forward over the stance foot. Two factors assist those with transfemoral amputations to stabilize the prosthetic knee joint. First, the prosthesis's design causes its knee joint axis to lie behind the force vector produced by ground reaction. Second, the prosthetic ankle's considerable stiffness prevents the shank from moving forward as long as body weight is directed through the foot's solid keel portion. Even prostheses with ankle mechanisms that permit some motion are stiff enough to retard the shank's forward movement, preventing any tendency for the prosthetic knee to bend during midstance and terminal stance.

To gain this advantage, persons with transfemoral amputations must sustain body weight on the prosthesis in late stance. If prosthetic stance is roughly equal in duration to the intact limb, the gait pattern will have a rhythmic cadence and fairly equal step and stride lengths. The tendency to walk with unequal step lengths, especially early in the rehabilitation process, can be attributed to a relatively short step with the nonamputated limb. When a new prosthesis wearer is unable or unwilling to sustain a sufficiently long period of stance on the prosthesis, swing phase of the nonamputated limb is curtailed and stride length is reduced.

A relatively brief stance duration may be the result of muscle weakness in the residual limb, most frequently in the hip abductors and hip extensors. A second cause that therapists should investigate is pain. Finally, imbalances of muscle length and joint excursion can limit the amount of time an individual can bear weight on the prosthesis during the gait cycle. Chief among these length imbalances is hip flexor tightness. Hip flexor muscles must elongate during terminal stance to allow apparent hip extension. If hip flexors are contracted and the residual hip joint's ROM is limited toward extension, compensatory strategies must be used and gait deviations become apparent. Slight tightness of hip flexors may cause excessive lumbar lordosis in late stance; although this accomplishes the motor task of forward progression and adequate step length, over time this strategy may lead to lower back dysfunction and pain. If tightness significantly limits hip extension excursion, then the stride length of the swing leg is compromised and abnormally short, and a rapid weight shift occurs from the prosthetic limb to the intact limb.

Contracture of hip flexors occurs when the muscles remain immobile in shortened position for periods of time. Unfortunately, the medical conditions and comorbidities among those with dysvascular or neuropathic amputation limit activity and mobility, placing those with transfemoral amputation at significant risk of developing flexion and abduction contracture. Long periods of sitting or lying in bed with the affected limb elevated cause the hip flexors' resting length to decrease. Some degree of tightness of the residual limb hip flexors occurs, even if the individual has been consistent with a preprosthetic hip extensor strengthening and "prone lying" stretching exercise program, when gait training with a transfemoral prosthesis commences.

Transfemoral amputation surgery creates muscle imbalance between hip adductor muscle groups and the gluteus maximus. Even a relatively long transfemoral amputation sacrifices a large portion of the hip adductor musculature.[18,19] Because these muscles produce hip adduction and internal rotation, their absence permits shortening over time in the muscles that produce hip abduction and external rotation. A principle abductor-external rotator is the gluteus maximus. Because the antagonistic adductor muscles can no longer effectively passively or actively oppose nor restrain the gluteus maximus, its resting length decreases. Similar shortening is likely to occur in the posterior portion of the gluteus medius. The fiber orientation of the gluteus medius near the hip joint parallels that of the gluteus maximus. The result is that those with transfemoral amputations frequently demonstrate a combination of hip flexion, abduction, and external rotation contractures.

When not wearing a prosthesis, an individual with a shortened gluteus maximus may sit with the residual limb abducted and externally rotated away from the midline. Although this strategy enlarges the functional base of support for sitting balance, those with shortness of the gluteus cannot adduct the hips and bring their thighs together upon request. A patient whose gluteus maximus is shortened instead flexes the lumbar spine and tilts the pelvis posteriorly in order to effectively extend the residual hip joint. The hip extension permits the gluteus maximus to elongate when the hips adduct.

Gluteus maximus shortness may also be evident when walking with the prosthesis. During terminal stance, the pelvis typically rotates forward on the side opposite the stance limb. This pelvic rotation contributes to the nonamputated limb's step and stride lengths. In rotating forward on the side opposite the amputation, pelvic movement produces internal rotation at the residual hip joint. Internal hip joint rotation elongates the gluteus maximus and other hip external rotators so that passive tension develops in the muscles during terminal stance. A shortened gluteus maximus can develop enough passive tension that it causes the residual hip joint to rotate externally during this phase of the gait cycle.

Therapists may detect limitation in two ways. The prosthetic foot rotates externally during terminal stance. This is most obvious if full body weight has not shifted onto the prosthesis or if weight shifts away from the prosthesis prematurely during midstance or terminal stance. Alternatively, the entire prosthesis may rotate inward on the residual limb over the course of several steps, even if there is appropriate weight bearing on the prosthesis. If a shortened gluteus maximus produces passive tension that rotates the residual hip externally during terminal stance, the residual limb may itself rotate externally *inside* the prosthetic socket. During gait, this appears to be relative inward rotation of the socket on the residual limb. Over the course of several steps, the toe of the prosthesis points more medially with each step. At the least, this prosthetic alignment is not cosmetic. If the "in toeing" is extreme, the prosthetic knee joint's axis rotates in space so that ground reaction and inertial forces no longer initiate knee flexion necessary for an effective prosthetic swing phase. Additionally, internal rotation of the prosthetic

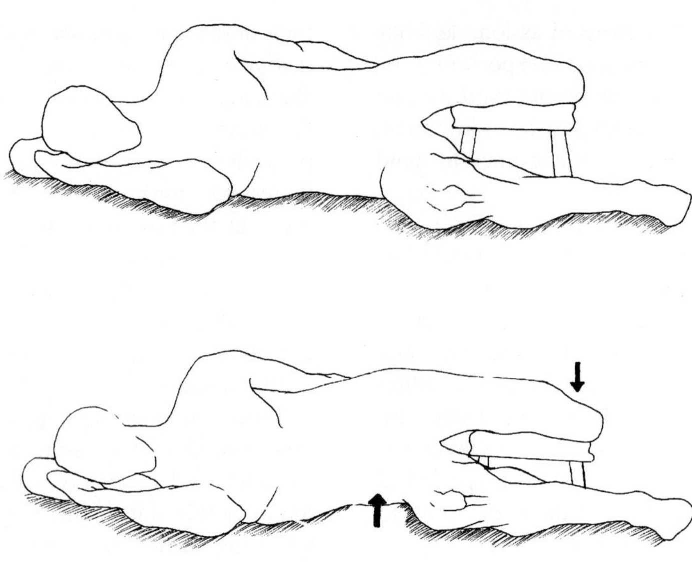

Figure 29-9
Active or isometric contraction of the medial residual limb against a low stool can counteract the tendency toward shortening of the gluteus maximus and address muscle strength imbalance between adductor and abductor muscle groups in the residual limb.

socket moves its anterior brim medially. Because the medial brim is relatively high, this migration toward the sensitive groin region may cause discomfort during gait.

Gluteal shortening can be avoided or reversed by maintaining strength in the residual hip adductor musculature. One strategy to accomplish this is performed in sidelying on the intact side (Figure 29-9).[17,20,21] The residual limb is positioned in extension on a short, padded stool, and the nonamputated hip and knee are slightly flexed to balance in sidelying. By pushing the residual thigh's medial surface downward into the stool, an individual with amputations can activate the residual adductor muscle mass against considerable resistance and attempt to lift the pelvis slightly from the surface on which the patient rests. The exercise addresses the strength imbalance between the hip adductors and abductors. It can reverse the tendency toward hip abductor tightness by maintaining strength in the hip adductors in an ROM where they are relatively short.

Preswing: Preparing for Swing Phase

Preswing, which concludes the stance phase of the gait cycle, is a period when many muscle groups of the trunk and lower extremities are active. The way in which a wearer of transfemoral prostheses coordinates movement during preswing determines the quality of movement exhibited during the swing phase. Flexion of the prosthetic knee unit must begin during preswing so that the prosthesis's overall length shortens sufficiently during early swing for effective toe clearance. If the prosthetic knee is not flexed adequately during preswing, there is a functionally longer limb to advance during swing and the toe of the prosthetic foot (which cannot actively dorsiflex) may drag or catch as the swing phase begins. This tendency is so dangerous and contributes so directly to falls and other mishaps that other compensatory strategies must be employed to advance the prosthetic limb. Such strategies include "hip hiking" (elevating the pelvis on the side of the amputation), abducting or circumducting the prosthesis (moving it in an arc away from midline during swing), or "vaulting" (arising on the toe through ankle plantar flexion) on the contralateral stance foot.

Patients' success in initiating preswing knee flexion depends on four factors: (1) the use of hip flexors; (2) the initiation of forward pelvic rotation; (3) the timing of heel rise; and (4) the controlled shifting of weight from the prosthesis to the nonamputated limb.

In normal gait at comfortable walking speed, walkers with intact lower extremities initiate knee flexion without having to activate the hamstrings to produce knee flexion. They do, however, quickly and forcefully activate their hip flexors to lift the limb from the floor; this is the second most important contribution of propulsive energy to the gait cycle. Patients with amputations must learn to activate the hip flexors forcefully inside the prosthetic socket as if they are "kicking" a ball with the front of the thigh. A rapid but brief concentric activation of these muscles accelerates the prosthesis's socket portion and, through reaction forces at the prosthetic knee, produces knee flexion. Indeed, studies of gait patterns of those with transfemoral amputation demonstrate that this strategy is the most important source of propulsive energy for effective prosthetic gait.[22]

Hip flexion, however strong, may not be enough by itself to flex the prosthetic knee and permit advancement of the prosthesis. Simultaneous forward movement of the pelvis on the side of the amputation must also occur. The pelvis's forward movement influences the location and orientation of the ground reaction force, which is generated by the body segments' weight and inertial forces. Laboratory studies demonstrate that the ground reaction force vector inclines forward during preswing from its point of origin where the foot contacts the floor.[23] Forward pelvic rotation contributes to the vector's forward inclination, causing it to fall behind the knee joint and produce knee flexion.

Another important event that initiates preswing knee flexion in the typical gait pattern is "heel rise." In an anatomically intact limb, the heel actually rises from the floor before preswing, at around 35% of the gait cycle during terminal stance.[16] As the anatomical ankle gradually dorsiflexes during midstance, the plantar flexor muscles elongate under eccentric action. Gradually, the plantar flexors develop enough force that their action becomes isometric and they prevent further ankle dorsiflexion. When this occurs, the lower leg's continued advance over the foot pulls the heel from the floor. "Heel rise" then inclines the leg's tibial portion forward and flexes the knee in a closed chain.

Persons with transfemoral amputations cannot employ this mechanism to begin flexing the prosthetic knee. Instead of ankle plantar flexors, they have a prosthetic "ankle" that resists dorsiflexion because it is stiff and inflexible. For the prosthetic heel to rise, the ground reaction force must pass in front of the prosthetic foot's keel. This event's timing depends on prosthetic alignments that influence the length of the prosthesis's heel and toe levers. A prosthesis with an excessively long toe lever produces a late heel rise; as a result, individuals with this type of prosthesis have difficulty initiating knee flexion and may complain that they feel as if they are walking uphill. (Conversely, prostheses with short toe levers will permit premature heel rise and knee flexion, a precarious situation known as "drop-off.")

Finally, the new prosthesis wearer must learn to control and take advantage of proper weight shift, body position, and posture during preswing. Initiation of knee flexion during preswing depends on a properly located ground reaction force. A therapist who understands the mechanics of preswing can focus fruitfully on the way that the person learning to use the prosthesis controls the transition of body weight late in stance. The person must be able to completely shift body weight onto the prosthetic foot in early stance, maintain weight bearing throughout the full stance period, and control the rate at which the weight's center of pressure moves anteriorly toward the end of the prosthetic keel in terminal stance and preswing.

Therapists are adept at training individuals new to prosthetic use to shift weight onto an involved or prosthetic limb during loading response. Training patients to maintain that weight shift and remove weight gradually during preswing is more challenging. A variety of "cross-over walking" or "braiding" is a part-task training technique that embodies an appropriate weight shift. Cross-over walking begins by balancing on the sound limb. Next, the individuals step forward and across the midline with the prosthesis, crossing it in front of the sound limb by simultaneously flexing and adducting the hip and rotating the pelvis forward on the prosthetic side (Figure 29-10).[20] In the next cycle of the activity the prosthesis is the stance limb, while the sound limb steps.

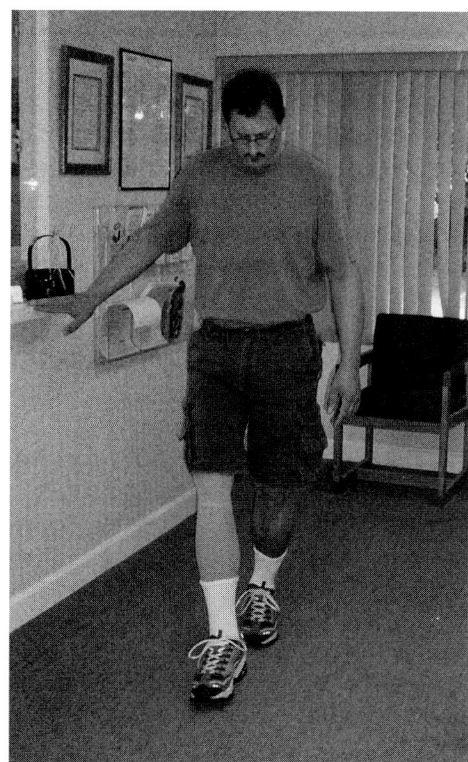

Figure 29-10
Cross-over walking can be used to facilitate control of pelvic and hip position as the prosthetic limb is loaded and unloaded during the activity.

Cross-over walking facilitates activity in stance limb hip abductor muscles at the same time that controlled pelvic rotation must occur on the swing side. Therapists can manually guide the pelvis through its requisite forward rotation on the prosthetic side. The activity must be performed in an erect posture, without flexion of the trunk or hips. Standing near a wall, with hands placed on the wall at shoulder height, provides a safe environment in which to practice the activity, in the clinic or as part of a home program.

CASE EXAMPLE 3

An Adolescent with a Long Transfemoral Amputation Due to Osteosarcoma of the Proximal Tibia

P. J. is a 14-year-old self-described "computer geek" diagnosed with grade 2 osteosarcoma of the proximal tibia 4 months ago. Because the tumor extended into the tibial plateau, limb-sparing surgery was not possible. His oncologist recommended a long transfemoral amputation. P. J. underwent 4 weeks of chemotherapy before amputation to "shrink" the tumor, a 3-week "break" for surgery, and then an additional 4 weeks of chemotherapy in the postoperative-preprosthetic period.

Although his residual limb healed well, P. J. had difficulty with nausea and thrush during his chemotherapy, losing almost 15 lb from his already slender frame. He spent much of his early postoperative time resting in his father's recliner with his lower limbs abducted and externally rotated, entertaining himself with his laptop computer and Playstation. He returned to school 1 month ago, initially attending half-days. After full days of school, he needed to take a nap when he came home. Two weeks ago, he received his training prosthesis, with an ischial-ramal containment socket, total elastic suspension belt, four-bar polycentric knee, and dynamic response foot. Although he can ambulate with his prosthesis using axillary crutches independently for up to 300 feet, he prefers using a rented wheelchair to get around at school, noting that walking is "exhausting."

When observing his gait, the outpatient therapist notes an effective initial contact and progression into midstance on the prosthetic side; however, the time spent in midstance to preswing is significantly less than that of the intact limb. Forward pelvic progression is compromised. Out toeing (external rotation) of the prosthetic foot during terminal stance is obvious, and the swinging intact limb has a shortened stride length. The therapist also notes that P. J. has difficulty initiating knee flexion in preswing and demonstrates a late heel rise. The therapist decides to reassess muscle performance and range of motion of the residual hip. When P. J. removes his prosthesis and sits on the edge of the mat, the therapist notes his residual limb is abducted away from the midline. P. J. has difficulty bringing his limbs to midline, moving into a strong posterior tilt when he tries to do so.

Questions to Consider

- What tests and measures would be appropriate for assessing muscle performance (strength, length, power, and endurance) of both P. J.'s intact and residual limbs? How might these tests or measures need to be modified because of the length of his residual limb? If modified, how will this affect the validity and reliability of the test or measure?
- Given the therapist's observations, what are the likely contributors to the gait difficulties that P. J. is experiencing? What findings are expected during the examination and evaluation?
- Considering his age, medical diagnosis, overall physical condition, and motivation, what is an estimation (prognosis) for improvement in the quality and functionality of P. J.'s ambulation with his prosthesis? Will he be able to remediate or correct the impairments contributing to his gait dysfunction or will he need to accommodate or adapt to "permanent" impairments? What are the immediate and long-term goals for this boy?
- What types of interventions are recommended to address the impairments that examination and evaluation have identified? In what combination might you use manual therapy, strengthening and endurance exercise, and gait training? What is the appropriate frequency and intensity for each component of intervention that you recommend? Which interventions require "hands on" physical therapy in the clinic? Which interventions can be incorporated into a home exercise program? How much time will be required to achieve P. J.'s goals?
- How will the efficacy of the interventions included in the plan of care be assessed? How frequently should muscle performance be reassessed? What other indicators of improvement could be monitored? What incentives could be created for this sedentary boy to become more physically active and achieve the optimal outcome of his prosthetic rehabilitation?

USING THE PROSTHESIS FOR ACTIVITIES OF DAILY LIVING

Although walking safely and efficiently with their prosthesis on level surfaces is a baseline mobility task that persons with transfemoral amputations are eager to master, other tasks are equally as important for resuming normal daily tasks and leisure activities. These include getting up and down from the floor, stepping over obstacles, ascending and descending curbs and stairs, negotiating on inclines and uneven terrain, and being able to walk quickly when the situation demands. Fear of falling (and being unable to get back up) during these types of activities often leads a person with transfemoral amputation to limit activity, in an effort to avoid a fall; this fear of falling can be as or more disabling than the limitations of the actual amputation. Practicing these tasks in the relatively controlled environment of a rehabilitation setting helps those new to prosthetic use build confidence and gain mastery of the more complex, but necessary, mobility tasks.

Facing Fear of Falling

The concern about falling that many individuals with transfemoral amputations have early in rehabilitation is understandable, given the impact that the loss of the anatomical ankle and knee has on the efficiency of postural responses. Many persons with transfemoral amputations experience an unanticipated fall at some point during rehabilitation or after discharge from their gait training program. This concern becomes problematic when it undermines confidence that is necessary to begin walking on inclines, stairs, and uneven terrain. Some therapists advocate teaching those new to prosthetic use how to fall as part of their rehabilitation program, in order to confront and decrease their fearfulness.

Because most persons with transfemoral amputations are older adults, with a number of interacting medical conditions, actual practice of falling techniques may entail greater risks than potential rewards. Having a "plan of action" to implement should a fall occur is another effective way to tackle fear of falling.

Learning How to Fall

Forward falls, even practice falls on a treatment mat from a kneeling position, produce large forces as the upper extremities contact the ground. Keeping the elbows and shoulders slightly flexed provides shock absorption as the upper extremities are suddenly loaded; however, extended wrists are at risk of ligamentous injury or osteoporotic fracture. An alternative technique involves "jackknifing," in which rapid hip flexion propels the center of mass backward so that contact with the ground is made with the buttocks, followed by a roll *backward* onto rounded back and shoulders.

If therapists do not wish to expose older individuals to the risks of practice falls, they can at least advise them how best to protect themselves should they fall. The most effective response to an irrecoverable loss of balance when wearing a transfemoral prosthesis is to bend at the waist while shifting body weight toward the nonamputated side. Falling toward the nonamputated side reduces the risk of injury should the prosthesis twist or turn during descent or landing. Instead, the impact of the fall is absorbed on the nonamputated side, first on the hip and then on the shoulder.

Therapists may alleviate some concern about falling by helping individuals with amputations develop a strategy to arise from the floor in the event that they unexpectedly fall. First, the person who has fallen should stop a moment and "take stock" to determine if the fall has resulted in injury. The person should try to regain calm in an anxiety-producing situation. Getting up immediately from the floor is unnecessary. The individual should also be empowered to "take charge" and direct others who may offer assistance.

Those who can learn how to get down to the floor in a controlled manner while wearing their prostheses are usually better able to understand how to "reverse" the process to return to standing. It may be helpful to have the therapist or a peer with amputation first demonstrate the sequence of movements. New prosthesis wearers can then be assisted or guided through the sequence with judicious verbal and tactile cues. While mastering this task, they develop various movement skills that can be applied to other movement problems they encounter during daily activities (e.g., how to kneel on the prosthetic knee; how to arise from kneeling; how to move among kneeling, sidesitting, and sidelying postures).

Assuming and Rising from a Kneeling Position

To learn to descend to the floor from a standing position, the first action is to lean on a stable piece of furniture to support and balance some of the body weight through the upper extremities. While balancing on the nonamputated leg, the individual prepares to kneel on the prosthetic knee using quick hip extension against the posterior wall of the socket to position the prosthetic foot as far behind him or her as possible. Using the arms for support and eccentric control of the intact limb's knee and hip, the prosthetic knee is then lowered toward the ground so that it is directly under the trunk. The individual is now in a "half-kneeling" position, with the prosthetic knee down and the knee and hip of the intact limb flexed to 90 degrees while the foot remains in contact with the floor. Maintaining upper extremity support, the individual carefully shifts weight toward the side of amputation. When the intact limb is sufficiently unweighted, it can be moved into a full kneeling position, next to the prosthetic one.

Once the person is in a kneeling position, the therapist may choose to continue the sequence until the patient is lying on the floor or to have the patient reverse directions and rise from kneeling at this point. The latter may be appropriate for those with limited endurance, as well as those with cognitive impairment who might more readily learn if novel movement sequences contain fewer steps.

To return to standing from a kneeling position, weight is momentarily shifted onto the prosthetic knee, which rests on the floor, using upper extremity support on the nearby, stable piece of furniture. Once the intact limb is sufficiently unweighted, rapid hip and knee flexion is used to move it forward into a half-kneel, with the foot flat on the floor. Bending at the waist, leaning into the furniture for upper body support, the individual then extends the sound hip and knee, to move upward toward standing. Once the sound limb is extended fully, hip flexion is used to bring the prosthesis forward until the prosthetic foot is slightly behind the sound foot.

Those who perform this technique next to a chair or bed can use it to regain a sitting position if they should be on the floor for any reason, including after a fall. Standing completely erect is unnecessary; as soon as the pelvis is slightly above the seating surface, the upper extremities and sound limb can be used to gently "propel" the amputated pelvis onto the seat. Once realigned into a symmetrical seated position, the individual can then rise to standing from sitting. In most instances, any person who can maneuver toward a piece of furniture and attain a kneeling posture can rise without assistance.

Moving Down to the Floor

To be confident that they can arise from the floor after a fall, new prosthesis wearers should practice not only the transitions between kneeling and standing postures but also the complete sequence (Figure 29-11), all the way down to the floor. This includes transitions among kneeling, sidesitting, and supine positions.

To move from a supported kneeling position into sidelying, the first action is to move the hand on the nonamputated side to the floor, positioned approximately 12 inches

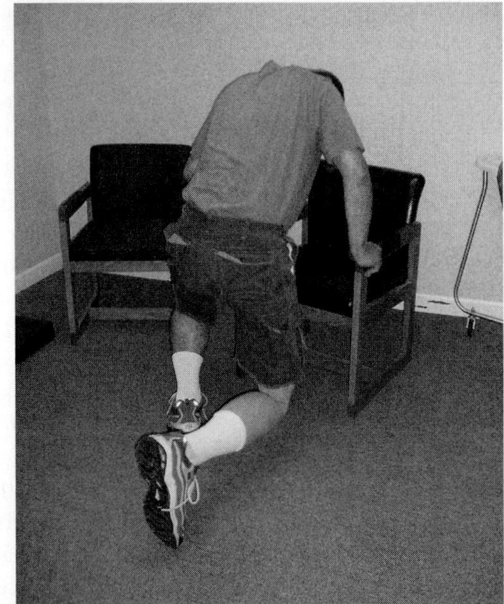

A

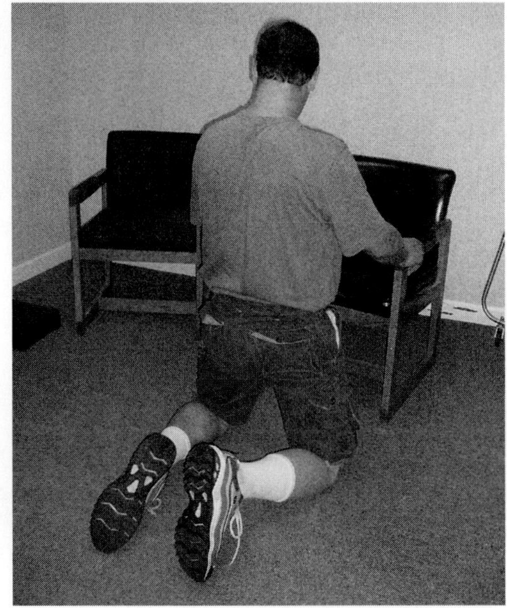

B

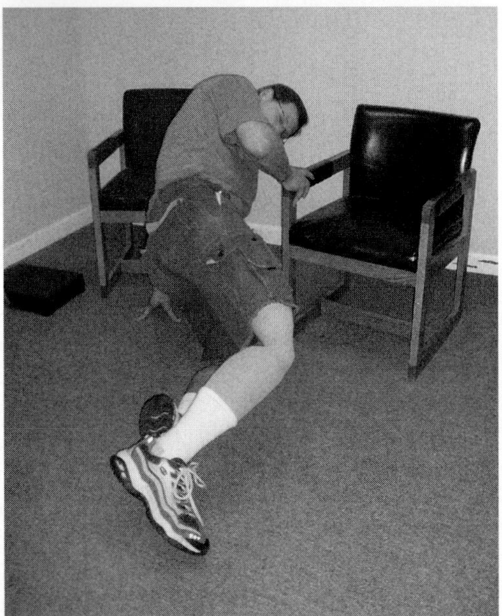

C

Figure 29-11

A, *In learning to transition between standing and lying on the floor, the individual supports body weight by leaning on a piece of furniture and using eccentric activity of the intact limb to lower the prosthetic knee. After shifting weight onto the prosthesis, the intact limb is lowered into kneeling, and the hands are transferred to the floor.* ***B,*** *The patient then lowers the pelvis, moving into sidesitting on the hip of the intact limb.* ***C,*** *Finally, the patient uses eccentric activity at the shoulder to lower the trunk into sidelying.*

lateral to and slightly in front of the nonamputated knee. The therapist can then use tactile cues (e.g., tapping near the sound limb's greater trochanter area) to prompt a controlled lowering of the sound hip toward the hand on the floor, into a sidesitting position. At this point, the other hand is lowered to the floor, and body weight rests on both hands and the thigh and buttock of the nonamputated limb.

To move toward sidelying, there must be a controlled flexion of the elbow on the nonamputated side of the body so that weight can be shifted onto the forearm, accompanied by a controlled lowering of the upper trunk. Eccentric horizontal adduction at the shoulder will then allow the individual to ease into a sidelying position. From this position (to simulate completely the effects of a fall), the individual can roll backward into a fully supine position.

Rising from the Floor

To get up from the floor, the motor sequence is reversed (Figure 29-12). First, the individual with amputation rolls into sidelying on the nonamputated side of the body from either a supine or prone position. Next, the individual moves to a sidesitting posture by flexing the hips and knees in both limbs and supporting upper body weight first on the outstretched arm, then on the forearm, and finally on the hand. From this sidesitting position, with weight borne on the side opposite the prosthesis, the individual maneuvers himself or herself close to a piece of furniture on which hands can be placed for support. Once so positioned, the individual moves from sidesitting to kneeling.

Some individuals may need to move first to quadruped position, sharing some part of their body weight on each of

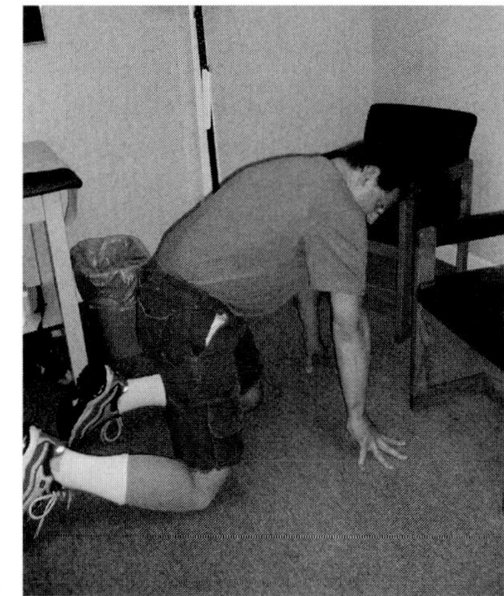
A

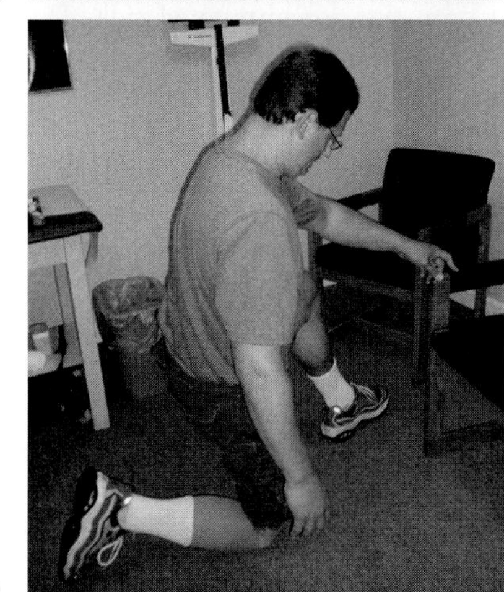
B

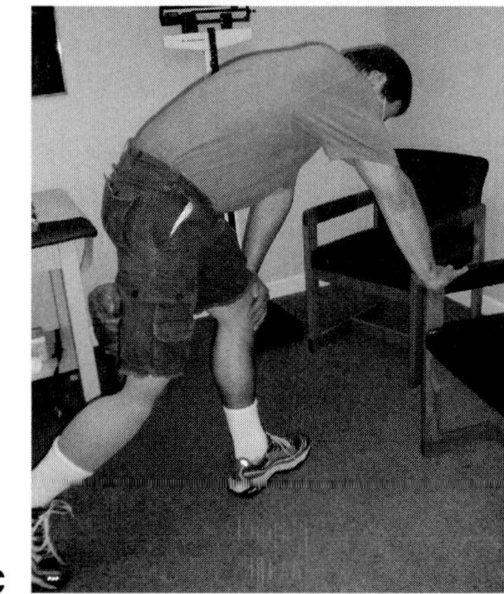
C

Figure 29-12
*To return to standing from the floor, many patients first move into sidesitting position and then into quadruped position (**A**), with the majority of weight borne on the intact limb and upper extremities. Using nearby furniture, they then move into kneeling, shift weight onto the prosthesis, and move the intact limb forward into half-kneeling position (**B**). They move their trunk up and forward over the intact foot using hip extensors and upper extremities, and then bring the prosthesis underneath their center into a stable standing position (**C**).*

their four extremities. Once balanced, they can place a hand on a chair, sofa, or wheelchair. They use this extremity to straighten the upper body and kneel while facing the piece of furniture. Shifting weight onto the prosthesis, they move the intact limb forward to assume a half-kneel and finally extend the sound hip and knee to rise from half-kneel toward standing.

Rising from and Sitting on Furniture

Persons who must wear a transfemoral prosthesis stand from and sit on a chair much as they would were they not wearing the appliance. The loss of the anatomical knee means that the transfemoral prosthesis, unlike its transtibial counterpart, cannot provide any assistance or support body weight during transfers. Instead, individuals with amputations must rely on the intact (nonamputated) limb, their arms, and, frequently, an assistive device during this transitional activity.

Early in the rehabilitation process, most individuals with transfemoral amputations prefer to sit in chairs with a surface height of at least 16 or 17 inches from the floor. They also prefer chairs with stable armrests that can be effectively used for upper extremity support when rising from or returning to a seated position. Because wheelchairs have both an appropriate seat height and stable armrests, many individuals with amputations prefer them to other chairs in their homes, often to the consternation of family members. Therapists can advise family members how to choose or modify chairs for their loved ones with amputations to use. The height of a household chair that is otherwise adequate can be modified by fastening a 2- × 4-inch wooden beam across the bottom of its rear legs. This provides a stable base and raises the rear of the seating surface. This modification alone eliminates much of the disadvantage that low chair surfaces present. Family members can elevate other surfaces on which persons with amputations sit by purchasing devices like raised toilet seats or foam wheelchair seat cushions.

To prepare to stand from a chair, the individual with an amputation must first move the pelvis forward on the sitting surface. The strategy that is usually recommended is a series of "push ups" against the armrests, accompanied by a forward scoot of the pelvis. This strategy effectively positions the trunk in a slight forward lean, ready to shift weight from the ischium to the feet in preparation to stand. Although a forceful lean against the back of the chair slides the pelvis forward on the seat, this strategy leads to a "semi-reclined" position of the trunk, with the center of mass far behind the feet. It can be difficult to return to upright trunk position and develop the controlled forward momentum for effective weight shift onto the feet.

For those who wear pants or slacks, a simple environmental cue might help them determine if they have moved far enough (but not too far) forward on the seating surface;

at the point where they are no longer able to see the seat between their thighs, it is likely that their ischial tuberosities are in the optimal (but still stable) position to rise from sitting.

Once forward in the chair, the sound (nonamputated) foot should be positioned on the floor so that it is almost under the pelvis, as close as possible to the vertical projection of the body's center of mass. This preparation helps individuals with transfemoral amputations achieve a stable posture for standing with a relatively small forward shift in body weight.

A person who relies on a walker for balance in standing may place it in front of the chair from which he or she is preparing to rise. Pushing directly *downward* on the armrests of the chair with both arms (or one armrest and the center of the walker) is the safest strategy when rising from a chair. When both arms are on the walker, the temptation is to pull upward, making the walker unstable; as a result it is difficult to control motion and remain balanced when shifting weight forward or backward. At least one hand must be positioned on the seating surface, whether it be a chair, bed, toilet, or the seat of a car.

No hardfast rule exists for which hand to place on the walker and which to leave on the seat surface. Individuals with transfemoral amputations discover which hand is most efficient as the primary support on the chair or seating surface, given their own strength and hand dominance, as well as the conditions of the environment in which they are functioning. The relative height of the chair's armrests may influence this decision. Individuals may elect to prepare to stand by rotating their upper body toward the nonamputated lower extremity; this positions the arm on that side of their body to push on the seat surface.

Should therapists need to analyze this task to advise patients, they can draw an analogy to the use of unilateral assistive devices, such as various types of canes. Patients with amputations generally hold their canes in the hand opposite the hip joint they want to assist. They may do well to stabilize the hand on the side opposite the hip joint that requires more assistance during this activity. Because a transfemoral prosthesis cannot be used during the transition to standing, it may be most beneficial to assist the hip joint muscles on the nonamputated side. This reasoning suggests that patients will be more successful if they place the hand on the side of the amputation on a stable surface like the chair, wheelchair, or toilet seat.

Reasonable arguments exist for using either hand. Therapists might do well to let those with transfemoral amputations sort through the various strategies to determine what will work most efficiently for them. They can experiment with different preparatory postures, varying not just their hand positions but their pelvic and trunk postures as well. However, they ultimately align their bodies in preparation. Rising to standing is accomplished by flexion of the hip and forward lean of the body to shift weight onto the sound (nonamputated) limb. Initially maintaining the forward inclination of the trunk, they rise up and forward into standing using a combination of hip and knee extension in the nonamputated limb, along with upper extremity support. As patients approach nearly erect standing posture, they may even use their prostheses for balance, positioning them under their bodies.

Persons who wear transfemoral prostheses may sit safely on furniture by following many of the same principles (Figure 29-13). Approaching the chair, they first back up until they can feel the seat on the back of their intact thigh. They may turn slightly toward the nonamputated side and reach for the armrest on that side. Next, they position the prosthetic foot slightly in front of their intact foot and shift their weight onto the nonamputated side. This maneuver permits them to control their descent using the muscles on the sound limb, and it permits unlocking of any stance control mechanism on the prosthetic knee joint. Even if patients walk using a locked knee, this strategy can place the prosthesis where it will not interfere as they use the sound limb to lower the body. At least one hand should be placed on the seating surface (armrest or edge of the bed, chair, or toilet) to assist descent. A slight forward lean will help to direct the pelvis backward onto the seat.

The therapist must be aware of the characteristics of the prosthetic knee joint when helping a new prosthetic wearer to master transitional activities. Certain prosthetic knees contain a polycentric linkage mechanism that maintains an extensor moment to stabilize the knee during midstance. This extensor moment persists until body weight is shifted forward over the prosthetic toe. Although this produces a more natural gait pattern by permitting knee flexion to begin during preswing, it may make it difficult to flex the knee when preparing to sit. The knee mechanism cannot be unlocked by shifting body weight away from the prosthesis, the strategy that unlocks a standard weight-activated friction knee. Instead, some portion of the body weight must be maintained on the prosthesis and shifted toward the prosthetic toe to unlock the knee just before sitting down.

To accomplish this, the individual can turn slightly toward the nonamputated side while maintaining some weight on the prosthesis, simultaneously rotating the pelvis forward on the amputated side. This pelvic rotation complements the turning in the upper body and shoulder girdle and permits the individual to shift some weight forward to the prosthetic toe. With practice, the timing of pelvic rotation allows the individual's weight to reach the prosthetic toe just as his or her hand reaches the chair. As body weight moves over the prosthetic toe, sufficient flexor moment exists at the polycentric knee to unlock and allow flexion. The prosthesis will no longer be able to support the individual, who must be ready to control descent into the chair using upper extremity support and the muscles of the nonamputated limb.

A

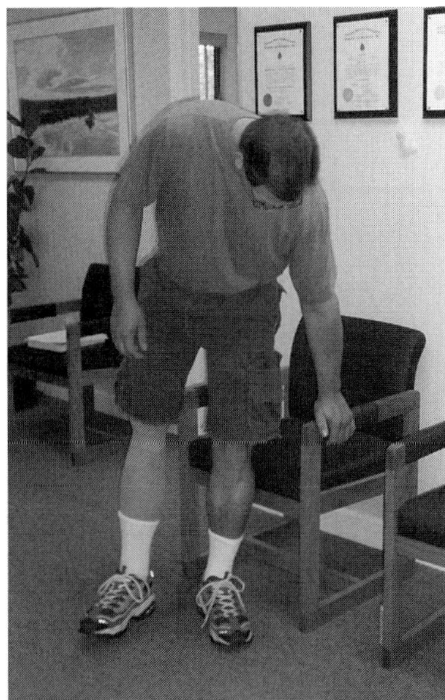

B

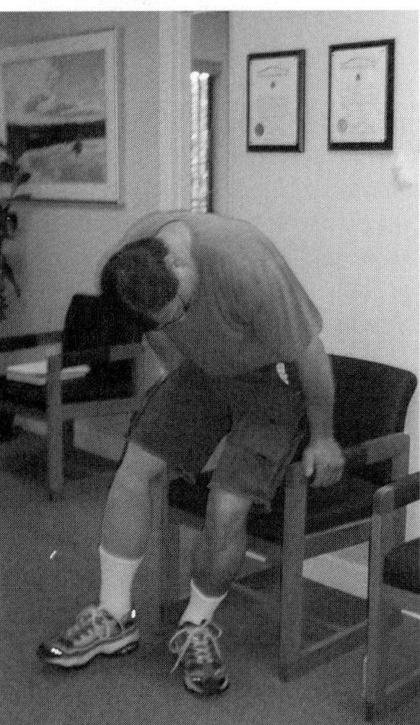

Figure 29-13

*In order to move safely from standing into sitting, the prosthetic knee must flex. For those with weight-activated prosthetic knees, turning slightly toward the intact limb **(A)** unloads the knee enough to allow flexion to occur **(B)**. Those with knees that require weight through the prosthetic toe to unlock use a similar technique, but they must maintain some body weight on the prosthesis. In either case, the prosthesis cannot help to control descent into the chair; this is accomplished with eccentric activity of the intact limb and supporting upper extremities.*

CASE EXAMPLE 1B

An Older Person with Dysvascular Transfemoral Amputation

T. C. has been using her prosthesis for 3 weeks, donning it over her "workout shorts" and rising to standing with moderate assistance from one person. She can walk on level surfaces with a rolling walker for distances up to 300 feet with supervision (and occasional augmented verbal feedback) from her therapist, granddaughter, or certified nursing assistant. Although she has practiced ambulation with bilateral axillary crutches (and can manage holding one of the parallel bars quite well), she feels much more secure with the rolling walker. She can monitor fit appropriately, stopping to apply additional sock ply whenever she senses "loosening" of socket fit. She is determined to return to her apartment and resume independent living and volunteer and leisure activities. However, fear of falling remains a significant concern. She has decided that the best way to address this fear is to figure out how to get up from the floor, so that she will know what to do if and when a fall occurs. Her granddaughter and best friend agree and plan to attend therapy sessions to learn how to assist her with this important task.

Questions to Consider

- What muscle groups and types of muscle performance are important for the motor tasks of rising to standing and rising from the floor? How are these two functional activities similar or different? What exercises or activities can be incorporated into T. C.'s daily program to target muscle performance in a way that best matches the activity of key muscles necessary for these two functional activities?
- What are the "steps" or components of each of these functional mobility tasks? How does the need for body stability, body transport, and object manipulation change or interact during the course of these activities? How might the therapist adapt or control the environment to assist mastery of these motor tasks?
- How can the principles of motor learning (e.g., practice conditions, type and timing of feedback) be applied to help T. C. master these two important motor tasks? How might the therapist assess progression toward mastery of these tasks?
- What resources and impairments will influence whether T. C. can safely accomplish these two motor tasks? What must she, her granddaughter, and her neighbor understand about the tasks to ensure her safety while rising to standing from sitting or from the floor? How might the therapist incorporate her "helpers" into the motor learning process?

Ascending and Descending Curbs and Stairs

Most persons who wear transfemoral prostheses must negotiate stairs one at a time using a step-to pattern; few develop the strength and coordination necessary to use a more natural, "step-over-step" approach. They learn to ascend leading with their intact limb and descend leading with the prosthetic limb.

To ascend a single curb or step, without a handrail, the transfemoral prosthesis wearer should squarely approach a curb and prepare to ascend by shifting body weight onto the prosthesis and assistive device (if used), and then step up with the intact (nonamputated) limb. To descend, the process is reversed. Placing the assistive device midway on the step below, the individual should shift weight onto the intact (nonamputated) limb and use eccentric control of that limb to lower the prosthesis to the step below. Once appropriately placed, weight is shifted onto the prosthesis, and the intact limb steps down, next to the prosthesis, on the same step.

Prosthesis wearers who will routinely ascend a number of stairs to enter their home or move from room to room should consider installing a sturdy handrail, positioned on the side of the staircase closest to the amputated limb as they ascend. By facing sideways toward the handrail, they may be able to ascend the stairs without an assistive device. Facing the handrail and using both hands for support, they lead with the nonamputated limb, which they always place "uphill" of the prosthetic one. They ascend a single step with the sound limb, then elevate the pelvis on the side of the residual limb, placing the prosthesis on the stair next to the sound limb (Figure 29-14).

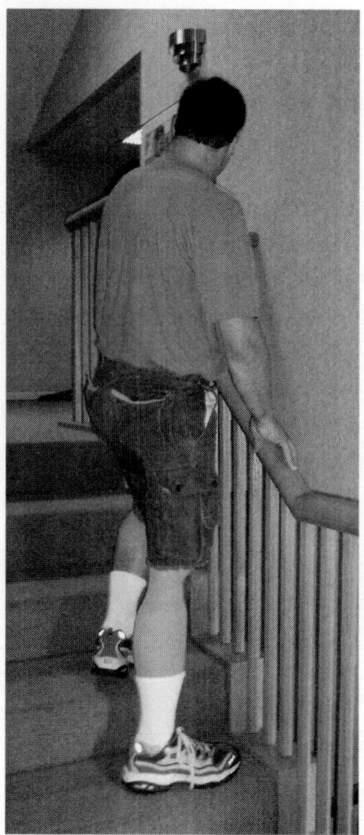

Figure 29-14
One strategy that can be used when learning to ascend stairs without an assistive device is to face the railing with the sound (nonamputated) limb "uphill," stepping up with the sound limb and then bringing the prosthetic limb up to the same step. To descend, the process is reversed, with the prosthetic limb "downhill" lowered to the step below, leaving enough space for a subsequent step down with the sound limb.

The sequence is reversed to descend. Facing the handrail, prosthesis wearers find that the prosthetic limb is "downhill" of the sound one, so that they descend a stair by first placing the prosthesis on the step below (see Figure 29-14). This sidestepping technique keeps the center of pressure through the middle of the prosthetic foot. This foot position locates the resulting ground reaction force far enough forward that it is unlikely to pass behind the prosthetic knee joint and disturb its stability. Once appropriately positioned, weight is shifted onto the stable prosthesis, and the sound limb is moved onto the step next to the prosthetic foot. Depending on the stairs' depth and width, individuals must experiment with foot placement, leaving enough space for the nonamputated limb as they step and position the prosthesis.

Although this sidestepping technique is safe and provides encouragement for new prosthesis wearers who confront stairs for the first time, it is inadequate for the various settings in which they must walk. They must also learn to address stairs using an assistive device.

In general, the safest assistive device for those using a transfemoral prosthesis on stairs is a cane. Although there are techniques for using a walker on stairs, they require that individuals support one hand on a handrail and the other on a walker placed sideways on the stair. The walker's stability depends on the downward force on the walker's "uphill" handle. The force must be applied so that its line of application falls within the walker's base of support. Although clients may perfect this technique in a controlled situation, on a set of three or four practice steps in a clinic, the same technique applied on an entire flight of stairs elsewhere may be disastrous. It may be difficult to produce the necessary downward force within the walker's base of support on steps with a different pitch or dimension, making it less stable and increasing the risk of falls.

A cane is held in the hand opposite the prosthesis to enlarge the available base of support. To ascend a flight of stairs, the basic idea is to have the cane "accompany" the prosthesis, positioned on the same step. After weight is shifted onto the prosthesis and cane, the individual stabilizes the prosthetic limb by extending the hip within the prosthetic socket, then steps up with the nonamputated limb. Elevation of the pelvis is used to lift the prosthesis up to the step, next to the nonamputated limb. Depending on the individual's postural control, the cane can be moved simultaneously or remain on the lower step until the prosthesis is positioned.

To descend, the sequence is reversed. The cane is first placed on the "downhill" step in anticipation of the prosthesis occupying that step as well. Using eccentric control of the nonamputated limb, the prosthesis is then lowered to the next step. The knee of the prosthesis must be stabilized, by extension of the residual limb hip within the socket to ensure stability before the intact limb steps down. Once the prosthesis is appropriately positioned and stable, weight shift onto the prosthesis allows the intact limb to be moved onto the step.

The individual descending the stairs must maintain an upright posture with a slight forward motion of the pelvis as he or she prepares to lower the intact limb. An erect posture produces a ground reaction force that is positioned anteriorly to the prosthetic knee, keeping it extended. If instead the individual "sits back" on the prosthesis before stepping down with the nonamputated limb, the position of the ground reaction force moves behind the prosthetic knee, creating a flexion moment that may cause the prosthetic knee to buckle.

Individuals who are strong, skilled, and brave can learn to descend stairs "step over step," using a modification of the basic step-to technique. The individual begins the sequence by placing the prosthesis on the next stair below, positioning the prosthetic foot's heel close to the stair edge so that the prosthetic toes overhang the edge. This position denies the foot the anterior support that ordinarily prevents the prosthetic shank from inclining forward, a motion that flexes the prosthetic knee. The individual must compensate for this lack of support by extending the residual hip joint forcefully inside the prosthetic socket to keep the prosthetic knee in extension. Shifting the weight onto the prosthesis, instead of placing the nonamputated limb next to the prosthesis, the patient advances it beyond the step's edge. Just as the nonamputated limb approaches the next stair, the individual "lets go" of the active hip extension that heretofore was applied within the socket, perhaps even flexing the hip joint slightly. As a result, the prosthetic knee rapidly flexes or "jackknifes," such that the nonamputated limb can land on the lower stair. To lower the prosthesis, the individual must be able to flex the residual limb within the socket with sufficient force to swing the prosthesis forward and place the prosthetic heel on the edge of the next lowest stair, and then repeat the process.

Ascending stairs "step over step," on the other hand, is difficult for individuals wearing transfemoral prostheses. The patient must be able to place the prosthesis on the upper step, then develop the force necessary to propel the body's center of gravity over that spot. This may be achieved if the individual can use the upper extremities to move the upper body by means of one or, better, two handrails. Otherwise, the patient must activate the residual gluteal muscles to develop a hip extensor moment that is sufficient to extend both the hip joint and, in a closed chain, the prosthetic knee joint. Those with any but the longest residual limbs find this difficult. Nevertheless, such an activity, performed in a controlled environment, might be a reasonable training technique for those who wish to improve not just residual limb strength but coordination and timing.

Managing Inclines, Slopes, Ramps, and Uneven Terrain

Ramps and uneven surfaces that slope upward are challenging because they cause the prosthetic shank to lean posteriorly. This creates an extensor moment at the prosthetic knee joint and slows the forward progress over the prosthetic foot. To ascend facing directly forward, an individual wearing a transfemoral prosthesis can take only a relatively short step with the prosthetic limb, and must contend with the unpleasant sensation of being forced backward, down the incline. This problem may be solved by extending the hip joint more forcefully to press the residual thigh into the socket's posterior wall. The patient may also lean the trunk forward slightly to overcome the angle of the incline. Those with short residual limbs may have insufficient lever arms, and those with relatively weak musculature may not be able to generate sufficient force to ascend facing directly forward.

Many transfemoral prosthesis wearers adapt the strategy used in stair climbing to ascend modest inclines or ramps by turning slightly to the side so that the prosthesis is relatively "downhill" and leading with the intact (nonamputated) limb (Figure 29-15). On extremely steep surfaces, the wearer turns to an angle 90 degrees from directly forward, ascending by sidestepping upward with the intact limb, and then following with the prosthesis. Even a slightly angled orientation affords the advantage of positioning the nonamputated limb in advance of the prosthetic one. This technique also compensates for the prosthetic ankle's stiffness and inability to dorsiflex. It permits more symmetrical step lengths with either limb without encountering difficulty in shifting weight onto the prosthesis.

Descending inclines or ramps presents a different problem: As the walking surface's downward angle permits the front of the prosthetic foot to drop, it produces a forward angulation in the prosthetic shank and a tendency to flex the prosthetic knee. Patients who are new to transfemoral prostheses lack confidence that they can overcome this knee flexion and may hesitate to commit weight to their prostheses. By "leading" with the prosthesis or placing it ahead of the sound limb in a manner similar to the one they use when descending stairs, patients can grade their weight shift onto the prosthesis and gain confidence in their ability to control the prosthetic knee. They must learn to anticipate and appropriately time the strong hip extensor activity necessary to extend the prosthetic knee when the prosthesis is on a downward slope. Those with weak hip extensor muscles or short residual limbs who have difficulty generating enough force can compensate by turning toward the amputated side as they descend moderate slopes and inclines (see Figure

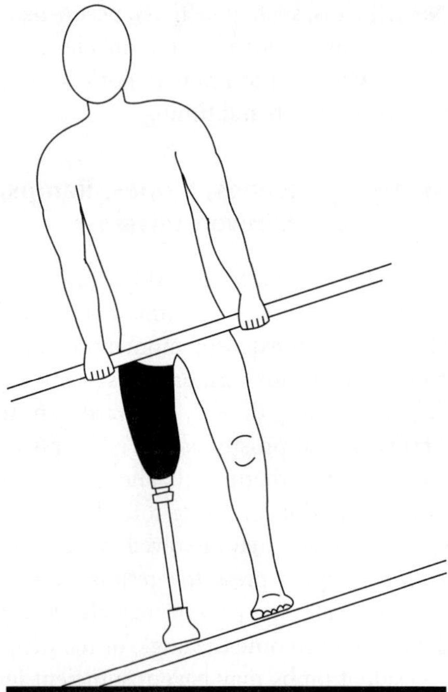

Figure 29-15
Turning somewhat sideways when ascending a ramp, leading with the sound limb, is often more comfortable than facing directly forward because it minimizes the impact of the extension moment at the knee created by the upward incline. Similarly, many individuals with transfemoral amputations feel more secure descending sideward, leading with the prosthesis, as this minimizes the destabilizing flexion moment and sense of being propelled forward created by the downward incline.

29-15). This orientation permits the prosthesis to lead the other side and reduces the flexion moments at the knee. On steep or extreme slopes, individuals might choose to turn completely to the side, using a side step to negotiate their way down a hill, leading with the prosthesis, or to descend by taking a series of short steps.

Other challenges that require thought and practice include uneven ground and avoiding obstacles or unsafe surfaces while walking by stepping around or over them. Many individuals can step over a small hole, bump, or object in their path by treating the obstacle as if it were a curb or step they must ascend. Using this approach, they face the obstacle with the prosthetic foot positioned slightly behind the sound foot (Figure 29-16). This foot position produces a ground reaction force that falls anteriorly to the prosthetic knee joint axis and stabilizes it in extension. As long as some weight remains on the prosthesis, this extensor moment helps individuals maintain balance as they step over the obstacle with the nonamputated limb. Once they have done so, they must forcefully flex the residual hip inside the prosthetic socket to "whip" the prosthesis forward over the obstacle.

Patients may hesitate to use this technique if the ground is sloped or if they do not trust their ability to stabilize the prosthetic knee as they bear full weight on the prosthesis. An alternative is to move over an obstacle in a less direct manner by modifying the sidestepping pattern described for ramps or inclines. During advanced gait training, patients approach the obstacle sideways with the nonamputated limb nearest it. Shifting their body weight onto the prosthesis once again, they flex the sound hip, swinging the sound limb forward and over the obstacle. After shifting weight to the sound limb (now on the other side of the obstacle), quick hip flexion swings the prosthesis up and over the obstacle. With experience, patients can pivot on the sound limb as they bring the prosthesis over the obstacle. They can then swing the prosthesis through, stepping onto it in a continuous motion as they move away from the obstacle.

Picking Up Objects from the Floor

Most people with intact lower extremities bend their knees and use eccentric control to reach objects that they have dropped on the ground. Those who wear transfemoral prostheses find it frustrating when they cannot easily pick up objects because of stability concerns. One strategy they may use to reach such objects is to shift their body weight to the nonamputated limb, then to step backward with the prosthesis (Figure 29-17). When the prosthetic foot is positioned slightly behind the nonamputated one, and weight is borne on both extremities, the ground reaction forces stabilize the prosthetic knee in extension. The stable prosthesis can help individuals maintain balance as they bend at the waist and reach for the object while flexing the nonamputated limb at the hip and knee.

This technique requires considerable strength in the nonamputated limb. Those who lack this strength can be successful if they apply what they learned in connection with kneeling on the floor. Although some individuals can learn to kneel without upper extremity assistance, most will reach the floor most easily if they can place their hands on a piece of furniture for balance. In either case, they balance on the nonamputated leg, then extend the residual hip quickly within the prosthesis to place the prosthesis as far behind them as possible. Flexing the trunk and the hip and knee joints on the nonamputated side, they gently lower the prosthetic knee joint to the floor and share their body weight between it and the nonamputated limb. In this position, they can retrieve the object, then prepare to arise once again from kneeling to standing. They do so by shifting their upper body's center of mass over the nonamputated limb by inclining their trunk in the direction of the knee on that side. Simultaneously, they extend the hip and knee joints to arise.

Moving Quickly and Running

Most patients who wear transfemoral prostheses first learn to move more quickly by skipping rather than running. This

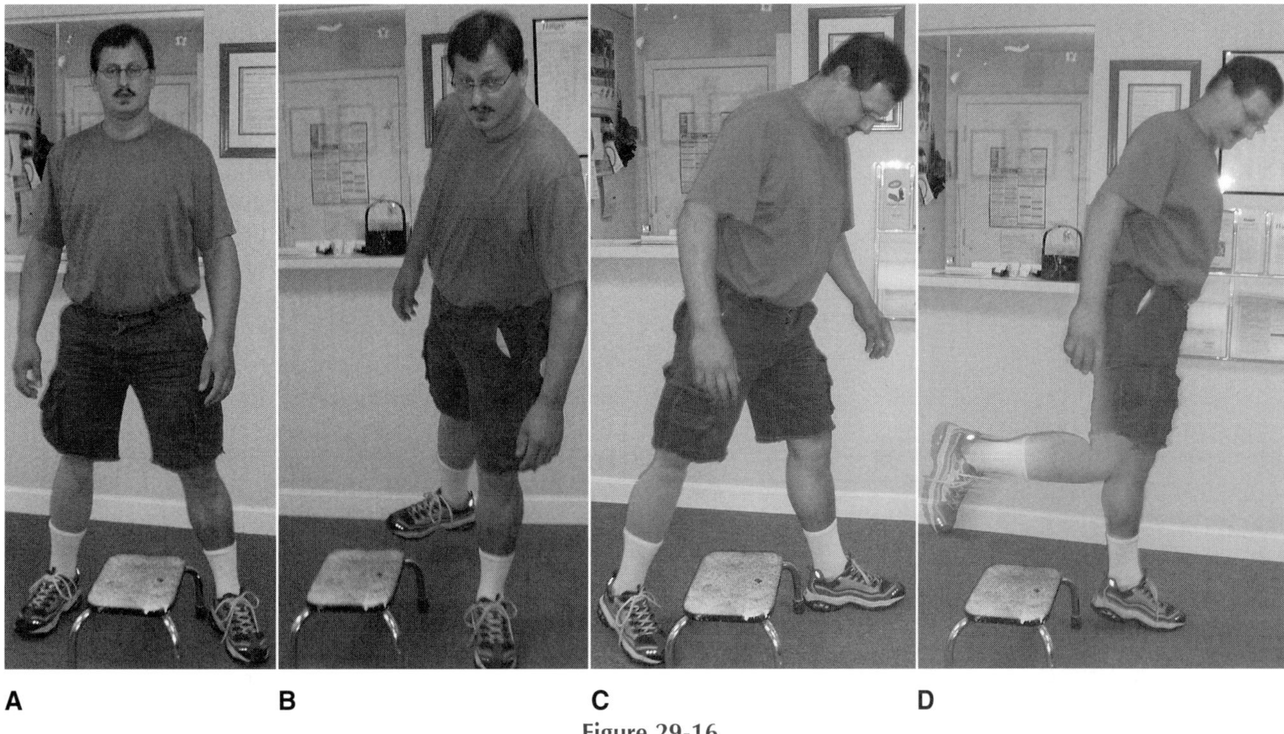

A B C D

Figure 29-16

*To clear obstacles on the ground, most individuals wearing transfemoral prostheses step over them with the sound limb (**A**), shift weight onto the sound limb, and then circumduct the prosthesis to clear the object (**B**). Some individuals will use an alternate strategy to step over relatively low obstacles, first stepping over with the sound limb (**C**), then forcefully flexing the hip on the prosthetic side to bend the prosthetic knee (**D**). Some individuals find that a slight turn sideways, bringing the sound limb closest to the object, reduces the difficulty of this task.*

movement, familiar from childhood games, involves taking two steps (actually hops) on the sound limb for each step with the prosthesis. The extra step gives the prosthesis time to swing through and be in a position to accept weight when it touches the ground.

The sequence begins by first stepping forward with the nonamputated limb. After shifting their weight to that limb, patients hop forward on it while they simultaneously begin swinging the prosthesis forward. They land on the prosthesis when the knee joint is fully extended. They support their body weight on the prosthesis momentarily, then transfer the weight immediately to the nonamputated limb so that they may repeat the sequence.

DETERMINING READINESS FOR THE DEFINITIVE PROSTHESIS

Patients with transfemoral amputations are ready to make the transition from the initial (temporary) prosthesis to a definitive (permanent) prosthesis when their residual limb's volume has stabilized, a process that typically takes 3 to 6 months. During this time, the limb's volume decreases gradually and may even fluctuate from day to day or between morning and afternoon during a single day. By adding or subtracting prosthetic socks, those with transfemoral amputation can maintain a proper fit between the socket and residual limb. When the number of prosthetic socks needed remains stable for a number of weeks, then it is likely time for a patient to return to the prosthetist and be fitted for a new prosthesis.

One obvious advantage of a definitive prosthesis is its improved appearance; a cosmetic cover conceals the hardware that must remain visible and accessible on a temporary prosthesis so that the prosthetist may adjust its alignment. A second advantage is an improvement in socket fit, if only because months of change in the residual limb's shape have likely compromised its intimate contact with the temporary prosthetic socket. A third advantage involves weight. The prosthetist will replace some of the temporary unit's heavier adjustable hardware with lighter or more streamlined components. This weight reduction may be minimal, however, depending on the cosmetic finishing and the inclusion of heavier components like a hydraulic knee mechanism.

If the residual limb's volume has not stabilized, moving to a definitive prosthesis ahead of schedule offers no advantage. Neither does the definitive prosthesis markedly improve the walking pattern for a patient who has not used the period of training to improve strength, ROM, and gait technique.

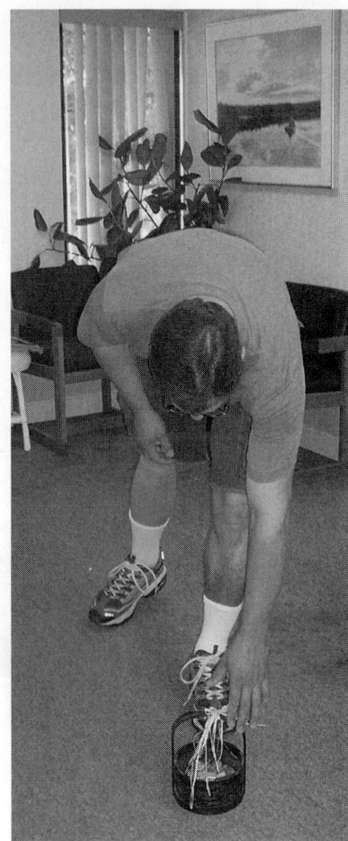

Figure 29-17

To retrieve an object from the floor, many patients wearing transfemoral prostheses position themselves close to the object, use a forceful hip extension to place the prosthesis (with an extended knee) behind them, and then reach for the object using eccentric control of the sound limb and upper extremity support on an assistive device or furniture (if available).

SUMMARY

Many patients with transfemoral amputations can learn to effectively use their prostheses to walk and perform usual daily activities. The best predictors of rehabilitation potential are preamputation ambulatory status and overall health, rather than surgical level. Individuals who are new to prosthetic use must master a number of key activities and tasks during the rehabilitation process. They must be able to safely and efficiently don and doff the prosthesis, ensure appropriate fit by adding or removing prosthetic socks, and adjust suspension. They must develop the strength and muscular control to effectively use prosthetic components during each subphase of walking, becoming confident and competent in shifting weight onto and off of the prosthesis and controlling the prosthetic knee joint. They may have to address strength and length imbalances of the residual limb that are consequences of the amputation surgery or of inactivity. They must develop the endurance and postural control necessary for active, functional prosthetic use. The primary goal of rehabilitation is to help individuals wearing transfemoral prostheses walk with a gait pattern that is energy efficient and cosmetic, using the least cumbersome assistive device possible. In addition to walking and changing direction on various level surfaces, those new to walking with a prosthesis must discover how best to navigate uneven terrain, ramps and inclines, curbs and stairs, and in crowded and busy environments. Because the risk of falling, although quite real, can lead to a disabling fear of falling, the opportunity to practice getting down to and rising from the floor can be empowering for those who wear transfemoral prostheses. Successful rehabilitation not only helps patients develop skills and abilities necessary to work, care for themselves, and participate in leisure activities but enhances quality of life and is tremendously rewarding for both individuals and therapists.

REFERENCES

1. Cruz CP, Eidt JF, Capps C, et al. Major lower extremity amputations at a Veterans Affairs hospital. *Am J Surg* 2003;186(5):449-455.
2. Moore TJ, Barron J, Hutchinson F, et al. Prosthetic usage following major lower extremity amputation. *Clin Orthop* 1989; Jan(238):219-224.
3. DeLuccia N, Pinto MA, Guedes JP, Albers MT. Rehabilitation after amputation for vascular disease: a follow up study. *Prosthet Orthot Int* 1992;16(2):124-128.
4. Davies B, Datta D. Mobility outcome following unilateral lower limb amputation. *Prosthet Orthot Int* 2003;27(3): 186-190.
5. Pinzur MS, Littooy F, Daniels J, et al. Multidisciplinary preoperative assessment and late function in dysvascular amputees. *Clin Orthop* 1992;Aug (281):239-243.
6. Penington G, Warmington S, Hull S, Freijah N. Rehabilitation of lower limb amputees and some implications for surgical management. *Aust N Z J Surg* 1992;62(10):774-779.
7. Cutson TM, Bongiorni DR. Rehabilitation of the older lower limb amputee: a brief review. *J Am Geriatr Soc* 1996;44(11): 1388-1393.
8. Kapp S. Suspension systems for prostheses. *Clin Orthop* 1999;April(361):55-62.
9. Northwestern University Medical School Prosthetics. Above-knee training. *Lower-Limb Prosthetics for Therapists.* Chicago: Northwestern University Medical School Prosthetics—Orthotics Center, 1989. pp.17-1-17-6.
10. May BJ. Assessment and treatment of individuals following lower extremity amputation. In O'Sullivan SB, Schmitz TJ (eds), *Physical Rehabilitation: Assessment and Treatment,* 4th ed. Philadelphia: F.A. Davis, 2001. pp. 619-644.
11. Schmitz TJ. Preambulation and gait training. In O'Sullivan SB, Schmitz TJ (eds), *Physical Rehabilitation: Assessment and Treatment,* 4th ed. Philadelphia: F.A. Davis, 2001. pp. 411-444.
12. Winstein CJ, Gardner ER, McNeal DR, et al. Standing balance training: effect on balance and locomotion in hemiparetic adults. *Arch Phys Med Rehabil* 1989;70(10):755-762.
13. Schmidt RA. Motor learning principles for physical therapy. In *Contemporary Management of Motor Control Problems:*

Proceedings of the II-STEP Conference. Alexandria, VA: Foundation for Physical Therapy, 1991. pp. 49-64.

14. Winstein CJ. Designing practice for motor learning: clinical implications. In *Contemporary Management of Motor Control Problems: Proceedings of the II-STEP Conference.* Alexandria, VA: Foundation for Physical Therapy, 1991. pp. 65-76.
15. Saunders JB, Inman VT, Eberhart HD. The major determinants in normal and pathological gait. *J Bone Joint Surg* 1953;35A(3):543-558.
16. Inman VT, Ralston HJ, Todd F. *Human Walking.* Baltimore: Williams & Wilkins, 1981. pp. 41-61.
17. Eisert O, Tester OW. Dynamic exercises for lower extremity amputees. *Arch Phys Med Rehab* 1954;35(11):695-704.
18. Gottschalk FA, Karoush S, Stills M. Does socket configuration influence the position of the femur in above knee amputation? *J Prosthet Orthot* 1989;2(1):94-102.
19. Gottschalk F. Transfemoral amputation: biomechanics and surgery. *Clin Orthop* 1999;April(361):15-22.
20. Gailey RS, McKenzie A. Prosthetic Gait Training Program for the Lower Extremity Amputees. Miami: University of Miami Department of Orthopedics, 1991.
21. May, BJ. Lower extremity prosthetic management. In *Amputations and Prosthetics: A Case Study Approach,* 2nd ed. Philadelphia: F.A. Davis, 2002. pp. 160-214.
22. Winter DA, Sienko S. Biomechanics of below-knee amputee gait. *J Biomech* 1988;21(5):361-367.
23. Cerny K. Pathomechanics of stance: clinical concepts for analysis. *Phys Ther* 1984;64(12):1851-1859.

30

Prosthetic Options for Persons with High-Level and Bilateral Amputation

JOHN W. MICHAEL

LEARNING OBJECTIVES

On completion of this chapter, the reader will be able to do the following:

1. Discuss the relative frequency of high-level and bilateral lower limb amputations.
2. Describe the importance of a multidisciplinary clinical team and coordinated rehabilitation care on functional outcomes for this group of patients.
3. Recognize the implications of the different causes of amputation for this group of patients.
4. Identify the two primary biomechanical limitations of hip disarticulation and higher level prostheses.
5. Estimate the relative energy cost of ambulation with high-level or bilateral limb loss.
6. Recognize the basic modifications to independence training for this patient population.

Although relatively uncommon in the developed world, high-level and bilateral lower limb amputations present unique rehabilitation challenges. Such a significant limb loss presents a substantial challenge to the patient, the prosthetist, and other rehabilitation professionals. Successful prosthesis fitting is often time consuming and difficult, but for many individuals with high or bilateral amputation, prostheses can serve a useful purpose by increasing functional independence and mobility. This chapter summarizes key concepts from the clinical and research literature.

HIGH-LEVEL LOWER LIMB LOSS

The first part of this chapter focuses on options for patients with a unilateral high-level limb absence, which is an amputation at or above the hip joint. Hip disarticulation and transpelvic and translumbar losses have been estimated to comprise fewer than 2% of all amputations in the United States.[1] As a result, only those clinicians associated with specialty centers, such as major trauma hospitals, have the opportunity to see significant numbers of such cases. Most prosthetists, therapists, and physicians see only a handful of patients with such high-level loss in a practice lifetime. One result of treating each high-level patient as one of a kind is that many differing approaches can be found in the literature.

Etiology

Although vascular impairment and neuropathy, whether or not they are associated with diabetes mellitus, are the most common causes for lower limb loss in the developed world, these risk factors rarely lead to high-level amputation.[2] Dysvascular and neuropathic symptoms are generally most pronounced in the distal (peripheral) limb, leading to nonhealing ulceration, infection, gangrene, and ablation. The trunk and a portion of the upper thigh are usually spared even in the presence of severe peripheral vascular disease. The assumptions about healing, cardiovascular limitations, and tolerance of activity derived from the experience with patients with dysvascular amputation do not apply to those with high-level amputation. Most patients with high-level amputation are relatively healthy and have reasonable cardiopulmonary reserves, excellent cognition, and a strong desire to attempt prosthetic fitting. Most patients with hip disarticulation or other high-level amputation should be offered the opportunity for prosthetic fitting and rehabilitation.

Many high-level amputations are performed for a tumor of the femur, such as osteosarcoma, although the frequency of tumor-related high-level amputation is decreasing with advances in limb-salvage procedures and more effective chemotherapy and radiation therapy.[3-5] Patients who require amputation because of tumor can be divided into two groups: those with benign or fully contained tumors who require no further oncological intervention and those undergoing chemotherapy and radiation after amputation.

Those with benign or fully contained tumors are typically in excellent physical condition after the amputation, eager to return to their former lifestyle as much as possible, and ready for early prosthetic fitting. The benefits of early prosthetic fitting are well established and are both physical and psychological.[3,6] Early mobilization and single-limb gait training on the contralateral limb with an appropriate assistive device are recommended to reduce the risk of deconditioning, which occurs even after a few days of hospitalization.[7]

The rehabilitation and prosthetic management of patients requiring chemotherapy or radiation therapy may have to be adapted or delayed depending on the patient's physical condition, energy level, tolerance of activity, and healing of the surgical site.

Biomechanics

Although, historically, loss of the entire lower limb assumed the use of locked joints in the prosthesis, ample clinical evidence is available that locked prosthetic joints are seldom necessary. Since the 1950s, free-motion hip, knee, and ankle joints for hip disarticulation and transpelvic prostheses have become the norm. The Canadian design hip disarticulation prosthesis was introduced by Colin McLaurin,[8] and the biomechanics of this prosthesis were clarified by Radcliffe in 1957.[9] These same biomechanical principles are also used in the functional design of prostheses for patients with higher level amputation.

In essence, the high-level prosthesis is stabilized by the ground reaction force (GRF), which occurs during walking.[10] For example, when standing quietly in the prosthesis, the person's weight-bearing line falls posterior to the hip joint, anterior to the knee joint, and anterior to the ankle joint. The resultant hip and knee extension moments are resisted by mechanical hyperextension stops of the prosthetic hip and knee joints, and the dorsiflexion moment is resisted by the stiffness of the prosthetic foot (Figure 30-1). This same principle permits the patient with paraplegia using bilateral Scott-Craig knee-ankle-foot orthoses to stand without external support.[11]

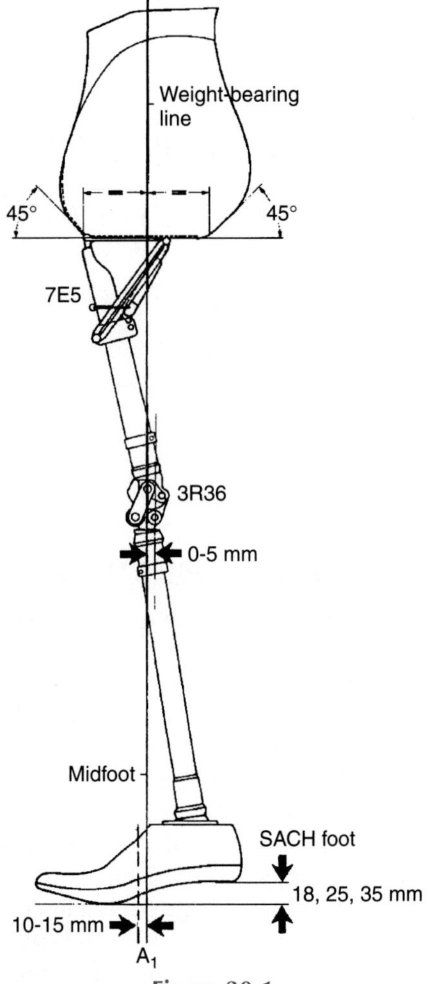

Figure 30-1
Static balance with a high-level lower limb prosthesis is achieved when the GRF passes posterior to the hip joint and anterior to the knee and ankle joints. The resulting extensor moments at the hip and knee, and dorsiflexion moment at the ankle, make the prosthesis stable. Mechanical stops in the prosthetic joints prevent further movement, and the patient is able to stand without exertion. SACH, *Solid-ankle, cushion heel. (Courtesy Otto Bock Orthopedic Industry, Inc., Minneapolis, Minn.)*

Ambulation with a high-level prosthesis also relies on the GRF (Figure 30-2). When an experienced prosthetic wearer walks with an optimally aligned hip disarticulation or transpelvic prosthesis, the dynamic gait is surprisingly smooth and consistent. Patients with hip disarticulation or transpelvic amputations who have sufficient balance and strength can learn to walk without any external aids, although the use of a cane is also common.

The basic functions of the GRF during ambulation with one type of high-level prosthesis can be summarized as follows. At initial contact, as the prosthetic heel touches the ground, the GRF passes posterior to the ankle axis, the heel cushion compresses, and the foot is lowered to the ground. At the same time, an extension moment is created at the prosthetic knee as the GRF passes anterior to the knee joint axis (see Figure 30-2, *A*). By midstance, alignment stability is maximal as the GRF passes posterior to the prosthetic hip joint axis and anterior to the prosthetic knee joint axis, just as it does during quiet standing (see Figure 30-2, *B*). As forward progression continues into preswing, the GRF moves posterior to the knee joint axis, allowing the knee to bend passively to facilitate swing phase foot clearance while weight is being shifted onto the opposite limb (see Figure 30-2, *C*).

Two major biomechanical deficits are inherent with hip disarticulation and transpelvic prostheses. First, the prosthetic limb is always fully extended at midswing because of the loss of active hip flexion. As a result, the length of the

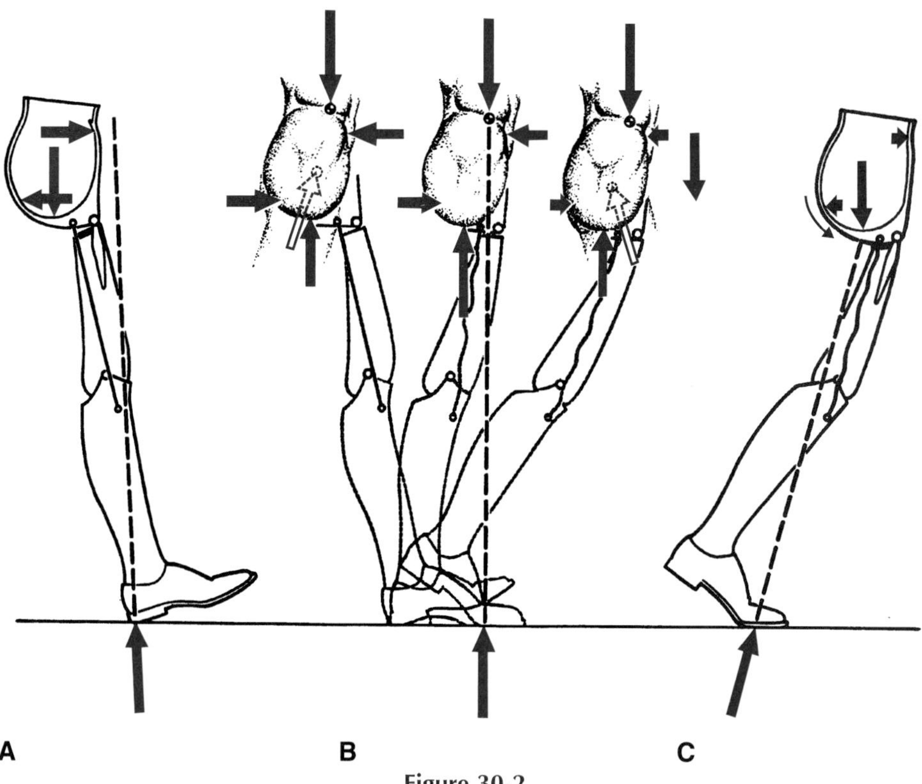

Figure 30-2

*The GRF at initial contact. From loading response through midstance (**A**) and terminal stance (**B**) and just prior to preswing (**C**) of the gait cycle for patients using a unilateral high-level prosthesis. Once properly aligned, the prosthesis will move in a consistent, predictable fashion and permit slow but steady ambulation. The patient uses trunk motion to initiate and control prosthetic movements. (From Van der Waarde T, Michael JW: Hip disarticulation and transpelvic management: prosthetic considerations. In Bowker JH, Michael JW [eds],* Atlas of Limb Prosthetics: Surgical, Prosthetic, and Rehabilitation Principles, *2nd ed. St. Louis: Mosby–Year Book, 1992. pp. 539-552.)*

prosthesis is typically shortened slightly, compared with the remaining limb, to assist in toe clearance during the swing phase of gait. The consequence of this strategy, however, is a second biomechanical deficit: a limb length discrepancy.[12]

Component Selection

The earliest hip disarticulation prosthesis designers insisted on locking all prosthetic joints. Later, proponents of free-axis joints for hip disarticulation prostheses advocated the use of only basic components, such as a single-axis knee and ankle. In recent years, a strong consensus has emerged that, to meet the patient's functional needs and goals fully, components for patients with hip disarticulation and transpelvic amputations should be selected for the same reasons and with the same criteria as for those with transfemoral and transtibial amputation.[13,14]

Choosing a Prosthetic Foot

All prosthetic feet have been successfully used at these high levels. Nonarticulating designs are often chosen because of their dependability, durability, and low maintenance; these designs rarely require servicing as a result of wear and tear. Single-axis feet (which allow the patient to quickly attain a stable foot-flat position) are used when enhanced knee stability is a concern. Multiaxial and dynamic response designs are usually reserved for higher-activity individuals who appreciate the added mobility of such components.[15]

Choosing a Prosthetic Knee Unit

The prosthetist selects a particular knee unit on the basis of the patient's functional needs. Because of the biomechanical stability of these prostheses, locked knee designs are rarely necessary. Locked knee designs have two additional drawbacks: they must be unlocked before sitting, and they may increase the risk of injury in the event of a fall. When stability is a primary concern, stance control or polycentric knees may be most appropriate. Single-axis knees, when properly aligned, also work well. The prosthetist might choose a pneumatic or hydraulic knee unit to provide fluid swing phase control for patients who are active and want the ability to change cadence.[14] Most recently, quite encouraging clinical results have been reported with a microprocessor-controlled, hydraulic stance and swing control knee, allowing active individuals to descend stairs foot-over-foot with a hip disarticulation prosthesis for the first time.[16]

Choosing a Prosthetic Hip Joint

The majority of patients with hip disarticulation benefit from a free-motion hip joint, although locking joints are still sometimes chosen for those with quite limited ambulation capabilities. Much effort has been made to provide some measure of active hip flexion motion in these prostheses because that would reduce or eliminate the key biomechanical deficits previously noted. In prior decades, modification of the hip joint by adding a coil spring mechanism that induced hip flexion when the prosthesis was unweighted was tried with some success, but maintenance and breakage of the spring precluded widespread acceptance. More recently, a flexible carbon fiber thigh "strut" that functions as a leaf spring has been used clinically in selected cases. Initial reports suggest that this approach increases cadence and that the improved swing clearance achieved by better prosthetic hip and knee flexion eliminates the need to shorten the prosthesis.[17] The use of vertical shock-absorbing shin elements and knees with stance flexion features is also being explored, with encouraging clinical acceptance.

Torque Absorbers

With the loss of three major biological joints of the lower limb, a corresponding loss of the body's ability to compensate for rotary motions inherent in gait occurs. For this reason, many prosthetists strongly recommend that a torque-absorbing device be included in these high-level prostheses. Torque absorbers typically improve both stride length and comfort by absorbing transverse forces that would otherwise be transmitted to the socket as skin shear.[18] Incorporation of a lockable turntable above the prosthetic knee is also suggested to facilitate common daily activities such as dressing and entering an automobile (Figure 30-3).

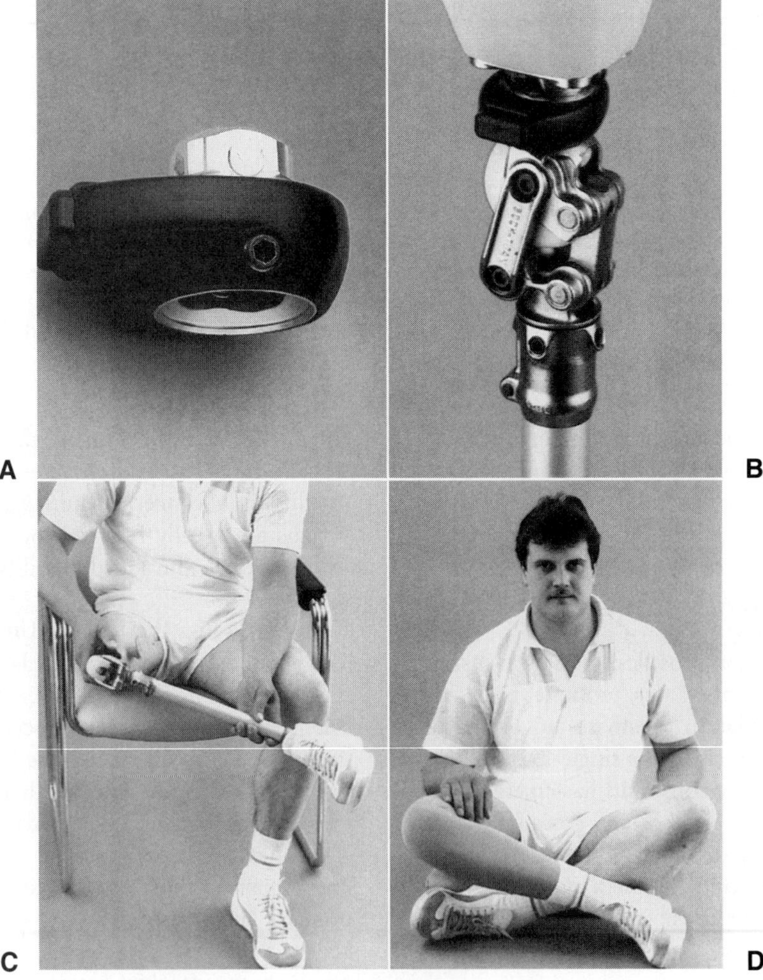

Figure 30-3

*A lockable turntable (**A**) positioned in the prosthesis above the prosthetic knee (**B**) makes dressing, entering an automobile, and similar daily tasks much easier for individuals with high-level amputation (**C** and **D**). A torsion adapter absorbs the torque forces generated during gait and decreases the stress on both the patient's skin and the prosthetic components. Such ancillary components should always be considered for patients with high-level amputations. (Courtesy Otto Bock Orthopedic Industry, Inc., Minneapolis, Minn.)*

Energy Consumption

The major unresolved drawback to prosthetic fitting for those with high-level amputation is the tremendous increase in effort required to control a prosthetic limb with passive joints. Walking with a hip disarticulation or transpelvic prosthesis is much like controlling a flail biological leg. The concentration and energy required to ambulate makes short distance ambulation much more practical than distance walking for all but the most vigorous adult wearers.

Gait studies suggest that the use of a hip disarticulation prosthesis requires approximately 200% more effort than unimpaired walking.[19] This is approximately the same effort required when using axillary crutches in single-limb gait. Because single-limb amputation with crutches tends to be faster than walking with a hip disarticulation prosthesis, the relatively high rejection rate of such prostheses is not surprising.

Most rehabilitation professionals believe that any patient with an amputation who is physically and mentally capable of prosthetic use should, if interested, be fitted with an initial prosthesis. This recommendation is particularly true for those with high-level amputation who may feel "cheated" and become depressed if their clinical teams do not allow them to try prosthetic ambulation.

Socket Design

A variety of socket designs have been described in the clinical literature. The most critical factors for successful use are careful fitting and secure suspension, regardless of which socket design is selected. For patients with hip disarticulation, encapsulation of the ascending pubic ramus may add stability, although not every patient is able to tolerate a proximal trimline in the perineum.[10,20] Flexible thermoplastic or silicone materials within a rigid laminated frame are more comfortable and increasingly popular than the more common hard plastic sockets (Figure 30-4).[21-23]

Suspension is achieved by carefully contouring the socket just proximal to the iliac crests whenever possible. When the patient is obese or has no ileum, shoulder straps may be necessary to minimize swing phase pistoning of the prosthesis.

The transpelvic socket must fully enclose the gluteal fold and perineal tissues and completely contain the soft tissues

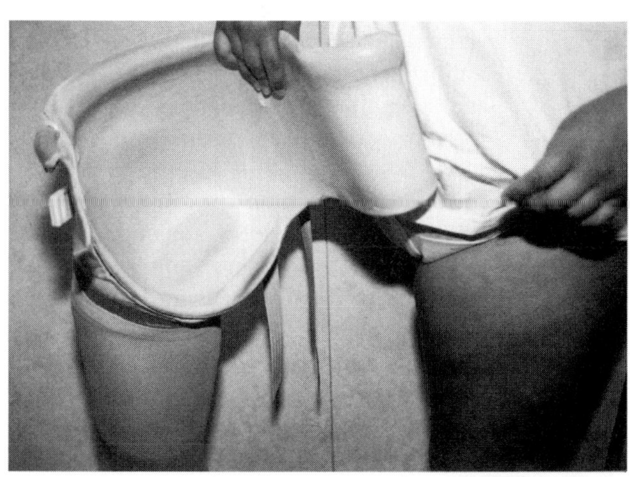
A

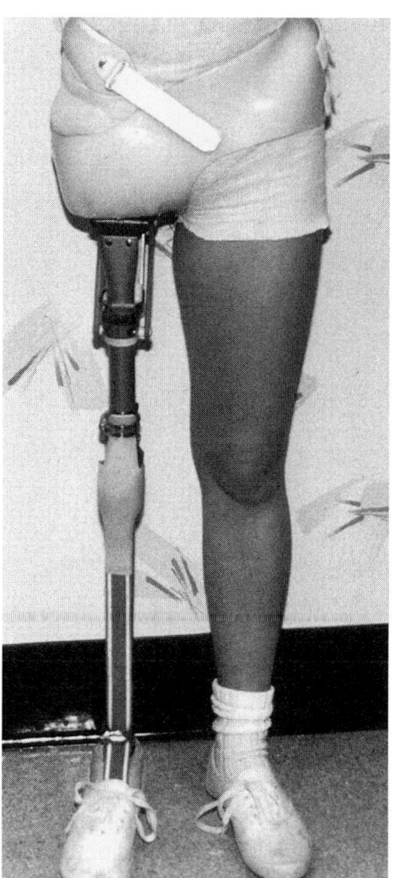
B

Figure 30-4

*The interior of a hip disarticulation socket (**A**) fabricated from flexible silicone rubber. Note the contouring of the proximal brim to encase the crest of the ileum. Thermoplastic sockets (**B**) are also used for hip disarticulation prostheses. (From Michael JW. Component selection criteria: lower limb disarticulations.* Clin Prosthet Orthot *1988;12[3]:99-108.)*

on the amputated side. Full enclosure provides comfortable weight bearing on the residual limb tissues despite the absence of hemipelvis. Early transpelvic sockets extended upward to contain the lower ribs.[24] Clinical experience has shown that this may not always be necessary for relatively muscular or lean individuals. Failure to contain the transpelvic residuum adequately results in obvious protrusion where the trimlines are insufficient. Prosthetists modify the positive plaster model of the transpelvic residuum to incorporate a diagonally directed compressive force in the socket design to support and contain transpelvic tissues and eliminate the risk of perineal shear and tissue breakdown.[25]

For patients with translumbar amputation, weight bearing is achieved with a combination of soft tissue compression and thoracic rib support. Because of the loss of more than half of the body mass in this amputation, weight-bearing tolerance is better than might be expected. Designs that allow the patient to vary the compression by adjustable straps are often useful.[26]

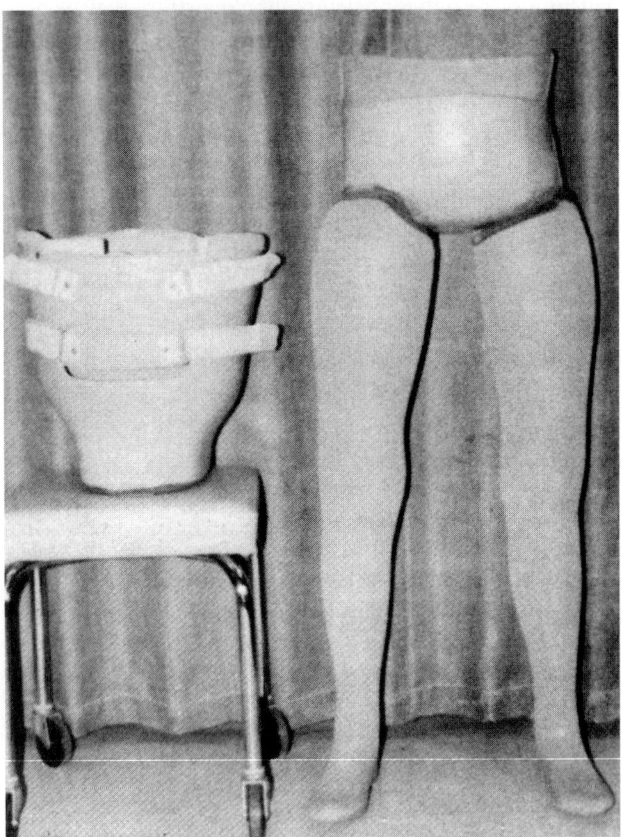

Figure 30-5
For patients with translumbar amputation, a laminated adjustable socket provides a stable base for sitting balance and wheeled stability (left). *The socket can be positioned within an outer shell with bilateral prosthetic limbs* (right) *for cosmesis in sitting and for limited prosthetic ambulation. (From Gruman G, Michael JW: Translumbar amputation: prosthetic considerations. In Bowker JH, Michael JW [eds],* Atlas of Limb Prosthetics: Surgical, Prosthetic, and Rehabilitation Principles, *2nd ed. St. Louis: Mosby–Year Book, 1992. pp. 563-568.)*

Patients with translumbar amputation require a socket for effective seating and wheeled mobility (Figure 30-5). Many patients with translumbar amputation successfully progress to ambulation for short distances with a prosthesis and choose to wear prosthetic limbs to enhance their cosmetic appearance and self-image. Long-term follow-up demonstrates positive prosthetic outcomes; return to work or school is usually a realistic goal.[27] For most patients, polycentric knees provide sufficient stability for the household ambulation typical of this population, making locking joints unnecessary.

Rehabilitation Outcomes after High-Level Amputation

Despite the obvious challenges that face patients with high-level amputation, a substantial percentage are able to manage a prosthetic device with appropriate training and long-term follow-up. Although the rate of prosthetic use varies, the trend is toward increasing functional use of a prosthesis.[3,28,29] Fitting by an experienced prosthetist with the support of a specialty clinical team is believed to enhance the likelihood of success.

CASE EXAMPLE 1

A Patient with Traumatic Hip Disarticulation

J. S. is a 20-year-old man with a traumatic hip disarticulation amputation caused by a motorcycle accident 2 weeks ago. His residual limb is healed but complicated by multiple skin grafts and insensate areas in the abdominal region from the amount of trauma. He is eager to return to college as quickly as possible to avoid having to repeat this semester's courses but must walk several blocks to various buildings on the small, hilly campus. He has a lean, athletic build and demonstrates excellent balance and strength when ambulating on his remaining limb with bilateral forearm crutches.

Questions to Consider

- What additional information might be gathered to help determine J. S.'s potential to use a hip disarticulation prosthesis? How does his medical history and reason for amputation affect his rehabilitation prognosis?
- How should J. S.'s readiness to be fit with a prosthesis be determined? What tests and measures should be used?
- What major concerns or challenges will J. S., his prosthetist, and rehabilitation team face in fitting his hip disarticulation prosthesis?
- What options for socket and suspension will the team likely consider for J. S. given his functional needs and prognosis?

- What factors will influence the choice of knee units for J. S.'s prosthesis? What type of knee should be recommended? Why?
- What factors will influence the choice of a prosthetic foot for J. S.'s prosthesis? What type of foot should be recommended? Why?
- How should rehabilitation goals be prioritized as J. S. begins his prosthetic training? How should his rehabilitation progress? How should the efficacy of intervention be assessed to determine how well the goals have been met?

Recommendations

On the basis of findings during the evaluation and discussion with J. S. about his current functional needs and ultimate prosthetic goals, the team recommends an initial endoskeletal prosthesis with a foam-lined thermoplastic socket that includes additional gel padding in the region of the tender grafted skin, a microprocessor-controlled stance and swing control hydraulic knee, dynamic response foot, and torque absorber. The clinical team considered first providing a less complex knee but decided against that option because it would require training to use a less responsive prosthesis, then subsequent retraining with the microprocessor knee more appropriate for his projected functional abilities, thereby increasing the duration of his rehabilitation program.

Intensive inpatient therapy focuses on ambulation first within the parallel bars and then with his forearm crutches to facilitate J. S.'s return to campus. He will continue with outpatient therapy until his gait has matured and will likely learn to ambulate with no balance aids. When his socket no longer fits because of normal postoperative atrophy, he will receive a new custom socket and protective covering for the prosthesis but will continue to use the same functional components originally provided for as long as they are functionally appropriate for his needs.

BILATERAL LOWER LIMB LOSS

The loss of both lower limbs complicates the rehabilitation process, especially if the loss occurs simultaneously.[30] In North America, simultaneous bilateral loss is infrequent; such cases are typically the result of traumatic transportation or industrial accidents or electrocution. In the developing world, simultaneous limb loss is more frequent; in areas of armed conflict and postwar zones, roadside bombs and landmines are a major cause.[31] Fortunately, most patients with traumatic amputation are healthy and strong and generally have a good prognosis for the successful use of prostheses.

Because vascular disease affects both limbs, patients with a single dysvascular amputation face a significant risk of eventual bilateral limb loss. An incidence as high as 50% for contralateral limb loss over a 5-year period has been reported.[32] Clinical follow-up suggests that successful use of a unilateral prosthesis increases the likelihood of success with bilateral artificial limbs. For this reason, early fitting after initial amputation is strongly advocated, even when amputation of the opposite limb seems imminent.[33]

Training the patient who has lost both lower limbs is quite similar to training the person who requires only one artificial limb. One major difference is that using two artificial limbs is physically more difficult, so the pace of advancement is slower and must be individualized according to the patient's strength, balance, and ability. Breaking down complex skills into small incremental tasks that can be more readily mastered is generally useful.

Because no contralateral sound limb can be depended on, patients with bilateral loss can be expected to walk slowly and cautiously, often with a relatively wide-based gait that maximizes their sense of stability. Balance aids are common but not universal. Environmental barriers such as ramps, hills, irregular surfaces, and curbs or stairs present special challenges that must be identified and overcome. Specific training in sitting down, rising from a chair, falling in a controlled manner, and recovering from a fall are all important tasks to be mastered. Transfer with and without artificial limbs is also an important skill to foster independence.

Training, like prosthetic fitting, must be individualized for each patient, taking into account physical condition, biomechanical loss, and prosthetic characteristics. The reason for the amputations influences the pace and type of training; otherwise healthy individuals who sustain traumatic limb loss may be able to advance rapidly unless skin trauma is present on the residual limbs.[34]

Energy Cost

The effort required to use a unilateral prosthesis increases in direct proportion to the level of amputation: the longer the residual limb, the lower the energy cost of walking with a prosthesis.[35] Saving as much functional limb length as possible is therefore an axiom in amputation surgery. Although preservation of the anatomical knee joint is important for patients with unilateral amputation, it is a critical consideration when bilateral limb loss is present: When at least one biological knee joint remains, the chances for practical ambulation significantly increase.[36]

Energy cost of ambulation is also related to the reason for limb loss.[37] In general, patients with dysvascular amputation have lower energy reserves and expend more effort walking than those with traumatic amputation (Figure 30-6). Long-term use of bilateral transfemoral prostheses is uncommon, but not impossible, for elderly patients with dysvascular amputation.[38] In contrast, a significant number of those with traumatic bilateral transfemoral amputation successfully use prostheses long term.[39] Patients with bilateral transtibial

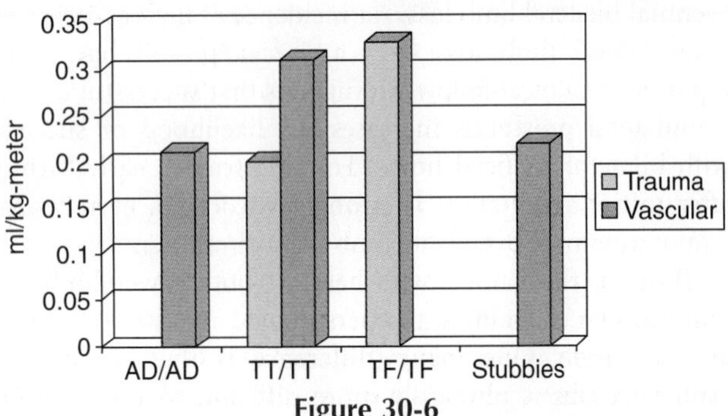

Figure 30-6

The energy (oxygen) cost of ambulation with bilateral prosthesis compared for patients with ankle disarticulation (AD), *transtibial amputation* (TT), *and transfemoral amputation* (TF) *when using traditional transfemoral prostheses and stubbies (simplified prostheses consisting only of the transfemoral sockets attached to a stable base, without any prosthetic knee). Note that energy costs increase as the level of amputation moves proximally. Energy cost is also higher in dysvascular amputation compared with traumatic amputation. Ambulation requires less effort for patients with at least one anatomical knee joint than for those with bilateral transfemoral amputation. Preservation of an anatomical knee joint increases likelihood of independence in ambulation. (Modified from Waters RL: The energy expenditure of amputee gait. In Bowker JH, Michael JW [eds],* Atlas of Limb Prosthetics: Surgical, Prosthetic, and Rehabilitation Principles, *2nd ed. St. Louis: Mosby-Year Book, 1992. pp. 381-387.)*

ambulation tend to do well with prostheses regardless of reason for amputation. Interestingly, bilateral transtibial prostheses require less effort than a unilateral transfemoral prosthesis; this finding emphasizes the importance of retaining biological knee function whenever possible.

Component Selection

Selection of components for patients with bilateral lower limb amputation is made by the same guidelines as for unilateral limb absence; no special bilateral components exist. The prosthetist should consider both prostheses together rather than simply generate a "right-side" and a "left-side" prescription recommendation. Prosthetists generally recommend that the same ankle-foot device be used on both sides so that gait mechanics will be consistent, but this is not an absolute necessity. Some patients ambulate best with different prosthetic feet, depending on the level of amputations, the length and condition of the residual limbs, the nature of their preferred activities, and other individual characteristics.

The range of physical differences between one patient with bilateral lower limb loss and another makes each new fitting a unique challenge. During the dynamic alignment procedure, a brief clinical trial with the recommended components is often helpful in confirming suitability for a specific individual before the prescription details are finalized. This trial is particularly helpful for experienced ambulators, who commonly develop strong preferences for a specific component after walking with it for many years.

Bilateral Transtibial Amputations

In North America, a solid-ankle, cushion heel prosthetic foot is often chosen for patients with bilateral transtibial amputation because such feet offer predictable standing balance. Most patients with bilateral amputation are concerned about falling backward. The prosthetist often chooses to use a slightly stiffer heel resistance to minimize the risk of backward falls. When concern about forward falls also exists, the prosthetist may also choose to use a slightly stiffer keel to offer additional resistance to falling forward. Patients classified as limited ambulators, those with poor postural responses, and those who walk with a very slow cadence often find this approach useful.

Active patients walk well with elastic keel and dynamic response feet or with multiaxial designs as long as they have sufficient strength and postural responses to manage these flexible components. Theoretically, single-axis feet are designed to generate an abrupt hyperextension moment at midstance, which loads the cruciate ligaments of the residual limb. In practice, little evidence exists that this loading is harmful; some patients with bilateral transtibial amputation prefer single-axis feet, choosing them over solid-ankle or dynamic response designs. Patient preference is an important consideration in prosthetic prescription; preference is even more critical for patients with bilateral amputation who literally have no "good foot" to stand on other than prosthetic devices. If a patient expresses a definite dissatisfaction with a particular foot during the fitting process, an alternative component should be tried before proceeding further.

The consideration of ancillary components, such as torque absorbers or shock-absorbing pylons, is important for all patients with bilateral amputation. Because patients with bilateral amputation must bear all their body weight on prosthetic devices all the time, components that increase comfort or protect the skin are particularly appropriate.

Lessening the weight of the prostheses, particularly at the ankle-foot area, is also important because lighter-weight prostheses are easier to control and increase acceptance of the device. Whenever possible, heavier components should be placed as close to the socket as possible.[40]

Bilateral Transfemoral Amputation

Because patients with bilateral transfemoral amputation have lost both anatomical ankles and knees, postural responses are compromised. For this reason, one of the primary goals of prosthetic prescription is stability in the stance phase of gait. One of the most effective prosthetic components for stance phase stability during level walking is a polycentric knee unit. For those patients who have the potential to walk at varying speeds, the addition of fluid swing phase control is recommended. Hydraulic stance and swing control units are also quite successful for this population. In recent years, microprocessor-controlled hydraulic knees offering both stance and swing phase control have been well received clinically by this population, and many experts believe this technology offers more reliable stability and better mobility under real-world conditions than strictly mechanical knee mechanisms.[41]

The risk of injury in a fall is greater if locking or stance control knees are used in both prostheses. For patients with significant stability issues, a locking or stance control knee may be used on one side. Because single-axis knees are stabilized by muscle control and postural responses at the hip, bilateral single-axis knees are often difficult to use safely in older adults with dysvascular amputation. Bilateral single-axis knees may be appropriate for small children because their short stature reduces the balance required to manage such components.

Ankle-foot components that emphasize stability and standing balances are typical for this group with bilateral loss. Solid-ankle designs predominate. Articulating designs are used less often; only those with very long transfemoral residual limbs and good muscle strength are typically able to control the added mobility provided by articulating ankle components. Many patients with bilateral transfemoral amputation use crutches or canes to assist with balance and postural control. Single-axis or multiaxial feet become easier to control if the patient leans forward slightly, shifting the center of gravity forward, so that the weight line falls anterior to the ankle axis at all times, eliminating the risk of falling backward.

Ancillary components, such as torque absorbers, often make walking easier and more comfortable for patients with bilateral transfemoral amputation. Some evidence exists that including components that permit controlled transverse rotation improves the gait kinematics of patients who wear two lower limb prostheses.[42] Locking rotation devices make many activities of daily living easier to accomplish.[43] Because the weight of such ancillary components must be considered, the perception of the artificial limb feeling heavy is minimized if the devices are positioned as far proximally within the prosthesis as possible.

Transfemoral-Transtibial Amputation

For patients with one transfemoral and one transtibial amputation, the preservation of one biological knee makes prosthetic use much easier and successful ambulation more likely.[44] For most patients, the transtibial side is the propulsive and balance limb and the transfemoral side supplements these functions. On the basis of these functional differences, the prosthetist may choose to use different prosthetic feet. When the transfemoral amputation is relatively short, for example, a single-axis foot and stance control knee might be recommended for the transfemoral prosthesis, whereas a dynamic response foot might be used in the transtibial prosthesis.

Socket Designs and Suspension

The person with bilateral lower limb loss is constantly bearing full weight on artificial limbs while walking or standing. All options to increase skin protection and comfort should be actively considered, and suspension must be as secure as possible. A soft insert and flexible sockets may be used to enhance comfort during wear and reduce the likelihood that shear forces will be problematic for the skin. Suction suspension, with silicone sleeves or inserts as necessary, minimizes pistoning during swing and should be considered for the majority of patients with bilateral amputation.

Cotton or wool prosthetic socks are often used as an interface between the residual limbs and the sockets when suction suspension is not feasible. In that event, supracondylar wedge or cuff suspensions are typically used in transtibial prostheses; Silesian belts are often used in transfemoral designs. Because most patients with bilateral amputation use a pair of prostheses, suspension belts are usually integrated into a single assembly. Because thigh corsets with metal side joints, hip joints and pelvic bands, and waist belts can be cumbersome for donning and doffing, they are typically avoided unless absolutely necessary.

Ischial containment sockets are as effective for patients with bilateral amputation at the transfemoral level (of one or both limbs) as they are for patients with a single transfemoral amputation. Patients who have previously worn a quadrilateral transfemoral socket, and those who are limited ambulators, may be satisfied with a traditional quadrilateral design. Total contact of the residual limb in the socket is important for both ischial containment and quadrilateral socket skin integrity.

The loss of both feet and both knees makes the use of bilateral transfemoral prostheses quite challenging. For many adults with acquired limb losses, an initial fitting with sockets attached to special rocker platforms may be advocated to facilitate initial gait training (Figure 30-7). Such "stubbies" require less energy and balance than full-length prosthetic limbs and give the patient new to bilateral prostheses the best chance for successful ambulation.[45] Once the patient is able to balance effectively on the stubbies, the prostheses can be converted to use artificial feet with solid pylons, which are gradually lengthened to increase the height of the prostheses. If the patient is able to manage full-length prostheses, prosthetic knees can be incorporated and definitive prostheses with full components provided.

Not all patients with bilateral transfemoral amputation choose to pursue ambulation with prostheses. Some are unable to build the necessary muscular strength or postural control for a safe gait. Others find the energy cost of ambulation with prostheses excessive. In these cases, patients

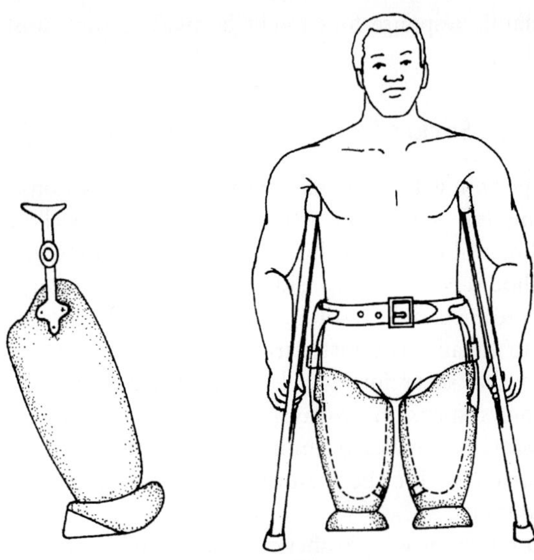

Figure 30-7

A pair of shortened prostheses, sometimes called stubbies, for early gait training for patients with bilateral traumatic transfemoral amputation. In these prostheses, patients can develop postural control without having to worry about the stability of prosthetic knee units. (From May BJ: Assessment and treatment of individuals following lower extremity amputation. In O'Sullivan SB, Schmitz TJ [eds], Physical Rehabilitation: Assessment and Treatment, *3rd ed. Philadelphia: F.A. Davis, 1994. pp. 392.)*

choose wheelchair mobility as a much less strenuous means of mobility and willingly adopt wheelchair use for the independence it provides.

Many patients with bilateral transfemoral amputation find a wheelchair most practical for long-distance mobility and use their limbs for walking short to moderate distances at home and work. Some patients accept the stubbies for long-term use, particularly if these devices allow them to remain independent in their home setting. Others choose to use their stubbies at home because they take less effort but wear full prostheses in public.

CASE EXAMPLE 2

A Patient with Bilateral Lower Extremity Amputations Caused by Chronic Dysvascular/Neuropathic Disease

R. W. is a 72-year-old woman who recently underwent an elective right transtibial amputation because of infection associated with diabetic neuropathy. Her residual limb is well healed and not unduly edematous, and she is eager to return to the condominium she shares with her daughter. Five years previously, R. W. underwent left transfemoral amputation after failed femoral-popliteal bypass surgery and has been a successful full-time prosthesis wearer until hospitalization for the recent amputation.

Questions to Consider

- What additional information might be gathered to help determine R. W.'s potential to use prostheses for her new right transtibial and existing left transfemoral residual limbs? How does her medical history and reason for amputation affect her rehabilitation prognosis?
- How should R. W.'s readiness to be fit with a transtibial prosthesis be determined? What tests and measures should be used to make this determination?
- What major concerns or challenges will R. W., her prosthetist, and rehabilitation team face in fitting the new transtibial prosthesis?
- What options for socket and suspension will the team likely consider for R. W.'s new transtibial and transfemoral prostheses, given her functional needs and prognosis?
- What factors influence the choice of knee units for R. W.'s transfemoral prosthesis? What type of knee should be recommended? Why?
- What factors influence the choice of a prosthetic foot for R. W.'s transtibial and transfemoral prostheses? What type of foot should be recommended for each prosthesis? Why?
- How should rehabilitation goals be prioritized as R. W. begins her prosthetic training? How should rehabilitation be assessed? Should the wearing schedules for her new transtibial limb be similar to or different from her transfemoral limb? Why or why not? How should the efficacy of intervention be assessed to determine how well the goals have been met?

Recommendations

Although her age and comorbidities make the use of two artificial limbs challenging, R. W. is a good candidate for bilateral fitting because of her motivation and proven success with a prior prosthesis. Her existing transfemoral prosthesis is well worn and no longer fitting optimally, so the prosthetic rehabilitation team recommends that two new prostheses be prescribed.

The transtibial prosthesis will provide primary balance and propulsion and enable her to rise from a seated position, applying significant forces to her residual limb. Her initial transtibial prosthesis will include a roll-on locking liner for suspension and a soft insert to protect the residual limb and provide added mediolateral stability at the knee through its supracondylar contours. She will use lightweight, solid-ankle dynamic response prosthetic feet on both artificial limbs because she prefers these components and has found them both stable and functional with her unilateral prosthesis.

Her new transfemoral prosthesis will be similar to what she has successfully worn, with a roll-on locking liner for suspension and a flexible ischial containment socket within a rigid frame for weight bearing and rotational stability. The roll-on suspension permits donning from a seated position, which is particularly advantageous for people with bilateral amputations. Initially, R. W. will wear an auxiliary elastic suspension belt for added security and rotational control.

Her unilateral prosthesis incorporated a single-axis knee with pneumatic swing control, but she will require a more mechanically stable design for bilateral stability. Because of cardiopulmonary restrictions and the loss of her second leg, the clinical team does not believe she will vary her walking pace as widely now, so the weight of a pneumatic swing control unit is no longer necessary. R. W. will receive a stable polycentric knee in her new prosthesis and undergo gait training for several weeks.

Although she is eager to have her endoskeletal prostheses finished with protective covers that make them appear more lifelike, this fabrication step will be deferred until after she has completed gait training and mastered the use of bilateral artificial limbs. R. W.'s prosthetist will see her periodically to reevaluate the alignment of both prostheses as her gait pattern matures, making small alignment changes in response to her changing needs and balance. Once her gait pattern has stabilized, the final fabrication will be completed.

R. W. will also be prescribed a wheelchair with a posteriorly offset axle, which she will use for traversing long distances. Training in wheelchair transfers and mobility will also be an important part of her rehabilitation.

SUMMARY

Individuals with high-level or bilateral lower limb amputations are rare in the developed world. In North America, they are believed to represent fewer than 5% of all persons with amputation.[46] Given these statistics, most prosthetists and therapists have limited opportunity to work with patients with such significant levels of limb loss. Although successful prosthetic training and rehabilitation for these patients are challenging, a large body of clinical information about managing such cases is available in the literature. This chapter has highlighted the key principles involved in rehabilitation of the person with high-level or bilateral lower limb amputations.

Surgical technique during the amputation largely determines the potential for long term ambulation.[47] Gentle handling of soft tissues and careful preservation of all functional joints and bony length are essential. Anchoring functioning muscles to bone (myodesis) at their normal resting length is strongly encouraged whenever possible.

The socket design and suspension methods chosen for patients with high-level or bilateral amputation should incorporate strategies to protect the skin and maximize patient comfort, especially for individuals with bilateral amputation. Components reflect each individual's need for stability and responsiveness at the ankle-foot, knee, or hip joint level.[48] Ancillary components to make the prosthesis more comfortable and easier to manage are advocated.

Although patients with bilateral transfemoral amputation caused by vascular disease often have difficulty mastering dual prosthetic devices, long-term use of functional prostheses is a realistic goal for patients with traumatic or tumor-related amputation who are otherwise healthy.[49] With appropriate fitting and rehabilitation, many patients with hip disarticulation and transpelvic amputations continue to use their prostheses definitively. Even patients with translumbar amputation are able to return to productive education or work activities with an appropriate prosthesis for sitting or limited ambulation.

Despite the obvious physical and psychological challenges faced by patients with high-level or bilateral lower limb amputation, prosthetic rehabilitation must always be considered and is often successful, especially when offered by an experienced clinical team in a supportive setting.[43] Although the sequelae from amputations of this magnitude present significant challenges, advances in surgical technique, prosthetic design and components, and rehabilitation contribute to successful outcomes for patients with high-level and bilateral amputation.

REFERENCES

1. Glattly HW. A preliminary report on the amputee census. *Artif Limbs* 1963;7(1):5.
2. Stern PH. The epidemiology of amputations. *Phys Med Rehabil Clin North Am* 1991;March-April(67):145-157.
3. Ferrapie AL, Brunel P, Besse W, et al. Lower limb proximal amputation for a tumor: retrospective study of 12 patients. *Prosthet Orthot Int* 2003;27(3):179-185.
4. Katrak P, O'Connor B, Woodgate I. Rehabilitation after total femur replacement: a report of 2 cases. *Arch Phys Med Rehabil* 2003;84(7):1080-1084.
5. Belthur MV, Grimer RJ, Suneja R, et al. Extensible endoprosthesis for bone tumors of the proximal femur in children. *J Pediatr Orthop* 2003;32(2):230-235.
6. Burgess E, Romano RL. The management of lower extremity amputees using immediate postsurgical prostheses. *Clin Orthop* 1968;March-April(57):137-146.
7. Cutson T, Bongiorni D, Michael JW. Early management of elderly dysvascular below-knee amputees. *J Prosthet Orthot* 1994;6(3):62-66.
8. McLaurin CA. The evolution of the Canadian-type hip disarticulation prosthesis. *Artif Limbs* 1957;4:22-28.
9. Radcliffe CW. Biomechanics of the Canadian-type hip disarticulation prosthesis. *Artif Limbs* 1957;4:29-38.
10. Stark G. Overview of the hip disarticulation prosthesis. *JPO J Pract Orthod* 2001;13(2):50-53.
11. Lehmann JR, Wareen CG, Hertling D. Craig-Scott orthosis: a biomechanical and functional evaluation. *Arch Phys Med Rehabil* 1976;57(9):438-442.
12. Van der Waarde T, Michael JW. Hip disarticulation and transpelvic management: prosthetic considerations. In Bowker JH, Michael JW (eds), *Atlas of Limb Prosthetics: Surgical, Prosthetic, and Rehabilitation Principles,* 2nd ed. St. Louis: Mosby-Year Book, 1992. pp. 539-552.

13. Michael JW. Component selection criteria: lower limb disarticulations. *Clin Prosthet Orthot* 1988;12(3):99-108.
14. Michael JW. Prosthetic knee mechanisms. *Phys Med Rehabil State Art Rev* 1994;8(1):147-164.
15. Michael JW. Prosthetic feet: options for the older client. *Top Geriatr Rehabil* 1992;8(1):30-38.
16. Stinus H. Biomechanics and evaluation of the microprocessor controlled C-leg exoprosthesis knee joint. *Z Orthop Ihre Grenzget* 2000;138(3):728-782.
17. Littig DN. Gait patterns in the unilateral hip disarticulation. *AAOP Proc* 1995;42.
18. Knoche W. Welche vorteile bringt der einbau eines torsionsadapters in beinprosthesn? *Orthop Tech* 1979; 30:12-14.
19. Huang C-T. Energy cost of ambulation with Canadian hip disarticulation prosthesis. *J Med Assoc State Ala* 1983;52(11):47-48.
20. Sabolich J, Guth T. The CAT-CAM HD: a new design for hip disarticulation patients. *Clin Prosthet Orthot* 1988;12:119-122.
21. Madden M. The flexible socket system as applied to the hip disarticulation amputee. *Orthot Prosthet* 1987;39(4):44-47.
22. Zaffer SM, Braddom RL, Conti A, et al. Total hip disarticulation prosthesis with suction socket: a report of two cases. *Am J Phys Med Rehabil* 1999;78(2):160-162.
23. Carlson JM, Wood SL. A flexible air-permeable prosthesis for bilateral hip disarticulation and hemicorporectomy amputees. *JPO J Pract Orthod* 1998;10(4):110-115.
24. Hampton F. A hemipelvectomy prosthesis. *Artif Limbs* 1964;8(1):3-27.
25. Hampton F. Northwestern University suspension casting technique for hemipelvectomy and hip disarticulation. *Artif Limbs* 1966;10(1):56-61.
26. Carlson MJ. A double socket prosthesis design for bilateral hip-to-hemi corporectomy amputation levels. *AAOP Proc* 1997.
27. Gruman G, Michael JW. Translumbar amputation: prosthetic considerations. In Bowker JH, Michael JW (eds), *Atlas of Limb Prosthetics: Surgical, Prosthetic, and Rehabilitation Principles,* 2nd ed. St. Louis: Mosby–Year Book, 1992. pp. 563-568.
28. Shurr DR. Hip disarticulation prostheses: a follow up. *Orthot Prosthet* 1983;37(3):50-57.
29. McAnelly RD, Refaeian M, O'Connell DG, et al. Successful prosthetic fitting of a 73-year old hip disarticulation amputee patient with cardiopulmonary disease. *Arch Phys Med Rehabil* 1998;79(5):585-588.
30. Rommers GM, Vos LDW, Groothoff JW, et al. Clinical rehabilitation of the amputee: a retrospective study. *Prosthet Orthot Int* 1996;20:72-78.
31. Korver AJH. Amputees in a hospital of the International Committee of the Red Cross. *Injury* 1993;24(9):607-609.
32. Anderson SP. Dysvascular amputee: what can we expect? *J Prosthet Orthot* 1995;7(2):43-50.
33. Sener S, Uygur F, Yakut Y, et al. Quality of life of rehabilitated lower limb amputees [abstract]. *Physiotherapy* 1995;81:455.
34. Atesalp AS, Ereler K, Gur E, et al. Bilateral lower limb amputations as a result of landmine injuries. *Prosthet Orthot Int* 1999;23:50-54.
35. Waters RL. The energy expenditure of amputee gait. In Bowker JH, Michael JW (eds), *Atlas of Limb Prosthetics: Surgical, Prosthetic, and Rehabilitation Principles,* 2nd ed. St. Louis: Mosby-Year Book, 1992. pp. 381-387.
36. Schuling S, Greitemann B, Seichter C. Gehfahigkeit Beidseits beinamputierter nach prosthetischer versorgung. *Z Orthop* 1994;132(3):235-238.
37. Pinzur MS, Gold J, Schwarz D, et al. Energy demands in walking for dysvascular amputees as compared to level of amputation. *Orthopaedics* 1992;15(9):1033-1037.
38. Moore TJ, Barron J, Hutchinson F, et al. Prosthetic usage following major lower extremity amputation. *Clin Orthop* 1989;Jan(238):219-224.
39. Dougherty PJ. Long-term follow-up study of bilateral above-knee amputees from the Vietnam war. *J Bone Joint Surg* 1999;81A:1384-1390.
40. Bach TM. Optimizing mass and mass distribution in lower limb prostheses. *Prosthet Orthot Aust* 1995;10(2):29-35.
41. Gutfleisch O. Peg legs and bionic limbs: the development of lower extremity prosthetics. *Interdisciplinary Science Reviews* 2003;28(2):139-149.
42. Schmidl H. Torsionadapter im kunstbein aus der sicht des technikers und des amputierten. *Orthop Tech* 1979;30:35-38.
43. Torres MM, Esquanazi A. Bilateral lower limb rehabilitation: a retrospective review. *West J Med* 1991;154(4):583-586.
44. Kruger LM. Stubby prostheses in the rehabilitation of infants and children with bilateral lower limb deficiencies. *Rehabilitation* 1990;29(1):12-15.
45. Torres MM. Incidence and causes of limb amputations. *Phys Med Rehabil State Art Rev* 1994;8:1-8.
46. Murdoch G, Jacobs NA, Wilson AB. *A Report of ISPO Consensus Conference on Amputation Surgery.* Copenhagen, Denmark: ISPO Copenhagen, 1992.
47. Lehneis HR, Ekus L, Fields G, et al. Prosthetic management of the cancer patient with high-level amputation. *Orthot Prosthet* 1981;35(2):10-28.
48. Collin C, Wade DT, Cochrane GM. Functional outcome of lower limb amputees with peripheral vascular disease. *Clin Rehabil* 1992;6:13-21.
49. Saadah ESH. Bilateral below-knee amputee 107 years old and still wearing artificial limbs. *Prosthet Orthot Int* 1988; 12:105-106.

31

Rehabilitation for Children with Limb Deficiencies

JOAN E. EDELSTEIN

LEARNING OBJECTIVES

On completion of this chapter, the reader will be able to do the following:

1. Relate developmental milestones to the habilitation of children with congenital limb deficiency and rehabilitation of those with amputation.
2. Describe how prostheses can be designed to accommodate longitudinal and circumferential growth so that fit remains comfortable and the child can attain maximum function.
3. Outline the ways a clinician can address psychosocial concerns for infants, toddlers, school-aged children, and adolescents.
4. Compare prosthetic options for children of various ages who have upper or lower limb deficiencies.
5. Specify the training goals for children of various ages fitted with upper and lower limb prostheses.
6. Design a habilitation program for an infant born with multiple limb deficiencies.

A baby girl whose left hand is missing, a boy who caught his foot in a powered lawn mower, and an adolescent recovering from osteogenic sarcoma of the distal femur have different skeletal, neuromuscular, learning, and psychosocial challenges from those of adults with amputation. Children share some rehabilitation issues with adults, particularly the basic components of the prosthesis and the essential elements of postoperative care. Other considerations, however, are unique to children. Because children are smaller than adults, the choice of prosthetic components is not as broad. Children grow and develop through the rehabilitation process. In addition, young people legally, financially, and emotionally depend on adults for their medical, surgical, and rehabilitation care.[1]

Comprehensive management of children with limb deficiencies requires that clinicians consider the causes of limb deficiency, the relation of developmental milestones to prosthetic selection and use, and the psychosocial factors that affect children. Specific issues regarding children with upper limb, lower limb, and multiple amputations require clinicians to design effective rehabilitation programs. Care of the infant born with a limb anomaly is *habilitation*, whereas management of an infant or child who undergoes amputation because of trauma or disease is *rehabilitation*. Unless the distinction is relevant, however, *habilitation* and *rehabilitation* are used interchangeably in this chapter. Similarly, *limb deficiency* is used to designate both congenital and acquired limb absence. The overall goal of physical therapy is to facilitate the normal developmental sequence and prevent the onset of secondary impairments and functional limitations such as contractures, weakness, and dependence in self-care.[1]

COMPREHENSIVE CONSIDERATIONS IN CHILDHOOD

The philosophy of this chapter is that the child with a limb deficiency is first and foremost a child, with the beauty, delight, and promise inherent in all young people.

Classification and Causes of Limb Deficiencies

The International Organization for Standardization approved a system of limb deficiency classification in 1989.[2] Congenital limb anomalies are described anatomically and radiologically as *transverse*, in which no skeletal elements exist below the level of normal development, or *longitudinal*, in which a reduction or absence of elements is present within the long axis of the limb, with normal skeletal elements usually present distal to the affected bone (Figure 31-1). This system replaces older terms, such as *phocomelia* (distal segments attached to the torso), *amelia* (complete absence of a limb), and *hemimelia* (partial absence of a limb).

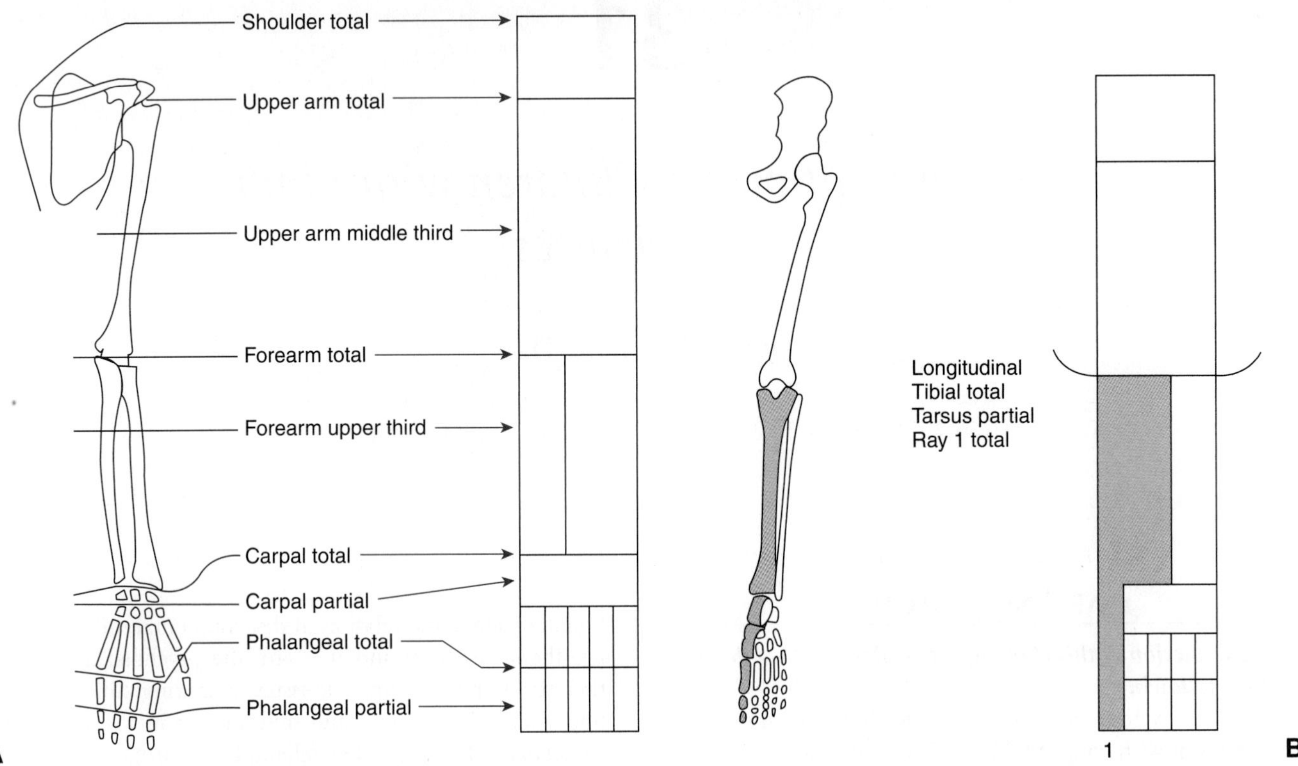

Figure 31-1

A, *The International Organization for Standardization/International Society for Prosthetics and Orthotics classification system for upper extremity transverse congenital limb deficiency. Lower extremity transverse deficiencies are named in a similar fashion. Levels can also be described by the name of the absent primary bone.* ***B,*** *An example of a lower extremity transverse congenital limb deficiency. The shaded area represents missing segments. Upper extremity transverse deficiencies are described by a similar strategy. (Reprinted from Murdoch G, Wilson AB [eds],* Amputation: Surgical Practice and Patient Management, *Oxford, UK: Butterworth Heinemann, 1996. pp. 352.)*

Limb deficiency in childhood is caused by congenital deficiency, trauma, cancer, and disease. In the total U.S. population, peripheral vascular disease among adults accounts for more than 80% of amputations, with a greater than 25% rate of increase in the latter half of the twentieth century. Rates of trauma- and cancer-related amputations are declining, whereas the incidence of congenital deficiencies remains stable.[3] A recent survey of all children with lower leg deficiencies in The Netherlands indicated 73% with congenital deficiencies and 27% with amputations due to malignancies (9%), trauma (8%), infection (4%), and other pathoses (6%).[4]

Among those with congenital limb anomalies, transverse deficiency of the upper limb, especially the left extremity, is the most common.[5] McGuirk and associates[6] found the overall prevalence of limb deficiency among 161,252 newborns to be 0.7 per 1000 births. Thirty percent of the defects were caused by genetic factors, 4% by teratogens, 35% by vascular disruption, and 32% by an unknown cause.[6]

Long-term follow-up study of the Childhood Cancer Survivor Study, which is composed of 14,054 individuals who have survived for 5 or more years after cancer treatment, indicates that osteosarcoma or Ewing's sarcoma of the lower limb or pelvis is the most common tumor; the median age at diagnosis is 14 years.[7] Some patients with tumor are treated by various limb-sparing procedures, and others undergo amputation. Long-term outcome is similar, although more patients with amputation used walking aids and were less satisfied with their status as children.[8,9]

Developmental Milestones

Infants develop motor skills in a predictable sequence, with well-established milestones that mark achievement of important functional abilities. In the absence of cerebral maldevelopment or malformation, the infant born with a limb anomaly or a young child who undergoes amputation demonstrates physical control at approximately the same time as an unaffected child does. Limb deficiency, however, often alters how the developmental tasks and activities are performed. For example, the 5-month-old infant who has only one intact leg will develop a distinctive style of crawling. Therapists who conduct initial evaluations of these children focus on muscle strength, range of motion, gross motor patterns, coordination, attention span, and interests.

The rate of neuromuscular development varies widely in all children, not just those with limb deficiency. Chronological age cannot provide a complete picture of a child's developmental level. In this chapter, milestones pertaining to upper and lower limb development are related to habilitation of children with limb disorders.

Children with limb deficiencies, regardless of cause, tend to have a lower energy output than unaffected children of the same age because of the energy demands of prosthesis use. Consequently, physical conditioning programs are important to enhance general health and endurance. Play and games increase coordination and improve strength. Children need to engage in active sports. Swimming is particularly beneficial because it does not traumatize the limbs and does not require a prosthesis; nevertheless, some children may be reluctant to display an anomalous limb.

Accommodating Growth

All children grow, regardless of congenital anomalies or amputations. Prosthetic planning should incorporate measures to maintain comfortable socket fit and symmetrical limb length. The preschool-aged child may need a new prosthesis almost yearly. Those in grade school often require a new prosthesis every 12 to 18 months, and teenagers outgrow prostheses every 18 to 24 months.[10]

Longitudinal growth is typically more rapid than circumferential growth, a troublesome fact for children with lower limb deficiency. Reconstructive surgery, especially circular (Ilizarov) fixation, suits children with minimal length discrepancy, whereas amputation remains preferable for those with severe limb loss.[11] Too short a lower limb prosthesis disturbs the quality and efficiency of gait and substantially increases energy cost. In contrast, an upper limb prosthesis that is slightly short will probably not present a noticeable asymmetry and will have little effect on bimanual activities. Endoskeletal prosthetic components facilitate lengthening and substitution of more sophisticated components.

Vigorous play causes considerable wear of the mechanical parts of prostheses. These parts are also vulnerable because of their small size and the sand, grass, and mud in which children often play. Children are likely to wear out prostheses from everyday use before circumferential growth necessitates a change. Signs of an outgrown socket include a tendency of the residual limb to slip out of the socket, pain or skin reddening caused by socket tightness, and a flesh roll around the margin of the socket. Socket liners are a convenient way to accommodate circumferential growth; as the child grows, liners can be removed. Alternatively, the prosthesis can be fitted with several layers of socks; the child eventually wears fewer socks to accommodate the added residual limb girth.[12] Flexible sockets fitted to extra-thick frames are another way to accommodate growth. To fit the larger residual limb, a new flexible socket is made and material is ground from the frame.[13,14]

Prosthetic alignment should complement the immature skeleton and joint capsules. For example, infants usually have genu varum, which becomes genu valgum by the third year.[12] Children with amputations through the bony diaphysis or metaphysis may have terminal bony overgrowth (Figure 31-2). As these children grow, terminal periosteal new bone may protrude beneath the terminal subcutaneous tissue and skin. Without treatment, a bursal sac forms and the skin becomes ecchymotic and hemorrhagic. The underlying bone then ruptures the bursal sac, and infection can occur.[10] Overgrowth is a particular problem when the adolescent growth spurt begins. Customary treatment is excision of the periosteal sac, transection of the distal 2 to 3 cm of bone, and primary closure of the incision. Children may require this procedure several times during the growth period.[15] Another approach is continuous skin traction, which can be used to maintain skin and soft tissue coverage over the distal end of the residual limb until skeletal growth is complete. The difficulties of keeping distal force on the limb day and night usually preclude this method. Disarticulation preserves the distal epiphyseal plate and thus is not associated with overgrowth.

In children with limb deficiencies, as in adults with amputation, availability of near normal range of motion is an important determinant of effective prosthetic use. For children, active therapeutic exercise designed to increase joint excursion is preferable to passive stretching, especially in the presence of congenital contracture.[16]

Postoperative Care

Postoperative care is simpler for young children who undergo amputation than for adolescents and adults. Ordinarily the residual limb presents little or no edema and the wound heals rapidly. Phantom pain can occur and is associated with the extent of preoperative pain.[15,17] Approximately one fourth of those with congenital limb deficiency or amputation before the age of 6 years have phantom sensation, with far fewer reporting phantom pain.[18,19] A pain diary may help older children and adolescents cope with phantom pain from traumatic limb loss.[20]

Psychosocial Factors in Habilitation and Rehabilitation

Habilitation amounts to more than selecting a suitable prosthesis and devising appropriate training. All children have personalities that develop along with their physical growth. Optimal emotional development occurs when parents and clinicians promote wholesome interactions. The essential message is that the child has a unique personality and that independence commensurate with age can be fostered.

Infants

Infants learn trust when their basic needs are met.[21] The baby with limb anomaly has as much need for trusting, responsive care as does the infant with normal limbs. If the family cannot accept the infant's appearance, the baby may have difficulty trusting others. For successful habilitation, parents must replace the expectation of a "perfect" infant

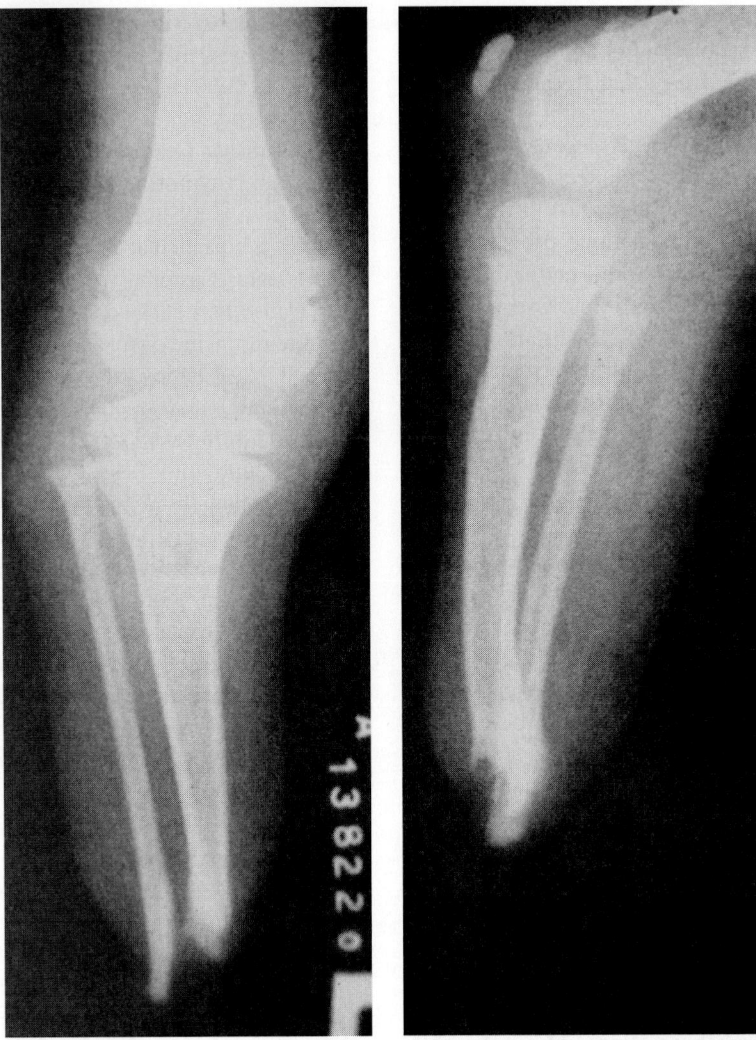

Figure 31-2

Bony overgrowth of the fibula in the transtibial residual limb of a 7-year-old child. In the original amputation surgery, the length of the fibula was originally slightly less than that of the tibia. (Courtesy J. E. Edelstein.)

with the reality of a baby who has a limb deficiency. Infants are susceptible to the anxieties of parents and others who interact with them. The birth of an infant with a limb deficiency can be a period of intense emotion. Because such a birth is a rare event in any hospital, medical staff may react with shock and feelings of helplessness and revulsion. Mothers have described the atmosphere of the delivery room as being "electrified" as staff react with silence or disgust.[22] Parents characterize the first few weeks after birth as nightmarish, a bad dream from which they want to wake. They believe they are alone with a unique and hopeless problem when questions go unanswered or evaded. Mourning for the loss of the ideal child is part of the coping process.[10] Parents are bombarded by the emotions of the child's grandparents, siblings, and other family members who comment and influence habilitation.

Although the newborn is too young for prosthetic fitting, early referral to a specialized clinic is highly desirable. The core team is composed of a pediatrician, physical therapist, occupational therapist, and prosthetist. The team should be able to draw on the expertise of psychologists, social workers, orthopedists, and engineers, depending on the needs of the child and family.[10] Effective clinical team management involves the family in rehabilitation decisions and weighs management recommendations in light of the immediate impact on the child's welfare and the long-term consequences on his or her appearance and function as an adult. An important resource for clinicians is the Association of Children's Prosthetic-Orthotic Clinics (6300 North River Road, Suite 727, Rosemont, IL 60018-4226). The association, founded in 1958, has held an annual interdisciplinary conference since 1972.

The clinical team can help parents realize they and their baby are acceptable. Families need time to talk about their feelings and obtain answers to their questions.[22] The team's approach considers motives such as hiding the deformity, maximizing function, and learning the parents' style of dealing with unexpected events. Team members should be empathetic to the parents' shock and grief, which can bear little relation to the amount of the infant's disability.[10] Some parents resist holding the baby, avoid direct contact, or withdraw into silence. When clinicians hold the baby, parents usually realize that the infant really is lovable. Rather than denying any difference, the team fosters the attitude that, yes, they know the child is different, but they recognize and accept the baby for what he or she is and what he or she can do.

CASE EXAMPLE 1A

A Newborn with Congenital Transradial Limb Deficiency

Mr. and Mrs. M. anticipated the birth of their second child with great eagerness. Mrs. M. had excellent prenatal care and had an easy pregnancy. The couple prepared their 2-year-old daughter for her new role as "big sister," encouraging her to feed her dolls bottles and push them in a stroller. Their daughter also moved to a junior bed with a coverlet that she chose. Mr. and Mrs. M. repainted the crib and hung new curtains in the nursery. The grandparents flew to town to await the birth and to help care for the older child and the new baby.

S. M. was born a few days later in the local hospital. She was a healthy, term infant with lusty lungs. The obstetrical nurse wrapped her in a receiving blanket and presented her to her proud parents. Mrs. M. was wheeled to her room for an overnight stay. Once settled in her room, Mr. and Mrs. M. unwrapped the baby, only to discover a left transradial limb deficiency. Mrs. M. shouted to the nurse on duty that someone had made a mistake. The nurse checked identification bracelets and confirmed that S. M. was indeed her daughter. Both Mr. and Mrs. M. were distraught that the baby's left hand was missing. In his grief and anger, Mr. M. threatened the nurse, medical staff, and hospital administration with legal action. Mrs. M., meanwhile, was silent, turning her head to the wall, refusing food and medication. Discharge to home with the baby is planned for the next morning.

Questions to Consider

- Given Mrs. M.'s depression and Mr. M.'s anger, how should the attending physician and nursing staff proceed?
- What should the social worker or psychologist do to provide appropriate guidance for the parents?
- How might the grandparents and older sister help Mr. and Mrs. M. when they return home with their new daughter?
- What is the most constructive response the physical therapist can give when first meeting S. M. and her parents?
- How can the physical therapist and occupational therapist facilitate positive immediate and long-term family interaction?

Families may be interested in seeing pictures or examples of the type of prosthesis that the child will probably use. Expectations regarding the extent of prosthetic restoration, however, may be unrealistic. Parents should understand what prosthetic and surgical possibilities exist so they can make rational decisions for their child. Infants usually receive the first prosthesis at approximately 6 to 9 months of age.[12,16,23-25] Some parents find it difficult to accept the prosthesis, believing that it draws attention to the limb deficiency.

The team can also help parents of children who undergo amputation because of trauma or disease cope with feelings of guilt and shock. Team members assist the family in realizing that they were not negligent in protecting the child against injury or not recognizing symptoms of a disease process early enough to prevent amputation.

In addition to clinical team management, families benefit from participating in peer support groups in which they can share concerns, exchange information, and observe children of various ages playing with and without prostheses. Some groups publish newsletters that share information with those who live too far from the meeting site. *Reach* is a newsletter published by the British Association of Parents Concerned with Children with Upper-Limb Anomalies (Reach Head Office, 25 High Street, Wellingborough, Northamptonshire, NN8 4J2, England). The Amputee Coalition of America (900 East Hill Avenue, Suite 285, Knoxville, TN 37915) is a peer advocacy organization that produces a magazine, monographs, and videos; has annual conferences; and offers Internet support (NLLICinfo@amputee-coalition.org). The organization also operates the National Limb Loss Information Center, which sponsors a youth activities program, national peer network, and limb loss education and awareness program, among other activities.

Parental acceptance of and active cooperation in the training program are the most important factors in its success and largely determine whether the child regards the prosthesis as a tool in daily activities.[10] Families need to learn skin care, prosthetic operation, maintenance, and the capabilities and limitations of the prosthesis. Outpatient training is preferable to avoid homesickness, which can interfere with the child's learning. In addition, the constant presence of one or both parents during therapy sessions enables the entire family to learn about prosthetic use and maintenance.[24] Putting a prosthesis on an active child is a skill that takes time for parents to master. Scheduling appointments after naps and meals is generally more productive than attempting to coerce a tired and upset child to participate in therapy. Clinicians need to recognize that infants have short attention spans and therefore should incorporate many brief activities in the treatment session.

Therapists who treat infants need to interpret nonverbal indications of comfort or discomfort and satisfaction or dissatisfaction with the prosthesis. For example, the infant who coos, smiles, and engages in play is probably content with the prosthesis and the function it offers, whereas a cranky, crying child may be contending with pinching or other pressure concentration from an ill-fitting socket. As with all patients, the clinician must frequently examine the child's skin, with particular attention to persistent redness, which indicates high pressure, and irritation, which may signal dermatitis.

CASE EXAMPLE 1B

A Child with Congenital Transradial Limb Deficiency

S. M. eats heartily, allows her older sister to sprinkle talcum powder on her, and is developing normally. She smiles and gurgles when someone approaches her. By 6 months she is sitting independently and can use both arms to clutch stuffed toys. She grabs the railings of her crib, attempting to pull herself to standing. The physical therapist recommended that the family take S. M. to a rehabilitation center that specializes in caring for children with amputations. At the center, Mr. and Mrs. M. overcame their initial hesitation and now participate enthusiastically in a peer support group, in which a dozen parents of children with limb deficiency trade advice and provide emotional support.

Mr. and Mrs. M. are concerned about unwelcome comments regarding their daughter's appearance, both with an empty sleeve and with the possibility of a hook terminal device. They tried to persuade the clinical team to provide S. M. with an infant passive mitt, which would disguise the anomaly. The therapist showed Mr. and Mrs. M. that the mitt has no prehensile capability. One of the members of the support group extolled the virtues of a myoelectric hand, so Mr. and Mrs. M. then argued that S. M. should be provided with "only the best," regardless of cost. Support group members pointed out that S. M. was too small for myoelectric fitting but might be a candidate in another year or two. S. M. is fitted with a simple transradial prosthesis consisting of infant voluntary-opening hook, wrist unit, socket, and infant harness. The prosthesis does not have a cable.

Questions to Consider

- What activities in the clinic would help S. M. acclimate to her new prosthesis?
- What activities would be appropriate for a home program for the first week after prosthetic fitting?
- What types of bimanual activities can be accomplished with a transradial prosthesis with a passive hand rather than a cable-controlled terminal device?
- What toys can be recommended to the grandparents that will help S. M. incorporate the prosthesis in her play time?
- How can the prosthesis facilitate S. M.'s physical and psychological development?

Toddlers

Toddlers must develop self-control to acquire the autonomy necessary to cope with their environment. The interval between 1 and 3 years of age is characterized by the development of language and functional communication, assertion of independence, and interpersonal control.[22] Children as young as 3 years should be informed of any impending surgery, whether to revise a congenital anomaly or treat a disease or injury. Doll play can help the child understand surgery and rehabilitation.[26,27] Special dolls that depict amputations at various levels, with and without prostheses, are available through Hal's Pals for Challenged Kids (PO Box 3490, Winter Park, CO 80482).

Children must resolve feelings of deprivation and resentment that accompany the visible alteration of their bodies.[10] Mobility, control, exploration, initiative, and creativity are prime emotional developmental milestones for older toddlers and young school-age children.[21] Parents and professional staff should encourage the child's independence. Facile use of a prosthesis can help children maximize their psychological potential. Children compare themselves with others and ask, "Where is my other hand (or leg)?" Children form two body images, one with and the other without the prosthesis. Parents should be able to give a simple and truthful answer, clearly stating that the child will not grow another hand, saying something like "you were born this way."[10] Similarly, children who undergo amputation need a realistic answer to the question, "What happened to you?"

The child may engage the parent in a power struggle regarding prosthetic wearing. A firm yet gentle approach with a range of acceptable choices usually enables the child to incorporate autonomy needs while gaining prosthetic proficiency.[22]

The clinical team should value the parents' comments about their child and involve the family in all aspects of care. The waiting room should have a variety of safe toys to make visits more pleasant. Parents should be present during the child's examination and prosthetic fitting to increase communication and thereby reduce anxiety and maximize effectiveness of the prosthetic prescription and fitting process.[22]

School-Aged Children

School-aged children need to become industrious,engaging in planning and executing tasks. The upper or lower limb prosthesis can be instrumental in fostering this important psychological task. [21] At this age, teachers, scout masters, clergy, and other adults are part of the child's social milieu. The clinical team can help prepare the child and family for these encounters.

In group experiences, the child may have to deal with feelings of social devaluation. The teacher or other group leader is in a position to bolster the child's sense of self-worth. The first encounter at school or camp can be the occasion when the child displays the prosthesis and demonstrates its function. The presentation usually dispels the

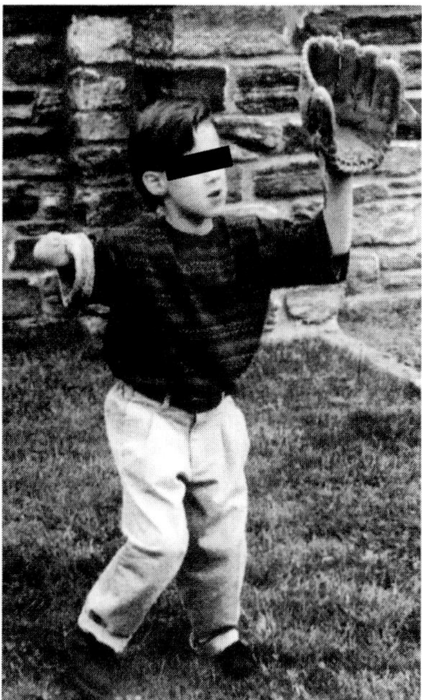

A

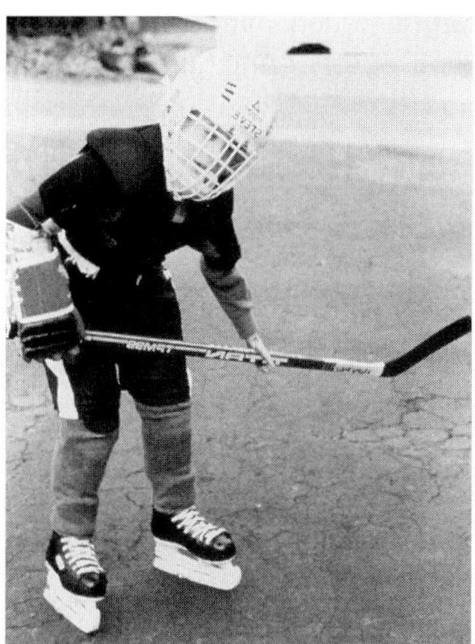

B

Figure 31-3

*Participation in sports and other organized activities such as softball (**A**) and hockey (**B**) fosters physical, psychological, and social development for children with limb deficiency just as it does for those with intact limbs. (Courtesy J. E. Edelstein.)*

mystery of the appliance and shows that the prosthesis is simply a tool that makes it easier for its wearer to engage in certain activities. The teacher should be aware of the appearance of the residual limb, the child's function with and without the prosthesis, any environmental or programmatic adaptations that the child may need, and how to cope with prosthetic malfunction. Anticipating awkward situations helps develop coping strategies. For example, in a circle game, classmates may be reluctant to hold hands with a child who wears an upper limb prosthesis. If the teacher holds the child's terminal device (hook or mechanical hand), the other students are likely to realize that it is not scary or unacceptable to do so. School officials may be concerned about the ability of a child with a prosthetic leg to maneuver in the classroom and playground. Classmates' natural curiosity should be dealt with through honest, simple answers. Although teasing is inevitable, the young child who feels secure understands that taunts are merely crude expressions of interest.

Among school-aged children with limb deficiencies, demographic variables (such as age, sex, socioeconomic status, and degree of limb loss) are not significant predictors of self-esteem. In contrast, social support, family functioning, self-perception, and microstressors affect the child's adaptation handicap. Perceived physical appearance is strongly predictive of general self-esteem.[28]

Many school-aged and older children respond favorably to scouting, camping, and other group recreational activities. Sports programs, such as skiing, horseback riding, and track events, are fun and give children with disabilities pride in athletic achievement (Figure 31-3).

Older Children and Adolescents

Adolescents face the critical step of developing a satisfying identity within themselves and with their peer groups. The teenager may select times when prosthetic wear is not desirable, for example, eschewing an upper limb prosthesis during a football game or discarding the leg prosthesis when swimming or playing beach volleyball. Adults should nurture young adults so they develop sufficient self-esteem to make satisfying decisions about when to use or remove the prosthesis. Teenagers with limb loss must cope with being visibly different. Young adults have to adapt to a culture designed for those who do not have a disability and must evaluate whether people relate to them as individuals or as people with handicaps.[29] During adolescence, feelings such as "Why did this happen to me?" are often intensified. Adolescents constantly reexamine their body image; group showering after physical education class may be especially stressful for those with limb loss. Other developmental concerns in which limb loss plays a role are choosing a vocation and obtaining a driver's license. The clinical team needs to be sensitive to concerns about privacy, confidentiality, and independence.[22]

Adolescents with bone cancer who undergo an amputation typically pass through a stage of initial impact when they learn that the treatment plan includes amputation. This news may be met with despair, discouragement, passive acceptance, or violent denial. Informing the adolescent of the rehabilitation process and the achievements of others can be helpful. The next stage is retreat, during which the adolescent experiences acute grief. Anger may be part of the coping process. The goal of grieving is giving up hope of retrieving the lost object. The staff can reinforce the patient's strengths and encourage maximal independence. The third stage is acknowledgment, when the adolescent is willing to participate in rehabilitation and has incorporated the changed appearance into his or her body image. Reconstruction, the final stage, involves the return to developmentally appropriate activities, such as school, sports, camp, and dating.[29]

CASE EXAMPLE 2

An Adolescent with Osteogenic Sarcoma

E. K., who is 15 years old, is scheduled tomorrow to have surgical ablation of his right arm at the level of the humeral epicondyles to remove an osteogenic sarcoma. Six months ago he fractured his right radial head. Although the fracture healed well, he noticed persistent tenderness at the elbow with a firm mass that was increasing in size. His physician referred him to an orthopedist. After a series of bone scans and biopsies, the orthopedist confirmed the diagnosis of osteogenic sarcoma and recommended immediate amputation. E. K. and his parents refused the surgery and traveled to four clinics in the surrounding states seeking advice regarding treatment of the tumor. They explored alternate methods of treatment, including herbal preparations to shrink the sarcoma, en bloc resection with implantation of an endoprosthetic elbow joint, and amputation of the arm distal to the epicondyles. After meeting with the clinical team at the children's medical center and speaking with several patients who had had surgery and rehabilitation, they reluctantly agreed to amputation during his summer vacation.

An excellent student, E. K. is also the shortstop on his high school varsity baseball team and plays the tuba in the marching band. For the past two summers he has been a counselor at a sports- and computer-oriented camp. The family is committed to devoting all its financial and emotional resources to enable E. K. to resume a full agenda of academic and recreational activities. E. K. has compiled considerable information regarding prostheses from the Internet.

Questions to Consider

- What postoperative management would foster wound healing and enable E. K. to become accustomed to a prosthesis?
- How can the occupational therapist and physical therapist help E. K. cope with loss of his dominant hand?
- Compare the advantages of a cable-controlled prosthesis with a prosthesis having a myoelectrically controlled terminal device and cable-controlled elbow unit.
- What terminal device would be most suitable for E. K.?
- How can the clinical team guide E. K. when he returns to school in September?
- In what recreational activities can E. K. engage after his amputation?

REHABILITATION AND PROSTHETIC DECISION MAKING

Not all children with limb deficiency benefit from prostheses. With certain upper limb anomalies, the remaining portion of the limb is more functional than it would be if it were covered by a prosthesis.[10,30] Children who are born with bilateral arm absence generally use their feet to play and can do almost everything they need to without using complicated and heavy prostheses.[24] In one large study, approximately half of the children with unilateral congenital deficiencies and two thirds of those with amputation received prostheses. By the age of 12 years, two thirds of those who had prostheses were still using them.[31]

Rehabilitation of Children with Upper Limb Amputation

Because functional use of an upper limb prosthesis often involves control of a terminal device, the prosthetic design and the rehabilitation program should be appropriate for the child's level of motor, cognitive, and perceptual development.

Infants

Prosthetic fitting and training should complement an infant's development. Although a prosthesis usually is not fitted until babies are at least 6 months of age, earlier developmental accomplishment paves the way for successful prosthetic use.

The average 2-month-old infant can hold objects with both hands. The baby who lacks one or both hands typically attempts to hug a stuffed animal with the forearms or upper arms, capitalizing on the tactile sensitivity of the skin. The normal 3-month-old can bring grasped objects to the mouth. Three months is also the age when babies attempt two-handed prehension, although this skill is not perfected until the child attains sitting balance at 6 to 9 months.[1]

The 4-month-old infant props on the forearms, shifts weight to reach, and usually enjoys shaking noisy rattles by using rapid elbow flexion and extension. An important developmental step is reached at approximately the same age when the child can manipulate objects with one hand while the other hand stabilizes the toy. Simultaneous sitting and manipulating are still challenging at this age.[1] Increased trunk strength enables the baby to reach unilaterally and bilaterally. Bilateral coordination at 4 months allows the infant to reach objects at the midline.[32] Two-handed holding of a bottle typically occurs at approximately 4.5 months.

By the fifth month, the infant can transfer toys from one hand to the other and is thus aware of the usefulness of holding objects.[32] The infant's dominant interest is in getting food; exploring surroundings; and making social contact with those who feed, hold, and provide care. Holding a large ball encourages the infant to clasp objects between the arms. Manipulating blocks or beads promotes stabilization of proximal body parts to allow fine movements with distal parts. Although a baby with intact limbs can get to the quadruped position and shift weight from side to side,[32] the infant who is missing one or both arms will probably find that crawling is impossible and will have difficulty coming to a sitting position and pulling to a standing position.[16]

Six months is generally considered the optimal age for upper limb prosthetic fitting.[10] The baby with unilateral amputation has achieved good sitting balance, can free the sound hand for manual activities while sitting, and is actively engaged in exploring the environment. The prosthesis restores symmetrical limb length and enables the infant to hold stuffed animals and similar toys at the midline. The prosthesis also accustoms parents to the concept that a prosthesis will likely be a permanent part of their child's wardrobe. Fitting can assuage parental guilt or shame regarding their infant's abnormal appearance by replacing negative reactions with a constructive device that enhances the baby's development. Many parents seek a prosthetic hand to disguise the limb anomaly. Early fitting provides experience that will be the basis for the young person's later decision regarding whether to continue with prosthetic use. Fitting before the age of 2 years appears to reduce the likelihood of the child's rejecting the prosthesis.[33]

Some clinicians advocate fitting a simple prosthesis between the ages of 3 and 6 months.[23,34] The rapid growth of younger infants, however, makes the maintenance of socket fit difficult. In addition, a younger baby may find the prosthesis a hindrance during rolling maneuvers. Infants who are much older than 6 months may resist a prosthesis that deprives them of using the tactile sensation at the end of the residual limb. Initial fitting after 2 years tends to result in greater rejection of the prosthesis because by then the child has developed compensatory techniques.[34]

At 8 months, most babies sit while manipulating objects with both hands by using gross palmar grasp and controlled release. A prosthesis aids in clasping large objects and stabilizing smaller ones while the sound hand explores them.[35] By 15 months, most children can place a pellet in a small container and use crayons for scribbling and a spoon for feeding. These skills can also be performed with a prosthesis.

Babies are usually fitted with a passive prosthesis, that is, one that does not have a cable or other operating mechanism. The terminal device may be a hook or a passive mitt. The hook is covered with pink or brown resilient plastic to disguise its mechanical appearance. The plastic also blunts the impact of the hook as infants explore with it, swiping themselves and others in the vicinity. The hook may be a voluntary-opening design, without a cable. Parents can place a rattle or other object in the hook to acquaint the baby with prehension on the deficient side. Some infants have a voluntary-closing hook on the first prosthesis; in the absence of a cable, the hook holds the toy secured with tape or a rubber band. A few children start with the Child Amputee Prosthetics Project (Los Angeles, Calif.) terminal device, which functions in the voluntary-opening mode. The three options offer little difference in function. A fourth terminal device option is the infant passive mitt. The mitt has a less mechanical appearance than other terminal devices but has no prehensile function; consequently, few objects can be taped or otherwise secured to it for the amusement of the baby. The absence of a hooked configuration hampers use of the mitt when the baby attempts to pull to standing at the side of the crib or playpen. Whatever the design, the terminal device is fitted into a wrist unit at the distal end of the socket.

The thermoplastic socket is custom molded to a plaster model of the child's residual limb. It is worn over a cotton sock that protects the skin from pressure concentration. A snug fit is needed around the humeral epicondyles to stabilize the prosthesis on the child's residual limb. Depending on the rate of growth, changes may be needed every 2 to 4 months. If the anomaly is comparable to transhumeral amputation, the first prosthesis usually does not have an elbow unit even if the anomaly is comparable to transhumeral amputation.

Regardless of the level of limb loss, the prosthetic socket is suspended on the infant's torso by a harness, which typically has more straps than an adult harness. The toddler harness inhibits the infant's attempts to remove the prosthesis, whether deliberately or inadvertently during rolling and crawling.

Clothing problems arise when a prosthesis is worn. The rigid parts of the prosthesis eventually wear holes in clothing. Shirts and blouses worn over the prosthesis should be loose fitting; raglan sleeves are preferable to sleeves set at the natural shoulder line, which can interfere with cable operation.

Training the infant fitted with a passive prosthesis usually begins with two sessions in a 1-week period and then at periodic follow-up appointments. The first session should be held when the baby is well rested and content. The therapist or parent puts the prosthesis on the baby, who is then placed on the floor with various toys. The therapist encourages the parents to play with and handle the baby while the infant is wearing the prosthesis. The baby may ignore the prosthesis because its socket eliminates the sense of touch and because the length of the prosthesis feels awkward. Parents should present large toys that require the use of both arms. The basic prosthesis allows the infant to cuddle a teddy bear, swat at a mobile and similar hanging toys, and use both upper limbs for rolling and crawling. Training involves instructing the parents and other caregivers to gain familiarity with the prosthesis, care for the infant's skin by making certain that the socket and harness do not exert undue pressure, and provide toys that require bimanual prehension (Box 31-1). Placing a rattle in the terminal device is another way of acquainting the infant with grasp on the side of limb deficiency. At the end of the session, the therapist and parent remove the prosthesis to inspect the child's skin for signs of irritation from the socket or harness. Parents learn how to apply the prosthesis and how to encourage full-time wear except during baths, naps, and bedtime. The baby may be rather awkward when sitting and moving while adjusting to the weight of the prosthesis. Toys suitable for the infant's developmental level, such as large balls, dolls, stuffed animals, balloons, xylophones, and other noisy and colorful objects, provide incentives for enjoying the prosthesis. Parents can put a mallet or other toy in the hook so that the infant can obtain pleasure from using the prosthesis. Push and pull toys are appropriate when the child is able to stand and cruise.[36,37]

Parents may be concerned when children catch the prosthesis on chair and table legs or use it to strike themselves or others; children recover balance readily, though, and peers are usually able to defend themselves successfully. Printed instructions, augmented by audiotapes or videotapes, are useful guides for the family.

At the second training session a few days later, the therapist can review the parents' experiences. Donning and doffing the prosthesis should be reviewed. Initially, the infant may tolerate the prosthesis only for a few minutes. It should be frequently applied during the day. Eventually, the child should be able to wear it most of the day, except when sleeping and bathing.

Subsequent follow-up sessions focus on the adequacy of prosthetic fit and the child's readiness for the addition of a cable to the prosthesis, substitution of a myoelectrically controlled prosthesis for a passive one, or, in the case of the child with transhumeral amputation, the addition of an elbow unit.

Toddlers

Control cables may be added to traditional, body-operated prostheses when the child is between the ages of 15 and 18 months. Active control may not become reliable until the toddler is approximately 2.5 years of age, when the understanding of cause and effect is established (Figure 31-4).[24] Readiness for the cable is indicated when the child wears the prosthesis full time, can follow simple instructions, has an attention span of at least 5 minutes, and will allow the therapist and prosthetist to handle him or her. A toddler who resists instruction from someone other than the parent may be too immature to learn to control the prosthesis.

If the prosthesis has a voluntary-opening hook, it should be fitted with a half- or a quarter-width rubber band to facilitate opening. The tension in the terminal device should be sufficient to let the child hold objects but not so great that opening the hook is difficult. Young children appear to use the voluntary-closing hook with as much ease as the more traditional voluntary-opening terminal devices. Goals of prosthetic training for toddlers are summarized in Box 31-2.

Training should be conducted in a quiet setting. The therapist and child sit at a low table with toys that require bimanual grasp, such as large beads and a string with a rigid tip. For the child with unilateral amputation, the terminal device serves to hold an object, such as a bead, while the child threads the string through the bead. The therapist is on the child's prosthetic side, holding the child's forearm at 90 degrees of elbow flexion, the optimal position of cable operation. This position also keeps the terminal device and the grasped object within view. The adult moves the child's forearm forward, flexing the shoulder, tensing the cable, and causing the hook to operate. When the arm is moved back

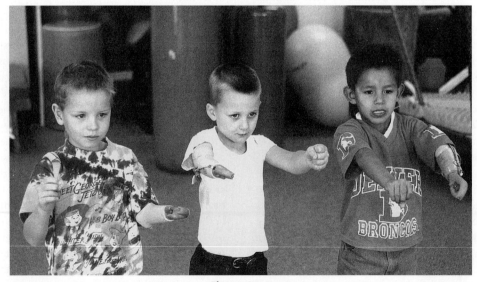

Figure 31-4
This group of children is learning that shoulder flexion produces terminal device operation because flexion tenses the control cable. (Courtesy T.R.S., Inc., Boulder, Colo.)

Box 31-1 *Prosthetic Training Goals for Infants*

Therapy sessions are designed to increase the infant's
- Comfort with the prosthesis
- Wearing tolerance
- Ability to clasp large objects
- Ability to use the prosthesis to aid in sitting and crawling

Parents of an infant with a prosthesis should do the following:
- Apply and remove the prosthesis correctly
- Care for the child's skin
- Care for the prosthesis
- Recognize and report to the clinical team any problems with the prosthesis or child

Box 31-2 *Prosthetic Training Goals for Toddlers*

Therapy sessions are designed to increase the toddler's
- Control of the terminal device
- Control of the elbow unit
- Use of the prosthesis in bimanual prehension
- Use of the prosthesis in functional activities

Parents of toddlers with prostheses should do the following:
- Provide toys that require bimanual prehension
- Encourage use of the prosthesis as an assistive device
- Inspect the skin to determine whether the prosthesis causes undue irritation

(shoulder extension), the terminal device changes position. A voluntary-opening hook opens with shoulder flexion, whereas a voluntary-closing hook closes with shoulder flexion. The child is encouraged to help with the control motion. With either design, the initial training involves placing a toy in the hook and encouraging the child to discover how to keep it in place. With a voluntary-opening hook, the child simply relaxes to allow the rubber bands or springs to keep the hook fingers closed. The voluntary-closing hook requires that the wearer exert tension on the control cable by the harness to keep the hook closed. Children use the same control motions as do adults, namely shoulder flexion or shoulder girdle protraction for terminal device operation. The toddler may revert to the earlier practice of opening the terminal device with the sound hand; eventually he or she will find that cable operation is more efficient, allowing more complex play maneuvers.

The natural inclination of the child is to reach for objects with the sound hand. To provide the child the necessary practice with the prosthesis, the therapist or parent should offer large objects or toys that require bimanual grasp to operate (Figure 31-5). Another technique to encourage prosthetic use is to have the child hold one object in the sound hand and another in the prosthesis. For example, two hand bells make twice as much sound as one. With some children, prosthetic training merely involves using the terminal device as a stabilizer rather than as a prehensile tool; for example, the child may lean the prosthesis onto a replica of a mailbox while placing objects in the slot with the sound hand. The prosthesis also serves to stabilize paper while the child draws and colors pictures.

Although children as young as 18 months have been fitted with myoelectrically controlled transradial prostheses,[38] those who are at least 3 years of age have an easier time learning to contract the appropriate flexors and extensors to close and open the hand (Figure 31-6). The prosthesis is relatively heavy, susceptible to breakdown, and needs more

A

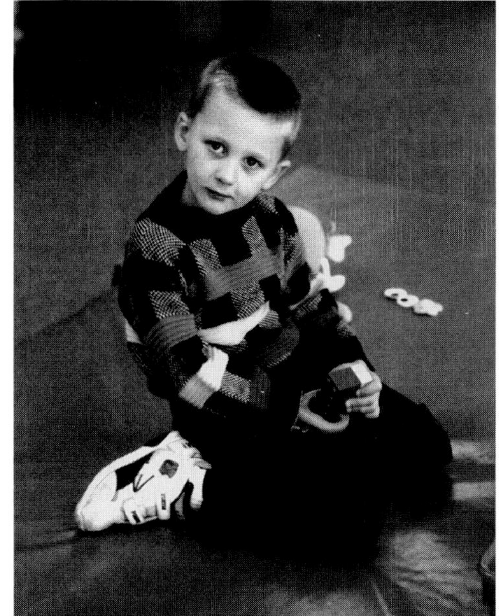

B

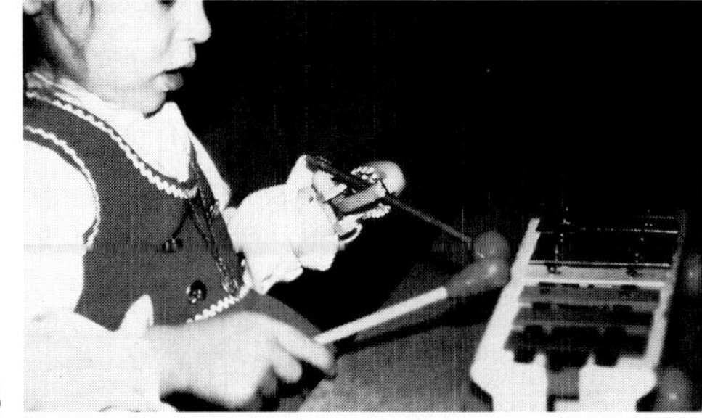

Figure 31-5
A, *Large objects or toys such as Duplo (Lego Systems, Inc., Enfield, Conn.) blocks that require bimanual prehension allow the child the opportunity to incorporate the prosthesis in functional activities. (Courtesy T.R.S., Inc., Boulder, Colo.)* ***B,*** *Other activities that encourage use of both upper extremities, such as playing a xylophone, can also be incorporated in the prosthetic program. (Courtesy J. E. Edelstein.)*

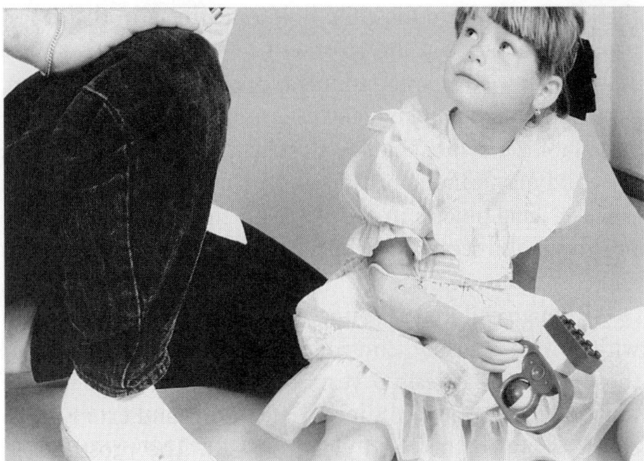

Figure 31-6
Young children can learn to contract the forearm muscles to operate the myoelectrically controlled terminal device. (Courtesy Otto Bock Orthopedic Industry, Inc., Minneapolis, Minn.)

maintenance than does a cable-operated device.[24] To prepare the child for a somewhat heavier myoelectric prosthesis, weight should be gradually added to the passive prosthesis. Rudimentary training begins with practice with the prosthesis off the arm. At first, the therapist may place an electrode on the sound forearm and ask the child to flex and extend the wrist to close and open the fingers of the prosthetic hand. The therapist then places an electrode on the forearm on the amputated side and encourages the child to discover that contraction of the forearm musculature on that side achieves the same results. Motorized toys can be used to help the child practice deliberate contraction of flexors and extensors to cause an electric train, for example, to go backward and forward, depending on which electrode is stimulated. When the child gains reasonable proficiency, the prosthetic socket can be made with the electrodes embedded in it. Care must be taken to achieve and maintain snug fit so that the electrodes are in constant contact with the skin.[39]

Practice to gain prosthetic proficiency is the same whether the prosthesis is cable or myoelectrically controlled. The beginner experiences many instances of dropping objects while learning the amount of muscle contraction or tension on the cable needed to maintain suitable terminal device closure. The ability to close the terminal device around an object develops before active release. Grasping an object from the tabletop is difficult. Children attempting to put objects into their mouths discover that the change in shoulder position alters the tension on the control cable. Similarly, children who drop toys and try to retrieve them from the floor discover how to hold the shoulder to maintain adequate cable tension. Those who are wearing myoelectrically controlled prostheses also notice that the prosthesis is easier to operate in some positions of the forearm than in others.

Practice in opening and closing the terminal device can involve moving pegs on a board. Tossing a beanbag is useful for teaching terminal device opening, as is playing cards. Cutting paper is another satisfying activity. The child holds the paper in the terminal device and uses the scissors in the sound hand. Prosthetic training should acquaint the child with objects of various textures, sizes, and shapes. Resilient foam toys are easier to grasp than are those made of rigid plastic, wood, or metal. Playing with sewing cards, nested barrels, and snap-apart beads; removing a toy from a drawstring bag; opening a zipper; removing loose clothing; opening small boxes of raisins; opening and closing felt-tipped pens; and playing the xylophone entice the child to attempt grasping, holding, and releasing motions with the terminal device.[35] Moving checkers or other markers from one location to another on a game board is a good drill. The prosthesis is helpful when swinging and climbing on the playground, rolling a wheelbarrow or doll carriage, jumping rope, and riding a tricycle. Children with unilateral amputation usually regard the intact limb as the dominant one. Many children with unilateral amputation refer to the prosthesis as the helper, which correctly identifies its role as a device that assists the intact hand.

Functional training depends on the child's ability to reach the mouth, waist, hips, feet, and perineum. Feeding, dressing, writing, and personal hygiene are incorporated at the appropriate times. Thirty-month-old children can throw and catch a ball, start uncomplicated dressing, and eat with a spoon with little spillage. Children play in sand, earth, and water and engage in rough and tumble activities, which can damage the prosthesis and the skin. Daily inspection and attention to minor problems help avoid major prosthetic repairs and skin disorders.

A 2-year-old with transhumeral amputation may have a prosthesis with an elbow unit, although mastery of the elbow-locking cable is unlikely to occur before the third birthday. Strategies to self-manage donning and doffing the prosthesis can be introduced to children as young as 3 years. They find removing the prosthesis easier than applying it.

At 3 years of age, the child may begin to be curious about the rotational possibilities of the wrist unit. Objects of various shapes within reach oblige the child to turn the terminal device in the wrist unit to the suitable position. Most objects can be manipulated with the terminal device in the pronated position; however, thin disks are more easily managed with the terminal device in midposition, and small balls are best cradled in the terminal device when it is rotated to the supinated position. Holding the handlebars of a tricycle or manipulating hand controls in other wheeled toys helps the child learn how to use terminal device rotation in the wrist unit (Figure 31-7). Prosthetic activities for the toddler should include eating, drinking, dressing, and managing crayons and other writing implements. Three-year-olds blow soap bubbles, pull up pants, pull a belt through loops in pants, and fill a cup with water from a spigot.[35]

Throughout the toddler phase, work periods should alternate with free play that may or may not involve the prosthesis. Weekly training sessions are effective. Parents should inspect the axilla; persistent redness indicates that the harness is applying undue pressure. The home program should include written suggestions regarding activities to promote bimanual prehension, instructions concerning the care of the prosthesis and the care of the child's skin, terminology pertaining to parts of the prosthesis, and ideas regarding clothing that will not impede prosthetic function.

School-Aged Children

An important consideration for the growing child is a socket large enough for comfortable fit and adequate prosthetic control.

The 4-year-old child is usually coordinated enough to grasp fragile objects without breaking or crushing them. With a voluntary-opening hook, the child must maintain tension on the control cable to prevent the hook fingers from snapping shut. A voluntary-closing terminal device necessitates application of gentle tension on the cable rather than forceful shoulder motion. With a myoelectrically controlled hand, the child must minimally contract flexors so that the fingers close on the object without undue pressure. Four-year-olds can pour from containers, peel a banana, sharpen a pencil with a hand-held sharpener, sew, hammer nails, and apply adhesive bandages (Figure 31-8). The average 5-year-old can open a milk container and sweep with a brush and dust pan.[35] Goals of prosthetic training for school-aged children are summarized in Box 31-3.

A

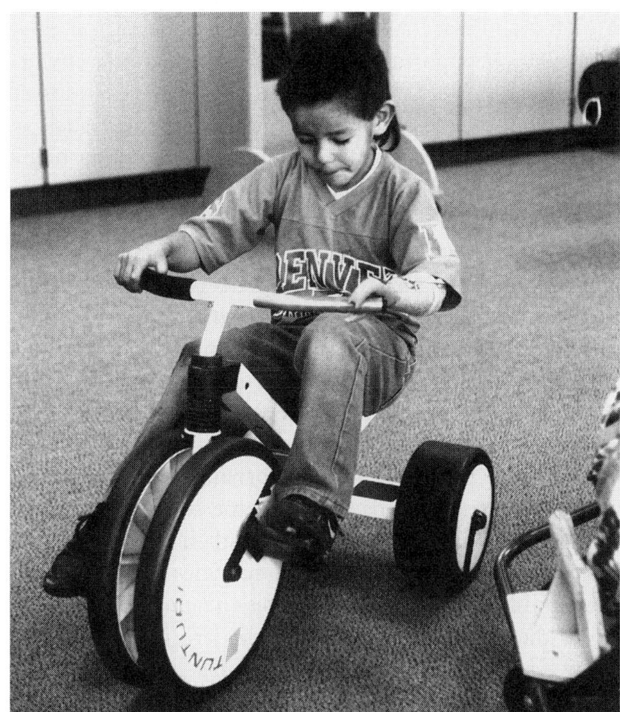

B

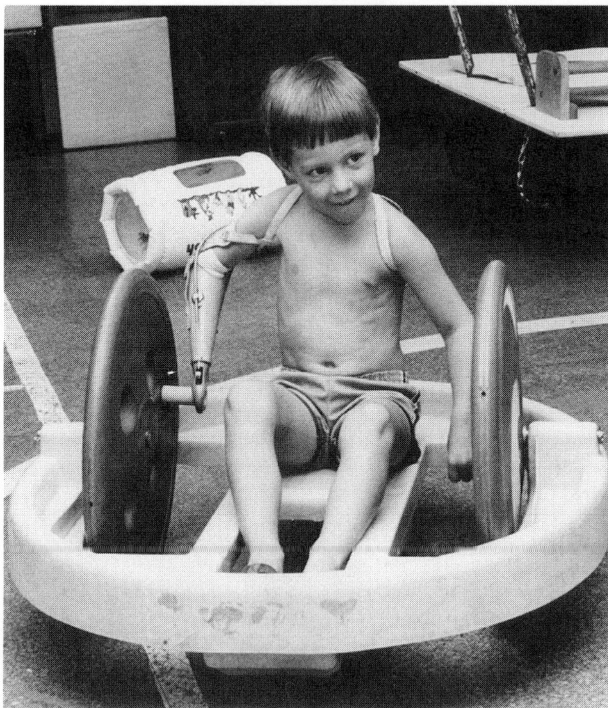

Figure 31-7

*Riding a tricycle (**A**) or other wheeled toy (**B**) provides excellent practice for using the prosthesis to assist the sound hand. (Courtesy T.R.S., Inc., Boulder, Colo.)*

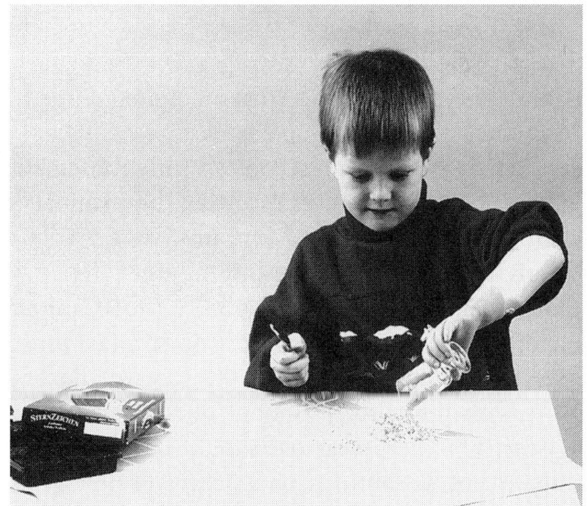

Figure 31-8

Preschool- and school-aged children develop manipulation skills as they incorporate their prosthesis in fine motor activities. Emptying a glass requires that the child generate the appropriate myoelectric signal to the forearm flexors to hold the container while positioning the limb to pour. (Courtesy Otto Bock Orthopedic Industry, Inc., Minneapolis, Minn.)

Box 31-3 *Prosthetic Training Goals for School-Aged Children*

Therapy sessions assist the school-aged child to do the following:

- Maintain proper prosthetic fit
- Grasp firm and fragile objects without dropping or crushing them
- Open and close the terminal device reliably
- Don and doff the prosthesis independently
- Dress independently
- Recognize when the prosthesis needs repair or alteration

Parents of school-aged children with prostheses should do the following:

- Encourage the child's independence in daily activities and play

The pediatric prehension assessment provides a standard clinical assessment of children with transradial amputation by objectively scoring activities of daily living that require repetitive use of a terminal device. Three test batteries correspond to age groups of 2 to 3 years, 4 to 5 years, and 6 to 7 years. In test 1, the child is asked to string four large beads, open four 35-mm film cans, separate three nested screw-top barrels, assemble 10 interlocking beads, and separate a five-piece notched plastic block. In test 2, the child uses a sewing card, strings 10 small beads, sticks an adhesive bandage to the table, cuts a paper circle and glues it to another paper, and opens a small package of tissues. In test 3, the child is asked to cut modeling plastic with a knife and fork, cut paper, discard 5 playing cards from a hand of 10 cards, lace a shoe and tie a bow, and wrap a book.[35]

Children in elementary school are often fascinated by card games. Maintaining several cards in the terminal device and then releasing the desired card involves a gradation of tension on the control cable for prostheses equipped with a voluntary-opening or -closing terminal device. Card playing is more difficult with a myoelectrically controlled prosthesis because the child must contract the forearm flexors and extensors with the correct amount of force at the appropriate time.[40-42] The 5-year-old should be independent in dressing, except for buttons, shoelaces, and pullover shirts and sweaters.[1] Compared with their peers, children who wear a unilateral transradial prosthesis may be slightly delayed in the development of bimanual functional skills, regardless of the age of prosthetic fitting; the delay may be attributable to the insensate and relatively rigid mechanical characteristics of the prosthesis.[43]

The child also needs to learn how to take care of the prosthesis, keep it clean, and ask for help when parts malfunction. Skin inspection is an essential part of training.

Older Children and Adolescents

Many older children are able to incorporate the prosthesis in school activities. Sports prostheses, such as those with a terminal device designed to hold a basketball, give wearers more opportunities to participate in group activities (Figure 31-9). Teenagers may find that playing a musical instrument is pleasurable. Simple adaptations, such as fingering a trumpet with the sound hand and supporting it with the prosthesis, can open a world of enjoyment to the musician.[44] Older adolescents should have vocational exploration, vocational assessment, and, when indicated, job training. Obtaining a driver's license is a meaningful event for most teenagers. The use of a prosthesis does not influence the capacity to drive, although those with upper limb deficiency are more likely to use adaptive devices when driving than those with lower limb deficiency.[45]

Some adolescents with unilateral limb deficiency seek escape from parental control by abandoning their prostheses, preferring to manage with the intact limb. A few young people ultimately resume prosthetic wear on a full-time or occasional basis. Certain activities are more easily accomplished without the prosthesis or cannot be done with a prosthesis. For example, prostheses are not worn when showering. Individuals with transradial amputation may prefer to stabilize objects in the antecubital fossa, using elbow flexion, rather than use a prosthetic terminal device. Sometimes simple equipment adaptation facilitates one-handed performance, such as the use of a book holder, guitar

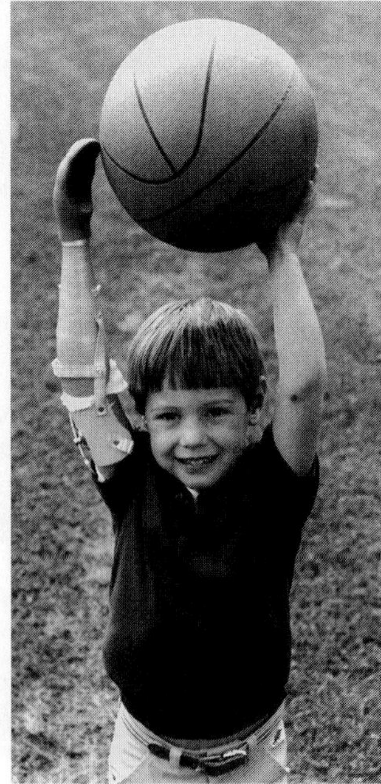

Figure 31-9
A variety of terminal devices are available for use in sports and recreational activities. This flexible mitt is shaped to enable participation in activities that require catching, manipulating, or throwing balls. (Courtesy T.R.S., Inc., Boulder, Colo.)

pick, or camera grip. Some people become quite facile with the remaining upper limb, learning to hit a baseball, use a keyboard, and fold laundry with one hand.[30]

Functional outcome evaluation of children fitted with unilateral upper prostheses is aided by the Prosthetic Upper Extremity Functional Index administered to parents and older children.[46] Long-term follow-up of children with unilateral transradial deficiency indicates that approximately 40% use a passive prosthesis, 40% use a voluntary-closing terminal device, and 15% use a myoelectrically controlled prosthesis.[47] Of those trained to use a myoelectrically controlled prosthesis, most report satisfaction with it even though many do not wear it.[48]

Rehabilitation of Children with Lower Limb Loss

The care of children with lower limb deficiencies is similar to that described for those with upper limb deficiencies. Management should suit the patient's developmental stage so that prosthetic use fosters achievement of key milestones. Parents serve as the primary instructors of their children, with the guidance of the physical therapist and other members of the clinical team. Early referral to a clinical team is equally important for the family with a child who has a lower-limb amputation or limb deficiency. Peer support is also valuable for parents who need to share concerns, suggestions, and camaraderie with others who have to cope with a similar situation.

Infants

Achievement of sitting balance in the infant is the major guide to lower-limb prosthetic fitting.[2] The average age when babies accomplish independent sitting is 6 months. Sitting depends on postural control and antigravity muscle strength. Sitting balance and trunk stabilization are also important for freeing the hands to explore the environment.[32,35] The goals of rehabilitation of infants with lower limb malformation or amputation are summarized in Box 31-4.

Box 31-4 *Prosthetic Training Goals for Infants with Lower Limb Deficiency*

Therapy sessions are designed to facilitate the infant's
- Comfort with the prosthesis
- Wearing tolerance
- Ability to stand by leaning against a table
- Ability to cruise around furniture
- Ability to walk with and without support from a doll carriage or other supporting toy

Parents of infants with lower limb prostheses should do the following:
- Apply and remove the prosthesis correctly
- Care for the child's skin
- Care for the prosthesis
- Recognize and report any problems with the prosthesis

Infants who are 5 to 7 months of age discover the mobility possibilities of crawling and creeping, moving from supine to four-point and sitting positions, and moving to the hands and knees from the sitting position.[49] Crawling involves the alternate action of the opposite arms and legs in a manner similar to walking. Hip extensors strengthen during crawling and kneeling. Rocking on four points before launching into crawling is another important precursor to walking.

Most babies are able to overcome gravity to pull up to a standing position and rise from kneeling to standing at approximately 8 months. When pulling to a standing position, the baby expends great energy bouncing and actively disturbing balance. Bouncing gradually gives way to shifting weight from side to side. The initial standing posture is wide based, with the hips abducted, flexed, and externally rotated. The base accommodates the child's new center of gravity position, which is higher than when crawling. Maintaining upright posture depends on sufficient maturity of the visual, proprioceptive, and vestibular systems.

Although the 7-month-old displays stepping movements when supported, cruising along furniture does not become a preferred mode of locomotion until the child is approximately 10 months old. Cruising is usually the first form of independent walking and builds strength of the hip abductors. The typical nondisabled child stands alone at approximately 11 months and walks alone at 12 months.[50] The urge to walk is the culmination of the endless pulling and standing activity that has occupied the baby for several preceding months.

Prosthetic fitting aims to facilitate the child's attainment of motor milestones. The infant who is missing a lower limb should have prosthetic restoration at approximately 6 months, when the baby has enough trunk control for sitting and is ready to pull to a standing position. A simple prosthesis fosters symmetrical sitting balance and aids the baby's attempts to pull to standing. In addition, the prosthesis equalizes leg length, adds weight to the anomalous side, and obviates the tendency to compensate with a one-legged standing pattern (Figure 31-10). Reducing the weight asymmetry inherent in limb deficiency facilitates rotational control of the trunk. The prosthesis enables standing and walking. Otherwise, the world is circumscribed by the confines of the stroller or playpen, and the deficiency becomes a source of shame to be hidden. Fitting before 6 months is undesirable because the prosthesis might hinder the baby's efforts to turn from prone to supine position and back again.

The first prosthesis includes a solid-ankle, cushion heel (SACH) foot and, for the child with transfemoral amputation, a locked-knee unit. The SACH foot is the smallest foot manufactured. Rubber-soled shoes give the infant more traction and are therefore preferable to leather-soled shoes. The prosthesis must be comfortable when the baby stands,

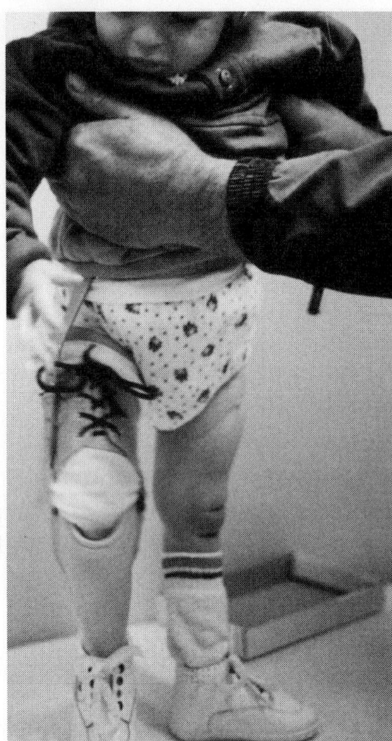

Figure 31-10

This toddler's transtibial prosthesis has a thigh cuff suspension with orthotic knee joints and a SACH foot. This choice of suspension system ensures the prosthesis will remain securely on the limb as the child alternates between sitting and standing during busy play activities. (Courtesy J. E. Edelstein.)

sits, squats, crawls, and climbs. By 3 years, most children can manage an unlocked knee.[12]

Useful equipment for working with young children with lower limb deficiency includes a play table, an elevated sandbox, a floor mat, a rolling stool, a full-length mirror, steps, and a ramp. During the first training session, the therapist and parent confirm that the prosthesis fits comfortably, without redness of the residual limb. Most of the handling of the child should be done by the parent, rather than the therapist, so that the family gains confidence in managing the child at home. A child-sized table and rolling and stacking toys should be available. The parent should encourage the child's standing on both feet by first supporting the trunk and then gradually reducing the support. The young child gains prosthetic tolerance and standing balance by being near the table. Initially, the child may lean the torso against the table while manipulating the toys. Eventually, the child will move along the periphery of the table to place objects in the desired location. The table enables the infant to gain prosthetic tolerance, cruise, move to and from to the floor, and play with the toys on the floor and on the table. Playing with toys on the table requires the use of both hands, thus enabling reliance on standing balance. The SACH foot causes the center of standing pressure to be more posterior than is the case with the anatomical foot.[51] Toys should be moved to places on the table where the child has to reach in different directions, shifting weight.

When first learning to walk with a prosthesis, the child moves as if maneuvering on a slippery surface, being rather cautious about balance. Initially, the child takes small steps and has a wide base, keeping the trunk upright and arms abducted. The new prosthetic wearer resembles normal peers who begin walking with increased hip and knee flexion, full-foot initial contact, short stride, increased cadence, and relative foot drop on the sound side in swing phase.[52-56]

At home, a sturdy table that is chest high to the child encourages standing balance and cruising during play with toys placed on the table. Raised sandboxes, blocks, finger paints, and pans of water with floating toys all promote standing balance. A playpen is a good environment to enable the baby to pull to standing, cruise the perimeter, and sit when he or she wishes. Balls are useful in prosthetic training. Kicking the ball requires balance on one leg and flexion of the other leg. The baby starts by holding on to a stable object with both hands, then with one, and eventually letting go. Throwing a ball requires good balance and usually sustains the infant's interest. Wheeled toys, such as a doll carriage, enable the child to walk with the prosthesis with a modicum of support. Independent ambulation is encouraged by placing toys where the child must take a few steps to reach them.

Young children frequently revert to crawling and sitting on the floor as they grow accustomed to the prosthesis. Falling is seldom a problem, inasmuch as the child generally lands on the buttocks as an anatomically normal child would. When the child falls or tries to retrieve a toy on the floor, the parents and therapist should let the child explore the movement and not be overly protective. Just as other children learn to walk by supporting themselves on furniture, the child who wears a prosthesis should have the same experience to develop confidence. Parallel bars, walkers, and harnesses are seldom advisable for children with unilateral amputation or bilateral transtibial amputation, although some fearful children may benefit from their use.[57,58]

Because the prosthesis imposes weight-bearing loads on portions of the leg not ordinarily used for this purpose, gradually building tolerance to prosthetic wear is important so that skin over weight-bearing areas can adjust to the pressure. During the first week most infants tolerate 1 hour of wear, after which the prosthesis should be removed and the skin examined. After a 10- to 15-minute rest period, the prosthesis can be reapplied for another hour. Signs of fatigue, limping, and the avoidance of standing on the prosthesis indicate that the prosthesis is irritating and should be removed. The infant with a transfemoral prosthesis should be checked to determine whether skin near the proximal part of the prosthesis is irritated by urine or feces, which may leak from the diaper.

Toddlers

By 15 months, toddlers are upright and mobile. The heel-toe sequence replaces flat-foot contact during the second year.

Box 31-5 *Prosthetic Training Goals for Toddlers with Lower Limb Deficiency*

Goals of rehabilitation for toddlers with lower limb deficiency include the following:

- Full-time wear of the prosthesis, except for bathing and sleeping
- Use of the prosthesis in age-appropriate ambulatory activities

Parents of toddlers with lower limb prostheses should do the following:

- Encourage use of the prosthesis
- Provide toys and equipment that require age-appropriate activities
- Inspect the skin to determine whether the prosthesis causes undue irritation

Box 31-6 *Goals for School-Aged Children and Adolescents with Lower Limb Deficiency*

In later childhood and adolescence, rehabilitation includes the following:

- Monitoring and maintaining proper prosthetic fit
- Inspecting the skin
- Donning and doffing the prosthesis independently
- Dressing independently
- Engaging in the full range of ambulatory activities with the prosthesis
- Recognizing when the prosthesis needs repair or alteration

Parents of school-aged children and adolescents with lower limb prostheses should do the following:

- Encourage the young person's independence
- Provide opportunities for sports participation

Neurological maturation, changes in physique, and improved strength are evident as the child's base of support narrows and stability improves.[54] Muscular activity has matured into the adult pattern.[55] Goals for rehabilitation (Box 31-5) reflect the developmental activities of a preschool-aged child.

Another developmental milestone expected of all children, including the child with a prosthesis, is running, which is met between 2 and 4 years of age. The flight phase (double float), the period when both feet are off the ground, occurs by strong application of propulsive force during late stance. The prosthetic foot offers much less energy storage and release compared with the gastrocnemius. Consequently, the child with a prosthesis adopts an asymmetric running gait that emphasizes propulsion on the sound side. Two-year-olds can kick a ball accurately, steer a push toy, and jump.[49] As with running, jumping with a prosthesis is primarily an action of the sound side. Games of throwing and catching a ball or beanbag and tossing darts help the toddler refine balance with the prosthesis.

The 3-year-old wearing a transfemoral prosthesis can usually control an articulated knee unit.[15] The child will probably leap, jump, gallop, climb stairs step over step, and ride a tricycle. The youngster with a prosthesis has an easier time if the tricycle pedal has a strap to secure the prosthetic foot. Jumping from a step and hopping are other toddler stunts. Playground equipment, such as a jungle gym, slide, swing, seesaw, sandbox, and tunnels, is enticing. Children with unilateral transtibial amputation achieve an almost normal gait and have no difficulty in climbing inclines and stairs.[24] Opportunities for kneeling, managing various types of chairs, and getting to and from the floor are additional elements in rehabilitation. The child will need help in removing and donning the prosthesis.

School-Aged Children and Adolescents

By 4 years of age, most children can descend stairs step over step, ride a bicycle, and roller skate.[15] Skates that clip on the shoe are preferable to shoe skates; the latter require that the prosthetic foot accommodate the height of the heel in the shoe skate. Five-year-olds skip rope and play dodge ball. Accurate kicking demonstrates balance on one foot while transferring force to the ball.[50] By age 6 years, most children can don and doff the prosthesis independently.[15] They can start, stop, and change direction with ease as well as skip and hop for long distances.[49] The child moves toward independence in prosthetic management as well, taking more responsibility for donning and doffing, skin inspection, and maintenance of the prosthesis (Box 31-6).

Children who undergo lower limb amputation after 5 years may respond favorably to balance and gait training similar to that appropriate for adults. Physical therapy emphasizes balance, weight shifting, control of the prosthetic foot, and, in the case of the child with transfemoral amputation, the knee unit.

CASE EXAMPLE 3

A Child with Traumatic Transfemoral Amputation

P. J., who is 4.5 years old, was riding his bicycle on the street in front of his home at twilight when an automobile turned the corner and struck him. In the police statement, the driver said he did not notice the child. P. J.'s father rushed him to the local hospital, where the boy was admitted to have his leg and thigh wounds debrided and dressed. Despite meticulous care at the hospital, the thigh wound became necrotic. The attending pediatrician arranged a consultation with the surgeon, who advised amputation at the transfemoral level immediately proximal to the femoral condyles. The family consented to the surgery, which proceeded uneventfully.

P. J.'s amputation wound was covered with an Unna dressing and healed rapidly. He is scheduled to come to the prosthetic clinic this morning.

Questions to Consider

- Describe the postoperative program that will enable P. J. to achieve the most rapid rehabilitation.
- What components (foot, shank, knee unit, socket, and suspension) would suit P. J. in his first prosthesis?
- Outline the steps in training P. J. to use his prosthesis.
- In addition to walking on level surfaces, what other activities should the physical therapist include in the initial rehabilitation program?
- How will P. J. resume riding his bicycle?
- What knee unit would suit P. J. when he enters junior high school?

Sports are particularly useful to develop self-esteem as well as strength and coordination.[59,60] Most children with amputations take part in physical education classes at school, sometimes with modified activity.[15] To withstand extremely high stresses, the prosthesis needs carbon acrylic or graphite reinforcement.[3] The child should understand that shoes must always be worn; the plantar surface of most prosthetic feet is not durable enough to withstand abrasion by a sidewalk, and the alignment of the foot is intended for a shoe.

Some activities are more easily performed without a lower limb prosthesis or do not require a prosthesis. Children should learn how to use crutches as an alternate mode of locomotion when the prosthesis is being repaired. Bathing is facilitated either by sitting on the shower floor or by using a sturdy bath seat. Most people prefer to swim and scuba dive without a prosthesis. They hop or use crutches to get from the dressing room to the water's edge. Sports prostheses, such as a swimming prosthesis with a fin in place of the foot, can be constructed. Bicycling, skiing, and mountain climbing are other sports that can be enjoyed with or without a prosthesis.[30]

Rehabilitation of Children with Multiple Limb Amputation

Babies who have anomalies of one or both upper limbs, together with lower limb deficiency, generally do best by being fitted first with simple lower limb prostheses to foster sitting balance. The introduction of upper and lower limb prostheses simultaneously is apt to overwhelm the infant. Upper limb prostheses should be provided after lower limb prostheses.

When both upper limbs are anomalous, a simple bilateral fitting counteracts the tendency toward development of positional scoliosis. The baby with bilateral upper limb deficiency should receive prostheses after independent walking is established; otherwise, prostheses make it more difficult to crawl, move about on the floor, and pull to standing with the chin for support. Those with bilateral upper limb deficiency become quite skillful with foot prehension.[61] The extent to which foot use should be encouraged is controversial. Foot prehension is so rarely observed in public that the child may experience unwanted stares. Nevertheless, feet have the tactile sensation and considerable dexterity that prostheses lack. Children with bilateral longitudinal deficiencies have partial or complete hands; they would be encumbered by wearing prostheses. Functional activities with and without prostheses should be introduced according to the physical and emotional maturity of the child. Adaptive aids may be required for some functions, such as personal hygiene.[62]

Infants with trimembral or quadrimembral limb deficiency move about by rolling along the floor. They need opportunities to look at objects and manipulate toys with their mouths and their residual limbs. Most infants develop good sitting balance and can scoot along on their buttocks. Because of the drastic reduction in body surface, these children can easily become overheated. They should be dressed very lightly to enable heat dissipation.

Toddlers with bilateral transfemoral limb deficiency may be initially fit with prostheses without knee units (Figure 31-11). Children with bilateral transfemoral amputations may require manually locking knees until they are 6 years or older.[3] They progress more rapidly after practice in the parallel bars if they have a pair of forearm or axillary crutches. Depending on the length of the residual limbs, children may

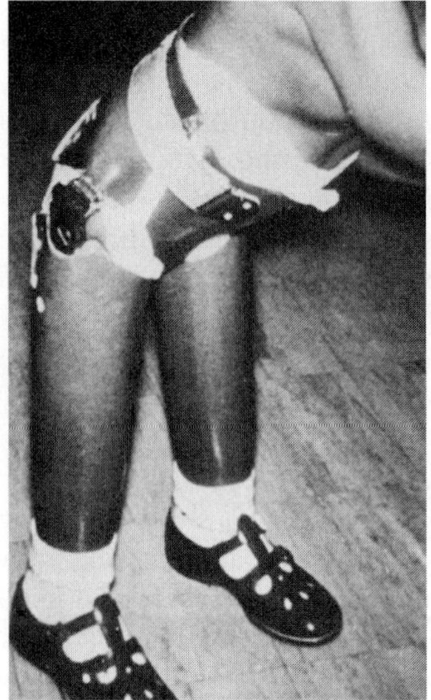

Figure 31-11
An infant or toddler with bilateral transverse transfemoral limb deficiency who is ready to pull to stand and cruise may be initially fit with prosthesis without knee units. (Courtesy J. E. Edelstein.)

eventually feel comfortable with a pair of forearm crutches or canes. Young children with bilateral transfemoral deficiency may walk indoors without any assistive devices; however, few are willing to venture outdoors and across streets without at least one cane. In adolescence, many find that a wheelchair provides more efficient mobility.

SUMMARY

Rehabilitation of children with limb deficiencies can be quite gratifying. The physical therapist, together with all members of the clinical team, should design the rehabilitation program to assist the child in achieving developmental milestones associated with maturing upper and lower limb function. Psychosocial factors govern the behavior of the child and family; team members need to recognize the basis for parental distress yet foster realistic expectations for the child's function while demonstrating that the child is lovable regardless of the condition of the limbs. Peer support is a helpful way of facilitating constructive response to the child.

REFERENCES

1. Stanger M. Limb deficiencies and amputations. In Campbell SK, Vander Linden DW, Palisano RJ (eds), *Physical Therapy for Children,* 2nd ed. Philadelphia: Saunders, 2000. pp. 370-397.
2. Day HJB. The ISO/ISPO classification of congenital limb deficiency. In Bowker JH, Michael JW (eds), *Atlas of Limb Prosthetics: Surgical, Prosthetic, and Rehabilitation Principles*, 2nd ed. St. Louis: Mosby-Year Book, 1992. pp. 743-760.
3. Dillingham TR, Pezzin LE, MacKenzie EJ. Limb amputation and limb deficiency: epidemiology and recent trends in the United States. *South Med J* 2002;95:875-883.
4. Rijnders LJ, Boonstra AM, Groothoff JW, et al. Lower limb deficient children in The Netherlands: epidemiological aspects. *Prosthet Orthot Int* 2000;24:13-18.
5. Jain S, Lakhtakia PK. Profile of congenital transverse deficiencies among cases of congenital orthopaedic anomalies. *J Orthop Surg (Hong Kong)* 2002;10:45-52.
6. McGuirk CK, Westgate MN, Holmes LB. Limb deficiencies in newborn infants. *Pediatrics* 2001;108:E64.
7. Nagarajan R, Neglia JP, Clohisy DR, et al. Education, employment, insurance, and marital status among 694 survivors of pediatric lower extremity bone tumors: a report from the Childhood Cancer Survivor Study. *Cancer* 2003;97:2554-2564.
8. Refaat Y, Gunnoe J, Hornicek FJ, et al. Comparison of quality of life after amputation or limb salvage. *Clin Orthop* 2002;397:298-305.
9. Nagarajan R, Neglia JP, Clohisy DR, et al. Limb salvage and amputation in survivors of pediatric lower extremity bone tumors: what are the long-term implications? *J Clin Oncol* 2002;20:4493-4501.
10. Blakeslee B (ed). *The Limb-Deficient Child.* Berkeley, CA: University of California, 1963.
11. Fixsen JA. Major lower limb congenital shortening: a mini review. *J Pediatr Orthop* 2003;12:1-12.
12. Cummings DR, Kapp SL. Lower-limb pediatric prosthetics: general considerations and philosophy. *J Prosthet Orthot* 1992;4(4):196-206.
13. Fishman S, Edelstein J, Krebs D. ISNY above-knee prosthetic sockets: pediatric experience. *J Pediatr Orthop* 1987;Oct(5): 557-562.
14. Fishman S, Berger N, Edelstein J. ISNY flexible sockets for upper-limb amputees. *J Assoc Child Prosthet Orthot Clin* 1989;24:8-11.
15. Boonstra AM, Rijnders LJ, Groothoff JW, et al. Children with congenital deficiencies or acquired amputations of the lower limbs: functional aspects. *Prosthet Orthot Int* 2000;24:19-27.
16. Setoguchi Y, Rosenfelder R. *The Limb-Deficient Child.* Springfield, IL: Thomas, 1982.
17. Krane EJ, Heller LB. The prevalence of phantom sensation and pain in pediatric amputees. *J Pain Symptom Mgt* 1995; 10(1):21-29.
18. Melzack R, Israel R, Lacroix R, et al. Phantom limbs in people with congenital limb deficiency or amputation in early childhood. *Brain* 1997;120:1603-1620.
19. Wilkins KL, McGrath PJ, Finley GA, et al. Phantom limb sensations and phantom limb pain in child and adolescent amputees. *Pain* 1998;78:7-12.
20. McGrath PA, Hillier LM. Phantom limb sensations in adolescents: a case study to illustrate the utility of sensation and pain logs in pediatric clinical practice. *J Pain Symptom Mgt* 1992;7(1):46-53.
21. Erikson EH. *Identity, Youth and Crisis.* New York: Norton, 1968.
22. Novotny M, Swagman A. Caring for children with orthotic/ prosthetic needs. *J Prosthet Orthot* 1992;4(4):191-195.
23. Challenor YB. Limb deficiencies in children. In Molnar GE (ed), *Pediatric Rehabilitation.* Baltimore: Williams & Wilkins, 1985. pp. 400-424.
24. Marquardt EG. A holistic approach to rehabilitation for the limb-deficient child. *Arch Phys Med Rehabil* 1983;64(6): 237-242.
25. Patton JG. Training the child with a unilateral upper-extremity prosthesis. In Atkins DJ, Meier RH (eds), *Functional Restoration of Adults and Children with Upper Extremity Amputation.* New York: Demos, 2004. pp. 297-316.
26. Letts M, Stevens L, Coleman J, et al. Puppetry and doll play as an adjunct to pediatric orthopedics. *J Pediatr Orthop* 1983;3(5):605-609.
26. Svoboda J. Psychosocial considerations in pediatrics: use of amputee dolls. *J Prosthet Orthot* 1992;4(4):207-212.
28. Varni JW, Setoguchi Y. Psychosocial factors in the management of children with limb deficiencies. *Phys Med Rehabil Clin North Am* 1991;2:395-404.
29. Boren HA. Adolescent adjustment to amputation necessitated by bone cancer. *Orthop Nurs* 1985;4(5):30-32.
30. Edelstein JE. Rehabilitation without prostheses. In Smith DG, Michael JW. Bowker JH (eds), *Atlas of Amputations and Limb Deficiencies*, 3rd ed. Rosemont, Ill: American Academy of Orthopaedic Surgeons, 2004. pp. 745-756.
31. Kuyper MA, Breedijk M, Mulders AH, et al. Prosthetic management of children in The Netherlands with upper limb deficiencies. *Prosthet Orthot Int* 2001;25:228-234.
32. Cech D, Martin S. *Functional Movement Development across the Life Span,* 2nd ed. Philadelphia: Saunders, 2001.

33. Postema K, van der Donk V, van Limbeek J, et al. Prosthesis rejection in children with a unilateral congenital arm defect. *Clin Rehabil* 1999;13:243-249.
34. Jain S. Rehabilitation in limb deficiency. 2: The pediatric amputee. *Arch Phys Med Rehabil* 1996;77(3 suppl):S9-S13.
35. Krebs D (ed). *Prehension Assessment: Prosthetic Therapy for the Upper-Limb Child Amputee.* Thorofare, NJ: Slack, 1987.
36. Krebs DE, Edelstein JE, Thornby MA. Prosthetic management children with limb deficiencies. *Phys Ther* 1991;71(12): 920-934.
37. Weiss-Lambrou R. *A Manual for the Congenital Unilateral Below-Elbow Child Amputee.* Rockville, MD: American Occupational Therapy Association, 1981.
38. Sorbye R. Myoelectric prosthetic fitting in young children. *Clin Orthop* 1980;May(148):34-40.
39. Glynn MK, Galway HR, Hunter G, et al. Management of the upper-limb–deficient child with a powered prosthetic device. *Clin Orthop* 1986;Aug(209):202-207.
40. Trost FJ. A comparison of conventional and myoelectric below-elbow prosthetic use. *Int Clin Information Bull* 1983;18:9-16.
41. Weaver SA, Lange LR, Vogts VM. Comparison of myoelectric and conventional prostheses for adolescent amputees. *Am J Occup Ther* 1988;42(2):87-91.
42. Edelstein JE, Berger N. Performance comparison among children fitted with myoelectric and body-powered hands. *Arch Phys Med Rehabil* 1993;74(4):376-380.
43. Thornby MA, Krebs DE. Bimanual skill development in pediatric below-elbow amputation: a multicenter, cross-sectional study. *Arch Phys Med Rehabil* 1992;73(8):697-702.
44. Edelstein J. Musical options for upper-limb amputees. In Lee M (ed), *Rehabilitation Music and Human Well-Being.* St. Louis: MMB Music, 1989.
45. Fernandez A, Lopez MJ, Navarro R. Performance of persons with juvenile-onset amputation in driving motor vehicles. *Arch Phys Med Rehabil* 2000;81:288-291.
46. Wright FV, Hubbard S, Naumann S, et al. Evaluation of the validity of the prosthetic upper extremity functional index for children. *Arch Phys Med Rehabil* 2003;84:518-527.
47. Crandall RC, Tomhave W. Pediatric unilateral below-elbow amputees: retrospective analysis of 34 patients given multiple prosthetic options. *J Pediatr Orthop* 2002;22:380-383.
48. Routhier F, Vincent C, Morissette MJ, et al. Clinical results of an investigation of paediatric upper limb myoelectric prosthesis fitting at the Quebec Rehabilitation Institute. *Prosthet Orthot Int* 2001;25:119-131.
49. Campbell SK. Understanding motor performance in children. In Campbell SK, Vander Linden DW, Palisano RJ (eds). *Physical Therapy for Children,* 2nd ed. Philadelphia: Saunders, 2000. pp. 3-45.
50. Tecklin JS (ed). *Pediatric Physical Therapy,* 3rd ed. Philadelphia: J.B. Lippincott, 1998.
51. Clark LA, Zernicke RF. Balance in lower limb child amputees. *Prosthet Orthot Int* 1981;5(1):11-18.
52. Higgins S, Higgins JR. The emergence of gait. In Craik RL, Oatis CA (eds), *Gait Analysis: Theory and Application.* St. Louis: Mosby, 1995. pp. 15-24.
53. Leonard EL. Early motor development and control: foundations for independent walking. In Smidt GL (ed), *Gait in Rehabilitation.* New York: Churchill Livingstone, 1990. pp. 121-140.
54. Stout JL. Gait: development and analysis. In Campbell SK (ed), *Physical Therapy for Children.* Philadelphia: Saunders, 1994. pp. 79-104.
55. Sutherland DH. *Gait Disorders in Childhood and Adolescence.* Baltimore: Williams & Wilkins, 1984.
56. Woollacott M, Shumway-Cook A (eds). *Development of Posture and Gait across the Life Span.* Columbia, SC: University of South Carolina, 1989.
57. Kitabayashi B. The physical therapist's responsibility to the lower extremity child amputee. *Phys Ther Rev* 1961; 41:722-727.
58. Radford J, Steensma J. The lower extremity toddler amputee: training procedures. *Phys Ther Rev* 1957;37:32-41.
59. Burgess EM, Rappopoort A. *Physical Fitness: A Guide for Individuals with Lower Limb Loss.* Baltimore: Department of Veterans Affairs, 1992.
60. Kegel B. Physical fitness: Sports and recreation for those with lower limb amputation or impairment. *Journal of Rehabilitation Research and Development Clinical Supplement no. 1.* Washington, DC: Department of Veterans Affairs, 1985.
61. Stoeker W. Foot skills and other alternatives to hand use. In Meier RH, Atkins DJ (eds). *Functional Restoration of Adults and Children with Upper Extremity Amputation.* New York: Demos, 2004. pp. 133-134.
62. Friedmann L. Functional skills training in multiple limb anomalies. In Atkins DJ, Meier RH (eds), *Comprehensive Management of the Upper-Limb Amputee.* New York: Springer-Verlag, 1988. pp. 150-164.

32

Prosthetic Options for Persons with Upper Extremity Amputation

JOHN R. ZENIE

LEARNING OBJECTIVES

On completion of this chapter, the reader will be able to do the following:

1. Compare and contrast prosthetic needs and expected functional outcomes for individuals with upper extremity amputations at various levels.
2. Compare and contrast the fitting and control issues for individuals with various etiologies of amputations and residual limb lengths.
3. Describe the factors that determine recommendations for prosthetic options (no prosthesis, passive prosthesis, body-powered prosthesis, externally powered systems, or hybrid prosthetic systems).
4. Compare and contrast options for donning and suspension of a prosthesis for individuals with upper extremity amputations of various levels.
5. Describe the biomechanical principles of transradial and transhumeral body-powered prosthetic control systems and the movement strategies necessary for control of electric terminal devices (TDs), elbow units, and other prosthetic components.
6. Explain the basic principles of myoelectric control, including determining electrode placement and the types of muscle contractions used to operate or switch among TDs, electric elbow units, and other electric prosthetic components.

IMPACT OF TECHNOLOGY

Prosthetic management of individuals with upper extremity amputations presents all allied health professionals, including prosthetists, with a set of unique challenges. For those wearing an upper extremity limb, the TD of the prosthesis is not covered or obscured by clothing in the same way that a lower extremity prosthesis is "hidden" by pants, socks, and shoes. By the virtue of its level, the person with upper extremity amputation must cope with not only physical appearance changes, but the loss of some of the most complex movement patterns and functional activities of the human body.

In addition, limb deficiency in the upper extremity deprives the patient of an extensive and valuable system of tactile and proprioceptive inputs that previously provided "feedback" to guide and refine functional movement.[1,2] Even the simplest tasks related to grasp and release become challenging. The ability to position prosthetic limb segments in space, as well as the ability to maintain advantageous postures needed to manipulate objects, challenge the medical community to continuously improve the functional and aesthetic outcomes of prosthetic replacement for patients in this population.[3-5]

Many of these challenges have been addressed with new and emerging technologies. These new technologies have made it possible, in some circumstances, to successfully "fit" a patient with high-level amputation who previously would have little or no reasonable expectation to succeed with traditional technology and fitting techniques.[2,6,7] Advanced socket interface designs and material science have afforded prosthetists the ability to offer stronger, more stable platforms for all levels of amputation, while in most cases saving substantial amounts of weight. Similarly, more innovative suspension strategies and interface mediums have increased the functional ranges of motion a patient can comfortably achieve.[8]

These advancements have had a profound and positive effect on the comfort, function, and compliance of both conventional body-powered and externally powered prosthesis at all levels of amputation. Further, the huge strides made in the externally powered arena have in large part been driven by these advancements and technological breakthroughs.

Length of the Residual Limb

Amputations to the upper extremity can be classified or named by the limb segments affected (Figure 32-1). The most distal are at the *partial hand* or *transcarpal* levels. Amputations that separate the carpal bones from the radius and ulna are referred to as *wrist disarticulations.* Amputations that occur within the substance of the radius and ulna are classified as *transradial* amputations. When the humerus is preserved but the radius and ulna are removed, the amputation is referred to as an *elbow disarticulation.* Those that leave more than 30% of humeral length are designated as *transhumeral* amputations. *Shoulder disarticulations* are those in which less than 30% of the proximal humerus remains. More proximal amputations that invade the central body cavity, resecting the clavicle and leading to derangement of the scapula, are described as forequarter amputations. In clinical prosthetic and rehabilitation practices, transradial and transhumeral amputations account for nearly 80% of all upper extremity amputations.[6]

All patients who have amputations of the upper extremity require a complete and thorough evaluation not only at the level of involvement but also of associated functional and physiological deficits associated with that specific amputation. For patients with partial hand amputations, the range of motion (ROM) of any remaining digits and the condition of the structural bones of the hand have a profound effect on the selection of possible prosthetic options. The inclusion or absence of an intact thumb also dictates the parameters of fitting.

For those with transverse amputations of the forearm, the length of the residual limb affects the amount of functional elbow flexion and forearm pronation and supination that will be retained independent of prosthetic intervention.[1] Articulations between the radius and the ulna along the entire forearm are necessary to provide for natural anatomical movements in supination and pronation; as the level of amputation moves proximally from the styloid process of the radius toward the elbow, the ability to perform and to use pronation and supination during functional activities is progressively lost (Figure 32-2). When the residual forearm is extremely short, all transverse motion is essentially lost, and it is difficult to gain any active functional forearm rotation for prosthetic use.

Amputations at the level of the elbow (elbow disarticulation) derive little functional benefit from the added length because the length of the limb limits options for cosmetic and functional placement of elbow units within the prosthesis, without substantially improving functional leverage.

Although the primary concern of surgeons who perform an upper extremity amputation is adequate closure of the wound, they must also consider the potential advantages of a fairly long lever arm, balanced by an understanding of the space requirements for prosthetic components. Provided that adequate skin and tissue viability are not compromised, consideration should be given to adequate room for a full array of prosthetic componentry.

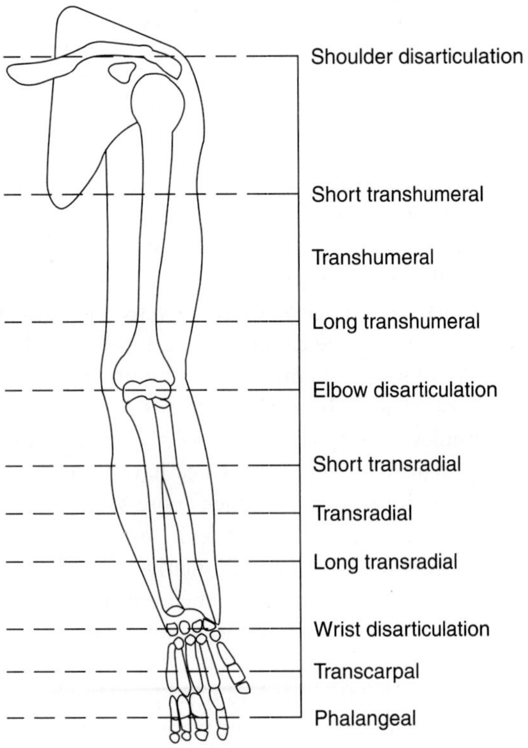

Shoulder disarticulation
Short transhumeral
Transhumeral
Long transhumeral
Elbow disarticulation
Short transradial
Transradial
Long transradial
Wrist disarticulation
Transcarpal
Phalangeal

Figure 32-1

Classification of upper extremity amputation and residual limbs. (From Murdoch G, Wilson AB. Amputation: Surgical Practice and Patient Management. *Oxford, UK: Butterworth, 1996. p. 308.)*

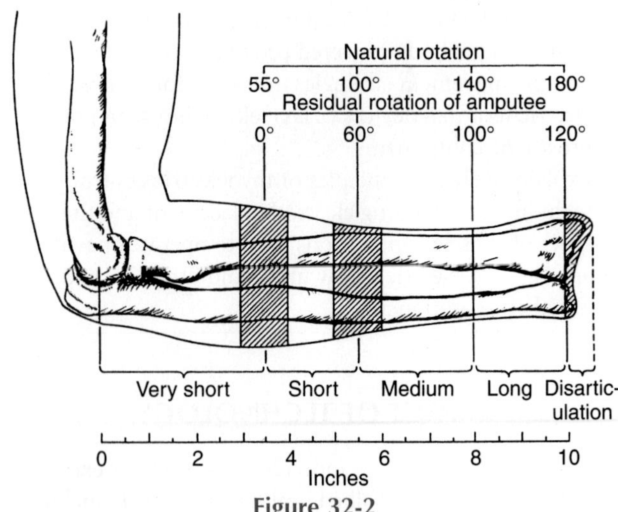

Figure 32-2

Potential for pronation and supination of transradial residual limbs of differing lengths. (From Taylor CI. The biomechanics of control in upper extremity prosthetics. Orthot Prosthet *1981;35:20.)*

Upper Extremity Prosthetic Component

Prosthetic components can be thought of as a means to replace lost functional capacity associated with the anatomical loss of limb segments. A TD is employed to replace grasp and release. An elbow mechanism is used to replace the humeral-ulnar articulation; a shoulder mechanism is placed proximally to provide humeral orientation in space at the shoulder disarticulation and scapulothoracic amputation levels. Rotators can be placed in the forearm of the prosthesis to substitute for pronation and supination or above the elbow unit to substitute for internal and external rotation of the shoulder as well.[9,10]

Partial Hand, Transcarpal, and Wrist Disarticulation

Until recently, patients with digit, partial hand, or transcarpal amputations were often offered passive (nonfunctioning) cosmetic prostheses (restorations).[11] Depending on the characteristics of the residual limb, a functional prehensile post might have been fabricated to regain some grasp and release capability of the affected limb. Recent advances in technology and microprocessors have made externally powered options more readily available (Figure 32-3).[12] These advances permit electric control despite the extremely distal amputation site.

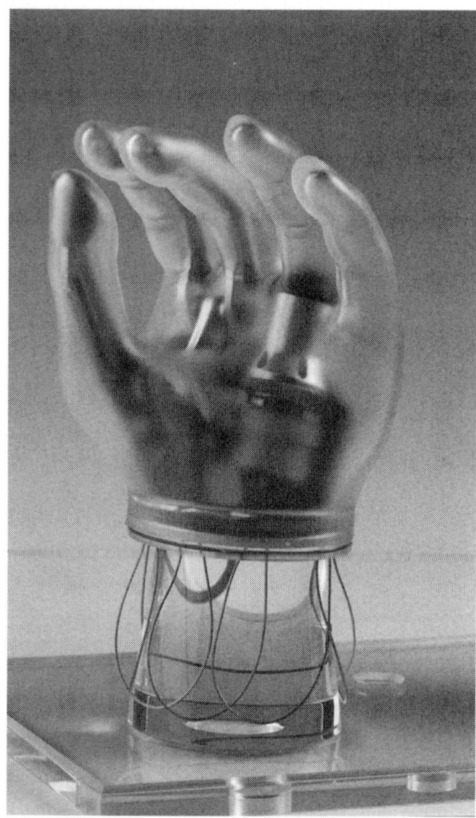

Figure 32-3
Example of an externally powered prosthetic hand used for individuals with a partial hand amputation or wrist disarticulation.

Consideration must be given preoperatively to any remaining functional digits. The status of sensation and mobility of these digits should not be understated. If functional range and sensation are inadequate, the surgeon considers a more proximal level of amputation.

The wrist disarticulation residual limb provides a long and functional lever for prosthetic use.[13] If the radial and ulnar styloid processes are preserved, then the prosthetist can use a positive suspension strategy over these prominences to keep the prosthesis stable suspended on the residual limb, making harnesses unnecessary. The disadvantage of wrist disarticulation, however, is limitation in room to fit a wrist and hand unit into a cosmetically acceptable prosthesis. If the styloid processes have been modified or removed during surgery, more aggressive proximal suspension strategies are necessary. In addition, the extra residual limb length leads to a difference in arm length once the wrist and prosthetic hand unit is in place, which might be cosmetically unacceptable to the patient. In such cases a more proximal amputation would allow for a full complement of prosthetic options.

Transradial and Transhumeral Considerations

For most adult transradial prostheses, nearly 8 inches of space is necessary beyond the distal residual limb for the prosthetic wrist rotator and TD or hand.[13] Similarly, at the transhumeral level, approximately 6 inches of space must be present beyond the distal residual limb to accommodate a mechanical elbow mechanism within the prosthesis.[14] For patients with a short residual humerus, a conventional (body-powered) prosthetic system may not be realistic, and even an externally powered prosthesis may be difficult or problematic to fit, suspend, and control. When the residual humerus is short, it may be necessary to treat a transhumeral amputation functionally as a shoulder disarticulation (Figure 32-4).

Positive models to fabricate any contemporary prosthesis can be secured with conventional plaster direct molding

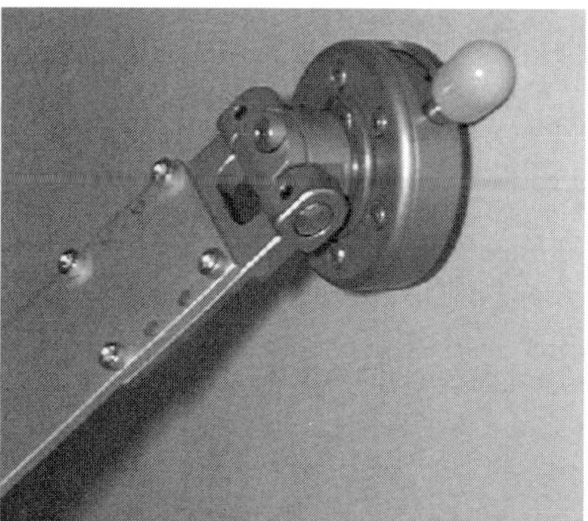

Figure 32-4
Example of a prosthetic shoulder joint used in individuals with a shoulder disarticulation or extremely short transhumeral residual limb.

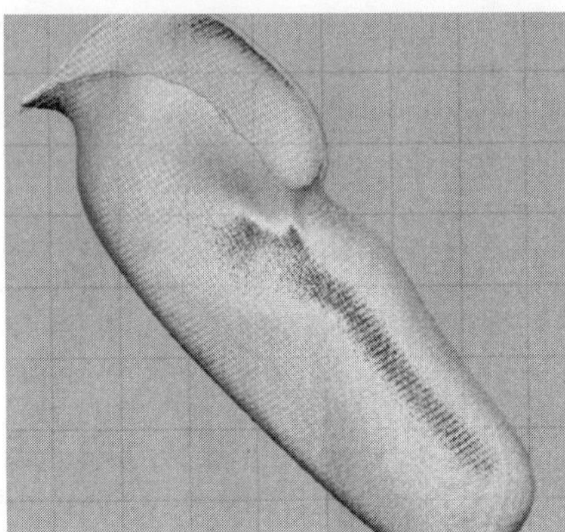

Figure 32-5

A computer-assisted design model of a transradial prosthetic socket. Note the aggressive anatomical contouring of the socket and the anteroposterior force system (between the anterior cubital fossa and olecranon) that will be used to suspend the socket on the residual limb. (Courtesy Advanced Arm Dynamics, Branford, Conn.)

techniques similar to those used for lower extremity amputations. Model acquisition and data collection are also possible using computer-aided design. Both direct contact and optical methods are finding ever-increasing utility in modern practice. This technology is particularly valuable as a means to quantify and document volume and shape changes, enhancing fit and function for optimal clinical outcomes (Figure 32-5).

ETIOLOGY OF UPPER EXTREMITY AMPUTATION

The etiology of upper extremity amputations varies widely. The earliest recorded use of limb prosthesis was that of a soldier who reportedly amputated his own limb around 484 BC.[16] One of the earliest known prostheses was fabricated of copper around 300 BC.[17] These early attempts at prosthetic management predate early surgical considerations for life-saving reasons by many decades. Ambrose Pare, whom many consider the father of modern orthopedic surgery, introduced early surgical techniques around 1529.[18] Public belief is that Pare performed the earliest UE amputation, an elbow disarticulation, late in 1536. The incidence and prevalence of UE amputation over the past several centuries is attributed to advances in the pharmacological and surgical management of disease, as well as trauma.[19] Upper extremity trauma related to industry, mechanized farming, and armed conflict has been the catalyst for medical and prosthetic advancements in the twentieth century.[6]

Of the approximately 54 million persons in the United States with disabilities, at least 10% have had amputations.[21] Although the exact number of patients with amputations is unknown, the number of patients with acquired and congenital amputations is significant. Of all persons with amputations, the number of patients with amputations to the upper extremity is small in comparison to all total amputations.[21] Compelling evidence suggests an estimated 10,000 new amputations to the upper extremity each year.[22] These numbers represent a large number of individuals who require prosthetic intervention.

The primary cause of acquired amputations is trauma.[6] Other causes of upper extremity amputation are the various sarcomas, as well as congenital limb deformities including amelias and phocomelias.[23-25] Amputations to address congenital limb deficiencies are most often performed on individuals younger than 15 years old, while amputation after traumatic injury is most often performed on those between 15 and 45 years old.[26] Seventy percent of all upper extremity amputations occur in persons younger than 64 years of age.[6,26] Because trauma is more likely to occur in the operation of machinery or in combat, many more amputations occur among males than females.[26]

PREPROSTHETIC CARE

All patients with upper extremity amputation, regardless of cause, require some degree of preprosthetic management. This is particularly essential with a recent amputation but includes even those persons who have worn prosthetic devices previously. Comprehensive preprosthetic and prosthetic management is a strong predictor of optimal rehabilitation outcomes.[27,28] After amputation surgery, facilitation of wound healing and effective pain management are the foundations for all other types of preprosthetic care. Care is most effective if coordinated through a multidisciplinary team—the prosthetist, surgeon, nurses, physical and occupational therapists, counselors, and others as necessary.[7]

Edema and Volume Control

Edema and volume control are additional key elements of preprosthetic care. If the wound site is adequately protected and bandaged, compressive wraps or shrinkers should be used as soon as possible. In most cases multidirectional shrinker garments are more effective than other methods, including elastic bandages.[29] Shrinkers appear to more efficiently control volume and shape the residual limb. When donned properly, shrinkers have far less tendency to migrate or shift position on the residual limb. In addition, shrinkers are more effective at creating the consistent distal toward proximal pressure gradient that is most effective. The compressive garment should terminate proximal to the joint above the amputation site when possible. With the transhumeral amputation, this requires the shrinker to include a modified shoulder cap. Such a device is rarely commercially available and usually requires custom fabrication on site. This additional effort has been shown to produce favorable results in comparison with shrinkers that terminate more distally.[28] Due diligence must be exercised to ensure that appropriate tension and compression gradients are achieved and maintained. Effective and timely volume management not only influences the residual limb volume and shape; many patients report that this compression is a surprisingly efficient tool in the management of phantom sensation.[29]

Skin Care, Desensitization, and Range of Motion

The services of a skilled therapist have proven invaluable in the areas of skin care, desensitization, and scar mobilization. Preprosthetic ROM and strengthening should be undertaken concurrently as tolerated. More information about preprosthetic care is found in Chapter 34.

Skin care can present some significant challenges, particularly when an individual has sustained a traumatic amputation. Chemical and electrical injuries with associated skin grafts can become problematic, particularly when irregular and uneven surface topography is present.[30] Maintaining skin integrity throughout both the fitting and postdelivery phase of rehabilitation is extremely important. The appropriate medical professional should carefully assess any postoperative open lesions. Blast and percussion injuries also present a complex array of socket interface and electrical conductivity issues.[31] This type of injury frequently displays an unusual soft tissue consistency. The tissue is unlike that of crushing, degloving (guatine) injuries. Tissues exposed to the enormous energy associated with blast injuries frequently respond to the outside compressive forces of shrinkers and preparatory sockets much more dramatically than do tissues injured by other sources. This phenomenon must be considered carefully, as its effects profoundly affect any rehabilitation plan.

The nature of any volume management protocol in and of itself begins the limb maturation and desensitization process simultaneously. Further and more focused efforts must be undertaken to assure that limb volume is both stabilizing and fostering a limb shape or contour that is favorable to donning, wearing, and operating a prosthetic device.[30] Limbs with large longitudinal contours or bulbous distal contours are least desirable. Residuum with insignificant tissue or skin coverage should also be avoided whenever possible. Ideally the residual limb is long enough to provide a functional lever arm but not so long as to preclude the use of a wide array of prosthetic components. Residual limbs with effective myodesis frequently display smaller myoelectric artifact without any apparent or material loss of volitional potential.

Preprosthetic ROM should be maximized regardless of the planned prosthetic intervention. Strengthening of the muscles about and proximal to the amputation is paramount. However, a more global approach to strengthening affords the patient a more expeditious and complete rehabilitation. These efforts to maximize ROM and increase volitional power should not overlook the secondary movers or accessory stabilizers. For patients with transradial amputations, for example, maximizing ROM and strength of pronation and supination is an important determinant of positive functional outcomes.

Adaptation Process

Patients and families facing amputation, whether congenital or acquired, adjust and cope with absence or loss of the limb differently.[32] The extent or level of involvement often has little to do with the complexity of the adaptation process. All persons must find ways to deal with the functional and aesthetic issues related to limb loss. Adaptation is an ongoing process rather than a specific event. In many cases the services of a qualified psychotherapist are valuable, providing the patient and caregivers are amenable to such intervention.

Most professionals agree that there is a fairly short window of opportunity within which the prospects for successful rehabilitation are greatest, although there is disagreement about the duration of this "optimal rehabilitation" period. In most circumstances the earlier a patient can be evaluated, fitted, and trained, the more likely a positive rehabilitation outcome occurs.[6] Malone and colleagues[27] suggest high levels of success with patients fit within the first 30 days following amputation. In addition, individuals fit with a prosthesis as early as possible return to work quickly, many within 4 months of injury.[6,27]

PROSTHETIC EVALUATION

Evaluation of all upper extremity amputations should include a complete documentation of the involved limb's ROM. Care should be exercised to identify both the active and passive ranges. Volitional muscle control should be evaluated and documented. Limb shape and contour, as well as tissue consistency, are important elements in the evaluation. Particular attention must be paid to any grafts, scars, or painful areas of the residuum. Pertinent medical history must be duly noted, as it may affect not only prosthetic development but all phases of the rehabilitation protocol.

This history must adequately address any injuries or pathoses on both sides of the body. For patients with high-level amputations, the prosthesis, regardless of configuration or power source, ultimately has some integrated components across one or both of the axilla, as well as the thoracic wall.

The objective of all prosthetic intervention should be to restore as much functional potential as possible.[33] This is best accomplished by using components, materials, and interface designs to most closely approximate the lost body segments and functions. The appropriateness of any design should address the patient's vocational, recreational, and aesthetic needs. The needs of most patients can be met with one or more prosthetic options.

PROSTHETIC OPTIONS

Depending on the patient's situation, the prosthetist and rehabilitation team can make a number of recommendations. These include not providing a prosthesis, providing a passive prosthesis or cosmetic restoration, designing a conventional body-powered system, or providing a sophisticated myoelectrically controlled prosthetic limb with multiple components.

No Prosthesis

A significant percentage of patients with upper extremity amputation elect not to use a prosthesis on a regular basis.[6] In many cases this decision can be traced to a poorly conceived or executed prosthetic device that was provided early in the patient rehabilitation process.[27] Some potential wearers report that the devices they have been exposed to are uncomfortable, heavy, and too slow during use or difficult to don and suspend.[6] The advent of advanced materials has enabled prosthetists to build lighter, stronger, and more comfortable systems, as well as extremely cosmetic restorations. Despite these advancements, not all individuals with amputations integrate a prosthesis into their body image. The prosthetist or rehabilitation team should follow patients who choose not to a prosthesis at regular intervals (often yearly) to ensure that their functional needs are being met. Given the rate of technological development, new components or devices are likely to become available to address problems the patient might have had at an earlier time.

Passive Prostheses and Restorations

This category of prosthesis consists of systems that do not possess the ability to actively position a mechanical elbow in space or actively provide grasp and release function, or both. The absence of these properties does not, however, render the prosthesis as passive as the name would suggest. These devices are extremely functional in terms of supporting objects or stabilizing items during bimanual tasks and activities, especially for young children with congenital deficiencies.[34,35] These systems most frequently have a self-suspending design and use a realistic hand as a TD. Suspension is achieved either with specific socket interface geometry or suction negative pressure. The absence of operational mechanical components generally results in fairly lightweight prostheses.

The finish of these devices varies widely. Production latex cosmetic gloves provide an extremely cost-effective medium for many patients. Many individuals, however, seek out more realistic restorations (Figure 32-6). These restorations require substantially greater investments in time and financial resources. This investment is most often rewarded with an extremely aesthetic, nearly imperceptible device. Silicone is the medium of choice for these cosmetic limbs, primarily because it is practically impervious to outside contaminants. Where latex readily stains and deteriorates in ultraviolet light, silicone does not mark and, for all practical purposes, is inert. Generally, the additional cost of silicone is mitigated by its superior cosmesis, durability, and increased coefficient of friction.

Conventional Body-Powered Systems

Conventional (body-powered) systems include any prosthesis that uses a control cable system to translate volitional muscle force and shoulder or arm movement to operate a TD or prosthetic elbow.[36] The patient must use specific strategies in order to effectively create enough excursion in the cable to control the TD or preposition the forearm in space. In

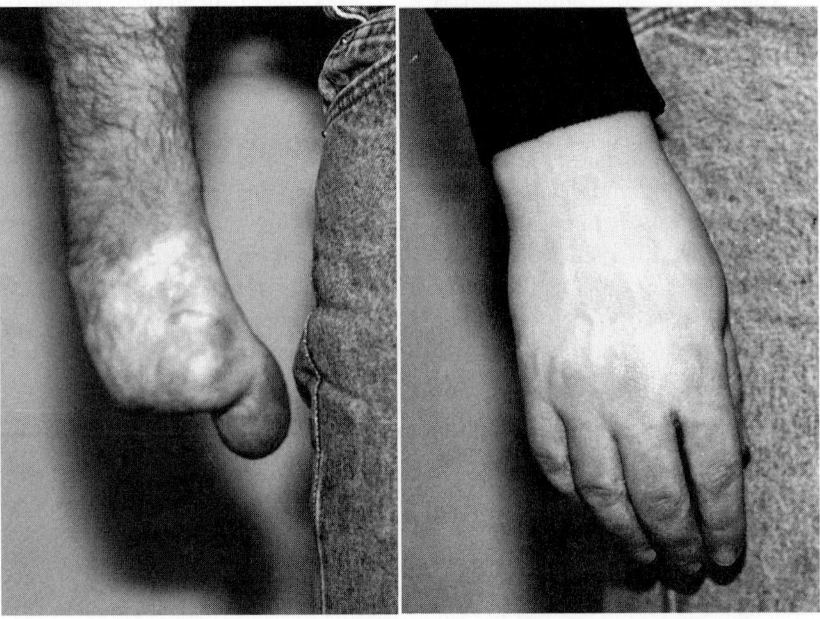

Figure 32-6
Example of a custom silicone passive prosthesis over a transcarpal (partial hand) residual limb. (Courtesy Michael Curtain.)

most instances the glenohumeral joint contributes the largest amount of excursion in conventional prosthetic control. Glenohumeral flexion typically has more than ample excursion and satisfactory power to provide useful motors for this type of control. Additional excursion can be achieved through scapular and biscapular abduction (scapular protraction). These secondary movements allow a well-trained and skilled prosthetic wearer to increase the functional *work envelope,* the space in which the wearer can effectively control the TD.

For most conventional upper extremity prostheses, the functional envelope is limited to a relatively small area below the shoulders, above the waist, and not far outward past shoulder width.[36] Many prosthetic wearers have significant difficulty with tasks that involve grasp-and-release tasks above the head or down near the feet. Because the control strategy involves generating cable excursion through flexion or protraction, or both, tasks and activities occurring behind the back are impossible. Despite these functional limitations, conventional prostheses have provided many patients with reliable and durable prosthetic systems.

Figure-of-Eight Suspension and Control Cable

The foundation of all conventional body-powered prostheses is a harnessing system that provides both a firm anchor for the control cables and, in many cases, a stable means of suspension. Most conventional systems use a figure-of-eight–style harness (Figure 32-7). The terminal ends of the figure-of-eight are formed by means of an axillary loop that is fit over the opposite shoulder, a control attachment cable, and an anterior suspension component on the amputated side. Most prosthetists recommend that the center of the figure-of-eight be positioned just below the seventh cervical vertebra and slightly toward the sound side.[36] The straps of the two axillary loops can be mobile by means of attachment to a circular ring or fixed with a sewn cross point. The use of a center ring often makes the donning process less difficult and appears to provide the most satisfactory ROM. Harnessing materials are most frequently constructed of medium weight Dacron webbing with both leather and plastic integrated components.

Cable Control for Self-Suspending Sockets

If the prosthetist recommends a self-suspending socket, the anterior suspension of a figure-of-eight harness is not necessary. In these instances a figure-of-nine harness, consisting mainly of the contralateral axillary loop, is used to minimize cumbersome harnessing while still maximizing a firm anchor for the control cable. Self-suspending sockets may be of an anatomically contoured design or that of a flexible silicone interface, with either a locking or suction valve mechanism.

Control and Suspension for Bilateral Prostheses

For patients with amputation of both upper extremities, careful clinical consideration must be given to achieving an easily donable and highly functional prosthetic system. Instead of using a traditional figure-of-eight harness with a contralateral axillary loop for each prosthesis, the two anterior suspension components are linked.[37] In this arrangement, the bilateral prosthetic system is effectively stabilized by the

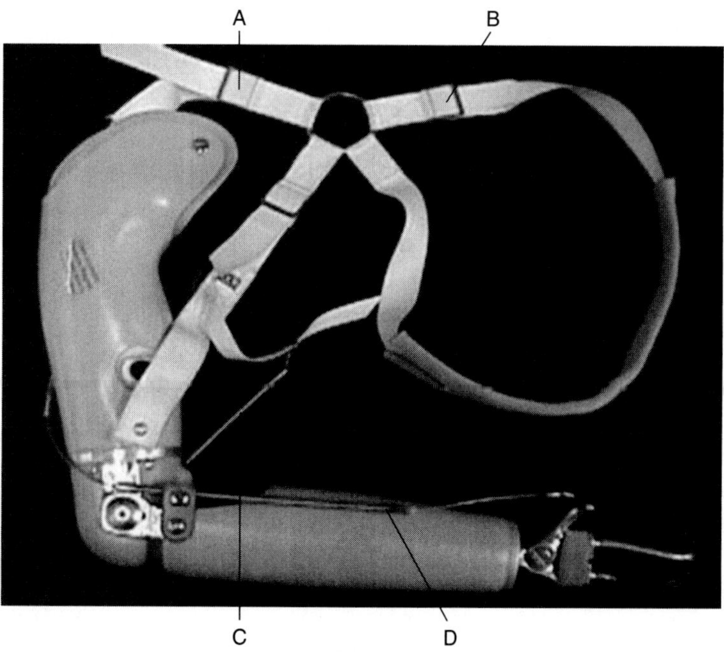

Figure 32-7

The figure-of-eight harness with posterior ring and cable control systems used in a conventional (body-powered) transhumeral prosthesis includes an anterior suspension loop (A), *the contralateral axillary loop* (B), *a cable to control locking and unlocking of the elbow mechanism* (C), *and a cable that will lift the forearm if the elbow unit is unlocked or operate the terminal device if the elbow unit is locked* (D).

equal counteracting forces from each prosthesis. On the basis of the patient's functional needs, the prosthetist may use either a single or dual ring system to maximize the efficiency of the conventional prostheses (Figure 32-8). The second ring in the system, mounted below the primary ring, is used exclusively for the control attachment straps. The more proximal ring is used for the anterior suspensor straps and, for patients with bilateral transhumeral residual limbs, the connection of elbow locking straps.

Some patients with bilateral amputations opt to use separate and completely independent harness systems for their prostheses, especially if they sometimes wear only one prosthesis or if their prostheses are dissimilar. An individual with bilateral transradial amputations, for example, might elect to use a conventional cable-driven system on the nondominant side and a self-suspending externally powered prosthesis on the dominant residual limb.

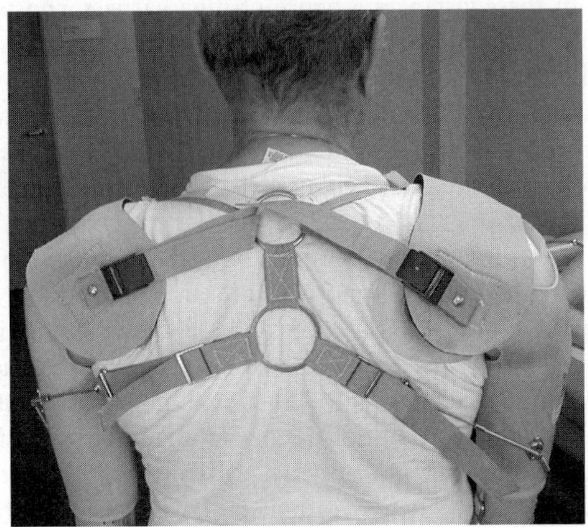

Figure 32-8
The harness system used for conventional (body-powered) bilateral transhumeral prostheses includes an upper ring that stabilizes the prostheses on the trunk and a lower ring that anchors the cable control systems.

Triceps Cuff in Conventional Transradial Prosthesis

Individuals with transradial amputations using a conventional harness suspension control the TD by means of a single cable.[36] In most instances a *triceps cuff* is used to secure the cable housing in an optimal position, as well as provide an integral link to the forearm section (Figure 32-9). Several mechanisms of connection are available between the triceps cuff and the forearm. Flexible Dacron hinges provide satisfactory suspension and ROM for most midlength transradial amputations. Steel cable hinges can be substituted in circumstances where extremely heavy axial loads can be expected (i.e., if a wearer must carry or move heavy objects at work). For those with short and extremely short transradial amputations, metal hinges provide better medial lateral stability at the elbow, as well as functional stop at full extension to protect the residual limb.

Cable Systems to Control a Prosthetic Elbow

Patients with transhumeral amputations need a dual cable system; an anterior cable controls the locking and unlocking of the elbow mechanism, while the other cable controls the TD (if the elbow is locked) or moves the prosthetic forearm (if the elbow is unlocked).[38] The second (longer) cable that attaches to the TD requires a split cable housing system. The proximal portion of the housing is attached to the humeral section, while the distal portion is attached at a location and height anterior to the elbow center.

Most elbow mechanisms have multiple locking positions at equally spaced intervals moving from full extension to

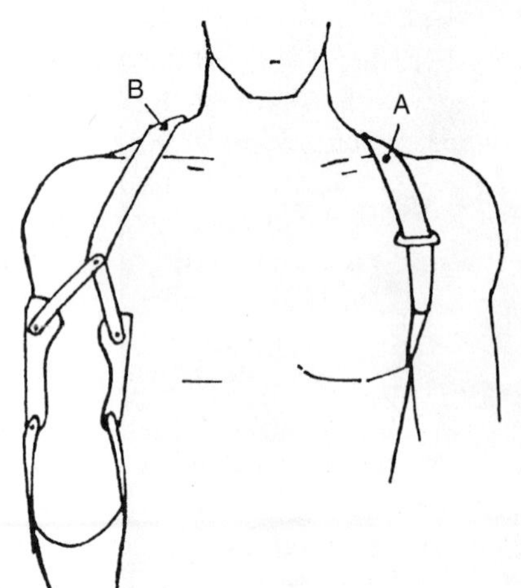

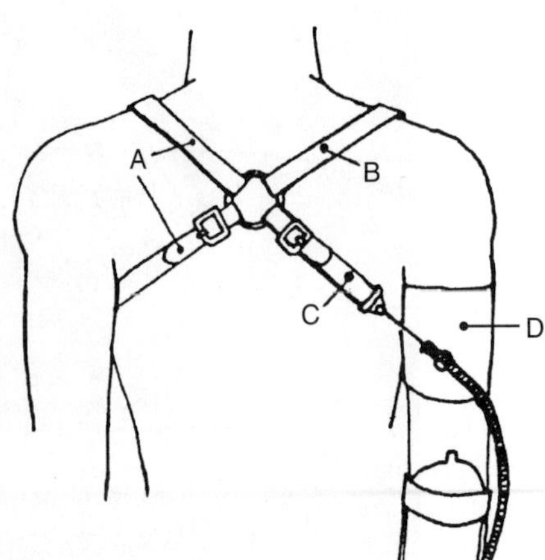

Figure 32-9
Anterior and posterior view of a figure-of-eight harness system for a transradial prosthesis, with the axillary loop (A), the anterior support strap that provides stability during a downward pull (B), the attachment strap for cable control of the terminal device (C), and the triceps pad that anchors the control cable in the most effective position (D). (Modified from the Northwestern University Printing and Duplicating Department, Evanston, Ill., 1987.)

flexion. The locking mechanism is most frequently activated using a rapid and forceful shoulder extension and abduction (Figure 32-10). When the elbow mechanism is "locked" in any given position, this quick down and back movement elongates an anterior cable that releases the lock; subsequent shoulder flexion or scapular abduction (protraction) affecting the posterior cable repositions the prosthetic forearm in space. This happens because the cable running to the TD is aligned anterior to the axis of rotation of the elbow mechanism; when the elbow is unlocked, tension through this cable causes the forearm to rise in flexion. When the forearm reaches the desired inclination for the task at hand, another quick down and back motion will reengage the lock. Once the elbow mechanism is locked, cable control is transferred to the TD, and subsequent shoulder flexion or protraction operates the prosthetic hook or hand. Because this control strategy is always sequential in nature, careful consideration and assessment must be given to the force excursion ratio. Failure to maximize these criteria results in incomplete elbow flexion or incomplete TD control.

Cables and Cable Housings

For both transradial and transhumeral prostheses, the cable and housings should traverse as straight a path as practical. An abrupt or sharp radius creates excessive and unnecessary drag as the cable passes through the housing. The mechanical efficiency of the system is critical to successful operation, particularly for those patients with limited strength or ROM.[39] Steel cable has been used successfully for many years in prosthetic practice. Steel cable is available in several thicknesses in order to meet the needs of all types of users. Clearly the heaviest cables are well suited to heavy work applications and are often used for individuals wearing prostheses for both upper extremities.

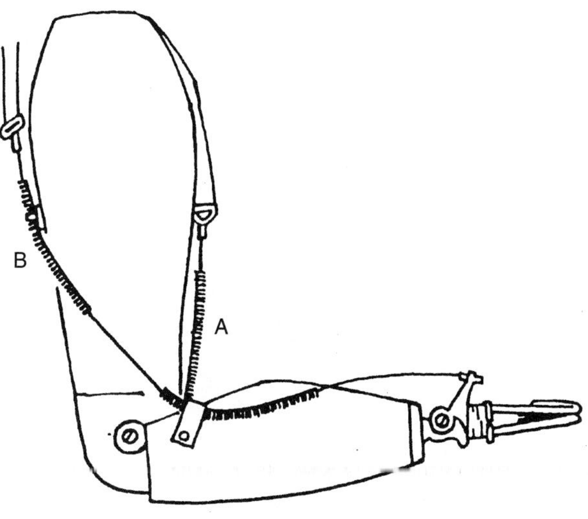

Figure 32-10
Dual control cable and lift loop of a conventional (body-powered) transhumeral prosthesis. Quick and forceful downward and backward shoulder motion operates the elbow locking and unlocking mechanism via the anterior cable (A). The second cable system (B) operates the terminal device if the elbow is locked or lifts the forearm if the elbow is locked. This occurs because the TD control cable is positioned anterior to the axis of the mechanical elbow joint. (Modified from Northwestern University Printing and Duplicating Department, Evanston, Ill., 1987.)

Low-friction linings are often added to the interior surfaces of the cable housing in order to improve the mechanical efficiency.[40] This technique effectively decreases the coefficient of friction of the stainless cable as it passes through the metal cable housing. Typically the low friction linings wear and require replacement before cable failure.

Recently, nonmetallic cable media with both high strength and low coefficients of friction have become available; these improve mechanical efficiency and daily wear characteristics of the prosthetic system.[41] When nonmetallic cables are used with low coefficient linings, the result is often an extremely smooth and highly efficient cable system. These nonmetallic cable alternatives are not mechanically wedged to the attachment hardware used at each end of a prosthetic cable system. Instead, cable connections are made by using highly specialized knots that provide a reliable connection with a smooth profile. Should a nonmetallic cable fail, it is possible for the wearer (with some assistance) to complete emergency repairs without returning the facility. Further, nonmetallic cables do not leave dark residue and stains typically associated with steel cables.

Although these nonmetallic cables are every bit as strong as their steel counterparts, one important drawback is that they do not provide any indication that the cable is nearing the end of its service life. Conversely, steel cables typically become rough and begin to drag as the individual strands of the cable part. Despite this single drawback, nonmetallic cables are strongly recommended in most clinical applications. Further consideration should be given to provide all patients with additional backup cables for times when immediate access to prosthetic repair services is not available.

TERMINAL DEVICES FOR CONVENTIONAL PROSTHESES

The TDs most often used for conventional body-powered prostheses are either a hook or hand (Figures 32-11 and 32-12).[36,42] Both are available as a *voluntary opening* system (the TD is closed at rest, and the wearer opens the hand by means of the cable) or as a *voluntary closing* system (the TD is open at rest, and the wearer closes the hand by means of the cable). Each configuration has its own inherent strengths and weaknesses.

Voluntary opening devices enable the wearer to apply volitional force and excursion of the cable (using shoulder flexion or abduction) to open the TD. Once tension is released from the cable system, the object being grasped

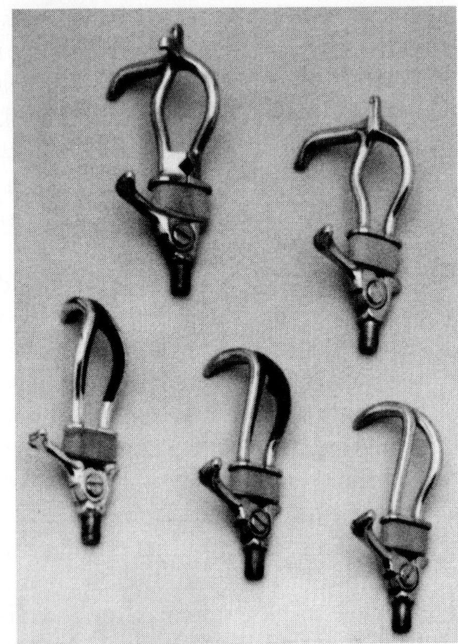

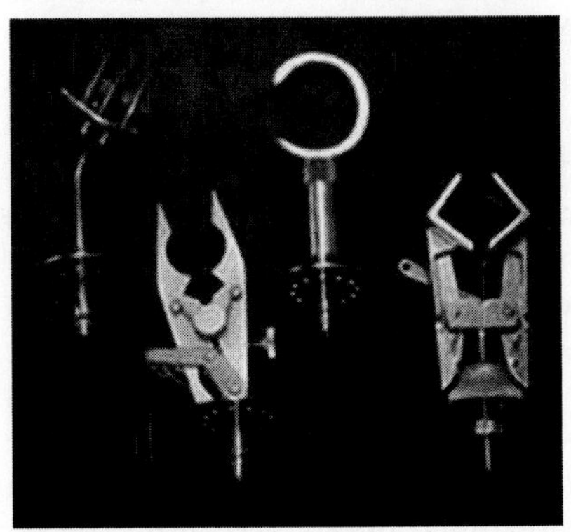

Figure 32-11

A, *Various conventional "hooks" are available to meet the functional needs of individuals using conventional (body-powered) prostheses. The top row of these voluntary opening terminal devices, designed for children, has a "thumb post," as well as coated grip surfaces that are held closed by rubber bands at the base of the hook. Adult hooks are available in a number of configurations to meet the functional and vocational needs of the wearer.* ***B,*** *Terminal devices have also been designed for occupations that require stabilizing objects, carrying objects, or holding cylindrical or spherical objects.*

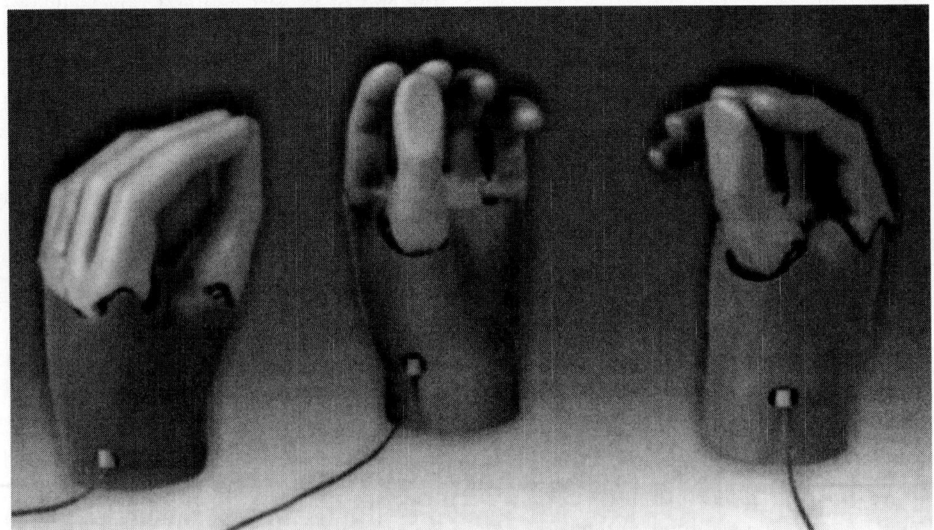

Figure 32-12

Examples of mechanical hands for a conventional (body-powered) prosthesis. Tension of the cable opens the hand to grasp an object using a mechanical "three jaw chuck" grasping pattern. Release of tension on the cable passively holds an object between the thumb and first two digits. To release a held object, the wearer applies tension to the cable once again, to open the mechanical hand. The fourth and fifth fingers are passive and prepositioned in slight flexion but are not part of the grasp and release function of the mechanical hand.

is "trapped" in the device, allowing the wearer to position the object in space as the task demands. The prehensile force (grip strength) is dictated by some external closing mechanism, most frequently springs or elastic bands (see Figure 32-11). Significant prehensile forces can be generated by using multiple layers of elastic bands or multiple springs but must be matched to the wearer's ability to create and sustain cable excursion. Because grip strength is determined by the number of elastics or springs used, it is constant and cannot be voluntarily modified when handling heavy or fragile objects. The mechanical inefficiency and friction inherent in a cable control system increase the force necessary to open the TD above the closing force achieved by the rubber bands or spring systems. Finding the right combination of external closing mechanism strength and user's motor control and excursion for the many different daily functional tasks can be challenging. Several manufacturers market voluntary opening prehensors with settings the wearer can adjust to light or forceful grip strength.[43]

In voluntary closing TDs, the volitional force and excursion supplied by the wearer closes the TD from its normally open position.[44] The key advantage of a voluntary closing TD is the ability to volitionally grade prehensile force, adapting it to the characteristics of the object to be held.[45] When a voluntary closing TD is used, significantly higher forces can be applied through the cabling system. In fact, with most voluntarily closing TD and cable systems, voluntary prehensile force is limited only by the motor powers available from the wearer or by discomfort of the residual limb. In this control strategy the patient must maintain both excursion and power in order to retain the object in the TD.

Voluntary closing devices are not often chosen for individuals with transhumeral amputations because the limited cable excursion available to them is also being used to preposition the forearm in space. Functionally, much of the cable excursions would be used to close the TD so that less would be available to move the forearm. Although those with transhumeral amputation frequently have adequate motor control to position the forearm in space, many are quite challenged to produce enough excursion to effectively operate the elbow throughout full ranges of motion while maintaining a graded prehension of the TD. These actions become even more challenging if the residual transhumeral limb is relatively short. The external passive closure of a voluntary opening TD tends to be more functional for these individuals. Because cable excursion is typically limited for those with bilateral amputations, voluntary opening devices are also the TDs of choice if bilateral conventional prostheses are recommended.

Socket Configurations

The transhumeral and transradial prosthetic sockets used in contemporary prosthetic practice have evolved from nonanatomically and functionally based designs to highly contoured, skeletally correct and intimately fitting designs. A significant portion of these anatomically contoured socket advancements have come as a direct result of changes in material technology. Until recently, upper extremity prosthetic sockets were fabricated using thermal setting resins for structural integrity and finish. By nature these materials were hard and did not yield effectively to changes in muscle contour as the wearer used the limb in functional activities. With the advent of moldable thermoplastics and advanced anatomically contoured socket designs, improvements in intimacy of fit and functional ROM have been achieved.

Most contemporary upper extremity prosthetic sockets use some type of flexible interface with a rigid frame exterior. The interface material is often composed of a high silicone content elastomer. These elastomers have dramatically improved patients' perceptions of fit and function with regard to comfort.

Transradial Self-Suspending Sockets

Many patients with transradial amputations are now fit with self-suspending sockets that both increase functional ROM during activity and, more importantly, improve wearer acceptance and compliance.[6] Highly specialized bone and muscle contour promote effective control in both conventional body-powered and myoelectrically controlled prostheses. Historically, self-suspending transradial sockets encase the medial and lateral humeral condyles to provide suspension.[36] The nature of this medial-lateral compression inherently decreased ROM, particularly in terminal flexion. New designs are becoming less dependent on the condyles and are using higher anteroposterior forces between the anterior fossa and olecranon of the elbow to achieve suspension. This strategy increases the wearer's ability to fully extend the elbow.

Advances in Donning Techniques

As the intimacy of socket designs has increased, so has the need for more effective donning techniques. Historically, cotton stockinettes or elastic bandages were adequate for drawing tissue into prosthetic sockets and allowed for satisfactory donning. Because these materials have high coefficient friction, they can be difficult to pull from the socket. High friction also can be fairly abrasive on the wearer's residual limb. A new generation of pull socks made of low-friction cloth have been developed (Advanced Arm Dynamics, Guilford, Conn.). Many have coatings impregnated into the cloth during manufacture to allow for effective, nonabrasive donning of intimately contoured prosthetic sockets. With the initial tension as it is first pulled through the opening in the socket, the pull sock encases the soft tissue of the residual limb as if it were a cylindrical cone. As the pull sock is drawn through the opening, it positions the soft tissue of the residual limb as intended by the contour of the socket. These donning tools have also enabled some individuals with bilateral amputations to independently don aggressive self-suspending sockets.

Advances in Transhumeral Socket Design

Whereas the traditional transhumeral prosthesis had an over-the-shoulder cap socket design, recent advances in socket design have resulted in sockets with laterally trim lines below the acromion process. The additions of anterior and posterior stabilizer extensions that cross toward the midline on the amputated side provide superior rotational stability.

CASE EXAMPLE 1

An Individual with Traumatic Transradial Amputation

P. C., 34, sustained a severe crush injury to his left hand, wrist, and lower forearm when a rock wall he was building in his backyard collapsed as he was working on it. The team at the trauma center determined that he was not a candidate for limb salvage and recommended transradial amputation. Now it is 8 weeks after the surgery. P. C. has been consistent with compression of his residual limb and his upper extremity home exercise program. He is referred for prescription of a transhumeral prosthesis. Clinical examination reveals a well-healed incision, with a skin graft over the anterior surface of the cubital fossa and residual limb. Tissue density is relatively firm. Touch and pressure sensation is slightly diminished in the area of the skin graft. P. C. can fully extend his elbow but lacks the final 25 degrees of elbow flexion. He has minimal pronation and supination ability in his residual limb. Shoulder range of motion and strength are within normal limits. The residual limb measures 16 cm from the lateral epicondyle to the distal end and 12.5 cm from the cubital fold to the distal end.

P. C. is right-hand dominant. He works as a self-employed building contractor, with a small business focused on home remodeling. He lives with his wife and three elementary school–aged children in a three-story Victorian home that he is in the process of rehabilitating. He is an avid water skier in the summer and downhill skier in the winter. P. C. is apprehensive about his ability to return to work and support his family.

Questions to Consider

- Given the condition and function of his residual limb, what type of socket and interface might the team might recommend for P. C. from among available options? Why would these be the optimal choices? What factors are likely to influence clinical decision making in this case?
- Given his employment and vocational interests, what type of suspension and control system might the team recommend for P. C. from among available options? Why would these be the optimal choices? Will a conventional cable control system allow P. C. the "work envelope" required for his job as a builder? Given his skin condition, would a myoelectrically controlled prosthesis be possible? How would the team determine this?
- Given his employment and vocational interests, what type of terminal device (or hand) and wrist unit might the team recommend for P. C.? Why would these be the optimal choices? What are the benefits and drawbacks of a "quick disconnect" wrist unit and having activity-specific terminal devices?

Recommendations

After much discussion P. C. and the team decide that a self-suspending transradial prosthesis with a flexible socket in a rigid frame is most appropriate. Given his role as a builder and the need to work overhead and have sufficient grip force to hold and manipulate lumber and other building materials, the team recommends a myoelectrically powered prosthesis with a power wrist control unit and a Griefer as a terminal device to be used in his work setting. P. C. inquires whether terminal devices might be interchangeable so that he can have a prosthetic hand with a silicone glove to wear when he is not at work.

EXTERNALLY POWERED SYSTEMS

All externally powered systems share a single common denominator: an *electric power cell* that provides electrical current to prosthetic components (Figure 32-13, *A* through *C*).[46] Cell technology has dramatically improved in the past decade. Traditional technology involved rechargeable nickel cadmium batteries that, in addition to environmental concerns on disposal, are vulnerable to a memory effect. Cell memory effect occurs when batteries are charged before reaching a fully discharged state. As batteries incur greater and greater amounts of memory, the maximal charge the battery accepts decreases. As maximal charge decreases, so does the maximal time a patient can expect service from the battery. As a practical matter, a patient cannot reasonably be expected to use the battery until full discharge is achieved, and therefore a rechargeable battery in this state is impractical.

As the medium that promotes electrical charge in prosthetic batteries has changed, memory effect has been virtually eradicated. Batteries made with lithium, lithium ion, and lithium polymer have no memory effect and supply significantly higher amounts of current, while simultaneously decreasing the weight of the battery. An active prosthetic user can now use an externally powered prosthesis more than a full day on a single charge. Because lithium-based cells are smaller and lighter, they are also less challenging to "fit" cosmetically into the prosthesis.

Other than having an electric cell, externally powered prostheses may have little in common with each other by classification. Electric TD componentry is available in many forms, including hooks, hands, and specially developed work tools. These tools can be oriented in space using electric

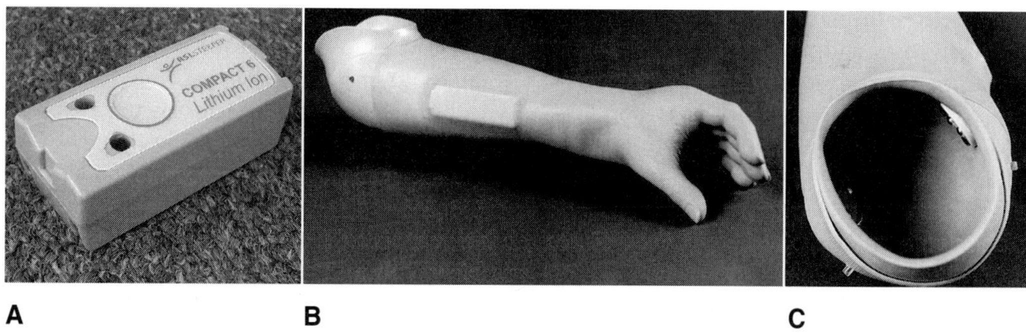

A B C

Figure 32-13

*An example of a lithium power cell used in a myoelectric prosthesis (**A**). This cell must be fit somewhere within the prosthesis (**B**) to power terminal devices and other prosthetic components, on the basis of signals received by the myoelectrodes (**C**) embedded in the walls of the socket.*

rotators that can substitute effectively for lost pronation and supination.[9]

Electric and electronic elbow mechanisms are also readily available. These mechanisms provide powered flexion and extension at the elbow joint (Figure 32-14). Substitution for internal and external rotation of the shoulder is more difficult. Most systems integrate a passive friction humeral rotator; this allows the patient to reposition the distal extremity in the desired amount of internal or external rotation.[10] Although actively powered humeral rotation has been problematic in terms of design and function, much research and development is under way.

For patients with exceptionally short transhumeral limbs and shoulder disarticulation, most prostheses use a mechanical device to replace the shoulder joint that can be passively prepositioned.[47] Electrically actuated locks are available for clinical use and provide an effective means of locking the position of the humerus relative to the midline of the body for individuals with high-level amputations.

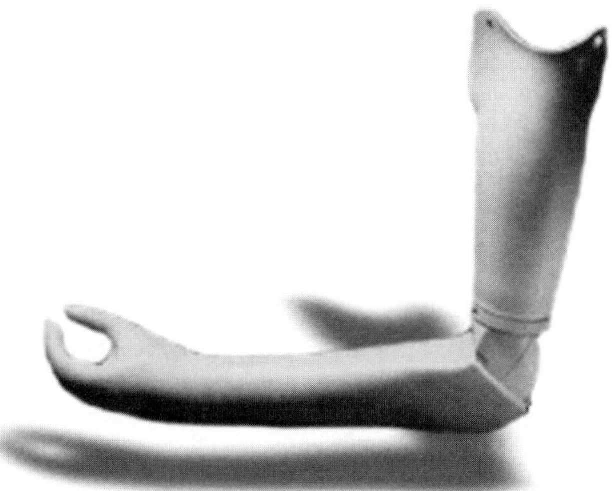

Figure 32-14

An example of a myoelectrically controlled transhumeral prosthesis with electric elbow and hand. The socket brim has anterior and posterior "wings" to stabilize the prosthesis on the residual humerus. Myoelectrodes over the residual biceps are used to flex the elbow or close the hand, while those over the residual triceps extend the elbow or open the hand. Quick cocontraction of biceps and triceps will switch control from elbow to hand mode.

DECISION MAKING

The decision process on what input devices will provide control to externally powered components is a complex one. Full assessment and evaluation of the available motors, ROMs, electromyographical signal, signal separation, and limb length and skin integrity must be considered.[48] The choice of input devices for externally powered devices represents a broad and wide-reaching array of control strategies that allow nearly all patients the opportunity to successfully control a prosthesis. The most common and preferred means to control a prosthesis is with the electromyographic (EMG) signal. This technology uses the small electrical potentials generated by contraction of the residual muscles to operate one or more devices. Modern circuitry and sophisticated filters allow most patients, even those with small signals, the potential for reasonable control.

MYOELECTRIC CONTROL SYSTEMS

Ideally the prosthetist tries to identify two independent signals in a set of physiologically paired (agonist and antagonist) muscles. The wearer can activate these signals over a wide spectrum of contraction intensity to use them as electrode sites. For those with transradial limbs, electrodes are typically positioned over flexor muscle residuum in the forearm to control grasp (closing of the TD) and the extensor muscle residuum to control release (opening of the TD).[49] Many patients who, with sufficient training, master independent contraction of these muscle groups are candidates for even more sophisticated control.

The prosthetist selects the most appropriate myoelectrodes from the many sizes and numerous configurations that are manufactured. The prosthetist also chooses electrodes on the basis of whether they require a remote or nonremote placement of the preamplification electronics. In selecting the myoelectrode and preamplification system, the prosthetist must carefully consider the location, function, and components (TD, elbow, locking mechanism, and rotators) to be used. Because nonremote sensing electrodes house the preamplifier in the bundle of the electrode, less space is necessary to house electronics in the prosthesis. Placing the preamp close to the electrode, however, increases the risk that perspiration will disrupt electronic function. Electrode selection should consider the amount of soft tissue present on the residual limb, the presence or absence of scar tissue, and the material medium with which the interface will be constructed.

Many components can interpret large or small, fast or slow muscular contractions and respond prosthetically in a *proportional* fashion, linking speed and force of device operation to speed and amplitude of muscle contraction under the myoelectrode site.[49] This graded control enables a patient to develop extremely precise speed and grip strength strategies. The well-developed independent control of antagonistic muscles also is a prerequisite for mode selection, which uses different types of contraction of the same muscle groups for dissimilar tasks. Many patients wearing a transradial myoelectrical prosthesis use a quick cocontraction of forearm muscle residuum to switch between control of the hand and the wrist unit. For those with transhumeral prostheses, quick cocontraction of shoulder flexors and extensors is used to switch between control of the electronic elbow and hand. Effective mode selection with cocontraction requires a patient to fire antagonistic muscles above a predetermined threshold at nearly the same instant.[49] Many patients find this technique challenging as control training begins. Mode selection is based on nearly simultaneous timing of contraction of agonistic and antagonistic muscles. Early in training, however, many new myoelectric prosthetic users focus on forcefulness of contraction in an effort to increase amplitude of the signal, rather than on producing the desired quick cocontraction.

If a patient struggles or is unable to master cocontraction mode selection, alternative strategies are always available. The prosthetist can use programmable controllers to allow complex muscle activity not generally associated with everyday tasks as the mode selection trigger. Additionally, many systems allow the user a default mode (usually to the TD) to which the mode selector reverts after a predetermined time interval.

Programmable microprocessors have had an additional impact on prosthetic fitting; they allow the prosthetist to experiment with multiple strategies without having to replace hardware. Before programmable microprocessors were available, myoelectric components were secured for individual patients without the benefit of real-time clinical assessment. Microprocessor control has allowed the prosthetist to maximize the patient's rehabilitation potential within a single hardware construct. Enormous benefit is also derived from the ability to save, recover, and manipulate software configurations easily and quickly with immediate patient feedback. This allows prosthetic users to experiment with a strategy for control and then progress to alternative strategies with the luxury of returning to the precise original strategy and settings quickly. Programmable controllers allow individuals with recent amputations to maximize their current physiological control and then progress to significantly more complex and involved strategies without having to replace components or relinquishing a prosthesis for modification.

Three basic approaches are used to program the microprocessor. In the first approach, adjustments to electronics are made through a direct connection to a laptop or similar computer using a graphical interface. Wireless interface communication or the implementation of coding plugs enables efficient assessment and modification of control strategies. For some individuals with new amputations who are candidates for early postoperative fitting, a myoelectrically controlled TD may be integrated in a rigid dressing immediately after surgery. The psychological and physiological benefits of early fitting have been well demonstrated.[27]

ALTERNATIVE CONTROL STRATEGIES

If effective myoelectric control is too difficult to master for a patient immediately after amputation surgery (or is inappropriate because of concomitant problems), the prosthetist may opt to use *switch control* as an alternative means of operating electric prosthetic components.[50] Switch control does not require myoelectric sensors against the skin. In addition, switch control of functional grasp and release can be mastered fairly readily by most new prosthetic users, without the appreciable training time required for myoelectric systems. Switch control systems require extremely small movement to trigger—typically an excursion in millimeters and a force in fractions of pounds.[51] This makes it much more functional than early postoperative devices with body-powered components that required larger cable excursions to operate TD or lock or unlock the prosthetic elbow. The small excursion and light force required to engage switch control makes prosthetic use feasible for individuals with limited ROM or strength. This technique allows for early intervention with limited exposure to the stresses on the recently amputated residual limb on the prosthetic wall. It also allows new users to develop functional grip strength within a short time. When switches are used to trigger externally powered prosthetic components, however, proportional control (graded action where the action of the device is proportional to the effort made to trigger its operation) is not possible.

Several other control systems are available as well. *Force sensitive resistors* (FSRs, also called *touch pads*) have found

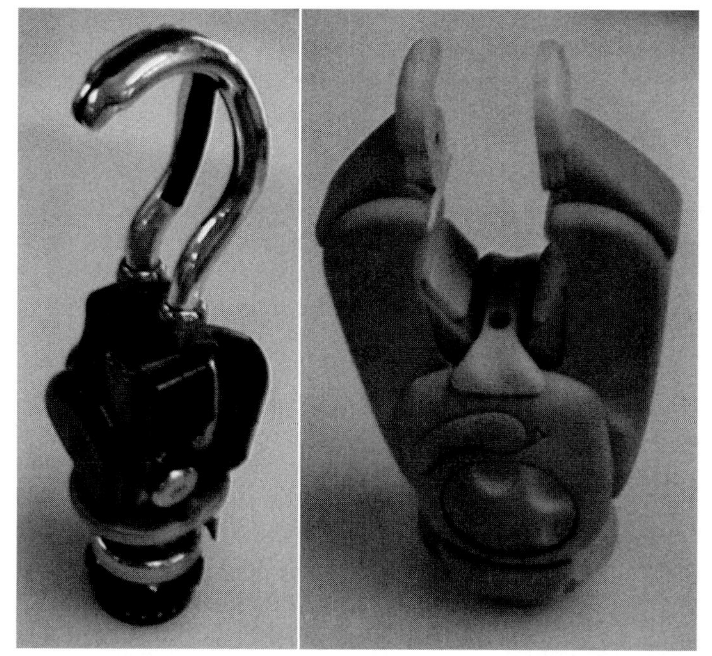

Figure 32-15

***A** and **B**, Examples of terminal devices that allow proportional control of grasp on the basis of muscle contraction speed at the myoelectrode site or the use of programmable microprocessor controllers.*

great utility as a primary control driver in instances when other signals are not readily available. FSRs are designed to interpret surface pressure on the pad and supply a resultant proportional output. Because these devices are extremely flat and small in diameter, they are well suited for applications such as residual limb buds in children with congenital limb deficiencies. Special consideration must be given, however, to the location and preparation of sites in which an FSR is to be used. These devices can become problematic if the base on which they are placed is not perfectly flat. Even a small radius can cause the conductive gel inside the sensor to fail. The location must be placed strategically to allow any perspiration to settle away from the sensor. Failure to adequately address this strategic locating of the device may cause the FSR to fail.

In addition to being used in early postoperative fittings, switches can also be used in definitive prostheses. Although most switches are activated by pulling a cable or strap, other applications are activated by depressing a lever or button. Some switches are complex in nature because they have numerous functions that are dictated by the position of the switch. Most switches do not have the capacity to provide proportional output to control electric components. The absence of proportionality can be viewed as a limiting factor in many switch control applications.

To achieve true proportionality, a servo-resistor or other sensing resistor would be necessary. These devices interpret the travel (excursion) applied to the system and translate this input quantitatively with predetermined electrical outputs. These devices can also translate force simultaneously or independently with excursion to create a proportional output.

Proportional control of all electrically powered devices (especially of elbows and the TDs) has enabled patients to achieve unprecedented levels of fine motor control and speed variability for skilled activity.[52,53] Technology has enabled this proportional control to further expand the functional envelope of the prosthesis, with higher-speed drive motors and clutches that allow extremely responsive and rapid control (Figure 32-15). When proportional control is coupled with circuitry designed to create and maintain stable prehensile patterns within the TD, wearers can achieve increasingly complex and sophisticated tasking patterns.

ELECTRIC TERMINAL DEVICES

Electric TDs are available in many configurations; the most commonly used is an electric hand (Figure 32-16).[54] Most hands are available in an array of sizes, from those designed to fit young children with congenital limb deficiencies to those that fit adults with traumatic amputations. Most hands use a "three jaw chuck" grasping pattern of the thumb and first two digits. The remaining fingers (digits four and five) follow passively but in a similar pattern to the active first two digits opposing the thumb. Significant grasp pressures can be achieved with most electromechanical hands; in fact, pressures can be so significant that patients must be cautioned during early training about the amount of force possible. In myoelectric prostheses with proportional control, maximum grip strength is achieved with corresponding maximum input signal generated by forceful muscle contraction.

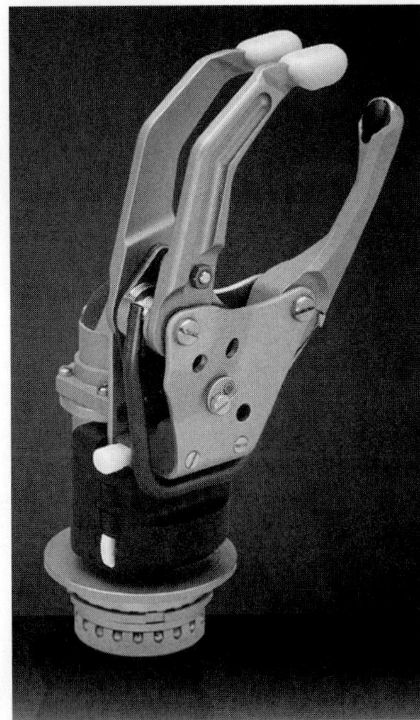

Figure 32-16
The internal mechanism of an externally powered prosthetic hand. The "three jaw chuck" allows functional grasp. The terminal device can be finished with a prosthetic glove that includes passive prosthetic fingers for third, fourth, and fifth digits.

Proportionality of input signal translates to both the speed of finger movement and the terminal force applied to the object being grasped. In a nonproportionally based system (such as simple switch control), maximum grip strength is achieved on a time-dependent basis. Recently, circuits have been added to provide slip control. This allows objects to be retained in the grasp without conscious control from patient input. Objects of a soft nature can also be manipulated more effectively without being crushed with such slip-sensing technology.

Although hands make up the majority of externally powered prostheses with TDs, other highly functional TDs are readily available.[54] These devices range from tools that closely resemble portable vices to terminal hardware that closely mimics the functional characteristics of an electric hook. Since most prostheses include a quick disconnect option for the TD, prosthetic wearers can easily change TDs to suit their functional demands. Many of the non–hand-type TDs can generate even greater forces than the corresponding hands. The geometries of the opening mechanism allow these alternative tools to easily grasp larger, cylindrical, and more irregularly shaped objects. The smaller tips of some of these tools allow patients to grasp smaller and flatter objects as well. When these alternative TDs are used, there is less obstruction of the visual field. As a result, many have better functional efficiency than possible with a prosthetic hand. To date no system is commercially available that satisfactorily replicates the lost proprioception and sensation of the fingers and anatomical hand. The size and location of the visual field blocked by the palmar surface of the hand and outstretched mechanical fingers has a significant impact on function.

TDs (hands and design tools) with wrist flexion potential can provide the patient with advantageous approaches for improved grasp. Wrist flexion also assists, in a small way, in restoring the visual field when using electromechanical hands.

Electric Elbow Components

A number of externally powered elbow components are commercially available, but many require that the prosthetist be specially trained in their implementation and usage.[55,56] Each of the commercially available electromechanical elbows uses proprietary signal processing and drive mechanisms to achieve design-specific functional attributes. In selecting an externally powered elbow unit, the prosthetist considers the specific functional needs of individual patients. The type of inputs necessary to control the elbow mechanism, the location of myoelectrodes, and the number of inputs necessary to control both the elbow and TD must be weighed in the decision on what elbow mechanism is most appropriate. Most commercially available elbow systems incorporate microprocessors that are compatible with a large array of input devices and can be programmed to use wrists and TDs from a large selection of manufacturers. Most prosthetists are no longer constrained to develop prosthetic recommendations from a single manufacturer product line; in fact, doing so often limits possibilities and therefore functional outcome.

Dual Control Strategies

Microprocessor control has assisted control strategies that can be better customized to individual patient needs.[49] The traditional control strategy for an individual using an externally powered transhumeral prosthesis might include one myoelectrode to capture EMG signals of the residual biceps and a second myoelectrode over the residual triceps. Assuming both signals are of satisfactory amplitude and differentiation, successful myoelectric control of two devices—an electrically powered elbow and an electrically powered TD—can be successfully achieved. In order to grasp an object, the patient purposefully contracts the biceps; an EMG signal from the biceps is programmed to promote elbow flexion. This physiologically correct application uses the biceps in a fashion similar to preamputation status. A signal is provided continuously until the forearm and elbow reach the desired position in space. The mechanism can be locked in this position by holding the elbow steady (no longer flexing or extending) through a predetermined and programmed time interval. The system then cycles to TD (hand) control, using the same to EMG inputs. The most commonly employed combination is contraction of the triceps to open the hand or extend the elbow and contraction of the biceps to close the hand or flex the elbow.

Sequential and Simultaneous Control Strategies

Myoelectric control of prosthetic pronation and supination can be added using an electric wrist rotator.[9] Under the constraints of a two-electrode system, the rotator is frequently controlled using a momentary contact switch mounted on the medial side of the humeral section, where it can be easily bumped against the body. In this configuration three inputs, two EMG and one switch, control forearm position in space, pronation, and grasp and release. This type of control strategy is often referred to as *sequential* because one task must be completed before the next is executed.

Recent developments in microcircuitry and microprocessors have made *simultaneous control* of more than one device possible. For simultaneous control, the same two myoelectrode EMG signals at the biceps and triceps are used. A wrist rotator and TD are also installed, but the momentary contact switch that previously controlled wrist position is removed. Instead, control of pronation and supination is triggered to the EMG inputs. Patients use their biceps to close the TD and pronate the prosthetic forearm and use the triceps to open the TD and supinate the prosthetic forearm. Mode selection, via cocontraction of the biceps and triceps, determines whether opening and closing of the TD or pronation and supination of the forearm will be triggered by subsequent EMG signal. Many individuals with UE amputations can master mode selection using this control strategy.

Simultaneous control of the elbow and TD can now be accomplished by adding a proportional input to the system. Great success can be achieved by inserting a linear potentiometer or strain gauge into the harnessing of the transhumeral prosthesis. As the wearer generates excursion in either humeral flexion or scapular protraction, the input device translates this movement or force into a usable signal to control position in space of the elbow mechanism. This makes both nonsequential and simultaneous control of the TD and elbow possible. This is advantageous as a patient can approach an object by bringing the forearm into the appropriate position while concurrently opening the hand in preparation for grasp.

The combination of greater TD speeds and long battery life enables myoelectrically controlled upper extremity prosthetic wearers to control multiple devices through ever-increasing functional planes. They can do so over time durations compatible with most everyday needs. The number of combinations of myoelectrodes and control strategies becomes limitless as more manufacturers develop modular componentry that is compatible with most commercially available systems.

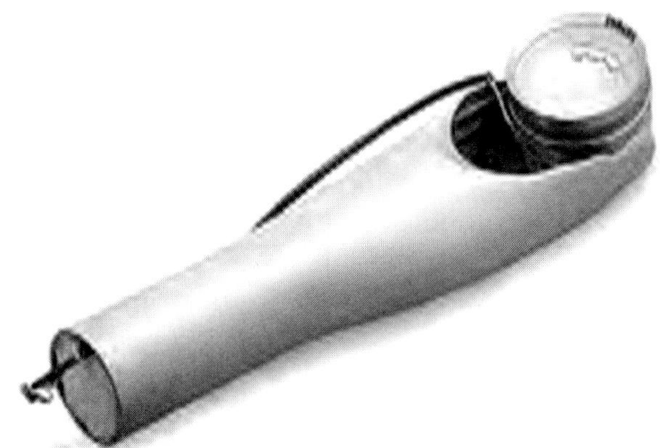

Figure 32-17
This hybrid transhumeral prosthetic system includes a myoelectrically controlled elbow and a cable for body-powered operation of the terminal device.

HYBRID PROSTHESES

For some individuals, the integration of technology from both the conventional and externally powered systems provides the greatest potential for functional outcome. Prosthetic systems can be configured to use an electrically powered elbow with a body-powered mechanical TD (Figure 32-17) or an electrically powered TD with a nonpowered elbow. Compelling arguments can be made for both control strategies; the ultimate decision for componentry and control systems must be based on a patient's ability to use proprioceptive feedback from the cable system, as well as available inputs for the electromechanical system. Consideration should also be given to the motivating factors to use a hybrid. Frequently, hybridized systems are sought because insufficient range or strength is available to provide complete functional control at the elbow joint and TD with conventional systems. This may be the result of a frozen shoulder, an unstable joint that is vulnerable to frequent subluxation, or shoulder disarticulation (Figure 32-18). If the musculature in the residual limb can generate satisfactory EMG signals despite the more proximal shoulder involvement, then myoelectric control of the TD can be achieved despite impairments limiting the strong volitional movements at the shoulder necessary to control a conventional system. Placement of the forearm in space can then be assisted using a large variety of spring-assisted or forearm-balancing mechanical devices. These technologies allow patients with varying degrees of functional capacity to be fitted successfully with components from two different arenas.

Activity-Specific Prostheses

Most of this chapter's discussions have revolved around functions that relate to activities of daily living and vocational pursuits. Most individuals with upper extremity

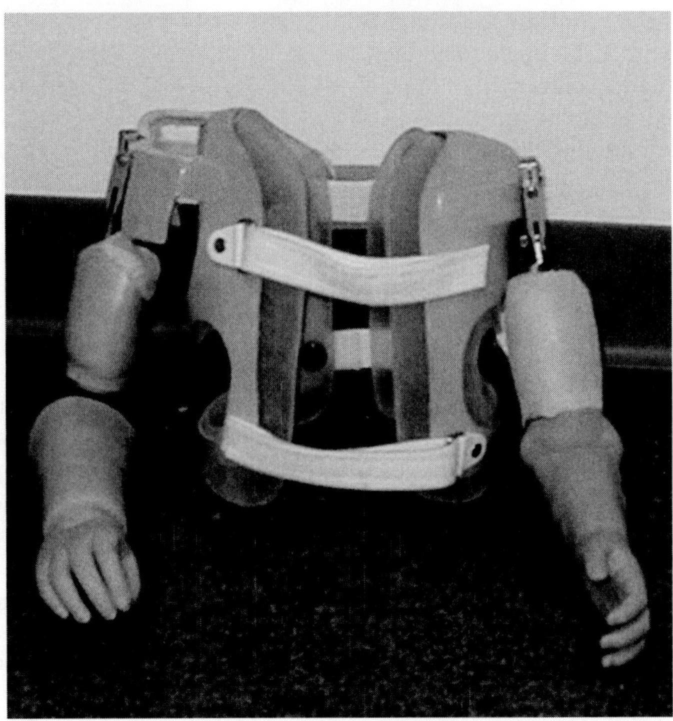

Figure 32-18
Example of a hybrid prosthesis designed for an individual with bilateral shoulder disarticulation as a result of trauma. Suspension is provided by a thermoplastic "jacket." A conventional shoulder joint is used on the right, while a myoelectric system incorporated on the left controls elbow motion, forearm rotation, and operation of the terminal device operation on the left.

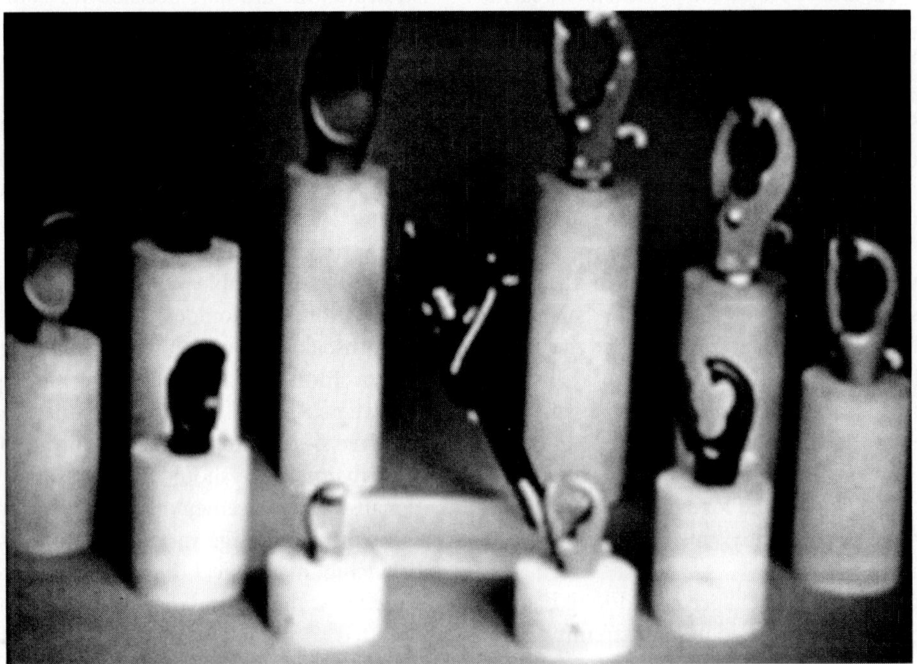

Figure 32-19
Examples of terminal devices that might be used for vocational and leisure activities. Passive terminal devices (left) *are often chosen for young children or for individuals involved in sports that require ball handling. Voluntary closing terminal devices* (right) *allow graded prehension for various skilled activities.*

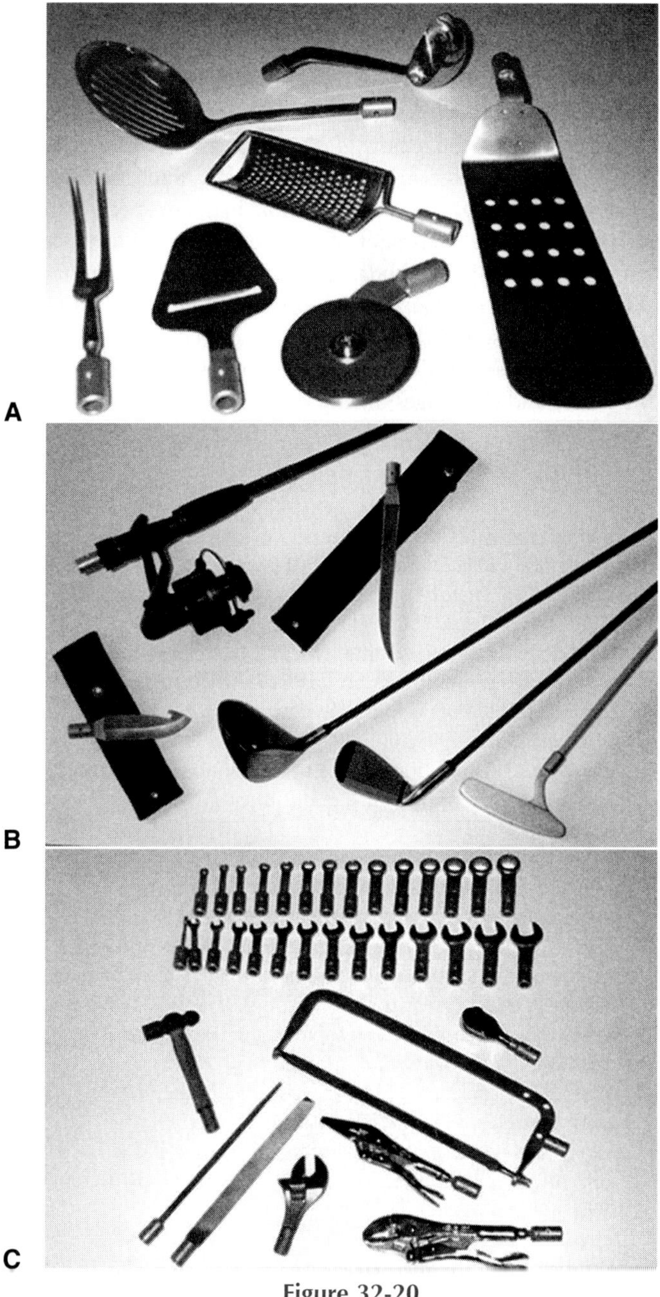

Figure 32-20

Examples of activity- or function-specific terminal devices that can be used in a prosthesis with "quick disconnect" attachment for the terminal device: ***A,*** *a variety of kitchen utensils and cooking tools,* ***B,*** *devices for leisure and sport activities such as fishing and golf, and* ***C,*** *carpentry and mechanical tools such as hammers, files, pliers, wrenches, ratchets, and saws. The prosthetic wearer disconnects the conventional terminal device or prosthetic hand and attaches the tool temporarily while involved in a given activity.*

amputations want to be involved in various pursuits beyond activities of daily living and vocational activities, just as they were before their amputations. A number of unique prosthetic applications, as well as adaptations and assistive tools for an existing prosthesis, can effectively address the recreational and avocational desires of individual patients.[57] Although conventional wisdom suggests that these pursuits not proceed until complete maximal rehabilitation has occurred with the primary prosthetic device, this is not always the case; being able to return to an important avocational activity might be a major motivating factor in rehabilitation. However, few patients have the financial resources for specialized prostheses for vocational and avocational activities. Most prosthetists make every attempt to implement activity-specific devices within the primary prosthetic design. Because the array of activities in which persons participate is limitless, so too is the creation of specific tools and adaptations to accommodate these needs. Quick-disconnect wrists allow for a myriad of options in place of the existing TD. Commercial application of TDs can include nearly any imaginable adaptation for sport and recreational pursuits (Figures 32-19 and 32-20). Specific challenges such as exposure to the elements, vibration, and impact may require more significant modification to ensure acceptable durability to the device.

CASE EXAMPLE 2

An Individual with Traumatic Transhumeral Amputation

E. S., 29, has been employed since high school in maintenance and mechanics and is responsible for cleaning and repairing the presses during the night shift at a paper manufacturing plant. Six months ago, while cleaning a press that had been improperly shut down, the sleeve of his sweatshirt became entangled in a press. His right arm was drawn into the press almost to the level of the axilla before his coworker could activate the safety stop mechanism. The crush and degloving injuries were so severe that the only option was amputation at a short transfemoral level. In addition, steady traction on his arm while being drawn into the press damaged his brachial plexus, and E. S. has significant weakness in residual muscles controlling his shoulder. His residual arm measures 14 cm from acromion to distal end. Range of motion (ROM) is limited by 50% in shoulder flexion, extension, and abduction. For 4 months, he has been wearing a body-powered–dual-cable control prosthesis suspended with a figure-of-eight harness, including a locking elbow and voluntary opening hook, but is not satisfied with the functional level this prosthesis allows him. He has developed signs of axillary compression (sensory impairment) in his intact left upper extremity. He is referred for evaluation for a myoelectrically controlled prosthesis.

Since the accident, E. S. has been living with his sister and her family, but he is eager to return to his own home, a cabin on a lake several hours from the rehabilitation and prosthetic center where he has been receiving care. He is seriously considering returning to college to study electrical engineering or material sciences, with the goal of becoming a prosthetist.

Questions to Consider

- Given the condition and function of his residual limb, what type of socket and interface might the team recommend for E. S. from among available options? Why would these be the optimal choices? What factors are likely to influence clinical decision making in this case?
- Given his brachial plexus injury and contralateral axillary compression, what type of suspension and control system might the team recommend for the patient E. S. from among available options? Why would these be the optimal choices? How would the team determine if a myoelectrically controlled prosthesis would be possible? Should other options for external power also be considered?
- What type of prosthetic elbow, wrist unit, and terminal device (or hand) and wrist unit might the team recommend for E. S.? Why would these be the optimal choices? What are the benefits and drawbacks of each unit?

Recommendations

E. S. has not been able to fully use his initial prosthesis effectively because of inadequate cable excursion due to limitations in ROM and strength. His effort to maximize cable excursion has resulted in compression injury of his remaining arm, compromising function of his left hand. The team determines that there is sufficient myoelectric signal to operate a power elbow, forearm rotator, and TD or hand. They recommend his harness suspension system be replaced with a custom-fit shoulder saddle to avoid further compression in the left axilla. The prosthesis will have a flexible socket with rigid frame; electrodes will be incorporated into the walls of the socket. A linear potentiometer will be used to provide full ROM of the prosthetic elbow, with simultaneous myoelectric control of the TD.

SUMMARY

Prosthetic rehabilitation of persons with upper extremity amputations is both challenging and rewarding. Success is often difficult to measure purely in clinical terms; however, maximizing individual functional potential and providing the appropriate amount of technology to assure acceptable outcomes are highly predictive of success. In addition to understanding the patient's needs, consideration of the needs and expectations of spouses, children, and extended family is also important. Once the patient's requirements are completely understood, careful and thoughtful rehabilitation plans can be developed. An effective prosthetic prescription will detail (1) the power source and control system (conventional or externally powered) that will operate prosthetic components, (2) the elbow design (for transhumeral or higher amputations), (3) the socket type and interface medium, (4) the appropriate TD (hook, hand, or specialized tools), and (5) the alignment of components. Each of these five categories can be subdivided into additional criteria-based items, the number of divisions based upon the complexity of the case and the clinical resources that are available. Following these guidelines will eliminate unnecessary difficulties and challenges during the design process.

REFERENCES

1. Baumgartner RF. Upper extremity amputation and prosthetics. *J Rehabil Res Devel* 2001;38(4):vii-x.
2. Childress DS. Historical aspects of powered-limb prostheses. *Clin Prosthet Orthot* 1985;9(1):2-13.
3. Millstein SG, Heger H, Hunter GA. Prosthetic use in adult upper limb amputees. *Prosthet Orthot Int* 1986;10(1):27-34.
4. Durance J, O'Shea P. Upper limb amputees: a clinical profile. *Int Disabil Study* 1988;10(2):68-72.
5. Sherman RA. Utilization of prostheses among US veterans with traumatic amputation: a pilot survey. *J Rehabil Res Dev* 1999;36(2):100-108.
6. Atkins DJ, Heard DC, Donovan WH. Epidemiologic overview of individuals with upper limb loss and their reported research priorities. *J Prosthet Orthot* 1996;8(2):2-11.
7. Vacek KM. Transition to a switch activated 3-S transhumeral prosthesis: a team approach. *J Prosthet Orthot* 1998;10(3):56-60.
8. Daly W. Clinical application of roll-on sleeves for myoelectrically controlled transradial and transhumeral prostheses. *J Prosthet Orthot* 2000;12(3):88-91.
9. Sears HH, Shaperman J. Electric wrist rotation in proportional control systems. *J Prosthet Ortho*t 1998;10(4):92-98.
10. Ivko JJ. Independence through humeral rotation in the conventional transhumeral prosthetic design. *J Prosthet Orthot* 1999;11(1):20-22.
11. Michael JW. Partial hand amputations: prosthetic and orthotic management. In Bowker JH, Michael JW (eds), *Atlas of Limb Prosthetics: Surgical, Prosthetic, and Rehabilitation Principles*, 2nd ed. St. Louis: Mosby-Year Book, 1992. pp. 217-226.
12. Weir RF, Grahn EC, Duff SJ. A new externally powered myoelectrically controlled prosthesis for persons with partial hand amputations at the metacarpals. *J Prosthet Orthot* 2001;13(2):26-33.
13. Burkhalter WE, Hampton FL, Smeitzer JA. Wrist disarticulation and below elbow amputation. In *American Academy of Orthopedic Surgeons, Atlas of Limb Prosthetics.* St. Louis: Mosby, 1981. pp. 183-191.
14. Fryer CM, Michael JW. Body powered components. In Bowker JH, Michael JW (eds), *Atlas of Limb Prosthetics*, 2nd ed. St. Louis: Mosby,

15. Meier RH, Atkins DJ. *Functional Restoration of Adults and Children with Upper Extremity Amputation.* New York: Demos Medical Publishers, 2004.
16. Fliegel O, Feuer SF. Historical development of lower extremity prostheses, *Arch Phys Med Rehabil* 1966;47(5):275-285.
17. Magee R. Amputation through the ages: the oldest major surgical operation. *Aust N Z J Surg* 1998;69(9):675-678.
18. Wilson AB. History of amputation surgery and prosthetics. In Bowker JH, Michael JW (eds), *Atlas of Limb Prosthetics: Surgical, Prosthetic, and Rehabilitation Principles,* 2nd ed. St. Louis: Mosby, 1992. pp. 3-13.
19. Robinson KP. Historical aspects of amputation. *Ann R Coll Surg Engl* 1991;73(3):134-136.
20. Gregory-Dean A. Amputations: statistics and trends. *Ann R Coll Surg Engl* 1991;73(3):137-142.
21. *Digest of Data of Persons with Disability; Mathematical Policy Research.* Washington DC: US National Institute on Disability and Rehabilitation Research, January 1992.
22. Torres MM. Incidence and causes of limb amputations. *Phys Med Rehabil: State Art Rev* 1994;8:1-8.
23. Kay HW, Newman JD. Relative incidences of new amputation, *Orthot Prosthet* 1975;29(2):3-16.
24. Nielsen CC. Issues affecting the future demands for orthotists and prosthetists. A study prepared for the National Commission on Orthotic and Prosthetic Education, November 1996.
25. McDonnell PM, Scott RN, McKay LA. Incidence of congenital upper limb deficiencies. *J Assoc Child Prosthet Orthot Clin* Spring 1988;23:8-14.
26. Leonard JA, Meier RH. Prosthetics. In DeLisa JA (ed), *Rehabilitation Medicine: Principles and Practice.* Philadelphia: J.B. Lippincott, 1993. pp. 330-345.
27. Malone JM, Flemming LL, Robertson J, et al. Immediate, early, and late postsurgical management of upper-limb amputation. *J Rehabil Res Dev* 1984;21(1):33-41.
27. Burrough SF, Brook JA. Patterns of acceptance and rejection of the upper limb prosthesis. *Orthot Prosthet* 1991;39(2): 40-47.
28. Manella KJ. Comparing effectiveness of elastic bandages and shrinker socks for lower extremity amputees. *Phys Ther* 1981;61(3):334-337.
29. Halburt J, Crotty M, Cameron ID. Evidence for the optimal management of acute and chronic phantom pain: a systematic review. *Clin J Pain* 2002;18(2):84-92.
30. Hunter GA. Amputation surgery of the arm in adults. In Murdock G, Wilson AB (eds), *Amputation: Surgical Practice and Patient Management.* Oxford UK: Butterworth-Heinemann, 1996. pp. 305-312.
31. Robinson KP. The problem amputation stump. In Murdock G, Wilson AB (eds). *Amputation: Surgical Practice and Patient Management.* Oxford UK: Butterworth-Heinemann, 1996. pp. 285-299.
32. Pucher I, Kickinger W, Frischenschlager O. Coping with amputation and phantom limb pain. *J Psychosom Res* 1999;46(4):379-383.
33. Dykes WG. Biomechanics and prosthetics. In Murdock G, Wilson AB (eds), *Amputation: Surgical Practice and Patient Management,* Oxford UK: Butterworth-Heinemann, 1996. pp. 334-341.
34. Michael JW. Prosthetic considerations during the growth period. In Murdock G, Wilson AB (eds), *Amputation: Surgical Practice and Patient Management.* Oxford UK: Butterworth-Heinemann, 1996. pp. 232-240.
35. Thornby MA, Krebs DE. Bimanual skill development in pediatric below-elbow amputation, a multicenter cross sectional study. *Arch Phys Med Rehabil* 1992;73(8):697-702.
36. Brenner CD. Prosthetic principles: wrist disarticulation and transradial amputation. In Bowker JH, Michael JW (eds), *Atlas of Limb Prosthetics: Surgical, Prosthetic, and Rehabilitation Principles,* 2nd ed. St. Louis: Mosby-Year Book, 1992. pp. 241-251.
37. Miguelez JM. Management of the bilateral upper limb deficient individual. *J Proceed* (an online journal of the American Academy of Orthotists and Prosthetist). Retrieved 2001, at http://www.oandp.org.
38. Smith DJ, Michael JW, Bowker JH (eds), *Atlas of Amputation and Limb Deficiencies,* Rosemont, IL: American Academy of Orthopaedic Surgeons, 2004.
39. Carlson LB, Veatch BD, Frey DD. Technical forum: efficiency of prosthetic cable and housing. *J Prosthet Orthot* 1995;7(3): 96-99.
40. Sammons F. The use of low-friction housing liner in upper extremity prostheses. *Bull Prosthet Res* 1983;10(4):77-81.
41. Exparza W, Ivko JJ. Technical note: friction free cable system; alternative cable system for transhumeral level conventional prosthesis. *J Prosthet Orthot* 1997;9(3):135-136.
42. Billock JN. Upper limb terminal devices: hand versus hooks. *Clin Prosthet Orthot* 19(2):57-65.
43. Frey DD, Carlson LE, Ramaswamy V. Voluntary opening prehensors with adjustable grip force. *J Prosthet Orthot* 1995;7(4):124-130.
44. Radocy B. Voluntary closing control: a successful new design approach to an old concept. *Clin Prosthet Orthot* 1986;10(2):82-86.
45. DeVisser H, Herder JL. Force-directed design of a voluntary closing hand prosthesis. *J Rehab Res Dev* 2000;37(3): 261-271.
46. Heger H, Millstein S, Hunter GA. Electrically powered prostheses for the adult with an acquired upper limb amputation. *J Bone Joint Surg* 1985;67B:278-281.
47. Miguelez JM. Critical factors in electrically powered upper extremity prosthetics. *J Prosthet Orthot* 2002;14(1):36-38.
48. Sears HH. Approaches to prescription of body powered and myoelectric prostheses. *Phys Med Rehabil Clin North Am* 1991;2(2):1047-1051.
49. Speigel SR. Adult myoelectric upper limb prosthetic training. In Atkins DJ, Meier RH (eds), *Comprehensive Management of the Upper Limb Amputee.* New York: Springer-Verlag; 1989
50. Berbrayer D, Farraday WT. Switch-activated electrically controlled prosthesis following a closed head injury: a case study. *J Prosthet Orthot* 1994;6(2):48-51.
51. Upper limb electronic technology moves forward. *O&P Bus News* 20-23, December 1999.
52. Eledstein JE, Berger N. Performance comparison among children fitted with myoelectric and body powered hands. *Arch Phys Med Rehabil* 1993;74(4):376-380.
53. Stein RB, Walley M. Functional comparison of upper extremity amputees using myoelectric and conventional prostheses. *Arch Phys Med Rehabil* 1983;64(6):243-248.
54. Heckathorne C. Components for adult externally powered systems. In Bowker JH, Michael JW (eds), *Atlas of Limb*

Prosthetics, 2nd ed. St. Louis: Mosby-Year Book, 1992. pp. 151-174.

55. Sears HH, Andrews JT, Jacobsen SC. Experience with the Utah arm, hand and terminal device. In Atkins DK (ed), *Comprehensive Management of the Upper Limb Amputee.* New York: Springer Verlag, 1989. pp. 194-210.
56. Williams TW. Use of Boston elbow for high level amputees. In Atkins DK (ed), *Comprehensive Management of the Upper Limb Amputee.* New York: Springer Verlag, 1989. pp. 211-226.
57. Rubin G. Devices enable persons with amputation to participate in sports. *Arch Phys Med Rehabil* 1983;64(1):37-40.

33

Rehabilitation for Persons with Upper Extremity Amputation

MARGARET WISE

LEARNING OBJECTIVES

On completion of this chapter, the reader will be able to do the following:

1. Compare the role and goals of rehabilitation in adult patients with new upper extremity amputation in the acute, preprosthetic, initial prosthetic training, and advanced skill phases of rehabilitation.
2. Identify the key components of examination and evaluation for patients with new upper extremity amputation in each of the phases of rehabilitation.
3. Discuss factors, including those in the psychosocial and affective domains, that influence the prognosis for successful prosthetic training for patients with upper extremity amputation.
4. Suggest an appropriate plan of care for patients with new amputation in each of the phases of rehabilitation, including wound and skin care, pain and edema management, and strategies to enhance range of motion and strength.
5. Discuss the pros and cons of the six prosthetic options the team and family consider in prosthetic planning.
6. Identify therapeutic activities and interventions to facilitate functional independence in activities of daily living.
7. Explain the process of selection of electrode placement and functional training for patients with electrically controlled upper extremity prostheses.

Hands can do all kinds of things…change a tire, bake a pie, fly a kite or catch a fly, plant a seed and help it grow, point the way for feet to go...Rough hands, smooth hands, plump hands, thin hands like wrinkled apple skin. Hands can do most anything…wear a ring, wear a glove, most important...hands can love![1]

EDITH BAER

REHABILITATION AFTER UPPER EXTREMITY AMPUTATION

Human hands are wonderfully complex sensory and motor organs, capable of interpreting and interacting with the environment. The fine manipulative skills and intricate grasp patterns of the hand cannot be duplicated. When a hand is lost, the ability to perform normal daily tasks is greatly changed. Although a prosthesis cannot duplicate hand function, it can help substitute for basic grasp in the performance of normal daily activities and help maintain bilateral hand function.

This chapter discusses the treatment of adults with amputations, including aspects of acute care, preprosthetic care, basic prosthetic training, and advanced functional skills training. Working with patients with upper limb amputation can be quite rewarding for therapists, who must draw on manual and orthopedic skills, functional skills for training activities of daily living, and counseling skills to respond to psychosocial needs.

INCIDENCE AND CAUSES OF UPPER EXTREMITY AMPUTATION

The primary cause of upper limb amputations is trauma, most commonly crush injuries, electrical burns that occur at work, or, in times of war, traumatic injuries sustained in combat. Congenital anomalies, infections, and tumors are other causes of amputation. Because upper extremity amputations are typically occupation related, they primarily occur in young adults between the ages of 20 and 40 years; the ratio of men to women is 4:1. Dillingham[2] reports approximately 18,500 new upper extremity amputations per year. Just fewer than 2000 of these are at wrist level or higher. The ratio of upper extremity amputations to lower extremity amputations is 1:9.[2-4]

CLASSIFICATION AND FUNCTIONAL IMPLICATIONS

The remaining part of the amputated limb is referred to as the *residual limb*. The broad categories used to describe levels of upper extremity amputation include *transphalangeal, metacarpal-phalangeal, transcarpal, wrist disarticulation (styloid), transradial, elbow disarticulation, transhumeral, humeral neck, shoulder disarticulation,* and *intrascapulothoracic* (Figure 33-1).[2]

Functionally speaking, the more proximal the level of amputation, the greater the loss of range of motion (ROM) and strength that results. Of particular importance are the loss of supination and pronation in amputations approaching the mid-forearm and the loss of shoulder rotation as the amputation approaches the axillary fold. Although a longer residual limb provides better mechanical advantage for prosthetic use, limb length does not always correspond to better prosthetic function. The length of the residual limb in an elbow disarticulation or long transhumeral length amputation, for example, limits the space available for an electric elbow unit and affects both cosmesis and function of the prosthesis.

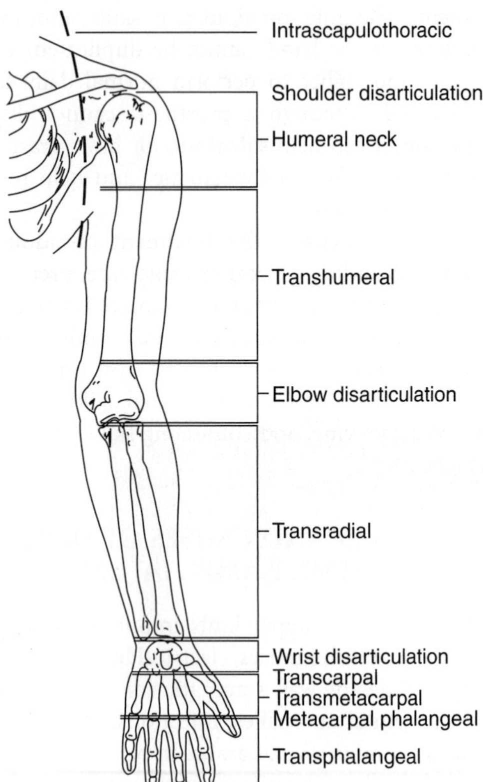

Figure 33-1
The upper extremity residual limb is described by the bony limb segment at which amputation occurred. (Modified from Kottke F, Lehman JF [eds]. Krusen's Handbook of Physical Medicine and Rehabilitation, *4th ed. Philadelphia: Saunders, 1990. pp. 1011.)*

STAGES OF REHABILITATION

The rehabilitation of individuals with upper extremity amputation can be divided into four phases: acute care, preprosthetic rehabilitation, basic prosthetic training, and advanced functional skills training. Although certain goals and activities are unique to each phase, the ultimate goal is to enhance function so that patients with upper extremity amputation can return to the activities and lifestyles most important to them.

Acute Care

Often the most pressing issue in the first days to weeks after traumatic upper extremity amputation is saving the patient's life. The patient may return to the operating room several times for surgeons to clean the wound or perform revision surgery. The patient usually has intravenous lines for antibiotics and pain medications; special infection control procedures may also be in place. The patient may not be fully alert or even have full recollection of what took place the first week or two after injury.

The initial goals of therapy may be quite basic and must be modified to be appropriate to the patient's medical status. Goals of the *acute phase of rehabilitation* include the following:

- To perform a screening evaluation to identify immediate priorities and help predict eventual outcome
- To develop rapport with the family and patient
- To control pain effectively
- To promote wound healing
- To establish a strategy for effective edema control
- To preserve as much passive ROM of the residual limb as possible

Screening Evaluation

Even though the patient may not be able to participate fully during an evaluation, the therapist can begin to gather information to guide the early rehabilitation process. Important facts to discern are the patient's medical status, presence of associated injuries, wound status, ROM, and whether a myodesis (when remnants of major muscles are surgically attached to the bone) or myoplasty (when muscle remnants of the antagonist muscles are sutured to each other) was performed on major antagonist muscle groups during surgery. This basic information helps the therapist develop an intervention plan for early care to facilitate further rehabilitation as the patient's medical status improves.

Rapport

During the acute care stage, when the patient's condition is likely to be quite serious, the family suddenly faces many difficult issues and often experiences emotional crisis. Establishing rapport with and providing necessary support to the family are key elements of the acute care stage. Family members may be struggling with questions such as, "How did this happen?" "Why did it happen?" and "What can the future hold?" The family may be overwhelmed by all the medical procedures being performed on their loved one. The therapist should take time to talk with the family, hear their concerns, and explain the goals for the current stage of rehabilitation as well as the long-range prognosis. During this period of crisis, neither the family nor the patient is ready to hear details about all types of prostheses available, but rather may be comforted to know that general prosthetic plans are being made and that the clinical team is working to help achieve a positive outcome that includes a bright future. Rapport with patients can be developed as they become more alert.

Pain Control

During this early phase, pain is primarily controlled by intravenous medication. Strong pain medication may influence the patient's affect and attitude; often the apparent anger and unwillingness to cooperate shown by patients with traumatic amputation is associated with the pain medication being used. Effective edema control also contributes to pain management. During these first few days, when many professionals are treating the patient day and night, sleep is often interrupted. Coordination of schedules with nursing helps maintain rest periods, which in turn may have a positive effect on pain management.

Wound Healing

Early wound healing and volume and edema control go hand in hand. Wound care protocols may vary depending on physician preference but generally include keeping the wound clean and dry. If a skin graft has closed the wound, the limb must be positioned to prevent tension over the suture lines (Figure 33-2). Initial bandage changes may be quite painful for the patient. During the acute period, some physicians prescribe pain medications before bandage changes. Unless contraindicated, a nonadherent dressing such as Xeroform (Kendall, Mansfield, Mass.) or Adaptic (Johnson & Johnson, New Brunswick, N.J.) can be used directly over the wound and then covered with sterile bandages. Soaking adherent areas with saline can ease removal of the dressing.

Edema Control

Effective edema control helps reduce the chance of adhesion formation along the healing suture line and aids in wound healing and management of pain. Edema may initially be controlled by bulky bandages and elevation. When the patient is able to tolerate pressure, elastic bandages may be applied in a figure-of-eight style, with gentle compressive pressure over the distal end that gradually tapers proximally. Ideally, the bandage should continue up and over one joint proximal to the amputation (e.g., above the elbow in transradial amputation) (Figures 33-3 and 33-4). The positioning of intravenous lines may limit the length of wrap. Elastic wraps must be frequently checked for proper placement and compression; close communication with nurses involved in the patient's care can facilitate this. As wounds heal and are able to tolerate greater compression, elastic wraps are replaced with a "shrinker" or a roll-on liner.

Range of Motion

After injury, patients tend to hold their residual limbs in a position of comfort; arms are typically adducted toward the body, with forearms supinated and elbows flexed. Soft tissue contractures begin to develop if the limb is consis-

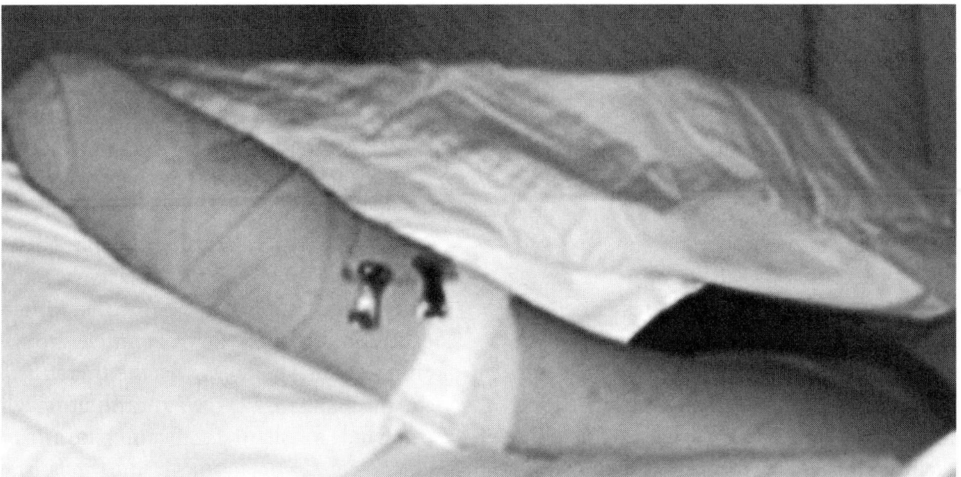

Figure 33-2

In the days after amputation surgery, the transradial residual limb is wrapped in a compressive dressing and a slightly elevated position is maintained to manage edema and control pain. Note the fully extended elbow.

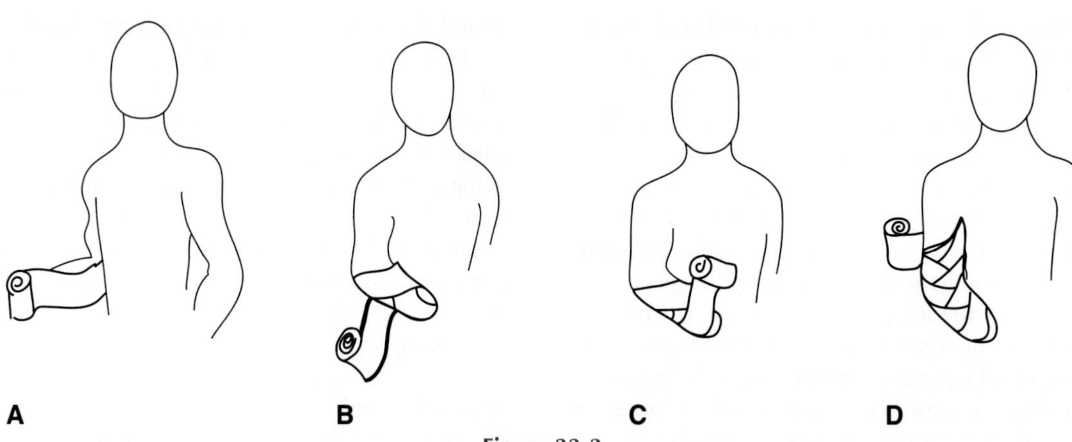

Figure 33-3

*To apply a compressive wrap to a transradial residual limb, the patient anchors the elastic bandage between the elbow and trunk and wraps it around the distal end of the limb (**A**). Next, a series of overlapping figure-of-eight layers of the wrap (**B** and **C**) are applied, creating a distal-toward-proximal pressure gradient. The wrap should continue proximally for several inches above the elbow joint (**D**).*

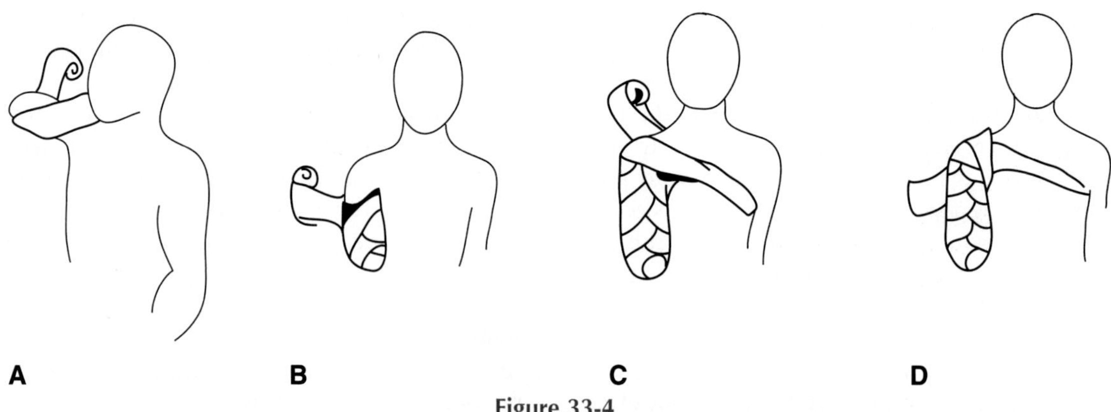

Figure 33-4

*To apply a compressive wrap to a transhumeral residual limb, the patient anchors the elastic bandage between the chin and clavicle and wraps it over and behind the distal end of the residual limb (**A**). Once the initial figure-of-eight layer is applied to anchor the end of the bandage, the patient continues to apply overlapping layers, creating a distal-toward-proximal pressure gradient (**B**). The wrap continues up and over the shoulder (**C**), over the anterior chest wall under the contralateral axilla, and then around the back, over the residual shoulder and under the axilla, before being secured in place (**D**).*

tently held in this position for even 1 to 2 weeks. In patients with transhumeral amputation, limitations of shoulder flexion, abduction, and external rotation are likely to occur. For those with transradial amputation, limitations in elbow extension and pronation are also likely to develop.

Early passive ROM exercise to gently elongate tissues of joints most at risk of contracture formation is essential and can be carefully performed even when intravenous lines are in place. Passive stretching should be performed slowly and gently, just to the point where the therapist begins to feel tension on the muscle or the patient begins to feel pain. Generally, with acute injuries, performing passive ROM twice daily is sufficient to increase motion. If, however, progress is not being made within 2 weeks, the therapist should consider static splinting as an adjunct to passive ROM.

CASE EXAMPLE 1

A Patient with Bilateral Traumatic Amputation of the Forearm

T. M. is a 17-year-old high school soccer player who underwent traumatic amputation of his right and left forearms when the sleeves of his winter jacket became caught in the blades of a running snow blower that had jammed, then suddenly released, as he was trying to clear the mechanism. T. M. was home alone when the accident occurred and had significant blood loss before he was able to reach a neighbor's home for assistance. At the local hospital, tourniquets were placed to control blood loss, wounds were flushed and cleaned, intravenous fluids with antibiotics and packed red blood cells were begun, and morphine was administered. T. M. was made ready for emergency transfer to the nearest trauma center.

On arrival at the trauma center, he was immediately taken to surgery for debridement and closure of his wounds. His parents arrived at the trauma center while he was in surgery. The right transradial residual limb has 3 inches of radius and ulna preserved and required a split-thickness skin graft to close (the donor site was the anterior right thigh). The left transradial residual limb had 7 inches of bone preserved and was closed without skin graft.

Two days have passed since T. M.'s surgery, and he is recovering in the surgical intensive care unit. His white blood cell count and temperature are moderately elevated. His residual limbs are in bulky dressings with elastic compressive wraps, with significant serosanguinous drainage noted at dressing changes. A morphine pump is being used for pain management. T. M. is currently receiving supplemental oxygen by nasal cannula and is sleeping fitfully. On questioning, he is semialert, oriented to family members and place, but not to others or time.

Questions to Consider

- What tests and measures are most appropriate to include in the screening evaluation at this point in the acute phase of T. M.'s care? What is the evidence of reliability and validity of these screening instruments? How will the information collected guide the development of a plan of care for this young man?
- What immediate concerns will T. M.'s parents likely express? In what ways can the team help establish an effective relationship with T. M. and his parents in these early days of care? What information is most important to help the family cope with this crisis situation and prepare for the days ahead? How will the rehabilitation team assess the family's understanding of the situation and need for emotional support?
- What specific intervention strategies should the rehabilitation team use to address issues of pain control, limb volume and edema, and wound healing in the next 2 to 5 days? How should patient and family education be best integrated with these strategies? How should the team assess whether these strategies are effective?
- What specific range of motion is most important to target for this young man with a short transradial residual limb on the right and a long transradial residual limb on the left, anticipating the need for bilateral prostheses in his future? What upper extremity joints are most at risk of contracture formation and why? What specific intervention strategies should the therapists initiate to preserve as much functional range of motion as possible? How might pain, medications, and level of consciousness influence the potential development of soft tissue contractures?
- What postsurgical complications is the team most likely to be concerned about? What are the warning signs of these complications? What members of the team are responsible for monitoring the development of these complications?
- What influence will immobility and pain have on T. M.'s ability to learn, endurance and physiological function, and emotional status during this early phase of rehabilitation?

Preprosthetic Rehabilitation

In many facilities, only when wound closure has occurred can patients with new upper extremity amputation be referred for rehabilitation care. During the preprosthetic therapy phase, the patient's medical condition is often stable enough to allow a more active role in care. Much must be accomplished during this phase.

Goals for the preprosthetic rehabilitation include the following:

- Establish good rapport and trust with the patient and family
- Complete a comprehensive evaluation to guide the team in determining an appropriate prosthetic plan
- Shape and control volume of the residual limb effectively
- Minimize adhesive scar tissue
- Desensitize the limb in preparation for prosthetic wear
- Achieve full ROM in remaining joints of the residual limb
- Strengthen the muscles of the residual limb to maximize potential for effective prosthetic use
- Provide appropriate intervention for rehabilitation of associated injuries
- Help the patient develop some independence in performing basic activities of daily living

Rapport

In the acute phase of care, when the patient is quite ill, rapport is primarily established with family members. These relationships can help facilitate trust between the therapist and the patient during the early preprosthetic period. Upper extremity amputation is a major traumatic event that affects the family as well. As all those involved grapple with the changes and challenges they are facing, the rehabilitation team encourages them to express their hopes, concerns, and fears.

Psychological counseling is considered an integral part of the early rehabilitation program and should be made available for the family and the patient.[5] Some patients may benefit from talking to individuals with amputations of a similar level. Speaking with peer counselors can be helpful; however, rehabilitation professions should screen potential peer counselors carefully. Some individuals who sustained amputations in previous years might not have had a good rehabilitation experience or have not had the benefit of more recent prosthetic design and components. A professional should be sure that peer counselors are offering current information and are emotionally well adjusted.

Comprehensive Evaluation

Before prosthetic options are discussed, a comprehensive evaluation is required. In specialized centers a team that includes the therapist, the prosthetist, the surgeon or physician, and the psychologist or counselor completes the evaluation. In other facilities the therapist and prosthetist are responsible for completing a comprehensive assessment.

The preprosthetic comprehensive evaluation begins with gathering of preliminary or background data, including the following:

- The cause and date of amputation
- Any associated injuries that might influence the rehabilitation process
- Hand dominance
- All medications the patient is currently taking

The evaluation continues with an assessment of the psychosocial environment as a resource for rehabilitation and eventual discharge. The therapist assesses the following patient characteristics:

- The availability of family and other support systems
- Living situation
- Level of education
- Prior occupation and leisure interests

The therapist then considers the condition of the residual limb, documenting the following:

- The presence and description of any phantom limb sensation
- The presence and description of any pain the patient is experiencing
- The length of the residual limb
- The presence of any edema, measured by limb circumference
- Skin condition and the presence of scar tissue or soft tissue adhesion
- Detailed ROM of the residual limb to identify any contractures that may have developed during the acute care phase
- Evaluation of upper extremity strength
- Evaluation of possible sites for placement of electrodes for myoelectrical control

The comprehensive evaluation concludes with a consideration of mobility and functional status, including the following assessments:

- Posture and skeletal alignment as a result of the missing limb
- Pertinent limitations of the lower extremity
- Postural control (static, anticipatory, and reactionary balance)
- Current and potential abilities to perform
- Activities of special interest to the individual, e.g., self care, work, leisure activities

If the patient previously used a prosthesis, a prosthetic history also includes the type of prosthesis used, how long the prosthesis was worn each day, and how the prosthesis was used in work and leisure activities. The team should determine the patient's opinions regarding the positive and negative aspects of a previous prosthesis as well as any different or additional functions that the patient wants to achieve.

Edema Control and Limb Shaping

As the patient's medical status improves, bulky bandages are removed and the patient becomes more mobile. The patient must continue to use some type of compression on the limb nearly 24 hours a day, removing it only for wound care and bathing. At this point, elasticized shrinker socks or a roll-on liner may replace the elastic figure-of-eight bandages because they are more convenient and provide more consistent compression (Figure 33-5). For those with transradial residual limbs, the shrinker should extend at least 2 inches above the elbow. For those with transhumeral residual limbs, the sock extends as high as possible on the humerus with a strap going across the chest to anchor it in place.

As limb volume decreases, the shrinker sock should be made smaller (leaving the seam on the outside of the sock) or replaced with a smaller size garment so that it still compresses the residual limb. If shrinker socks are not available or the patient is not yet able to tolerate the compressive force provided by a shrinker, tubular elastic bandaging, such as Compressogrip (Knit-Rite, Kansas City, Kan.) or Tubigrip (Seton Healthcare Group, Oldham, England), is an alternative. Typically a double layer of bandage is worn, with the layer underneath longer and extending 2 inches further proximally than the second layer.

Edema can further be reduced through soft tissue mobilization and retrograde massage. Soft tissue mobilization around areas of adherent tissue through gentle friction massage in circular clockwise and counter-clockwise motions helps enhance circulation and increase flexibility. Ending treatment with retrograde massage with gentle stroking techniques in the direction of lymphatic flow also helps control edema.[6] Heat modalities may be useful as a preparation for subsequent massage and active exercises.

Elevation, while still important, becomes more difficult to enforce with a mobile patient. A strategy that encourages elevation as well as active participation in care involves encouraging the patient to extend the arm overhead while in the shower, participate in dressing, and use the arm as an assist during other functional activities. Raising the residual limb over the head and performing isometric contractions of remaining musculature at least once an hour during the day is also helpful (Figure 33-6).

Management of the Incision and Scar

When the incision lines are adequately closed and stitches have been removed, scar management becomes a primary concern. When adherent scar tissue forms, the tissue of the residual limb does not move freely. Adherent scar tissue near the end of the bone is a particular problem that may lead to

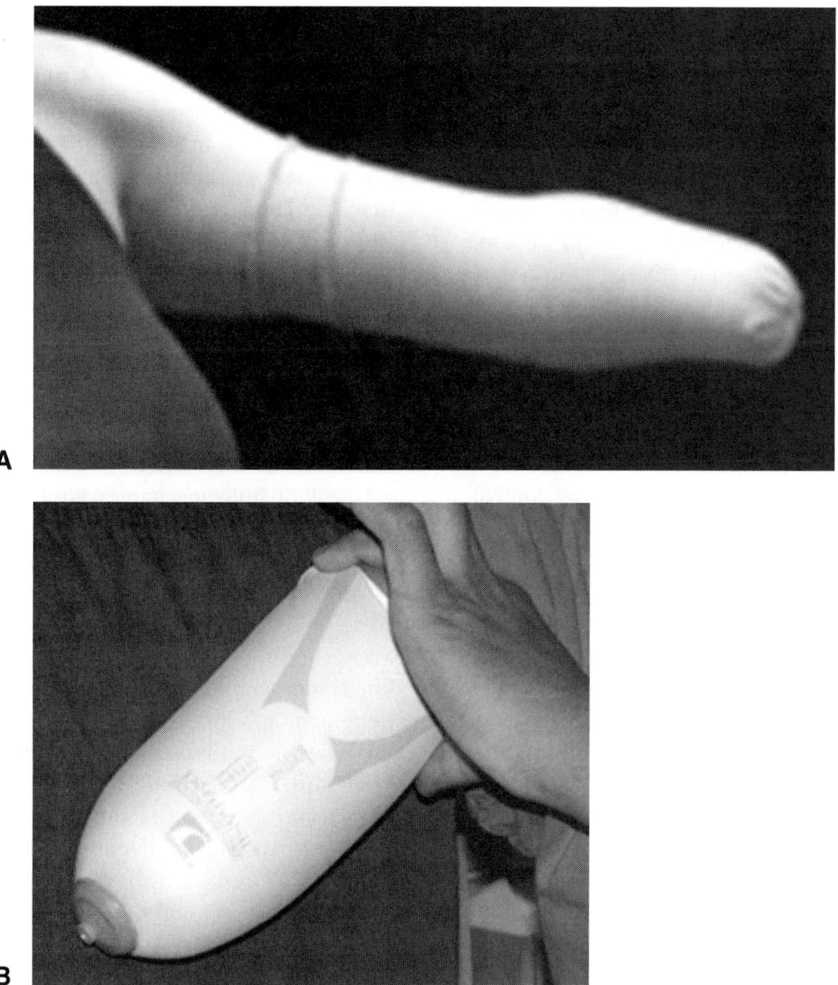

Figure 33-5
*An appropriately applied commercially available transradial (**A**) and transhumeral (**B**) elasticized shrinker garment.*

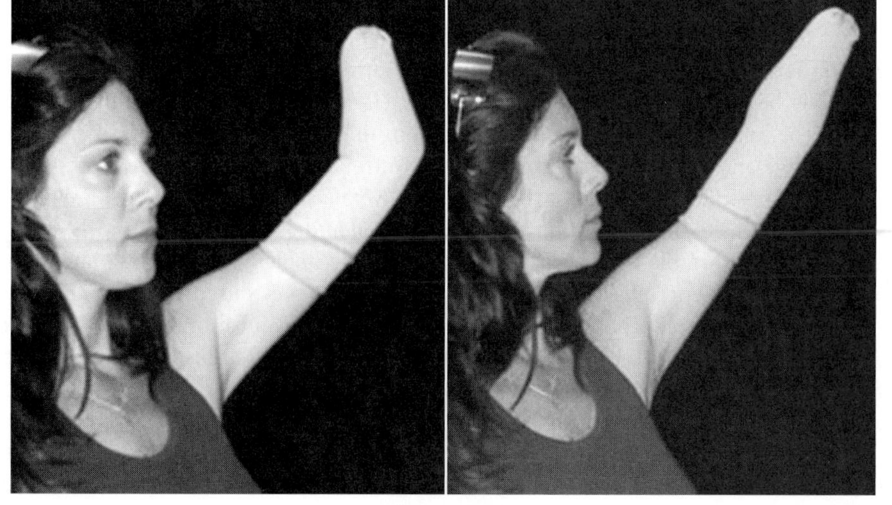

Figure 33-6
*In the preprosthetic stage of rehabilitation, patients with transradial amputation are able to take a more active role in their program, such as active ROM (**A**) and isometric exercise (**B**), emphasizing elbow extension as a strategy to minimize risk of elbow flexion contracture.*

skin breakdown because of traction across the scar when the prosthesis is worn. Scar tissue adherence can be minimized by active ROM and gentle friction massage. Circular massage directly over the incision line, with pressure increasing as tolerated, is a way of minimizing adherent scar formation. A slightly sticky cream or oil, such pure lanolin or vitamin E oil, is preferred so the scar can be more easily mobilized over underlying tissue. Silicone gel sheeting can also be used under bandages to apply pressure directly over the scar to deter adherent scar formation.

Desensitization

Persons with recent amputation often have altered sensation or dysesthesias, including incisional pain, phantom sensation, phantom pain, and hypersensitivity. *Incisional pain* is treated with pain medications and effective edema control. Incisional pain typically subsides as the wound heals and begins to mature and stabilize.

Phantom sensation is a normal phenomenon experienced by most patients with recent amputation. Patients typically report that they "feel" all or part of their amputated limbs. Some describe a pulling, tingling, or burning sensation in the missing limb. Most describe the feeling of a tight fist or a tight band around the arm. Phantom sensation is usually more annoying than painful. Many patients are hesitant to discuss these sensations for fear of sounding "crazy." For this reason, the likelihood of experiencing phantom sensation should be discussed with the patient as early in the rehabilitation process as possible. As rehabilitation progresses to more motion and prosthetic use, phantom sensation typically decreases to a point at which it is not significantly annoying, but it does not usually disappear entirely.

Phantom pain does not occur in all patients, but when it does it is extremely problematic. Unlike phantom sensation, phantom pain is a pathological condition that may persist long after amputation, hindering functional prosthetic use and lifestyle. A number of treatments have been suggested, including heat, desensitization techniques, limb revision, and neurosurgery. None has been shown to work consistently. Other issues that may be confused with phantom pain include proximal nerve damage and neuromas, which may require limb revision or neurosurgical intervention.[7,8]

Hypersensitivity is increased sensitivity to stimuli. Light touch is often particularly uncomfortable for the patient with a hypersensitive residual limb. Hypersensitivity can be effectively treated with a systematic and structured program that includes firm massage, various textures stroked on the limb, submersion of the residual limb in various graded media (e.g., dried beans, rice, and popcorn), vibration, transcutaneous electrical nerve stimulation, and increased functional use of the residual limb during daily activities.[9]

Enhancing Range of Motion

Having as close to full upper extremity ROM as possible allows the patient to use the prosthesis to its full capability. Elbow flexion contracture and loss of supination and pronation are common occurrences in patients with transradial amputation. Patients with transhumeral amputation may lose scapula mobility and all shoulder motions, especially external rotation and horizontal adduction. Interventions such as heat modalities, soft tissue mobilization, gentle stretching, and active ROM exercise can often quickly improve motion in patients with recently developed tissue tightness and ROM restriction. Long-term contractures may require static or dynamic splinting or casting and may take weeks to resolve.

The possible loss of lower extremity ROM caused by immobility and reduced activity during the acute and early rehabilitative phases of care should also be addressed. Limitations in lower extremity range may affect balance and impede good body mechanics. For those with bilateral upper extremity amputation, good balance and lower extremity ROM are essential for the performance of most basic and instrumental activities of daily living.

Strengthening

When the wound has healed and pain is decreasing, strengthening is initiated for all muscles of the residual limb and for major muscle groups of the other extremity. For intact musculature, initial strengthening may be achieved through isometric contraction. The patient usually quickly progresses to active resistive exercises by using manual resistance, weight cuffs, elastic bands, weight machines, and functional activities.

Management of Concurrent Injuries and Limitations

Traumatic upper extremity amputations seldom occur in isolation. When an upper extremity is caught in a press or other apparatus, the injured person struggles to get out of the machine by pulling and twisting and even using other extremities to extricate the arm from the machine. The patient can have obvious injuries such as fractures and soft tissue and muscle damage. Other injuries are often present but are not obvious on initial investigation. Painful and limiting rotator cuff injuries on the injured limb or the contralateral shoulder are not uncommon.

Myofascial trigger points are almost always present. Travell and Simons[10] describe a myofascial trigger point as a "hyperirritable locus within a taut band of skeletal muscle, located in the muscular tissue and/or its associated fascia. The spot is painful on compression and can evoke characteristic referred pain and autonomic phenomena." For patients with upper extremity amputation, trigger points are often found bilaterally in the upper trapezius, rhomboids, and teres minor muscles. Individuals with transradial amputations may have trigger point pain in the wrist and finger flexors or extensors. Those with transhumeral amputations may have trigger point pain in all three portions of the deltoid. All associated injuries must be treated so the patient can more fully participate in prosthetic training.

Basic Training in Activities of Daily Living

When the dominant hand is amputated, most persons with unilateral amputation choose to change hand dominance for activities requiring fine coordination and manipulative skills, such as writing and eating. Drawing, craft activities, and games can all contribute to developing hand coordination and change of hand dominance.

Patients with an upper extremity amputation must remain as independent as possible in basic or survival functional skills such as eating, dressing, and hygiene, but not rely solely on one hand. Reminding the patient that the task will become easier with the prosthesis helps establish an expectation that the patient will soon be using two "hands." Remaining bimanual is important for ease of performance and for minimizing risk of overuse syndrome of the remaining extremity.

CASE EXAMPLE 2

A Patient with Transhumeral Amputation

R. O. is a 37-year-old automobile mechanic who underwent a transhumeral amputation of the right upper extremity 3 weeks ago after he sustained a crush injury when a car slipped off the jack while he was changing its tire in a neighbor's driveway, pinning him at the elbow. While struggling to get out from under the vehicle, he seriously strained his right rotator cuff. At this point, all surgical drains and sutures have been removed, and the wound has closed except for a 1/4-inch area medially that continues to leave slight signs of clear drainage on the nonadherent dressing. R. O. is currently using a double layer of elasticized Tubigrip (Seton Healthcare Group, Oldham, England), for volume control. He reports a sensation of a tight constrictive cuff around his "missing" right elbow and a somewhat unpredictable shooting "electric" sensation into his missing forearm and hand. He tends to hold his residual limb diagonally across his lower chest. R. O. experiences pain in his right shoulder with movement in all planes.

Active and passive range of motion (ROM) is evaluated with R. O. in the supine position. Active ROM at the shoulder is currently 0 to 90 degrees of flexion, 0 to 70 degrees of abduction, 0 degrees of internal rotation, and 0 to 25 degrees of external rotation. His shoulder and residual limb can be passively moved into 115 degrees of flexion, 90 degrees of abduction, 10 degrees of internal rotation, and 40 degrees of external rotation.

R. O. is having a difficult time imagining how he will be able to return to work to support his young family (a wife and two preschool-aged children). He is discouraged and impatient with his postoperative pain and phantom sensation. He is reluctant to allow his residual limb to be moved, passively or with active assistance, toward any end ROM at the shoulder because of impingement pain. He is discouraged with the skill level he has reached in self-care with his nondominant left upper extremity.

Questions to Consider

- What are R. O.'s most immediate educational and support needs now that he has begun the early rehabilitative, preprosthetic period of care? What strategies would help strengthen rapport with R. O., help him understand the next steps in the process, and enhance his outlook and motivation?
- What tests and measures are most important to use in the comprehensive examination and evaluation of R. O.'s residual limb and potential for prosthetic rehabilitation? What is the evidence of reliability and validity of these measures? How will the results of the assessment influence immediate and long-term therapeutic goals?
- Given the length of his residual limb and the status of his incision line, what specific strategies for volume control, edema, and limb shaping should be recommend at this time? How should effectiveness of the recommended volume control and limb shaping interventions be assessed? What are the indicators of readiness for prosthetic fitting?
- Given the status of his incision line, what strategies are now appropriate to reduce likelihood of scar formation along the incision line? Why is expecting R. O. to be responsible for this aspect of his care important?
- Given the dysesthesia that R. O. is currently experiencing, what interventions might be used to help his residual limb become less hypersensitive to sensory stimulation? What is the evidence of efficacy of the interventions available? Why is addressing dysesthesia important, on both a functional and psychological level, for patients such as R. O. with recent amputation?
- Given his current level of discomfort and the concurrent rotator cuff dysfunction, what contractures are most likely to develop at R. O.'s shoulder? Considering his hopes to return to work as an auto mechanic, what shoulder motions would be most important to preserve and enhance in preparation for prosthetic training? What specific strategies should be used to accomplish this?
- What impact might a rotator cuff injury have on R. O.'s potential to use a prosthesis successfully? How should the severity of his rotator cuff impairment be assessed? What strategies could be used to improve the function of his shoulder, given the acuity of his rotator cuff injury?
- What types of muscle performance are most important to address at this point? What strategies should be used to address strength, power, and control of the various types of muscle contraction that R. O. will need to use his prosthesis effectively?
- What basic activities of daily living skills should be priorities for functional training at this point? What

strategies should be used to enhance motor learning of skilled activity with his left (nondominant) hand? How might his residual limb be incorporated during these functional activities?

Determining a Prosthetic Plan

Evaluations by therapists, prosthetists, and other team members determine prosthetic options that can be discussed with the patient and family. Factors such as the patient's strength, ROM, handedness, and other physical findings as well as career, vocational pursuits, and long-term goals are important determinants of an individual prosthetic plan. The patient, family, and team members decide from the following options:

1. No prosthesis
2. A *passive prosthesis* to meet the patient's need for cosmesis and function
3. A *body-powered prosthesis* to meet the patient's functional needs
4. An *externally powered prosthesis* (also called an electric prosthesis) to meet the patient's functional needs
5. A *hybrid prosthesis* (combination body-powered and externally powered) to allow the patient to reach optimal levels of function
6. One or more *activity-specific prostheses* to allow the patient to reach optimal levels of function

The prosthetist and therapist discuss the pros and cons of the various control schemes available to operate the prosthesis with the patient and family, with the goals of selecting the control schemes that will allow the patient to become the most functional. The prosthetist may begin fabrication of the prosthesis as the therapist and patient work to achieve important preprosthetic goals. At this point the patient and family see more fully the patent-centered team in action. Involvement of the patient and family from the beginning of the rehabilitation process helps the patient accept and participate in the needed training and eventually accept the prosthesis.

Motions Required to Operate a Body-Powered Prosthesis

If plans are to use a body-powered prosthesis, strengthening shoulder joint and shoulder girdle musculature in both upper extremities is important. For maximal use of the prosthesis with minimum effort, the patient must be able to isolate muscle function with subtle, fluid motion to operate a body-powered prosthesis efficiently. The patient needs to be able to perform one or more of the following motions, through as large a ROM as possible:

- Shoulder protraction or biscapular abduction
- Shoulder flexion
- Shoulder depression, extension, and abduction

The additional motions of elbow flexion and extension, forearm supination and pronation, and shoulder internal and external rotation should also be strengthened. Patients with very high levels of amputation or those with brachial plexus injuries may need to use chest expansion to operate the prosthesis. Chest expansion involves having the patient inhale deeply to expand the chest and then slowly exhale.

Muscle Requirements for a Myoelectrical Prosthesis

When a muscle contracts, it generates an electromyographic signal. The electromyographic signals produced by contracting muscles can be detected by surface electrodes placed in the socket of the prosthesis and are used to control mechanical functions of the prosthesis. Whenever possible, with adults, two separate muscles are used to operate the prosthesis.[11] The therapist is often called on to work with the prosthetist in selecting the most appropriate electrode sites. For those with transradial amputation, the sites most often selected are over the muscle bellies of the wrist flexors and extensors. For those with transhumeral residual limbs, the most frequently used sites for electrode placement are over the biceps and triceps.

Selecting Electrode Sites

An optimal electrode site for a myoelectrically controlled prosthetic component has seven characteristics.[12] First, the site must be located over superficial muscles, preferably not over heavy adipose tissue or graft sites. Second, the patient must have sufficient muscle strength to activate the prosthesis without undue fatigue. Third, the sites must use motions reasonable to learn and relate to normal movement (e.g., wrist extensors for opening the TD and wrist flexors for closing the TD for grip). Fourth, the site must use muscles that the patient can control independently of other motions. Fifth, the site must use muscles that, when activated, will not interfere with, or inhibit, normal activity. Sixth, if dual control is desired, the sites must use two sets of muscles that the patient can physiologically contract together as well as independently of each other. Finally, the electrode sites must be able to be contained within the critical constraints of the socket.

Precise electrode placement makes it easier for a patient to use a myoelectrical prosthesis. The therapist palpates the most likely spot while the patient contracts the desired muscle to test for strength and consistency of the contraction. Once a potential site is located, the skin is cleaned and moistened with water and a surface electrode is positioned over the muscle, parallel to the muscle fibers. The electrode is connected to biofeedback equipment, such as a Myolab (Motion Control) or the Myoboy (Otto Bock HealthCare, Vienna, Austria) (Figure 33-7). The strength of the signal can be read from the meter, and precise electrode placement is adjusted as necessary. Once the electrode site is determined for one muscle, the second electrode site is found over the antagonist in a similar manner.

Control Site Training

Once the best electrode sites have been located, the patient must learn to control consistency of muscle contraction. For effective use of a myoelectrically controlled prosthesis, good muscle control is more important than overall strength of contractions. During control site training, the patient should learn three patterns of muscle activation:

1. To contract one muscle (muscle A, agonist) to a specific level, while leaving the other (muscle B, antagonist) at rest or in a quiet state
2. To contract muscle B to a specific level while leaving muscle A at rest or in a quiet state
3. To perform quick and equal co-contractions of muscles A and B

Biofeedback equipment, or muscle trainers, greatly facilitate this training to master effective, efficient muscle control. Once patients can consistently produce isolated muscle signals on command without undue fatigue, they are ready to proceed with myoelectrical prosthetic training.

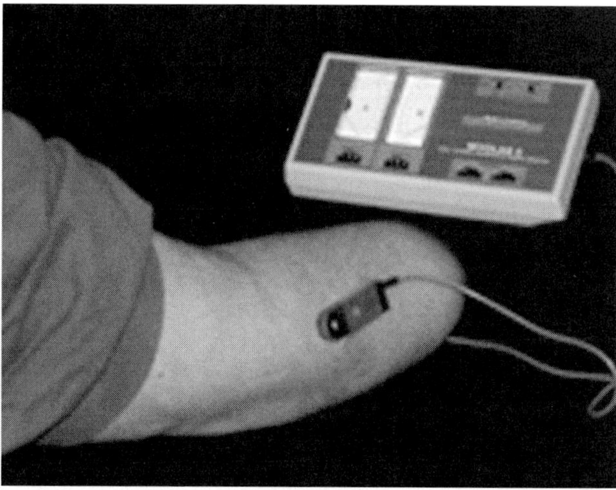

Figure 33-7
Surface electrodes are used to locate potential myoelectrical control sites and provide biofeedback to help patients master the types of contractions necessary to control actions of the terminal device, wrist unit, and forearm motion and elbow lock (for those with transhumeral limbs).

Basic Prosthetic Training

When the patient receives the prosthesis, the basic prosthetic training phase of care begins. Goals in basic prosthetic training include the following:

- To become independent in skin care of the residual limb
- To increase wearing tolerance of the prosthesis to a period functional for the individual
- To become independent in donning and doffing the prosthesis
- To understand the function and operating schemes of various prosthetic components
- To develop necessary skills to use and control the prosthesis effectively during functional activities
- To incorporate the prosthesis effectively in activities of daily living

Learning to operate the basic controls of a body-powered prosthesis is, of course, different from learning to operate a myoelectrically controlled prosthesis. Once basic operations are mastered, however, training methods of using the prosthesis are fairly similar.

Skin Care

Most therapists prefer that the patient wear a t-shirt under the harness of a body-powered prosthesis, especially in early prosthetic training, to prevent skin irritation when learning to operate the cable systems. As skin tolerance develops, the t-shirt becomes optional. For the externally or myoelectrically powered prosthesis, direct contact must be made between the skin and electrode sites. Regardless of the control system being used, the residual arm and axilla must be washed daily with mild soap and water, and the socket of the prosthesis must be wiped clean with a damp cloth. The harness should be removed and cleaned as needed. Patients using a body-powered prosthesis often wear prosthetic socks as an interface between the skin and socket surface. A fresh, clean sock should be used each day; in hot weather, the sock may need to be changed several times per day. For those using a myoelectrical prosthesis, the electrodes may need to be cleaned several times each day to ensure effective contact between control site and the electrode. Although skin pliability is important, the application of moisturizers or lotions before donning the prosthesis is generally not recommended and is contraindicated with a myoelectrical prosthesis. New prosthetic users must understand that skin irritation, if not quickly addressed, may lead to a prolonged period out of the prosthesis. New users are counseled to notify the physician, prosthetist, or therapist as soon as any rash or signs of infection are noted.

Wearing Tolerance

In early prosthetic training, the prosthetic wearing period is typically limited to 30 to 45 minutes at a time. After each wearing period, the prosthesis is removed and skin condition carefully examined. Areas of redness (reactive hyperemia) that persist for more than 20 minutes after the residual limb is out of the socket may indicate areas of high pressure; the prosthetist should be consulted for possible modification of the socket. For those wearing a body-powered prosthesis, the skin of the sound axilla must also be examined. Until skin tolerance is developed, padding placed in the axillary region under the harness may increase comfort and allow longer wearing time. Wearing time is gradually increased, according to the patient's tolerance, skin condition, and need for prosthesis use.

Donning and Doffing

Full prosthetic use includes independence in donning and doffing. Both body-powered and myoelectrical prostheses

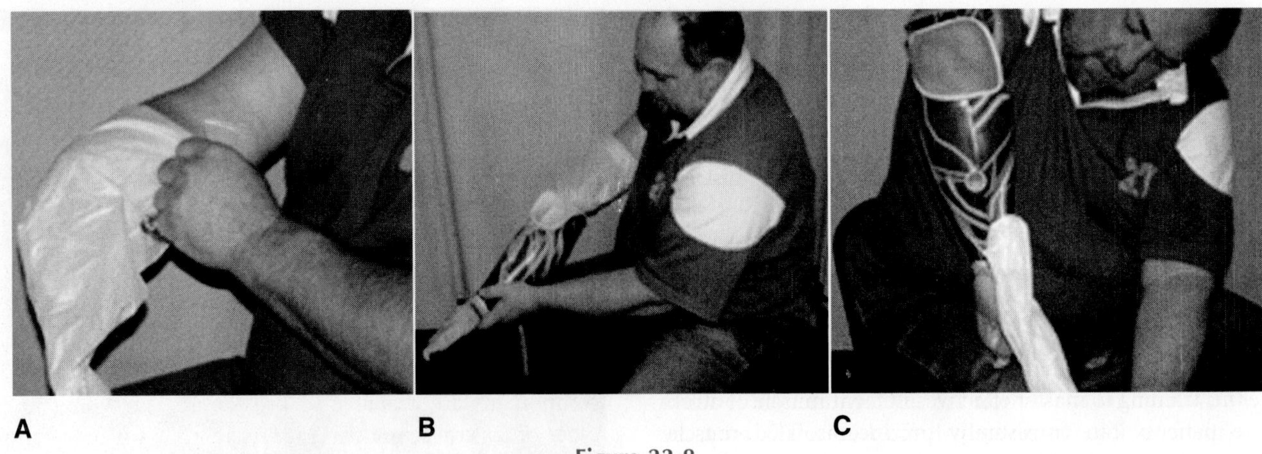

Figure 33-8

*This patient is donning his myoelectrical transradial prosthesis. First, he positions his pull-in sleeve on the residual limb (**A**), leaving a distal "tail" that he will thread through the distal opening in the socket (**B**). Once his limb is positioned in the socket, he gently tugs the sleeve out through the opening so that total contact between skin and socket surface is achieved (**C**).*

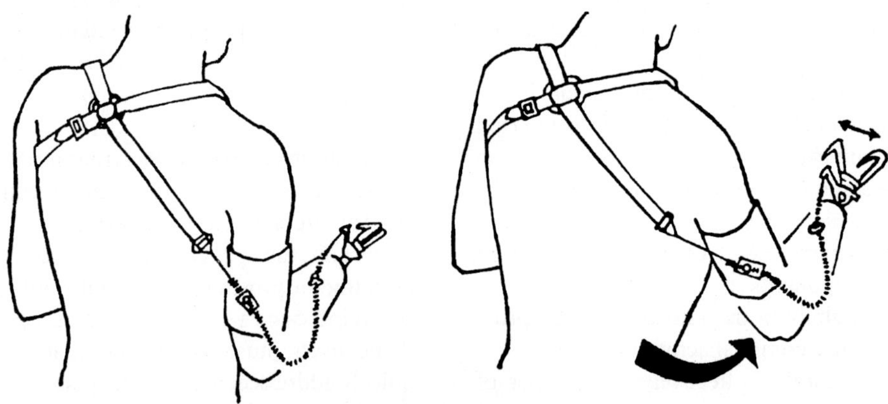

Figure 33-9

The harness and cable system of a body-powered transradial prosthesis. Glenohumeral flexion and scapular abduction (protraction) increase tension on the control cable to operate this voluntary-opening TD during activities performed away from the center of the body. Bilateral scapular (biscapular) abduction increases cable tension for fine motor activities performed near the midline or closer to the trunk. The same motion would allow graded prehension in a voluntary-closing terminal device. (Modified from Northwestern University Printing and Duplicating Department, Evanston, Ill., 1987.)

can be donned by either the push-in or pull-in method. Unless a roll-on line with pin lock is used, the pull-in method is the preferred method for several reasons (Figure 33-8). It offers the advantage of distributing tissue equally in the socket; equal and consistent tissue placement is especially important for those using an electrically powered prosthesis. Pulling-in to the socket is accomplished in the following manner:

1. The patient applies a low-friction sleeve (often made of parachute-type material) over the residual limb.
2. The distal end of the sleeve is positioned through a "pull hole" in the wall of the prosthesis.
3. The patient then gently pulls each side of the sleeve, equally and repeatedly, until the sleeve completely comes out of the pull hole and the arm is pulled into the socket.

Alternative methods of donning may be required for patients with high levels of amputation. Those with very high bilateral transhumeral amputation may need special equipment for independence in donning and doffing. Some individuals with very high bilateral amputation may decide that the effort required to don the prostheses independently is worth the energy expenditure.

Control of the Body-Powered Prosthesis

In the body-powered prosthesis, forces generated by gross body motions are translated through the harness and cable system to activate the forearm and terminal device (TD) (Figure 33-9). The individual with transradial amputation only needs to learn to operate the TD. In short, any motion that puts tension on the cable operates the TD (either hook or hand). In voluntary-opening TDs, tension on the cable opens the TD and either rubber bands or springs close the TD. The addition of rubber bands or springs increases pinch power. In voluntary-closing TDs, the TD remains open until tension is applied on the cable; then the device closes in proportion to the amount of tension on the cable.

Control movements to operate the TD for the transradial prosthesis include shoulder flexion on the sound side, shoulder flexion of the amputated side, or biscapular abduction (shoulder protraction).

Individuals with long transradial limbs typically retain active forearm supination and pronation; this active movement can be used to position the TD for function. If active movement is lost or severely limited, the TD must be passively rotated in the wrist unit. Wrist flexion units are typically operated manually; the patient changes the angle of the TD with the other hand.

The patient with transhumeral amputation must be able to control the TD, forearm motion (flexion and extension to lift and reach), and the elbow locking and unlocking mechanism. When the elbow component in a transhumeral prosthesis is locked, the TD operates exactly as the TD in the transradial prosthesis does—by using shoulder flexion or biscapular abduction and shoulder protraction. When the elbow component is unlocked, however, tension on the cable created by these movements causes the forearm of the prosthesis to flex. When tension on the cable gradually releases (by using eccentric contraction of these muscles) the elbow returns to extension.

The elbow component of a transhumeral prosthesis is locked or unlocked with a combination of motions, unlike the motion used to operate the TD. This motion is simultaneous humeral abduction, extension, and depression—a quick "down and back" motion of the arm. The use of a very different movement strategy helps ensure that the elbow component will not unintentionally unlock during functional activities with the TD.

To position the TD optimally for the functional task at hand, passive motion (either with the intact limb or pressure against a stable surface) is used to rotate the TD in the wrist unit. Similarly, internal and external rotation of the forearm of the prosthesis is passively controlled by rotation at the elbow turntable. Consider a carpenter wearing a transhumeral prosthesis who wants to hold a nail steady on a piece of lumber while working at his bench. First, he might catch his hook on the edge of the bench and rotate it to a proper position to hold the nail. Then, with the elbow of his prosthesis unlocked, he uses biscapular abduction to flex the forearm of his prosthesis into the desired position to accomplish his task. Finally, he locks the elbow to hold the forearm in proper position so that he is able to control opening of the terminal device to grasp the nail. A new prosthetic user may have to think carefully and perform each of these motions deliberately, but an experienced prosthetic user could perform all these motions in a matter of seconds.

Control of the Electric Prosthesis

Electric prostheses can be controlled in a variety of ways. Depending upon the patient's physical and cognitive presentation, the prosthetist may choose from surface electrodes, touch pads, switches, rockers, and other input services. Myoelectric control is often used to operate the prosthesis. Control of the myoelectric prosthesis involves deriving myoelectrical signals from the voluntary contraction of muscles. Surface electrodes implanted in the walls of the prosthetic socket record electrical signals generated by muscle contraction. These signals are processed and used to control mechanical functions of the prosthesis. A wide variety of components are available to prosthetists, providing many types of control schemes.[13] (See Chapter 32 for more information about myoelectrical control system options.) The therapist must consult with the prosthetists on every patient regarding the exact controls used so that the best functional outcome can be achieved. The patient with a long transradial amputation usually retains control of some supination and pronation of the forearm. The patient with a shorter forearm amputation requires a wrist rotation unit to achieve forearm supination or pronation. Several options exist for control of wrist and forearm rotation. The wrist unit can be passively positioned by using the intact hand to position the terminal device for task-specific function. Alternately, the wrist rotator can be myoelectrically controlled. For active myoelectrically controlled wrist rotation, the individual with a transradial amputation must switch from hand (or other TD) mode to wrist mode. One way to accomplish this is for the individual to quickly and simultaneously contract forearm flexors and extensors. Once the unit is in wrist mode, contraction of the extensors rotates the hand into supination and contraction of the flexors rotates the wrist into pronation. When strength of contraction signal is at issue, control schemes can be altered because muscles with the most consistently reliable control should operate the function deemed most important.

Patients with transhumeral myoelectric prostheses have to manage the additional complexity of controlling the forearm (for flexion and extension) and the elbow (for lock and unlock function) as well as the TD and wrist rotator. Commonly used transhumeral control schemes use contraction of the biceps and triceps to operate the prosthetic TD and forearm. When the elbow unit is locked, contraction of one muscle opens the terminal device. Contraction of the opposite muscle signals closure of the TD. When the elbow is unlocked, contraction of the control muscle flexes the forearm. The speed of operation is matched to the rapidity and strength of the myoelectric signal generated by muscle contraction. Graded prehension and elbow motion is possible with practice.

Engineers have realized the complexity of motions the prosthesis must perform for fluid, functional upper extremity motion. They are working with prosthetists, therapists, and patients to develop new components and control schemes for more functional prostheses. Nowhere is this more obvious than recent changes seen in the transhumeral prosthesis. Currently, most prostheses require the elbow unit to be locked in order to operate the terminal device. Manufacturers are now working to develop newer types of transhumeral prostheses to allow simultaneous control of the hand and forearm for more normal grasp. It is anticipated that the future will hold even more exciting developments that will help the individual with upper limb amputation to function more independently at home, at work, and in leisure activities.

Skills Training

Once the patient understands how to operate all the components, all individual movements should be put together for functional prosthetic use. Similar training principles are used whether the control system is body powered or myoelectrical. The new prosthetic user must learn how to control the terminal device selectively so that it is opened just enough to grasp the intended object while maintaining just enough tension on the muscle or cable to hold the object without squeezing it. Another fundamental skill to master is the ability to operate the terminal device at various levels and in various positions. These positions may include tasks requiring the elbow to be flexed to 90 degrees while the arm is held at the side of the body; tasks requiring a forward or upward (above waist height) motion for grasping, lifting or carrying; and tasks requiring picking objects up from a lower surface, such as the floor.

The new prosthetic user needs to practice how to position the TD in advance to prevent unnecessary or awkward movements. This involves actively or passively turning the TD for efficient grasp and positioning the elbow at the correct angle for the task.

The new user needs opportunities to practice bimanual activities, such as transferring objects from one hand to the other. A variety of activities may be used to help the patient develop gross coordination skills; these may include turning pages in a book, throwing a beanbag, and spooning or pouring uncooked rice.

Many functional activities, such as grooming and cooking, require fine coordination and control of the prosthesis. Training activities to develop fine coordination skills can include stacking 1-inch blocks, playing cards, stringing small beads, or working leather crafts.

Using the Prosthesis in Activities of Daily Living

After learning basic control moves, the patient is ready to begin incorporating prosthetic use in activities of daily living, such as the following:

- Cutting food, buttering bread, using a utensil to eat different types of food
- Opening and closing various types of packages, boxes, containers, and jars
- Putting toothpaste on a toothbrush, cleaning and clipping fingernails, holding a hair dryer while styling hair
- Tying shoelaces, fastening the zipper on a jacket, and holding pants in place while fastening them

CASE EXAMPLE 3

A Patient with Bilateral Upper Extremity Amputation after Electrocution

E. H. is a 19-year-old college freshman studying to become a marine biologist. Six months ago, he participated in a school project on a boat with an instructor and other students to measure lake depth and take samples of underwater plants. The day before, the local power company had begun stringing power lines that extended over the edge of the lake and inadvertently left these wires lower than intended. E. H. was using an aluminum pole to measure water depth and accidentally touched these live wires with the pole. He was immediately electrocuted, rendered unconscious, and fell into the water. The other students pulled him from the lake and resuscitated him in approximately 4 minutes. He was medically evacuated to the trauma center, where he was found to have burns on both hands and forearms. The entrance wound, where the electrical current entered his body, was in his right (dominant) hand. The exit wounds were in his left forearm and thigh. As result of the burns and subsequent tissue damage, amputation was necessary on the right side at the mid-transradial level and on the left at mid-humeral level; he received a skin graft on his left thigh and left arm.

E. H. was hospitalized for 2 months near his home and then discharged to live with his family (parents and brother) and receive outpatient therapy. At the time of discharge, in addition to bilateral upper extremity range of motion limitations, E. H. had severe balance deficits and limited lower extremity strength and flexibility bilaterally. He was completely dependent in activities of daily living.

Three months later he is referred to an outpatient prosthetic center for prosthetic fitting and therapy to train to use his prostheses to become as independent as possible, including returning to school to pursue his career in marine biology. E. H.'s wounds are well healed. His arms are well contoured, show minimal edema, and have few adhesions and full range of motion. Hip flexion is limited to 85 degrees, extension to neutral. He is able to stand on the right foot for 20 seconds and the left for 5 seconds. Because of inactivity, E. H. is 40 pounds overweight. E. H. receives his prostheses 3 weeks after beginning prosthetic rehabilitation.

Questions to Consider

- What is the stage of E. H.'s rehabilitation? What tests and measures are appropriate at this time? What is his prognosis for prosthetic use and return to functional independence at home and school? What are the most important goals that he needs to accomplish in his early prosthetic rehabilitation? How will his goals change as prosthetic rehabilitation progresses? How many weeks will likely be required?

- What effect will his impairments and limitations in balance and lower extremity range of motion have on upper extremity prosthetic training and future activities of daily living skills? How might interventions to address these impairments and functional limitations be incorporated in the plan of care?
- What factors should be considered when planning prosthetic options? What are the pros and cons of body-powered or electrically controlled prostheses for E. H.? Will one type of prosthesis meet his needs? Why or why not?
- Should his initial prosthetic training be unilateral or bilateral? Why? If beginning training with a single prosthesis, which should be targeted? Why? What basic components should be recommended for each of his prostheses?
- How can the team assist E. H. in learning to use his electrical hands or hooks? What control motions are needed for the right (transradial) side? What motions are needed for the left (transhumeral) side? How might E. H. progress from simple activity to more complex and realistic activities with his terminal devices to facilitate learning while minimizing frustration?
- What effect does elbow function have on hand positioning? How will elbow function affect the use of his transradial prosthesis? What is the sequence that E. H. needs to master to control elbow function of his transhumeral prosthesis? What kinds of activities would help him master elbow control in both single-limb and bimanual tasks? How would training tasks be graded to ensure success?
- Are E. H.'s goals of returning to college to study marine biology realistic? What problems might he face?

ADVANCED FUNCTIONAL SKILLS TRAINING

The full understanding of all components and the ability to operate them to the fullest extent are necessary before discharge from therapy. For example, using the forearm and hand for fluid reach and grasp and walking with a near-normal arm swing are possible. Although prosthesis use in self-care and basic activities of daily living is important, the ability of the patient to function in all aspects of life is more important. The real reason patients will continue to use their prostheses is to do things that are important to them, such as household chores, household maintenance, child care, vocational activities, and recreational activities (e.g., playing golf, bowling, hunting, fishing, bicycling).

SUMMARY

New advances in prosthetics are achieved every year, resulting in better socket design, increased comfort, reduced weight, advanced componentry, and better cosmesis. These changes have resulted in better patient satisfaction and increased use. Patients deserve prostheses that meet their needs and fit well; they also deserve comprehensive training. Working with patients to help them return to functional lives can be a challenging and rewarding experience for the prosthetist, therapist, and other team members. Most patients can become independent in all functional activities.

REFERENCES

1. Baer E. *The Wonder of Hands.* New York: MacMillan, 1992.
2. Dillingham TR. Rehabilitation of the upper limb amputee. In Dillingham TR, Belandres RV (eds), *Rehabilitation of the Injured Combatant,* Washington, DC: Office of the Surgeon General, Department of the Army, 1998. pp. 33-73.
3. Atkins DJ, Meier RH. *Comprehensive Management of the Upper-Limb Amputee,* New York: Springer-Verlag, 1989.
4. Olivett BL. Conventional fitting of the adult amputee. In Hunter J, Mackin E, Callahan A (eds), *Rehabilitation of the Hand and Upper Extremity,* 4th ed, St. Louis: Mosby, 1995. pp. 1223-1240.
5. Desmond D, MacLachlan M. Psychosocial issues in the field of prosthetics and orthotics. *J Prosthet Orthot* 2002;14(1):19-21.
6. Colditz JC. Therapist's management of the stiff hand. In Hunter J, Mackin E, Callahan A (eds), *Rehabilitation of the Hand and Upper Extremity,* 5th ed. St. Louis: Mosby, 2002. pp. 1021-1049.
7. Brown PW. Psychologically based hand disorders. In Hunter J, Mackin E, Callahan A (eds), *Rehabilitation of the Hand and Upper Extremity,* 5th ed. St. Louis: Mosby, 2002. pp. 9-19.
8. Shenaq S, Meier R, Brotzman B, et al. The painful residual limb: Treatment strategies. In Atkins DJ, Meier RH (eds). *Comprehensive Management of the Upper-Limb Amputee,* New York: Springer-Verlag, 1989. pp. 72-78.
9. Waylett-Rendall J. Desensitization of the traumatized hand. In Hunter J, Mackin E, Callahan A (eds), *Rehabilitation of the Hand and Upper Extremity,* 4th ed. St. Louis: Mosby, 1995. pp. 693-700.
10. Travell JG, Simons DG. *Myofascial Pain and Dysfunction, The Trigger Point Manual.* Baltimore, MD: Williams & Wilkins, 1983.
11. Hubbard S. Myoprosthetic management of the upper limb amputee. In Hunter J, Mackin E, Callahan A (eds), *Rehabilitation of the Hand and Upper Extremity,* 4th ed. St. Louis: Mosby, 1995. pp. 1241-1252.
12. Proceedings from the University of New Brunswick's Myoelectric Controls/Powered Prosthetics Symposium, Fredricton, New Brunswick, Canada, August 25-27, 2002.
13. Lake C, Miguelez JM. Comparative analysis of microprocessors in upper limb prosthetics. *J Prosthet Orthot* 2003;15(2):48-63.

RECOMMENDED READING

Daly W. Clinical application of roll-on sleeves for myoelectrically controlled transradial and transhumeral prostheses. *J Prosthet Orthot* 2000;12(3):88-91.

Jones LE, Davidson JH. Save that arm: a study of problems in the remaining arm of unilateral upper limb amputees. *J Int Soc Prosthet Orthot* 1999;23(1):55-58.

Kisner C, Colby LA. *Therapeutic Exercise Foundations and Techniques,* 3rd ed. Philadelphia: F.A. Davis, 1996.

Miguelez JM, Miguelez MD. The Micro Frame: the next generation of interface design for glenohumeral disarticulation and associated levels of limb deficiency. *J Prosthet Orthot* 2003;15(2):66-71.

Muzumdar A (ed). *Powered Upper Limb Prostheses, Control, Implementation and Clinical Application.* Berlin, Germany: Springer-Verlag Berlin Heidelberg, 2004.

Smith D, Michael J, Bowker J, et al (eds). Atlas of Amputations and Limb Deficiencies: Surgical, Prosthetic, and Rehabilitation Principles, 3rd ed. Alexandria, VA: American Academy of Orthopaedic Surgeons, 2004.

Soltanian H, de Bese G, Beasley R, et al. Passive hand prostheses. In Brown RE, Neumeister MW (eds). *Hand Clinics: Mutilating Hand Injuries,* vol 19. Philadelphia: Saunders, 2003. pp. 177-183.

Supan T. Active functional prostheses. In Brown RE, Neumeister MW (eds). *Hand Clinics: Mutilating Hand Injuries,* vol 19. Philadelphia: Saunders, 2003. pp. 185-191.

Index*

*Note: Page numbers followed by *f* indicate figures; *t*, tables; *b*, boxes.

D

G

H

K

L

N

O

P

Q

R

S

T

U

V